Rehabilitation of the Aging and Elderly Patient

Rehabilitation of the Aging and Elderly Patient

Editors

Gerald Felsenthal, M.D.

Chief, Department of Rehabilitative Medicine
Sinai Hospital of Baltimore
Clinical Professor
Department of Epidemiology and Preventive Medicine
University of Maryland School of Medicine
Associate Professor
Department of Rehabilitation Medicine
The Johns Hopkins University School of Medicine
Baltimore, Maryland

Susan J. Garrison, M.D.

Associate Professor
Department of Physical Medicine and Rehabilitation
Baylor College of Medicine
Medical Director, Rehabilitation Center
The Methodist Hospital
Houston, Texas

Franz U. Steinberg, M.D., F.A.C.P.

Emeritus Professor of Clinical Medicine
Washington University School of Medicine
Staff Physician and Co-Director
Resident Physician Training
Physical Medicine and Rehabilitation
Department of Rehabilitation
The Jewish Hospital of St. Louis
St. Louis, Missouri

Williams & Wilkins

BALTIMORE • PHILADELPHIA • HONG KONG
LONDON • MUNICH • SYDNEY • TOKYO

A WAVERLY COMPANY

Editor: John P. Butler
Managing Editor: Linda S. Napora
Copy Editor: Dorothy E. Shiffler
Designer: Wilma E. Rosenberger
Illustration Planner: Ray Lowman
Production Coordinator: Charles E. Zeller

Accurate indications, adverse reactions, and dosage schedules for drugs are provided in this book, but it is possible that they may change. The reader is urged to review the package information data of the manufacturers of the medications mentioned.

Printed in the United States of America

Library of Congress Cataloging in Publication Data

Rehabilitation of the aging and elderly patient / editors, Gerald
 Felsenthal, Susan J. Garrison, Franz U. Steinberg.
     p. cm.
   Includes index.
   ISBN 0-683-03125-2
   1. Aged–Rehabilitation. 2. Aged, Physically handicapped–
 Rehabilitation. I. Felsenthal, Gerald. II. Garrison, Susan J.
 III. Steinberg, Franz U., 1913–
   [DNLM: 1. Aging–physiology. 2. Geriatrics. 3. Rehabilitation–
 in old age. WT 100 R34533 1993]
 RC953.5.R45 1993
 618.97′03–dc20
 DNLM/DLC   92-48558
 for Library of Congress   CIP

                                        94 95 96 97
                                     2 3 4 5 6 7 8 9 10

Preface

Rehabilitation of the Aging and Elderly Patient was conceived as a response to the urgent medical and social needs of both the elderly population and the younger, though aging, disabled population. The numerical growth of the elderly now exceeds that of any other age group in the United States; the cost of their care has become a major health care problem. Furthermore, younger disabled persons experience the physiologic changes of aging in addition to their original impairments. Often, the price of survival for aging and elderly patients is a permanent disability that impairs function and diminishes independence. It is imperative that health care professionals meet the challenge of keeping these populations fit and functional as long as possible in order to maximize our health care dollars and other resources. Therefore, with the help of our chapter authors, we have edited a book dedicated to our patients who are aging with a disability and those who are growing older, thereby sustaining impairments and disabilities.

The emphasis in *Rehabilitation of the Aging and Elderly Patient* is the maintenance and restoration of function; this is not simply another text on geriatric medicine. The aging and impairment of organ systems influence general fitness and endurance; accordingly, rehabilitation goals and treatment must be modified.

However, obstacles to rehabilitation are not only physical, but also attitudinal, financial, and social; all aspects must be addressed in order to maintain or restore function. The rehabilitation program must include realistic functional goals, established with the patient and family and appropriate for the patient's functional setting.

The first section of the book discusses general aspects and pathophysiology of human aging. The second section deals with the assessment and management of specific impairments and disabilities of both the older patient and the younger impaired patient who is aging. Chapters on the rehabilitation team; rehabilitation settings; the working elderly; research; outcome studies; legal aspects; ethical considerations, and the education of students, resident physicians, and fellows comprise the remaining three sections.

The editors wish to express their sincere appreciation to the contributing chapter authors. Without their expertise and cooperation, this book would not have been feasible. Moreover, we wish to thank our families and our secretaries for their understanding, support, and assistance during the preparation of this book.

Gerald Felsenthal
Susan J. Garrison
Franz U. Steinberg

Contributors

Michael A. Alexander, M.D.
Clinical Associate Professor
Department of Rehabilitation Medicine
Jefferson Medical College
Philadelphia, Pennsylvania
Chief of Rehabilitation
Alfred I. du Pont Institute
Wilmington, Delaware

Bill Allen, J.D.
Medical Humanities Program
University of Florida College of Medicine
Gainesville, Florida

J. Michael Anderson, M.D.
Active Staff
Department of Rehabilitation Medicine
Sinai Hospital of Baltimore
Clinical Assistant Professor
Department of Epidemiology and Preventive Medicine
University of Maryland School of Medicine
Baltimore, Maryland

Sunanda Apte-Kakade, M.D.
Staff M.D., Miland E. Knapp Rehabilitation Center
Associate Physician, Department of Physical Medicine and
  Rehabilitation
Hennepin County Medical Center
Assistant Professor, University of Minnesota
Department of Physical Medicine and Rehabilitation
Minneapolis, Minnesota

John R. Bach, M.D.
Assistant Professor of Physical Medicine and Rehabilitation
University of Medicine and Dentistry of New Jersey—New
  Jersey Medical School
Newark, New Jersey

John D. Banja, Ph.D.
Associate Professor of Rehabilitation Medicine
Assistant Professor of Community and Preventive Medicine
Emory University School of Medicine
Atlanta, Georgia

Donna H. Butler, D.O.
Department of Rehabilitation Medicine
Sinai Hospital of Baltimore
Clinical Assistant Professor
Department of Epidemiology and Preventive Medicine
University of Maryland School of Medicine
Baltimore, Maryland

Gary S. Clark, M.D.
Clinical Associate Professor of Rehabilitation Medicine
State University of New York at Buffalo
Head, Department of Rehabilitation Medicine
Buffalo General Hospital
Buffalo, New York

Nancy D. Cobble, M.D.
Rocky Mountain Multiple Sclerosis Center
Colorado Neurological Institute
Englewood, Colorado

Joel A. Delisa, M.D.
Professor and Chairman
Department of Physical Medicine and Rehabilitation
University of Medicine and Dentistry of New Jersey—New
  Jersey Medical School
Medical Director and Chief Medical Officer
Kessler Institute for Rehabilitation
Chairman, Physical Medicine and Rehabilitation
St. Barnabus Medical Center
West Orange, New Jersey

Paul T. Diamond, M.D.
Assistant Professor
Department of Physical Medicine and Rehabilitation
University of Virginia Health Science Center
Charlottesville, Virginia

Ann S. DuChane, M.S., C.C.C.Sp.
Supervisor of Speech-Language Pathology
Franklin Square Hospital
Instructor, Department of Rehabilitation Medicine
The Johns Hopkins University School of Medicine
Baltimore, Maryland

Daniel Dumitru, M.D.
Associate Professor
Department of Rehabilitation Medicine
University of Texas Health Science Center at San Antonio
San Antonio, Texas

Alberto Esquenazi, M.D.
Director, Gait and Motion Analysis Laboratory and Regional
  Amputee Rehabilitation Center
Moss Rehabilitation Hospital
Assistant Professor, Department of Rehabilitation Medicine
Temple University School of Medicine
Philadelphia, Pennsylvania

Avital Fast, M.D.
Chairman, Department of Rehabilitation Medicine
St. Vincents Hospital
Professor of Rehabilitation Medicine
New York Medical College
New York, New York

Gerald Felsenthal, M.D.
Chief, Department of Rehabilitation Medicine
Sinai Hospital of Baltimore
Clinical Professor
Department of Epidemiology and Preventive Medicine
University of Maryland School of Medicine
Associate Professor
Department of Rehabilitation Medicine
The Johns Hopkins University School of Medicine
Baltimore, Maryland

Steven V. Fisher, M.D.
Medical Director, Miland E. Knapp Rehabilitation Center
Chief, Department of Physical Medicine and Rehabilitation
Hennepin County Medical Center
Associate Professor
Department of Physical Medicine and Rehabilitation
University of Minnesota
Minneapolis, Minnesota

Loren M. Fishman, M.D.
Director
Department of Physical Medicine and Rehabilitation
Flushing Hospital Medical Center
Flushing, New York
Clinical Assistant Professor
Department of Rehabilitation Medicine
Albert Einstein College of Medicine
Bronx, New York

Kathleen Fox, Ph.D., M.H.S.
Assistant Professor
Division of Gerontology
Department of Epidemiology and Preventive Medicine
University of Maryland School of Medicine
Baltimore, Maryland

Janet C. Frank, M.S.
Assistant Director for Programs
UCLA Multicampus Program in Geriatric Medicine and
    Gerontology
UCLA School of Medicine
Los Angeles, California

Gerald W. Friedland, M.D.
Professor of Radiology
Stanford University
Chief, Radiology Service
Department of Veterans Affairs Medical Center
Palo Alto, California

Walter R. Frontera, M.D., Ph.D.
Associate Professor
Department of Physical Medicine and Rehabilitation
University of Puerto Rico School of Medicine
San Juan, Puerto Rico
Director, Center for Sports Health and Exercise Sciences
    (A combined project of the Puerto Rico Olympic Commit-
    tee and the University of Puerto Rico Medical Sciences
    Campus)
Albergue Olimpico
Salinas, Puerto Rico
Clinical Associate Professor
Department of Rehabilitation Medicine
Tufts University School of Medicine
Boston, Massachusetts

Joseph J. Gallo, M.D., M.P.H.
The Johns Hopkins University School of Hygiene and Public
    Health
Baltimore, Maryland

Gail L. Gamble, M.D.
Consultant
Department of Physical Medicine and Rehabilitation
Mayo Clinic and Mayo Foundation
Assistant Professor of Physical Medicine and Rehabilitation
Mayo Medical School
Rochester, Minnesota

Fae H. Garden, M.D.
Assistant Professor
Department of Physical Medicine and Rehabilitation
Baylor College of Medicine
Houston, Texas

Susan J. Garrison, M.D.
Associate Professor
Department of Physical Medicine and Rehabilitation
Baylor College of Medicine
Medical Director, Rehabilitation Center
The Methodist Hospital
Houston, Texas

Arthur M. Gershkoff, M.D.
Clinical Assistant Professor
Department of Rehabilitation Medicine
Thomas Jefferson University
Attending Physiatrist
Magee Rehabilitation Hospital
Philadelphia, Pennsylvania

Martin A. Goins, M.D.
Chairman, Department of Otolaryngology
Sinai Hospital of Baltimore
Assistant Professor
Department of Otolaryngology and Head and Neck Surgery
The Johns Hopkins University School of Medicine
Baltimore, Maryland

Erwin G. Gonzalez, M.D.
Director, Department of Physical Medicine and
    Rehabilitation
Beth Israel Medical Center
Professor of Rehabilitation Medicine
Mount Sinai School of Medicine
New York, New York

Carl V. Granger, M.D.
Professor of Rehabilitation Medicine
Director of Center for Functional Assessment Research
School of Medicine and Biomedical Sciences
State University of New York at Buffalo
Buffalo, New York

Jim Grigsby, M.D.
Rocky Mountain Multiple Sclerosis Center
Colorado Neurological Institute
Englewood, Colorado

Lauro S. Halstead, M.D.
Director, Post Polio Program
National Rehabilitation Hospital
Clinical Professor, Department of Medicine
Georgetown University School of Medicine
Washington, D.C.

Norman C. Hursh, Sc.D.
Associate Professor and Director of Vocational Evaluation
Department of Rehabilitation Counseling
Boston University
Boston, Massachusetts

Sudesh Sheela Jain, M.D.
Assistant Professor
Clinical Physical Medicine and Rehabilitation
University of Medicine and Dentistry—New Jersey Medical
    School
Director, Amputee Service
Kessler Institute for Rehabilitation
Administrative Director
Department of Physical Medicine and Rehabilitation
St. Barnabas Medical Center
West Orange, New Jersey

Fran E. Kaiser, M.D.
Geriatric Research Education and Clinical Center
VA Medical Center
Division of Geriatric Medicine
St. Louis University Medical Center
St. Louis, Missouri

Karen J. Kalupa, O.T.R.
Supervisor, Occupational Therapy
Health Span Mercy Hospital
formerly, Supervisor, Occupational Therapy
Miland E. Knapp Rehabilitation Center
Minneapolis, Minnesota

Claudia H. Kawas, M.D.
Assistant Professor
Department of Neurology
The Johns Hopkins University School of Medicine
Baltimore, Maryland

Jeffrey Lafferman, M.D.
Department of Medicine
Levindale Hebrew Geriatric Center and Hospital
Baltimore, Maryland

Judy C. Lane, M.D.
Rehabilitation Associates of Colorado, Inc.
Englewood, Colorado

Stephen S. Lefrak, M.D.
Professor of Medicine
Respiratory and Critical Care Division
Department of Medicine
Washington University School of Medicine
The Jewish Hospital of St. Louis
St. Louis, Missouri

James A. Leonard, Jr., M.D.
Clinical Associate Professor
Associate Chairman
Department of Physical Medicine and Rehabilitation
Medical Director
Division of Orthotics and Prosthetics
The University of Michigan Medical School
Ann Arbor, Michigan

Margaret R. Lie, M.D.
Consultant
Department of Physical Medicine and Rehabilitation
Mayo Clinic and Mayo Foundation
Associate Professor of Physical Medicine and Rehabilitation
Mayo Medical School
Rochester, Minnesota

Jay Magaziner, Ph.D., M.S. Hyg.
Associate Professor
Division of Gerontology
Department of Epidemiology and Preventive Medicine
University of Maryland School of Medicine
Baltimore, Maryland

S. Van McCrary, Ph.D., J.D., M.P.H.
Medical Humanities Program
University of Florida College of Medicine
Gainesville, Florida

Kevin M. Means, M.D.
Associate Professor
Department of Physical Medicine & Rehabilitation
University of Arkansas for Medical Sciences
Medical Director
Falls and Mobility Disorders Program
Assistant Chief
Physical Medicine & Rehabilitation Service
John L. McClellan Department of Veterans Affairs Medical
    Center
Little Rock, Arkansas

Carol N. Meredith, Ph.D.
Assistant Professor
Division of Clinical Nutrition
Department of Internal Medicine
University of California, Davis
Davis, California

Jan R. Miller, M.D.
Rocky Mountain Multiple Sclerosis Center
Colorado Neurological Institute
Englewood, Colorado

Lawrence S. Miller, M.D.
Medical Director, Comprehensive Rehabilitation Services
St. Joseph's Medical Center
Director, Geriatric Rehabilitation Services at UCLA
    Medical Center
Clinical Professor of Medicine
UCLA
Burbank, California

Arshag D. Mooradian, M.D.
Professor of Internal Medicine
Director of the Division of Endocrinology and Metabolism
St. Louis University School of Medicine
St. Louis, Missouri

John E. Morley, M.B., B.Ch.
Geriatric Research Education and Clinical Center
VA Medical Center
Dammert Professor of Gerontology
Director, Department of Internal Medicine
Division of Geriatric Medicine
St. Louis University Medical Center
St. Louis, Missouri

Maureen R. Nelson, M.D.
Assistant Professor of Physical Medicine and Pediatrics
Department of Physical Medicine and Pediatrics
Baylor College of Medicine
Chief, Physical Medicine and Rehabilitation
Texas Children's Hospital
Houston, Texas

Patricia Nelson, M.D.
Instructor of Medicine
Respiratory and Critical Care Division
Department of Medicine
Washington University School of Medicine
The Jewish Hospital of St. Louis
St. Louis, Missouri

John J. Nicholas, M.D.
Professor and Chairman
Department of Physical Medicine and Rehabilitation
Rush-Presbyterian-St. Luke's Medical Center
Chicago, Illinois
Rehabilitation and Medicine Clinics, Inc.
Wheaton, Illinois

Jeffrey B. Palmer, M.D.
Associate Professor and Director
Electrodiagnostic Laboratory
Departments of Rehabilitation Medicine and Otolaryngol-
    ogy—Head and Neck Surgery
The Johns Hopkins University School of Medicine
Baltimore, Maryland

Beverly Parker, M.D.
Staff Geriatrician
Medical Director, Clinical Research Unit
Department of Veterans Affairs Medical Center
Boise, Idaho
Clinical Instructor of Medicine
University of Washington School of Medicine
Seattle, Washington

Inder Perkash, M.D.
Professor of Urology and Functional Restoration
The Paralyzed Veterans of America
Professor of Spinal Cord Injury
Stanford University
Chief, The Spinal Cord Injury Service
Department of Veterans Affairs Medical Center
Palo Alto, California

Horace M. Perry III, M.D.
Geriatric Research Education and Clinical Center
VA Medical Center
Division of Geriatric Medicine
St. Louis University Medical Center
St. Louis, Missouri

John B. Redford, M.D.
Distinguished Professor
Department of Rehabilitation Medicine
University of Kansas Medical Center
Kansas City, Kansas
Chief of RMS
VA Medical Center
Kansas City, Missouri

Marcel A. Reischer, M.D.
Affiliate Staff
Department of Rehabilitation Medicine
Sinai Hospital of Baltimore
Baltimore, Maryland

Aaron N. Rosenberg, M.D.
Associate Professor
Department of Orthopedics
Rush Medical College of Rush University
Chicago, Illinois

Felicia D. Sankey, M.D.
Assistant Professor
Department of Physical Medicine & Rehabilitation
University of Arkansas for Medical Sciences
Staff Physician
Physical Medicine & Rehabilitation Service
John L. McClellan Department of Veterans Affairs Medical
    Center
Little Rock, Arkansas

Donald E. Shrey, Ph.D.
Associate Professor and Director of Disability Management
Department of Physical Medicine and Rehabilitation
University of Cincinnati Medical Center
Cincinnati, Ohio

Hilary Siebens, M.D.
Assistant Clinical Professor
Department of Medicine/Geriatrics/Physical Medicine and
    Rehabilitation
Assistant Medical Director
Department of Rehabilitation Medicine
Cedars-Sinai Medical Center
Los Angeles, California

Andrew J. Silver, M.D.
Geriatric Research Education Clinical Center
VA Medical Center
Geriatric Medicine
St. Louis University School of Medicine
St. Louis, Missouri

Mehrsheed Sinaki, M.D., M.S.
Consultant
Department of Physical Medicine and Rehabilitation
Mayo Clinic and Mayo Foundation
Professor of Physical Medicine and Rehabilitation
Mayo Medical School
Rochester, Minnesota

Henry A. Spindler, M.D.
Affiliate Staff
Department of Rehabilitation Medicine
Sinai Hospital of Baltimore
Baltimore, Maryland

Barry D. Stein, M.D.
Department of Rehabilitation Medicine
Sinai Hospital of Baltimore
Clinical Assistant Professor
Department of Epidemiology and Preventive Medicine
University of Maryland School of Medicine
Baltimore, Maryland

Franz U. Steinberg, M.D., F.A.C.P.
Emeritus Professor of Clinical Medicine
Washington University School of Medicine
Department of Rehabilitation
The Jewish Hospital of St. Louis
St. Louis, Missouri

M. G. Stineman, M.D.
Assistant Professor of Rehabilitation Medicine
Department of Rehabilitation Medicine
University of Pennsylvania Medical Center
Philadelphia, Pennsylvania

Elaine Thompson, Ph.D., P.T.
Assistant Professor
Department of Physical Therapy
Beaver College
Glenside, Pennsylvania

Richard E. Verville, J.D.
Partner
White, Fine and Verville
Washington, D.C.

Robert E. Vestal, M.D.
Chief, Clinical Pharmacology and Gerontology Research
    Unit
Associate Chief of Staff for Research and Development
Department of Veterans Affairs Medical Center
Boise, Idaho
Professor of Medicine
Adjunct Professor of Pharmacology
University of Washington
Seattle, Washington

Stanley F. Wainapel, M.D., M.P.H.
Medical Director
Jewish Guild for the Blind (Adult Day Services)
Associate Professor of Clinical Rehabilitation Medicine
Columbia University College of Physicians and Surgeons
New York, New York

Nicolas E. Walsh, M.D.
Professor and Chairman
Department of Rehabilitation Medicine
University of Texas Health Science Center at San Antonio
San Antonio, Texas

Nirandon Wongsurawat, M.D., F.A.C.P.
Professor of Internal Medicine
St. Louis University School of Medicine
Physician-In-Charge of Medicine
Jefferson Barracks VA Medical Center
St. Louis, Missouri

Gary M. Yarkony, M.D.
Attending Physican and Director of Spinal Cord Injury
    Rehabilitation
Rehabilitation Institute of Chicago
Midwest Regional Spinal Cord Injury Care System
Assistant Professor
Department of Rehabilitation
Northwestern University Medical School
Adjunct Assistant Professor
Pritzker Institute for Medical Engineering
Illinois Institute of Technology
Chicago, Illinois

Sheryl Itkin Zimmerman, Ph.D.
Assistant Professor
Division of Gerontology
Department of Epidemiology and Preventive Medicine
University of Maryland School of Medicine
Baltimore, Maryland

Contents

SECTION I

GERONTOLOGY: GENERAL ASPECTS

1
Biology of Aging

Arshag D. Mooradian

The aging phenomenon has been the subject of human interest since the dawn of civilization. This is partly because of a basic human need to explain the unknown and partly because of pragmatic reasons to prolong life and/or avoid the degenerative changes of aging. From the perspective of the health care professional, some knowledge of the age-related biologic changes would help optimize health care delivery. It is, therefore, not surprising that a modern textbook on geriatric rehabilitation should include a chapter on the biology of aging.

Intrinsic to the problem of defining aging is the lack of reliable biomarkers that will allow us to identify premature aging syndromes more reliably and help predict future morbidity. In this chapter, a brief description of various theories of aging will be presented, the available potential biomarkers of aging will be discussed, and the age-related changes in physiologic parameters will be reviewed.

THREE THEORIES OF AGING

The quest for the "Fountain of Youth" has been associated with a proliferation of theories of aging. Theories are based on population studies, organ system changes, or cellular studies (1, 2) (Table 1.1).

Population-based Theories

There are two types of population-based theories. Type I theories are based on the generalized rate of living theory. The life span of various species is correlated with various indices of rate of living and development, such as age at sexual maturation, brain weight, or metabolic rate (3, 4). It is suggested that the life span-energy potential (i.e., the total energy spent over the life span) is constant for all animal species. Since caloric intake increases metabolic rate, the observation that food restriction prolongs life can be taken as indirect evidence supportive of this theory. However, experiments in laboratory animals have failed to demonstrate a lasting effect of food restriction on the metabolic rate (5).

Type II population-based theories assume that aging is the result of collagen cross-linking. This set of theories is currently disfavored since animal species with differences in life span may have similar collagen composition (1, 2).

Organ System-based Theories

This set of theories relates aging to changes in certain organ systems, particularly the endocrine and immune systems. Relevant to these theories is the notion of a "pacemaker" of aging. None of the age-related changes in hormonal secretion has been causally related to aging. Similarly, none of the age-related changes in the immune system cause aging. Restoration of impaired immune functions in aged animals does not prolong the life span (6). It is more likely that the age-related changes in the immune system are secondary phenomena. Currently, there is no experimental evidence to support these theories.

Cellular-based Theories

This set of theories is currently the most popular. Recent experimental findings support cellular-based

Table 1.1. Theories of Aging[a]

Population-based theories
Type I: Rate of living theory; correlations between life span of species and metabolic rate, age at sexual maturation, body weight, or brain weight
Type II: Collagen theories; currently disfavored
Organ system-based theories
Role of the immune system
Role of the endocrine system
"Pacemaker" of aging
Cellular-based theories
Somatic–mutation theory
Orgel's error–catastrophe theory
Free radical damage
DNA or DNA-binding protein alterations

[a] Adapted from Mooradian AD. Molecular theories of aging. In: Morley JE, Glizk Z, Rubenstein LZ, eds. *Geriatric Nutrition. A Comprehensive Review.* New York, NY: Raven Press; 1990: 11–18 and Hart RW, Turturo A. Theories of aging. *Rev Biol Res Aging.* 1:5–17, 1983.

theories of aging. As a group, these theories date back to 1891 when Weismann suggested "wear and tear" theory (7). According to this theory, senescence is the result of wearing down of somatic cells. This concept gained considerable momentum when Hayflick and Moorhead demonstrated that diploid cells in culture have a limited potential to replicate (8). The finite replicative capacity of cultured fibroblasts correlates with the life span of different species. Fibroblasts isolated from the turtle, which has a long life span, are capable of replicating more times than fibroblasts isolated from mice, which have a short life span. The finite lifetime of cultured fibroblasts also correlates with the age of the donor. Older individuals have fibroblasts that tend to undergo fewer doublings in vitro compared to fibroblasts isolated from younger individuals (9).

The somatic–mutation theory and the error–catastrophe theory are interrelated cellular-based theories. These theories assume that the error frequency within a cell increases with time until it reaches a threshold catastrophic level that ushers the onset of cellular senescence. Most of the available data do not support these theories. Induction of cellular errors by supplying inappropriate amino acids does not cause cellular senescence. In addition, despite the methodological difficulties in studying the phenomenon, it appears that the frequency of cellular errors does not increase with age (10, 11).

The free radical theory of aging is a very popular theory (12). Normal mitochondrial respiration or autooxidation of biomolecules such as flavins and catecholamines is the source of a host of free radicals. Radiation damage and environmental toxins often enhance free radical generation. This is one way by which environmental factors could modulate the intrinsic rate of aging. The biochemically active radicals can damage DNA and alter the structural and functional integrity of biological membranes. The administration of antioxidants, however, does not prolong life span. The earlier encouraging findings of life span extension in mice treated with antioxidants have been attributed to inadvertently occurring relative food restriction. In one study, supplementary vitamin E (an antioxidant) reduced the age-related accumulation of cardiac lipofuscin without altering the life span of the animals (13, 14). It is possible that the failure of antioxidants to prolong life span is due to the inability to deliver these chemicals to the critical sites of free radical generation at sufficient concentrations. The reader is referred to an elegant review of the pros and cons of the free radical theory of aging written by Dr. R. Sohal (15).

Age-related alterations in DNA or DNA binding proteins have been the subject of intense research. These changes may underlie most of the biochemical basis of aging (16). Changes in DNA structure and transcribability occur with age. Decreased DNA digestibility with

alkali and urea has been proposed as a potential biomarker of aging (17, 18). Increased thermal stability of DNA in aged animals has been documented in several studies (19). Perhaps the most dramatic age-related change in DNA function is "leaky" expression of genes. There is an age-related derepression of viral and globin-related mRNA in the brain and liver (20), and tyrosine hydroxylase expression is increased with age (21). For certain genes, these observations are attributed to an age-related decrease in methylation status, which will allow the expression of suppressed genes (22). For the majority of changes in genomic function, however, the underlying mechanisms are totally unknown. A recent tantalizing observation related cellular senescence in vitro to chromosome one (23). When these studies are confirmed, it will facilitate the search for the set of genes that govern cellular replication or senescence.

DETERMINANTS OF LIFE EXPECTANCY AND LIFE SPAN

Life expectancy refers to the average number of years of life expected at a given age. Life span is the maximal attainable age for a given species. The latter is the x-axis intercept of population survival curves (24) (Fig. 1.1). The shape of these curves is influenced by the degree of relevance of aging to death. Thus, when the probability of death is independent of age, the survival curve is exponential, i.e., the percentage of individuals dying at any age is constant (curve a). On the other hand, when age is the sole determinant of death, the survival curve is rectangular (curve c). The survival curves of all mammalian species are intermediate between these two extreme hypothetical curves. Thus, death, in reality, is the result of a composite of factors related to aging and environmental hazards.

With the advent of technology and the improvements in health care over the last century, the life expectancy of human beings has been extended without a change in life span. This is referred to as the rectangularization of the survival curves. Although genetic fac-

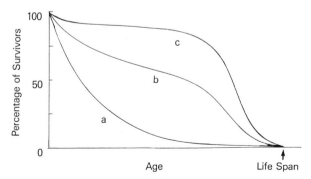

Figure 1.1 Hypothetical population survival curves. Life span is the intercept with x-axis. Adapted from Kirkwood TBL, Holliday R. The evaluation of aging and longevity. *Proc R Soc Biol Lond. 205:531–546, 1979.*

tors are probably the most important determinants of life expectancy, factors such as good dietary habits, exercise, and avoidance of radiation exposure have important modulating effects. The only intervention, however, that has been consistently shown to improve life span in experimental animals is dietary restriction. Although for maximal benefit this intervention should be started early in life, it appears that restriction of calories without malnutrition is beneficial in rats even when it is started in midlife (25–28). In addition to extending the life span, caloric restriction results in delay in the emergence of age-related physiologic, biochemical, and immunologic changes and retards the emergence of neoplasms (25). Caloric restriction, however, invariably results in growth retardation and, as such, its applicability to humans is unknown.

Interestingly, a recent study reported that a pharmacologic manipulation, namely treatment of rats with deprenyl, significantly increases life expectancy and life span (29). This drug, an inhibitor of monoamine oxidase subtype B, is being used extensively in patients with Parkinson's disease. It is quite premature, however, to recommend this drug to the general population as the "Fountain of Youth." Other interventions, such as consumption of antioxidants (vitamins C and E), superoxide dismutase, and gerovital-H3, have not withstood the test of time, and elderly patients should be educated as to the lack of efficacy and potential harm of some of these agents (25).

PHYSIOLOGIC CHANGES WITH AGE

A variety of changes in organ system functions occur with age. Some of these changes are related to aging; the others are secondary to life-style and diseases common in the elderly. In the following section, the physiologic changes in individual organ systems will be summarized, and their possible relevance to the rehabilitation of patients with chronic diseases will be discussed.

Cardiovascular System

The effect of age on the cardiovascular system has been extensively studied (30). Age-related changes in this system are summarized in Table 1.2. Although the literature is still controversial, it appears that aging, per se, does not alter cardiac output or cardiac index (cardiac output divided by surface area). This is true even with increasing exercise load. Heart rate, especially during exercise, is lower in the elderly. The normal cardiac output, despite the reduced heart rate, is, therefore, the result of increased stroke volume with age. Left ventricular size is also increased with age. Thus, stroke volume is increased with age, even though the ejection fraction is reduced. It appears that the heart in older subjects

Table 1.2. Age-related Changes in the Cardiovascular System

Increased
Stroke volume
End-diastolic volume
End-systolic volume
Systolic blood pressure
Normal
Cardiac output
Myocardial contractility (or mildly decreased)
Decreased
Heart rate
Ejection fraction

utilizes Frank-Starling forces. Maintenance of normal cardiac output is often at the expense of modestly increased left ventricular end-diastolic pressure. This observation suggests that, although cardiac output may be maintained in the healthy elderly, they are more likely to develop early dyspnea with exertion. Overall, it appears that pulmonary or musculoskeletal changes or motivational factors are more important than are cardiovascular factors in limiting the exercise ability of the healthy elderly.

It is noteworthy, however, that most elderly patients under medical care, and especially those in rehabilitation wards, are those who have not aged successfully. In this subgroup of patients, cardiovascular changes are more pronounced. Many have increased systolic blood pressure, increased workload of the heart, decreased cardiac output, and increased left ventricular end-diastolic pressure. The significant limitations of cardiovascular reserve should be taken into account when prescribing an exercise program for these patients. In addition, subclinical coronary artery disease is common in this patient population, and vigorous physical rehabilitation programs can precipitate cardiac arrests, which appear to occur most commonly in the gymnasium and during practice sessions using the parallel bars (31). Fortunately, most of these patients with cardiac arrests can be successfully resuscitated if they have appropriate medical supervision; however, care should be taken to avoid the situation in the first place.

Central Nervous System

It is widely believed that the central nervous system (CNS) undergoes dramatic changes with aging, to the extent that some unscrupulous people have used the words senility and aging interchangeably. This misperception is most likely based on the increased prevalence of age-related degenerative diseases of the CNS, such as Alzheimer's disease. The age-related changes in the CNS function are usually modest (32). These include decreased speed of brain processing during performing verbal or manual tasks, increasing difficulty of learning new skills, and mild loss of memory (32). Brain mass, as assessed by computerized tomographic scans, is also reduced with age (33). Overall intelligence, however, is not significantly altered. Diabetic elderly patients appear to be at higher risk for decreased cognitive abilities (34, 35).

Patients with CNS changes require additional attention to make sure that they understand and follow the instructions given during a rehabilitation program. Compliance with prescribed medications should be monitored carefully and recommendations should be reinforced through an ongoing education program.

Pulmonary Function

The age-related changes in pulmonary function are summarized in Table 1.3. The partial pressure of arterial oxygen (PaO_2) declines steadily with age, while $PaCO_2$ is not significantly altered (36). Decreased lung compliance, increased chest wall stiffness, and weaker respiratory muscles account for most of the age-related changes in pulmonary functions. With age, vital capacity is reduced, while functional residual capacity, residual volume, and closing volume are increased. The expiratory flow rates such as FEV_1 (forced expiratory volume at 1 second) and midmaximal flow (MMF) are also reduced with age. These changes are probably more important than the changes in the cardiovascular system in limiting exercise capacity of the elderly. Obviously, pulmonary aging is accelerated in chronic smokers who are exposed to increased free radical damage of the lungs. Elderly patients with chronic obstructive lung disease pose a special challenge for rehabilitation programs. Special breathing exercises, such as blowing against pursed lips, will increase respiratory muscle strength and help reduce respiratory fatigue.

Renal Function

Aging is associated with significant structural changes in the kidney. Although medullary mass is relatively preserved, there is usually a marked atrophy of cortical mass (37, 38). Decreased renal blood flow and increased intrarenal shunting of blood may contribute to the functional changes in the kidney. Hyalinization of the glomeruli is usually focal and segmental, and nephronal units are decreased. Since the structural changes occur in all the segments of the nephron (i.e., the glomerulus and the tubules) it is not surprising that the age-related declines in the various renal functions occur in parallel (38). Thus, with age, the following parameters are decreased: renal plasma flow, glomerular filtration rate, sodium retention and excretion, potassium and acid load excretion, and sensitivity to antidiuretic hormone (ADH). Longitudinal studies of renal function have made two important observations that may well be applicable to a variety of age-related changes in organ function; one is that age-related decline in renal function is not a universal phenomenon (39). Some individuals do not have reduced renal function with age. The second tantalizing observation is that age-related decline in renal function is often exponential, i.e., the functional decline is accelerated with age.

The reduced renal function with age has important clinical implications. The dosage of a variety of drugs known to be eliminated through the renal route should be adjusted for renal function. It should be emphasized that serum creatinine (Scr) measurements in the elderly underestimate the degree of renal function impairment. Estimation of creatinine clearance (Cr. Cl.) from the Cockroft-Gault equation (40), though not always accurate, is clinically useful.

$$Creatinine\ (Cr)\ clearance = \frac{140 - age \times body\ weight\ (kg)}{Scr\ (mg/dL)\ \times 72}$$

Multiply the result by 0.85 for women.

Digestive System

The age-related changes in the oral cavity and the rest of the gastrointestinal tract (41) are summarized in Table 1.4. The oral cavity undergoes significant changes with age. Some of the changes are secondary to disease, poor hygiene, and smoking habits. Loss of teeth and decreased chewing efficiency are common among the elderly. The salivary flow rate is reduced, although the histologic changes in salivary glands with age are modest (42). The swallowing mechanism is usually not altered with age. On the other hand, patients with dis-

Table 1.3. Age-related Changes in Pulmonary Function

Vital capacity declines linearly from age 20 to 80; 26 mL/yr for men and 22 mL/yr for women
Total lung capacity (TLC) remains constant
Residual volume increases from 20% of TLC to 35% at age 60
Arterial PO_2 decreases (A–aO_2 difference increases) secondary to ventilation–perfusion mismatch. CO diffusion capacity is also decreased
Elastic recoil decreases, closing volume increases
Maximum voluntary ventilation (FEV_1) and maximum expiratory flow rate decrease

Table 1.4. Age-related Changes in the Digestive System

Oral/dental changes: Loss of teeth, decreased salivation, decreased taste.
Esophagus: Decreased frequency of peristaltic waves and increased frequency of tertiary contractions in a subgroup of patients; delayed lower esophageal sphincter relaxation. Only modest decrease in amplitude of contractions
Stomach: Normal motility; atrophy of glands. Achlorhydria is a disease
Small intestine: Normal transit; some villous atrophy
Colon: Decreased motility
Liver/pancreas: Large reserve, changes are clinically insignificant

eases affecting oral musculature, such as stroke or Parkinson's disease, pose special challenges for the speech pathologist in a rehabilitation ward. Alterations in the taste sensation are usually modest and of little clinical significance. However, when the patient is prescribed a drug that can alter taste sensation, the older patient may be at higher risk for refraining from food intake. Loss of the hedonic qualities of food can be an important component of the anorexia of aging.

Although older patients with diabetes and neurologic diseases have abnormal esophageal motility, in healthy elderly the only change seen is decreased amplitude of esophageal contractions.

Age-related changes in the stomach include some glandular atrophy and decreased acid output; pepsin secretion remains normal. Whereas hypochlorhydria is common, achlorhydria should be regarded as disease (e.g., pernicious anemia). Decreased stomach acidity interferes with the absorption of certain drugs, such as ketoconazole, and may contribute to decreased iron absorption.

Gastric motility is not altered with age. Small intestinal transit time is also not altered, although the absorptive surface area may be reduced. In contrast, aging is associated with reduced colonic motility, which contributes to the problem of constipation in the elderly (41).

Age-related changes in the function of other digestive organs such as the liver and the pancreas are usually of no clinical significance (41). In general, the mass of these organs and the blood flow are reduced. Pancreatic trypsin secretion may be reduced, while the flow of pancreatic fluid and bicarbonate secretion are not altered. The vast reserve capacity of these organs accounts for the lack of clinical effects of the modest changes that occur with age.

Overall, the digestive function is well preserved with age. The absorption rate (i.e., per unit time) of some drugs and nutrients may be altered in a subgroup of patients, but the total cumulative absorption is usually unaltered.

Hematopoietic and Immune Systems

Healthy elderly have normal measurements on complete blood count (CBC). Thus, aging does not alter the hematocrit, hemoglobin levels, red blood cell indices, white blood cell count and distribution, nor platelet counts (43). Studies in laboratory animals have not found a major age-related change in the distribution of hematopoietic progenitor cells. In humans, especially in a subgroup of patients, it appears that some of the progenitor cells are reduced (43). The amount of active bone marrow is reduced with age and so is the functional reserve. In general, hematopoietic response to bleeding or infection is brisk but may not be sustained. Anemia in

the elderly should not be attributed to aging, and appropriate workup is necessary to determine the underlying pathology.

The production and consumption of certain components of the complement cascade may be decreased, yet this is the system that is least affected with age.

The immune system undergoes significant changes with aging (44). Thymic involution is a universal phenomenon. T-cells and the distribution of the T-cell subtypes are usually more affected than are B-cells. Immunoglobulin response to simple T-cell-independent antigens, such as pneumococcal vaccine, is maintained better than the response to complex T-cell-dependent antigens, such as the tetanus or influenza vaccines. Macrophage function and the chemotactic or phagocytic activity of polymorphonuclear cells are usually well maintained, although intracellular bactericidal activity may be reduced. These changes are aggravated in the presence of protein malnutrition (43). Age-related alterations in the immune system may account for the increased susceptibility to and the increased severity of infections in the elderly. It should be noted, however, that the opportunistic infections commonly associated with immunodeficiency are not common in the elderly patient populations.

Endocrine System

A variety of changes in the endocrine system occur with age (45) (Table 1.5). The basal and stimulated plasma norepinephrine levels are increased, while beta adrenergic receptor stimulation in cardiovascular systems is

Table 1.5. Age-related Changes in the Basal Levels of Plasma Hormones[a]

High
Parathyroid hormone
Insulin
Glucagon
Norepinephrine
Vasopressin
Thyroid stimulating hormone (TSH)
Luteinizing hormone (LH)
Follicle stimulating hormone (FSH)
Normal
Epinephrine
Cortisol
Thyroxine (T_4)
Growth hormone
Thyroid stimulating hormone (TSH)
Low
Triiodothyronine (T_3)
Active renin
Dehydroepiandrosterone (DHEA)
Aldosterone
Insulin-like growth factor-1 (IGF-1)
Testosterone

[a] Adapted from Mooradian AD, Morley JE, Korenman SG. Endocrinology in aging. *Disease-a-Month.* 34(7):398–461, 1988.

decreased (45). The plasma epinephrine level is not altered. Of the adrenal gland hormones, cortisol level in the plasma is normal, while aldosterone level and adrenal androgens, especially dehydro-3-epiandrosterone, are reduced. The reduced plasma aldosterone secretion is probably secondary to reduced active renin levels (45).

Age-related glucose intolerance is manifested by an increase in postprandial blood glucose levels, while fasting levels are changed minimally (46).

Thyroid function tests are usually not altered with age, with the possible exception of a modest decrease in serum triiodothyronine (T_3) levels (45). Thyroid disease, however, especially hypothyroidism and palpable nodules, is common in the elderly. Of the pituitary hormones, growth hormone secretion is reduced and may contribute to some of the age-related changes in body composition. On the other hand, serum vasopressin level is increased, while renal responsiveness to this hormone is reduced (45).

The most dramatic endocrine change with aging is the loss of ovarian steroid secretion in women at menopause. Testosterone secretion in men undergoes a more gradual decline with age (47, 48). It remains to be seen if some of the age-related changes in body composition and the musculoskeletal system can be attributed to changes in hormonal secretion.

Body Composition and Musculoskeletal System

Body weight increases in men until the sixth decade and thereafter declines gradually. In women, body weight increases until the seventh decade (49). With age, there is a loss of lean body mass, primarily muscle mass, with preferential accumulation of adipose tissue (50). Intracellular fluid volume and total body water decrease with age, while extracellular fluid volume is maintained. Within the intracellular compartment, however, the increase in plasma volume is counterbalanced with a decrease in interstitial volume.

The changes in body composition have important clinical implications. With the increase in adipose tissue mass, the half-life of lipid soluble drug elimination is increased in the elderly.

Although the total muscle mass is decreased with age, certain muscle groups, especially those that are not very dependent on life-style such as the diaphragm and cardiac muscle, do not show a significant loss of mass. This suggests that muscle groups that are used in regular exercises would also not undergo a major loss in mass with age.

Another component of the age-related loss of lean body mass is bone loss (51). This is the result of an imbalance between bone formation and bone resorption. Hormonal and nutritional factors play an important role in bone loss, but other variables, yet unidentified, are probably as important.

Degenerative changes of the joint may not be distinguishable from age-related changes, and it may well be that the former are a manifestation of accelerated aging.

The changes in musculoskeletal system with age can pose important limitations on the rehabilitation potential of the elderly patient.

BIOMARKERS OF AGING

One of the major difficulties in gerontologic research is the lack of specific and quantifiable markers of biologic aging. The possible benefits of such markers include standardization of studies in aging populations and possible prediction of future morbidity and mortality (52). The age-related physiologic changes described in the previous section meet only one criterion of biomarkers, namely correlation with age of the individual. In this respect, perhaps the age-related change in dark adaptation is the best predictor of age. However, the direct relationship between these changes and the aging process is not clear. The racemization of amino acids in long-lived proteins, such as dentin of the tooth, correlates with the age of the tooth (52). However, an identical process occurs in in vitro incubations, and the biologic significance of these changes is not clear. Glycation of proteins and the formation of advanced glycation end products (AGE) have been suggested as markers of aging. This hypothesis also explains the premature aging that occurs in diabetes. Recent studies, however, have failed to find increased AGE in lens proteins with age (53). We have recently found that alkali-induced DNA unwinding rate correlates with the age of the donor (17). Interestingly, this change occurs prematurely in diabetic patients (17). Longitudinal studies are needed to determine if this observation is a valid biomarker of aging.

SUMMARY

The determinants of aging and life span are still unknown. More research, focusing on the identification of biomarkers of aging and models of premature aging, is needed. A myriad of physiologic changes occur with age. Some of these are the result of diseases that are common in the aged, while others may be a direct consequence of tissue aging. Although the changes in many organ systems may be clinically insignificant because of large reserve capacity, there is a clear age-related decrease in adaptation to perturbations in function. Perhaps the best marker of aging can be referred to as "homeostenosis," indicating reduced reserve capacity and poor adaptive responses to environmental and endogenous challenges to the biologic functions. Given these limitations, restoration of function through rehabilitation of older individuals can be a unique challenge.

References

1. Mooradian AD. Molecular theories of aging. In: Morley JE, Glizk Z, Rubenstein LZ, eds. *Geriatric Nutrition. A Comprehensive Review.* New York, NY: Raven Press; 1990:11–18.
2. Hart RW, Turturo A. Theories of aging. *Rev Biol Res Aging.* 1:5–17, 1983.
3. Cutler RG. Nature of aging and life maintenance processes. In: Cutler RG, ed. *Interdisciplinary Topics in Gerontology, IX.* New York, NY: Kerger; 1976:83–133.
4. Sacher G. Evaluation of the entropy and information terms governing mammalian longevity. In: Cutler RD, ed. *Interdisciplinary Topics in Gerontology, IX.* New York, NY: Kerger; 1976:69–82.
5. McCarter RJ, McGee JR. Transient reduction of metabolic rate by food restriction. *Am J Physiol.* 257:E175–E179, 1989.
6. Hirokawa K, Sato K, Makinodan T. Restoration of impaired immune functions in aging animals. V. Long term immunopotentiating effects of combined young bone marrow and newborn thymus grafts. *Clin Immunol Immunopathol* 22:297–304, 1982.
7. Weismann A. The duration of life. In: Poulton EB, Schonland S, Shipley AE, eds. *Essays on Heredity and Kindred Biological Problems.* Authorized translation 2nd ed. Oxford, England: Clarendon Press; 1981:1–92.
8. Hayflick L, Moorhead PS. The serial cultivation of human diploid cell strains. *Exp Cell Res.* 25:585–621, 1961.
9. Hayflick L. The cellular basis of biological aging. In: Finch CE, Hayflick L, eds. *Handbook of the Biology of Aging.* New York, NY: Van Nostrand; 1976:159–188.
10. Bozcuk AN. Testing the protein error hypothesis of aging in drosophila. *Exp Gerontol.* 11:103–112, 1976.
11. Hoffman GW. On the origin of the genetic code and the stability of the translation apparatus. *J Mol Biol.* 86:349–362, 1974.
12. Harman D. The aging process. *Proc Natl Acad Sci USA.* 78:7124–7128, 1981.
13. Blackett AD, Hall DA. The effects of vitamin E on mouse fitness and survival. *Gerontology.* 27:133–139, 1981.
14. Blackett AD, Hall DA. Vitamin E. Its significance in mouse aging. *Age Ageing.* 10:191–195, 1981.
15. Sohal RS. The free radical theory of aging: A critique. *Rev Biol Res Aging.* 3:431–449, 1987.
16. Kirkwood TBL. DNA mutations and aging. *Mutation Research (DNAging).* Pilot Issue:7–13, 1988.
17. Hartnell JM, Morley JE, Mooradian AD. Alkali-induced white blood cell DNA unwinding rate is reduced in healthy elderly. A potential biomarker of aging. *J Gerontol Biol Sci.* 44:B125–B130, 1989.
18. Hartnell JM, Storric MD, Mooradian AD. The tissue specificity of the age-related changes in alkali-induced DNA unwinding. *Mutation Research.* 219:187–192, 1989.
19. Bardyshev GD, Zhelabovskaya SM. Composition, template properties and thermostability of liver chromatin from rats of various ages at deproteinization by NaCl solutions. *Exp Gerontol.* 7:321–330, 1972.
20. Ono T, Cutler RG. Age-dependent relaxation of gene expression. Increase of endogenous murine leukemia virus-related and globin-related RNA in brain and liver of mice. *Proc Natl Acad Sci USA.* 75:4431–4435, 1978.
21. Wareham KA, Lyon MF, Glenister PH, Williams ED. Age-related reactivation of an x-linked gene. *Nature.* 327:725–727, 1987.
22. Wilson VL, Jones PA. DNA methylation decreases in aging but not in immortal cells. *Science.* 220:1055–1057, 1983.
23. Sugawara O, Oshimura M, Koi M, Annab LA, Barrett JC. Induction of cellular senescence in immortalized cells by human chromosome 1. *Science.* 247:707–709, 1990.
24. Kirkwood TBL, Holliday R. The evaluation of aging and longevity. *Proc R Soc Biol Lond.* 205:531–546, 1979.
25. Schneider EL, Reed JD. Life extension. *N Engl J Med.* 312:1159–1168, 1985.
26. Masoro EJ. Biology of aging. Current state of knowledge. *Arch Intern Med.* 147:166–169, 1987.
27. Masoro EJ. Nutrition and aging. A current assessment. *J Nutr.* 115:842–848, 1985.
28. Mooradian AD. Nutritional modulation of life span and gene expression. In: Morley JE, Moderator, Nutrition in the elderly. *Ann Intern Med.* 109:890–904, 1988.
29. Knoll J. The striatal dopamine dependency of life span in male rats. Longevity Study With (-)Deprenyl. *Mech Ageing Dev.* 46:237–262, 1988.
30. Lakatta EG. Health, disease and cardiovascular aging. In: *America's Aging: Health in an Older Society.* Washington, DC: National Academy Press; 1985:73–104.
31. Redford JB. Geriatric rehabilitation. In: Ruskin AP, ed. *Current Therapy in Physiatry. Physical Medicine and Rehabilitation.* Philadelphia, Pa: WB Saunders; 1984:90–99.
32. Katzman R, Terry R. Normal aging of the nervous system. In: Katzman R, Terry R, eds. *Neurology of Aging.* Philadelphia, Pa: Ft. Davis Co. Publishers; 1983:15–49.
33. Jacoby RJ, Levy R, Dawson JM. Computed tomography in the elderly: The normal population. *Br J Psychiatry.* 136:249–255, 1982.
34. Mooradian AD, Perryman K, Fitten J, Kavonian G, Morley JE. Cortical function in elderly non-insulin dependent diabetic patients: Behavioral and electrophysiological studies. *Arch Intern Med.* 148:2369–2372, 1988.
35. Mooradian AD. Diabetic complications of the central nervous system. *Endocrine Reviews.* 9:346–356, 1988.
36. Knudson RJ. Aging of the respiratory system. *Curr Pulmonol.* 10:1–24, 1989.
37. Goldman R. Aging of the excretory system in kidney and bladder. In: Finch CE, Hayflick L, eds. *Handbook of the Biology of Aging.* 1st ed. New York, NY: Van Nostrand Reinhold Co; 1977:409–431.
38. Meyer BR. Renal function in aging. *J Am Geriatr Soc* 37:791–800, 1989.
39. Rowe JW, Andres R, Tobin JD, et al. The effect of age on creatinine clearance in man. A cross-sectional and longitudinal study. *J Gerontol* 31:155–163, 1976.
40. Cockcroft DW, Gault MH. Prediction of creatinine clearance from serum creatinine. *Nephron.* 16:31–61, 1976.
41. Nelson JB, Castell DO. Aging of the gastrointestinal system. In: Hazzard WR, Andres R, Bierman EL, Blass JP, eds. *Principles of Geriatric Medicine and Gerontology.* New York, NY: McGraw-Hill; 1990:593–608.
42. Mintz GA, Mooradian AD. Age-related morphologic changes in rat sublingual salivary glands. *Gerontology.* 6:137–144, 1988.
43. Lipschitz DA, Udupa KB. Age and the hematopoietic system. *J Am Geriatr Soc.* 34:448–454, 1986.
44. Yoshikawa TT, Norman DC. Aging and clinical practice. In: *Infectious Diseases.* New York, NY: Igakushoin; 1987.
45. Mooradian AD, Morley JE, Korenman SG. Endocrinology in aging. *Disease-a-Month.* 34(7):398–461, 1988.
46. Morley JE, Mooradian AD, Rosenthal MH, Kaiser FE. Diabetes mellitus in the elderly: Is it different? *Am J Med.* 83:533–544, 1987.
47. Morley JE, Korenman SG, Mooradian AD, Kaiser FE. UCLA Grand Rounds: male sexual dysfunction in the elderly. *J Am Geriatr Soc.* 34:1014–1022, 1987.
48. Mooradian AD, Morley JE, Korenman SK. The biological actions of androgens. *Endocrine Review.* 8:1–28, 1987.

49. Andres R. Mortality and obesity: the rationale for age specific height-weight tables. In: Andres R, Bierman EL, Hazzard WR, eds. *Principles of Geriatric Medicine.* New York, NY: McGraw-Hill; 1985:311–318.

50. Forbes GB. The adult decline in lean body mass. *Hum Biol.* 48:161–173, 1976.

51. Morley JE, Gorbien MJ, Mooradian AD, Silver AJ, Brickman AS, Kaiser FE. UCLA Geriatric Grand Rounds: osteoporosis. *J Am Geriatr Soc.* 36:845–859, 1988.

52. Mooradian AD. Biomarkers of aging: Do we know what to look for. *J Gerontol Biol Sci* 45:B183–B186, 1990.

53. Patrick JS, Thorpe SR, Baynes JW. Nonenzymatic glycosylation of protein does not increase with age in normal human lenses. *J Gerontol.* 45:B18–B23, 1990.

2

Demography and Epidemiology of Disabilities in the Aged

Sheryl Itkin Zimmerman, Kathleen Fox, and Jay Magaziner

The numbers and proportion of aged people in the population are increasing dramatically. Accompanying this growth are escalating needs for care, resulting from more persons surviving to older ages. This chapter describes the changing demography of the aged population in the United States and provides estimates of the numbers and proportion of older persons with significant disabilities. To accomplish these objectives, demographic projections will employ US Census and mortality data. Disability estimates will derive from national studies of older persons in the community and institutions.

Disability typically refers to the functional limitations that follow illness. Although there are many ways of defining disability in individuals and populations (1–3), it is *not* our intention to select any one approach or to review this field. Instead, we will describe disability in five important functional domains: physical, instrumental, cognitive, affective, and social. We selected these functional domains because they are important aspects of the quality of life (4), and all have been measured in national studies using standardized techniques.

DEFINING THE AGED POPULATION

Most gerontologists agree that the aging process begins at birth, continues until death, and varies greatly in the rate of change for individuals and body systems (5). Although it is objective, the passing of time since birth (chronological age) is not a particularly precise marker of aging nor an accurate index for the beginning of old age. A more sensitive indicator would take account of each person's functional abilities along multiple dimensions. This perspective has been referred to as functional age. Given the many aspects of functioning, its variability across individuals, and measurement difficulties, this concept has not received much attention. While acknowledging its limitations, chronological age is the marker of choice, and age 65 typically is con-

sidered the start of old age (6). Nonetheless, it is important to recognize the significance of functional ability for the aged and the high degree of heterogeneity among those 65 years of age and older.

Historical changes in birth rates and life expectancy are resulting in dramatic increases in the numbers and proportion of those aged 65 years and older. As shown in Table 2.1, shifts in life expectancy have been dramatic. For example, a female born in 1900 could expect to live only 48 years, compared with a female born today who might live almost 80 years. The gains for men have been slightly less dramatic, increasing from 46 years in 1900 to 72 years in 1990. Similarly, a female who reached age 65 in 1900 could expect to live to age 77, and today could expect to become 85 years of age; men reaching age 65 in 1990 might live until age 80. Accompanying these increases in life expectancy has been a noticeable variation in health and functional well-being. This variability has resulted in the recognition of three groups of older persons: the young-old (ages 65–74 years), a group in relatively good health; the old-old (ages 75–84 years), a group whose health is beginning to decline; and the oldest-old (ages 85 + years), a group of survivors who are in the poorest health (7, 8).

GROWTH OF THE OLDER POPULATION: DEMOGRAPHIC CHANGES

At the beginning of this century, those 65 years and older numbered 3 million and represented 4% of the total population (Table 2.2). In 1990, over 30 million Americans were 65 years of age or older and represented approximately 12.7% of the US population. By the year 2000, 35 million Americans are expected to be 65 years or older; and by 2050, this number is expected to surpass 67 million, almost 22% of the total US population.

Within the older population, these increases will be most pronounced among the oldest-old, those 85 years

Table 2.1. Life Expectancy at Birth and Age 65 by Gender: United States, 1900–2050[a]

Year	At Birth		At Age 65	
	Male	Female	Male	Female
1900	46.3	48.3	11.5	12.2
1950	65.6	71.1	12.8	15.0
1960	66.6	73.1	12.8	15.8
1970	67.7	74.8	13.1	17.0
1980	70.0	77.4	14.1	18.3
1985	71.2	78.2	14.6	18.6
1990	71.6	79.2	15.0	19.5
2000	72.9	80.5	15.7	20.5
2010	73.8	81.5	16.1	21.2
2020	74.2	82.0	16.5	21.7
2030	74.6	82.5	16.8	22.1
2040	75.0	83.1	17.1	22.6
2050	75.5	83.6	17.4	23.1

[a] Sources: National Center for Health Statistics. *Health, United States, 1986.* (14) Spencer G, US Bureau of the Census. Projections of the population of the United States, by age, sex, and race: 1983 to 2080. *Current Population Reports.* Series P-25, No. 952, May 1984.
Adapted from US Senate Special Committee on Aging. (9)

and older. This group, which today numbers 3.3 million and represents 1.3% of the population, numbered only 123,000 in 1900. By 2000 they will number 4.9 million; and by 2050, 16 million Americans will be ages 85 years and older. This anticipated increase of more than 380% from 1990 to 2050 is particularly significant when one considers the accompanying declines in functionality and the associated demands for health care by this segment of the aged population.

MORTALITY, DISEASE, AND DISABILITY AMONG THE AGED

The 10 leading causes of death among the aged are show in Table 2.3 (9). For those 65 years and older, the leading causes of death are heart disease, malignant neoplasms, and cerebrovascular disease. Despite the attention typically given to disease as a cause of death, of additional importance is the occurrence of disease and related disability before death. In general, the occur-

Table 2.2. Actual and Projected Growth of the Older Population: United States, 1900–2050 (Numbers in Thousands)[a]

Year	All Ages	65+ Years		65–74 Years		75–84 Years		85+ Years	
		Number	%	Number	%	Number	%	Number	%
1900	76,303	3,084	4.0	2,189	2.9	772	1.0	123	0.2
1930	122,775	6,634	5.4	4,721	3.8	1,641	1.3	272	0.2
1960	179,323	16,560	9.2	10,997	6.1	4,633	2.6	929	0.5
1990	249,657	31,697	12.7	18,035	7.2	10,349	4.1	3,313	1.3
2020	296,597	51,422	17.3	29,855	10.1	14,486	4.9	7,081	2.4
2050	309,488	67,411	21.8	30,114	9.7	21,263	6.9	16,034	5.2

[a] Sources: Spender G, US Bureau of the Census. Projections of the population of the United States, by age, sex, and race: 1983 to 2080. *Current Population Reports.* Series P-25, No. 952, May 1984.
US Bureau of the Census. Tabulated from Decennial Censuses of Population, 1900 to 1980.
US Bureau of the Census. Estimates of the population of the United States, by age, sex, and race: 1980–1986. *Current Population Reports.* Series P-25, No. 1000, February 1987.
Adapted from US Senate Special Committee on Aging. (9)

Table 2.3. Death Rates for Ten Leading Causes of Death Among Older People, by Age: 1984 (Rates per 100,000 Population in Age Group)[a]

Cause of Death (per 100,000)	65+ Years	65–74 Years	75–84 Years	85+ Years
All causes	5,103	2,848	6,398	15,223
Diseases of the heart	2,186	1,103	2,749	7,251
Malignant neoplasms	1,042	835	1,272	1,604
Cerebrovascular diseases	476	177	626	1,884
Chronic obstructive pulmonary diseases	199	141	270	331
Pneumonia and influenza	182	54	216	883
Diabetes	95	59	126	217
Accidents	87	50	107	257
Atherosclerosis	83	17	88	488
Nephritis, nephrotic syndrome, nephrosis	58	27	76	201
Septicemia	41	20	52	142
All other causes	654	365	816	1,965

[a] Source: National Center for Health Statistics. Advance report of final mortality statistics, 1984. *Monthly Vital Statistics Report 35,* No. 6, Supplement (2), September 1986.
Adapted from US Senate Special Committee on Aging. (9)

rence of acute conditions decreases with advancing age, while that of chronic conditions increases. Furthermore, the disability that follows both acute and chronic conditions increases with advancing age (10). The leading chronic conditions and associated disability are shown in Table 2.4. The three most prevalent conditions among the aged are arthritis, hypertension, and heart disease.

As expected, increases in disability accompany these chronic conditions, which accumulate with advancing age (11–13).

The presence of multiple chronic diseases limits activities for persons 65 years of age and older. Thirty-nine percent of the aged had some limitation of activity in 1986 because of chronic health conditions. Sixteen

Table 2.4.   Number of Leading Chronic Conditions per 1000 Persons and Percent with Activity Limitations Due to Chronic Disease by Age: United States, 1985[a]

	All Ages[b]	Under 18 Years	18–44 Years	45–64 Years	65+ Years
Chronic Conditions (per 1000)					
Arthritis	28.6	2.2	52.1	268.5	472.8
Hypertension	125.1	2.3	64.1	258.9	414.5
Hearing impairment	90.7	19.2	49.8	159.0	294.4
Heart condition	82.6	21.2	40.1	129.0	304.5
Orthopedic impairment	112.6	33.2	125.3	160.6	170.8
Sinusitis	139.0	59.6	164.4	184.8	154.5
Cataracts	25.0	2.1	1.8	24.4	164.0
Diabetes	26.2	1.9	9.1	51.9	103.8
Visual impairment	36.4	10.8	32.8	43.7	96.5
Tinnitus	26.1	0.7	15.0	49.8	91.7
Activity Limitation (%)					
None	86.0	94.9	91.6	76.6	60.4
Limitation, not in a major activity	4.5	1.5	2.8	5.9	15.5
Limitation in a major activity	9.5	3.7	5.7	17.5	24.1

[a]Source: US Dept of Health and Human Services. Current Estimates from the *National Health Interview Survey, United States, 1985.* Series 10, No. 160, September 1986.
Adapted from Magaziner J. (10)
[b]Data are presented as rates/percents per age group.

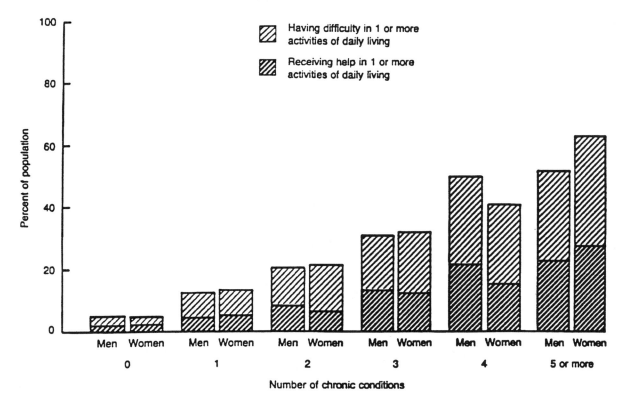

Figure 2.1.   Age-adjusted prevalence of men and women 60 years of age and older having difficulty and receiving help in 1 or more activities of daily living, by number of chronic conditions: United States, 1984. Source: National Health Interview Survey, Supplement on Aging, 1984. Adapted from Guralnik et al. (12).

percent were limited by health problems, but not in a major activity. Figure 2.1 shows a clear, graded increase in the proportion of disabled elderly with no chronic conditions to those with five or more chronic conditions. Approximately 10% of the 65 and older age group were unable to undertake major life activities because of health problems (14).

While some argue that morbidity and the disability that accompanies it eventually will be delayed until the very end of life and thereby compressed into a relatively short period of time (i.e., compression of morbidity), evidence for this view is limited (15, 16). It is generally agreed that within the next 50 years we will continue to witness increasing amounts of disability in the aged, especially among the oldest-old segment.

RESIDENTIAL SETTING OF THOSE WITH DISABILITIES: COMMUNITY OR INSTITUTION?

Persons in need of long-term assistance for their disabilities (i.e., the long-term care population) will require this aid both in institutional and community settings. Contrary to popular belief, only 5% of the aged reside in nursing homes, while 70% to 80% of those with significant disabilities requiring long-term care reside in the community (17). Assuming there are no significant changes in long-term care policies that would increase the number of nursing home beds, it is expected that the number of community-dwelling aged who require long-term care for their disability will increase substantially into the next century (Fig. 2.2).

EPIDEMIOLOGY OF DISABILITY

To provide an overview of the current disability status of older persons in the United States, we have derived estimates from published reports of disability for several functional domains. We restricted ourselves to national studies of community-dwelling and institutionalized aged conducted since 1980. Some estimates vary slightly from study to study, primarily depending on the definition of functioning employed. We provide current estimates of functioning relying on standard measurement approaches, derived from the following studies.

National Health Interview Survey (NHIS), Supplement on Aging

The NHIS is a large continuing survey of the civilian noninstitutionalized population of the United States, conducted by the National Center for Health Statistics. Each year the US Bureau of the Census interviews people in approximately 42,000 households to learn about their health and use of health care. In 1984, a Supplement on Aging was added to the NHIS to obtain information about older people living in the community. The objective of the supplement was to characterize the health and social status of people ages 55 years and over in the United States (18).

National Nursing Home Survey (NNHS)

The 1985 NNHS is a nationwide sample survey of nursing and related care homes, their residents, and staff. It is designed to provide comprehensive informa-

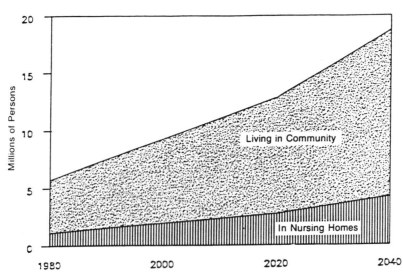

Figure 2.2.   Older Americans in need of long-term care, 1980–2040. Source: Senate Special Committee on Aging, Developments in Aging: 1984, 99th Cong., 1st sess., 28 February 1985, S. Rept. 99-5. Reprinted from US Senate. *Developments in Aging: 1984, Vol. 1. A* *Report of the Special Committee on Aging.* Washington, DC: US Government Printing Office; 1985. Adapted from Kingson ER, Hirshorn BA, Cornman JM: (17)

tion about people using long-term care and about the facilities in which they reside (19).

National Institute of Mental Health Epidemiologic Catchment Area Program (NIMH ECA)

From 1980 to 1984, the NIMH ECA program surveyed households and institutions in five catchment areas to estimate the prevalence of mental disorders in the United States. These areas were Los Angeles, California; New Haven, Connecticut; Baltimore, Maryland; St. Louis, Missouri; and Durham, North Carolina. Although data were not derived from a national probability sample, differing geographic and demographic compositions of these communities help make the results generalizable (20).

Established Populations for Epidemiological Studies of the Elderly (EPESE)

The EPESE studies began in 1980 in three locations: New Haven, Connecticut; Iowa and Washington Counties, East Central Iowa; and East Boston, Massachusetts. The goals of the project are to identify predictors of mortality, hospitalization, and long-term care placement and to assess risk factors for disease and disability (21).

FIVE FUNCTIONAL DOMAINS OF DISABILITY

As indicated earlier, we will focus on five major functional domains to describe disability: physical, instrumental, cognitive, affective, and social. For each domain, we first will describe the functional status of community-dwelling older persons, followed by a description of those residing in nursing homes.

Physical Activities of Daily Living

Physical disability often is measured in terms of functional limitations in the ability to perform everyday activities of daily living (ADLs). These activities include bathing, dressing, grooming, using the toilet, eating, walking, and transferring from a bed or chair.

COMMUNITY AGED

Data from the Supplement on Aging to the 1984 National Health Interview Survey (NHIS) show that approximately 2 million people (7.6% of those ages 65 years and older who were living in the community) were receiving help with one or more of the basic ADLs (22). An additional 4 million people (15%) were functionally limited, but received no help (23). Nine percent of the community aged had difficulty performing one of the seven physical ADLs. Approximately 5% had difficulty

with two activities; 3% had difficulty with three activities; and 6% had difficulty performing four or more physical ADLs. The aged were more likely to have problems walking than with any other activity; almost 19% had difficulty walking. In decreasing order, difficulty bathing and getting outdoors were each experienced by approximately 10%; 8% had difficulty getting on and off a bed or a chair; 6% experienced difficulty dressing; and 4% had difficulty using the toilet. Approximately 6% of the noninstitutionalized population ages 65 years and older were incontinent on a daily basis, and an additional 5% experienced it less often. Eating was the activity least often causing a problem; only 2% reported difficulties (23, 24).

As seen in Figure 2.3, the proportion of persons having difficulty performing these activities increased dramatically with age. The proportion dependent among persons ages 75 to 84 years was approximately double that for persons 65 to 74 years (23–25). The proportion dependent among the oldest-old was two to three times that of the 75 to 84-year-old group. Persons ages 85 years and older constituted a substantially disproportionate share of all persons dependent in physical functioning. Although representing only 7% of the aged, they constituted 18% to 26% of those dependent in personal care activities and 27% of those dependent in mobility (24).

INSTITUTIONALIZED AGED

The previous figures understate limitations in physical functioning because many of the most dependent aged were institutionalized in nursing homes (24, 25). The 1985 National Nursing Home Survey (NNHS) indicated that 30.4% of nursing home residents ages 65 years and older were dependent in six ADL functions. Only 7.6% of the elderly residents were independent in all ADLs. In reference to specific activities, 91% were dependent in bathing; 78% were dependent in dressing, and 63% required assistance toileting and transferring (Table 2.5). Twenty-six percent of the residents were walking with assistance, and an additional 47% were bedbound or chair-bound (19, 22).

Instrumental Activities of Daily Living

Instrumental ADLs assess ability related to home management by obtaining information about tasks such as shopping for personal items, preparing meals, managing money, using the telephone, and doing light housework (e.g., washing dishes).

COMMUNITY AGED

In general, the aged experienced more difficulty with instrumental activities than with physical activities. Twenty-seven percent (7 million persons) were functionally limited in instrumental activities; 22% (5.9 mil-

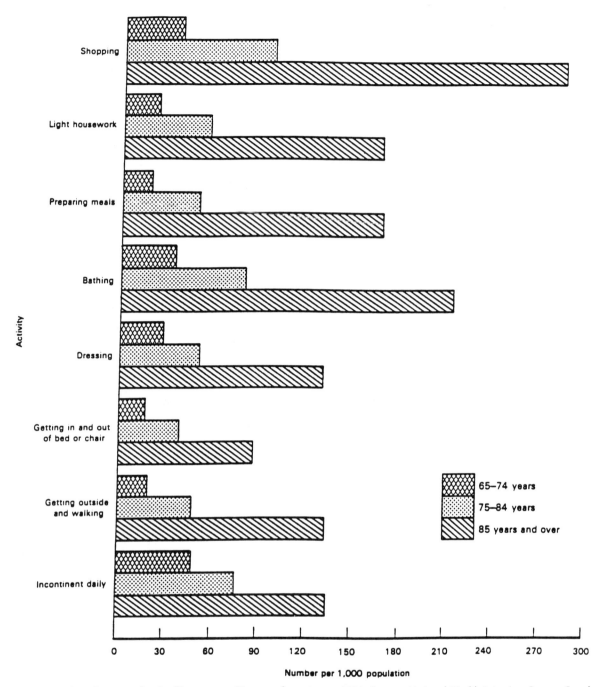

Figure 2.3. Proportion of community-dwelling persons 65 years of age and older dependent in selected activities by age group: United States, 1984. Source: National Health Interview Survey, Supplement on Aging, 1984. Adapted from Fulton et al. (24).

lion) received help with activities such as preparing meals, managing money, and using the telephone. Heavy housework was the instrumental ADL most likely to require assistance, with difficulties experienced by approximately 6.3 million persons (24%) (Table 2.6). Similarly, shopping presented difficulty for 11% of the aged because of the strength, stamina, and transportation required to accomplish this task (23, 24).

INSTITUTIONALIZED AGED

Between 65% and 78% of aged nursing home residents were dependent in select instrumental ADLs (Table 2.7). Overall, 86% of residents received help with these activities. Seventy-five percent required help with care of personal possessions; 78% needed assistance securing personal items, and 65% received help to use the

Table 2.5. Percent Distribution of Nursing Home Residents 65 Years of Age and Older by Selected Physical Functioning Status, According to Age: United States, 1985[a]

Functional Status	65+[b] Years	65–74 Years	75–84 Years	85+ Years
Bathing				
Independent	9.0	15.2	9.7	6.1
Requires assistance	91.0	84.8	90.3	93.9
Dressing				
Independent	22.4	29.8	24.1	18.3
Requires assistance (includes those who do not dress)	77.6	70.2	75.9	81.7
Mobility				
Independent	26.4	39.6	30.4	18.4
Requires assistance	26.3	20.4	24.7	29.6
Chairfast	40.8	33.7	38.7	45.1
Bedfast	6.5	6.3	6.1	6.9
Transferring				
Independent	37.4	47.9	40.3	31.3
Requires assistance	62.6	52.1	59.7	68.7
Using the toilet				
Independent	36.8	43.4	39.7	32.0
Requires assistance	51.1	45.8	47.8	55.9
Does not use toilet	12.1	10.8	12.6	12.1

[a] Source: National Nursing Home Survey, 1985.
Adapted from Hing E, Sekscenski E, Strahan G. (19)
[b] Data are presented as rates/percents per age group.

Table 2.6. Percent Distribution of Community-Dwelling Persons 65 Years of Age and Older Who Have Difficulty Performing Selected Instrumental Activities of Daily Living, According to Age: United States, 1984[a]

Age	Preparing Meals	Shopping	Managing Money	Using Telephone	Doing Heavy Housework	Doing Light Housework
65 years and older[b]	7.1	11.3	5.1	4.8	23.8	7.1
65–74 years	4.0	6.4	2.2	2.7	18.6	4.3
75–84 years	8.8	15.0	6.3	6.0	28.7	8.9
85 years and older	26.1	37.0	24.0	17.5	47.8	23.6

[a] Source: National Health Interview Survey, National Center for Health Statistics, 1984.
Adapted from Dawson et al. (23).
[b] Data are presented as rates/percents per age group.

Table 2.7. Percent Distribution of Nursing Home Residents by Selected Instrumental Functioning Status, According to Age: United States, 1985[a]

	Under 65 Years	65+ Years	65–74 Years	75–84 Years	85+ Years
Does not receive help	24.9	14.0	18.6	15.6	11.0
Receives help	75.1	86.0	81.4	84.4	89.0
Care of personal possessions	60.4	75.2	69.9	74.1	78.0
Handling money	66.5	76.5	70.7	75.1	79.8
Securing personal items	62.4	78.1	72.1	75.9	82.0
Using the telephone	47.9	64.7	58.8	64.0	67.3

[a] Source: National Nursing Home Survey, 1985.
Adapted from Hing et al. (19).

telephone. Similar to the community aged, the rates of persons requiring assistance were consistently higher for the oldest-old than for other aged residents (19, 22).

Cognitive Functioning

Persons ages 65 years and older have significantly higher rates of severe cognitive impairment than those of any younger age group (20). Not surprisingly, Alzheimer's disease is the leading cause of cognitive impairment among the elderly (9). Dementia is one of the four conditions considered to be most important in the causation of disability among the aged (other causes are cancer, ischemic heart disease, and arthritis and other musculoskeletal problems). By the year 2060, the number of elderly persons with disabilities attributable to dementia is projected to be 1.6 million (26).

COMMUNITY AGED

Data from the National Institute of Mental Health Epidemiologic Catchment Area (NIMH ECA) program indicated that 5% of the community-dwelling aged were severely cognitively impaired. The rate increased sharply with advancing age from 2.9% for the young-old, to 6.8% for the old-old and 15.8% for the oldest-old (20). Examining less severe deficits in cognitive functioning, the Established Populations for Epidemiologic Studies of the Elderly (EPESE) project found that approximately 50% to 75% of the community aged made at least one error on a standard mental status evaluation (21). The 1984 Supplement on Aging to the NHIS examined memory problems; 15% of persons had frequent problems remembering, and only 26% never had difficulties. As anticipated, memory deficits increased with age. More than one quarter of the oldest-old reported an increase in the frequency of memory problems over the preceding year (27).

INSTITUTIONALIZED AGED

Cognitive impairment is one of the principal reasons for institutionalization (9). The prevalence of dementia in nursing homes is much higher than among community-dwelling aged, ranging from 47% to 56% (28). The 1985 NNHS reported that 50% of aged nursing home residents had a diagnosis of organic brain syndrome, including Alzheimer's disease. Increases with age were evidenced as 38% of residents ages 65 to 74 years, 49% of those 75 to 84 years, and 56% of those ages 85 years and older were diagnosed with dementia (29). An important component of cognitive impairment is its relationship to functional limitations. In 1985, more than 60% of aged nursing home residents had cognitive deficits that impaired their ability to perform ADLs (9).

Affective Functioning: Depression

Detecting affective disorders among the aged is problematic. Rates tend to be lower for this population than for younger persons, but it is likely that cognitive impairments preclude the ability to make accurate assessments (20). In addition, rates often reflect only primary depressions. These estimates are misleading because the aged are more at risk for secondary depressions than is any other age group; they suffer from more physical illness and take more medications. Compared to younger persons, suicide is a more frequent cause of death among the aged. In 1984, the suicide rate for white elderly men was four times the national rate (41.6 vs. 11.6 per 100,000) (9).

COMMUNITY AGED

The NIMH ECA program detected depression among less than 1% of the community-dwelling aged (20). Depressive symptomatology, however, often is reported at much higher rates, as great as 15% (9). Almost one half of the EPESE sample reported two or more symptoms indicative of depression, with older persons reporting more depressive symptomatology than did younger individuals (21). As with cognitive disorders, persons exhibiting major functional impairments tend to report more symptoms of depression (30).

INSTITUTIONALIZED AGED

The NNHS found that 11% of the institutionalized elderly were depressed. The prevalence of depressive disorders decreased with age, from 14% for those ages 65 to 74 years, to 13% for persons 75 to 84 years, and 8% for those ages 85 years and older (29). Similar to the community-dwelling aged, depressive symptoms were more prevalent than clinical diagnoses. Twenty-five percent of persons with dementia exhibited depres-

Table 2.8. Percent Distribution of Community-Dwelling Persons 65 Years of Age and Older by Living Arrangement, According to Age and Family Composition[a]

	Living Arrangement		
	Alone	Couples	Others
Age			
65–74 years	24	64	12
75–84 years	39	43	18
85 + years	45	22	33
Family Composition			
No children	27	13	22
One child	19	17	17
Two or more children	54	70	61

[a] Sources: Bureau of the Census, 1987.
National Health Interview Survey, Supplement on Aging, National Center for Health Statistics, 1984.
Adapted from Kasper JD. (35).

sive symptomatology, as did 21% of those with no cognitive impairment (unpublished data from the NNHS).

Social Functioning

Social support is related to disease outcome. Persons with fewer social attachments (such as widows or those with no children) and less interaction die at a higher rate and are more likely to feel depressed (31, 32). In general, the majority of aged persons do not consider themselves to be socially isolated; they perceive their level of social contact to be adequate. Only 1% have unmet social interaction needs; an additional 2% are at high risk for developing unmet needs. As evidenced in other functional areas, this risk increases with age (33).

COMMUNITY AGED

The majority of aged men are married (75%), whereas only 38% of aged women are married; most women are widowed (51%). The sex difference in marital status is due to the male's shorter life span and his greater tendency to choose a younger spouse and to remarry if he is widowed (9). Of all community aged, 54% reside with a spouse; 16% live with others, and 30% live alone. Eight million aged persons live alone, the majority of whom are widowed, female, and average 75 years of age (34). Table 2.8 shows age-related differences in the living arrangements of community-dwelling aged. Most people ages 65 to 74 years are married and reside with a spouse (64%); most of those ages 85 years and older live alone (45%) (35).

Living arrangement also relates to family composition. Although more than one half of those who live alone have two or more children, 27% have no children, a proportion higher than that for those who live with others (35). The Supplement on Aging to the NHIS found that these persons were not isolated or lacking social interaction, however. Eighty-nine percent of those living alone had either children, siblings, or both. Most lived near family with whom they had frequent contact, and approximately 90% reported that they had talked to or seen relatives or friends during the previous two weeks. Only 5% of the aged living alone had no social contacts during that time. Social integration was evidenced further by reports that one half of those persons who live alone had attended a religious service during the prior two weeks, and one quarter had attended a group event, such as a movie (34).

INSTITUTIONALIZED AGED

There is a variance between the social supports of community-dwelling and institutionalized persons. At the time of admission, 16% of nursing home residents surveyed by the NNHS were married, and 63% had children (36). Not surprisingly, the availability of informal social support networks to provide care for the elderly affected their likelihood of institutionalization. Seventy-eight percent of residents were admitted to nursing homes because they required more care than household members could provide (19). Living alone placed persons at greater risk of entering a nursing home; 14% of persons living alone who required assistance entered a nursing home within two years, compared to 8% of impaired persons who resided with a spouse (35).

IMPLICATIONS FOR THE FUTURE

Impairments in physical, instrumental, cognitive, affective, and social functioning are evidenced among the aged. As this proportion of the population grows, more persons will require assistance in these functional domains. This increase has significant implications for health care delivery. For example, assuming that the level of disability and use of nursing home beds remains stable, the current 1.3 million residents may be succeeded by a need for up to 5.9 million nursing home beds by the year 2040 (28). The even larger segment of the aged requiring care in the community will increase more dramatically. Assessment and treatment of the aged will require more time and consume more health care resources. To address this escalating need, primary care providers can become more skillful in recognizing early signs of disability. Interdisciplinary treatment provided by more specialists trained in medicine, psychiatry, rehabilitation medicine, physical therapy, occupational therapy, social work, and other areas will be needed to assess and manage the multiplicity of functional impairment among the aged. Finally, the most effective long-term solution to decrease functional impairments is a continued focus on the prevention and cure of diseases that cause the greatest disability among the aged.

References

1. Nagi SZ. Some conceptual issues in disability and rehabilitation. In: Sussman MB, ed. *Sociology and Rehabilitation*. Washington, DC: American Sociological Association; 1965.
2. Verbrugge L. Disability. *Rheumatic Dis Clin North Am*. 16(3):741–761, 1990.
3. World Health Organization. *International Classification of Impairments, Disabilities and Handicaps*. Geneva: WHO; 1980.
4. Bergner M. Quality of life, health status, and clinical research. *Med Care*. 27:S148–156, 1989.
5. Eisdorfer C. Some variables relating to longevity in humans. In: Ostfeld AM, Gibson DC, eds. *Epidemiology of Aging*. Washington, DC: Government Printing Office; 1977. US Dept of HEW publication NIH 77–711.
6. Neugarten BL, Datan N. Sociological perspectives on the life cycle. In: Baltes PB, Schaie KW, eds. *Life-Span Developmental Psychology: Personality and Socialization*. New York, NY: Academic Press; 1973.
7. Neugarten BL. Age groups in American society and the rise of the young-old. *Ann Am Acad Political Social Sciences*. September:187–198, 1974.

8. Rosenwaik I. A demographic portrait of the oldest-old. *Milbank Mem Fund Q.* 63:187–205, 1985.

9. US Senate Special Committee on Aging. *Aging America: Trends and Projections, 1987–88 ed.* Washington, DC: US Dept of Health and Human Services; 1988.

10. Magaziner J. Demographic and epidemiologic considerations for developing preventive strategies in the elderly. *Md Med J.* 38:115–120, 1989.

11. Fredman L, Haynes SG. An epidemiologic profile of the elderly. In: Phillips H, Gaylord S, eds. *Aging and Public Health.* New York, NY: Springer Publishing Co; 1985.

12. Guralnik JM, LaCroix AZ, Everett DF, and Kovar MG. Aging in the eighties: The prevalence of comorbidity and its association with disability. *National Center for Health Statistics, Advance Data* No. 170, May 26, 1989.

13. Soldo BJ, Manton KG. Health status and service needs of the oldest old: current patterns and future trends. *Milbank Mem Fund Q.* 63:286–319, 1985.

14. National Center for Health Statistics. *Health, United States, 1987.* Washington, DC: US Governmentt Printing Office; 1988.

15. Fries JF. Aging, natural death, and the compression of morbidity. *N Engl J Med.* 303:130–135, 1980.

16. Schneider EL, Brody JA. Aging, natural death and the compression of morbidity: another view. *N Engl J Med.* 309:854–856, 1983.

17. Kingson ER, Hirshorn BA, Cornman JM. *Ties that Bind: The Interdependence of Generations.* Washington, DC: Seven Locks Press; 1986.

18. Kovar MG. Aging in the eighties: preliminary data from the Supplement on Aging to the National Health Interview Survey, United States, January–June 1984. *National Center for Health Statistics, Advance Data* No. 115, May 1, 1986.

19. Hing E, Sekscenski E, Strahan G. The National Nursing Home Survey; 1985 summary for the United States. *Vital & Health Stat.* Series 13, No. 97, 1989.

20. Regier DA, Boyd JH, Burke JD, et al. One month prevalence of mental disorders in the United States. *Arch Gen Psychiatry.* 45:977–986, 1988.

21. Cornoni-Huntley J, Brock DB, Ostfeld AM, Taylor JO, Wallace RB, eds. *Established Populations for Epidemiologic Studies of the Elderly: Resource Data Book.* Bethesda, Md: 1986. National Institutes of Health; NIH publication 86-2443.

22. Kovar MG, Hendershot G, Mathis E. Older people in the United States who receive help with basic activities of daily living. *Am J Pub Health.* 79:778–779, 1989.

23. Dawson D, Hendershot G, Fulton, J. Aging in the eighties: functional limitations of individuals age 65 and over. *National Center for Health Statistics, Advance Data* No. 133, June 10, 1987.

24. Fulton JP, Katz S, Jack SS, and Hendershot GE. Physical functioning of the aged, United States, 1984. *Vital & Health Stat.* Series 10, No. 167, 1989.

25. Cornoni-Huntley JC, Foley DJ, White LR, et al. Epidemiology of disability in the oldest old: methodologic issues and preliminary findings. *Milbank Mem Fund Q.* 63:350–376, 1985.

26. Manton KG. Epidemiological, demographic, and social correlates of disability among the elderly. *Milbank Mem Fund Q.* 67:13–58, 1989.

27. Cutler SJ, Grams AE. Correlates of self-reported everyday memory problems. *J Gerontol.* 43:S82–S90, 1988.

28. Schneider EL, Guralnik JM. The aging of America. *JAMA.* 263:2335–2340, 1990.

29. Strahan GW. Mental illness in nursing homes: United States, 1985. *Vital & Health Stat.* Series 13, No. 105, 1991.

30. Berkman LF, Berkman CS, Kasl S, et al. Depressive symptoms in relation to physical health and functioning in the elderly. *Am J Epidemiol.* 124:372–388, 1986.

31. Blazer DG. Social support and mortality in an elderly community population. *Am J Epidemiol.* 115:684–694, 1982.

32. Goldberg EL, Van Natta P, Comstock GW. Depressive symptoms, social networks and social support of elderly women. *Am J Epidemiol.* 121:448–456, 1985.

33. Branch LG, Jette AM. The Framingham disability study: I. Social disability among the aging. *Am J Public Health.* 71:1202–1210, 1981.

34. Kovar MG. Aging in the eighties, age 65 years and over and living alone, contacts with family, friends, and neighbors. *National Center for Health Statistics, Advance Data* No. 116, May 9, 1986.

35. Kasper JD. *Aging Alone-Profiles and Projections.* Baltimore, Md: The Commonwealth Fund; 1988.

36. Hing E. Use of nursing homes by the elderly: preliminary data from the 1985 National Nursing Home Survey. *National Center for Health Statistics, Advance Data* No. 135, May 14, 1987.

SECTION II

PATHOPHYSIOLOGY OF HUMAN AGING

3

The Aging Respiratory System

Patricia Nelson and Stephen S. Lefrak

As aging occurs, the respiratory system undergoes a measurable decline in physiologic function. This age-related loss is influenced both by the life-style of the individual and by his or her environment. The regular performance of physical exercise, lifetime inhalation of cigarette smoke and other pollutants, and recurrent respiratory illness may differentially affect the rate of decline of lung function. The most important consequence of the age-related changes that occur is the reduction in the physiologic reserve of the respiratory system, especially the reserve for alveolar gas exchange. The functional capacity (or physiologic reserve) of healthy young persons is in marked excess over the amount required to meet their metabolic needs, even under stress. Because elderly individuals have a reduced physiologic reserve, they are more vulnerable to stresses and injuries. Despite this reduction in physiologic reserve, respiratory symptoms such as inappropriate shortness of breath or cough are always attributable to disease and should not be ascribed to aging.

Table 3.1 is a summary of five functional divisions of the respiratory system and the changes that occur with aging. Each of these areas will be discussed separately and in more detail in this chapter. Reviews of normal respiratory physiology may be helpful in understanding the changes that occur (1–3). In addition, the effects of aging on respiration during sleep and on airway reactivity will be discussed.

RESPIRATORY BELLOWS

The respiratory bellows consists of the thoracic cage, the diaphragm, the accessory muscles of respiration, and the intercostal muscles. Together these components provide the mechanical forces necessary for efficient ventilation.

Thorax

The thoracic cage stiffens with advancing age (4). This rigidity can be attributed to calcification of the costal cartilages and articulations between the vertebrae and ribs. In addition, the chest often becomes barrel-shaped. This change, once termed senile emphysema, is due to an increase in spinal dorsal kyphosis and thoracic anteroposterior diameter resulting from degenerative changes in the intervertebral discs. Because of chest wall stiffening, the work demanded of the respiratory muscles in moving the thoracic cage increases with age and may be 30% greater at age 60 than at age 20 (5).

Respiratory Muscles

The strength of the respiratory muscles appears to decrease with age. The maximal expiratory and inspiratory pressures generated by young subjects are greater than those generated by elderly subjects of ages 75 to 90 years (6, 7). In addition, during maximum voluntary ventilation measurements, positive and negative swings in esophageal pressure, which estimate changes in intrathoracic pressure, decline progressively with age (8). Although the mechanisms leading to this decrease in muscle strength are not known, extrapolation of data gathered on aging skeletal muscles suggest that, in expiratory muscles, it may be related to a reduction in muscle fiber number and size. Expiratory intercostal muscles appear to be 20% smaller in fiber cross-sectional area after 50 years of age due to a reduction of both slow-twitch and fast-twitch muscle areas (9). Conversely, inspiratory intercostal muscles maintain a constant fiber size with aging. The reason for the loss in inspiratory muscle strength is not known.

Furthermore, the function of the diaphragm is impaired during aging due to a change in its configuration (10). The muscle fibers of the diaphragm become flatter and shorter, increasing its radius of curvature. This alteration decreases the tension that the diaphragm can generate and the effectiveness with which this tension is converted into the pressure differential necessary to ventilate the lungs. This change in configuration probably occurs because the functional residual capacity (the amount of air remaining in the lungs after a quiet exhalation) increases with age. In addition, the diaphragm

Table 3.1. Functional Divisions of the Respiratory System and Effects of Aging[a]

Functional Division	Function	Responsible Organs or Tissues	Comments	Effect of Aging
Respiratory Bellows	Generation of "pumping" forces	Diaphragm, accessory muscles of respiration, rib cage, and chest wall	Influenced by level of physical conditioning	Decreased muscle strength and effectiveness; increased stiffness
Conducting Airways	Transportation of gas to lung parenchyma	Mouth, trachea, bronchi, subsegmental bronchi, terminal bronchioles	Includes all airways from mouth to level of respiratory bronchiole	Minimal changes
Lung Parenchyma	Exchange of alveolar gas	Alveolar ducts, alveoli, pulmonary capillary bed, lung interstitium	For greatest efficiency, local ventilation and perfusion must be closely matched	Changes resembling ventilation–perfusion mismatching, decreasing arterial oxygen tension
Ventilation Control	Regulation of ventilation	Medulla and pons, carotid and aortic bodies	Adjust frequency and depth of tidal breathing to achieve appropriate arterial Po_2 and Pco_2 with minimal energy expenditure	Decreased responsiveness to hypoxemia and hypercarbia
Cardiovascular System	Gas transport to the tissues	Heart and vascular system	Cardiovascular system is always the limiting factor for gas transport in exercising elderly normals	Decreased maximal output

[a] From Gracy DR, ed. *Pulmonary Disease in the Adult.* Chicago, Ill: Year Book Medical Publishers; 1981. By permission of Mayo Foundation.

contour may be modified because of the changes in the chest wall mentioned earlier.

CONDUCTING AIRWAYS

The conducting airways consist of the air passages from the mouth to the respiratory bronchioles. With aging, these airways undergo calcification of their cartilage and hypertrophy of the bronchial glands. Despite these changes, airway resistance to air flow does not increase with aging. An increase in compliance, or distensibility, of both the lungs and small airways may account, in part, for the preservation of airway resistance (11). In addition, large airways, such as the trachea, may increase in diameter with aging (12), which would decrease their resistance to flow. As will be discussed later, increased airway compliance may also result in compression of the airways during forced maximal expiration and contribute to a decrease in maximal expiratory flow rates.

LUNG PARENCHYMA

In this chapter, lung parenchyma is considered that portion of the lung tissue involved in respiratory gas exchange. This includes airways distal to the terminal bronchiole, the pulmonary capillary bed, and the lung interstitium.

Distal Airspaces

The number of alveoli in the lung reaches approximately 200 million to 300 million by the eighth year of life and then remains constant throughout life. After the age of 30 years, the alveolar ducts undergo progressive dilation, and alveolar duct volume increases (13). Since the alveolar number is constant, the average surface area of the lung must decrease. These alterations result in a decrease both in alveolar surface area and in the percentage of parenchymal air contained in the alveoli with increasing age. As a result, the internal surface area of the lung which is 70 m² to 80 m² at age 20 years, thereafter decreases at a rate of 0.27 m²/yr (14). Microscopically, the alveolar ducts and respiratory bronchioles enlarge at the expense of the surrounding alveoli, which become more shallow and broad (Fig. 3.1). This process of alveolar duct enlargement has been called ductectasia to distinguish it from emphysema in which destruction of the alveolar septa occurs. Although several investigators (15, 16) have reported loss of septa in the distal airspaces of aged lungs (lesions indistinguishable from emphysema), this finding is infrequent in elderly nonsmokers and does not appear to be statistically significant when accounting for smoking history. The mechanism behind these changes is not known, but the effects of repeated mechanical stress, environmental pollutants

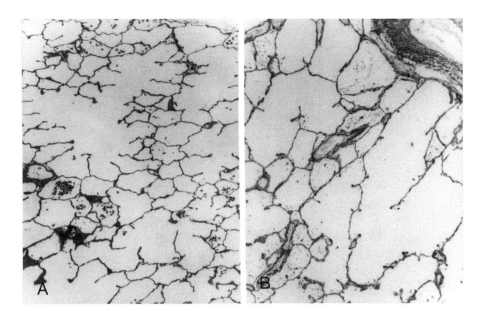

Figure 3.1 Histologic changes in aging lung. (A) Normal lung of a 36-year-old woman. **(B)** Normal lung of a 93-year-old woman. The alveolar ducts are dilated, and shortening and loss of interalveolar septa are observed. From Gracy DR. *Pulmonary Disease in the Adult.* Chicago, Ill: Year Book Medical Publishers; 1981. Reproduced by permission of Mayo Foundation.

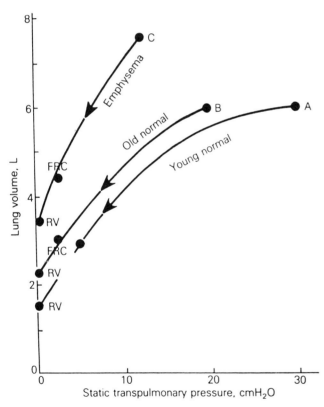

Figure 3.2. Pressure–volume curves for the lungs of young (A) and old (B) asymptomatic nonsmoking women, compared with that for patients with emphysema (C). The static pressure–volume curve is shifted to the left in elderly subjects although less so than in emphysematous subjects. At a given lung volume, there is a loss of elastic recoil pressure with age, but no change in the slope of the relationship between pressure and volume (pulmonary compliance). From Fishman AP. *The Lungs in Later Life.* New York, NY: McGraw Hill; 1982. Reproduced with permission of McGraw Hill, Inc.

such as cigarette smoke, and infection may, in combination with the aging process itself, produce them.

Elastic Recoil and Connective Tissue of the Lung

The natural tendency of the lung to retract inward, reducing its volume, is termed elastic recoil. This retractile force is the result of two forces acting on the lung parenchyma: retractive forces produced when connective tissue elastin is stretched and surface tension forces produced at the curved air–fluid interfaces of the small airways and alveoli. Elastic recoil pressure varies with lung volume. If alveolar pressure is measured at different lung volumes, a pressure–volume curve, which reflects static elastic recoil, can be plotted. In both elderly individuals and those with emphysema, this curve is shifted to the left (Fig. 3.2) compared to that of healthy young subjects (17). This indicates that, for a given lung volume, elastic recoil is decreased in aged and emphysematous lungs. However, in elderly subjects, the shift is less than in emphysematous subjects, and the slope of this curve, the static pulmonary compliance, does not change.

The explanation for the loss of elastic recoil in aged lungs is not clear. Although pleural elastin content increases with age, parenchymal elastin content does not change, and collagen content appears to decrease (18). Qualitative changes in lung elastin and collagen and changes in the location and orientation of individual fibers may account for some of the decrease in elastic recoil. In addition, the loss of surface area in the aged lung, discussed previously, reduces the curved gas-liquid

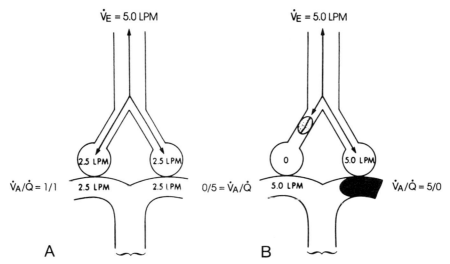

Figure 3.3. Diagrammatic representation of ventilation and perfusion matching. An "ideal" two-compartment lung with exact matching of alveolar ventilation and perfusion ($\dot{V}_A/\dot{Q}$) is shown in **(A).** The total minute ventilation ($\dot{V}_E$) of 5.0 L/min is equally divided among the alveoli, as is the total perfusion $\dot{Q}$, resulting in a $\dot{V}_A/\dot{Q}$ equal to 1.0. In **(B),** a totally imperfect lung is shown. The right bronchus is occluded by a peanut, and the blood supply to the left unit is completely occluded by a blood clot. The result is that all the ventilation is distributed to the left unit and all the perfusion is distributed to the right unit. The right unit with a $\dot{V}_A/\dot{Q}$ of 0/5 functions as a physiologic shunt and the left unit with a $\dot{V}_A/\dot{Q}$ of 5/0 functions as a physiologic dead space. No gas transfer occurs despite the fact that the total ventilation and perfusion received by the lung is normal. Similar processes of disordered gas exchange occur as the lung ages or becomes diseased, but not to such an extreme. From Gracy DR. *Pulmonary Disease in the Adult.* Chicago, Ill: Year Book Medical Publishers; 1981. Reproduced by permission of Mayo Foundation.

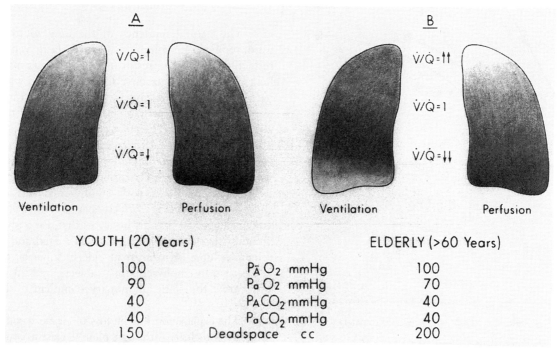

YOUTH (20 Years)		ELDERLY (>60 Years)
100	$P_{\bar{A}}O_2$ mmHg	100
90	P_aO_2 mmHg	70
40	$P_{A}CO_2$ mmHg	40
40	P_aCO_2 mmHg	40
150	Deadspace cc	200

Figure 3.4. Differences in ventilation and perfusion matching in young and elderly adults. The lungs are divided into three zones: apex, midzones, and base. The midzones of the lungs of both the young and old subjects demonstrate relatively well matched ventilation and perfusion. In young lung **(A),** the apex is relatively overventilated with respect to perfusion, and this region contributes minimal amounts to dead space. The basilar areas in the young lungs are relatively overperfused with respect to ventilation and functionally contribute areas of minimal shunt. This basic pattern is maintained in the elderly **(B),** but the degree of ventilation–perfusion mismatching is much greater, primarily because of changes in regional ventilation. The lung apices are more overventilated with respect to perfusion, and the lung bases are more overperfused with respect to ventilation. The effects of these phenomena on gas exchange are tabulated below the diagrams. From Gracy DR. *Pulmonary Disease in the Adult.* Chicago, Ill: Year Book Medical Publishers; 1981. Reproduced by permission of Mayo Foundation.

interface of the distal airways and alveoli. This reduces the surface tension forces and will reduce the total elastic recoil pressure of the lungs.

Alveolar Gas Exchange

Alveolar gas exchange depends on efficient perfusion of the alveolus with capillary blood and its simultaneous matched ventilation with inspired air. The amount of ventilation relative to perfusion is expressed as the ventilation–perfusion ($\dot{V}A/\dot{Q}$) ratio for a given lung region. Close matching of $\dot{V}A/\dot{Q}$ throughout the entire lung is required for efficient removal of carbon dioxide and oxygenation of venous blood (Fig. 3.3A). If a region receives decreased ventilation relative to perfusion (decreased $\dot{V}A/\dot{Q}$), then this region becomes a physiologic shunt. Gas exchange, in particular oxygenation of the blood, will be inefficient as a result of the relatively overperfused alveolus (Fig. 3.3B). If a decrease in perfusion relative to ventilation occurs (increased $\dot{V}A/\dot{Q}$), then that alveolus receives an excess of inspired air, and gas exchange is also inefficient. This creates physiologic dead space or wasted ventilation and may result in a rise in carbon dioxide tension (Fig. 3.3B) unless homeostatic mechanisms are effective.

In normal young subjects, ventilation and perfusion in the lung as a whole are evenly matched. In the upright position, basilar regions of the lung receive more perfusion relative to ventilation, whereas apical regions receive less perfusion relative to ventilation. These regional differences in $\dot{V}A/\dot{Q}$ result from the effect of gravity on pulmonary artery blood flow and the pleural pressure gradient. In the elderly, these differences are magnified as small airway closure occurs in basilar areas of the lung during tidal breathing because of the loss of elastic recoil and alveolar surface tension. In addition, in the up-right position inspired gas is distributed preferentially to the lung apices rather than the lung bases (Fig. 3.4), which remain well perfused. Both closure of the small airways and unequal distribution of ventilation in the elderly increase regional ventilation–perfusion mismatching, causing a decline in arterial oxygen tension (19). In the supine position, ventilation–perfusion mismatching increases further, and arterial oxygen falls even lower. In normal aging, the decrease in arterial oxygen tension is approximately 4 mm Hg per decade after age 20 years (Fig. 3.5) (20).

Unlike the decline in the arterial partial pressure of oxygen, arterial carbon dioxide tension does not change during aging. Although ventilation–perfusion mismatching and an increase in dead space occurs, the elderly have an increased minute ventilation which offsets the more inefficient removal of carbon dioxide. In addition, the elderly have decreased metabolic activity and carbon dioxide production at rest resulting from a decline in muscle mass. These act to offset the effect of increased dead space on alveolar carbon dioxide exchange.

Ventilatory Control

Ventilation is closely controlled to maintain stable arterial tensions of carbon dioxide and oxygen throughout a wide range of physiologic conditions and stresses. The minute ventilation is the product of the depth and rate of respiration. It is controlled by a complex system of afferent and efferent signals whose function is integrated in the respiratory control center located in the medulla and pons. The primary mediators of minute ventilation are the partial pressures of carbon dioxide and oxygen in arterial blood and signals from mechanoreceptors in the lung and chest wall. The tension of car-

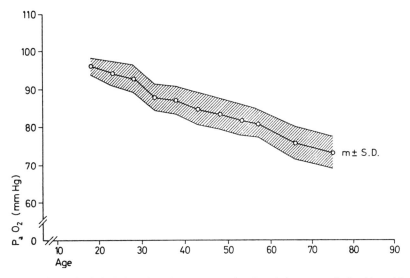

Figure 3.5. PaO₂ mean values and standard deviations in relation to age. From Sorbini CA, Grassi V, Solinas E, et al. Arterial oxygen tension in relation to age in healthy subjects. *Respiration.* 25:3–13, 1986. Reproduced with permission of S. Karger AG, Basel.

bon dioxide is monitored primarily by chemosensors in the medulla. These chemosensors detect changes in carbon dioxide tension by reacting to corresponding changes in pericellular pH that occur when carbon dioxide interacts with water to form a weak acid. Sensors that monitor oxygen tension are located in specialized neural tissue in the carotid and aortic bodies, which provide afferent output to the respiratory center.

Under normal conditions, ventilation is well matched to metabolic demands. During periods of exercise or stress in which carbon dioxide production and oxygen consumption increase, arterial blood gases remain stable. In young adults, a fall in the alveolar oxygen tension to 40 mm Hg causes the minute ventilation to increase approximately five times over the basal level. In contrast, in the elderly, the ventilatory response to hypoxia is reduced by approximately 51% and the central response to hypercapnia by about 41% (Table 3.2) (21, 22). The response of the ventilatory rate to arterial blood gas disturbances is normal, but elderly subjects show a diminished increase in tidal volume in response to both hypoxemia and hypercapnia. Although the elderly have a decrease in compliance of the respiratory system and in respiratory muscle strength, these changes do not account for the decreased ventilatory response. Peterson and colleagues (22) found that ventilatory responses, as reflected by occlusion pressure (the change in mouth pressure during the first 0.1 second of inspiration against an occluded airway), are depressed by about 50% in the elderly under both hypoxic and hypercapnic conditions. These measurements are unaffected by the compliance of the respiratory system. When corrected for respiratory muscle strength, the occlusion pressure responses were still decreased in the elderly, suggesting that decreased ventilatory drive, or neural output from the respiratory center, is responsible for the diminished increase in tidal volume to hypoxemic and hypercapnic stimuli.

Table 3.2. Age Contrasted Response to Hypoxemia and Hypercapnia[a,b]

Physiologic Stimulus	Ventilatory Response	
	Young Adults	Elderly Adults
Hypoxemia (PaO_2 40 mm Hg)[c]	40 L/min	10 LPM
Hypercapnia[d]	3.4 L/min/mm Hg	2.0 L/min/mm Hg
	Cardiac Frequency Increase (%)	
Hypoxemia (PaO_2 40 mm Hg)	34.1	11.5
Hypercapnia ($PaCO_2$ 55 mm Hg)	15.0	−0.9

[a]From Gracy DR. *Pulmonary Disease in the Adult.* Chicago, Ill: Year Book Medical Publishers; 1981.
[b]Data from Kronenberg RS, Drage CW. Attenuation of the ventilatory and heart rate responses to hypoxia and hypercapnia with aging in normal men. *J Clin Invest.* 52:1812–1819, 1973.
[c]Values given are the mean level of minute ventilation observed in response to the hypoxic stimulus.
[d]Values given are the mean increase in minute ventilation that was observed for each millimeter of mercury rise in alveolar PCO_2.

The mechanoreceptors in the lung and chest wall also affect minute ventilation. In young adults, signals based on displacement of the lungs and chest wall while breathing against resistive and elastic loads are more important in detecting lung volume changes than is the amount of respiratory muscle force generated against these loads (23). Young subjects can reproduce a control tidal volume fairly accurately while breathing against a series of elastic and resistive loads if the load is mild to moderate in scale. Elderly subjects are more sensitive to cues related to respiratory muscle force rather than volume. They perceive a change in the force required to overcome a ventilatory load as a change in volume more than do younger subjects. Therefore, ventilatory drive and perception of lung volume are more dependent on respiratory force in the elderly (Fig. 3.6).

Because the elderly have less ventilatory drive to hypoxic or hypercapnic stimuli combined with more tenuous alveolar gas exchange, they are more susceptible to development of ventilatory failure following an insult that raises carbon dioxide production (such as fever or postoperative states) or increases physiologic dead space or shunt (such as pulmonary embolism, congestive heart failure, pneumonia, or atelectasis). If their lung becomes less compliant because of one of the above conditions, their work of breathing may increase, thereby increasing the respiratory force necessary to achieve a given tidal volume. They may be more likely to breathe at smaller lung volumes and faster respiratory rates and thus further impair the efficiency of alveolar gas exchange.

PULMONARY FUNCTION STUDIES IN THE ELDERLY

Lung Volumes

Many of the physiologic changes discussed in the previous sections can be detected by measurements obtained in the pulmonary function laboratory. An interpretation of lung volumes is shown in Figure 3.7. The total lung capacity is the total volume of air that the lungs can hold following a maximal inhalation. The residual volume is the volume of gas remaining in the lungs after a maximal exhalation. The vital capacity is the total volume of air that can be exhaled following a maximal inhalation. Together, the residual volume and vital capacity equal the total lung capacity. The total lung capacity remains constant with aging (Fig. 3.8). Although elastic recoil of the lung parenchyma decreases in the elderly, the chest wall becomes more rigid thereby preventing a decrease in the maximal volume of the thorax.

The residual volume increases with age (Fig. 3.8), most likely due to early airway closure in the dependent portions of the lungs. Airway patency is determined by the transmural pressure, the pressure across the airway

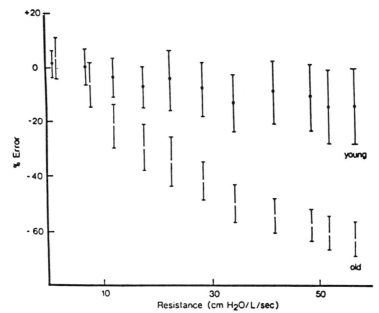

Figure 3.6. Error in tidal volume reproduction during resistive loading of increasing severity in young (closed circles) and older (open circles) subjects. Percent error is derived from the difference in volume between a test breath against a resistive load and control breath (unloaded breath), expressed as percentage of the control breath volume. Bars represent mean values ± standard error. From Tac M, Altose MD, Cherniak NS. Effects of aging on sensation of respiratory force and displacement. *J Appl Physiol.* 55:1437, 1983. Reproduced with permission of the American Physiological Society, Bethesda, Md.

wall. Transmural pressure depends on lung elastic recoil, the tension of the airway wall, and the pressure within the airway. Since elastic recoil decreases with age, the transmural pressure decreases and the airways close at higher lung volumes, resulting in a higher residual volume. This effect is most pronounced at the lung bases because the effect of gravity on the pleural pressure gradient is greatest at the bases in the upright individual. Additional factors that may contribute to the increase in residual volume are the decrease in chest wall compliance and the decrease in respiratory muscle strength that occur with aging. These two components of the respiratory bellows system create the "squeezing" force that can be applied to the pleural cavity during exhalation. As this force diminishes with aging, the amount of air remaining in the lungs after a maximal exhalation increases.

Corresponding to the increase in residual volume is a decrease in vital capacity (recall that the total lung capacity, which does not change with aging, is the sum of the vital capacity and residual volume). The decrease in vital capacity is about 20 mL per year after age 20 years. The functional residual capacity, which is the volume at which the outward forces of the chest wall are balanced by the inward recoil forces of the lung after a passive exhalation, increases in the elderly for reasons similar to those causing the increase in residual volume (Fig. 3.9).

Airflow

Under normal circumstances, the rate of airflow during inspiration is predominantly dependent upon muscular effort. Since respiratory muscle strength decreases in the elderly, maximal inspiratory flow decreases with aging.

Expiratory flow rates at high lung volumes (>70% of the vital capacity) also are dependent on respiratory muscle strength. At lower lung volumes, however, airflow rates are less effort dependent. Once maximal airflow rate is established by the initial forced expiratory effort, flow rate at any given lung volume will depend on both the elastic recoil pressure and resistance within the airways. During forced exhalation, a point is reached in which the positive pleural pressure will equal or exceed the pressure within the airway and cause dynamic compression of the airway. This point, the equal pressure point (EPP), is the site of airflow limitation (Fig. 3.10). Because elastic recoil pressure decreases in the elderly, the EPP occurs closer to the alveolus. At a given lung volume, dynamic airway closure occurs earlier and expiratory flow rate is less in the elderly when compared to younger subjects. Accordingly, the one-second forced expiratory volume (FEV_1) and forced vital capacity (FVC) are decreased in elderly subjects relative to younger counterparts (Fig. 3.11).

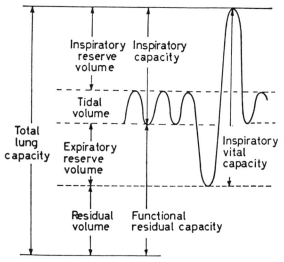

Figure 3.7. The total lung capacity and its subdivisions. The four primary lung volumes are: *(a)* tidal volume (TV)—the volume of gas exhaled during a quiet average exhalation, *(b)* residual volume (RV)—the volume of gas remaining in the thorax following a maximal exhalation, *(c)* expiratory reserve volume (ERV)—the maximum volume of gas that can be exhaled following a quiet normal exhalation, and *(d)* inspiratory reserve volume (IRV)—the maximum volume of air that can be inhaled after a quiet normal inspiration. There are four lung capacities that are derived by combining two or more of the primary lung volumes: *(a)* total lung capacity (TLC)—the total volume of air in the thorax at maximum inhalation. It is the sum of the four primary lung volumes. *(b)* Functional residual capacity (FRC)—the volume of gas remaining in the chest following an average exhalation at rest. It is the sum of the expiratory reserve volume and residual volume. *(c)* Vital capacity (VC)—the maximum volume of gas that can be exhaled from the thorax following a maximal inhalation. It represents the difference between the total lung capacity and residual volume. *(d)* Inspiratory capacity (IC)—the maximum volume of air that can be inhaled following a quiet normal exhalation. It is the sum of tidal volume and inspiratory reserve volume.

The mechanism of flow limitation may be better explained by wave speed propagation theory (24, 25). Although complicated, this theory states that flow in compliant tubes, such as the airways, will depend on the intrinsic properties of the airways, the properties of the gas within them, and their stiffness, as well as their cross-sectional area. There is a maximal speed of flow that is determined by these properties. When this wave speed is reached, flow is limited, and increasing effort will not result in an increase in expiratory flow. Elastic recoil pressure is important in determining the transmural pressure across the airway. Thus, it affects the stiffness of the airways, as well as establishes the driving pressure for flow. As elastic recoil pressure decreases with aging, the airways will be less stiff, and driving pressure will decrease. Therefore, maximum expiratory flow decreases with increasing age.

AIRWAY RESPONSIVENESS AND AIRWAY CLEARANCE

When the airways are subjected to a chemical stimulus, such as an irritating gas, they often constrict via reflex. This bronchoconstriction can be measured as an increase in airway resistance and a decrease in expiratory flow rate. FVC and FEV_1 will fall. The increase in airway resistance is due to an increase in bronchial smooth muscle tone. The airway's smooth muscle will also constrict in response to a number of mediators, such as histamine, leukotrienes, and certain neural peptides. These mediators are believed to be present in increased amounts in subjects with chronic airway inflammation, such as smokers and asthmatics.

In normal subjects, inhalation of a bronchoconstricting substance, such as methacholine, produces little change in airway resistance unless very high concentra-

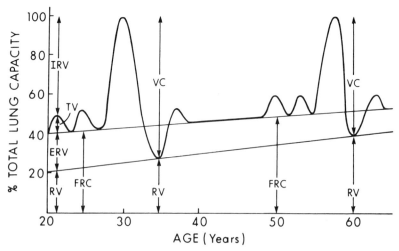

Figure 3.8. Effects of aging on lung volumes and capacities. Total lung capacity does not change with age. Residual volume (RV) and functional residual capacity (FRC) increase with age. Consequently, vital capacity (VC) and inspiratory capacity (IC) decrease with advancing age. From Gracy DR. *Pulmonary Disease in the Adult.* Chicago, Ill: Year Book Medical Publishers; 1981. Reproduced by permission of Mayo Foundation.

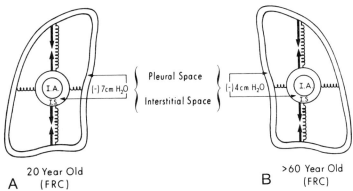

A 20 Year Old (FRC)

B >60 Year Old (FRC)

Figure 3.9. Changes in elastic recoil pressure with aging. The elastic recoil of the lung is represented by the coiled springs. The relative recoil force of the springs is represented by the thickness of the arrows. It is this recoil force that accounts for the negative pressure in the pleural space and in the interstitial space (IS) surrounding the intraparenchymal airways (IA). The 20-year-old lung (**A**) had a distending or transmural pressure of 7 cm water across the airways at functional residual capacity (FRC). Because of the loss of recoil pressure with aging, the 60-year-old lung (**B**) has a pressure of only 4 cm water across the airways. This decreased transmural pressure across the airways contributes to the instability of these airways compared to those of the young and favors early airway closure. The pressures given are approximately correct but are given only for illustrative purposes. From Gracy DR. *Pulmonary Disease in the Adult.* Chicago, Ill: Year Book Medical Publishers; 1981. Reproduced by permission of Mayo Foundation.

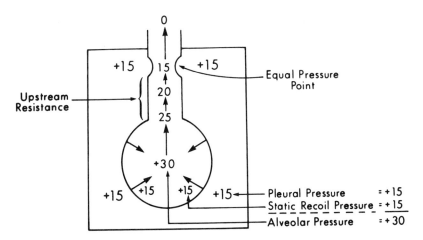

Figure 3.10. Diagrammatic representation of the equal pressure point (EPP). In this model of the EPP the lungs and airways are represented as a single unit enclosed in the thorax. During a forced exhalation, the alveolar pressure (30 cm water) is equal to the sum of the pleural pressure (15 cm water) and the static recoil pressure (15 cm water) of the lungs at that point. As gas flows from the alveolus toward the mouth, the pressure decreases along the airway. At some point, the pressure in the airways will equal the pressure surrounding them (15 cm water), and the EPP will be reached. At different lung volumes, the EPP will change. At equivalent lung volumes, the lungs of aged individuals have reduced recoil pressure, and the EPP is displaced toward the alveolus when compared to the lungs of young normal subjects. From Gracy DR. *Pulmonary Disease in the Adult.* Chicago, Ill: Year Book Medical Publishers; 1981. Reproduced by permission of Mayo Foundation.

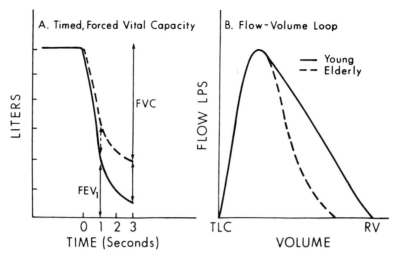

Figure 3.11. Diagrammatic comparison of the timed forced vital capacity (FVC) and flow volume loop of an elderly and young person. In both methods of measurement, the subject fully exhales with maximal effort from total lung capacity. In **(A)**, the FVC is recorded as lung volume in liters as a function of time. The forced expiratory volume exhaled in one second (FEV_1) is shown as a measurement of flow rates. The elderly person has a reduced FEV_1 and FVC when compared to the young person. In **(B)**, the FVC is recorded as flow rate in liters per second (LPS) as a function of lung volume. The flow–volume loop demonstrates that at any lung volume, an elderly subject's maximum expiratory flow rate is less than that of a young subject. The elderly person's flow-volume loop also assumes a convex shape at low lung volume, which may result from loss of lung recoil or from intrinsic changes in the small airways. From Gracy DR. *Pulmonary Disease in the Adult.* Chicago, Ill: Year Book Medical Publishers; 1981. Reproduced by permission of Mayo Foundation.

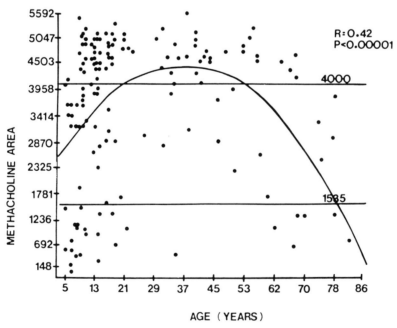

Figure 3.12. Methacholine responses in individuals 5 to 86 years of age. Results >4999 indicate normal responses. Values<1535 indicate responses that are >250 breath units of methacholine and would indicate airway hyperreactivity in adults. The best fitting curve is superimposed. From Hopp RJ, Bewtra A, Nair NM, et al. The effects of age on methacholine response. *J Allergy Clin Immunol.* 76:611, 1985. Reproduced with permission of Mosby Year Book, Inc., St. Louis, Mo.

tions are used. In the elderly, who have no history of airway disease, smaller doses of methacholine are required to produce an increase in airway resistance (Fig. 3.12) (26). This finding suggests that bronchial smooth muscle reactivity differs between elderly and young adults or that the accessibility of particulate matter to the bronchi and the initiation of a bronchoconstricting stimulus differ. Furthermore, the elderly have a decreased number of cilia and a thicker mucus blanket lining their airways. In addition to decreasing the effectiveness of cough, these alterations may modify the clearance and distribution of particles in the airways of the elderly.

In contrast to the increased airway responsiveness due to inhalation of methacholine, an opposite effect is seen when the elderly are exposed to an irritant gas such as ozone. Young adults show decrements in FVC and FEV_1 after inhalation of ozone that exceed those seen in the elderly. In a study by Drechyler-Parks and coworkers (27), elderly subjects complained more of upper airway irritation by the ozone, whereas younger subjects experienced more symptoms of lung irritation. The distribution of ventilation and therefore the distribution of inhaled gases differs in young and elderly adults (28). This may account for the disparity in their responses to ozone.

SLEEP

Ventilatory responses in young subjects during sleep depend predominantly on changes in carbon dioxide tension. Despite the decreased responsiveness of the elderly to hypercarbia, discussed earlier, their mean ventilation during sleep does not differ significantly from that of younger adults. The pattern of ventilation in the elderly, however, is much more irregular than in young adults (29). The elderly tend to have more fragmented sleep and frequent nocturnal awakenings. Thirty-five percent to 40% have repetitive periodic apneas and increasing periods of hypoxemia during sleep (30). Although apneic spells are terminated by an arousal from sleep, the number of arousals are not always associated with an apneic spell. Therefore, while apneas and arousals are correlated, apnea is not the only mechanism that leads to sleep fragmentation in the elderly. Other reasons for fragmented sleep and disordered breathing patterns in the elderly are hypothesized but still unclear.

CARDIOVASCULAR RESPONSES AND EXERCISE

Despite the decline in maximal ventilatory capacity with age, oxygen delivery by the cardiovascular system, rather than oxygen uptake by the respiratory system, is the limiting factor in determining maximal oxygen consumption. After about age 20 years, a progressive decline in maximal heart rate and cardiac output occurs (31, 32). Regular physical activity can improve maximal oxygen uptake and slow the rate of decline in cardiovascular function, but it will not prevent this decline from occurring (33). The cardiovascular response to blood gas abnormalities is also diminished in the elderly. Kronenberg and Drage (21) have shown (Table 3.2) that, when severe hypoxemia or hypercapnia is acutely induced, aged subjects show a response in heart rate only one third that of the control group and fail to respond at all to hypercapnia.

Because of the decrease in functional capacity of the cardiovascular system, elderly individuals are less able to perform aerobic work, especially when stressed. If they become ill and have an increased metabolic demand for oxygen, their cardiovascular system cannot meet this demand as well as that of a younger individual. Oxygen delivery to the tissues may consequently suffer.

SUMMARY

Despite the gradual decline in the functional reserve of the respiratory system with aging, the healthy individual, even when he or she reaches an advanced age, has no respiratory symptoms. However, because the functional respiratory reserve is markedly reduced, disease processes that stress this system can have sudden and sometimes disastrous consequences in the elderly. In addition, elderly patients who are developing respiratory failure may not manifest such usual clinical signs as tachypnea and tachycardia because of their blunted ventilatory and cardiac responses to blood gas derangements. One must be aware of the respiratory fragility of the elderly patient and institute early measures to prevent medical complications from developing. Recommended steps are: (a) avoid inactivity and prolonged periods of time in the recumbent position, (b) provide early and vigorous respiratory care, (c) lessen metabolic demands (such as fever), (d) closely monitor arterial blood gases, (e) administer ventilatory support as early as indicated, and (f) observe the patient closely for subtle signs of impending respiratory failure such as mental status confusion or slight mental status changes.

References

1. Murray JS. *The Normal Lung*. Philadelphia, Pa: WB Saunders; 1986.
2. Bates DV, et al. *Respiratory Function in Disease*. 3rd ed. Philadelphia, Pa: WB Saunders; 1989.
3. Cherniak RM, Cherniak L, Naimari D. *Respiration in Health and Disease*. 2nd ed. Philadelphia, Pa: WB Saunders; 1972.
4. Mittman C, Edelman NH, Norris AH, et al. Relationship between chest wall and pulmonary compliance and age. *J Appl Physiol*. 20:1211–1216, 1965.
5. Turner JM, Mead J, Wohl ME. Elasticity of human lungs in relation to age. *J Appl Physiol*. 25:664–671, 1968.
6. Black LF, Hyatt RE. Maximal respiratory pressures: normal val-

ues and relationship to age and sex. *Am Rev Resp Dis.* 99:696–702, 1969.

7. Noseda A, Van Muylem A, Estenne M, Yernault JC. Inspiratory and expiratory lung pressure–volume curve in healthy males and females. *Bull Eur Physiopathol Respir.* 20:245–249, 1984.

8. Cook CD, Mead J, Orzalsi MM. Static volume–pressure characteristics of the respiratory system during maximal efforts. *J Appl Physiol.* 19:1016–1022, 1964.

9. Mizuno M. Human respiratory muscles: fibre morphology and capillary supply. *Euro Respir J.* 4:587–601, 1991.

10. Rochester DF. Respiratory disease: attention turns to the air pump. *Am J Med.* 68:803–805, 1980.

11. Knudson RJ, Clark DF, Kennedy TC, et al. Effect of aging alone on mechanical properties of the normal adult human lung. *J Appl Physiol.* 43:1054–1062, 1977.

12. Gibellino F, Osmanliev DP, Watson A, Pride NP. Increase in tracheal size with age: implications for maximal expiratory flow. *Am Rev Resp Dis.* 132:784–787, 1985.

13. Thurlbeck WM, Angus GE. Growth and aging of the normal human lung. *Chest.* 67(suppl 2):3–7, 1975.

14. Thurlbeck WM. Internal surface area of non-emphysematous lungs. *Am Rev Resp Dis.* 95:765–773, 1967.

15. Azcuy A, Anderson AE Jr, Foraker AG. The morphological spectrum of aging and emphysematous lungs. *Ann Intern Med.* 57:1–17, 1962.

16. Pump KK. The aged lung. *Chest.* 60:571–577, 1971.

17. Pride NB. Pulmonary distensibility in age and disease. *Bull Eur Physiopathol Resp.* 10:103–108, 1974.

18. Andreotti L, Bossotti A, Cammelli D, Aiello E, Sampognaro S: Connective tissue in aging lung. *Gerontology.* 29:377–387, 1983.

19. Holland J, Milic-Emili J, Macklin PT, et al. Regional distribution of pulmonary ventilation and perfusion in elderly subjects. *J Clin Invest.* 47:81–92, 1968.

20. Sorbini CA, Grassi V, Solinas E, et al. Arterial oxygen tension in relation to age in healthy subjects. *Respiration.* 25:3–13, 1968.

21. Kronenberg RS, Drage CW. Attenuation of the ventilatory and heart rate responses to hypoxia and hypercapnia with aging in normal men. *J Clin Invest.* 52:1812–1819, 1973.

22. Peterson DD, Pack AI, Silage DA, Fishman AP. Effects of aging on ventilatory and occlusion pressure responses to hypoxia and hypercapnia. *Am Rev Resp Dis.* 124:387–391, 1981.

23. Tack M, Altose MD, Cherniak NS. Effects of aging on sensation of respiratory force and displacement. *J Appl Physiol.* 55:1433–1440, 1983.

24. Dawson SV, Elliot EA. Wave-speed limitation on expiratory flow—a unifying concept. *J Appl Physiol.* 43:498–515, 1977.

25. Mead J. Expiratory flow limitation: a physiologist's point of view. *Fed Proc.* 1980, 2771–2775.

26. Hopp RJ, Bewtra A, Nair NM, et al. The effects of age on methacholine response. *J Allergy Clin Immunol.* 76:609–613, 1985.

27. Drechsler-Parks DM, Bedi JF, Horvath SM. Pulmonary function responses of older men and women to ozone exposure. *Exp Gerontol.* 22:91–101, 1987.

28. Edelman NH, Mittman C, Norris AH, Shock NW. Effects of respiratory pattern on age differences in ventilation uniformity. *J Appl Physiol.* 24:49–53, 1968.

29. Shore ET, Millman RP, Silage DA, et al. Ventilatory and arousal patterns during sleep in normal young and elderly subjects. *J Appl Physiol.* 59:1607–1615, 1985.

30. Knight H, Millman RP, Pack AI, et al. Clinical significance of sleep apnea in the elderly. *Am Rev Resp Dis.* 136:845–850, 1987.

31. Stanford BA. Exercise and the elderly. *Exer Sport Sci Rev.* 16:341–379, 1988.

32. Mahler DA, Cunningham LN, Curfman GD. Aging and exercise performance. *Clin Geriat Med.* 2:433–452, 1986.

33. Seals DR, Hazberg JM, Hurley BF, et al. Endurance training in older men and women. 1. Cardiovascular response to exercise. *J Appl Physiol.* 57:1024–1029, 1984.

34. Lefrak SS, Campbell EJ. Structure and function of the aging respiratory system. In: Gracy DR, ed. *Pulmonary Disease in the Adult.* Chicago, Ill: Year Book Medical Publishers; 1981.

35. Peterson DD, Fishman AP. The lungs in later life. In: Fishman AP, ed, update. *Pulmonary Diseases and Disorders.* New York, NY: McGraw Hill; 1982.

4

Exercise in the Rehabilitation of the Elderly

Walter R. Frontera and Carol N. Meredith

POPULATION OVERVIEW

Demographics

By the year 2020, there will be 52 million Americans over the age of 65. Life expectancy will be 82 years for women and 74.2 years for men, and 6.7 million persons will be over 85 years of age. These figures show a rapid increase in the total number of older Americans, especially in the number of the oldest-old (1). Numerous studies have described the physiology and metabolism of persons aged between 60 and 75 years (the young-old), but it is the old-old (aged 75 to 85 years) and the oldest-old (aged over 85 years) who absorb most of the nursing home care, acute health care, and ancillary health and social services devoted to the elderly. Persons of advanced old age make up a little-known biologic entity, as this is their first appearance in substantial numbers in the history of humanity.

As a population advances from early old age to advanced old age, its composition changes. The oldest Americans are mostly women (1), and the elderly nursing home population is 75% female. Compared to men, women throughout old age have less strength and endurance (2), are more likely to be disabled (3), have a greater tendency to fall and fracture bones (4), but are more likely to survive after trauma (5). Older women are 50% less likely to have an able-bodied spouse to provide help with home care and thus require more assistance by social services (6). Figure 4.1 shows the increase in the proportion of elderly men and women needing help with activities of daily living (7). The use of exercise in preserving or increasing muscle mass, bone mass, and physical function has only recently begun to be explored in older women, yet rehabilitation may show the greatest benefits in this group.

Biologic Characteristics

The elderly have special biologic characteristics that affect their need and capacity for exercise; however, the plasticity of the motor system to adapt to a training load

appears to be maintained into the tenth decade of life in humans (8) and also in very old rats (9).

VARIABILITY

The population becomes more diverse at older ages (10). Measurements or interventions must consider that older persons are less homogeneous than are their younger counterparts. They have each undergone different physiologic changes in response to unique genetic endowments and accumulated effects of a lifetime of different habits of eating, smoking, drinking, or exercising, in addition to having a history of different diseases and accidents. Variability demands carefully designed programs for exercise, adapted to each individual.

BODY COMPOSITION

Aging is accompanied by a gradual loss of lean tissue and an increase in fat, even in the absence of obe-

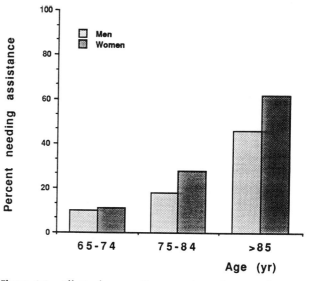

Figure 4.1. Effect of age on the percentage of men and women needing assistance with activities of daily living, while living at home or in an institution. Adapted from Schneider EL, Guralnik JM. The aging of America: impact on health care costs. JAMA. 263:2335–2340, 1990.

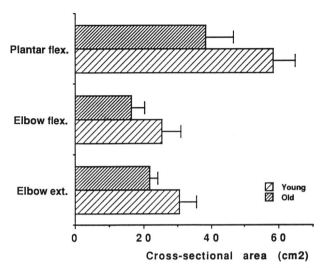

Figure 4.2. Decline in cross-sectional area of various limb muscles (plantar flexors, elbow flexors, elbow extensors), measured by computerized tomography at the site of greatest girth, in old men compared to young men. Adapted from Rice CL, Cunningham DA, Patterson DH, Lefcoe MS. Arm and leg composition determined by computed tomography in young and elderly men. *Clin Physiol.* 9:207–220, 1989.

sity. The decline in muscle mass and bone mineral in part reflects lower physical activity and endocrine changes (10, 11). Total body muscle mass (12, 13), limb muscle volume (14), cross-sectional area (CSA) of limb muscles, muscle fiber area, and fiber number (15–17) are all reduced with age. Figure 4.2 shows the cross-sectional area of arm and leg muscles in young and old men, with a significantly lower muscle size for the older group (14).

Lower muscle mass is a major factor in the diminished strength of elderly men and women (14, 18). Other changes in the contractile function of aged muscles are longer twitch contraction, slower rate of relaxation, and increased fatigability (16, 19, 20). Age alters the sarcoplasmic reticulum, decreasing Ca^{+2}-ATPase and impairing the efficient metabolism of Ca^{+2} (21).

Weakness of the lower limbs affects gait and balance. Weakness of the upper body has little effect on ambulation but can impair the performance of many necessary daily activities. Upper body weakness, defined as the inability to lift 10 pounds, has been described in over half of free-living healthy women over the age of 75 (2).

Loss of bone mineral increases the risk of fracture, usually as a result of a fall, which is an important cause of disability in the elderly, especially women. Osteoporosis leading to kyphoses and pain will reduce voluntary activity, which in turn can further reduce functional capacity.

HABITUAL ACTIVITY

Walking distance declines with age and tends to be lower in women than men, although there are regional and cultural differences. American women in their sixties walk an average of 10 km/wk (22). Walking at least one mile (1.6 km) three times a week (i.e., 4.8 km/wk) is associated with a lower risk of bone fracture in free-living elderly (23).

Walking activity correlates with a larger food intake and helps ensure the adequate provision of essential nutrients and water (22). The decreased energy expenditure of housebound or institutionalized elderly persons may be one of the causes of lower appetite, leading to chronic low food intake and eventual undernutrition (24), which can be exacerbated by periods of illness and even lower food intake (25). Undernutrition affects muscle contractile properties (26) and prolongs convalescence and rehabilitation in the elderly (27).

Greater habitual activity is associated with lower morbidity and mortality in middle-aged persons (28), in persons over 70 years old (29), and in persons over 80 years old (3). Psychosocial factors such as diminished autonomy and lack of social support can lead to inactivity, physiologic changes, and a consequent increase in passivity and morbidity (30). Programs to increase moderately vigorous rehabilitation regimens may improve health and capacity for independent living in the elderly by increasing strength and endurance, maintaining healthier body composition and metabolism, and improving nutrition.

CHRONIC DISEASE

The number of chronic conditions increases with age and is associated with an increased number of prescribed drugs taken daily. While conditions such as noninsulin-dependent diabetes, atherosclerosis, cardiovascular disease, and osteoporosis can be ameliorated by a physical exercise program, they also increase the hazards of exercise, requiring a careful evaluation and monitoring of the patient and an adaptation of the rehabilitation regimen.

MOTOR DISABILITY IN THE ELDERLY

Ambulation

The ability to walk safely indoors and outdoors is vital for independent living. In persons with low functional capacity or who are bound to a wheelchair, strength as well as endurance determine the capacity for independent movement (31). Among free-living, healthy older persons, impaired strength is more prevalent than impaired walking ability, especially in women (2). In young persons, ambulation is not related to strength, but in the deconditioned older person, walking speed is related to the strength of the knee extensors (8) and gastrocnemius (32). To be active in a city environment, older persons must be able to walk at a speed greater than 1.4 m/s, which is the minimum speed required to safely cross an intersection. However, the average walking speed of persons in their seventies is reduced to 1.1 ± 0.2 m/s for women and 1.2 ± 0.2 m/s in men (34). Older persons spending a lot of time outdoors are also those who are capable of walking fast (33).

In women in their 70s, there is a relationship between strength of the knee extensors and the height of a step climbed without a handrail (34). The use of public transportation and entry into many buildings requires climbing steps, demanding a certain minimum strength of the lower limbs in addition to aerobic capacity. When strength and endurance fall below the threshold necessary for moving about outdoors, it is likely that an older person will become housebound and even less active, further decreasing functional capacity.

Falls and Fractures

An important cause of death and disability in the elderly is falling and bone fractures (Fig. 4.3). Each year about one third of elderly persons living at home suffers a fall. Falling, even when it does not produce an injury, affects behavior. In the 6 months following a fall, voluntary activity declines, probably because of the fear of falling again (35). Injuries occur in 10% to 20% of falls (5). Falling is related to hip weakness, poor balance, postural sway, and medications (36). Falls are more common in persons with lower grip strength (37), suggesting that weakness of some or all muscles is one of the causes of falling. Falling is more common in women, who are also more likely to suffer a fracture from the fall; and fall injuries increase with age, as shown in Figure 4.3 (5). Postural sway does not improve with exercise training (38), but medications can sometimes be adjusted, and strength can be increased with rehabilitation.

In institutionalized patients aged an average 87 years, a reduction in certain medications (such as diuretics) and enrollment in exercise programs to improve strength and mobility led to a lower frequency of falls and length of hospitalization in the subsequent 2 years (39).

The incidence of hip fracture is increasing in the United States (40). Although mortality rate during hospitalization has declined, long-term prospects for regaining mobility are worse. Changes in hospital reimbursements have discouraged prolonged rehabilitation programs of fracture patients. Duration of hospitalization after hip fracture has decreased from 17.9 days in 1982 to 8.6 days in 1985, mainly because of a 50% decline in the days devoted to physical therapy (41). At the same time, the proportion of patients discharged to nursing homes has increased from 21% to 48%, and those receiving nursing home care 6 months after discharge have increased from 13% to 39% (41). A walking speed above 0.15 m/s on discharge from hospital appears to differentiate between the capacity for independent living and long-term hospital care (42). Other predictors of ambulation 1 year after fracture are younger age, better health and physical function before the fracture occurred, and less depression (43). With adequate physical therapy of hip fracture patients, 66% of those over the age of 80 years could return home within a year, and 62% of a group aged over 91 years gained independent ambulation using an assistive device (44). Programs to maintain physical strength and endurance in the healthy elderly may help prevent falls and fractures and improve the rate of return to ambulation if a fracture occurs, even in the oldest-old.

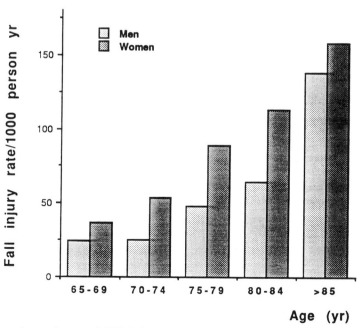

Figure 4.3.   Effect of age and gender on the rate of fall injuries per year. Adapted from Sattin RW, Huber DAL, DeVito CA, Rodríguez JG, Ros A, Bacchelli S. Stevens JA. Waxweiler RJ. The incidence of fall injury events among the elderly in a defined population. *Am J Epidemiol.* 131:1028–1037, 1990.

Detraining Effects of Immobility and Inactivity

Inactivity ranges from a sedentary life-style with no episodes of moderate or vigorous exercise to the complete immobility of the bedridden. The results of inactivity on the musculoskeletal system at any age are a loss of muscle and bone mass, loss of cardiovascular fitness, weakness, and joint contractures. Bedrest causes more severe problems: cardiac output decreases; orthostatic intolerance may occur; blood volume declines; micturition becomes difficult; incontinence is more likely, and breathing requires a greater effort (45). It is clear that bedrest in young persons causes changes that are similar to the aging process (11).

In young persons, inactivity and bedrest change metabolism, body composition, and function within a few days or weeks, while recovery is a slower process, taking weeks or months. In healthy young men, a week of bedrest reduces muscle mass, lowers glucose tolerance, and increases insulin secretion (46). Mineral content of the spine decreases at a rate of 0.9% per week during bedrest (47). The loss of muscle strength can be as high as 5% per day (45), especially in the leg muscles. Muscle fibers lose length, oxidative capacity, and contractile proteins. Absence of loading and decreased motion of the joints leads to contractures and changes similar to osteoarthritis. Motor coordination decreases, with an increase in postural sway when the person stands up.

The metabolic and functional effects of bedrest have not been studied in the healthy elderly, but they are likely to be more severe and difficult to reverse than in the young. In middle-aged men, after 10 days of bedrest, cardiovascular fitness was restored by everyday activity, but only after 30 days (48). In a group of mostly middle-aged patients, the recovery of vertebral bone mineral density after bedrest took more than 4 months (47). Older persons could require more than simple habitual activity in order to recover body composition and function after an episode of bedrest, and early and regular rehabilitation therapy may be indicated.

The psychologic effects of bedrest may be more detrimental in older persons, who already suffer sensory deprivation. Bedrest leads to impaired perception and affective changes such as anxiety, fear, and depression (45). Resuming ambulation and daily activities after being severely deconditioned and psychologically affected by bedrest is likely to be a daunting prospect for the older patient.

Studies of institutionalized elderly persons show that immobilization is not widely recognized as a hazard to physical and mental health. A study of nonambulatory elderly residents of a nursing home showed that, in 85% of cases, immobility was not mentioned in either nursing or physician problem lists (49). Physical restraint and/or sedation of elderly persons has been shown to damage social functioning and to increase morbidity and mortality (50). Nearly all nursing homes in the United States use physical restraints on 25% to 50% of their residents, usually to prevent wandering, self-damage, or acts of aggression in mentally impaired patients (50). A recent study of nursing homes has shown that the use of sedatives and restraints has been increasing, to the point that 40% to 50% of residents in skilled nursing homes have their mobility restricted by these means (51).

EXERCISE PHYSIOLOGY AND PRACTICAL APPROACHES TOWARD REHABILITATION TRAINING

Strength: Physiology and Training

Reduction in strength with age has been attributed to one or more of the following changes (16): (a) a loss of muscle mass due to smaller and fewer muscle fibers, (b) a loss of motor neurons, (c) a change in muscle architecture, such as fiber length and angle of pennation, which cannot be measured in vivo, (d) a defect in the excitation–contraction mechanism, including energy supply, and (e) psychosocial changes leading to a reduced capacity to activate otherwise normal motor units.

Muscle strength in the elderly is associated with the capacity to perform activities of daily living, as shown in Figure 4.4 (52). The absolute levels of force needed to perform an activity vital for independent living, such as standing from a sitting position, are lower than normal strength at a younger age but can become near maximal efforts at an older age. This loss of reserve function means that there is a dangerously small margin between maximal strength and the threshold for adequate performance of daily activities. After minor surgery, illness, or bedrest, an elderly person may be deconditioned to the point of being unable to live independently.

Strength training can lead to major improvements of function in the elderly. A small strength gain in severely deconditioned persons can get them from being just unable to move independently to just being able to do so, with a marked increase in function. Improvements in muscle strength with heavy resistance training of the knee extensors have improved tandem gait speed and functional mobility even in persons in their nineties (8).

Strength training is an important component of traditional rehabilitation programs. A typical exercise prescription for training large muscle groups such as the extensors and flexors of the knee and elbow is shown in Table 4.1. Since 1970, several studies have examined how this type of therapeutic exercise affects the morphology and function of skeletal muscles in older men and women, as summarized in Table 4.2. In two studies (53, 54) training consisted of static (isometric) exercises; another three (55, 56, 57) used low resistance exercises, and the

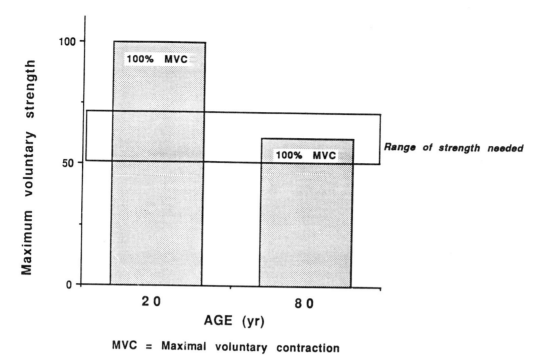

MVC = Maximal voluntary contraction

Figure 4.4   Effect of age on the estimated percentage of a maximal voluntary contraction (%MVC) of the quadriceps muscles required to raise a healthy woman from a low, armless chair. A 20-year-old woman uses less than 75% of her maximum strength. An 80-year-old woman uses all her strength to rise slowly and is unable to rise quickly from a low chair. Adapted from Young A. Exercise physiology in geriatric practice. *Acta Med Scand.* Suppl. 711:227–232, 1986.

Table 4.1.   Typical Exercise Prescriptions for Strength[a] and Aerobic Training[b]

Variable	Strength	Aerobic
Type of exercise	Dynamic (free-weights, variable resistance)	Walking, cycling, rowing, swimming, dancing
Muscle groups	Any	Large
Frequency	2–3 times/wk	3–5 times/wk
Duration of muscle activity	9 s/contraction (3 s each for the concentric, the static, and the eccentric phase)	20–60 min
Sets and repetitions	1–3 sets of 8–12 repetitions	—
Intensity	60%–80% of 1 RM	60%–90% of maximal heart rate or 50%–85% of Vo₂max
Rest periods	2–3 s between repetitions, 2 min between sets	None

[a]This description does not include circuit weight training programs characterized by low resistance (40%–60% of 1 RM) and a larger number of repetitions (15–30).
[b]All training sessions should start with a 10–15 minute warm-up period and flexibility exercises and finish with a 10 minute cool-down period.

remaining six studies (8, 21, 58–61) used an adaptation of the original progressive resistance exercises designed by DeLorme in the 1940s (62).

As Table 4.2 shows, strength training effectively increases the strength of various aged muscles, using a variety of training regimens. Static and dynamic strength [one repetition maximum (1 RM) and isokinetic peak torque] increase markedly with training. The percentage gain in strength per day of training in various studies ranges from 0.2% to 5.1%. As has also been described in young subjects, the results were most dramatic when training and testing methods used the same type of muscle contraction and/or the same equipment. The relationship between torque and velocity of contraction changes after training. This means that the strength-trained older person can attain faster velocity at an equal level of torque.

Table 4.2. Adaptations to Strength Conditioning in Older Men and Women[a]

Variable	Range of Reported Improvements
Strength	
Static	↑ 13 to 72%
1 RM	↑ 9 to 227%
Isokinetic	↑ 7 to 29%
Strength gain/day	
Static	↑ 0.3 to 4%
1 RM	↑ 3 to 5%
Isokinetic	↑ 0.2 to 0.5%
Isokinetic work	↑ 18 to 21%
Torque-velocity curve	↑ Velocity at a given torque
Muscle size	
Cross-sectional area (CT scan)	↑ 9 to 12%
Type I fiber area	↑ 31 to 38%
Type II fiber area	↑ 26 to 52%
Mean fiber area	↑ 27%
Turnover of muscle protein (from urinary 3-methylhistidine)	↑ 41%
Muscle fiber type distribution	No change
Integrated electromyographic activity	↑ 23%
Muscle membrane Na-K pumps	↑ 40%
Sarcoplasmic reticulum Ca^{+2}-ATPase	Decrease with age is prevented
Aerobic power ($\dot{V}O_2$max)	↑ 0 to 6%
Maximum exercise heart rate	No change
Maximum exercise blood pressure	No change
Hemoglobin concentration	No change
Blood volume	No change
Capillary density per fiber	↑ 15%
Oxidative enzyme activity (citrate synthase)	↑ 30%

[a]Data from references 8, 21, 53–61.

A greater capacity for isokinetic work allows the older person to cover a greater distance with a similar level of force production. Thus, the mechanical behavior of the muscle is sensitive to the overload associated with the training program.

Functional adaptations were accompanied by morphologic changes in some studies. A significant increase in muscle cross-sectional area, determined with computerized tomography, and in type I and type II fiber areas, measured in muscle biopsy samples, accompanied the gains in strength. Although earlier reports had questioned the capacity of older human muscles to hypertrophy (61), studies using more sophisticated measurements of muscle area show that the older person retains the capacity to respond to stimuli that increase muscle mass (8, 58, 59). Also, the increased excretion of 3-methylhistidine in the urine after training indicates active turnover of muscle contractile proteins (59). The fiber type distribution in hypertrophied muscles does not change after training.

Gains in strength do not correlate with changes in muscle size, but are in themselves heterogeneous according to the method used for measurement. Other mechanisms may contribute to the development of a stronger muscle, including increased integrated electromyographic activity (IEMG), a learning effect, synchronization of motor units, reflex potentiation, supraspinal facilitation, or inhibition of inhibitory influences (63). Peripheral adaptations in the muscle (such as change in fiber architecture, increased density of contractile proteins, and adaptations in connective tissue may help function (63). Strength training prevents the decrease with age of the enzyme Ca^{+2}-ATPase in the sarcoplasmic reticulum (21). This enzyme is responsible for the active transport of Ca^{+2} ions released during muscle stimulation back into the sarcoplasmic reticulum, and its greater activity may allow a faster relaxation. The normalization of the electrolyte environment in the muscle cell is also favored by the increased concentration of Na-K pumps that occurs with strength training in the elderly (64). These subcellular mechanisms may help delay fatigue.

In older men, strength training has been associated with changes in some, but not all, of the determinants of aerobic capacity ($\dot{V}O_2$max). Strength training in the elderly has no effect on the central determinants of aerobic capacity such as maximal heart rate and blood pressure, hemoglobin concentration, and blood volume (65). Increases in capillary density and oxidative enzyme activity in the trained muscle have been reported in older men who showed increased VO_2max after twelve weeks of strength training (65). Others, however, have reported no change in VO_2max) with strength training (60), probably due to differences in the exercise prescription and the initial level of fitness.

Aerobic Exercise

MAXIMAL OXYGEN UPTAKE

The maximal oxygen uptake (VO_2max) is the amount of oxygen that can be transported in the blood and utilized in the muscles during maximal exercise while breathing air at sea level. Physiologically, VO_2max is the product of cardiac output and the arteriovenous oxygen difference (a-vO_2 difference), integrating central and peripheral organs and systems for supplying oxygen to active muscles. VO_2max is a measurement accepted by the World Health Organization as a quantitative index of cardiovascular health. The transport of oxygen from the atmosphere to the mitochondria involves a series of steps: lung ventilation, diffusion across the alveolar–capillary membrane, binding to hemoglobin and circulation in the blood, diffusion from the capillaries to the mitochondria in muscle, and incorporation as the final electron acceptor in the electron transport chain.

All of the steps in the oxygen transport chain are influenced by age (66), explaining the common observation that VO_2max declines with aging (67, 68). The decline in maximal heart rate and the loss of muscle mass deserve special attention. Since cardiac output is the product of heart rate and stroke volume, heart rate has been consistently identified as a cause of lower central response to maximal exercise (68, 69). On the other hand, the loss of muscle mass may account for almost half of the age-associated decline in VO_2max in untrained men and women (13). The importance of each factor may depend on the person's training status. In untrained healthy elders, an increased stroke volume compensates for a lowered heart rate, maintaining exercise cardiac output (70). On the other hand, in master athletes, a reduction in both heart rate and stroke volume contribute to lower cardiac output (71). In both populations the a-vO_2 difference is decreased. Maintaining an active lifestyle moderates the age-related decline in VO_2max. Aerobic capacity declines 9% per decade in untrained men, but only 5% in trained subjects (68). These findings suggest that the age-related decline in aerobic capacity is due, at least in part, to a sedentary life-style. The importance of external factors to human aging has been recognized by researchers in the field. Rowe and Kahn have stated that the effects of the aging process have been exaggerated, and modifying effects of diet, exercise, personal habits, and psychosocial factors have been underestimated. (30).

ENDURANCE AND FUNCTIONAL CAPACITY

Endurance can be defined as the time that a person can maintain either a static force or a power level involving a combination of concentric and/or eccentric muscular contractions. The stress submaximal exercise imposes on a patient, and, therefore, the endurance or tolerance for that exercise intensity, depends on how much energy is needed to successfully perform the task in relation to the patient's maximal capacity. When analyzing aerobic activities, this level of exercise intensity is commonly expressed as a percent of VO_2max. It follows that the age-related decline in VO_2max must be associated with a reduction in endurance for a given exercise intensity. This situation is similar to that illustrated in Figure 4.4 for muscle strength. In the elderly, a common activity such as walking a city block may demand an effort that is close to maximal aerobic capacity, making it difficult to maintain for a long time. At these exercise intensities, active muscles fatigue and the balance between myocardial oxygen supply and demand may be altered, resulting in ischemia.

ADAPTATIONS TO AEROBIC TRAINING

A typical exercise prescription recommended by the American College of Sports Medicine (72) and followed in many studies is presented in Table 4.1.

A summary of the adaptations to various aerobic training programs is shown in Table 4.3, based on several recent studies. These data, involving submaximal and maximal testing, show that the trainability of elderly persons is similar to that of younger individuals. Submaximal testing may be preferred because when prescribing exercise for this population the important information is probably the response of the heart and circulation to quite modest effort (73). On the other hand, it may be hazardous to predict maximal aerobic capacity from submaximal measurements of heart rate. There is some evidence that the optimum sensitivity and specificity of electrocardiographic interpretation is obtained with tests that are carried to more than 85% of maximum oxygen intake.

Changes in ventilation, cardiac function, circulation, and muscle metabolism can be examined at submaximal and maximal intensities of exercise. When tested at submaximal intensities, but at the same absolute power output as before training, minute ventilation (VE) is reduced (74), suggesting a more efficient ventilation in the trained state. After training, the cardiovascular response to submaximal exercise is different, as cardiac output does not change (75) but becomes more efficient. The decreased heart rate, which lowers the myocardial oxygen demand, is compensated by a larger stroke volume (75, 76). This increase in stroke volume is related to a larger

Table 4.3. Adaptations to Aerobic Conditioning in Older Men and Women[a]

Variable	Range of Reported Improvements
Ventilation	
During submaximal exercise[b]	
Minute ventilation (V_E)	↓ 9 to 15%
During maximal exercise	
Minute ventilation (V_E)	↑ 20 to 30%
% Maximal voluntary ventilation (MVV)	↑ 16%
Cardiac function	
During submaximal exercise	
Heart rate	↓ 9 to 20 beats/min
Stroke volume	↑ 8%
Cardiac output	No change
During maximal exercise	
Heart rate	No change
Stroke volume	↑ 6 to 28%
Cardiac output	↑ 0 to 34%
Circulation	
Total hemoglobin	↑ 7%
Blood volume	↑ 8%
Systemic vascular resistance during submaximal exercise	↓ 5 to 18%
Leg blood flow during maximal exercise	↑ 42%
Muscle metabolism	
Fiber type distribution	No change or increased type IIA
Capillary density	No change
In vitro oxidative capacity	↑ 128%
Oxidative enzyme activity	↑ 0 to 45%
Glycogen stores	↑ 10 to 28%
Mitochondrial number, mean volume, and volume fraction	No change
During submaximal exercise	
Arteriovenous O_2 difference	No change
Blood lactate	↓ 21 to 44%
During maximal exercise	
Arteriovenous O_2 difference	↑ 14.0%
Integrated Response	
Submaximal V_{O_2}	No change
V_{O_2}max	↑ 11 to 30%

[a]Data from 56, 60, 74–82, 89–91.
[b]Submaximal: comparison made at same absolute power output.

blood volume, greater blood flow to the exercising muscles, and a lowered systemic vascular resistance (75, 77). Finally, since cardiac output and a-vO_2 difference do not change, oxygen consumption of skeletal muscles exercising at a submaximal intensity remains the same after training.

During maximal exercise, V_E increases (78). Trained elderly persons can use a larger proportion of the ventilatory reserve [% of maximal voluntary ventilation (MVV)] compared to untrained persons (74). Maximal heart rate does not change, and maximal stroke volume has been reported to show either a nonsignificant change (75) or a significant increase (79). Adaptations in maximal cardiac output have been reported to be similar to the changes observed in stroke volume (75, 79). On the other hand, the a-vO_2 difference during maximal exercise increases with training (75). Therefore, even with no significant increase in cardiac output, peripheral adaptations take place that can explain the increase in

V_{O_2}max in older men and women after training (60, 78). Capillary density has not been reported to change, but improved oxygen extraction may be due to increased activity of muscle oxidative enzymes (78, 80). Unchanged mitochondrial volume and number after training suggest that adaptations in oxidative capacity occur within the existing mitochondrial volume fraction (81). No change in muscle fiber type distribution or increase in the percentage of type IIA (fast twitch oxidative) fibers have been reported (56, 81).

With training, a previously stressful activity becomes easy to carry out. There are two explanations for this. First, submaximal oxygen consumption, and therefore the absolute energy cost of submaximal activity, does not change with training, although a higher V_{O_2}max has been attained. This means that a trained older person has increased endurance for submaximal exercise, and this increases the capacity for most activities of daily living. Second, improvements in the efficiency of movement can lower the energy cost of an activity and improve endurance even if maximal aerobic capacity remains low (76).

Two additional adaptations to an aerobic training program are associated with greater endurance. Training increases muscle glycogen stores and lowers blood lactate accumulation at submaximal power output, favoring the prolongation of muscle activity. Larger glycogen stores improve the availability of fuel for muscle contraction (78, 80). A lower blood lactate accumulation indicates a smaller contribution from the less efficient anaerobic pathways for energy production (80, 82). High lactate levels, increased H^+ production, and decreased pH in the cellular environment are all associated with muscular fatigue. With training, these changes are delayed or occur at a higher absolute power output.

Precautions and Contraindications

Patients in this age group should undergo a comprehensive health evaluation before starting a strength or aerobic training program. The American Heart Association (83) and the American College of Sports Medicine (72) recommend that the conditions listed in Table 4.4 be considered contraindications to exercise. After initiating the training program, signs and symptoms presented in Table 4.5 should be considered when evaluating the appropriateness of the quantity and quality of exercise.

Many strength training programs include a static component, and clinicians frequently express concern because of the excessive pressor response to static exercise when compared with dynamic exercise. However, the cardiovascular adjustments that occur during exercise are influenced more by the amount of muscle activated than by the type of contraction (84). If properly designed and supervised, strength training has been shown to be safe even in frail nursing-home residents aged over 86 years (8). Risks are minimized by using proper weight-lifting techniques that avoid straining and the Valsalva maneuver. In recent studies, circuit weight training has been successfully used in the rehabilitation of cardiac and coronary disease-prone patients with minimal complications (85); this form of strength training has a greater aerobic component.

Detraining

In young subjects, the cessation of strength training rapidly leads to a decrease in strength. After 24 weeks of strength training in young men, maximal isometric force declined 11.4% by 4 weeks of no training (86). Preliminary studies in very old persons after 8 weeks of strength training show a 32% loss of maximum dynamic strength after 4 weeks of no training (8).

In young endurance-trained subjects, the cessation of exercise leads to lower cardiovascular endurance, a decrease in the activity of oxidative enzymes in skeletal muscle, and greater perceived exertion during submaximal exercise carried out only 12 days after stopping training (87). In middle-aged men after a period of training, VO_2max is back to initial low values when measured 15 weeks after resuming a sedentary life-style (88).

These findings suggest that rapid detraining also occurs in the elderly and that programs of strength and aerobic training or rehabilitation must be constantly maintained to prevent deterioration of functional capacity.

Table 4.4. Reasons for Deferring Exercise[a]

Unstable angina
Resting SBP over 200 mm Hg or resting DBP over 100 mm Hg
Hypertension with exercise: SBP over 250, or DBP over 120
Moderate to severe aortic stenosis
Acute systemic illness, active infectious disease, or fever
Uncontrolled atrial or ventricular dysrhythmias
Uncontrolled tachycardia (greater than 100 bpm)
Symptomatic congestive heart failure
Third degree heart block
Active pericarditis or myocarditis
Endocarditis
Recent embolism
Thrombophlebitis
Resting ST segment displacement (greater than 3 mm)
Active or uncontrolled metabolic disorders: hyperthyroidism, adrenal insufficiency, gout, or diabetes
Orthopedic problems that would prohibit exercise
Uncontrolled rheumatic diseases
Severe anemia
Adverse environmental conditions (high temperature and high relative humidity, significant air pollution)
Recent (less than 3–4 hours) large meals
Cerebral dysfunction (vertigo)
Certain drugs (decongestants, anorectics, atropine)

[a] Modified from American College of Sports Medicine. The recommended quantity and quality of exercise for developing and maintaining cardiorespiratory and muscular fitness in healthy adults. *Med Sci Sports Exerc.* 22:265–274, 1990 and American Heart Association. *Exercise Testing and Training of Individuals with Heart Disease or at High Risk for Its Development: A Handbook for Physicians.* 1975.

Table 4.5. Signs and Symptoms of Excessive Effort[a]

Angina
Ataxia, light-headedness, confusion
Nausea and vomiting
Leg claudication
Pallor, cyanosis
Dyspnea persisting for more than 10 minutes
Inappropriate bradycardia
Prolonged fatigue after exercise
Insomnia
Prolonged tachycardia after exercise
Weight gain due to fluid retention (heart failure)
Orthopedic problems aggravated by exercise

[a] Modified from American College of Sports Medicine. The recommended quantity and quality of exercise for developing and maintaining cardiorespiratory and muscular fitness in healthy adults. *Med Sci Sports Exerc.* 22:265–274, 1990 and American Heart Association. *Exercise Testing and Training of Individuals with Heart Disease or High Risk for Its Development: A Handbook for Physicians.* 1975.

SUMMARY

Clinical and experimental studies show that exercise training is feasible and effective even in advanced old age. Conversely, immobility accelerates the aging process. Therapeutic exercise may prolong independence and health of the free-living elderly and improve recovery of elderly inpatients. There is increasing physiologic evidence that elderly muscles respond well to rehabilitation exercise, but recent trends show that rehabilitation of elderly inpatients during convalescence is being reduced in many hospitals. Physical movement must be recognized as a key factor for the maintenance and improvement of health in the elderly.

The authors are grateful to Diane Hardy for assistance in preparing this manuscript.

References

1. US Bureau of the Census. Estimates of the population of the United States by age, sex, and race: 1980 and 1985. Washington, DC: Government Printing Office; 1986.
2. Jette AM, Branch LG. The Framingham Disability Study: II. Physical disability among the aging. *Am J Pub Health.* 71:1211–1216, 1981.
3. Harris T, Kovar MG, Suzman R, Kleinman JC, Feldman JJ. Longitudinal study of physical ability in the oldest-old. *Am J Pub Health.* 79:698–702, 1989.
4. Prudham D, Evans J. Factors associated with falls in the elderly: a community study. *Age Ageing.* 10:141–146, 1981.
5. Sattin RW, Huber DAL, DeVito CA, et al. The incidence of fall injury events among the elderly in a defined population. *Am J Epidemiol.* 131:1028–1037, 1990.
6. Davis MA, Randall E, Forthofer RN, Lee ES, Margen S: Living arrangements and dietary patterns of older adults in the United States. *J Gerontol* 40:434–442, 1985.
7. Schneider EL, Guralnik JM. The aging of America: impact on health care costs. *JAMA.* 263:2335–2340, 1990.
8. Fiatarone MA, Marks EC, Ryan ND, Meredith CN, Lipsitz LA, Evans WJ: High-intensity strength training in nonagenarians. *JAMA* 263:3029–3034, 1990.
9. Klitgaard H, Marc R, Brunet A, Vandewalle H, Monod H. Contractile properties of old rat muscles: effect of increased use. *J Appl Physiol.* 67:1401–1408, 1989.
10. Minaker KL, Rowe J: Health and disease among the oldest old: a clinical perspective. *Health and Society.* 63:324–349, 1985.
11. Bortz WM. Disuse and aging. *JAMA.* 248:1203–1208, 1982.
12. Cohn SH, Vartsky D, Yasumura S, et al. Compartmental body composition based on total-body nitrogen, potassium, and calcium. *Am J Physiol.* 239:E524–530, 1980.
13. Flegg JL, Lakatta EG. Role of muscle loss in the age-associated reduction in VO_2max. *J Appl Physiol.* 65:1147–1151, 1988.
14. Rice CL, Cunningham DA, Paterson DH, Lefcoe MS. Arm and leg composition determined by computed tomography in young and elderly men. *Clin Physiol.* 9:207–220, 1989.
15. Aniansson A, Hedberg M, Henning GB, Grimby G. Muscle morphology, enzymatic activity, and muscle strength in elderly men: a follow-up study. *Muscle & Nerve.* 9:585–591, 1986.
16. Larsson L, Grimby G, Karlsson J. Muscle strength and speed of movement in relation to age and muscle morphology. *J Appl Physiol.* 46:451–456, 1979.
17. Lexell J, Taylor CC, Sjostrom M. What is the cause of the ageing atrophy? *J Neurol Sci.* 84:275–294, 1988.
18. Frontera WR, Hughes VA, Lutz K, Evans WJ. A cross-sectional study of muscle strength and mass in 45 to 78 year old men and women. *J Appl Physiol.* 71:644–650, 1991.
19. Davies CTM, Thomas DO, White MJ. Mechanical properties of young and elderly human muscle. *Acta Med Scand.* 711(suppl):219–226, 1986.
20. Vandervoort AA, McComas AJ. Contractile changes in opposing muscles of the human ankle joint with aging. *J Appl Physiol.* 61:361–367, 1986.
21. Klitgaard H, Ausoni S, Damiani E. Sarcoplasmic reticulum of human skeletal muscle: age-related changes and effect of training. *Acta Physiol Scand.* 137:23–31, 1989.
22. Cauley JA, LaPorte RE, Sandler RB, Schramm MM, Kriska AM. Comparison of methods to measure physical activity in postmenopausal women. *Am J Clin Nutr.* 45:14–22, 1987.
23. Sorock GS, Bush TL, Golden AL, Fried LP, Breuer B, Hale WE. Physical activity and fracture risk in a free-living elderly cohort. *J Gerontol.* 43:M134–M139, 1988.
24. Silver AJ, Morley JE, Strome LS, Jones D, Vickers L. Nutritional status in an academic nursing home. *J Am Geriatr Soc.* 36:487–491, 1988.
25. Rammohan M, Juan D, Jung, D. Hypophagia among hospitalized elderly. *J Am Diet Assoc.* 89:1774–1779, 1989.
26. Jeejeebhoy KN. Muscle function and nutrition. *Gut.* 27:25–39, 1986.
27. Bastow MD, Rawlings J, Allison SO. Benefits of supplementary tube feeding after fractures of the neck of the femur: a randomised control trial. *Br Med J.* 287:1589–1592, 1983.
28. Blair SN, Kohl HE, Paffenbarger RS, Clark DG, Cooper KH, Gibbons LW: Physical fitness and all-cause mortality: a prospective study of healthy men and women. *JAMA.* 262:2395–2401, 1989.
29. Kaplan GA, Seeman TE, Cohen RD, Knudsen LP, Guralnik J. Mortality among the elderly in the Alameda County Study: behavioral and demographic risk factors. *Am J Pub Health.* 77:307–312, 1987.
30. Rowe JW, Kahn RL. Human aging: usual and successful. *Science.* 237:143–149, 1987.
31. Sawka MN, Glaser RM, Laubach LL, Al-Samkari O, Suryaprasad AG. Wheelchair exercise performance of the young, middle-aged, and elderly. *J Appl Physiol.* 50:824–828, 1981.
32. Bassey EJ, Bendall MJ, and Pearson M. Muscle strength in the triceps surae and objectively measured customary walking activity in men and women over 65 years of age. *Clin Sci.* 74:85–89, 1988.
33. Isaacs B. Clinical and laboratory studies of falls in old people. *Clin Geriatr Med.* 1:513–524, 1985.
34. Aniansson A, Rundgren A, Sperling L. Evaluation of functional capacity in activities of daily living in 70-year-old men and women. *Scan J Rehab Med.* 12:145–154, 1980.
35. Vellas B, Cayla F, Bocquet H, dePemille F, Albarede JL. Prospective study of restriction of activity in old people after falls. *Age and Ageing.* 16:189–193, 1987.
36. Robbins AS, Rubenstein LZ, Josephson KR, Schulman BL, Osterweil D, and Fine G. Predictors of falls among elderly people: results of two population-based studies. *Arch Intern Med.* 149:1628–1633, 1989.
37. Wickham C, Cooper C, Margetts BM, Barker DJP. Muscle strength, activity, housing and the risk of falls in elderly people. *Age and Ageing.* 18:47–51, 1989.
38. Crilly RG, Willems DA, Trenholm KJ, Hayes KC, and Delaguerriere-Richardson LFO. Effect of exercise on postural sway in the elderly. *Gerontol.* 35:137–143, 1989.
39. Rubenstein LZ, Robbins AS, Josephson KR, Schulman BL, Osterweil D. The value of assessing falls in an elderly population:

a randomized clinical trial. *Ann Intern Med.* 113:308–316, 1990.

40. Rodríguez JG, Sattin RW, Waxweiler RJ. Incidence of hip fractures, United States, 1970–83. *Am J Prev Med.* 5:175–181, 1989.

41. Fitzgerald JF, Fagan LF, Tierney WM, Dittus RS. Changing patterns of hip fracture care before and after implementation of the prospective payment system. *JAMA.* 258:218–221, 1987.

42. Friedman PJ, Richmond DE, Baskett JJ. A prospective trial of serial gait speed as a measure of rehabilitation in the elderly. *Age and Ageing.* 17:227–235, 1988.

43. Mossey JM, Mutran E, Knott K, Craik R. Determinants of recovery 12 months after hip fracture: the importance of psychosocial factors. *Am J Public Health.* 79:279–286, 1989.

44. Kauffman TL, Albright L, Wagner C. Rehabilitation outcomes after hip fracture in persons 90 years old and older. *Arch Phys Med Rehabil.* 68:369–371, 1987.

45. Harper CM, Lyles YM. Physiology and complications of bed rest. *J Am Geriatr Soc.* 36:1047–1054, 1988.

46. Shangraw RE, Stuart CE, Prince MJ, Peters EJ, Wolfe RR. Insulin responsiveness of protein metabolism in vivo following bedrest in humans. *Am J Physiol.* 255:E548–E558, 1988.

47. Krolner B, Toft B. Vertebral bone loss: an unheeded side effect of therapeutic bed rest. *Clin Sci.* 64:537–540, 1983.

48. DeBusk RF, Convertino VA, Hung J, Goldwater D. Exercise conditioning in middle-aged men after 10 days of bed rest. *Circulation.* 68:245–250, 1983.

49. Selikson S, Damus K, Hamerman D. Risk factors associated with immobility. *J Am Geriatr Soc.* 36:707–712, 1988.

50. Folmar S, Wilson H. Social behavior and physical restraints. *Gerontologist.* 29:650–653, 1989.

51. Commission on California State Government Organization and Economy. Skilled nursing homes: care without dignity. Report 109, State of California, 1991.

52. Young A. Exercise physiology in geriatric practice. *Acta Med Scand.* 711 (suppl):227–232, 1986.

53. Kauffman TL. Strength training effect in young and aged women. *Arch Phys Med Rehabil.* 66:223–226, 1985.

54. Liemohn WP. Strength and aging: an exploratory study. *Int J Aging Hum Devel.* 6:347–357, 1975.

55. Agre JC, Pierce LE, Raab DM, McAdams M, Smith EL. Light resistance and stretching exercise in elderly women: effect upon strength. *Arch Phys Med Rehabil.* 69:273–276, 1988.

56. Aniansson A, Gustafsson E. Physical training in elderly men with special reference to quadriceps muscle strength and morphology. *Clin Physiol.* 1:87–98, 1981.

57. Larsson L. Physical training effects on muscle morphology in sedentary males at different ages. *Med Sci Sports Exerc.* 14:203–206, 1982.

58. Brown AB, McCartney N, Sale DG. Positive adaptations to weight-lifting training in the elderly. *J Appl Physiol.* 69:1725–1733, 1990.

59. Frontera WR, Meredith CN, O'Reilly KP, Knuttgen HG, Evans WJ: Strength conditioning in older men: skeletal muscle hypertrophy and improved function. *J Appl Physiol.* 64:1038–1044, 1988.

60. Hagberg JM, Graves JE, Limacher M, et al. Cardiovascular responses of 70–79-yr-old men and women to exercise training. *J Appl Physiol.* 66:2589–2594, 1989.

61. Moritani T, deVries HA. Potential for gross muscle hypertrophy in older men. *J Gerontol.* 35:672–682, 1980.

62. Delorme TL. Restoration of muscle power by heavy resistance exercise. *J Bone Joint Surg.* 27:645–667, 1945.

63. Rutherford OM, Jones DA. The role of learning and coordination in strength training. *Eur J Appl Physiol.* 55:100–105, 1986.

64. Klitgaard H, Clausen T. Increased total concentration of Na-K pumps in vastus lateralis muscle of old trained human subjects. *J Appl Physiol.* 67:2491–2494, 1989.

65. Frontera WR, Meredith CN, O'Reilly KP, Evans WJ. Strength

66. Timiras PS. *Physiological Basis of Aging and Geriatrics.* 1st ed. New York, NY: Macmillan Publishing Co; 1988.

67. Dehn MM, Bruce RA. Longitudinal variations in maximal oxygen intake with age and activity. *J Appl Physiol.* 33:805–807, 1972.

68. Heath GW, Hagberg JM, Ehsani AA, Holloszy JO. A physiological comparison of young and older endurance athletes. *J Appl Physiol.* 51:634–640, 1981.

69. Higginbotham MB, Morris KG, Williams RS, Coleman RE, Cobb FR. Physiologic basis for the age-related decline in aerobic work capacity. *Am J Cardiol.* 57:1374–1379, 1986.

70. Rodeheffer RD, Gerstenblith G, Becker LC, Flegg JL, Weisfeldt ML, Lakatta EG. Exercise cardiac output is maintained with advancing age in healthy human subjects: cardiac dilatation and increased stroke volume compensate for a diminished heart rate. *Circulation.* 69:203–213, 1984.

71. Rivera AM, Pels AE III, Sady SP, Sady MA, Culliname CM, Thompson PD. Physiological factors associated with the lower maximal oxygen consumption of master runners. *J Appl Physiol.* 66:949–957, 1989.

72. American College of Sports Medicine. The recommended quantity and quality of exercise for developing and maintaining cardiorespiratory and muscular fitness in healthy adults. *Med Sci Sports Exerc.* 22:265–274, 1990.

73. Shephard RJ. Safety of exercise testing—The role of the paramedical exercise specialist. *Clin J Sport Med.* 1:8–11, 1991.

74. Yerg JE II, Seals DR, Hagberg JM, Holloszy JO. Effect of endurance training on ventilatory function in older individuals. *J Appl Physiol.* 58:791–794, 1985.

75. Seals DR, Hagberg JM, Hurley BF, Ehsani AA, Holloszy JO. Endurance training in older men and women. I. Cardiovascular responses to exercise. *J Appl Physiol.* 57:1024–1029, 1984.

76. Badenhop DT, Cleary PA, School SF, Fox EL, Bartels RL. Physiological adjustments to higher- or lower-intensity exercise in elders. *Med Sci Sports Exerc.* 15:496–502, 1983.

77. Martin WH, Kohrt WM, Malley MT, Korte E, Stoltz S. Exercise training enhances leg vasodilatory capacity of 65-yr-old men and women. *J Appl Physiol.* 69:1804–1807, 1990.

78. Meredith CN, Frontera WR, Fisher EC, et al. Peripheral effects of endurance training in young and old subjects. *J Appl Physiol.* 66:2844–2849, 1989.

79. Makrides L, Heigenhauser GJF, McCartney N, Jones NL. Physical training in young and older healthy subjects. In: Sutton JR, Brock RM, eds. *Sports Medicine for the Mature Athlete.* 1st ed. Indianapolis, Ind: Benchmark Press Inc; 1986.

80. Suominen H, Heikkinen E, Liesen H, Michel D, Hollman W: Effects of 8 weeks' endurance training on skeletal muscle metabolism in 56–70-year-old sedentary men. *Eur J Appl Physiol.* 37:173–180, 1977.

81. Orlander J, Aniansson A. Effects of physical training on skeletal muscle metabolism and ultrastructure in 70–75-year-old men. *Acta Physiol Scand.* 109:149–154, 1980.

82. Seals DR, Hurley BF, Schultz J, Hagberg JA. Endurance training in older men and women. II. Blood lactate response to submaximal exercise. *J Appl Physiol.* 57:1030–1033, 1984.

83. American Heart Association. *Exercise Testing and Training of Individuals with Heart Disease or at High Risk for Its Development: A Handbook for Physicians.* 1975.

84. Lewis SF, Taylor WF, Graham RM, Pettinger WA, Schutte JE, Blomqvist CG. Cardiovascular responses to exercise as functions of absolute and relative workload. *J Appl Physiol.* 54:1314–1323, 1983.

85. Stewart KJ. Resistive training effects on strength and cardiovascular endurance in cardiac and coronary prone patients. *Med Sci Sports Exerc.* 21:678–682, 1989.

86. Hakkinen K, Alen M, Komi PV. Changes in isometric force and

relaxation time, electromyographic and muscle fiber characteristics of human skeletal muscle during strength training and detraining. *Acta Physiol Scand.* 125:573–585, 1985.

87. Coyle EF, Martin WH, Bloomfield SA, Lowry OH, Holloszy JO. Effects of detraining on responses to submaximal exercise. *J Appl Physiol.* 59:853–859, 1985.

88. Siegel W, Blomqvist G, Mitchell JH. Effects of a quantitated physical training program on middle-aged sedentary men. *Circulation.* 41:19–29, 1970.

89. Benestad AM. Trainability of old men. *Acta Med Scand.* 178:321–327, 1965.

90. Frontera WR, Evans WJ. Exercise performance and endurance training in the elderly. *Top Geriatr Rehab.* 2:17–32, 1986.

91. Niinimaa V, Shephard RJ. Training and oxygen conductance in the elderly. II. the cardiovascular system. *J Gerontol.* 33:362–367, 1978.

5
Endocrine and Metabolic Disorders

Horace M. Perry III, John E. Morley, and Fran E. Kaiser

Endocrinologic disorders represent some of the most treatable conditions commonly present among older persons. In addition, the decrease in normal growth hormone and sex hormone values that occur with aging may play a role in the pathogenesis of the frailty syndromes often present in older persons. One of the important aspects of endocrinology in older persons is the need to be able to distinguish the effects of intercurrent disease from those of aging *per se*. An example of this would be the euthyroid sick syndrome where illness results in a decrease in thyroid hormones as a physiologic compensatory mechanism to decrease the person's energy expenditure. Older persons often receive multiple drugs that can alter hormonal values, e.g., beta-blockers increase serum thyroxine levels and diuretics decrease serum testosterone levels.

With advancing age, there is a decrease in suppressor T-cell activity, an increase in autoantibodies, and a propensity to develop autoimmune disease. This can interact with the decreased functional capacity of endocrine organs that occurs with advancing age to produce endocrine organ failure. The prevalence of neoplasia increases in older persons, and some endocrine organs are no exception. The most malignant form of thyroid disease, anaplastic carcinoma, occurs most commonly in older persons. Also, it must be remembered that nonendocrine malignancies can result in ectopic hormone production and syndromes such as the syndrome of inappropriate antidiuretic hormone (ADH) production.

A classical feature of disease associated with aging is atypical or nonspecific presentations. Apathetic thyrotoxicosis is a well-recognized example of an atypical presentation. Nonspecific presentations such as delirium or dementia are commonly seen in older persons with hypothyroidism or hypoadrenalism. Pheochromocytoma or hyperthyroidism can present as unexplained weight loss. Atypical and nonspecific presentations tend to be the rule rather than the exception in older persons with endocrine disease.

Finally, it must be remembered that normal values may change with advancing age. Thus, it appears that

Table 5.1. Major Serum Hormonal Changes Seen with Aging

Hormone	Effect
Growth hormone	Decreased
Insulin growth factor I	Decreased
Prolactin	Increased
Thyroxine	Unchanged
Triiodothyronine	Decreased
TSH	Normal or mild increase
Bioavailable testosterone	Decreased (male)
Estradiol	Decreased (female)
Gonadotropins	Normal or increased
Cortisol	Unchanged
Dehydroepiandrosterone	Decreased
Aldosterone	Decreased
Norepinephrine	Increased
Epinephrine	Unchanged
Parathyroid hormone	Increased
Calcitonin	Decreased
Arginine vasopressin	Increased
Atrial naturetic factor	Increased
Insulin	Increased

an ideal cholesterol level for a person over 70 years of age may be as high as 240 to 280 mg/dL (1), which is higher than the recommended level for younger persons. Table 5.1 presents some age-related hormonal changes.

This chapter will explore some of the unique aspects of the endocrine system and aging. In particular, we will concentrate on those aspects that may interact with the older patient undergoing rehabilitation.

GROWTH HORMONE MENOPAUSE

Numerous studies have demonstrated that with advancing age there is a decrease in growth hormone secretion (2). In particular, there is a decreased responsiveness of growth hormone secretion at the pituitary level when stimulated by growth hormone-releasing hormone. Animal studies have suggested that this is due to excessive somatostatin release from the hypothalamus. Somatostatin inhibits growth hormone release from the pituitary.

Growth hormone causes the release of insulin growth factor I (IGF-I) (somatomedin C) from the liver. There is a decrease in IGF-I levels with aging. This is even more marked in older persons with protein energy malnutrition.

Rudman (3) has suggested that a growth hormone "menopause" occurs with aging. Many effects of growth hormone are in the opposite direction to those commonly observed with aging. Growth hormone decreases adipose mass and increases muscle and bone mass; kidney, liver and spleen size; renal blood flow, and glomerular filtration rate. In addition, growth hormone improves thymic and immune functions. Based on these findings, there have been a number of studies of the utility of growth hormone administration in older persons.

Marcus et al. (4) demonstrated that 7-day administration of growth hormone increased IGF-I levels, nitrogen retention, sodium excretion, and glucose, insulin, phosphate, parathormone, osteocalcin, 1,25-dihydroxycholecalciferol, and urinary calcium levels, while decreasing cholesterol and triglyceride levels. Rudman et al (5) found that a low dose of growth hormone can be safely administered for 6 months to persons over 60 years of age. This resulted in an increase in IGF-I and lean body mass. Unfortunately, neither of these studies examined the effect of growth hormone on muscle strength or other aspects of potential frailty, e.g., balance or gait.

Two other studies examined the role of growth hormone administration to malnourished older persons (6, 7). Both of these studies showed that growth hormone could result in weight gain, nitrogen retention, and possibly an increase in muscle mass. It seems reasonable that recombinant growth hormone may be useful during the initial therapy of protein energy malnutrition. The potential role of growth hormone or IGF-I in the management of muscle weakness and other aspects of frailty remains to be explored.

THYROID DISEASE

Many older persons appear to be hypothyroid. Symptoms of hypothyroidism are identical to a number of physiologic changes in aging or common complaints of older persons (Table 5.2). Recently, Mooradian (8) has shown a decreased ability of thyroid hormone to produce mRNA transcription in older animals, suggesting that with aging there may be a specific defect in thyroid hormone action.

Hypothyroidism occurs in 4% to 5% of older persons, with another 14% having slightly elevated thyrotropin (TSH) levels and normal thyroid hormone levels, i.e., compensated hypothyroidism (9). Common causes of hypothyroidism in older persons are autoimmune dis-

Table 5.2. Common Changes Seen with Aging and Hypothyroidism

Dry skin
Poor tissue turgor
Hair loss
Cold intolerance
Fatigue
Anorexia
Constipation
Muscle weakness
Memory dysfunction

ease and thyroid ablation secondary to prior surgery or radioactive iodine. Up to 20% of older persons have elevated titers of thyroglobulin and microsomal antibodies. Titers of 1:64 or higher of antimicrosomal antibodies and mildly elevated TSH levels are highly predictive of subsequent development of hypothyroidism (10).

The signs and symptoms of hypothyroidism are often subtle and nonspecific. Clinical examination may detect as few as 1 in 10 persons with biochemical hypothyroidism. Dementia and/or delirium may be caused by hypothyroidism. Many older persons with hypothyroidism only complain of fatigue. Anorexia, depression, dyspnea, muscular weakness, and joint pain are other nonspecific presentations of hypothyroidism. Hypothyroidism can result in marked increases in creatinine phosphokinase (CPK) levels, including an increase in the MB band. This is because liver metabolism of CPK is inadequate in the absence of thyroid hormones. This can lead to hypothyroidism being misdiagnosed as a silent myocardial infarction.

The treatment for hypothyroidism is L-thyroxine. Replacement should start with a low dose (e.g., 25 μg) and should be increased slowly. Adequate replacement in many older persons, which is measured by the return of the TSH level into the normal range, is between 75 and 100 μg. Excessive thyroid hormone replacement can result in osteoporosis. Thyroid extract should not be used, as wide variations in biologic strength between different batches are commonly observed.

Hyperthyroidism occurs in 0.5% to 2% of older persons (11). Autoimmune (Graves') disease is the commonest cause, but multinodular and single nodule thyrotoxicosis are commoner in older than younger persons. In older persons the classical presenting features of hyperthyroidism may be absent, i.e., apathetic hyperthyroidism. These patients have weight loss, proximal muscle weakness, anorexia, heart failure, atrial fibrillation, and blepharoptosis instead of the more common exophthalmos.

The diagnosis of hyperthyroidism is made by demonstrating an elevation in thyroid hormone levels after correcting for abnormalities in the thyroid-binding globulin levels utilizing the T_3 resin uptake. The supersensitive TSH assays, which theoretically allow demonstration of suppressed TSH levels, lack adequate sensitivity or specificity in sick older persons to recommend its routine use. If thyroxine levels are near the upper limits of normal, measurement of triiodothyronine (T_3) by radioimmunoassay may make the diagnosis of T_3 toxicosis. This occurs in up to 10% of older persons with hyperthyroidism. Hyperthyroidism results in a suppressed TSH response to thyrotropin-releasing hormone (TRH). Unfortunately, aging alone, or in combination with illness, also results in a flat TSH response to TRH. For this reason TRH testing is only useful when a TSH response is present, which effectively rules out hyperthyroidism.

Treatment of hyperthyroidism in older persons consists of radioactive iodine ablation of the thyroid gland. In those without contraindication, short term use of beta-blockers may alleviate symptoms. Following ablative therapy, patients need to be carefully observed for the development of hypothyroidism.

A special situation occurs when an older person is ill and develops the euthyroid sick syndrome (12). Illness results in a decrease in the monoidinase that converts thyroxine to T_3, resulting in very low T_3 levels. With illness, there is also a decrease in thyroxine-binding globulin levels leading to an increase in T_3 uptake levels. Severe illness can also result in a decrease in thyroxine levels. This decrease is particularly marked in patients with renal failure. TSH levels may be normal, slightly increased, or decreased. Table 5.3 summarizes the findings in the euthyroid sick syndrome.

DIABETES MELLITUS

Approximately 18% of persons between 65 and 75 years of age have diabetes mellitus (13). Of these, almost 50% are unaware that they have diabetes, and elevated blood glucose levels are often ignored by physicians. Diabetics are at greater risk for institutionalization and have a greater risk for morbidity and mortality than nondiabetics.

Mortality from diabetic comas (Table 5.4) increases with advancing age. The predominant coma in older diabetics is hyperosmolar coma, which is particularly common in institutionalized residents with demen-

tia (13). Diuretics are a major precipitating factor of this form of coma. Approximately 10% of older persons with diabetic coma will present with ketoacidosis. Lactic acidosis occurs in older persons who are poorly insulinized and have a hypotensive episode such as that precipitated by a myocardial infarction.

Older persons are at greater risk for hypoglycemia than are younger ones (14). This is particularly true over the age of 85 years. Both oral sulfonylureas and insulin have an increased incidence of hypoglycemia in older persons. Besides age, numerous other factors predispose to hypoglycemia in older persons (Table 5.5). Chlorpropamide has an extremely long half-life and thus produces prolonged hypoglycemia. It also produces hyponatremia in older persons. For these reasons chlorpropamide should never be used in older persons.

Old age combined with diabetes appears to result in long-term complications (i.e., nephropathy, neuropathy, and retinopathy) that occur earlier than would be expected in younger persons (13). Diabetics with elevated glucose levels have a poorer outcome following a stroke than those whose glucose levels are better controlled (15). Older persons often have hypodipsia, which can, in combination with hyperglycemia, lead to dehydration (13). Diabetics can have a hyperosmolar diuresis, which can precipitate incontinence. Hyperglycemia has been associated with increased pain perception, such as that seen with painful neuropathies. Infections, in particular unusual infections such as tuberculosis, malignant otitis media (due to *Pseudomonas aeruginosa*), candidiasis, and mucormycosis, appear to be more common in diabetics.

Amputations occur most commonly in diabetics, and the majority of diabetic amputees are over the age

Table 5.4. Diabetic Comas

Hyperglycemic comas
  Hyperosmolar coma
  Ketoacidosis
  Lactic acidosis
Hypoglycemic comas

Table 5.5. Factors Predisposing to Hypoglycemia in Older Persons

Protein energy malnutrition
Abnormal liver and/or kidney function
Adrenocortical insufficiency
Acute illness
Cerebrovascular accidents
Drugs:
  Alcohol
  Salicylates
  Coumadin
  Haloperidol
  Imipramine
  H_2-receptor antagonists
  Chlorpropamide

Table 5.3. Biochemical Findings of Primary Hypothyroidism Compared with Euthyroid Sick Syndrome

	Primary Hypothyroidism	Euthyroid Sick Syndrome
Thyroxine (T_4)	D[a]	N or D
T_3 uptake	D	I
Triiodothyronine (T_3)	D	N or D
TSH	I	N
Reverse T_3	N or D	I
TSH response to TRH[a]	I	N or D

[a]N = normal; D = decreased; I = increased; TSH = thyrotropin-stimulating hormone; TRH = thyrotropin-releasing hormone.

of 65 years. A diabetic who has one amputation has a high likelihood of needing a second amputation. For this reason, diabetics and their physicians and caregivers need to pay meticulous attention to foot care. Foot infections need to be detected early and treated vigorously.

Cognitive dysfunction occurs in Type II diabetics with hyperglycemia (16). Animal studies suggest that the memory dysfunction is due to high glucose levels rather than to atherosclerosis or cerebral infarcts. This memory dysfunction has been shown to result in diabetics having a poorer recall of medication changes made by physicians than do age-matched controls. Thus, diabetics are at major risk for problems with compliance and should have their medication changes written down and be given memory aids, such as pill boxes.

Older diabetics have an increased prevalence of depression (17). Not only can depression cause major problems with compliance, but it is also highly correlated with mortality in older diabetics. For this reason, all older diabetics should be screened for depression utilizing the Yesavage Geriatric Depression Scale (18).

Falsely elevated levels of glycosylated hemoglobin have been reported to occur in older persons (19). For this reason, we recommend serum fructosamine levels to follow diabetic control in older persons. Serum fructosamine should be corrected for albumin or protein levels.

In general, unless an older person is grossly overweight, dietary management does not play a major role in the treatment of diabetics over 70 years of age. A nursing home study showed no detrimental effects of a regular nondiabetic diet on fasting glucose, glycosylated hemoglobin, plasma triglycerides, and cholesterol (20). Postprandial hypotension in older persons, which has been shown to be associated with falls, is triggered by glucose ingestion, suggesting that high carbohydrate diets should not be utilized in older persons (21). Megadoses of vitamin C can alter blood glucose levels (13). Diabetes mellitus produces hyperzincuria and zinc deficiency. Zinc deficiency has been associated with immune dysfunction and poor wound healing. This state should be considered in all older diabetics with poorly healing peripheral vascular ulcers or decubitus ulcers (22, 23).

Glucose disposal rate is related to maximum voluntary oxygen consumption in older persons. Preliminary studies have suggested that walking programs may produce benefits in persons with Type II diabetes mellitus. It should be noted that, while vigorous exercise improves glucose disposal, it also inhibits insulin release (24). Care of the feet and choosing adequate footwear are extremely important when recommending an exercise program to older diabetics. In addition, diabetic retinopathy can be associated with retinal detachment during very vigorous exercise.

Of the available oral sulfonylurea hypoglycemic agents, the first generation agent tolbutamide may be best suited to the very old, mild diabetic because of its extremely short half-life. In general, because of the decreased propensity to drug–drug interactions, the second generation agents (i.e., glipsizide and glyburide) appear to be the most suitable for the treatment of most young-old diabetics.

The biguanide metformin appears to have a relatively low incidence of lactic acidosis in older persons (25). Metformin does, however, cause gastrointestinal discomfort, weight loss, and malabsorption of vitamin B_{12} and folate. Overall, short-term studies have suggested that metformin may be an effective and safe agent in older persons who do not have liver or renal disease.

Insulin therapy can be safely used in older persons. Older diabetics with visual disturbances have been reported to make a 10% to 20% error when drawing up their insulin (13). Many older persons benefit from having their insulin syringes predrawn by a pharmacist. Alternatively, the use of special magnifiers may be useful for some persons.

We suggest that most older persons benefit from blood glucose control where no fasting glucose level is greater than 140 mg/dL and all glucose levels are below 200 mg/dL.

ADRENAL HORMONES

As both cortisol production and clearance rates decrease with advancing age, there is no change in serum cortisol levels (2). There is also minimal change in the cortisol response to corticotropin (ACTH). The ACTH response to corticotropin-releasing factor is unchanged with aging. Older persons tend to be more likely to fail to show normal cortisol suppression following an overnight dexamethasone suppression test. This is particularly true if the person is depressed, has dementia or unsuspected alcoholism, or is on phenylhydantoin.

Adrenal insufficiency is often missed in older persons because of its nonspecific presentations. Patients with fatigue, unexplained fever, hyponatremia, hyperkalemia, hypotension (or amelioration of hypertension), and hypoglycemia should be considered for the possibility of adrenocortical insufficiency. The causes of adrenocortical insufficiency in older persons include Addison's (autoimmune) disease, tuberculosis, adrenal hemorrhage, and cancer (e.g., secondary tumor from prostate cancer). In most cases the diagnosis can be made by utilizing the cosyntropin (synthetic ACTH) stimulatory test. The treatment is steroid replacement. Steroid replacement should not be administered in the afternoon or evening as steroids may interfere with sleep.

Older persons have a decrease in active renin and aldosterone levels. This increases the chances of an older person having hyperkalemia secondary to hyporeninemic hypoaldosteronism. This is particularly true in older persons with diabetes mellitus and mildly elevated creatinine levels. Beta-blockers and nonsteroidal antiinflammatory agents can precipitate hyperkalemia in older persons by blocking potassium secretion.

There is a marked decrease in dehydroepiandro-sterone (DHEA) secretion with advancing age. In animals, DHEA administration prolongs life span. Human studies have suggested that low levels of DHEA-sulfate may be predictive of cardiovascular mortality and hypercholesterolemia. In addition, in nursing home residents, low DHEA levels predict poor functional status (26). This is important, as animal studies suggest DHEA may play a role in cognition (27).

There is an increase in norepinephrine levels and no change in epinephrine levels with advancing age. With aging, there is a decrease in beta-adrenergic responsiveness due mainly to a postreceptor deficit. In addition, there may be a mild uncoupling of the platelet alpha-2-adrenergic receptor adenylate cyclase complex with advancing age. These alterations in catecholamines may play a role in the postprandial hypotension syndrome that is seen in older persons.

Pheochromocytomas occur as commonly in old as in young persons, but the diagnosis is more often missed in older persons. Any older person with malnutrition and failure of hypertension to improve with weight loss should be tested for a possible pheochromocytoma.

MENOPAUSE

The permanent cessation of menses (menopause) occurs at an average age of 51 years in women in the United States (28). The age at which menopause occurs is not altered by age at menarche, race, socioeconomic status, body build, number of pregnancies, or age at pregnancy, but smoking has been associated with an earlier onset of menopause. With aging, as the number of ova and follicles in the ovary decrease, estradiol (the major estrogen produced by the ovary) concentration diminishes and luteinizing hormone (LH) level rises. As granulosa and thecal cells of the ovary degenerate, follicle-stimulating hormone (FSH) level rises.

Menopausal symptoms can include hot flashes—a sudden sensation of heat and flushing, with or without sweating, which occurs in 65% to 76% of women who undergo spontaneous menopause—as well as symptoms of anxiety, insomnia, headaches, cognitive change, and vaginal dryness. The occurrence of hot flashes can last for long periods of time: 64% of 126 women had hot flashes for 1 to 5 years, 26% for 6 to 10 years, and 10% for more than 11 years (29). Up to 15% of postmenopausal women report hot flashes for as long as 16 years after menopause. Women with hot flashes tend to have lower body weights than those who are asymptomatic. Hot flash patterns differ in varying individuals and, while some studies suggest that fewer flashes occur during sleep, the perception of the flash may be greater at night (29). There is a close association between LH pulses and hot flashes, but flashes can occur in women without LH release. Norepinephrine, a catecholamine that causes vasoconstriction, diminishes during hot flashes, while epinephrine increases, resulting in increased blood flow (29). Neurotensin, another vasodilator, also increases, as do LH, growth hormone, and ACTH. The role of these hormones is not clear in the genesis of the flash.

Loss of estrogen can be associated with urogenital atrophy; burning; pruritus; dyspareunia (painful intercourse), and alterations in urination, including dysuria, increased frequency of urination, and nocturia (30).

Sexual dysfunction that may occur after the menopause cannot be completely linked to the hormonal changes that occur; however, the alterations in hormone levels do directly affect vaginal physiology—there is thinning of the vaginal epithelium and diminished vaginal blood flow, as well as an increase in vaginal pH and decreased vaginal lubrication. The role of estrogen and libido remains controversial. In perimenopausal women, there was no correlation of libido, sexual response, or sexual satisfaction with the ovarian hormonal profile (30). Lack of a partner, a partner's sexual dysfunction, health problems, or a decline in libido may all contribute to sexual dysfunction. The effect of hysterectomy (the second most common major surgery performed in the United States today, cesarian section being the most common) on sexuality may result in a reduction in libido and reduced orgasmic ability. Alternative procedures such as myomectomy, endometrial resection (for submucosal fibroids), or supracervical hysterectomies (which are thought to better preserve sexual function) should be considered and their risks and benefits weighed against those of a total hysterectomy with or without bilateral oophorectomy.

The hormonal alterations of the menopause create and foster a series of other health problems including ischemic heart disease and osteoporosis, however, hormonal replacement is protective. The mechanism(s) of estrogenic cardioprotective effects are not clear. High density lipoproteins (HDL) levels, "good" cholesterol, increase while low density lipoprotein (LDL) levels decrease. Estrogen may also stimulate production of prostaglandin I_2, a vasodilator. The use of a progestational agent in conjunction with estrogen can negate many of the positive effects on HDL. Osteoporosis (loss of bone mass) occurs rapidly after menopause. The finding that osteoblasts have estrogen receptors suggests that one of the primary factors in the occurrence of osteoporosis is the loss of estrogen (31, 32). Numerous studies have shown that estrogen therapy retards the loss of bone mass (33). Since the prevention of bone loss also reduces hip fracture risk, epidemiologic data have also shown that estrogen replacement therapy reduces hip fracture risk if treatment begins in the first few years following menopause (34).

It is generally felt that replacement therapy for osteoporosis should be lifelong. Hot flashes, vaginal dryness, and preventive effects against cardiovascular disease (or at least reduction of risk) will all improve with estrogen therapy. The risks of unopposed estrogen in those with an intact uterus include a risk of endometrial carcinoma. In those receiving estrogen along with a progestational agent, the risk of endometrial cancer is actually *less* than in those receiving no hormonal therapy. Data regarding breast cancer and estrogen therapy remain inconclusive, but breast cancer should remain a contraindication to estrogen therapy. Other contraindications include vaginal bleeding, estrogen-dependent tumors, and active thromboembolic disease.

The most efficacious timing/dose/type of hormonal replacement therapy remains elusive. It is important to remember that although transdermal estrogen is convenient, it does *not* eliminate the need for progesterone in women with an intact uterus. Furthermore, transdermal therapy does not confer the benefit of an improved HDL level. Generally, an oral dose of conjugated estrogen of 0.625 mg per day for 21 days and progesterone for 5 to 15 days per month (such as medroxyprogesterone acetate 5 to 10 mg/d) is used if a woman still has a uterus. There is no indication that progesterone has any benefit in those women who had a hysterectomy. No long-term studies of the effects or benefits of combination therapy exist, and, although data support the use of estrogen for the treatment of problems such as hot flashes and vaginal dryness, each woman needs to weigh the risks versus the benefit of such therapy (28).

TESTOSTERONE

With aging, changes in testicular, pituitary, and hypothalamic function occur. Testosterone, produced by the Leydig cells of the testis (which decrease in number with aging) falls (in most studies) as a function of aging (35). In the circulation, most testosterone is bound to sex hormone-binding globulin (SHBG) and to albumin. It has been shown that the testosterone bound to albumin is available for use by the body's tissue. Non-SHBG bound testosterone is the bioavailable (tissue available) moiety. Bioavailable testosterone (BT) falls with age.

The circadian variation of both testosterone and bioavailable testosterone is also lost with aging. Estradiol, a peripheral metabolite of testosterone, remains unchanged or increases with age. The clinical effects of these alterations (decreased testosterone and bioavailable testosterone) may result in many of the so-called "aging phenomena" of "normal" men. Loss of energy, diminished muscle mass, decreased bone mass, and diminished libido may occur, and the role of these changes and their contributions to the frailty of aging remains to be elucidated.

In many, but not all, studies of the response to the lower androgen concentrations of aging males and the testicular changes that occur, there is a rise of gonadotropins. However, in many healthy older subjects, as well as in those individuals with impotence, a low BT, testosterone, and LH concentration is found which suggests a population with abnormal responsiveness of the hypothalamic–pituitary axis (36). Also supporting an alteration of response in the hypothalamic–pituitary axis with aging is a decreased LH response to gonadotropin-releasing hormone (GnRH). Along with the age-related decrease in Leydig cell number, changes in Sertoli cells and sperm production also occur. FSH rises, and inhibin (another glycoprotein produced by Sertoli cells, which feeds back to inhibit FSH) falls.

The role of testosterone therapy in reversing aging changes remains to be seen. Testosterone should be reserved for those patients with hypogonadism, and at the present only testosterone patches or injections are recommended. Oral testosterone carries with it an increased likelihood of hepatotoxicity.

IMPOTENCE

With aging, there is an increased prevalence of impotence (the inability to get or maintain an erection sufficient for intercourse in 75% or more of attempts). It had been thought, until the past 10 years or so, that impotence was primarily a psychogenic disorder. However, in those over 60 years of age, about 90% of impotence is organic (37). Despite that, one cannot discount the impact of psychologic overlay—such as performance anxiety—that may occur. Erections seem to be dependent on approximately four major variables: (*a*) libido (sex drive), (*b*) adequacy of hormones, (*c*) vascular health and (*d*) neurologic processes. Impairment, even to a small degree, of one or more of these components, can affect erectile ability.

As can be seen in Table 5.6, impotence has a variety of causes, the most common of which appears to be vascular (37). Since the advent of Doppler studies, which can measure penile systolic pressure, these pressures can be indexed to brachial artery pressure to give a relative index of adequacy of the arterial system (penile-brachial pressure index). The importance of detection of penile vascular abnormalities is bolstered by the finding that abnormal penile-brachial pressure indices are predictive of the risks of myocardial infarction and/or cerebrovascular accidents. Furthermore, not only arterial disorders but also venous leakage or varicosities, as well as arterial–venous malfunctions, may be associated with the inability to obtain or maintain an erection.

Many medications, including antihypertensive agents (all classes), digoxin, and cimetidine, are associated with impotence (30). Impotence secondary to medication may be an important cause of noncompliance with drug therapy.

Table 5.6. Causes of Impotence

Vascular disorder
  Arterial
  Venous
  Mixed lesions
  Pelvic steal syndrome
Hormonal imbalance
  Primary or secondary hypogonadism
  Hypo/hyperthyroidism
  Hyperprolactinemia
Diabetes
  Multifactorial (vascular, neuropathic)
Neurologic injury
  Stroke
  Multiple sclerosis
  Spinal cord injury
  Autonomic/peripheral neuropathy
  Pelvic irradiation
Medications
  Antihypertensives (all)
  Cimetidine
  Digoxin
  Alcohol, methadone, heroin
  CNS depressants
  Antipsychotic drugs, tricyclics, monoamine oxidase inhibitors
Psychogenic concerns
  Anxiety
  Bereavement
  Depression

Hypogonadism (either primary testicular failure or secondary hypothalamic–pituitary hypogonadism) may also play a role in the pathogenesis of impotence. While erectile capability does not always appear to relate to a given hormone level, libido is clearly hormonally linked. In addition to libido, maintenance of energy level, bone mass, and muscle mass is linked to testosterone concentrations.

It is important in evaluating individuals with impotence not only to obtain a sexual history (in addition to the medical history) that takes into account duration of impotence, quality and duration of erections, and partner availability and interest, but also to conduct a thorough physical examination including evaluation of neurologic function (38). Evaluation of hormonal levels, including testosterone, bioavailable testosterone, luteinizing and follicle-stimulating hormones, prolactin, and thyroid functions is important. As mentioned, noninvasive vascular evaluation (penile Doppler studies) can be helpful. Nocturnal penile tumescence (NPT) studies are not especially helpful in older men, as abnormal NPT readings can occur despite the ability to have intercourse. Appropriate neurologic evaluation is quite difficult, as no "gold standard" study has evolved. Electromyographic pudendal or penile nerve conduction velocities and clinical assessment of peripheral or autonomic neuropathy are among the tools generally considered. At present, we limit evaluation to noninvasive clinical neurologic assessment.

Treatment options are based on the underlying etiology. Vasculogenic impotence may respond to intracorporal injections of papaverine with or without phentolamine or prostaglandin E_1. However, adverse effects such as priapism, bruising of the penis, and fibrosis may make this problematic in some individuals. Vacuum tumescent devices, while requiring some degree of manual dexterity, can be quite successful in improving erectile ability in a safe manner in those who have both vascular and/or neuropathic impotence. In this procedure, a hollow plastic cylinder with a pump is placed over the penis. The negative pressure from the vacuum pump results in increased blood flow to the penis. A constriction band is then placed at the base of the penis, and the plastic cylinder is removed. The band may be kept on for as long as 30 minutes and then should be removed. (39).

In hypogonadal men, testosterone therapy, using testosterone enanthate, testosterone propionate, or testosterone cypionate, should be given as intramuscular injections every 2 weeks. Oral testosterone causes an increased prevalence of adverse effects, such as hepatotoxicity, and thus should not be used. The use of testosterone scrotal patches will also improve hormonal levels, but is far more costly than testosterone injection. Adverse effects of testosterone therapy may include increased hematocrit, gynecomastia, water retention, and an increase in LDL cholesterol.

Penile prosthetic devices are relatively permanent cures, but some data suggest that the life span of a given device may be as short as 5 years. Complications such as erosion, infection, and scarring of the penis may occur.

Overall, with the advent of these therapeutic modalities, we are able to treat most men suffering from impotence, and therefore, it is imperative that the issue of sexual dysfunction be addressed in all older individuals.

PRIMARY HYPERPARATHYROIDISM

Primary hyperparathyroidism (HPT) is generally a disease of postmenopausal women. With the advent of routine serum multichannel analysis, the annual incidence of discovery of hypercalcemia due to HPT is two per thousand in individuals over the age of 60 years (40). Since only about 10% of these individuals undergo surgery, the prevalence rate must be significantly higher. Although it is not clear why, the classic presentation significant of hypercalcemia with "brown tumor" (osteitis fibrosa) does not appear to be as common now as previously. The best therapy for this classic disease is surgical removal of the parathyroid glands at the hands of an *experienced* surgeon (41). Many more individuals with minimal hypercalcemia (less than 11.5 mg/dL) and who are relatively asymptomatic are identified. Although there appears to be some controversy, most of these individuals may be observed. If they progress (hypercalcemia worsens, renal stones develop, or osteoporosis supervenes) surgery is recommended. Many do not progress (41, 42). On the other hand, if any of these signs already coexist with HPT, surgery should be recommended. Although this surgery is not emergent, it should be done as soon as convenient.

The etiology of HPT is not clear. Recently, a monoclonal origin of parathyroid adenoma has been reported for some Type 1 multiple endocrine neoplasms, but not for all hyperparathyroidism (43.)

The major endocrine differential diagnosis of hypercalcemia is hyperparathyroidism, cancer and familial hypercalcemic hypocalciuria. The latter is uncommon, does not benefit from surgery, and does not have significant sequelae once appropriately diagnosed (44). Cancer and HPT may be difficult to distinguish. New assays to detect the parathyroid hormone-related peptide (thought to cause hypercalcemia of malignancy) and intact (solid phase) parathyroid hormone are reported to distinguish well between these, although wide clinical experience is lacking at this time (45).

References

1. Kaiser FE, Morley JE. Cholesterol can be lowered in older persons: should we care? *J Am Geriatr Soc.* 38:84–85, 1990.
2. Mooradian AD, Morley JE, Korenman SG. Endocrinology in aging. *Disease-a-Month.* 34:395–461, 1988.
3. Rudman D. Growth hormone, body composition and aging. *J Am Geriatr Soc.* 33:800–807, 1985.
4. Marcus R, Butterfield G, Holloway L, et al. Effects of short term administration of recombinant human growth hormone to elderly people. *J Clin Endocrinol Metab.* 70:519–527, 1990.
5. Rudman D, Feller AG, Nagraj HS, et al. Effects of human growth hormone in men over 60 years old. *N Eng J Med.* 323:1–6, 1990.
6. Kaiser FE, Silver AJ, Morley JE. The effect of recombinant human growth hormone on malnourished older individuals. *J Am Geriatr Soc.* 39(3):235–40, 1991.
7. Binnerts A, Wilson JH, Lamberts SW. The effects of human growth hormone administration in elderly adults with recent weight loss. *J Clin Endocrinol Metab.* 67:1312–1316, 1988.
8. Mooradian AD, Deebaj L, Wong NC. Age related alterations in the response of hepatic lipogenic enzymes to altered thyroid states in the rat. *J Endocrinol.* 128(1):79–84, 1991.
9. Robuschi A, Safran M, Braverman LE, et al. Hypothyroidism in the elderly. *Endocrine Rev.* 8:142–153, 1987.
10. Rosenthal MJ, Hunt WC, Garry PJ, Goodwin JS. Thyroid failure in the elderly: microsomal antibodies as discriminant for therapy. *JAMA.* 258:209–213, 1987.
11. Bartels EC, Kingsley JWJ. Hyperthyroidism in patients over 60. *Geriatrics.* 4:333–340, 1949.
12. Morley JE, Slag MF, Elson MK, Shafer RB. The interpretation of thyroid function tests in hospitalized patients. *JAMA.* 249:2377–2379, 1983.
13. Morley JE, Mooradian AD, Rosenthal MJ, Kaiser FE. Diabetes mellitus in elderly patients: is it different? *Am J Med.* 83:533–544, 1987.
14. Morley JE, Perry HM. The management of diabetes mellitus in older individuals. *Drugs.* 41:548–565, 1991.
15. Olsson T, Vittanen M, Asplund K, Eriksson S, Hägg E. Prognosis after stroke in diabetic patients: a controlled prospective study. *Diabetologia.* 33:244–249, 1990.
16. Morley JE, Flood JF. Psychosocial aspects of diabetes mellitus in older persons. *J Am Geriatr Soc.* 38:605–606, 1990.
17. Naliboff BD, Rosenthal M. Effects of age on complications in adult onset diabetes. *J Am Geriatr Soc.* 37:838–842, 1989.
18. Yesavage JA, Brink TL, Rose TL. Development and validation of a geriatric depression screening scale: a preliminary report. *J Psychiatr Res.* 17:37–41, 1983.
19. Morley JE. Fructosamine or glycated hemoglobin. *J Am Geriatr Soc.* 37:911–912, 1989.
20. Coulston AM, Mandelbaum D, Reaven GM. Dietary management of nursing home residents with non-insulin dependent diabetes mellitus. *Am J Clin Nutr.* 51:67–71, 1990.
21. Jansen RWM, Peeters TC, Van Lier HJJ, Hoefnagels WHL. The effect of oral glucose, protein, fat and water loading on blood pressure and the gastrointestinal peptides: VIP and somatostatin in hypertensive elderly subjects. *Eur J Clin Invest.* 20:192–198, 1990.
22. Mooradian AD, Morley JE. Micronutrient in diabetes mellitus. *Am J Clin Nutr.* 45:877–895, 1987.
23. Kinlaw WB, Levine AS, Morley JE, Silvis SE, McClain CJ. Abnormal zinc metabolism in type II diabetes mellitus. *Am J Med.* 75:273–277, 1983.
24. Kahn SE, Larson VG, Beard JC, et al. Effect of exercise on insulin action, glucose tolerance and insulin secretion in aging. *Am J Physiol.* 258:E937–943, 1990.
25. Joseph Kutty S, Potter JM. Comparison of tolbutamide and metformin in elderly diabetic patients. *Diabetic Med.* 7:510–514, 1990.
26. Rudman D, Shetty KR, Mattson DE. Plasma dehydroepiandrosterone sulfate in nursing home men. *J Am Geriatr Soc.* 38:421–427, 1990.
27. Flood JF, Roberts E. Dehydroepiandrosterone sulfate improves memory in aging mice. *Brain Res.* 448:178–181, 1988.
28. Kaiser FE, Morley JE. The menopause and beyond. In Cassel CR, Reisenberg D, (eds). *Geriatric Medicine.* New York, NY: Springer-Verlag; 1990:279–290.
29. Feldman BM, Voda A, Gronseth E. The prevalence of hot flash and associated variables among perimenopausal women. *Res Nurs Health.* 8:261–268, 1985.
30. Cutler WB, Garcia CR, McCoy N. Perimenopausal sexuality. *Arch Sex Behav.* 16:225–234, 1980.
31. Erikssen EF, Colvard DS, Berg NJ. Evidence of estrogen receptors in normal human osteoblast-like cells. *Science.* 241:84–86, 1988.
32. Komm BS, Terpening CM, Benz DJ. Estrogen binding, receptor mRNA, and biologic response in osteoblast-like osteosarcoma cells. *Science.* 241:81–84, 1988.
33. Lindsay R. Estrogens, bone mass, and osteoporotic fracture. *Am J Med.* 91:5B, 10S–13S, 1991.
34. Law MR, Wald NJ, Meade TW. Strategies for prevention of osteoporosis and hip fracture. *Br Med J.* 303:453–459, 1991.
35. Morley JE, Kaiser FE, Johnson LE. Male reproductive function. In: Cassel CR, Reisenberg, eds. *Geriatric Medicine.* New York, NY: Springer-Verlag; 1990: 256–270.
36. Korenman SG, Morley JE, Mooradian AD, et al. Secondary hypogonadism in older men: its relation to impotence. *J Clin Endocrinol Metab.* 71:963–969, 1990.
37. Slag MF, Morley JE, Elson MK, et al. Impotence in medical clinic outpatients. *JAMA.* 249:1736–1740, 1983.
38. Drugs that cause sexual dysfunction. *Medical Letter.* 29:65–90, 1987.

39. Morley JE. Impotence. *Am J Med.* 80:897–905, 1986.
40. Heath HM III, Hodgson SF, Kennedy MA. Primary hyperparathyroidism incidence, morbidity and potential economic impact in a community. N. Engl J Med 302:189-193, 1980.
41. Bilezikian JP. Primary hyperparathyroidism. In Favus MJ, ed. *Primer on the Metabolic Bone Diseases and Disorders of Mineral Metabolism.* Richmond, Va: William Byrd Press; 1990.
42. Bilezikian JP. Surgery or no surgery for primary hyperparathyroidism. *Ann Intern Med.* 102:402–403, 1985.
43. Marx SJ. Genetic defects in primary hyperparathyroidism. *New Engl J Med.* 318:699–701, 1988.
44. Marx SJ, Stock JL, Attie MF, et al. Familial hypocalciuric hypercalcemia: recognition among patients referred after unsuccessful parathyroid exploration. *Ann Intern Med.* 92:351–355, 1980.
45. Nussbaum SR, Zahradnite RJ, Lavigne JR, et al. Highly sensitive two-site immunoradiometric assay of parathryrin and its clinical utility in evaluating patients with hypercalcemia. *Clin Chem.* 33:1364–1367, 1987.

6

Nutrition Needs and Deficiencies in Old Age

John E. Morley and Andrew J. Silver

Nutrition is the cornerstone of rehabilitation of many geriatric patients. Protein energy malnutrition has been demonstrated to be a major indicator of impending mortality both on rehabilitation units (1) and in nursing homes (2). Mild degrees of vitamin and mineral deficiency have been associated with cognitive dysfunction (3). Patients with hip fractures often have calcium and vitamin D deficiencies (4). Nutritional care plays a major role in the healing of decubitus ulcers. Patients with dysphagia following stroke are at particular risk for developing protein energy malnutrition. For these reasons, it is essential that the nutritional status of all older patients undergoing rehabilitation be carefully assessed and, where appropriate, active nutritional rehabilitation be instituted. In addition, consideration of primary prevention strategies to prevent the development of nutritional deficiencies needs to be considered in all older persons receiving rehabilitation.

PROTEIN ENERGY MALNUTRITION

Protein energy malnutrition is present in approximately 10% of older outpatients (5), 30% to 60% of hospitalized patients (6), and 20% to 50% of nursing home residents (7). Protein energy malnutrition can present as marasmus, kwashiorkor, or a mixture of both. Marasmus occurs when an inadequate supply of calories results in mobilization of skeletal muscle fat, and glycogen for energy and to maintain visceral protein levels within the normal range. Diagnosis of marasmus is made by the demonstration of weight loss, a decreased weight for height, a low midarm circumference, and/or low skinfold measurements. Immune function is often preserved early in the course of marasmus.

Kwashiorkor presents with a decrease in serum albumin and other visceral proteins. Serum albumin levels are normally above 4.0 g/dL in ambulatory older persons. When a person lies down, there is a redistribution of extracellular fluid, resulting in a decrement of serum albumin by 0.5 g/dL. Immune dysfunction, e.g., anergy, is usually present. Kwashiorkor is often precipitated by an acute infection or an intercurrent illness. In some cases, the patient may have a mixed picture of kwashiorkor and marasmus. Table 6.1 lists the standard for the diagnosis of protein energy malnutrition.

Besides producing generalized weakness and fatigue, protein energy malnutrition appears to have particularly deleterious effects on the hematologic and immune systems. Patients with protein energy malnutrition are particularly prone to develop anemia with features similar to the anemia of chronic disease, i.e., a normal to elevated serum ferritin and a low total iron binding capacity (10). In addition, there is a marked decrease in cell mediated immunity as demonstrated by a decreased mitogen response, decreased T-cell number, decreased helper cell number with an increase in T suppressor cells, and decreased natural killer cell activity (11). While B-cell number is normal, serum antibody production is decreased. Neutrophil function is also decreased. All of these changes decrease the ability of the person to resist infection. It should be noted that many of these changes are in the same direction as the changes in the immune system that occur with aging and that aging and protein energy malnutrition appear to interact synergistically to produce more severe deficits in immune function.

Table 6.1. Standard for the Diagnosis of Protein Energy Malnutrition

Less than 15% of average body weight, utilizing the age-related tables of Master, et al (8)

Five pound weight loss in less than 3 months; ten pound weight loss in 6 months or less

Midarm circumference at the 10th percentile or less, using the age-related tables of Frisancho (9)

Serum albumin less than 4.0 g/dL in ambulatory person and less than 3.5 g/dL in recumbent person

Etiology of Protein Energy Malnutrition

Less than one third of all protein energy malnutrition in older persons is due to cancer. The causes of protein energy malnutrition stretch from such simple factors as the failure to provide ethnically acceptable foods to older institutionalized individuals, and the inability of persons to carry out self-feeding or instrumental activities of daily living such as food preparation or shopping to complex metabolic disorders such as hyperthyroidism or pheochromocytoma. In many cases, a number of factors interact to cause weight loss. Some common causes of weight loss are listed in Table 6.2 (12).

A number of age-associated factors tend to lead to a mild decrease in food intake. These include a decrease in the sense of smell and, in some cases, the sense of taste. Visual impairment can further lead to a decreased appreciation of the hedonic qualities of food. Periodontitis, caries, edentulousness, and xerostomia are all conditions that commonly occur in older persons and can interfere with the mechanical ingestion of food. Animal studies have suggested that aging is associated with a decrease in the dynorphin (opioid) feeding drive and an increase in the satiety effect of the gastrointestinal hormone, cholecystokinin (13).

Psychologic factors are particularly important in weight loss in older persons (14). Diagnosis of depression is commonly missed in older persons. Treatment of depression with low doses of antidepressants can often dramatically reverse weight loss. In some cases of severe protein energy malnutrition associated with depression, electroconvulsive therapy may be lifesaving. Late-life paranoia can be associated with a refusal to eat. This condition is usually responsive to low doses of haloperidol. Patients with dementia require prolonged staff time for feeding, and this is often not available in hospitals or other institutions. Demented patients who are consistent pacers utilize large amounts of energy and require a large caloric intake. Recently, it has been recognized that a form of anorexia nervosa (called anorexia tardive) can occur in older persons. Women who have a history of anorexia nervosa as a child are particularly likely to have a recurrence with advancing age. In addition, abnormal attitudes to food ingestion have been identified in older persons with malnutrition (15). These may be precipitated by a desire for longevity related to the concept that caloric restriction may prolong life or be secondary to physician-initiated interventions such as low-cholesterol diet.

Patients with chronic obstructive pulmonary disease often develop weight loss related to both excess energy utilization and anorexia related to shortness of breath interfering with food ingestion. These persons often respond with weight gain when given six to eight small meals per day. Patients with dysphagia need to be carefully evaluated for weight loss and in many cases may need temporary insertion of a nasogastric or gastrostomy tube. Chronic intestinal ischemia, which may result in early satiety, can be treated with nitrates or calcium channel antagonists. A number of drugs, particularly digoxin and theophylline, can cause anorexia and/or nausea, which can lead to weight loss.

Management of Protein Energy Malnutrition

The secret of successful management of protein energy malnutrition is the early detection and treatment of the condition. Reversible causes of malnutrition, such as depression or hyperthyroidism, need to be treated. The possibility of drug-induced anorexia needs to be considered and medications adjusted appropriately. A careful history of attitudes to food intake needs to be obtained. Food preferences of the patient should be obtained and menus designed to support these preferences. Some patients respond well to being encouraged to eat as much as they like of a favored food, e.g., a candy bar. Patients with malnutrition who are receiving special medical diets, e.g., diabetic, low-fat, or low-salt, should have these discontinued whenever possible. Dietary supplements should be introduced as soon as a calorie count shows inadequate caloric intake. It is important to encourage relatives to become involved as part of the therapeutic team.

Early use of tube feeding can be crucial to obtain a good response. Tube feeding should be considered a temporizing measure and not necessarily a permanent one. Patients who reject long-term tube feeding should be encouraged to choose a time-limiting period of tube feeding to allow the exclusion of treatable disease. When

Table 6.2. Common Causes of Protein Energy Malnutrition in Older Persons

Social
  Poverty
  Difficulty with shopping
  Institutionalized foods/lack of ethnic qualities
  Eating in unattractive institutionalized environments
Psychologic
  Depression
  Dementia
  Late-life paranoia
  Anorexia nervosa/anorexia tardive
  Bereavement
Medical
  Drugs—digoxin, cimetidine, theophylline
  Dysphagia—cerebrovascular accident
  Parkinsonism
  Hyperthyroidism
  Pheochromocytoma
  Monilial esophagitis
  Ischemic bowel—abdominal angina
  Malabsorption syndromes
  Chronic obstructive pulmonary disease
  Medical diets—low-salt, low-fat

the gastrointestinal tract is intact, enteral feeding is preferred to parenteral feeding. Enteral feeding can be accomplished either by the transnasal approach or percutaneously, either by percutaneous endoscopic gastrostomy or surgically. For long-term feeding or when the patient regularly removes a nasogastric tube, percutaneous enteral feeding is generally the preferred method of nutrient administration. Bolus or nocturnal (intermittent) feeding may be preferred to continous feeding in patients undergoing rehabilitation, as these forms maximize the patient's independence. Parenteral feeding is utilized when obstruction, ileus, peritonitis, vomiting, gastrointestinal hemorrhage, or only limited small bowel areas for absorption are present.

Refeeding after a period of food deprivation can be associated with a number of complications (16). Mechanical problems are predominantly limited to clogging of the tube, particularly when medications are administered through small-bore tubes. Metabolic complications include water retention, which can worsen cardiac failure; hyperkalemia and hypokalemia; hyponatremia; hypomagnesemia, and hyperglycemia. Contaminated enteral feeding formula can result in severe gastroenteritis. Occasionally, a nasogastric tube can be mistakenly placed into the lung or mediastinum. Aspiration of formula feedings into the lungs and continuous aspiration of oral cavity secretions remain a serious problem in tubefed patients. This risk can be minimized by elevating the head of the bed, placing the tube in the duodenum, and possibly by utilizing a constant infusion pump. Diarrhea can be caused by intestinal atrophy and malabsorption, lactose deficiency, hyperosmolar feedings, pseudomembranous colitis secondary to antibiotic administration, and magnesium-containing antacids. Many commercially available formulas do not contain selenium and can thus result in selenium deficiency.

Finally, it should be recognized that recombinant growth hormone administration has been successfully used to treat severe protein energy malnutrition (17).

OBESITY

Early studies suggested an increase in adipose tissue in proportion to total body mass with advancing age (18). However, much of the increase in adiposity was due to the older group weighing substantially more than the younger group. Recently, Silver, et al (19) have found that there is a small increase in the percent of adipose tissue between 20 and 40 years of age and a marked decrease in adipose tissue in those over 80 years. With advancing age, a major change appears to be a shift of adipose tissue from peripheral to central sites (20).

Approximately 26% of males between 65 and 74 years of age are overweight as are 36% of females of the same age (21). It needs to be recognized that, with advancing age, underweight is more closely associated with

mortality than is obesity. Major problems associated with obesity in older persons are impaired functional status, increased surgical risk, decubitus ulcers, hypertension, diabetes mellitus, osteoarthritis, and sleep apnea.

Management of obesity in older persons begins with an exercise program. Dietary intervention is limited to those of over 130% of average weight, and in no case should the diet contain less than 1000 cal per day with adequate vitamin and mineral supplement. A behavior modification program should be carried out in conjunction with the above measures. Low and very-low calorie diets, anorectic and thermogenic drugs, and surgery are usually inappropriate in older persons.

FOOD AND COGNITION

Mild degrees of malnutrition have been associated with cognitive dysfunction in older persons (3). Studies in animals and humans have shown that feeding immediately after a task is learned enhances memory (22). Food consolidates memory retention by releasing the gastrointestinal hormone, cholecystokinin, which activates ascending nerve fibers in the vagus. These vagal fibers carry messages to the midbrain and from there to the amygdala. This ability of food to enhance memory may be particularly important in patients with Alzheimer's dementia who are losing weight.

FOOD-INDUCED HYPOTENSION

There is an increase in falling blood pressure following a meal in institutionalized subjects. Food in older persons has been demonstrated to induce a fall in both systolic and diastolic blood pressure (23). This fall in blood pressure is specifically induced by diets rich in carbohydrates. While the exact reason of the meal-associated hypotension is uncertain, it appears to be related to the elevated norepinephrine levels that occur with aging. In addition, older persons have a marked increase in atrionaturetic factor following a meal, which could lead to a diuresis that would prolong the hypotension.

LIPIDS

Cholesterol levels increase with advancing age, until 60 years of age in males and 70 years of age in females (24). High density lipoprotein levels remain inversely predictive of atherosclerotic heart disease with advancing age, but there is less evidence that total cholesterol levels are a risk factor in older persons (25). In fact, a number of studies have suggested that in older persons a low cholesterol level is highly predictive of increased mortality (26, 27). In institutionalized persons, a cholesterol level below 160 mg/dL is the single best predictor of death, presumably because it is also an excellent indicator of protein energy malnutrition (2). There is no study that has shown that intervention to lower cholesterol has any salutary effects on morbidity or mortality in older persons. As was previously pointed out, dietary intervention may precipitate protein energy malnutrition. A recent study has suggested that optimum mortality may be seen at cholesterol levels as high as 280 mg/dL. For this reason, intervention to lower cholesterol levels should be limited to those with serum cholesterol levels greater than 300 mg/dL and, where deemed necessary, drug therapy should be the management of choice (28).

Fish oils, such as eicosapentanoic and docosapentanoic acid, appear to decrease the risk of coronary artery disease by decreasing platelet adhesiveness and lowering triglycerides and LDL cholesterol (29). For these reasons, it would appear that there is minimal risk and potentially some benefit in suggesting to older persons that they increase their fish consumption to three to four times per week.

VITAMINS

Exact vitamin requirements for older persons remain uncertain in many cases and the revised recommended daily allowances (RDA) still fail to give recommendations for those over 70 years of age. In the older person, vitamin deficiencies often coexist with protein energy malnutrition and are corrected when the protein energy malnutrition is corrected. When vitamin deficiencies do exist, they are usually at a subclinical or biochemical level. Early clinical symptoms of vitamin deficiency tend to be nonspecific and include fatigue, irritability, impaired cognitive function, anorexia, and weight loss. In biochemical studies, deficiencies of specific vitamins range from 0 to 56%, and their prevalence is highly dependent on whether the person is free living, hospitalized, or in a nursing home (30, 31).

Vitamin A deficiency characteristically presents with night blindness and occasionally with follicular hyperkeratosis. However, most follicular keratosis in older persons is due to poor hygiene rather than to vitamin A deficiency. Patients with liver disease are particularly prone to developing night blindness, and this may require both vitamin A and zinc (which stimulates retinol binding protein synthesis in the liver) replacement. Epidemiologic studies have suggested a link between vitamin A and/or carotenoid intake and lung cancer.

Excessive intake of beta-carotene leads to an orange-yellow skin without sclera discoloration. In older persons the most common cause of yellow skin associated with hypercarotenemia is hypothyroidism. Persons taking doses of vitamin A in excess of 15,000 retinol equivalents (1 RE = 1 μg transretinol = 6 μg beta-carotene) can develop toxicity that includes malaise, headaches, hepatic dysfunction, and hypercalcemia. The hypercalcemia is due to the ability of vitamin A to convert

precursors of parathormone to release the active hormone from the parathyroid gland.

Vitamin D deficiency may be relatively common in older institutionalized persons due to a tendency for them to not be exposed to sunlight, decrease in the ability of ultraviolet light to produce cholecalciferol in older skin, and a decrease in 1,25 hydroxylase activity in the kidneys which produces the active 1,25 dihydroxy vitamin D. For these reasons, many older persons may benefit from taking 200 to 400 IU vitamin D per day.

Vitamin E is commonly taken as a supplement by older persons. This is predominantly because many believe that as an antioxidant it will reduce tissue damage by free radicals. The evidence that vitamin E has any effect on prolongation of life or morbidity is not available. Vitamin E has minimal toxic effects, although high doses may occasionally potentiate the effects of anticoagulants.

Alcoholism and diabetes mellitus can increase the chance that older persons will develop thiamine (vitamin B_1) deficiency. If a malnourished person is given a glucose infusion, it is prudent to administer a single dose (100 mg) of thiamine at the same time to prevent the precipitation of Wernicke's encephalopathy. Alternatively, in alcoholics or patients with liver disease who receive thiamine, glucose needs to be administered to prevent hypoglycemia from developing.

Riboflavin (B_2) and pyridoxine (B_6) deficiencies occur in coexistence with protein energy malnutrition. Phenothiazines may increase the propensity to develop riboflavin deficiency. Isoniazide, hydralazine, and estrogens increase pyridoxine metabolism. Nicotinamide deficiency is particularly prevalent in alcoholics and patients with carcinoid or who are receiving isoniazid. The classical finding of dermatoses on the sun-exposed area is very rare in older persons.

Up to 8% of older persons have folate deficiency, and 80% consume less than three quarters of the RDA. Alcoholism and diphenylhydantoin consumption are major risk factors for folate deficiency. A macrocytic anemia and a dementia syndrome are the commonest signs of folate deficiency.

Vitamin B_{12} deficiency can occur in 1% to 2% of persons overt 60 years of age and 4% to 5% of persons over 80 years of age. The major clinical manifestations are dementia, a macrocytic anemia, and subacute combined degeneration of the spinal cord. Vitamin B_{12} deficiency appears to be particularly common in patients with Alzheimer's disease, but at present there is no evidence that vitamin B_{12} replacement improves these patients' cognitive dysfunction. Patients with combined iron vitamin B_{12} deficiency may have a normocytic or microcytic anemia instead of the classic macrocytic anemia. The diagnosis of vitamin B_{12} deficiency is best made based on serum levels, although the exact interpretation of these levels remains problematic. It is probably not cost-effective to carry out a Schilling test in most older persons with vitamin B_{12} deficiency. Treatment is 100 μg of vitamin B_{12} given intramuscularly every month. During the first few days of vitamin B_{12} replacement, hypokalemia may develop, and this should be monitored for in the older person.

Vitamin C (ascorbic acid) is the most commonly used vitamin supplement, with some older individuals ingesting up to 20 g per day. Frank vitamin C deficiency (scurvy) is very rare. High dose vitamin C intake may precipitate diarrhea. Vitamin C use will cause false negative fecal and urinary occult blood tests, and, also, high doses (75 g/d) can interfere with serum glucose testing. Vitamin C may promote healing in patients with decubitus ulcers.

TRACE MINERALS

Many older persons are in a borderline zinc-deficient state. This is especially true of persons taking diuretics and those who have diabetes mellitus or cirrhosis of the liver. Patients with depressed serum zinc levels experience an accelerated healing of peripheral vascular and perhaps, decubitus ulcers, when zinc is replaced (30). Zinc deficiency causes problems with dark adaptation. High doses of zinc may slow the progression of macular degeneration (32). Zinc deficiency leads to impaired T-cell function (30). In some older males, zinc deficiency has been associated with low testosterone levels and impotence (30). A complete listing of the putative effects of zinc deficiency is given in Table 6.3.

Zinc supplementation may produce a copper-deficient anemia. Very high doses of zinc have been shown to inhibit immune function and to decrease HDL cholesterol. Despite these potential side effects, when zinc deficiency is suspected, it is recommended to conduct a therapeutic trial of zinc sulfate 220 mg three times per day. As the sulfate moiety can cause mild gastritis, zinc sulfate should always be given with meals.

Selenium forms part of the glutathione peroxidase molecule. Glutathione peroxidase functions to decrease the levels of hydrogen peroxides within cells and thus to limit free radical damage. Selenium deficiency may play a role in producing muscle weakness and pain, T and B-cell dysfunction, nail changes, anorexia, and possibly a cardiomyopathy (30). Selenium deficiency has been suggested to play a role in the pathogenesis of cancers, particularly those of the gastrointestinal tract. Selenium toxicity has occurred in those taking a health food supplement mistakenly containing 180 times more than the usual supplementary dose. These persons developed a garlic odor on their breath, nail changes, nausea, dizziness, sweating, and a peripheral neuropathy.

Copper metabolism is generally well preserved with aging. Copper deficiency can produce anemia and neutropenia and may be associated with osteoporosis, muscle weakness, and bleeding.

Chromium is combined biologically with dl-nicotinic acid-glutathione, and this complex appears to be necessary for maintenance of normal glucose tolerance. A controlled study has shown that chromium and nicotinic acid when taken orally resulted in a decrease of the response to a glucose load in older persons with a mild age-associated hyperglycemia (33).

Trace elements play an important role in the maintenance of tissue structure and many enzyme reactions. Despite this, little is known concerning the effects of aging on trace mineral metabolism and the potential role of trace minerals in the aging process and the diseases associated with it.

DRUG-NUTRIENT INTERACTIONS

In recent years it has become clear that drugs may interfere with nutrient absorption or increase nutrient demands. Equally, some nutrients may alter drug absorption and/or bioavailability. Drugs may also cause anorexia and/or nausea, thus precipitating malnutrition. Drugs and nutrients are particularly likely to produce these effects in older persons who may already be in borderline nutrient status and have poor adaptation mechanisms to a variety of stressors. Table 6.4 lists some of the more common drug/nutrient:nutrient/drug interactions in older individuals.

WATER

Water is arguably the most important of all nutrients. With advancing age, there is a decrease in both total body water and extracellular water. Older individuals have approximately a 25% decrease in thirst perception compared to younger persons. This appears to be predominantly due to a decrease in the mu opioid drinking drive system (34). In addition, many older persons, when hospitalized, are placed in situations where access to water is limited, e.g., in physical restraints or having limited mobility following a stroke. The addition of diuretics or laxatives further interferes with the ability of older persons to maintain themselves in an adequate

Table 6.3. Effects of Zinc Deficiency

Acrodermatitis enterohepatica
Slowed wound healing, e.g., peripheral vascular ulcers, decubitus ulcers
Diarrhea
Impaired night vision
Anorexia/hypogeusia
T-cell dysfunction
Cognitive impairment
Hypogonadism/impotence

Table 6.4.   Common Drug-Nutrient Interaction

Drug Effect on Nutrients	
Drug	Effect
Digitalis, theophylline ibuprofen, levodopa	Decreased caloric intake (anorexia)
Isoniazid	Nicotinamide and pyridoxine deficiency
Diuretics	Magnesium, potassium, trace mineral deficiency
Mineral oil, cholestyramine	Vitamins A, D, and K malabsorption

Nutrient Effect on Drugs	
Nutrient	Effect
Calcium	Hypercalcemia with hydrochlorothiazide
	Impaired iron absorption
Aminoride	Impaired levodopa absorption
Vitamin D	Increased digoxin sensitivity
Pyridoxine	Inhibition of levodopa effect
Vitamins E, K	Inhibition of coumadin effect
Vitamin C	Increased haloperidol effect

state of hydration. It should be remembered that adequate hydration is an excellent laxative.

All older persons should have their hydration status carefully assessed. A blood urea nitrogen (BUN) to creatinine ratio greater than 20:1 or postural hypotension should immediately suggest the possibility of dehydration. Physicians should regularly write a water prescription as part of routine admission orders (a minimum of 1 liter of extra fluids per day).

It should be remembered that, because of alterations in the hypophyseal-vasopressin system with advancing age, older persons may also develop hyponatremia. Tube-fed older persons are particularly prone to develop hyponatremia due to the low salt content of many of the feeding formulas. Serum sodium content needs to be regularly checked in older persons, and the health care team often needs to perform a delicate balancing act to maintain the proper sodium concentration in the older person.

NUTRITION AND DISEASE PREVENTION

It is an intrinsically attractive concept that nutritional modulation can slow down the aging process and prevent the development of morbidity. This concept has been fueled by the demonstrations in animals that dietary restriction can prolong life (35). Unfortunately, dietary restriction in older humans appears more likely to precipitate death by starvation rather than to prolong life. Overall, there have been few controlled studies assessing the benefits of nutrient manipulation in disease prevention in older individuals.

References

1. Sullivan DM, Patch GA, Walls RC, Lipschitz DA. Impact of nutrition status on morbidity and mortality in a select population of geriatric rehabilitation patients. *Am J Clin Nutr.* 51:749–758, 1990.

2. Rudman D, Mattson DE, Nagraj HS, et al. Antecedents of death in the men of a Veterans Administration nursing home. *J Am Geriatr Soc.* 35:496–502, 1987.

3. Goodwin JS, Goodwin JM, Gorg PJ. Association between nutritional status and cognitive functioning in a healthy elderly population. *JAMA.* 249:2917–2921, 1983.

4. Pierron RL, Perry HM III, Grossberg G, Morley JE, Mahon G, Stewart T. The aging hip. *J Am Geriatr Soc.* 38:1339–1352, 1990.

5. Miller DK, Morley JE, Rubenstein LZ, Pietruszka FM, Strome LS. Formal geriatric assessment instruments and the care of older general medical outpatients. *J Am Geriatr Soc.* 38:645–651, 1990.

6. Agarwal N, Acevedo F, Leighton LS, Cayten CG, Pitchumoni CS. Predictive ability of various nutritional variables for mortality in elderly people. *Am J Clin Nutr.* 48:1173–1178, 1988.

7. Silver AJ, Morley JE, Strome LS, Jones D, Vickers L. Nutritional status in an academic nursing home. *J Am Geriatr Soc.* 36:487–491, 1988.

8. Master AM, Lasser RP, Beckman G. Tables of average weight and height of Americans aged 65 to 94 years. *JAMA.* 172:658–674, 1960.

9. Frisancho AR. New norms for upper limb fat and muscle areas for assessment of nutritional status. *Am J Clin Nutr.* 34:2540–2545, 1981.

10. Lipschitz DA. The anemia of chronic disease. *J Am Geriatr Soc.* 38:1258–1264, 1990.

11. James SJ, Castle SC, Makinodan T. Modulation of age-associated immune dysfunction by nutritional intervention. In: Morley JE, Glick Z, Rubenstein LZ, eds. *Geriatric Medicine.* New York, NY: Raven Press; 1990:203–224.

12. Morley JE, Silver AJ. Anorexia in the elderly. *Neurobiol Aging.* 9:9–16, 1988.

13. Morley JE. Appetite regulation: the role of peptides and hormones. *J Endocrinol Invest.* 12:135–147, 1989.

14. Morley JE, Silver AJ, Miller DK, Rubenstein LZ. The anorexia of the elderly. *NY Acad Sci.* 575:50–59, 1989.

15. Miller DK, Morley JE, Rubenstein LZ, Pietreszka FM. Abnormal eating attitudes and body image in older undernourished individuals. *J Am Geriatr Soc.* 39:462–466, 1991.

16. Morley JE, Silver A, Fiatarone M, Mooradian AD. Nutrition and the elderly. *J Am Geriatr Soc.* 34:823–832, 1986.

17. Kaiser FE, Silver AJ, Morley JE. The effect of recombinant growth hormone on malnourished older individuals. *J Am Geriatr Soc.* 39:235–240, 1991.

18. Glick Z. Energy balance. In: Morley JE, Glick Z, Rubenstein

LZ, eds. *Geriatric Nutrition*. New York, NY: Raven Press; 1990:27–40.

19. Silver AJ, Guillen CP, Kahl MJ, Morley JE. Effects of aging on body fat. *Gerontologist*. 30:262A, 1990.

20. Fukagawa NK, Bandini LG, Young JB. Effect of age on body composition and resting metabolic rate. *Am J Physiol*. 259:E233–238, 1990.

21. Morley JE, Glick Z. Obesity. In: Morley JE, Glick Z, Rubenstein LZ, eds. *Geriatric Nutrition*. New York, NY: Raven Press; 1990:293–306.

22. Flood JF, Smith GE, Morley JE. Modulation of memory processing by cholecystokin: dependence on the vagus nerve. *Science*. 236:832–834, 1987.

23. Jansen RWMM, Peetcrs TL, VanLier HJJ, Hoefnagels WML. The effect of oral glucose, protein, fat and water loading on blood pressure and the gastrointestinal peptides VIP and somatostatin in hypertensive elderly subjects. *Eur J Clin Invest*. 20:192–198, 1990.

24. Anderson KM, Castelli WP, Levy D. Cholesterol and mortality: 30 years of follow-up from the Framingham study. *JAMA*. 257:2176–2180, 1987.

25. Castelli WP, Gassison RJ, Wilson PWF. Incidence of coronary heart disease and lipoprotein cholesterol levels: the Framingham study. *JAMA*. 256:2835–2838, 1986.

26. Forette B, Tortrat D, Wolmark Y. Cholesterol as a risk factor for mortality in elderly women. *Lancet*. 1:868–870, 1989.

27. Agnes E, Hansen PF. Fasting serum cholesterol and triglycerides in a ten year prospective study in old age. *Acta Med Scand*. 214:33–61, 1983.

28. Kaiser FE, Morley JE. Cholesterol can be lowered in older persons: should we care? *J Am Geriatr Soc*. 38:84–85, 1990.

29. Saunders TAB. Fish and coronary artery disease. *Br Heart J*. 57:214–219, 1987.

30. Morley JE, Mooradian AD, Silver AJ, Heber D, Alfin-Slater RD. Nutrition in the elderly. *Ann Intern Med*. 109:890–904, 1988.

31. Johnson LE. Vitamin disorders in the elderly. In: Morley JE, Glick Z, Rubenstein LZ, eds. *Geriatric Nutrition*. New York, NY: Raven Press; 1990:117–148.

32. Newsone DA, Swartz M, Leone NC, Elston RC, Miller E. Oral zinc and macular degeneration. *Arch Ophthalmol*. 106:192–198, 1988.

33. Urberg M, Zemmel MB. Evidence for synergism between chromium and nicotinic acid in the control of glucose tolerance in elderly humans. *Metabolism*. 34:196–199, 1987.

34. Silver AJ. Dehydration/sodium balance. In: Velas BJ, Albarede J-L, Guez D, eds. *Facts and Research in Gerontology*. Paris: Editeur Maloine; 1990:115–124.

35. Masoro EJ. Nutrition and longevity. In: Morley JE, Glick Z, Rubenstein LZ, eds. *Geriatric Nutrition*. New York, NY: Raven Press; 1990; 19–26.

7

Pharmacology and Aging

Beverly Parker and Robert E. Vestal

Clinical pharmacology is an important topic in the rational treatment of patients of all ages. It is particularly relevant in the elderly population because of the high prevalence of chronic diseases that cause them to be disproportionately large consumers of prescription and over-the-counter medications (1). In addition, many of the age-related changes in physiology, as well as the consequences of their pathologic conditions, make the elderly particularly susceptible to adverse drug reactions that range from minor to life-threatening in severity. The elderly are a particularly heterogenous population, and chronologic age frequently does not parallel physiologic age, further adding to the challenge of appropriate drug use.

In order to assist the clinician in providing optimum care, this chapter is designed to introduce some of the basic concepts of clinical pharmacology and relate them to the particular problems of the elderly population. In addition, a few specific categories of drugs with particular relevance to rehabilitation patients will be discussed in detail.

EPIDEMIOLOGY AND DEMOGRAPHY

As a result of escalating technology, advances in medical care and drug therapy, and general improvement in the standard of living in the western world, life expectancy at birth is at an all-time high. The elderly are the fastest growing segment of the population, particularly the very-old—that is, persons over the age of 85. In 1990, there were 31.5 million persons over age 65 in the United States (2). This age group now constitutes 12.6% of the population and is projected to increase to 65.6 million by the year 2030 when it will be nearly 22% of the total population. As mentioned above, the prevalence of symptomatic chronic disease increases with age, and the elderly currently account for 31% of all physician contacts and 25% to 30% of all dollars spent on medications (2). Approximately 40% of the drug dollars of the elderly are spent on nonprescription medications (3). It is estimated that two thirds of persons of either sex over the age of 65 in the United States use at least one over-the-counter medication. In particular, arteriosclerosis, hypertension, diabetes mellitus, osteoarthritis, osteoporosis and its complications, cataracts, glaucoma, dementia, depression, constipation, and malignancies are highly prevalent and provoke the use of the large majority of medications used by this population.

There are a number of social, economic, and physiologic changes in the elderly that affect their interaction with medications. These people tend to be socially isolated due to the loss of a spouse or other family members. Loss of transportation options due to physical disability also cuts down on interactions with the outside world. This predisposes them to depression and loss of mobility, as well as poor nutrition because of an inability to shop and lack of interest in proper eating habits. Lessened financial circumstances also contribute to inadequate health due to poor nutrition, inability to afford prescribed medications, or inability to afford a physician contact for diagnosis of health problems. In addition, these patients more frequently suffer from cognitive impairment, sensory deficits, and physical frailty, all of which make them less able to withstand a physiologic insult (illness or adverse drug reaction).

ADVERSE DRUG REACTIONS

Adverse drug reactions are a concern in the elderly, primarily because of the increased potential for morbidity in this population. Most of the studies to date have shown an increased incidence of adverse drug reactions in the elderly, and geriatric patients account for approximately 40% of all hospital admissions for this problem (4, 5). Age is not the only contributing factor; adverse drug reactions are associated with polypharmacy; extended exposure to medications; certain disease states such as dementia and renal or hepatic insufficiency, and a history of prior drug reactions (4). Adverse drug reactions are frequently misdiagnosed as exacerbations of existing diseases or a new disease, which prompts the health care provider to add more medications. It cannot be overemphasized that adverse drug reactions should be considered as a possible cause of any presenting symptom or sign. They should be suspected particularly in patients with delirium, incontinence, urinary or fecal retention, gait disorders, falls, sedation, fever, or postural hypotension. It is important to remember that many nonsystemic medications (intraocular, topical, or nonabsorbed enteric) may have significant systemic side effects and drug interactions.

DRUG INTERACTIONS

In general, it should be assumed that the elderly are equally or more susceptible to drug interactions than are younger patients. With the high incidence of polypharmacy, often from multiple providers, including prescription and nonprescription medications, the potential for drug interactions is immense (6). Most of these potential interactions remain clinically silent. Good studies of outpatients are lacking, but reviews of nursing home prescribing information reveal a high prevalence of potentially clinically significant drug interactions (7, 8). Certain drugs or classes of drugs are of particular concern because of overlapping side effect profiles, narrow therapeutic index, or potential for significant morbidity or mortality from the interaction (6). For example, drugs such as sedative hypnotics, narcotics, tricyclic antidepressants, antiparkinson drugs, and alcohol have the potential to cause additive central nervous system depression (9). Interactions involving medications such as digoxin, theophylline, and systemic anticoagulants must also be aggressively monitored because the outcome from such interactions is potentially fatal (9).

COMPLIANCE

Compliance is also a major issue in the appropriate pharmacologic management of the geriatric patient. It is very difficult to assess compliance independently in patients of any age, and the clinician is often forced to rely on the patients' history alone. Measurement of steady state plasma drug levels, monitored use of various pill box devices, and pill counts are only of limited usefulness and availability. Furthermore, they are time-consuming and may be expensive. Patient histories are often unreliable because of diminished memory or unwillingness of the patient to admit to noncompliance. Patients may be reluctant to reveal that they cannot afford a prescribed medication, that they cannot get the container open, or that they cannot remember to take or if they have taken a medication (10). In addition, the dosing form may preclude successful administration of medication. Examples include drugs requiring subcutaneous injection, rectal or vaginal insertion, or application to a distal extremity that the patient does not have

the flexibility to reach. Patients may be embarrassed or fearful of revealing inability to maintain compliance as this would be a threat to independent living. Ignorance of the drug names, the purpose of a given medication, and the appropriate dosing schedule are also implicated in noncompliance (10). The most common form of medication noncompliance is omission, which may account for up to 90% of all noncompliance and may be a cause of lack of therapeutic efficacy (10).

It is important to distinguish intentional nonadherence from noncompliance. Most studies estimate that 40% to 45% of elderly patients are noncompliant with their medication regimen, and one study found that intelligent nonadherence accounted for 70% of the instances of noncompliance (11). Patients often decrease drug dosages to decrease bothersome side effects and frequently are able to do so without a decline in clinical efficacy. It is important for the clinician to remember that clinical response is the goal and that compliance is best served by working as a partner with patients to develop a regimen that achieves the desired result without compromising the quality of life.

PHARMACOKINETICS IN THE ELDERLY

Pharmacokinetics is the study of the absorption, distribution, metabolism, and excretion of drugs and their metabolites in the body. Various pharmacokinetic models have been developed and mathematical relationships defined to provide information about the disposition of medications (12, 13). This increases our ability to prescribe rationally in both healthy and disease states based on known parameters such as clearance, elimination half-life, volume of distribution, metabolic pathways, and the presence or absence of clinically significant metabolites. This is particularly important when using drugs with a low therapeutic index.

Absorption

Absorption refers to the movement of drug from the site of administration to the vascular space. Both the rate and the extent of absorption must be considered. The rate of absorption will affect the duration, as well as the magnitude of, effect. Intramuscular injections and sustained release enteric formulations are generally given to provide a longer duration of effect with a minimum of steady state plasma level fluctuation. A continuous intravenous infusion will also achieve this, but is impractical or undesirable for outpatients and even for the majority of inpatients.

The extent of absorption is primarily dependent on the mode of administration and the pharmaceutical formulation of the drug. Intravenous administration is the accepted gold standard because 100% of the drug is delivered to the plasma compartment. Subcutaneous or intramuscular injection may deliver something less than 100% of the dose depending upon regional blood flow at the injection site and the chemical characteristics of the drug. Bioavailability of orally administered medication is dependent not only upon the extent of absorption across the intestinal mucosa but also upon the extent of presystemic or "first pass" metabolism in the liver. Many age-related alterations in the gastrointestinal tract have been described, including increased gastric pH, decreased splanchnic blood flow, decreased intestinal absorptive surface area, and altered bowel motility (Table 7.1) (13, 14). Both passive and active transport processes in the gastrointestinal tract are impaired, but these changes in the rate of absorption have little clinical importance (14). Available data indicate that the extent of drug absorption is unchanged by age. Other factors such as concomitant food intake, concurrent drug therapy, and disease states are much more clinically important than age alone.

Distribution

The distribution of drugs in the body is largely determined by the polarity of the drug. Nonpolar drugs are fat-soluble and distribute widely in tissues, particularly in adipose depots, and are far more likely to cross the blood-brain barrier. Polar drugs are water-soluble and are more likely to enter lean body tissue and less likely to cross into the central nervous system. With aging, there is a linear decline in total body water and lean body mass of 10% to 20% (3). At the same time, there is a concomitant increase in total body fat (Table 7.1) (13). Thus, the volume of distribution of fat-soluble drugs such as benzodiazepines and barbiturates tends to increase and that of water-soluble drugs such as ethanol, digoxin, and aminoglycoside antibiotics tends to decrease. However, results of various studies are often contradictory, and the majority of medications show no change in their apparent volume of distribution (13).

Distribution is also affected by the extent of plasma protein binding (14). With advancing age, there is a modest decrease in serum albumin, which is exacerbated by chronic disease states (15). This results in increased plasma levels of unbound drug. In turn, this can have significant clinical effects during the acute dosing of such drugs as meperidine, furosemide, theophylline, phenytoin, salsalate, and warfarin because it is the unbound drug that has physiologic activity (16). During chronic dosing of these drugs, however, the increased free drug level is diminished by an acceleration of the hepatic and renal metabolism and excretion of free drug: Alpha-1-acid glycoprotein levels are the same or even somewhat higher in the elderly, which leads to increased protein binding of drugs such as lidocaine and imipramine.

Distribution may also be affected by the physiologic alterations in regional blood flow with age, but blood flow has a more important influence on the metabolism and excretion of drugs.

Metabolism

Although small amounts of some drugs may be metabolized in organs such as the gut, lung, and kidney, metabolism in general may be considered to be hepatic (14). No changes in liver function tests have been demonstrated with age, but the metabolic activity of this organ is altered. Liver mass declines steadily with age after 50 years of age, and this loss is disproportionately large compared to the general loss of lean body mass (Table 7.1). In addition, there is a reduction in hepatic blood flow of 40% to 45% as a result of decreased cardiac output and a diminished proportion of that cardiac output coming to the liver (13). Studies in experimental animals have shown a decrease in microsomal enzyme activity and induction (13), but this has not been directly shown in man. In fact, recent studies with human liver microsomes failed to demonstrate age differences in microsomal enzyme activity. It appears that alterations in the metabolic capacity of the liver are primarily determined by genetic and environmental factors (such as cigarette smoking) and by liver blood flow and mass and that the influence of age alone is minimal. It also seems clear that the cytoplasmic enzyme biotransformation pathways are unaffected by age.

There are two physiologic patterns of hepatic metabolism. Drugs that are rapidly metabolized are said to have high intrinsic clearance, and the rate of their metabolism is largely dependent on hepatic blood flow. Drugs that are slowly metabolized are said to have low intrinsic clearance, and their metabolism is largely determined by the degree of protein binding and the intrinsic hepatic enzyme activity. Hepatic biotransformation of drugs is affected by various forms of malnutrition,

Table 7.1. Physiologic Changes with Aging That Alter Drug Disposition

Absorption
- ↑ Gastric pH
- ↓ Absorptive surface
- ↓ Splanchnic blood flow
- ↓ GI motility

Distribution
- ↑ Body fat %
- ↓ Lean body mass
- ↓ Body water
- ↓ Serum albumin
- ↑ Alpha-1-acid glycoprotein

Metabolism
- ↓ Hepatic blood flow
- ↓ Hepatic mass

Excretion
- ↓ Renal blood flow
- ↓ Glomerular filtration rate
- ↓ Tubular secretion

including vitamin, mineral, and trace element deficiencies; protein-calorie deficiency; and prolonged fasting, as well as by inducers and inhibitors of enzyme activity (16, 17). However, at this time further studies are needed before any firm conclusions can be reached regarding the effect of age alone on pharmacokinetic drug interactions.

Excretion

Changes in the human kidney with age have been extensively studied, and the effect on the elimination of drugs can be reliably predicted. There are steady decreases in the glomerular filtration rate; there is decreased tubular secretory function, and there is a decrease in renal blood flow (Table 7.1) (14). Creatinine clearance (Cv. Cl), which is a measure of glomerular filtration rate, decreases approximately 35% between the third and tenth decades of life and can be readily and accurately measured with a 24-hour urine collection and the determination of creatinine in serum and urine (13). Alternatively, it can be estimated by the following formula:

$$Cr\ Cl = \frac{(140 - age) \times weight\ (kg)}{72 \times serum\ creatinine\ (mg/dL)}$$

The result should be multiplied by 0.85 for females and be adjusted for lean body mass in the case of extreme obesity to avoid overestimates. It should be remembered that there is an age-related decline in creatinine production with the decrease in lean body mass, which may cause spuriously low serum creatinine levels in the face of clinically significant renal impairment (14). When practical, the use of peak and trough plasma levels is recommended.

PHARMACODYNAMICS

Pharmacodynamics refers to the physiologic effect of a given medication or combination of medications (12). It is measured by assessing the clinical response. The elderly have an apparent increased sensitivity to a number of medications as measured both by an increased duration of desired effect as well as an increased incidence of adverse reactions at standard dosages (7). Drugs with age-related pharmacodynamic changes include narcotic analgesics, benzodiazepines, systemic anticoagulants, digoxin, theophylline, lidocaine, and beta-blockers. The World Health Organization has recommended that reduced dosages of these medications be given in the elderly population (3). The mechanism for the increased sensitivity of the aged to these medications remains unclear due largely to inconsistent or incomplete information.

SPECIFIC DRUG CATEGORIES

Nonsteroidal Antiinflammatory Drugs

Nonsteroidal antiinflammatory drugs (NSAIDs) are used very commonly in the elderly, accounting for 5% to 6% of all outpatient prescriptions yearly (2). In addition to their use for inflammatory diseases such as rheumatoid arthritis and osteoarthritis, they are commonly used as nonspecific analgesics for a wide variety of conditions, often without supervision by a physician (18). NSAIDs, as a group, have a high potential for gastrointestinal irritation and erosion, antiplatelet activity, and renal insult (18). Nearly all of these medications undergo hepatic metabolism and then renal excretion of metabolites, although a few drugs are excreted by the kidney without prior biotransformation (19). The clearance of several NSAIDs and their metabolites, including salicylates, ibuprofen, ketoprofen, naproxen, and piroxicam, is reduced, and the elimination half-life of many of them is increased, which may lead to significant accumulation of the drug with standard dosing regimens (17). Variable and generally minor changes in protein binding and volume of distribution have been noted, but these changes have no known clinical significance (19).

It is unknown whether these changes in kinetics are responsible for the increased incidence of adverse reactions to NSAIDs in the elderly. It is recommended that initial doses of these medications be substantially reduced and that increases be titrated to patient response and side effects. Careful monitoring for renal insufficiency and gastrointestinal bleeding are of particular importance, as the potential morbidity from these problems is high. Only for the salicylates are plasma levels widely available and reliable, and toxic side effects (most commonly tinnitus) may occur even within the therapeutic range. The nonacetylated salicylates, such as salsalate, have the least problematic side effect profile as they have no platelet or gastrointestinal erosive effects at low to moderate doses (2 to 3.5 g per day).

Anticoagulants

A number of systemic anticoagulants are commonly used in the elderly population as the incidence of thromboembolic disease, as well as other conditions predisposing to thromboembolic disease, increases.

The most commonly used agents include warfarin, heparin, aspirin, and dextran. Other agents with antiplatelet activity in vitro, such as dipyridamole, sulfinpyrazone, and indomethacin, lack evidence of activity and efficacy in vivo. Warfarin acts by inhibiting the synthesis of the vitamin K-dependent clotting factors. Warfarin is 98% to 99.6% protein-bound, and thus its clinical activity is readily altered by other drugs that displace it from albumin (often antibiotics) (20). An intrinsic increase in sensitivity to warfarin has been shown in the elderly with lowered levels of vitamin K-dependent factors, even with similar warfarin plasma levels when compared to younger subjects (21). Thus, decreased warfarin doses and lower warfarin plasma levels would be needed to achieve desired levels of anticoagulation. Heparin acts by enhancing the activity of intrinsic antithrombin III, and this promotes clot lysis and discourages the formation of clot (20). Aspirin decreases platelet adhesiveness by interfering with the conversion of arachidonic acid to thromboxane A2 by the enzyme cyclooxygenase. These effects on the platelet are irreversible and thus will endure for the life of the platelet (20). Dextran has many effects on the clotting cascade, including dilution of circulating clotting factors, decreased platelet adhesiveness, and increased fibrin clot lysis (20).

Clinical indications for systemic anticoagulation include deep venous thrombosis, pulmonary embolism, chronic or paroxysmal atrial fibrillation, prosthetic cardiac valves, transient ischemic attacks, stroke in evolution, chronic or unstable angina, and postmyocardial infarction. The use of warfarin or heparin in transient ischemic attacks or coronary artery disease in the elderly lacks evidence of efficacy (20). Contraindications to anticoagulation are many, but age alone cannot be considered a contraindication for short-term or long-term anticoagulation (22). Absolute and relative contraindications include unexplained anemia, active peptic ulcer disease, uncontrolled or unexplained gastrointestinal bleeding, malignant hypertension, renal failure, hepatic failure, recent cerebrovascular accident (less than 6 months), recent spinal anesthesia, recent surgery (particularly intracranial), inability or unwillingness to be reliable or compliant with the medication and testing regimen, and high risk for falls or other trauma. The use of systemic anticoagulants in the elderly should be cautious and carefully monitored but should not be excluded without specific reason in a patient with an appropriate indication, as these conditions requiring anticoagulation have excessive morbidity and mortality if left untreated.

Narcotic Analgesics

Narcotic analgesics are widely used in the elderly inpatient and outpatient populations, accounting for 2.4% of all nonhospital prescriptions in 1988 (2). Meperidine is the seventh most commonly prescribed medication to hospitalized elderly, and morphine is 16th (2). The elderly generally have an increased sensitivity to the action of narcotics, most notably morphine and fentanyl (23). Morphine has been shown to offer a greater degree of pain relief and an increased duration of pain relief in the elderly when compared to the young (24). It has a decreased clearance and volume of distribution, but the elimination half-life is unchanged, and no increase in

respiratory depression has been demonstrated in the elderly (24). Meperidine has a variably decreased volume of distribution (4) and an increased free fraction, but the renal clearance of both the parent drug and the normeperidine metabolite is decreased (25). There is a direct correlation between creatinine clearance and normeperidine clearance. With repeated doses of meperidine, there is significant accumulation of both meperidine and normeperidine, and the potential for a serious adverse drug reaction escalates (25). For this reason, the use of regular or repeated meperidine dosing is not recommended in the elderly or others with any degree of renal impairment. Fentanyl also shows a marked decrease in clearance in the elderly, and it has been shown to cause increased central nervous system sensitivity, respiratory depression, tachyphylaxis, and hypertensive responses (23). Codeine seems to have declining efficacy in the elderly and causes much constipation.

Sedative Hypnotics

There are many drugs available with sedative properties. Primary sedative hypnotic drugs include the benzodiazepines, barbiturates, chloral hydrate, and ethanol. Secondary sedatives of interest in the elderly population include narcotics, antihistamines, and the tricyclic antidepressants. In the United States, the elderly are not disproportionate users of sedatives (26), but in this age group 70% of users are female. There is an increased prevalence of long-term use of sedatives with increasing age, and 75% of all users over the age of 65 years continue for longer than 1 year.

Benzodiazepines accounted for 60 million prescriptions or 4% of the total for 1988 (2). Other sedative hypnotics accounted for a further 2%. Approximately two thirds of benzodiazepine prescriptions are repeats, which reflects the high prevalence of long-term use. Although dependence and tolerance develop, dosages of benzodiazepines are rarely increased by patients. Elderly patients actually tend to spontaneously decrease both dose amount and dose frequency over time. These drugs have low abuse potential as there are no reinforcing affects seen, and recreational use is exceedingly rare (26). Overdosage is nonetheless a problem in the elderly who show increased central nervous system sensitivity and accumulation, particularly with drugs with longer elimination half-lives and active metabolites (27). Use of benzodiazepines with half-lives greater than 24 hours has also been associated with a substantially increased risk of falls, as well as increased risk of hip fracture as a result of these falls (28). Oversedation is rarely life-threatening unless there is an interaction with other sedative medication (26).

Indications for the use of sedative hypnotic medication include insomnia either associated with an anxiety neurosis, an abnormal situation or stress, or leading to behavior problems (29). The duration of effect of a benzodiazepine correlates more closely with the dose given than with the half-life of the drug. It is important to remember that 15% to 20% of patients will recover normal sleep patterns without treatment and that another one third will respond to placebo (29). Unless concomitant treatment is needed for an anxiety neurosis, these medications should be prescribed for periods not exceeding 2 to 4 weeks of sustained regular use. They can be safely used for extended periods for occasional treatment of insomnia.

Anticonvulsants

Because of accumulated injury and increased incidence of intracranial pathology that predisposes to seizure disorders, the anticonvulsants are commonly used in the elderly both therapeutically and prophylactically. Phenytoin is the most commonly prescribed drug in this category for all adults (2). There is no significant change in the half-life, the volume of distribution, or the clearance in the elderly (29). The half-life of phenytoin is long (average 22 hours with a range of 7 to 48 hours, in part depending upon dose), thus permitting once-daily dosing. It should be noted however that the hepatic metabolism of phenytoin is saturable; thus, plasma levels may increase abruptly with small increases in dose (29). No decrease in metabolic capacity has been shown definitively in the elderly. Phenytoin has a narrow therapeutic index, and acute toxic effects include ataxia, nystagmus, and hyperglycemia. Chronic side effects include gingival hyperplasia and hirsutism. It should be noted that oral absorption of phenytoin is significantly decreased by many enteral tube feeding preparations. Thus, plasma levels should be monitored regularly, and dose and/or feeding preparation changes should be made as needed. Levels should also be carefully monitored when tube feedings are discontinued to avoid toxicity; dose reductions may be required.

Carbamazepine is another highly effective anticonvulsant in the elderly. No pharmacokinetic changes have been demonstrated with age (30). It may also be used in the treatment of central pain syndromes such as thalamic pain or tic doulouveux. It does require twice daily dosing, as its half-life is only 15 hours.

Valproic acid shows some changes in the kinetics of the free drug, but total drug kinetics are unchanged with age (31). Phenobarbital is rarely recommended for use in the elderly because of problems with oversedation and paradoxical central nervous system excitation (31). Ethosuximide is effective only in petit mal forms of epilepsy, and these are rare in the elderly (31). In general, monotherapy is effective and preferred in the elderly. Plasma drug level monitoring should be utilized as needed to optimize dosing.

GENERAL PRESCRIBING PRINCIPLES

In general, the elderly are more sensitive to both the toxic and therapeutic effects of drugs and much attention should be given to the appropriate use of medications in this population (see Table 7.2).

1. *Drug history is essential.* As part of the initial evaluation of any patient an extensive drug history should be obtained. It is critical to know *everything* the patient is taking including prescription, nonprescription, topical, intraocular, intranasal, rectal, or vaginal preparations. Patients should be specifically questioned about habits such as smoking and alcohol, caffeine, and illegal or recreational drug use. It is also helpful to inquire about what other health care providers they see; this may prompt them to remember medications obtained from these providers of which you might otherwise have been unaware.

2. *Use no drug before its time.* As shown previously, the prevalence of patient symptoms in this population is nearly 100%, and many of them are vague or extremely nonspecific (1). Although it is not always possible, one should try to make a diagnosis before instituting any therapeutic intervention. An adverse drug reaction or drug interaction should always be considered in the differential diagnosis of any sign or symptom with which the patient presents, in order to avoid escalating iatrogenic problems. Nonpharmacologic methods of symptomatic relief should also be encouraged when appropriate, including behavior modification, physical therapy, biofeedback, and support groups.

3. *Use no drug beyond its time.* It is crucial for the physician to frequently and regularly review the medications used by patients and discontinue drugs that are no longer deemed necessary or appropriate. Simplification of the medication regimen when possible will both increase compliance and reduce the risk of an adverse drug reaction. When medications are discontinued or doses changed, patients should be encouraged to dispose of remaining doses to prevent inadvertent or intentional nonprescribed use of the medication at a later date.

4. *Know the drugs you use.* It is more effective to use a few drugs well than to use a large number of drugs without thoroughly understanding their pharmacologic properties. The explosive increase in the numbers of available medications has made it impossible to effectively know the entire pharmaceutical armamentarium available. It is not appropriate to assume that drugs in

Table 7.2. Prescribing Principles

Obtain a complete drug history
Use no drug before its time
Use no drug beyond its time
Know the drugs you use
Use the minimum dose needed
Encourage compliance
Watch for iatrogenic complications

the same therapeutic category will act the same even if their side effect profile is similar, as the cellular mechanism of action may be very different.

5. *Start low, go slow.* For many drugs it is appropriate to begin at doses well below the accepted therapeutic dose in the younger adult population. Titrate dosing to therapeutic response, and use the minimum dose needed for therapeutic efficacy. The use of plasma drug levels as well as periodic monitoring of renal function can be very helpful.

6. *Encourage compliance.* The most important factor in patient compliance is good communication between the patient and the physician. Improved compliance will result from better patient understanding of the medical regimen, and patients should be given understandable information regarding the name of the medication (both trade and generic), the reason they are on the medication, and the expected therapeutic effect and possible side effects. In addition, low frequency of dosing, appropriate formulation, lower cost when possible, and accessible containers have been shown to increase compliance. The use of assistive devices such as daily pill containers and tear off calendars may be helpful for some patients. Encourage the patient to report noncompliance, as changes may be necessary and possible without jeopardizing the therapeutic goal. You cannot assume that the patient is taking medications just because they have been prescribed.

7. *Be alert to iatrogenic complications.* The incidence of adverse reactions to drugs correlates with the number of medications prescribed, which in turn correlates with the severity of illness and the number of diagnoses. Thus, a drug may be the cause for unusual or new symptoms, which may have to be managed by discontinuing the offending agent.

It is important to remember that medications are only one part of the comprehensive care of the elderly patient and that clinical geriatrics has many other tools available for solving the problems with which these patients present.

References

1. Hale WE, Perkins LL, May FE, Marks RG, Stewart RB. Symptom prevalance in the elderly. An evaluation of age, sex, disease and medication use. *J Am Geriatr Soc.* 34:333–340, 1986.
2. Tomita DK, Kennedy DL, Baum C, Knapp DE, Anello C. *Drug Utilization in the United States: 1988.* Washington, DC: US Dept of Health and Human Services; 1989.
3. Vestal RE. Clinical pharmacology. In: Hazzard WR, Andres R, Bierman EL, Blass JP, eds. *Principles of Geriatric Medicine and Gerontology.* 2nd ed. New York, NY: McGraw-Hill; 1990.
4. Cusack BJ, Vestal RE. Clinical pharmacology: special considerations in the elderly. In: Calkins E, Davis PJ, Ford AB, eds. *Practice of Geriatric Medicine* Philadelphia, Pa: W.B. Saunders; 1986.
5. Nolan L, O'Malley K. Prescribing for the elderly: part I. Sensitivity of the elderly to adverse drug reactions. *J Am Geriatr Soc.* 30:329–333, 1982.
6. Lamy PP. The elderly and drug interactions. *J Am Geriatr Soc.* 34:586–592, 1986.
7. Ouslander JG. Drug therapy in the elderly. *Ann Intern Med.* 95:711–722, 1981.
8. Nolan L, O'Malley K. Prescribing for the elderly: part II. Prescribing patterns: differences due to age. *J Am Geriatr Soc.* 36:245–254, 1988.
9. Prescott LF. Clinically important drug interactions. In: Speight TM, ed. *Avery's Drug Treatment.* 3rd ed. Auckland: ADIS Press Ltd; 1987.
10. Morrow DM, Leirer V, Sheikh J. Adherence and medication instructions. *J Am Geriatr Soc.* 36:1147–1160, 1988.
11. Cooper JK, Love DW, Raffoul PR. Intentional prescription nonadherance (noncompliance) by the elderly. *J Am Geriatr Soc.* 30:329–333, 1982.
12. Vestal RE. Geriatric clinical pharmacology: an overview. In: Vestal RE, ed. *Drug Treatment in the Elderly.* Sydney: ADIS Health Science Press: 1984.
13. Vestal RE, Dawson GW. Pharmacology and aging. In: Finch CE, Schneider EL, eds. *Handbook of the Biology of Aging.* 2nd ed. New York, NY: Van Nostrand Reinhold: 1985.
14. Schumucker DL. Aging and drug disposition: an update. *Pharmacol Rev.* 37(2):133–148, 1985.
15. Greenblatt DJ, Sellers EM, Shader RI. Drug disposition in old age. *N Engl J Med.* 306(18):1081–1088, 1982.
16. Montamat SC, Cusack BJ, Vestal RE. Management of drug therapy in the elderly. *N Engl J Med.* 321:303–309, 1989.
17. Cusack BJ. Drug metabolism in the elderly. *J Clin Pharmacol.* 28:571–576, 1988.
18. Lamy PP. Renal effects of nonsteroidal antiinflammatory drugs. *J Am Geriatr Soc.* 34:361–367, 1986.
19. Woodhouse KW, Wynne H. The pharmacokinetics of nonsteroidal antiinflammatory drugs in the elderly. *Clin Pharmacokinet.* 12:111–122, 1987.
20. Shepherd, AMM. Anticoagulant therapy. In: Swift CG, ed. *Clinical Pharmacology in the Elderly.* New York, NY: Marcel Dekker Inc: 1987.
21. Routledge PA, Chapman PH, Davies DM, Rawlins MD. Pharmacokinetics and pharmacodynamics of warfarin at steady state. *Br J Clin Pharmacol.* 8:243–247, 1986.
22. Gurwitz JH, Goldberg RJ, Holden A, Knapic N, Ansell J. Age-related risks of long term oral anticoagulant therapy. *Arch Intern Med.* 148:1733–1736, 1988.
23. Shanks C. General anesthesia. In: Swift CG, ed. *Clinical Pharmacology in the Elderly.* New York, NY: Marcel Dekker Inc: 1987.
24. Kaiko RF, Wallenstein SL, Rogers AG, Grabinski PY, Houde RW. Narcotics in the elderly. *Med Clin North Am.* 66(5):1079–1089, 1982.
25. Odar-Cederlof I, Boreus LO, Bondesson U, Holmberg L, Heyner L. Comparison of renal excretion of Pethedine (Meperidine) and its metabolites in old and young patients. *Eur J Clin Pharmacol.* 28:171–175, 1985.
26. Woods JH, Katz JL, Winger G. Abuse liability of benzodiazepines. *Pharmacol Rev.* 39(4):251–413, 1987.
27. Cook PJ. Benzodiazepine hypnotics in the elderly. *Acta Psychiatr Scand.* 74 (suppl 332):149–158, 1986.
28. Ray WA, Griffen MR, Schaffner W, Baugh DK, Melton LJ. Psychotropic drug use and the risk of hip fracture. *N Engl J Med.* 316(7):363–369, 1987.
29. Castleden M, Swift CG. Hypnotics, sedatives and anticonvulsants. In: Swift CG, ed. *Clinical Pharmacology in the Elderly.* New York, NY: Marcel Dekker Inc: 1987.
30. Hockings N, Pall A, Moody J, Davidson VM, Davidson DLW. The effects of age on carbamazepine pharmacokinetics and adverse effects. *Br J Clin Pharmacol.* 22:725–728, 1986.
31. Perucca E, Grimaldi R, Gatti G, Pirracchio S, Frigo GM. Pharmacokinetics of valproic acid in the elderly. *Br J Clin Pharmacol.* 17:665–669, 1984.

8

Temperature Regulation in the Aged

Nirandon Wongsurawat

Healthy humans and other warm-blooded or homeothermic animals maintain a narrow internal temperature range independent of external conditions and physical activity. This is achieved by balancing heat gain and heat loss. In general, the nude body can indefinitely maintain a normal core body temperature in dry air with ambient temperature between 16°C and 54°C.

Extreme temperatures have had a major impact on human history since ancient times. The Old Testament refers to death while laboring in the heat in the fields. Heat was an important factor in the outcome of the Crusades. Napoleon failed miserably because of the severe winter; only a handful of his 12,000-man division survived the cold during their retreat from Russia. Cold was a major factor for United States casualties in the Korean War.

EFFECTS OF AGE ON CONSTANT BODY TEMPERATURE MAINTENANCE

In order to maintain a relatively constant body temperature, the rate of heat gain must be equal to the rate of heat loss. The person must be in heat balance. Thermoregulation operates almost entirely through centers in the hypothalamus. Heat gain is dependent on a number of factors, including ambient temperature, basal metabolic rate, muscle activity, and the effects of thyroxine and catecholamines to increase chemical thermogenesis. Body heat is lost by radiation, conduction, convection, and evaporation. Ambient temperature is an important factor affecting heat loss.

Elderly people are vulnerable to extreme changes in environmental temperature. This is due to impaired function of thermoregulatory processes (1–3). Although there is no significant difference in basal temperatures between young and old adults, the temperature-lowering effect of iced water is enhanced in the elderly (4). Drinking 9 ounces of iced water lowered oral temperature by 1.7°C for individuals over 60 years of age compared to 1.4°C for those 40 to 60 years and 0.9°C for those under 40 years of age. Several factors contribute

to the impairment of thermoregulatory function in the elderly. Decline in cardiopulmonary, neuromuscular, and gastrointestinal functions contributes to disturbances of the thermoregulatory mechanism (5). Use of multiple drugs also affects temperature regulation. Malnutrition, which often reaches endemic proportions in many institutionalized elderly, further interferes with the ability of these older adults to maintain their body temperature (6). Nutrition is an important factor in thermoregulation because 80% of the calories in the food of warm-blooded animals goes to maintain body temperature. The impairment of the thermoregulatory system in the elderly is likely to be responsible for the excess mortality in this population during extremes in the environmental temperature.

Aging is associated with decreased basal metabolic rate, which is partially related to the reduction in lean body mass. Catecholamines are major hormones capable of causing an immediate increase in metabolism. Sympathetic stimulation of brown fat activates lipase to break down triglycerides to glycerol and free fatty acids. Free fatty acids are then oxidized to carbon dioxide and water, releasing thermal energy. However, older humans have almost no brown fat, and beta-adrenergic responsiveness is also decreased with advancing age. Chemical thermogenesis can increase the rate of heat production by about only 10% in the aged compared with 100% in infants. Another mechanism of chemical thermogenesis is through the secretion of hypothalamic thyrotropin-releasing hormone, which stimulates the release of pituitary thyroid-stimulating hormone. There is a slight decline in triiodothyronine levels with age, although thyroxine levels remain normal. Thyroid economy in the elderly probably does not contribute to temperature dysregulation, except in the case of hypothyroidism or myxedema.

The insulator system of the body consists of the skin, subcutaneous tissues, and, especially, subcutaneous fat. Fat is an excellent insulator because it conducts heat only one third as efficiently as other tissues. Loss of subcutaneous fat, which is common with aging, decreases the insulation. In addition, weight loss, a common problem in older individuals, further decreases the total adipose tissue mass. Heat transfer from the body core to the exterior is regulated by blood flow to the skin. This is under control of the autonomic nervous system. To dissipate body heat, the sympathetic centers in the posterior hypothalamus are inhibited. This results in vasodilation of the skin blood vessels. The rate of heat transfer to the skin can be increased eightfold via this mechanism. To conserve body heat, the posterior hypothalamic centers are stimulated, causing cutaneous vasoconstriction. Approximately half of older individuals demonstrate abnormal peripheral blood flow responses to cooling and warming as compared to young controls. A longitudinal study has shown progressive deterioration of blood flow responses to variations in the thermal environment with advancing age (2). The failure of adequate blood flow responses to temperature with aging appears to be secondary to sympathetic nervous system malfunction.

Cold signals from the skin and spinal cord stimulate the motor center for shivering in the hypothalamus. Shivering is an effective mechanism to generate heat to prevent lowering of body temperature. During maximum shivering, muscular heat production can rise tenfold. One study (7) showed that with lowering of ambient temperatures shivering occurred in 30% of young subjects and in only 10% of older subjects. The shivering response is also less efficient in the elderly (8). This may be due to a loss of motor power in the muscle mass.

Heat loss from the body occurs through radiation, conduction, and evaporation. Radiation is the loss of heat in the form of electromagnetic infrared rays and accounts for approximately 60% of total heat loss. Conduction occurs mainly to the air adjacent to the body (15%) from which it is removed by air currents (convection). Clothing greatly decreases the loss of heat by conduction. However, when clothing becomes wet it loses its ability to prevent heat loss, as water increases the rate of heat transmission at least 20-fold. Evaporation accounts for 22% of heat loss. Loss of body heat by evaporation of sweat is regulated by the autonomic nervous system. Evaporation through sweating is an essential mechanism for heat dissipation when the ambient temperature is greater than the skin temperature. For each gram of water evaporated, 0.58 kilocalories of heat is lost. The body temperature threshold for the onset of sweating is increased, and the sweating activity is markedly decreased in the aged in comparison with the younger age groups (9).

Higher cortical centers are also involved in thermoregulation. Older individuals have impaired ability to recognize environmental temperature changes and, therefore, often fail to make the appropriate behavioral changes necessary to maintain their body temperature (10).

Numerous neurotransmitters have been putatively involved in the central regulation of body temperature (11). Prostaglandins appear to be in part the mediators of the pyrexial response to endogenous pyrogens such as interleukin-1 (11). A number of neuropeptides have been shown to modulate body temperature (12). Thyrotropin-releasing hormone acts within the preoptic nucleus of the anterior hypothalamus to produce hyperthermia independent of its ability to release thyroid hormones. Beta-endorphin has a biphasic effect on temperature. This effect is blunted with aging, possibly secondary to the reduction in the number of opioid receptor sites seen with aging. Age-related alterations in the neurotransmitter regulation of body temperature undoubtedly contribute to the impairment of the thermal homeostasis seen with advancing age.

HYPERTHERMIA

Over 1,700 deaths were attributed to the heat during the summer of 1980. Studies by the Center for Disease Control in St. Louis and Kansas City clearly demonstrated that the hyperthermia case rates rose steadily with increasing age (13). Heat stroke rates in persons 65 years or older were 35 times greater than that for the 19 to 44-year age group. There is also a definite inverse relationship of case rates with socioeconomic status. Persons without access to air conditioning were 50 times more likely to die from heat stroke than were those with air-conditioning.

Medical Conditions

Preexisting diseases common in the elderly are important factors that impair the response to increases in environmental temperature and therefore contribute to the excess mortality during heat waves. Ischemic heart disease, cerebrovascular disease, diabetes mellitus, and chronic lung disease have been identified as the major contributors to excess mortality. The death rate from cancer also increases when the temperature rises. Mortality due to hyperthermia depends more on the severity of preexisting diseases than the severity of heat stress.

Several drugs prescribed for common illnesses in geriatric patients predispose the elderly to heat stroke. These drugs (Table 8.1) generally act by impairing the sweat response, altering awareness of heat, decreasing cardiac output and extracellular fluid volume, and in-

Table 8.1. Drugs That Interfere with Temperature Regulation

Antiadrenergics (beta-sympathetic blockers)
Anticholinergics (parasympathetic blockers)
Diuretics
Monoamine oxidase inhibitors
Phenothiazines
Tricyclic antidepressants

ducing sodium depletion. Amphetamines act directly on the hypothalamus to increase body temperature.

Pathophysiology

The spectrum of heat illness ranges from heat cramps with normal body temperature, to heat exhaustion with still intact thermoregulation, to heat stroke with rapid rise of core temperature and failure of body heat regulation. Heat cramps and heat exhaustion are relatively common conditions with little morbidity, but heat stroke is a medical emergency with high mortality.

In a hot environment, if the air is dry and air currents are flowing, a healthy person can weather up to 65.5°C for several hours with no ill effects. If the humidity is 100%, the body temperature will begin to rise whenever the ambient temperature rises above 34°C. As long as the core temperature is 1°C or more above the skin temperature, body heat can continue to dissipate via vasodilation mechanism. Air convection can keep skin temperature low enough to allow this to continue up to about 32°C. In a warmer environment, especially when the temperature of the surroundings is greater than skin temperature, heat loss by radiation and conduction (convection) is not possible. The body gains heat by these mechanisms instead of losing heat to the environment. Under such conditions, the only way the body can dissipate heat is through sweat formation and evaporation of sweat to cool the skin. Even with maximal sweating, there is a limit at which the body can lose heat. Worse, the hypothalamus becomes less effective as it is excessively heated. Thus, a high body temperature tends to perpetuate itself. As the core temperature rises, hyperventilation ensues. Cerebral functions deteriorate from irritability to confusion, lethargy, and coma. When body core temperature rises above 41°C, parenchymal cells begin to be damaged by denaturation of proteins. Almost all cells are killed if the temperature rises to 50°C.

Heat Stroke

Heat stroke is a heat syndrome produced by overheating of the body core, generally over 40°C. This is a true medical emergency with mortality rate up to 80%. Thermoregulatory mechanism fails after exposure to high environmental temperature and humidity. There are two types of heat stroke, classic and exertional.

Classic heat stroke is the type most common in the elderly. It often develops during the first few days of a heat wave. Significant dehydration and anhydrosis are common features. Early manifestations are those of heat exhaustion, with headache, malaise, dizziness, anorexia, nausea, vomiting, and dyspnea. All of these symptoms are nonspecific. Central nervous system signs are first to appear and persist the longest. Generalized seizures occur in 60% of patients and loss of consciousness in 70%. Practically every neurologic abnormality has been described. The cerebellum is very sensitive to heat stress, and cerebellar ataxia may be the only permanent residual.

Cardiovascular response in the elderly is hypodynamic. Hypovolemia is usually present. Electrocardiographic (ECG) abnormalities include ST-segment depression, T-wave inversion, sinus tachycardia, premature ventricular contractions, and conduction defects. Hyperventilation, up to 60 breaths/min, is common because it helps increase heat loss. However, respiratory alkalosis may be a complication, and tetany and severe hypokalemia may develop.

Marked elevations of serum liver enzyme (aspartate aminotransferase lactate dehydrogenase) are common but residual hepatic damage is rare. Hematologic complications occur in up to 20% of heat stroke patients. Prothrombin and partial thromboplastin times (PT and PTT) are elevated. Fibrinogen levels are decreased. The platelet count may be low. The syndrome of disseminated intravascular coagulation, if it occurs, is usually mild.

Treatment

Diagnosis of heat stroke is generally uncomplicated. A rectal thermistor probe should be used to monitor core temperature. Regular glass thermometers are inadequate and can be dangerous in patients with seizures. All clothing should be removed. Cooling must be initiated immediately. The more rapid the cooling, the lower the mortality. The patient should be moved to a cool place, an air-conditioned room if possible. Ice-water bath is effective but a cumbersome method. Ice packs should be applied to neck, axilla, and inguinal area. The patient's skin should be kept wet and evaporation maximized by a fan. This method is as effective as an ice-water bath. Aspirin is of no value because the thermoregulatory setpoint is normal in heat stroke; the failure is in the mechanisms to eliminate heat. Other measures should include, where appropriate, endotracheal intubation, a Swan-Ganz catheter, and a urinary catheter placement. Intravenous fluids may be chilled prior to infusion. Cooling should be stopped when core temperature declines to 39°C to avoid hypothermia. There may be rebound hyperthermia 3 to 6 hours after cooling is stopped. Complete recovery has been reported in a patient with a core temperature of 46.5°C. Patients who once had heat stroke often have permanent impairment of thermoregulatory control. They become more susceptible to heat illness.

HYPOTHERMIA

Hypothermia is present when the body core temperature falls below 35°C. Accidental hypothermia develops when the body temperature decreases unintentionally to hypothermic levels. The elderly are especially vulnerable to this potentially fatal condition. Studies in Great Britain have shown that up to 10% of elderly people living at home had body temperatures near hypothermic level (7). However, a study in Maine failed to find a similar prevalence of borderline hypothermia in older Americans (14). The incidence of hypothermia in older patients (over 65 years) admitted to London hospitals during winter months was 3.6%. Mortality due to hypothermia in Great Britain has been reported to be as high as 80% (10). The annual incidence of hypothermia in the United States is about 60,000 (15). Approximately 700 deaths due to cold exposure take place here each year (16). Death rates of patients presenting with hypothermia increase with age. In persons 75 years of age or older, the risk of dying from hypothermia is five times that for younger groups (16).

Pathophysiology

Most patients with accidental hypothermia are admitted during the winter months because exposure is the most common cause of severe hypothermia. However, ambient temperature during nights of warmer months still can be significantly lower than body temperature. Therefore, hypothermia can be found in any month of the year. This is especially true for older people who may have an impaired capacity to feel cold. Hypothermia can also be found in association with a number of illnesses (Table 8.2).

Vasoconstriction of the blood vessels in the skin is the initial response to external cold to conserve heat. When conservation of heat fails to maintain body temperature, increased heat production becomes necessary. Shivering is an effective means to generate heat, but this mechanism cannot be maintained for a prolonged period of time. The early cardiac response is tachycardia and an increase in stroke volume. Along with an initial increase in cardiac output, the respiratory rate accelerated and oxygen consumption increases, reflecting a sharp rise in the metabolic rate.

Table 8.2. Etiologic Conditions Associated with Accidental Hypothermia

Exposure to cold
Neurologic conditions
   Stroke, head trauma, brain tumor, hypothalamic diseases,
     Wernicke's encephalopathy, cord transection, sarcoidosis,
     dementia
Metabolic conditions
   Hypothyroidism, starvation, hypopituitarism, diabetes mellitus,
     hypoglycemia, hypoadrenalism, anorexia nervosa
Drug-induced conditions
   Alcohol, phenothiazines, sedatives, general anesthetics,
     organophosphate, salicylates
Miscellaneous
   Old age, arthritis, immobility, uremia, carbon monoxide
     poisoning, heart failure, liver disease, sepsis, burns, psoriasis

As the body temperature falls further, shivering ceases. Muscular rigidity occurs at about 30°C. All major organ system functions begin to deteriorate. The heart rate and stroke volume decrease, and cardiac output drops. Cardiac rhythm becomes irregular. The ECG may provide an important diagnostic clue. Osborn waves, characterized by a widening of the base of QRS complex and a J point deflection, are pathognomonic (17). Osborn waves can be seen with hypothermia of any cause but do not herald ventricular fibrillation. They are present in 30% of hypothermic patients. Creatine phosphokinase (CPK-MB) may increase without myocardial infarct. At 28°C, myocardial irritability increases, and ventricular fibrillation becomes a major risk. Stimulation such as urinary catheterization, endotracheal intubation, and moving or handling of the patient may easily precipitate ventricular fibrillation. Most hypothermic patients die of ventricular fibrillation.

HYPERGLYCEMIA

Hyperglycemia is a common finding. This is due to the stimulation of catecholamine and glucocorticoids or glycogenolysis and gluconeogenesis. Insulin activity is inhibited during hypothermia. Renal clearance of glucose is reduced. All these revert with rewarming, and therefore hypoglycemia may suddenly develop during the treatment of hypothermia, especially if insulin is used to correct hyperglycemia on admission. Hypoglycemia may be a prominent feature upon admission in alcoholic and malnourished patients. Shivering may also have completely exhausted the already low levels of glucose stores.

RESPIRATORY EFFECTS

Cough reflex is depressed. Bronchorrhea, atelectasis, and pneumonia are common findings. Major respiratory depression leading to respiratory arrest occurs at about 25°C to 24°C. Reduced ventilation is due to a reduction of metabolic demand and the direct effect of cold on the respiratory center. Arterial blood gas measurements under standard conditions at 37°C should be corrected for the patient's temperature because the P_{O_2} and P_{CO_2} will be falsely elevated and pH will be factitiously low.

HYPOVOLEMIA

Hypovolemia may develop as a result of cold diuresis. Hemoconcentration and increased blood viscosity further compound the problem with tissue perfusion. Acidosis caused by hypoventilation is increased by lactate accumulation during shivering response and tissue hypoperfusion. Hypokalemia is commonly seen and may contribute to cardiac irritability especially at lower temperatures. Leukopenia and thrombocytopenia are secondary to sequestration in the liver and spleen. Clotting abnormalities and disseminated intravascular coagulation may develop around 20°C. Cerebral blood flow is reduced by 6% for each degree (Celsius) decrease in core temperature. This may result in a decline in mental status, ataxia, hyporeflexia, and mydriasis. Focal signs, seizures, and paralysis may also develop. At 19°C, the EEG becomes flat and the heart stops.

Clinical Presentation

Because the signs and symptoms of hypothermia are nonspecific and the lowest temperature registered by most standard thermometers is around 35°C, many hypothermic patients may not have their condition recognized. Therefore, it is important to keep this diagnosis in mind, especially in the elderly with cold skin, bradycardia, hypotension, sepsis, or in coma. The physiologic consequences of hypothermia are complex. A pulseless patient with ice-cold skin and without blood pressure may not yet be dead. No patients with profound hypothermia should be pronounced dead until they have been rewarmed to 36°C and remain unresponsive to resuscitation. One reported patient recovered completely while in the morgue.

Most patients are nonshivering on admission. Mental status varies from confusion to comatose to apparent death. The pupils may be dilated and sluggishly reactive. Muscular rigidity may be present. The skin is cold. There may be purpura or bullae over pressure-dependent areas. Bradycardia is common. Blood pressure may not be detectable. Bronchopneumonia may be present. Sepsis is a common cause of hypothermia in the elderly and carries a very high mortality rate (18). Elderly patients who develop hypothermia should be promptly treated as septic unless proven otherwise. The most critical physical finding, however, is a core temperature below 35°C. The diagnosis, therefore, requires a low-reading thermometer and a high degree of suspicion. Taking a rectal temperature with a low-reading thermometer should be a routine practice.

Laboratory investigation should include blood counts and coagulation parameters; electrolytes; liver, renal and pancreatic function; urinalysis; arterial blood gases; chest film, and ECG. Other studies are drug screening, skull films, blood culture, and postrewarming thyroid and adrenal function tests. Any number of laboratory results may be abnormal. Hyperglycemia, hypoglycemia, hypokalemia, metabolic acidosis, prolonged PT and PTT, azotemia, and evidence of acute pancreatitis are common findings. Atelectasis or pneumonia is frequently seen in the chest roentgenogram. Osborn waves, when present, are pathognomonic of hypothermia. Adrenal responsiveness to corticotropin (ACTH) stimulation may be spuriously decreased.

Treatment

Accidental hypothermia is a medical emergency, and patients should be treated in a hospital. Core (rectal) temperature should be continuously monitored. Patients must be handled very carefully and should have cardiac monitoring. Hypothermic patients are at high risk for ventricular fibrillation, which is resistant to defibrillation until the core temperature rises above 28°C. Cardiopulmonary resuscitation should continue as the patient is being rewarmed. Most drugs are ineffective in hypothermic patients and may result in later overmedication. Moderate acidosis improves with restoration of ventilation and rewarming. Sodium bicarbonate should be given in case of severe acidosis (pH < 7.25). Rewarming alone may adequately raise blood pressure in hypotensive patients; however, patients with prolonged hypothermia will require a large amount of volume replacement. Fluids should be warmed to 40°C. If supplemental oxygen is given, it should also be heated to 42°C. Severe hyperglycemia (>400 mg/dL) may be treated very carefully with insulin, and blood glucose levels must be monitored frequently. If myxedema is suspected, thyroxine may be given along with corticosteroid after appropriate laboratories studies have been drawn. Thiamine and glucose should always be given together if Wernicke's encephalopathy or hypoglycemia is suspected.

Rewarming to restore normal body temperature is the primary treatment. The cold, wet clothing must be removed, and the patient should be placed in a warm environment. Rewarming techniques range from passive to active to invasive rewarming. Passive rewarming with a blanket is adequate for mild hypothermia (above 32°C). With moderate hypothermia (29.4°C to 32°C) and stable cardiac status, patients should be actively but slowly rewarmed with electric blankets, warmed intravenous fluids, and heated humidified oxygen. Patients with more severe hypothermia and cardiac instability should be rapidly rewarmed by invasive means such as peritoneal dialysis with a dialysate temperature of 43.5°C. Peritoneal dialysis is the method of choice for profound hypothermia caused by drug overdoses, especially barbiturate intoxication.

SUMMARY

As is always the case, prevention is better than cure. Hyperthermia and hypothermia are preventable causes of death. Through active education programs, the public should be well informed about these conditions in extremes of environmental temperature. Special efforts should be made to reach persons at greatest risk, which include the elderly, poor, alcoholic, chronically ill, persons taking neuroleptic or anticholinergic drugs, and those confined in bed unable to care for themselves. Outreach to these vulnerable groups should reduce the morbidity and mortality from environmental hazards.

Acknowledgment. This work was supported by the Department of Veterans Affairs.

References

1. Wagner JA, Robinson S, Marino RP. Age and temperature regulation of humans in neutral and cold regulation. *J Appl Physiol.* 37:562–565, 1974.
2. Collins KJ, Exton-Smith AN, Fox RH, Macdonald IC, Woodward M. Accidental hypothermia and impaired temperature homeostasis in the elderly. *Br Med J.* 1:353–356, 1977.
3. Emslie-Smith D. Hypothermia in the elderly. *Br J Hosp Med.* 11:442–452, 1981.
4. Sugarek NJ. Temperature lowering after iced water: enhanced effects in the elderly. *J Am Geriatr Soc.* 34:526–529, 1986.
5. Collins KJ, Exton-Smith AN, James MH, et al. Functional changes in autonomic nervous responses with ageing. *Age and Ageing.* 9:17–24, 1980.
6. Morley JE, Silver A, Fiatarone M, et al. UCLA Grand Rounds: nutrition and the elderly. *J Am Geriatr Soc.* 34:823–832, 1986.
7. Fox RH, Woodward PM, Exton-Smith AN, et al. Body temperatures in the elderly: a national study of physiological, social and environmental conditions, *Br Med J.* 1:200–206, 1973.
8. Collins KJ, Easton JC, Exton-Smith AN. Shivering thermogenesis and vasomotor response with convective cooling in the elderly. *J Physiol.* 20:76, 1981.
9. Foster KG, Ellis FP, Dore C, et al. Sweat responses in the aged. *Age and Ageing.* 5:91–101, 1976.
10. Reuler JB. Hypothermia: pathophysiology, clinical settings and management. *Ann Int Med.* 89:519–527, 1978.
11. Lipton JM, Clark WG. Neurotransmitters in temperature control. *Ann Rev Physiol.* 48:613–623, 1986.
12. Morley JE, Levine AS, Oken MM et al. Neuropeptides and thermoregulation: the interactions of bombesin, neurotensin, TRH, somatostatin, naloxone and prostaglandins. *Peptides.* 3:1–6, 1982.
13. Lybarger JA, Kilbourne EM. Hyperthermia and hypothermia in the elderly: an epidemiological review. In: Davis BB, Wood WG, eds. *Homeostatic Function and Aging.* New York, NY: Raven Press; 1985:149–156.
14. Keilson L, Lambert D, Fabion D, et al. Screening for hypothermia in the ambulatory elderly: the Maine experience. *JAMA.* 254:1781–1784, 1985.
15. Dunlevy J. Hearing before subcommittee on public assistance and employment compensation of the House Committee on Ways and Means. 96th US Congress House Committee on Ways and Means; 1979:52–59.
16. National Center for Health Statistics. *Public Use Data Tapes–Mortality (1968–1980).* Hyattsville, Md: US Department of Health and Human Services; 1980.
17. Trevino A, Razi B, Beller BM, The characteristic electrocardiogram of accidental hypothermia. *Arch Intern Med.* 127:470–473, 1971.
18. Kramer MR, Vandijk J, Rosin AJ. Mortality in elderly patients with thermoregulatory failure. *Arch Intern Med.* 149:1521–1523, 1989.

SECTION III

ASSESSMENT AND MANAGEMENT OF THE DISABLED ELDERLY

9

Medical Evaluation, Assessment of Function and Potential, and Rehabilitation Plan

Franz U. Steinberg

Rehabilitation of the disabled elderly must be based on a thorough understanding of the patient's medical problems and functional deficiencies. Medical, functional, psychologic and social aspects are part of an effective rehabilitation program. It is not possible to surmise the patient's functional losses from the conventional medical data alone. Function needs to be assessed separately. On the other hand, success or failure of rehabilitation is greatly affected by the disease process underlying the disability. Therefore, a detailed medical evaluation is an important component in the work-up of an elderly patient who enters for a rehabilitation program.

AGING AND DISEASE

Aging alters the response to disease. The degenerative changes that are part of aging and the stress of previous diseases make the body respond to the same noxious stimuli in different ways. As time goes on, altered immune responses and general degenerative changes weaken the defense mechanisms and the ability of the aging body to cope with disease. Different functions decline with aging at different rates. The internal environment of the body, that is, core temperature, acidity of the blood, electrolyte content, and osmotic pressure, is controlled by homeostatic processes and varies little from youth to old age. However, as Shock (1) has found, the recovery of the homeostatic balance, once it has been disturbed by disease or environmental factors, is significantly delayed in old age. Thus, hypothermia, from which a young individual may recover promptly, may be fatal to an older person (see Chapter 8). Dehydration and fluid overload are difficult to correct in an elderly person because natural corrective mechanisms available to a younger person are considerably less effective in old age.

Shock (1) has also described the change in various body functions with aging. Functions that depend on only one organ system, such as blood glucose levels or nerve conduction velocity, show little change over a lifetime. On the other hand, functions that require the integrated activity of several organ systems, such as vital capacity, maximum breathing capacity, maximum oxygen uptake, and renal blood flow, show a marked decline with age.

Composition of body tissues changes considerably over a lifetime. Total intracellular water decreases by about 7% of body weight from youth to old age, probably because of a loss of cells. The amount of extracellular water remains constant. Body fat increases from 15% of body weight at age 30 years to 30% at age 80 years. This fact needs to be kept in mind when prescribing fat-soluble drugs because dosage and frequency of administration need to be kept on the low side.

Body weight increases slowly up to the age of 45 to 55 years and gradually declines thereafter. In women, the peak is reached later in life, and the decrease in older age is not as marked as it is in men. Individuals become shorter with advancing years. The validity of this observation is difficult to verify by cross-sectional data since succeeding generations seem to be taller than their predecessors. The loss of height is due to a progressive dehydration of the intervertebral discs and occasionally to the collapse of osteoporotic vertebrae. Span, the distance of fingertips to fingertips of horizontally raised arms, changes very little during a lifetime. This measurement is closely related to height, and a decrease of the height/span ratio indicates shrinkage of the spinal column.

Other skeletal abnormalities also develop with aging. The kyphosis of the thoracic spine increases. This is most marked in women with osteoporosis who have developed wedge fractures of the anterior portions of the vertebrae. In compensation, the neck tends to be held in extension. This posture leads to the shortening and thickening of the posterior cervical muscles while the anterior muscles are stretched and become atrophic. In the lumbosacral spine, the normal lordotic curve diminishes with age, and the low back appears flattened. The bony pelvis becomes wider both in aging men and women. The angle of the femoral neck to the femoral shaft becomes larger, resulting in a valgus deformity of the hips. In aging women, the knees may develop varus deformities leading to a narrow-based insecure gait. The arches of the fleet flatten causing callus formation on poorly padded bones. These postural changes in the very old evoke a picture of an old man or woman walking or standing with a stoop, the head pushed forward but the neck extended, the knees in varus position, the ankles turned outward, and the arches of the feet flattened.

Since a major part of the rehabilitation program consists of active exercises, it is important to review the functional changes of the aging heart. The structural proteins of the myocardium become stiffer, and there is an increase in collagen at the expense of muscle. As a result, the compliance of the ventricular wall is diminished. The myocardial cells are postmitotic and once lost cannot be replaced. They are stable and should last a lifetime, but they undergo progressive morphologic and biochemical changes. The collagen and elastic components are metabolically inert, but they undergo degenerative changes with age as well.

Aging arteries undergo thinning and fragmentation of the elastic lamellae with a gradual replacement by collagen. Lipids and calcium are deposited in the media of the arterial wall. As a result of these changes, the arteries become more rigid and less compliant. The elastic property of the normal aorta allows it to store one half of the stroke volume during systole and eject it gradually during diastole. Because of the loss of elasticity, this buffering effect declines with aging. In compensation for the decline of this buffering function, the volume of the aorta increases up to the age of 60 years. In later years, as the ability of the aorta to store blood during systole is further decreased, the systolic blood pressure rises, and the blood velocity is increased. These changes are contributory causes to hypertrophy of the left ventricular wall. The small arteries undergo atherosclerotic changes leading to narrowing of the lumen. The capillaries show thickening of the basal membranes with age, both in diabetics and nondiabetics (2).

The resting heart rate does not change with age (3). With progressive exercise, the heart rate rises very little in healthy elderly persons, but the maximal achievable heart rate declines steadily with advancing years. A rough formula gives the maximal heart rate as "220 − age." The exercise stroke volume, however, increases with age. By this mechanism, the cardiac output, which is the product of rate times stroke volume, remains relatively unchanged. The left ventricular ejection fraction, that is the volume of blood ejected by the left ventricle as related to the diastolic end volume, has become a sensitive clinical test to determine and quantify heart function. At rest it does not change with age, but at increasingly strenuous exercises there is an age-associated decrease of the ejection fraction (4).

With advancing age, the prevalence of heart disease increases steadily. Heart disease affects the patient's effort tolerance in various ways depending on the extent of the impairment. Therefore, every patient with heart disease needs to be evaluated individually before a rehabilitation program is initiated. Details are given in Chapter 21.

Pulmonary function also declines with age. There is a decrease of the elastic recoil of the lungs, even in absence of disease. The vital capacity declines, while the residual volume becomes somewhat larger. The airflow is affected by aging. Maximal voluntary ventilation, peak expiratory flow rate, and the 1-second forced expiratory volume decline with age.

The respiratory system undergoes structural and functional changes with age; however, in the absence of disease these changes do not interfere significantly with gas exchanges in aging individuals and with effort tolerance. (See Chapters 3 and 22.)

MEDICAL EVALUATION OF THE GERIATRIC PATIENT

The medical evaluation of an elderly patient is complicated by several factors. First, a geriatric patient may suffer from more than one disease. In a random sampling of 200 persons over the age of 65 years, Williamson (5) found a mean of 3.26 significant lesions in men and 3.42 in women (6). In over 2200 autopsies in the age range of 65 to 84 years, Howell (6) found an average of 7.02 significant lesions. Therefore, physicians cannot be satisfied with having diagnosed just one disease. A comprehensive search for additional problems must continue so that other diseases, if present, will be uncovered. Several diseases in the same person may have very different causes, but they will interact and affect the medical treatment, the prognosis, and the rehabilitation potential. Second, advancing age changes the response to disease. Pain, diagnostic for many diseases in the young, may be minimal or absent in the very old. Inflammatory disease or perforation of a viscus may produce little or no pain. A myocardial infarction may be painless and become manifest only by a circulatory collapse. Infections may not be suspected in a prostrate elderly patient because fever or leukocytosis may not be present.

Medical History

Taking the history of a geriatric patient may present a number of difficulties. If the patient is hard of hearing, effective communication will be difficult. It becomes a particular problem if the patient tries to hide the hearing defect and guesses on a question that he or she has not clearly understood. Other obstacles are memory defects or a mild confusion, which may not be obvious on first contact. Third, patients may fail to report certain symptoms since they may pass them off as signs of aging and therefore not worth mentioning (7). Furthermore, taking the history is complicated because it covers many years and many medical problems, and many patients tend to stray from one event to another and then back again, making it very difficult to establish a chronologic disease-oriented account. Taking an accurate history may take a great deal of time. However, it is an important task that should not be delegated to untrained personnel.

The physician should start by asking for the chief complaint, the symptoms that brought the patient to the physician. Frequently, there are other more significant symptoms that need to be pursued in more detail. Some patients relate an insignificant chief complaint to the physician because they may not wish to admit to themselves that they may have a serious medical problem.

Many medical terms need to be clarified because they may have a different meaning to the patient than to the medical profession. Indigestion, for instance, may mean heartburn, chest pain, or nausea. Terms such as dizziness, fainting, insomnia, diarrhea, and constipation may have to be clarified by a careful, detailed description. It is also important to determine what brings on certain symptoms, when a symptom first appeared, and what the patient does to obtain relief.

The past medical history needs to be explored with particular emphasis on diseases that may have left chronic sequelae or partial disabilities. When past events are investigated, memory defects may become a particularly serious impediment. In this case, family members need to be consulted, and old medical records may need to be reviewed.

The physician needs to gather information on all of the medication in use, whether medically prescribed or purchased over the counter. Many patients have difficulties remembering the names of drugs. In that case they should be asked to bring all their current medications with them for every office visit. Patients should be asked about the use of tobacco and about alcohol consumption now or in the past.

Nutritional deficiencies are common in the elderly. The physician should inquire about the patient's appetite, but the answers may be misleading because very often the patient is not aware that appetite and food intake are poor. The questions for this reason must be specific: what do you eat for breakfast, for lunch, for dinner? Specific questions will reveal if there is an adequate consumption of fruit, vegetables, proteins, and bulk. Understanding family members will be helpful in obtaining the correct information and remedying deficiencies. (See Chapter 6.) The history must also include salient social facts. A recent social decline may have a profound effect on the patient's physical well-being. A loss of a job or retirement causing a marked change of the daily routine, a recent change of the dwelling place, the death of a family member or close friend, or tension between patient and children may all cause depression and have a negative impact on the patient's well-being. Patients may find it difficult to discuss these problems; they have to be brought to light through tactful questioning.

Physical Examination and Laboratory Results

The physical examination of the elderly patient should be complete and thorough. In many aspects it does not differ from examinations performed on younger individuals. However, some important points need to be stressed (8).

The skin should be examined for excessive dryness, scratch marks, bruises, and petechiae. Patients who are rather immobile need to be examined for pressure marks or ulcers over weight-bearing areas.

Examination of the tongue and oral mucosa will give some clues about the state of nutrition and hydration. The condition of teeth and dentures needs to be assessed since poor mastication will contribute to nutritional deficiencies.

The neck is palpated for thyroid enlargement and nodules. The presence of lymph nodes should be noted. The carotid arteries are examined for bruits and excessive tortuosity. Female breasts should be examined, and mammograms should be done once a year.

The configuration of the chest should be noted. A significant anterior enlargement may be due to diminished elasticity of the costal cartilages. However, it does not as such indicate the presence of chronic obstructive pulmonary disease. The mobility of the diaphragm, as estimated by percussion in inspiration and expiration, should be noted. Fine rales over the bases of the lungs that disappear on coughing may indicate atelectases. In contrast, fine rales that appear after coughing indicate pulmonary congestion or infiltration of lung parenchyma by infection or other causes. Auscultation of the heart should be done both in sitting and supine position. In many elderly patients, systolic murmurs will be present over the aortic valve area. If the murmur peaks early and is not louder than 2/6, it is most likely caused by sclerotic changes of the aortic valvular ring and not clinically significant. Murmurs caused by aortic stenosis are louder and may be transmitted to the carotids. The second aortic sound may be diminished or absent in true stenosis of the aortic valve.

The abdomen is examined for masses, enlarged liver or spleen, and for areas of tenderness. The physician should palpate the abdominal aorta for an aneurysm. Aneurysms are usually larger than 3 cm and pulsate in the lateral direction as well as anteriorly. The diagnosis can be confirmed by an ultrasound examination. Aneurysms 6 cm wide or wider need to be evaluated by a vascular surgeon since they are at risk of rupture.

A rectal examination should be done on all males either with the patient standing or lying on his left side so that the prostate can be palpated. An enlarged, hard prostate or stony hard nodules suggest a malignancy and require further evaluation. (See Chapter 25.) Women should have a gynecologic examination once a year.

An examination of the lower extremities should include an evaluation of the arterial circulation. The femoral, popliteal, and pedal arteries are easily palpated. If no pulses can be felt in either of the two pedal arteries, a Doppler ultrasound examination should be performed. Attention must be given to discoloration of the skin and to atrophy of skin and nails indicating a chronically deficient arterial circulation. Usually the feet will feel cool to the touch, and the toes will blanch when the leg is elevated. (See Chapter 15.)

It is estimated that 30% to 40% of all initial visits by elderly patients to a physician's office are made because of musculoskeletal symptoms. For this reason, the examination must include an assessment of bones and joints. The extremities are examined for joint tenderness, tightness, and true loss of range of motion, with or without pain. The muscular system is assessed for weakness, spasticity, or atrophy. The spine is examined for deviations from the normal contour: abnormal lateral curvatures, an increase of kyphosis in the thoracic spine, and a decrease of the normal lordotic lumbosacral curve. Range of motion is checked in all segments of the spine, and deviations from normal are measured and noted. In elderly persons the cervical spine requires special attention since cervical spondylosis is a common and painful affliction. It may be the cause not only of neck pain but also of occipital headaches and pain and numbness in the arms.

A neurologic examination should be done on all patients who exhibit neurologic symptoms. On others, a screening examination may suffice. This includes an evaluation of speech and cognitive status. Deficits may have become obvious during the taking of the history. The extremities are tested for loss of muscle strength, tremors, spasticity, and rigidity. A sensory examination is done for touch and pinprick. Vibratory perception is tested over the ankle malleoli or big toes. Tendon reflexes are tested. It should be noted that ankle jerks may be unobtainable in the very old and that vibratory perception may be diminished or absent (9). Much of the screening can be done by assessing simple functions. The patient is observed while getting on and off the examination table. Gait abnormalities should be noted. (See Chapter 20.) The patient should be asked to stand on toes, heels, and one leg at a time. Patients should be able to get up from a firm chair with the arms folded across the chest. They should be able to hold the arms extended forward with the eyes closed. Significant abnormalities noted at the screening examination will require a more detailed evaluation (10).

Geriatric patients should be seen by an ophthalmologist once a year. They should be checked for glaucoma, cataracts, and retinal lesions.

Laboratory examinations should include a complete blood count, a blood sugar taken fasting or 2 hours after a meal, blood urea nitrogen, serum creatinine, cholesterol, and high and low density lipoproteins and triglycerides, if indicated. If the patient is known or suspected to have diabetes mellitus, a glycated hemoglobin determination will provide information on the state of the diabetic control over the preceding 8 to 12 weeks. More recently, the determination of serum fructosamine, a glycated amino acid has been recommended. It is easier to do than the glycated hemoglobin test and less expensive. It gives approximate information on the diabetic control over the preceding 2 to 3 weeks (11).

In males, a Prostate Specific Antigen test (PSA) should be done at least once as a baseline. It should be repeated if the patient develops symptoms of prostatism or if the gland appears enlarged and hard on rectal examination.

Geriatric patients should have at least one recent electrocardiogram in their record to serve as baseline if they should develop cardiac symptoms. Chest radiograms should be done at the physician's discretion, especially in heavy smokers. Asymptomatic lung cancers are discovered by such an examination in a phase when they will still respond to active therapy.

COMMON SYNDROMES

Elderly persons frequently seek medical care for complaints that are not specific to any one diagnostic category. These syndromes may be quite incapacitating; for this reason they require careful diagnostic attention.

Fatigue and Weakness

A sudden onset of fatigue and weakness in an older, usually vigorous individual may suggest an acute illness. In the very old and particularly in diabetics, a myocardial infarction may be painless, and extreme weakness, sometimes with syncope, may be its only manifestation. Other causes of extreme weakness of sudden onset may be anemia caused by occult blood loss or hemolysis, infections with little or no fever or other striking symptoms, "small strokes" without neurologic deficits, or adverse drug reactions.

A gradual and poorly defined onset of chronic fatigue requires a different approach. It may be the result of several causes such as anemia of various origins, congestive heart failure with reduced cardiac output, or hypoxia due to pulmonary disease. Another common cause is the excessive use of sedatives and particularly of hypnotics. Many old persons believe that they do not get enough sleep, but further investigation may show that their time asleep is quite adequate. Many hypnotics in common use are eliminated slowly and are responsible for daytime fatigue. Barbiturates are known to be poorly tolerated by the aged. Benzodiazepines are fat-soluble drugs, and, since in the elderly there is a relative increase of fat tissue, the volume of distribution of these medications is increased. This results in a prolongation of their half-life and an accumulation in the body. Some of the benzodiazepines have metabolites with the same sedative action as the parent drug. They also have a longer half-life resulting in an accumulation of the drug in the tissues and an ever increasing drowsiness and fatigue. This had been a common side effect of flurazepam (Dalmane) until its cause was recognized and the recommended nighttime dosage reduced.

Disorders of thyroid function must also be considered in elderly patients who complain of fatigue. Hypothyroidism is more common in the aged than is thyrotoxicosis. Hypothyroidism may have an insidious onset with mental and physical slowing, followed by cold intolerance, dry skin, and weight gain. An early diagnosis can be made by an increase of the thyroid-stimulating hormone level (TSH). In this fashion, the patient can be treated before all of the other signs and symptoms have become manifest.

An elderly thyrotoxic patient may not exhibit the abnormal hyperactivity seen in younger patients. To the contrary, the patient may be apathetic, and the condition is frequently misdiagnosed as old age depression. For details see Chapter 5.

If no abnormal physical findings are present, the cause of fatigue may be psychologic. The patient may be depressed or simply bored and seek refuge in frequent daytime naps. Some elderly people believe that their age requires a great deal of rest, and they increasingly cut down on activities. The physician, however, should encourage regular activities, preferably out of the patient's home, increased socialization, and the pursuit of old and new interests.

Muscular weakness must be distinguished from fatigue even though the patient may use these terms interchangeably. Muscle strength declines with old age but usually not to the point of seriously interfering with common day-to-day activities (12). Recent investigations have suggested that the muscle weakness of the very old and frail may be due to disuse and immobility rather than to a truly degenerative process. It has also been shown that even in the very old and very frail, muscles can be strengthened by a judicious and suitable exercise program (13). The small hand muscles become atrophic with a moderate weakening of the grip. Functionally more important is the common weakness of the pelvic girdle muscles making it difficult for the patient to get up from a chair without help. It also makes for an awkward and insecure gait and is responsible for falls. Weakness of the shoulder will make it difficult for patients to elevate the arms and to work on a high shelf.

It is obviously important to consider and rule out neurogenic or myogenic disease before any exercise program is started. Dermatomyositis/polymyositis is a disease of advancing years. It is frequently associated with malignancies especially in males. The weakness is predominantly in the proximal muscles.

Certain drugs may be responsible for muscle weakness. Corticosteroids if taken for an extended period of time are common offenders. Diuretics that may have caused hypokalemia may be responsible for muscle weakness. Other disorders that may give rise to muscular weakness are hypothyroidism and hyperthyroidism, hypercalcemia of any cause, and diabetic amyotrophy.

Objective muscle testing, repeated from time to time, is essential so improvement or deterioration can be monitored. Often this is not easy since muscle tests require the patient's cooperation. Functional testing such as having the patients hold their arms extended in front of them, arising from a chair, or stepping on and off a stool may be quite informative.

Dizziness

Dizziness is a common symptom that makes elderly patients seek medical care. Diagnosis and therapy may be vexing problems because objective findings may be absent, and the obtainable history may be vague. The physician needs to establish first what the patient means by dizziness. All too often, the patient's perception differs from the medical interpretation. A precise description of the symptoms remains the physician's primary and most valuable tool.

In 1989, Sloane and Baloh (14) published a report that established symptomatic categories and related them to the diagnoses of the underlying pathologies. This report was based on the study of 116 patients, 70 years of age or older. Forty-two percent presented with true vertigo, described as "an illusion of movement, usually of spinning." Dysequilibrium, described as a feeling of imbalance, was encountered in 28% of all cases. Both vertigo and dysequilibrium were reported in a small number of cases. Presyncopal lightheadedness was encountered in 13%. The remaining 17% were classified as "other." A subclassification of vertigo was "benign postural vertigo" (BPV). About one half of all vertigo cases fell into this category. Attacks of BPV are brought on by abrupt changes of position such as turning over in bed or coming up quickly from a supine position. These episodes generally last less than one minute and their frequency varies.

Two major diagnostic categories were established based on the anatomic location of the lesion: peripheral vestibular disorders and cerebrovascular disorders. The syndrome of benign positional vertigo made up 50% of the peripheral vestibular disorders. Patients with cerebrovascular disorders may exhibit all of the symptoms previously described. The lesion is almost always located in the posterior brain, usually in the vertebrobasilar circulation. Patients suffering from cerebrovascular dizziness are usually older. The symptoms can be quite variable. They are often associated with other abnormal signs characteristic of posterior circulation disorders. Fairly common are transient ischemic attacks (TIA) presenting with vertigo and lasting from a few minutes to a few hours. Other transient neurologic deficits within the posterior cerebral location are usually present. They include gait abnormalities, truncal ataxia, and a positive Romberg sign. Valuable diagnostic tests are electronystagmography, audiometry, and caloric or rotational testing of the vestibular response.

Some drugs, such as salicylates if taken in large dosages, quinidine, and phenytoin, may cause dizziness.

Headache

Migraine headaches usually disappear as the sufferer reaches old age. Only occasionally does one encounter an elderly patient who still has typical attacks of migraine. Occipital headaches may be caused by osteoarthritic changes in the cervical spine. Hypertension and vascular lesions may also be the cause of headaches.

Giant cell arteritis of the temporal arteries may be associated with severe throbbing headaches. It is a disease of middle or old age, and it needs to be considered in the differential diagnosis of headache with sudden onset. Tender and hardened arteries can often be palpated in the temporal area. The eyegrounds may show retinal hemorrhages and beginning optic atrophy. An important diagnostic sign is a markedly elevated erythrocyte sedimentation rate. An early diagnosis is mandatory and may need to include a biopsy of the temporal artery. It is very important to start treatment with adrenocortical steroids as soon as possible in order to prevent further deterioration of the eyesight.

Syncope

The physician is rarely present to witness a syncopal attack. The patient will usually not be able to contribute much information, and bystanders may be too excited to provide worthwhile observations.

This section will only discuss attacks of fainting from which the patient recovers fairly promptly without neurologic sequelae. Transient ischemic attacks do not fall into this category, since by definition they leave the patient with a temporary neurologic deficit. Many of the syncopal attacks in the elderly are due to atherosclerotic changes with narrowing of the major cerebral arteries or their branches. The circulation in the internal carotids can be further impaired by hyperextension of the neck such as when working on high shelves. Some elderly men complain that they become dizzy and faint when shaving. Cardiac disorders are common causes of fainting. It may be the only symptom of a myocardial infarction that had presented without pain. Dysrhythmias with an excessively rapid heart rate or a heart block with bradycardia are occasional causes. Gastrointestinal hemorrhages may be associated with fainting before the appearance of bloody or tarry stools provide a definite diagnosis. In diabetics on insulin a precipitous drop of the blood sugar may cause loss of consciousness. Epileptic seizures in the aged may be due to an idiopathic epilepsy that may have produced only a few attacks in a lifetime. Seizures that appear for the first time in old age may be due to a vascular lesion, a tumor, or subdural hematoma. Hyperventilation with alkalosis and tetany may cause fainting. It is a functional disorder that can occur in all age groups and may affect elderly men and women.

Depending on the cause, therapeutic management may have a considerable preventive value. However, if the attacks are too frequent, it may become inadvisable for the patient to continue living alone.

Orthostatic Hypotension

Orthostatic hypotension is defined as the drop of the systolic blood pressure by at least 20 mm Hg upon rising from a supine to an upright position, either to standing or sitting, and remaining in this position for 1 to 3 minutes. It is a common condition among the geriatric population. It may be caused by a variety of medical problems, one of which is heart disease, particularly when associated with reduced cardiac output. Orthostatic hypotension may be caused by blood loss or anemia of other causes, decreased blood volume due to dehydration in frail elderly persons, diabetes, and nutritional deficiencies with neuropathy. Central nervous system diseases with accompanying orthostatic hypotension are Parkinson's disease, Shy-Drager syndrome, brainstem and spinal cord lesions, and multiple cerebral infarcts. Medications that may precipitate orthostatic hypotension are phenothiazines, benzodiazepines, diuretics, antihypertensives, and levodopa.

Typical symptoms include lightheadedness when arising from a supine position, at times associated with vertigo. Syncope may occur, often leading to a disastrous fall. In otherwise healthy persons, orthostatic hypotension may be almost asymptomatic and be discovered only if the patient is specifically examined for postural blood pressure changes. Recent studies found the prevalence of orthostatic hypotension in normotensive elderly subjects to be less than 7% (15).

In the past, the cause of orthostatic hypotension was thought to be a malfunction of the baroreceptors located in the carotid sinus and the aortic arch. However, recently, investigators have found the pathophysiologic mechanism to be more complex. They also have discovered a paradoxical relationship of systolic hypertension in the aged to orthostatic hypotension (16, 17).

When an individual rapidly assumes an upright position after having been recumbent for some time, there is a shift of 500 mL to 700 mL of venous blood to the lower part of the body. This results in a decrease of venous return to the heart and thereby a reduction of the diastolic filling of the ventricles and the cardiac output. This inactivates the baroreceptors whose usual function is to lower the blood pressure when it has risen to high levels. In orthostatic hypotension there is the reverse effect. The inactivation of the baroreceptors causes a reflex stimulation of the sympathetic nervous system in the attempt to raise the blood pressure. This mechanism is quite effective in younger persons and in the well elderly. It may fail, however, in the presence of acute medical problems and in serious chronic circulatory dysfunction. It is noteworthy in this connection that sustained blood pressure elevations blunt the sensitivity of the baroreceptors. This explains why orthostatic hypotension can be a common complication of isolated systolic hypertension in the aged (16, 17).

The clinical correlation between these two conditions has been demonstrated by a large multicenter epidemiologic study, entitled "Systolic Hypertension in the Elderly Program" or SHEP (15). This study identified 4736 men and women, 60 years of age and older with isolated systolic hypertension. The subjects had resting systolic pressures of 160 mm Hg or above with a diastolic pressure of 90 mm Hg or below. The SHEP study found a prevalence of 17% of orthostatic hypotension, or 817 cases in their cohort of 4732 subjects with isolated systolic hypertension.

Another causal mechanism for the development of both systolic hypertension and secondarily of orthostatic hypotension is the increased rigidity of the aorta and other large arteries caused by the replacement of elastin in the arterial wall by collagen. The rigidity decreases the elastic recoil of the aorta during systole and thereby causes an elevation of the systolic blood pressure, an increased pulse wave velocity, and eventually a stiffness and thickening of the left ventricular wall. These structural changes in the heart and large arteries impair early and efficient ventricular filling. Enhanced contraction of the atria can still compensate for this impairment. However, a reduced venous return to the atria and to the ventricles when the patient is upright may reduce the cardiac output and result in a hypotensive episode (16).

In contrast to previously held opinions that isolated systolic hypertension is not harmful, the SHEP study indicates that the associated orthostatic hypotension may carry significant risks and that therapy may well be indicated.

Malnutrition and Anorexia

A sudden loss of appetite may be the presenting symptom of an acute illness such as an infection or congestive heart failure. Chronic diseases such as uremia, liver dysfunction, and malignancies may be accompanied by anorexia, often of insidious onset. Long-term anorexia may also be due to depression, but typical anorexia nervosa appears to be rare in old age. Poor eating habits with resulting chronic malnutrition may have developed earlier in life. They become more pronounced in old age when taste and smell sensations become blunted, taking away the pleasure of eating. Elderly people often do better with highly seasoned food. Nutritional needs and deficiencies are discussed in in Chapter 6.

Old persons may not be aware of their poor nutrition, and they may deny that there is a problem. A prescribed diet needs to be based on the patient's usual eating habits, and changes need to be made slowly so they will be accepted. The food should look appetizing. It should be served in reasonable amounts; a plate piled high with food may look discouraging to a person with poor appetite.

Alcoholism

A recent study has shown that moderate alcohol consumption reduces cardiovascular mortality in the middle-aged and aged (18). However, a study done by a Congressional Select Committee on Aging has revealed that nearly 2.5 million elderly Americans and one half of all nursing home residents suffer from alcohol-related problems. Among the elderly, the highest incidence of alcoholism is encountered in widowers above the age of 75 years. Late versus early-life onset of alcoholism has been studied recently (19, 20). The overall incidence of alcoholism declines with age even though new risk factors may develop. Alcoholics with late-life onset usually have serious psychologic problems such as the loss of a spouse or other family members and friends, loneliness, and changes in life-style and social circumstances. The alcohol problem is often not discovered until late because the patient may not wish to admit to his or her habit or may not even realize that he or she has developed a problem. Elderly men usually drink at home when alone and are not seen when intoxicated. Elderly women who live alone or are left alone at home much of a day may become alcoholics out of boredom and loneliness. They often become quite skillful in hiding their drinking habit.

Mental changes in elderly alcoholics are variable and hard to classify. Anxieties and phobias are common. The patients become forgetful, and their ability to concentrate diminishes. The differential diagnosis between alcoholic brain disorder and senile dementia of the Alzheimer type is difficult. Even computed tomography scans in patients with chronic alcohol-induced brain disease may closely resemble the changes seen in senile dementia of the Alzheimer type (21, 22).

The treatment of elderly alcoholics is complicated because of multiple physical disorders that may or may not be directly related to alcohol abuse. It has been established that these associated ailments, such as gastrointestinal disorders, liver disease, nutritional deficiencies, and neuropathies, must be treated as vigorously as alcoholism itself. Assessment and therapy in alcoholism of the elderly patient is a dual task in which internist and psychiatrist must cooperate (20).

Elderly persons have a reduced tolerance to alcohol as they do to other central nervous system depressant chemicals. Another serious complication is interaction with certain drugs. Several medications in the sedative or tranquilizer group, such as barbiturates, benzodiazepines, and propoxyphenes, are synergistic or additive with alcohol. The therapeutic effect of other drugs such as warfarin and tolbutamide are depressed by alcohol.

Treatment of alcoholism is difficult; it requires patience and the patient's cooperation. However, elderly alcoholics have a higher rate of success than do other age groups in shedding the alcohol habit once they have understood how damaging it is to their health and well-being.

ASSESSMENT OF PHYSICAL FUNCTION AND REHABILITATION POTENTIAL

Chronic disease and the disabilities caused by the disease process are the most common health problems of the aged. Chronic disease is not curable, but advances in medicine and surgery often succeed in keeping these disorders from seriously impairing the patient's life-style and in postponing the onset of late-life infirmity. Also, because of the remarkable progress of medical and surgical care, elderly patients now stand a good chance of surviving an acute illness or the acute complications of a chronic illness that might have been fatal decades earlier. However, all too often the price of survival is a disability that impairs function and threatens to deprive survivors of their independence. It is the mission of rehabilitation to minimize the loss of function and to keep the disability from becoming the cause of a social decline.

There is no firm and reliable correlation between the medical diagnosis and the severity of the resulting disability. Impairment and disability need to be evaluated separately by assessing the loss of function and independence in mobility and self-care.

The following sections will use the definitions of impairment, disability, and handicap as established by the World Health Organization in 1980 (23).

Impairment: Loss of abnormality of anatomic, physiologic or psychologic function. (Example: paralysis of one leg)

Disability: A restriction or lack of ability to perform an activity in the manner or within the range considered normal for a human being. (Example: unable to walk without mechanical aids)

Handicap: A disadvantage for a given individual, resulting from an impairment or disability, that limits or prevents the fulfillment of a role that is normal for the individual, considering age, sex and social and cultural factors. (Example: unable to return to his job as factory foreman)

In young or middle-aged subjects the assessment will have to be concerned not only with the patients' ability to care for themselves but also with the fulfillment of their occupational and social obligations. The assessment will be simpler for older individuals who have retired from their work. Their main concern will then be self-care and the maintenance of household duties. However, in the older disabled the task of assessing functional potentials may be made complicated by medical problems that may not permit strenuous rehabilitation activities.

Physical Medicine and Rehabilitation, a specialty dealing with physical disabilities, started developing methods of functional evaluation in the early 1950's. It became obvious that an assessment system needed to do more than just give a one-time record of the patient's functional status. If repeated in intervals, it would serve as a measure of the patient's progress and of the effectiveness of the rehabilitation program. This, in turn, would require a scoring system for the activities to be assessed. Furthermore, the evaluation instrument would need to be adapted to the population served since, for example, goals are different for elderly retired persons than for injured industrial workers. It soon turned out that no evaluation system was suitable for all rehabilitation services, and many institutions began to develop systems of their own. Feinstein (24), who searched the pertinent literature in 1986, found 43 indexes for evaluating activities of daily living, 15 which had been published in the preceding decade. It is clear that the multitude of assessment instruments makes communication with other rehabilitation professionals difficult.

It is not possible to describe the many assessment systems within the context of this chapter. Many of these systems have found use only in a limited number of rehabilitation facilities; they may differ from other instruments only by a few details needed to adapt to a particular patient population or to accommodate special interests of rehabilitation professionals. Readers who wish to study this topic in more detail are referred to a monograph by C. V. Granger and G. E. Gresham entitled "Functional Assessment in Rehabilitation Medicine" (25).

Pulses

Most assessment systems divide activities of daily living (ADL) into separate categories. For instance, Moskowitz and McCann developed an early assessment system called PULSES (26). In this system, P stands for general physical condition, U for function of upper extremities, L for function of lower extremities, S for sensory function, E for excretory function, and S for mental and emotional status. PULSES rates the various functions on a 4-grade scale. Grade 1 denotes normal function; grade 4 indicates the most severe impairment. Grades 2 and 3 are intermediate. Later rating systems have usually used the higher numbers to indicate the best performance and low numbers and 0 for the most severe impairments. Some investigators have divided the major categories into subcategories in order to be able to provide more details. Each subcategory is graded separately. The scores are averaged, and this average becomes the score for the major category. Thereafter, the point values of the functional categories are added, and the sum becomes the ADL score for the patient.

Kenny Self-care Evaluation

This system was used for the Kenny Self-Care Evaluation, developed by Schoening and coworkers at the Kenny Institute in 1965 (27, 28). This system has 19 major categories, and each category is subdivided into a variable number of subcategories. Each subcategory is rated on a scale of 0 to 4 depending on the level of independence with which the activity can be performed. The calculations are done as previously described. The value of the Kenny system lies in the separate scoring of subcategories and categories, thereby giving very detailed information on the patient's ADL performance. Schoening and his coworkers also emphasized that the Kenny Self-Care Evaluation can be used to quantitate nursing workload, which is in essence the reciprocal of the level of functional independence manifested by disabled patients. (27). Anderson used the Kenny System for the functional evaluation of stroke patients and found that it had a good predictive value with regard to future improvement (29).

Uniform Data System for Medical Rehabilitation

Granger and associates at the New York State University at Buffalo developed a system designed to document the severity of patient disabilities and to assess the outcome of medical rehabilitation. The system

was given the name "Uniform Data System for Medical Rehabilitation." Included was a procedure called "Functional Independence Measure" (FIM) to assess a patient's performance over time and the outcome of the rehabilitation program. FIM assesses 18 items dealing with self-care ability; sphincter control; mobility, including transfers, walking and wheelchair locomotion; communication, and social cognition. These items are graded on seven levels: 7 = Complete Independence, 6 = Modified Independence, 5 = Supervision or Setup, 4 = Minimal contact assistance; the patient does 76% to 99% of the effort, 3 = Moderate assistance; the patient requires some physical help but is able to do 50% to 75% of the effort, 2 = Maximal assistance; the patient does some ADL tasks but expends only 25% to 49% of the effort, and 1 = The patient is totally dependent in all aspects of ADL. (A copy of the "Guide for Use of the Uniform Data Set for Medical Rehabilitation" (and FIM) can be obtained by writing to the Buffalo General Hospital, State University of New York at Buffalo.)

One of the assets of the FIM is that the seven grades are clearly defined and set up separately for each ADL activity. There is some concern about the use of percentages in the delineation of the patient's active participation. These activities cannot be measured quantitatively, and there may be major discrepancies between institutions. The FIM system measures what the patient actually does and not what he or she could be expected to do considering medical diagnosis and impairment. The attending physician should, of course, try to determine the cause of any discrepancy between performance and reasonable expectations. The patient may be depressed or still too weak following an acute phase of his illness. In any case, the key of the FIM grading system is the degree of independence from assistance or supervision by another person.

The graded functions are disabilities not impairments. The Functional Independence Measure was intended to include only a minimum number of basic ADL functions that may underlie more complex activities. The system is not difficult to use. It is discipline-free, which means that it should be useful to geriatricians, neurologists, and rheumatologists, in addition to physiatrists (30).

Other ADL Evaluation Systems

Two other ADL evaluation systems need to be mentioned because they have taken a different approach from the ones previously discussed and because they have been used frequently in rehabilitation facilities; they are the Barthel Index and the Katz Index of ADL.

BARTHEL INDEX

The Barthel Index was first described in 1965 (31). It lists 10 ADL such as feeding, transfers, bathing, walking on level surface, ascending and descending steps, dressing, controlling bowels, controlling bladder, personal toilet (shave, clean teeth, comb hair, etc.), getting on and off the toilet. Each function is graded as 5, 10, or 15 points if done independently. If done only with help, it will usually be graded with 5 points less. An activity that could not be done at all is scored as 0. A person who could perform all the listed activities independently would have a score of 100. The point values attached to each activity are somewhat arbitrary. Granger adapted the Barthel Index for a comprehensive study of stroke patients; he also used it in comparison with the PULSES system (32). Granger found both systems useful in a study of over 300 severely disabled patients in 10 different institutions. He also noted that interrater variations were minimal.

KATZ INDEX

The Katz Index of ADL was developed by Sidney Katz and associates working with elderly women who were recovering from hip fractures at the Benjamin Rose Hospital in Cleveland (33). The patients were assigned to one of seven groups:

A. Independent in feeding, continence, transferring, going to toilet, dressing, and bathing.
B. Independent in all but one of these functions.
C. Independent in all but bathing and one additional function.
D. Independent in all but bathing, dressing, and one additional function.
E. Independent in all but bathing, dressing, going to toilet, and one additional function.
F. Independent in all but bathing, dressing, going to toilet, transferring, and one additional function.
G. Dependent in all six functions.

The scoring is based solely on the patient's independence in performing a function. Independent in this case means that it has to be done without assistance of any type and without supervision.

The Katz Index has raised a number of interesting theoretical points. The various activities from Group C on down are arranged in a hierarchial order. By this order, bathing is the most difficult activity, first lost and the last to recover. This is followed by dressing, then by going to toilet and then by transferring. Katz concluded that there is a definite order by which certain functions are lost and then regained as the patient recovers. There are questions about the validity of this premise. Katz has used an additional category of "Other" for patients whose functions do not fall into the hierarchial order that he had established. It is encouraging that out of Katz' original group of 1001 patients only 41 or 4% had to be classified as "Other" (25). Another advantage of the Katz

Index is that it does not use an arbitrary assignment of point values to given activities. The Katz Index has not included walking as an evaluated activity. However, Katz did his original study on patients recovering from hip fractures, and these subjects were at that time unable or not permitted to walk. Investigators who have since used the Katz Index have added ambulation as fully independent, partially independent (with mechanical aids or human assistance), or unable to walk.

The Katz Index can be used to assess improvement or deterioration of a patient's functional ability. If a function is lost or if a function returns, the patient can be easily demoted to a lower class or promoted to a higher one.

The Katz Index has been popular and used in many research studies. It has attracted clinical investigators who do not like the arbitrary assignment of points to given activities as in the Barthel Index. Donaldson (34) and Gresham (35) did studies comparing the sensitivity of the Barthel Index, the Katz Index, and the Kenny Self-Care Evaluation. They found the Kenny Evaluation to be the most sensitive to subtle changes and the Katz Index the least sensitive. In follow-up studies, the three indexes moved in parallel. The difference in sensitivity was small, indicating that essentially one system is as good as the other.

Instrumental Activities of Daily Living

For many individuals, additional and more complex activities need to be assessed. These are persons who live in the community and are independent in self-care. These activities have been named Instrumental Activities of Daily Living; they are vital for maintaining normal functions in the family and community. The individuals are tested for their competence in keeping their dwelling in order, either by doing the work themselves or by supervising others to do it for them. Included are activities such as cleaning, preparing meals, laundry, shopping, using the telephone, taking their medications, and managing money.

Information is obtained by interviewing the individual; at times a member of the family or a friend needs to be interviewed as well (36, 37). The individual's social life and his or her participation in out-of-the-home activities need to be assessed. Often a change in the person's life-style may be the first sign of a physical or mental decline. An elderly individual who no longer goes to concerts, theater, or church or who has become reluctant to visit friends or accept invitations is heading for some type of trouble. The interviewing of friends will be helpful in this regard since the elderly person may not admit to a change or may make light of it. The cause can be physical or psychologic. Early recognition is important so remedial steps can be taken.

Since functional assessments have become frequently used tools in rehabilitation, a number of papers have been published that take issue with the statistical methods used and with conclusions drawn from the data. An early paper was published in 1962 by two psychologists, Kelman and Willner, who had used various assessment procedures while studying populations in nursing homes (38). From this experience, they concluded that there was a lack of standardization of outcome criteria and of methods of measurement. They felt that the data collection was often unreliable because different examiners would obtain different information from the same patient, often depending on the patient's mood and his or her perception of the examiner's role and motivation in asking so many personal questions. This problem should be familiar to practicing physicians, but obviously it is quite disruptive when collecting material for a scientific study. The authors discussed many more procedural errors that they had encountered and delineated the way to make data collection and utilization more reliable. Kelman and Willner's paper has presented the theoretical and scientific standards on which functional assessment procedures have been built at that early phase and for years thereafter.

In 1986, Feinstein published a paper entitled "Scientific and Clinical Problems in Indexes of Functional Disability" (24). Feinstein, as previously mentioned, had searched the literature and had found 43 papers describing new indexes for rating self-care activities. He found several defects in the indexes that impaired the quality of data collection and data assessment. The most serious flaw was the failure to consider the patient's effort in the performance of a given activity. For instance, a cardiac patient may have chest pain when quickly climbing a flight of stairs to the second floor of his home. When he or she does it very slowly, there is no pain. The magnitude of the task has remained the same, but by reducing the speed the patient's effort is diminished and the activity can now be performed without adverse effects. Most rating systems do not take effort and speed of performance into consideration.

Most assessment systems rate an ADL activity by the level of independence at which the task is performed. This came about when various investigators found that the dependence-independence scale allows for fairly precise measurements. It gives no consideration, however, to the effort that the patient must make to initiate the task and the speed and ease with which it is performed. As an example, a patient who dresses without help from anyone will have a top score in the dressing category. However, difficulties in putting on shoes and socks may unduly prolong the time and tire him. If his wife puts on the shoes and socks, he will be no longer independent in dressing. Her assistance will save the patient time and effort, but his independence score will be decreased. Feinstein found only one paper, published in 1973, that included self-initiation and speed in its grad-

ing system (39). However, the inclusions made the calculations unduly complicated for routine clinical use.

A second deficiency cited by Feinstein is the failure to take the patient's wishes and personal rehabilitation goals into account. A woman recovering from a stroke may not be interested in arts and crafts training since she had done very little of it during earlier years. Her main interest may be to cook and bake and to experiment with new dishes. Physicians and therapists need to investigate the patient's interests during the initial assessment period and before a definite program has been put into effect. If emphasis is given to the patient's goals, good cooperation will be obtained. An apparently poor motivation may simply be a sign that the rehabilitation program does not meet the patient's interests and accustomed activities.

Most indexes are quite effective in assessing a patient's performance at a given point of time, but as Feinstein has pointed out they are not sensitive enough to discern changes over a span of time. Yet physicians and therapists need a measure to indicate if the patient is progressing or regressing. In some indexes the rating scale may be too coarse for the detection of subtle changes. Feinstein suggested that the best approach would be to construct "indexes of transition" to record the progress of single activities, functions, or symptoms whenever this appears desirable. Orthopedists, physiatrists, and therapists have for many decades used manual muscle strength testing for this purpose. In recent years, Mahler and associates have developed a transition index system for dyspnea (40), which appears to be quite effective. The system could be easily adapted for other symptoms or functions.

The growth of geriatrics as a clinical and academic field has created a great deal of interest in assessment tools to be used in the care of the elderly. The literature on this topic has become quite voluminous. The procedures used for the assessment of function of the elderly differ considerably from those used for the younger disabled rehabilitation patient. The elderly often suffer from various pathologic processes. The resulting impairments and disabilities may greatly differ from one patient to the other and for this reason require a careful analytic approach.

Geriatricians who have given a great deal of time and thought to this problem have concluded that the most accurate assessment can be done with elderly patients while temporarily hospitalized in a Geriatric Evaluation and Management (GEM) unit (41). Applegate and others (42) recommend that patients be "targeted" before admission to such a unit. This means that the patients should undergo a preliminary evaluation so that those who are too good and those who are too frail and ill will not be admitted. The GEM units are most effective if the evaluation is done by a team of physicians, therapists, and nurses who will be later involved in the rehabilitation of the patient. Applegate reports that only 20% of the patients who had been in a GEM unit needed posthospital institutional care, compared to 38% of those who were discharged from a general medical floor of the same hospital. The results for patients treated in an outpatient GEM unit were less favorable. Benefits of having elderly patients in a GEM unit included better medical diagnoses, more suitable posthospital placements, and an improved functional status.

Assessment programs should be carefully described, including the methods used, the types of patients who were assessed and also who did the assessing. Cohen (43) has recommended repetition of the most positive and best designed studies so results can be verified before they are disseminated.

Geriatric assessment indexes include evaluations of ADL, instrumental ADL, cognitive function, nutrition, and social functions. The emphasis varies with the investigator's main interest. Musculoskeletal functions are often assessed as well. They are the least satisfactory parts of the geriatric indexes. Some of the screening tests proposed are faulty and suggest an inadequate knowledge of muscle function and kinesiology. The authors would have benefited from reviewing the literature on this topic in the Physical Medicine and Rehabilitation literature, a specialty which has had more than 40 years of experience in this field, or they could have asked a physiatrist for assistance.

Recommendations

Functional assessments cannot be strictly quantitative because, unlike laboratory data, the activities, functions, and symptoms are not measurable in numbers. Even the most sophisticated statistical methods cannot correct for this inherent flaw. Investigators who are designing new indexes of functional evaluation should accept this limitation and not strive for mathematical perfection.

Grades of rating scales should be clearly defined and described. Different functional categories, for instance "dressing" and "bathing," need different grade descriptions for the rating scale. Independence for bathing needs to be defined differently than for dressing. This has been very effectively done in the FIM method. Assessment systems may require consultations with specialists in the respective fields.

Professionals who wish to set up a new index should first review the literature. There may be well-established and verified indexes that with slight modifications would satisfy the needs of the investigator. Whenever possible, functions should be tested at the involved body part itself and not at remote sites. In patients who tend to lose their balance and have fallen as a result, coordination should be assessed by examining the legs for ataxia, poor proprioception, and poor coordination instead of doing a paper and pencil test such as having the patient connect small numbered circles in numerical order and in a set period of time. The statistical correlation of this test with coordination tests of the lower extremities may be satisfactory. However, we are dealing with aging individuals, and many functions may have become somewhat deficient over time. This does not mean that there is a joint causal relationship from one to the other.

Timed testing should usually be avoided. Elderly patients may not do as well because the pressure of timing will make them nervous. Furthermore, elderly persons slow down in all their activities and, unless the slowing is excessive, it will interfere little with function. Only if an excessive amount of time is consumed in dressing or eating a meal may some corrective action be needed.

In conclusion, assessing a disabled patient and grading his or her performance of usual daily tasks should not be the only criterion for the admission to a rehabilitation program. Past medical history, current medical condition, and psychosocial status have to be considered carefully. It is important to remember that in the very old the learning capacity is often diminished. If a patient will not recall tomorrow what he or she learned today, he or she will not do well in a rehabilitation program.

REHABILITATION PROGRAM

This section will be limited to a discussion of the general aspects of geriatric rehabilitation. Assessment and rehabilitation planning for specific disabilities are covered in the various chapters in which these disabilities are discussed.

Patient Education

It is important to acquaint patients and families with the concept of rehabilitation as early as possible. They need to understand that with appropriate care some of the impaired functions may recover. They must also realize that uninvolved parts of the body can be trained to take over lost functions. It should be pointed out, as an example, that patients with a stroke and right-sided paralysis can be taught to write, type, and perform many other skilled activities with the left hand. Rehabilitation personnel should show a realistic but positive and hopeful attitude at all times.

Rehabilitation should be initiated early, and from the beginning it should be part of the overall medical program. Patients should be positioned properly and turned frequently to prevent skin breakdown. Rehabilitative measures that do not require much of the patient's active participation should be started within the first few days. Paralyzed limbs should be exercised early and splinted if necessary before contractures develop. Rehabilitation is not the third phase of medicine. It should be started early before prolonged immobilization has caused secondary complications.

This principle also applies to the care of the ambulatory elderly outpatient. It is estimated that approximately 35% to 40% of geriatric patients who seek medical attention do so because of musculoskeletal problems. These patients should have an early and thorough evaluation and receive preventive care in order to at least delay the onset of a more serious disability.

These examples show that there are significant preventive aspects to rehabilitation even though this application does not meet the dictionary definition of the word rehabilitation. It is important to emphasize this point in order to repudiate the previously held opinion that rehabilitation is prescribed as an afterthought when nothing else worthwhile can be done.

Rehabilitation Departments

The organization of patient care in institutional rehabilitation departments differs considerably from that of any other hospital department. The main difference is the use of a multidisciplinary team, an arrangement that is unique to rehabilitation medicine. Disabled patients require the one-to-one attention of different professionals such as physical, occupational, and speech therapists; nurses; psychologists, and social workers, all educated and certified in their fields of expertise. These professional health care specialists spend a great deal of time with individual patients and train them in the skills they must acquire. Obviously not every patient needs care from all of the team members, but many of them do. Each patient is discussed at a team conference once every week or two. The team members report to the physiatrist, the physician specialist in rehabilitation medicine, and to each other. The observations and opinions of the team members are taken into serious consideration for the future planning of the patient's program.

The physiatrist is the primary physician of patients hospitalized in a Rehabilitation Department. His or her function is to examine the patient, evaluate functional ability, and write the prescriptions for therapy. He or she must be the responsible coordinator of the patient's care. In many situations it will be necessary to have other physicians from different specialties in attendance as well. They will serve as consultants to the physiatrist; if the patient becomes seriously ill, the consultant will assume the role of the primary physician and, if necessary, transfer the patient to his or her service. The easy cooperation between specialties may be most important for elderly rehabilitation patients whose primary illness may not yet be under full control.

Rehabilitation as a specialty has found a slow acceptance by the medical profession. The multidisciplinary team structure was strange to the practicing physician who was accustomed to giving orders to nurses and seeing them carried out without discussion or formal conferences. The concepts that partial function could be restored to many paralyzed limbs and that patients could be taught to compensate for lost functions by substituting with other parts of the body seemed strange and unrealistic. Some physicians equate physical therapy with rehabilitation. This is a regrettable misconception. Physical therapy is a very important component of rehabilitation, but elderly disabled patients needs a full program to teach them to care for their personal needs as best as possible, to improve their communication by speech therapy if needed, to retrain bowel and bladder function, and to counteract discouragement and depression. A corollary to this misconception is the often expressed opinion, now supported by insurance companies, that elderly patients with stroke need not be in a rehabilitation center but could as well be taken care of in a nursing home. Many nursing homes have physical therapists, but they usually work part-time and are unable to give the individual patients the amount of time that they need. Very few homes have occupational therapists. Only a few nurses in nursing homes have had training in rehabilitation nursing, and their time is usually filled with the difficult and time-consuming care of frail and ill nursing home patients.

Another opinion frequently expressed is that the life expectancy of stroke patients is very short and that an expensive rehabilitation program is not cost-effective. This opinion is not supported by statistical data. Baker and associates (44) reported that 62% of 420 patients had survived to the seventh year after stroke. In 1973–1974 Anderson et al (29) studied 216 stroke patients who had been in the rehabilitation department between 1960 and 1970. Of these, 109 patients had died; 107 had survived, but only 79 (36.5% of the total population of 216) were available for study. The survival time of these patients ranged from 5 years to more than 15 years. Fifty percent were still alive 15 years after the stroke. Ford and Katz (45), who made an extensive search of the medical literature on the prognosis of stroke patients, found that the average survival after a stroke at the end of 5 years averaged 42%. All of these studies had been done on patients with stroke due to cerebral infarction.

A recent study by Fitzgerald et al (46) on hip fracture patients demonstrated the importance of an adequate rehabilitation program in the care of elderly disabled patients. The authors were specifically interested in the effect of the prospective payment system (PPS) of Medicare, which was enacted on January 1, 1984. The purpose of this system was to reduce the length of hospitalization of Medicare patients. The study was done on 338 patients with hip fracture, all managed in the same hospital. Of these, 149 patients were treated before implementation of the PPS, 189 after implementation. Before the implementation of PPS, hip fracture patients received intensive physical therapy and gait training in the hospital through the department of orthopedic surgery. After PPS implementation, they were discharged from the hospital earlier. The mean duration of hospital stay postimplementation of PPS was 12.6 days compared to 21.9 days before. The number of physical therapy sessions in the hospital decreased from 7.6 to 6.3 sessions. The average distance patients could walk at the time of discharge decreased from 28 m to 11 m. The confinement of hip fracture patients to nursing homes at the time of hospital discharge rose postimplementation from 38% to 60%. More importantly, the proportion of patients still in nursing homes one year later rose from 9% to 33% after PPS implementation. A subgroup of patients who were free of any coexisting conditions or complications showed similar results. It is clear that the outcome of care for hip fracture patients became worse after the implementation of PPS by Medicare. It appears that the discharge from the hospital occurred before the patients had received full benefits from physical therapy and that nursing home physical therapy was not adequate to restore satisfactory ambulation.

In general, recently disabled patients and, particularly, elderly patients need a certain length of time to adapt emotionally to their disability and to accept the need for rehabilitation. If rushed through an initial program without given time for this adaptation, they will not cooperate. They will not follow through with exercises they were asked to do at home, and they will not keep appointments for outpatient therapy. Patients need to have participated in rehabilitation activities for a reasonable period of time before they will appreciate their importance.

SCIENTIFIC ASPECTS OF REHABILITATION

Rehabilitation has greatly benefited from the progress in basic medical sciences that has taken place over the last few decades. When rehabilitation first became a medical specialty, many of the therapeutic modalities were applied more or less empirically. As the physiologic effects of heat, cold, and electricity were investigated, these modalities became better understood and were more appropriately applied. A great deal of progress has been made in neurophysiology, muscle function, and exercise physiology. These advances have provided physicians and therapists with a better understanding of normal and abnormal mobility of the human body. The result has been more effective methods designed to improve muscle strength, neuromuscular coordination, and the prevention and management of contractures and stiffness. We have learned that exercises have to be specific to the impairment and disability to be treated if best results are to be achieved and no harm to be done. There have been many technologic advances in the development of diagnostic and therapeutic

devices, such as isokinetic equipment that is useful for strengthening weakened muscles but can also serve as a dynamometer. Orthotics and prosthetics have developed useful and more comfortable braces and artificial limbs. There are now lightweight prostheses available for amputees in the geriatric age group. (See Chapter 33.) Occupational therapy has many new devices available to aid patients with impaired hand function. A whole new generation of wheelchairs has been created that are lighter in weight and easier to use. These devices also need to be selected with care to meet the specific requirements of the individual patient. Most of these advances have been engendered by the progress of scientific biomechanics. The application of biomechanic principles to the assessment of disability and the prescription of exercises and orthoses is essential to success.

The recognition that elderly people, when in acceptable health, can tolerate a fair degree of physical stress has led to the development of physical fitness programs for the aged. The physician who prescribes the program has to be able to determine how much exertion the patient can tolerate and what to prescribe so the effort will not exceed tolerable limits. Recent data have shown that even frail women in their eighties can tolerate suitably selected exercises and improve their fitness and sense of well-being (13). Another area in which rehabilitative measures can prevent progressive deterioration is early musculoskeletal problems encountered in many active elderly persons. It has now been recognized that the source of pain may be remote from the site of discomfort. For instance, knee pain may be caused by a lesion of the hip or the ankle. A careful assessment of the patient's posture and a thorough understanding of body mechanics will elucidate the source of the discomfort. Exercises, orthotic devices, or suitable shoes may relieve the problem.

Cognitive problems may seriously interfere with rehabilitation. Many psychiatrists and psychologists have developed a considerable expertise in this field. Instead of writing failures of rehabilitation off to "poor motivation," they may find that the patient is seriously depressed. Cognitive dysfunction that has recently developed may be due to circulatory disorders, infections, or poorly tolerated medications. Cognitive impairment due to organic disease may clear up with time and appropriate medical attention.

From the preceding discussion, it should be obvious that the scientific knowledgebase of Physical Medicine and Rehabilitation has grown considerably over the last 20 years. The reference list for this chapter lists a few texts and monographs for those who wish to pursue this topic further (47–50). In response to this growth in knowledge, the American Board of Physical Medicine and Rehabilitation has increased the required period of training for physiatrists to 3 years in an accredited residency plus 1 additional year of fundamental clinical education. This may be a year of Internal Medicine, Pediatrics, or Family Practice or a transitional program. Rehabilitation can no longer be practiced and taught by self-appointed experts who may have taken one or two short courses. Frank H. Krusen (51), one of the founders of Physical Medicine and Rehabilitation, has expressed this well: "Good rehabilitation is not a field for tyros. While rehabilitation should be everybody's interest, it cannot be everybody's business."

References

1. Shock NW. Systems integration. In: Finch CE, Hayflick C, eds. *Handbook of Biology of Aging.* New York, NY: Van Nostrand Reinhold; 1977.

2. Kilo C, Vogler N, Williamson JR. Muscle capillary basement membrane changes related to aging and diabetes mellitus. *Diabetes.* 21:881–905, 1972.

3. Hazzard WR, Andres R, Bierman E, Blass JP, eds. *Principles of Geriatric Medicine and Gerontology.* 2nd ed. New York, NY: McGraw Hill; 1990; Chapters 8, 44, 46.

4. Port S, Cobb FR, Coleman RE, Jones RH. Effect of age on the response of the left ventricular ejection fraction to exercise. *N Engl J Med.* 303:1133–1137, 1980.

5. Williamson J, et al. Old people at home, their unreported needs. *Lancet.* 1:1117–1120, 1964.

6. Howell TH. *A Student's Guide to Geriatrics.* 2nd ed. Springfield, Il: CC Thomas; 1970.

7. Fields SD. History-taking in the elderly: obtaining useful information. *Geriatrics.* 46(8):26–35, 1991.

8. Fields SD. Special considerations in the physical examination of older patients. *Geriatrics.* 46(8):39–44, 1991.

9. Steinberg FU, Graber AL. The effect of age and peripheral circulation on the perception of vibration. *Arch Phys Med Rehabil.* 44:645–650, 1963.

10. Morris JC, McManus DQ. The neurology of aging: normal versus pathologic change. *Geriatrics.* 46(8):47–54, 1991.

11. Morley JE. Fructosamine or glycated hemoglobin. *J Am Geriatr Soc.* 37:911–912, 1989. Editorial.

12. Aniansson A, Gustafasson E. Physical training in elderly men with special reference to quadriceps muscle strength and morphology. *Clin Physiol.* 1:87–98, 1981.

13. Fiatarone MA, Marks EC, Ryan ND, Meredith CN, Lipsitz LA, Evans WJ. High-intensity strength training in nonagenarians. *JAMA.* 263:3029–3034, 1990.

14. Sloane PD, Baloh RW. Persistent dizziness in geriatric patients. *J Am Geriatr Soc.* 37:1031–1038, 1989.

15. Applegate WB, Davis BR, Black HR, et al. Prevalence of postural hypotension at baseline in the Systolic Hypertension in the Elderly Program (SHEP) cohort. *J Am Geriatr Soc.* 39:1057–1064, 1991.

16. Lipsitz LA. Orthostatic hypotension in the elderly. *N Engl J Med.* 321:952–957, 1989.

17. Stern N, Tuck MC. Homeostatic fragility in the elderly. *Cardiol Clinics.* 4:201–211, 1986.

18. Scherr PA, LaCroix AS, Wallace RB, et al. Light to moderate alcohol consumption and mortality in the elderly. *J Am Geriatr Soc.* 40:651–657, 1992.

19. *Alcohol and Health.* Seventh Special Report to the US Congress from the Secretary of Health and Human Services, 1990. Rockville, Md.

20. Atkinson RM. Alcoholism in the elderly population. *Mayo Clin Proc.* 63:825–829, 1988. Editorial.

21. King MB. Alcohol abuse and dementia. *Int J Geriatr Psych.* 1:31–36, 1986.

22. Pfefferbaum A, Rosenbloom M. Brain CT changes in alcoholics: effects of age and alcohol consumption. *Alcoholism.* 12:81–87, 1988.

23. World Health Organization. *International Classification of Impairments, Disabilities, and Handicaps.* Geneva: WHO; 1980.

24. Feinstein AR, Josephy BR, Wells CK. Scientific and clinical problems in indexes of functional disability. *Ann Intern Med.* 105:413–420, 1986.

25. Granger CV, Gresham GE, eds. *Functional Assessment in Rehabilitation Medicine.* Baltimore, Md: Williams & Wilkins; 1984.

26. Moskowitz E, McCann CB. Classification of disability in the chronically ill and aging. *J Chronic Dis.* 5:342–346, 1957.

27. Schoening HA, Anderegg L, Bergstrom D. Numerical scoring of self-care status of patients. *Arch Phys Med Rehabil.* 46:689–697, 1965.

28. Schoening HA, Iversen IA. Numerical scoring of self-care status: a study of the Kenny self-care evaluation. *Arch Phys Med Rehabil.* 49:221–229, 1968.

29. Anderson E, Anderson TP, Kottke F. Maintenance of gains achieved during stroke rehabilitation. *Arch Phys Med Rehabil.* 58:345–352, 1977.

30. Granger CV. Health accounting—Functional assessment of the long-term patient. In: Kottke FJ, Lehmann JF, eds. *Krusen's Handbook of Physical Medicine and Rehabilitation.* 4th ed. Philadelphia, Pa: W. B. Saunders; 1990.

31. Mahoney FI, Barthel DW. Functional evaluation: the Barthel Index. *Maryland State Med J.* 14:61–65, 1965.

32. Granger CV, Albrecht GL, Hamilton BB. Outcome of comprehensive medical rehabilitation: measurement by PULSES Profile and the Barthel Index. *Arch Phys Med Rehabil.* 60:145–154, 1979.

33. Katz S, Ford AB, Moskowitz RW, et al. Studies of illness in the aged. The Index of ADL: a standardized measure of biological and psychosocial function. *JAMA.* 185:914–919, 1963.

34. Donaldson SW, Wagner CC, Gresham GE. A unified ADL form. *Arch Phys Med Rehabil.* 54:175–180, 1973.

35. Gresham GE, Phillips TF, Labi ML. ADL status in stroke: relative merits of three standard indexes. *Arch Phys Med Rehabil.* 61:355–358, 1980.

36. Lawton MP, Brody EM. Assessment of older people. Self-maintaining and instrumental activities of daily living. *Gerontologist.* 9:179–186, 1969.

37. Lawton MP, Moss M, Fulcomer M, Kleban MH. A research and service oriented multilevel assessment instrument. *J Gerontol.* 37:91–99, 1982.

38. Kelman HR, Willner A. Problems in measurement and evaluation of rehabilitation. *Arch Phys Med Rehabil.* 43:172–181, 1962.

39. Sarno JE, Sarno MT, Levita E. The functional life scale. *Arch Phys Med Rehabil.* 54:214–220, 1973.

40. Mahler DA, Weinberg DH, Wells CK, Feinstein AR. The measurement of dyspnoea. *Chest.* 85:751–758, 1984.

41. Rubinstein LZ, Stuck AE, Siu AL, Wieland D. Impacts of geriatric evaluation and management programs on defined outcomes: overview of the evidence. *J Am Geriatr Soc.* 39(suppl):8S–16S, 1991.

42. Applegate W, Deyo R, Kramer A, Meehan S. Geriatric evaluation and management: current status and future research directions. *J Am Geriatr Soc.* 39(suppl):2S–7S, 1991.

43. Cohen HJ. Commentary. *J Am Geriatr Soc.* 39(suppl)17S–18S, 1991.

44. Baker RN, Schwartz WS, Ramseyer JC. Prognosis among survivors of ischemic stroke. *Neurology.* 18:933–941, 1968.

45. Katz S, Ford AB, Chinn AB, Newill VA. Prognosis after stroke. A critical review. *Medicine.* 45:223–236, 1966.

46. Fitzgerald JF, Moore PS, Dittus RS. The care of elderly patients with hip fracture. Changes since implementation of the prospective payment system. *N Engl J Med.* 319:1392–1397, 1988.

47. Kottke FJ, Lehmann JF, eds. *Krusen's Handbook of Physical Medi-*

cine and Rehabilitation. 4th ed. Philadelphia, Pa: W. B. Saunders; 1990. Chapters 18, 19, 20.

48. Nordin M, Frankel VH, eds. *Basic Biomechanics of the Musculoskeletal System.* 2nd ed. Philadelphia, Pa: Lea & Febiger; 1989.

49. Shephard RJ. *Exercise Physiology.* Toronto: B. C. Decker; 1987.
50. Knuttgen HG, ed. *Neuromuscular Mechanism for Therapeutic and Conditioning Exercise.* Baltimore, Md: University Park Press; 1976.
51. Frank H. Krusen, ed. *Handbook of Physical Medicine and Rehabilitation.* 2nd ed. Philadelphia, Pa: W. B. Saunders; 1971:6.

10
Arthritis and Arthroplasties

John J. Nicholas and Aaron N. Rosenberg

ARTHRITIS

Arthritis, joint, and musculoskeletal diseases commonly affect older patients (1, 2). We all know this from the childhood board game "Uncle Wiggly" (whose "rheumatism" delayed one's game) and from numerous epidemiologic studies (3). Some forms of arthritis, joint, and musculoskeletal diseases occur *more frequently* in the elderly, and some forms of arthritis that occur more commonly in younger patients occur in older patients in a *different form*. Physicians providing rehabilitation to older patients must recognize these differences.

Other changes in the musculoskeletal joint system are related to aging and are not always clearly diseases. Osteoporosis of the axial and peripheral skeleton occurs often, especially in white, small, elderly females. It is not known how osteoporosis affects joints, but osteoporosis and osteoarthritis (OA) of the hip seem to exclude one another (4–6). Patients with osteoarthritis have a lower incidence of hip fracture than those with osteoporosis.

Available evidence also suggests that older patients are weaker, have less endurance, and have smaller muscle fibers than do younger patients (7). It is known that the elderly have fewer anterior horn cells (8–13). However, part of their weakness is due to a lower level of physical conditioning, since older patients can increase both strength and endurance following training programs (14, 15).

In addition, the joint range of motion (ROM) is diminished (16). Joint degeneration (OA) is not an obligatory concomitant of aging and is distinct from age-related joint changes (17, 18). Osteoarthritis occurs more frequently in the elderly, but it is not ubiquitous and is often unilateral. Changes in the staining of the articular cartilage, the growth of osteophytes, the thinning of cartilage, the increase in the metabolism of chondrocytes, the development of juxtaarticular cysts, and sclerosis are the pathologic changes found in OA. However, they do not occur in all joints, even to minor degrees, suggesting a process not directly related to increased age. The tendons, ligaments, and capsule surrounding joints lose elasticity as evidenced by a decrease in joint ROM and a sense of stiffness in older patients. Stiffness following sleep, prolonged sitting, or exercise is more common and prolonged in older patients, who describe it frequently, for example after prolonged sitting and driving to Florida on vacation from northern climates.

Physiatrists will do well to consider these phenomena when treating older patients. The presence of osteoporosis should be determined before prescribing flexion exercises, which load the spine and may cause compression fractures. ROM exercises should initially be of a few degrees only and done gently, not vigorously. Strengthening exercises must be designed to occur within the limited ROM and not stress osteoporotic limbs. Endurance exercises should be designed to avoid overuse of limited and/or damaged joints.

Osteoarthritis

Patients with OA often complain of unilateral or monarticular joint pain (multiple joint involvement is much less common). The pain is associated with use and weight bearing, and stiffness is noted following rest. Commonly involved joints include the knees and hips. The carpometacarpal (CMC) and metacarpophalangeal (MCP) joints of the thumbs, the distal interphalangeal (DIP) and, less commonly, proximal interphalangeal (PIP) joints of the fingers, the shoulders, and elbows are more rarely involved. The cervical and lumbar spines are almost always involved in older patients but are often asymptomatic. For that matter, OA of other joints may also *not* be associated with pain (19, 20). Treatment includes nonsteroidal antiinflammatory drugs (NSAID) and joint injections. Surgical treatments include joint replacement, osteotomy, and arthrodesis. Rehabilitation techniques include decreasing weight bearing on affected joints by the use of canes, crutches, walkers, and dieting. The prescription of shoe lifts for leg length discrepancies will correct biomechanical abnormalities due to shortening or lengthening of limbs following surgery or severe OA. It is my practice to try serial temporary shoe lifts until the patient feels comfortable, rather than prescribe a certain height on the basis of measurement of leg length. Older patients who are resistant to the use of visible aids for walking must be shown that they obtain pain relief, and then perhaps they will use canes in private, even if not in public.

Cervical collars may decrease pain in the neck from OA if it is associated with motion. Various adjustments must be tried so the patients will tolerate the brace by eliminating rubbing and avoiding excessive extension. Back braces are usually not as affective for OA of the spine as they are for acute herniated discs, which may occur even in elderly patients with osteoarthritic spinal stenosis. Thumb spicas decrease pain when they immobilize the CMC and MCP joints of the thumb with OA.

Joint injections are easily administered to the CMC and MCP joints of the thumb, the DIP joints of the fingers, the knees, elbow, and shoulder joint, but not the hips and spine. Injections are thought to help only if there is an inflammatory element to the pathology, but a trial must be made in order to see if an inflammatory element is present.

Probably, exercise will increase the strength of muscles around involved joints, particularly the hip and knee extensors (21). Certainly, increasing the strength of these muscles by diligent and persistent exercise will improve the muscular response after surgery. Excessive excursion of the joint during exercise will likely increase pain. So, therefore, either exercise that is isometrical at multiple angles of a hip or knee joint or exercise that is partially isometric and includes high resistance with few repetitions will allow the greatest increase in muscle strength with the least pain. It has recently been shown that exercising the knee with the hip in an extended rather than flexed position will diminish muscle weakness at the hip and knee and improve and even diminish pain for OA of the knee (22, 23).

Polymyalgia Rheumatica

Polymyalgia rheumatica (PMR) is a recently described disease characterized by widespread aches and pains with motion (rheumatism), minimal joint effusions, rarely hot joints on joint scans, and nearly constantly elevated sedimentation rates. Mild anemia, often very sudden onset, and depression are frequent. These symptoms may readily be confused with hypercalcemia, hypothyroidism, depression, and the onset of rheumatoid arthritis. The joints and muscles are not tender on examination, but the patient hurts when moving. NSAID and adrenocorticosteroids (steroids) immediately suppress the pain and allow resumption of motion and activities of daily living (ADL). However, treatment is required for a prolonged time (18 to 36 months), and, frequently, osteoporosis, spinal compression fractures,

cataracts, hypertension, diabetes, candida infections, and peptic ulcers, develop or become worse.

In addition, temporal arteritis (TA) and widespread giant cell arteritis may occur. TA requires even higher doses of steroids or cytotoxic drugs in order to prevent blindness and arterial occlusion in the arm, cerebral, or coronary circulations. Following these high doses, the complications of steroid treatment are even more likely to occur.

Exercise programs to maintain muscle strength, endurance, and ROM, particularly in the proximal muscles, may help. These muscles are affected by pain, which decreases motion, but they also become weak due to steroid myopathy and disuse. Activity should be monitored and walking urged to prevent osteoporosis. Shoulder contractures must be sought on examination and treated with persistent ROM exercises, heat or cold modalities, transcutaneous nerve stimulation (TENS), and, if available and with good compliance, a constant passive range of motion (CPROM) machine.

Gout And Pseudogout

Pseudogout is a term applied to arthritis that occurs in older patients' knees, elbows, wrists, and shoulders as a very acute inflammatory arthritis (Type II synovial fluid) which mimics gout. However, the synovial fluid examination reveals crystals of calcium pyrophosphate rather than monosodium urate—thus "pseudogout." The articular cartilage of these patients nearly always demonstrates calcifications on radiographs (chondrocalcinosis) and OA. Pseudogout in the elderly is usually an accompanying feature of aging or OA, but in younger patients a specific cause must be sought, for example hyperparathyroidism, hemochromatosis, or thyroid disease. Treatment with NSAID and/or joint injections of steroids usually terminates an attack promptly. Joint aspiration and synovial fluid analysis are required for an accurate diagnosis.

Physiatrists should be prepared to increase the strength about involved joints as one would do for OA. A sudden arthritis within the first 24 to 48 hours following a surgical procedure in an elderly patient should suggest pseudogout or gout.

Gout will present itself similarly to pseudogout, but with a predilection for the first metatarsal phalangeal joint. NSAID are given for acute attacks, and blood uric acid lowering agents (Anturane, Benemid, Zyloprim) are given to diminish the total body quantity of uric acid. Occasionally, both gout and pseudogout present as polyarticular arthritis resembling rheumatoid arthritis or systemic lupus erythematosus, but joint aspirations will distinguish these conditions.

If medical treatment and compliance with treatment are inadequate, the physiatrist will need to provide, at least on a temporary basis, walkers, crutches, specially fitted shoes, and, of course, muscle strengthening exercises to those joints that have been inflamed for prolonged periods and thus weakened.

Rheumatoid Arthritis

Rheumatoid arthritis (RA) occurs most commonly in young female adults or in children. It occurs less frequently in the elderly and when it does so, *it is different.* For example, young women are more commonly affected than men (2 or 3 to 1), but in the older adult the incidence is about equal between the sexes. Cecil and Kammerer (24) in 1951 reviewed 100 consecutive patients with onset RA after the age of sixty years. They found 90 cases had only mild radiographic changes, and 71 had "moderate or severe" functional disability. However, 55 had RA for 1 year or less and only 5 had subcutaneous nodules. The small joints of the hands were most frequently involved, *but* there was a striking frequency of shoulder involvement. Dordick (25), in 1956, described 50 consecutive cases of RA with the onset over age 60 years; 46 patients had mild radiographic abnormalities; the duration of the disease was relatively short, and hand and shoulder involvement was common.

Brown and Sones in 1967 (26) described 156 cases of RA with onset after age 65 years. Males and females were nearly equally involved, and shoulder pain was noted with increased frequency (26). Rheumatoid factor (RF) was positive in 13 out of 29 cases (45%). Ehrlich, Katz, and Cohen (27) in 1970 described 43 cases of RA with onset after age sixty years. The shoulders were involved unusually often (25 of 43 cases); subcutaneous nodules occurred in 6 out of 43. Radiographs of the patients revealed milder changes than in a younger group.

Terkeltaub et al (28) in 1983 compared 34 patients with RA onset after age 60 years with a younger group. They found a shorter duration of disease and lower incidence of RF in the older group. They noted greater functional capacity, and shoulder joints were *not* more frequently involved; but shoulder synovitis was "more impressive." The sex ratio was nearly equal.

Deal et al (29) in 1985 described 78 patients with RA onset after age 60 years. Shoulder involvement was more common at onset in the elderly. RF and subcutaneous nodules were less frequent at onset, and these authors claimed a better outcome for the older patients. They presented no description of functional assessment data.

In summary, RA is *different* in the elderly. The sex ratio is more equal, and the duration of the disease is, not surprisingly, shorter. Shoulder involvement is more striking, more frequent, and begins earlier, and x-ray findings (again not surprisingly) are less severe. My personal experience is that this disease is devastating to the

function of older patients in spite of the lower frequency of abnormalities on x-ray films, physical examination, and serologic testing. A comprehensive rehabilitation program including ADL evaluation is indicated. Rehabilitation treatment of these patients must be intensive, and social and psychiatric support for the patient and the family must be strong. Many of the treatments appropriate for younger patients with RA are, of course, applicable; but they must be applied with more persistence and patience on the part of the physiatrist, therapist, and patient. Older patients, for example, benefit from the use of crutches, canes, and walkers to relieve pain in weight-bearing joints, but they do not like these "badges of disability and age." Moist heat and hot baths relieve pain in inflamed joints but must be applied daily and frequently. Patients must be taught that the rehabilitation treatment, as well as medicines, must be used regularly and repeatedly to obtain improvement (30).

Inflamed joints cause weakness of the surrounding muscles and strengthening exercises must be prescribed. Exercises should be characterized by maximum force and minimum repetitions in order to avoid increasing inflammation. The use of assisted exercise by a therapist rather than use of weights and exercise machines may be necessary. The frequency and force involved must be individually prescribed so that joints do not flare up and so that joints are rested by the time of the next exercise session.

Recently, several authors have published data describing the effect of aerobic exercise in patients with apparently mild (but not well described RA (31–36). These authors report an increase in ADL activities, the sense of well-being, and aerobic functioning following treadmill or bicycle exercise. Caution must be employed when prescribing aerobic exercise to rheumatoid patients, however, because aerobic exercise may increase inflammation. In addition, the long-term effects of increased wear and tear from exercise on inflamed joints has not been clearly described. In experimental animals and clinical situations such as hemiplegia where inflamed joints are overused on the nonhemiplegic side, an increase in inflammation and severity of arthritis occurs following exercise (37–40).

Some older patients may be less accommodating to changes, new ideas, or new treatments. They have after all performed their ADL and run their lives for a long time in ways to which they are accustomed. The changes that must be made to adapt to RA, a persistent and pervasive disease, are harder for those with a long, established routine. Although they may not have as many demanding responsibilities, as for example the young housewife with three children, everyday ADL can be more demanding on available resources. The physician must enlist the patient's family as well as the patient in support of the treatment program and be persistent and patient in an effort to get the patient to follow the treatment program for what may be long-term results rather than short-term therapeutic victories. A brief period of hospitalization on a rehabilitation unit will provide the opportunity both for treatment and education of these patients.

Systemic Lupus Erythematosus

Numerous authors have described the clinical characteristics of systemic lupus erythematosus (SLE) of the elderly compared to those of younger patients. Joseph and Zarafonetis (41) noted five cases of SLE onset after age 50 (a) with renal disease, (b) with pulmonary tuberculosis obscured by steroids, (c) as a mild disease, (d) as deadly hemolytic anemia, and (e) as a perforated diverticulum on steroids. Foad et al (42) noted nine cases with onset after age 60 years, with an RA-like disease; less commonly, serositis; and included five with mild renal disease. Dimant et al (43) noted in 16 of 234 SLE patients over age 51 years that the older group had more discoid lupus, photosensitivity, and pulmonary fibrosis, and less oral ulcers, Raynaud's phenomena, cutaneous vasculitis, neuropsychiatric symptoms, leukopenia, hypocomplementemia, and marked proteinuria.

Baker et al (44) described 39 patients with SLE onset after age 50 years and found pleuritis and pericarditis to be the most common presenting manifestations. Pulmonary abnormalities were common and Raynaud's phenomena, neuropsychiatric disease, alopecia, and skin rash were less common. The older patients generally lived longer. Ballou (45) described 25 patients with SLE over the age of 55 years at diagnosis. Fewer of the older patients were black; they had less renal disease and CNS involvement; but skin and hematologic manifestations were similar. Hypocomplementemia occurred less often. However, serositis occurred more often in the older patients, and central nervous system (CNS) and renal disease were less common. MacDonald et al (46), on the other hand, reported 10 SLE patients with onset after age 50 years who had an unusually increased frequency of neurologic manifestations, including neuropathy and cerebritis. Catoggio et al (47) reported 13 female patients who developed SLE after 55 years of age and noted increased interstitial pulmonary disease and neuropsychiatric findings. Hashimoto et al (48) reported 21 cases between the ages of 50 and 81 years. These older patients had more renal disease and joint deformities, pleuritis, myocarditis, and thrombocytopenia, but proteinuria was less in older patients. Finally, Ward and Polisson (49), in a meta-analysis of older patients with SLE, found an increased frequency of serositis, pulmonary disease, and Sjögren's syndrome and a decreased frequency of Raynaud's phenomenon and alopecia.

In summary, the clinical and laboratory manifestations of SLE in the elderly are quite varied, but severe renal disease is less frequent and neuropsychiatric manifestations are fairly common. Rehabilitation for these patients will depend upon the extent and nature of the neuropsychiatric, neurologic, and other problems (for example: foot drop, paraplegia, hemiplegia, encephalitis, steroid-induced compression fractures, myopathy, and arthritis).

Aseptic necrosis of bone usually requires diligent diagnostic efforts. Joint replacement may ultimately be required, but the relief of pain with weight-bearing devices (crutches, canes, walkers) is an appropriate preliminary treatment. Deformities and disability, especially in the shoulders, and nonerosive deforming arthritis of the hands and fingers (Jaccoud's arthritis) will require treatment. Jaccoud's arthritis should be treated with work simplification and energy conservation techniques, ADL devices and aids, and dynamic splinting. Resting splints are not likely to cause any permanent correction of the ulnar deviation, MCP subluxation, or swan's neck and boutonniere deformities that are the hallmark of this condition. Surgical intervention is not complicated by thin osteoporotic bone in SLE as it is in RA.

Other Conditions

Hypertrophic pulmonary osteoarthropathy (HPOA or clubbing) probably occurs more commonly in older than younger patients. However, the causes in younger patients (congenital heart disease, arteriovenous shunts, alcoholic cirrhosis) are different from the causes in the elderly (bronchiectasis, pulmonary tuberculosis, lung or pleural cancer). NSAID relieve the pain of HPOA readily, but the cause must be assiduously sought as it is frequently fatal or frequently can be treated.

Neuropathic joints (Charcot's joints) may occur in both the old and young, but again the cause differs. Syringomyelia is more likely to occur in younger patients and tertiary syphilis and diabetes in the older patient population. Medical management is insufficient because prolonged and continued use and weight bearing will cause joint destruction to progress even if the pain has been diminished. Surgical joint replacement is not always successful.

Rehabilitation techniques include the prescription of canes, crutches, walkers, and wheelchairs. An attempt should be made to decrease weight bearing and the consequent trauma to Charcot foot and ankle joints. Custom-designed inserts and molded shoes should be carefully designed and applied in order to avoid skin breakdown and abrasions from protruding metatarsal (MT) heads and other bony prominences.

A patellar tendon-bearing orthosis relieves weight in the stance phase and then only if the orthosis keeps the heel from touching the bottom of the shoe. Frequently, a lift must be provided for the contralateral shoe, and the patient taught *not* to use a toe off gait. A rocker bottom added to the shoe may eliminate the toe off stage of gait and allow for more weight removal. This device is worth a try if carefully fitted at the patellar tendon and tibial flares.

Ischial weight-bearing orthoses may relieve weight on the hip joint but only if the patient sits on the ischial tuberosity and understands the function of the brace. A rocker bottom shoe and a lift (on the opposite side) are helpful. Again, the brace functions only if the patient avoids toe off. In soft tissue weight-bearing sockets—narrow mediolateral, ischial containment, Normal Shape Normal Alignment (NSNA), Contoured Adducted Trochanteric Controlled Alignment Method (CAT-CAM)—weight is not transmitted from above the hip joint to the ischial tuberosity and brace and thence to the floor. These sockets transmit weight from the hip joint to the thigh tissues to the floor. When the patient reaches the toe off phase of walking, his or her weight will be transferred from the heel attachment of the orthosis to the first metatarsal bone and then up the leg to the hip joint. Therefore, patients must be carefully trained, and the ischiald weight-bearing orthosis, like the patellar tendon weight-bearing orthosis, must be carefully fitted (50).

Many musculoskeletal problems of a nonsystemic nature occur frequently in the older population. Chard and Hazleman (51) described 100 geriatric English patients admitted to an acute hospital. Twenty-one had significant shoulder disease, including chronic rotator cuff rupture in seven; two had frozen shoulders; two had OA of the humerus; one had apatite-related shoulder arthritis, and six had stroke-related disease. The author commented that only 3 of 21 patients had sought medical care for these conditions. These were English patients, and it may be that in the American system there is more ready access to care and more ready physician response to patient complaints. However, physicians should be on the alert for these conditions in both inpatients and outpatients.

These conditions should be treated promptly and vigorously, as delay may prolong recovery and increase disability in the elderly. Tendinitis at the shoulder must be treated by prohibiting or decreasing the activity that caused it. NSAID and steroid injections around the tendon will help. Elimination of overuse, steroid injections into the posterior rotator cuff, NSAID, and surgical resection of the impinging acromion must be administered to the patient with x-ray and clinical signs of impingement. The frozen shoulder is often resistant to treatment in the elderly, and heat/cold, NSAID, and ROM exercises don't always do the job. Steroid injections into the shoulder joint seem to help some but not others and are worth a try. When all else fails, TENS used constantly, especially during ROM exercises, and a carefully fitted CPROM machine can give remarkable results. Compliance, however, must be complete and patient cooperation enthusiastic.

An older patient with the shoulder-hand syndrome or reflex sympathetic dystrophy must be examined for a Pancoast tumor. Stellate ganglion blocks given to the point of a change in skin temperature can be repeated until the patient can move his hand freely and then motion must be persistently maintained with *active* ROM exercise during the period immediately following the stellate block.

General Suggestions

The use of steroid injections in the elderly is not precluded by diabetes. Strengthening exercises are limited only by the participation of the patient. The use of ADL aids and devices and walking aids may be limited by patient acceptance but are no less effective. Compliance with treatment must be maintained and the causes of noncompliance sought by questioning. Older patients are no more likely to follow the advice of their physician than are younger patients. They are also, however, no less likely to benefit from treatment and even a partial decrease in their disability may make a considerable improvement in their everyday life. The arthritic and musculoskeletal conditions of the elderly *must not* be ignored or accepted as an inevitable and irremediable concomitant of old age.

ARTHROPLASTIES

Joint Arthroplasty

While much may be accomplished for the elderly arthritic patient in the operating room, a successful surgical procedure must be accompanied by appropriate physical therapy to achieve optimum patient function. Conversely, inappropriate postoperative management may lead to a poor result or significant complications. Thus, excellent communication between surgeon and physiatrist is necessary to optimize the result of arthritis surgery performed in the elderly.

Several principles should be kept in mind. Perhaps the foremost is the already mentioned need for excellent communication between patient, therapist, and surgeon. This may, and probably should, include preoperative evaluation. "The results of surgery are made before surgery" (52, p 498). Intimately influencing the problems of a chronically affected arthritic joint are the rest of the patient's resources: physical, mental, and social. The results of arthroplasty in a patient with monoarticular osteoarthritic hip disease and no other medical problems would be expected to differ from that of a frail multiarticular rheumatoid with multiple other medical problems. Appropriate preoperative assessment is frequently helpful and occasionally essential in providing an appropriate treatment plan when severe muscle atrophy and multiarticular involvement are present.

In the elderly, it is frequently noted that soft tissues are hard and that hard tissues are soft. This is another way of saying that osteopenia has rendered the bone weak and contracted periarticular tissues have lost their elasticity. These factors must be considered in the rehabilitation effort.

While arthroplasty is the most common form of surgical arthritis treatment in the elderly, occasionally, periarticular osteotomy may be performed to realign the lower extremity (53, 54). These procedures are useful in patients with good ROM and where altering the forces about the joint may be expected to decrease pain and improve function. Unless casting is involved, the postoperative requirements are to reestablish ROM and muscle strength, while minimizing weight bearing until osteotomy healing has occurred.

Most often, the elderly arthritic will require joint arthroplasty or replacement. Over the past 20 years, this procedure has become the most reliable and effective modality in the treatment of the arthritic joint. Most commonly replaced is the hip, followed by the knee, and much less frequently the shoulder and elbow. Due to the strong influence of the periarticular soft tissue contractures accompanying finger and wrist joint replacements, these are most frequently managed by the surgeon in conjunction with the occupational therapist and are beyond the scope of this discussion.

While the basic principles of postarthroplasty physiatric management have been well reviewed elsewhere (55), it is reasonable to reiterate certain fundamental concepts. The long-standing pattern of joint pain, muscle splinting, and contracture that frequently accompanies arthritis can lead to significant neuromuscular incoordination, which must be relieved by physiotherapy in the postoperative period. Of maximum importance, then, as an overall goal of rehabilitation, should be relief of pain. Gentle handling of the patient and consideration of operative soft tissue trauma should be kept in mind. A practical definition of pain has been given by Opitz (55), "The degree of discomfort that causes motor incoordination, such as unreasonable co-contraction of antagonist muscle groups." Avoidance of this co-contraction is a fundamental tenant of postarthroplasty therapy. It is thus advisable as a preliminary step to establish a relaxed passive range of motion (PROM). As a pain-free range is established, active-assisted exercises may be included. Muscle reeducation follows as a natural concomitant of teaching light functional ADL. As the active ROM (through a pain-free arc) returns to the maximal desired range, more active and aggressive strengthening activity may be pursued. Such activity must be designed to minimize stress on prosthetic parts and should be initially oriented toward increasing endurance.

It is important to keep in mind following arthroplasty that the patient may have other painful musculoskeletal conditions that may inhibit function. These must be carefully assessed and treated in conjunction with the recently operated part to achieve maximum functional recovery from the surgical procedure.

Hip Arthroplasty

After contemporary total hip replacement, the hip is a most forgiving joint and, even without formal rehabilitation, will generally provide adequate ROM and pain-free support. However, a satisfactory result may be greatly improved with appropriate rehabilitation (55–57).

Of prime concern to the postoperative rehabilitative effort is the type of surgical approach used and the method of fixation of the arthroplasty components. If the surgical approach required osteotomy of the greater trochanter or extensive muscle release, the repair involved may limit full weight bearing or active exercising of certain muscle groups (particularly the gluteus medius and minimus). In addition, components that are not cemented in place may rely on bony ingrowth stabilization, which takes up to 6 weeks to occur. Prior to that time, weight bearing should be minimized.

Discussion of therapy for the postoperative total hip patient must begin with a discussion of hip stability. For the hip to function appropriately, the femoral head must remain seated in the acetabulum. Three basic factors govern hip stability: component positioning, soft-tissue tension, and possible impingement of structures. Component position may be such that instability or dislocation will occur at extreme positions. This problem may be exacerbated by inadequate soft-tissue tension or impingement of the femur on the pelvis.

The most common positions of impingement and instability are: (a) 60 degrees of flexion, adduction, and internal rotation past neutral—dislocation posterior; (b) 90 degrees or greater flexion, adduction, and internal rotation past neutral—dislocation posterior; and (c) full extension, adduction, and external rotation—dislocation anterior. These positions may be noted in the following situations: (a) arising from bed or chair, moving to the contralateral side with the leg adducted and internally rotated; (b) toilet activities with a low seat, feet apart, knees together, or managing foot care in the same position; and (c) turning away from the operated hip in extension while lying in bed or standing.

It is most likely that the operating surgeon will have the best sense of where potential instability lies and should be consulted should any question arise. In any case, all instabilities have in common adduction of the hip, which should be avoided postoperatively unless a postoperative abduction contracture must be corrected.

In general, the rehabilitative effort consists of obtaining full ROM (preventing contracture, particularly flexion), strengthening the periarticular musculature (particularly gluteus medius and minimus), and gait training.

ROM exercises are important to prevent contracture, particularly flexion and external rotation. These may be countered by specific avoidance of inbed postures with the hip flexed and externally rotated. This position is generally one that relieves stress on the hip and is readily adopted by the postoperative patient. The patient should be reminded to keep the leg extended as much as possible. The tendency to externally rotate the limb may be countered by placing a rolled blanket under the greater trochanter or utilizing a "bunny boot" to keep the foot perpendicular to the bed.

After the initial 36 to 48 hours following surgery, the patient is allowed to stand and specific exercises are begun. Severely debilitated, elderly, or unmotivated patients may require little specific therapy directed at the hip and may require more general conditioning and gait training. All patients should be reminded to be cautious about avoiding positions of instability. The patient with good preoperative motion will generally recover motion with relative ease, while the patient with severe preoperative contracture requiring surgical release may require intensive stretching.

In the vast majority of cases, contracture will involve one or more components of flexion, external rotation, and adduction. Should adductor, external rotator, or iliopsoas release have been necessary at the time of surgery, therapy must be directed against recurrence. Precautions against hip instability are the boundary upon which ROM of motion exercises are carried out. In general, the abducted hip is safe from dislocation, and rotational stretching is quite safe in this position. Thus, crossing the leg, foot over thigh is quite safe (flexion, abduction, external rotation), while crossing thigh over thigh is much less so (flexion, adduction, neutral rotation).

Adduction is generally safe with the thigh in neutral rotation and extension. Abduction contracture, however, is rare and most commonly associated with trochanteric advancement. Adduction contracture is more common and may require aggressive stretching postoperatively.

ROM exercises should be graded and increased gradually as wound healing and patient tolerance increase. They should be performed while standing or lying but rarely while sitting. Sitting promotes flexion contracture, generally tires the hip, and should be limited to ½ hour sessions 3 or 4 times a day for the first 6 to 8 weeks after surgery.

Muscle strengthening must be initiated based on examination for specific muscle weakness. Most important for prevention of a postoperative abductor lurch are exercises to strengthen the abductors. These muscles may have been violated during the surgical approach, and before initiation of a vigorous strengthening program, it may be necessary to check with the surgeon involved. Alternatively, a trochanteric osteotomy may have been

performed and active abductor strengthening may need to be delayed to allow its healing. Supine abductor strengthening without resistance may generally be started early. More active exercises should be initiated only if the abductor muscle-trochanter complex is fully intact and can withstand intense contraction as judged by the operating surgeon.

Gait training may begin the day the patient first leaves bed. Assistive devices (usually crutches or a walker) will generally be required for the first several weeks to limit weight bearing (usually between 40 and 60 pounds) or assist in balance. The emphasis in gait training is to utilize full extension of the hip, to avoid "breaking the knee" in late stance phase, and to maintain symmetrical stride length. As confidence is acquired and if full weight bearing is allowed, the patient may walk with two or even one cane. A cane should continue to be used until all limp is gone.

Finally, stair climbing is taught, leading up with the nonoperated limb and down with the operated. Concomitantly, the patient should be instructed by occupational therapy in modifications necessary to accomplish all ADL. When independent in all exercises and able to ambulate and climb stairs independently, the patient is usually ready for discharge.

Most patients will go home with a raised toilet seat. This allows for toilet activities without the hip flexion required for a low seat. This may be discontinued at 6 weeks to 3 months in most cases but may be required for longer depending on the surgeon's assessment of hip stability. The restrictions of hip flexion, thigh adduction, and operative side lying may be lifted at a similar time. Most patients should be cautioned against deep squatting indefinitely and taught how to kneel on the ipsilateral knee to reach the ground if needed.

Knee Arthroplasty

Success following total knee arthroplasty is more dependent on appropriate postoperative management than is total hip arthroplasty. Of primary importance is the need for an adequate ROM (58, 59). At least 90 degrees ROM is required for activities such as sitting in a car, climbing stairs, and arising from a chair. Thus, during the first several postoperative weeks, the emphasis is on achieving this motion.

Recently, the concept of the continuous passive motion (CPM) device has been introduced to the rehabilitative effort following total joint arthroplasty, most commonly used at the knee. These devices are designed to offer passive motion to the joint with controls that allow setting of limits for flexion, extension, and the speed of the flexion/extension arc. In general, this device is utilized to increase the flexion arc on a gradually continuous basis. Five to 10 degree increments in flexion may be achieved every 6 to 12 hours while the patient rests in bed. A rule of thumb is that if the patient has been comfortable at the current level of flexion for several hours, the flexion of the machine may be increased. The most commonly seen problem with the CPM device is the tendency to develop flexion contracture (lack of full extension), and this must be carefully avoided. Most frequently, CPM is discontinued at night and the knee is rested in an immobilizer in extension to avoid flexion.

After surgery, the knee is usually immobilized for 48 hours in a bulky dressing. After the drains have been removed, the patient is allowed to assume an upright position, and stiff knee ambulation is begun. Crutches or a walker are used to protect the limb as long as needed to either allow for ingrowth of cementless components or until quadriceps function has recovered sufficiently to protect the knee.

Gentle active and active-assisted motion is initiated along with early ambulation. Short arc and isometric quadriceps and hamstring strengthening are utilized early (first week postoperative) to minimize tension on the capsular repair. Most surgeons avoid resistance strengthening of the quadriceps during the first 3 to 6 weeks after surgery in order to prevent patellar dislocation or capsular dehiscence.

Motion in the knee must not be gained at the expense of wound healing. Cold packs are frequently used after exercise to decrease wound inflammation and moist or dry heat prior to exercise to decrease tissue edema. Strengthening of periarticular musculature and gait training, while of great importance, may be improved upon at any time in the postoperative course. If, however, ROM has not approached 90 degrees by 3 weeks after surgery, manipulation of the knee under general anesthesia may be required. Hence, ROM of the knee takes priority over all other physiotherapy considerations. An experienced therapist will be able to assist in determining the need for manipulation. Some patients will develop a firm end point in flexion quite short of 90 degrees and no improvement without manipulation seems possible, while others will have a softer end point and show slow but gradual progress. Such information may be of help in deciding to reanesthetize the patient for purposes of manipulation.

Full extension is also important for excellent knee function. Permanent flexion contracture renders gait and standing more fatiguing. If extension is full passively and not actively, this will usually clear with several months of quadriceps strengthening exercise. Permanent flexion contracture may be a result of poor surgical technique, constraints imposed by morbid anatomy not correctable at the time of surgery, or poor postoperative rehabilitation technique. As always, communication with the operative surgeon will help set the guidelines for postoperative expectation.

Stability of the knee is governed by the intrinsic constraint of the prosthesis plus additional support by the ligamentous structures about the knee: medial and lateral collateral ligaments, posterior cruciate ligament, and the intact extensor mechanism. Any apparent instability should be reported to the surgeon immediately. Occasionally, bracing may be required.

Gait training should incorporate appropriate assistive devices to maintain balance and appropriate weight bearing. Most total knee arthroplasty patients may bear full weight on the limb, but patients with major bone grafting or a prosthesis requiring bone ingrowth may need to limit weight bearing for variable periods of time after surgery.

Eventually, reestablishment of the normal "knee flexion wave" (full extension at heel strike, flexion in midstance, reextension at toe off) during stance phase may be expected. As the quadriceps gains strength and the patient regains confidence and balance, the patient may be weaned from assistive devices.

Discharge should be avoided prior to reaching the 90 degree flexion and full extension goal. Once there goals are reached and the patient can manage level gait, stairs, and an independent exercise program, he or she is ready for discharge.

Shoulder and Elbow Arthroplasty

In general, rehabilitation of the shoulder must be individualized, depending on the underlying condition and the surgeon's estimate of prosthetic stability and full stability of bony or soft tissue repairs required at the time of surgery (52). The shoulder joint is intrinsically less stable than the knee or hip. In some patients with significant preoperative defects, more limited postoperative goals are employed, with emphasis aimed at maintaining joint stability and achieving muscle control over a limited motion arc. During the first 2 weeks after surgery, a passive or gentle active-assisted ROM program is initiated, with isometric exercises introduced during the third week. More active exercises are begun at the fourth week and, depending on stability, may be upgraded to active resistance.

In patients with more limited goals, it is important to reduce motion for many weeks to allow for scar formation to assist in the generation of joint stability. While only one upper extremity may be incapacitated and the patient otherwise independent, the need for prolonged supervised rehabilitation is often found in these more complex cases. As always, the surgeon's guidelines should be strictly adhered to in order to achieve optimal results. In some patients, final ROM may be limited by the status of muscle or capsular tissue repair, and final goals should be arrived at with the operating surgeon. In general, the anterior shoulder capsule and musculature are divided to achieve joint exposure and so external rotation is limited to the point determined intraoperatively to be short of rupturing these tissues (or causing suture line dehiscence). If the anterior deltoid is removed from the clavicle for exposure, active forward flexion and lateral abduction may need to be delayed until this tissue repair is mature.

In general, the final goal should be to achieve sufficient internal rotation to allow for toilet hygiene, with abduction and forward flexion sufficient to bring the hand to the back of the head and the mouth, and external rotation sufficient to allow for ease in donning and doffing clothing.

The elbow generates less concern for stability. Nonetheless, active resistance exercise is best avoided for 4 to 6 weeks after surgery while ROM is achieved. At the elbow, flexion is the most important function and, in general, should allow the hand to reach the mouth. Limited extension is least debilitating at this joint and is of less concern.

Continuous passive motion devices are available for the upper extremity and may prove useful in rehabilitation of the elbow and shoulder joint. At the elbow, as at the knee, the wound should not be sacrificed for motion. Wound healing problems in these subcutaneous joints may lead to disastrous complications, so evidence of marginal wound necrosis, drainage, or increased inflammation should lead to placing the joint at rest until these problems have subsided.

Regardless of the joint involved, the most basic principle in postoperative rehabilitation remains communication. Patient, therapist, physiatrist and surgeon must allow for full and free communication to optimize the results that may be obtained in the management of the elderly. Each has specific knowledge and skills, which when fully shared, will allow the patient the greatest possibility for restoration of full function.

References

1. Bergstrom G, Bjelle A, Sorensen LB, Sundh V, Svanborg A. Prevalence of symptoms and signs of joint impairment at age 79. *Scand J Rehabil Med.* 17:173–182, 1985.
2. Bergstrom G, Aniansson A, Bjelle A, Grimby G, Lundgren-Lindquist B, Svanborg A. Funtional consequences of joint impairment at age 79. *Scand J Rehabil Med.* 17:183–190, 1985.
3. Garis HR. *Uncle Wiggly Game.* Springfield, Mass: Milton Bradley Co; date unlisted.
4. Weintroub S, Papo J, Ashkenazi R, Tardiman SL, Salama R. Osteoarthritis of the hip and fractures of the proximal end of the femur. *Acta Orthop Scand.* 54:261–264, 1982.
5. Osteoarthrosis and fractures of the upper end of the femur. *Br Med J.* December 23:686–687, 1972.
6. Dequeker J. The relationship between osteoporosis and osteoarthritis. *Clin Rheum Dis.* 11:271–296, 1985.
7. Shephard RJ. *Physiology and Biochemistry of Exercise.* New York, NY: Prager Publishers; 1982.
8. Jennekens FGI, Tomlinson BE, Walton JN. Histochemical aspects of five limb muscles in old age—an autopsy study. *J Neurol Sci.* 14:259–276, 1971.
9. Tomlinson BE, Irving D. The number of limb motor neurons in the human lumbosacral cord throughout life. *Neurol Sci.* 34:213–219, 1977.
10. McComas ARM, Upton REPS. Motorneuron disease and aging. *Lancet.* December 29:1477–1480, 1973.
11. Kawamura Y, Okazaki H, O'Brien PC, Dyck PJ. Lumbar motoneurons of man I: number and diameter histogram of alpha and gamma axons of ventral root. *J Neurol Pathol Exp Neurol.* 36:853–860, 1977.
12. Kamamura YP, O'Brien H, Okazaki P, Dyck J. Lumbar motoneurons of man II: the number and diameter distribution of and intermediate-diameter cytons in "motor neuron columns" of spinal cord of man. *J Neurol Pathol Exp Neurol.* 36:861–870, 1977.
13. Howard JE, McGill KC, Dorfman LJ. Age effects on properties of motor unit action potentials: ADEMG analysis. *Ann Neurol.* 24:207–212, 1988.
14. Sidney KH, Shephard RJ. Frequency and intensity of exercise training for elderly subjects. *Med Sci Sports.* 10(2):125–131, 1978.
15. Fiatarone MA, Marks EC, Ryan ND, Meredith CN, Lipsitz LA, Evans WJ. High-intensity strength training in nonagenarians, effects on skeletal muscle. *JAMA.* 263:3029–3034, 1990.
16. Svanborg A. Practical and functional consequences of aging. *Gerontology.* 34(suppl 1):11–15, 1988.
17. Thonar EJ, Bjornsson S, Kuettner KE. Kuettner K, et al, eds. *Age-Related Changes in Cartilage Proteoglycans: Articular Cartilage Biochemistry.* New York, NY: Raven Press: 1986:273–287.
18. Mankin HJ. Kelly WH, Harris ED Jr, Ruddy S, Sledge CB, eds. *Pathogenesis of Osteoarthritis Textbook of Rheumatology.* Philadelphia, Pa: W.B. Saunders; 1989:1488, 1490.
19. Cobbs S, Merchant WR, Rubin TR. The relation of symptoms to osteoarthritis. *J Chron Dis.* 5:197–204, 1957.
20. Gresham GE, Rathey UK: Osteoarthritis in the knees of aged persons. Relationship between roentgenographic and clinical manifestations. *JAMA.* 233:168–170, 1975.
21. Chamberlain MA, Care G, Harfield B. Physiotherapy in osteoarthritis of the knees. *Int Rehabil Med.* 4:101–106, 1982.
22. Fisher N, Prendergast DR, Gresham G, Calkins EC. The effect of muscle rehabilitation on the muscular and functional performance of patients with osteoarthritis of the knees. *Arch Phys Med Rehabil.* 72:367–374, 1991.
23. Fisher N, Pendergast DR, Calkins EC. Maximal isometric torque of knee extension as a function of muscle length in subjects of advancing age. *Arch Phys Med Rehabil.* 71:729, 1990.
24. Cecil RL, Kammerer WH. Rheumatoid arthritis in the elderly. *Am J Med.* April:439–445, 1951.
25. Dordick JR. Rheumatoid arthritis in the elderly. *J Am Geriatr Soc.* 4:588–591, 1951.
26. Brown JW, Sones DA. The onset of rheumatoid arthritis in the aged. *J Am Geriatr Soc.* 15:873–881, 1967.
27. Ehrlich GE, Katz WA, Cohen SH. Rheumatoid arthritis in the aged. *Geriatrics.* February:103–113, 1970.
28. Terkeltaub R, Esdaile J, Decary F, Tannenbau H. A clinical study of older age rheumatoid arthritis with comparison to a younger onset group. *J Rheumatol.* 10:418–424, 1983.
29. Deal CL, Meenan RF, Goldenberg DL, et al. The clinical features of elderly-onset rheumatoid arthritis. *Arthritis Rheum.* 28:987–994, 1985.
30. Gerber LH, Hicks JE. Rehabilitation management of rheumatic diseases. In: *Handbook of Rehabilitation Rheumatology.* Atlanta, Ga: American Rheumatism Association; 1988:82–90.
31. Minor MA, Hewett JE, Webel RR, Anderson SK, Kay DR. Efficacy of physical conditioning exercise in patients with rheumatoid arthritis and osteoarthritis. *Arthritis Rheum.* 32:1396–1405, 1989.
32. Harkcom TM, Lampman RM, Banwell BF, Caston CW. Therapeutic value of graded aerobic exercise training in rheumatoid arthritis. *Arthritis Rheum.* 28:32–39, 1985.
33. Semble EL, Loeser RF, Wise CM. Therapeutic exercise for rheumatoid arthritis and osteoarthritis. *Semin Arthritis Rheum.* 20:32–40, 1990.

34. Lyngberg K, Danneskiold-Samsoe B, Halskov O. The effect of physical training on patients with rheumatoid arthritis: changes in disease activity, muscle strength and aerobic capacity, a clinically controlled minimized cross-over study. *Clin Exp Rheum.* 6:253–269, 1988.

35. Nordemar R, Ekblom B, Zachrisson L, et al. Physical training in rheumatoid arthritis: a controlled long-term study I. *Scand J Rheumatol.* 10:17–23, 1981.

36. Nordemar R. Physical training in rheumatoid arthritis: a controlled long-term study II. Functional capacity and general attitudes. *Scan J Rheumatol.* 10:25–30, 1981.

37. Bland JH, Eady WM. Hemiplegia and rheumatoid arthritis. *Arthritis Rheum.* 11:72–79, 1968.

38. Glynn JJ, Clayton MH. Sparing effect of hemiplegia on tophaceous gout. *Ann Rheum Dis.* 35:534–535, 1976.

39. Thompson M, Bywaters EGL. Unilateral rheumatoid arthritis following hemiplegia. *Ann Rheum Dis.* 21:370–377, 1962.

40. Palmosk MJ, Brandt KD. Immobilization of the knee prevents osteoartritis after anterior chuciate ligament transection. *Arthritis Rheum.* 25:1201–1208, 1982.

41. Joseph RR, Zarafonetis CJD. Clinical onset of lupus erythematosus in the older age group. *J Am Geriatr Soc.* 787–799, 1964.

42. Foad BSI, Sheon RP, Kirsner AB. Systemic lupus erythematosus in the elderly. *Arch Intern Med.* 130:743–746, 1990.

43. Dimant J, Ginzler EM, Schlesinger M, Diamond HS, Kaplan D. Systemic lupus erythematosus in the older age group: computer analysis. *J Am Geriatr Soc.* 27:58–61, 1979.

44. Baker SB, Rovira JR, Campion EW, Mills JA. Late onset systemic lupus erythematosus. *Am J Med.* 66:727–732, 1979.

45. Ballou SP, Khan MA, Kushner I. Clinical features of systemic lupus erythematosus. *Arthritis Rheum.* 25:55–60, 1982.

46. McDonald K, Hutchinson M, Breshihan B. The frequent occurrence of neurological disease in patients with late-onset systemic lupus erythematosus. *Br J Rheum.* 23:186–189, 1984.

47. Catoggio LJ, Skinner RP, Smith G, Maddison PJ. Systemic lupus erythematosus in the elderly: clinical and serological characteristics. *J Rheum.* 11:175–180, 1984.

48. Hashimoto H, Tsuda H, Hirano T, Takasaki Y, Matsumoto T, Hirose S. Differences in clinical and immunlogical findings of systemic lupus erythematosus related to age. *J Rheum.* 14:497–501, 1987.

49. Ward MM, Polisson RP. A meta-analysis of the clinical manifestations of older-onset systemic lupus erythematosus. *Arthritis Rheum.* 32:1226–1232, 1989.

50. Lehman JF. Lower extremity orthotics. In: Redford JB, ed. *Orthotics, Etc.* Baltimore, Md: Williams and Wilkins; 1986:327–337.

51. Chard MD, Hazleman BL. Shoulder disorders in the elderly (a hospital study). *Ann Rheum Dis.* 46:684–687, 1987.

52. Neer CS. *Shoulder Reconstruction.* Philadelphia, Pa: W. B. Saunders; 1990:498.

53. Insall JN. *Surgery of the Knee.* New York, NY: Churchill Livingstone; 1984:551–586.

54. Bombelli R, Andrew TA, Flanagan JP. *Intertrochanteric osteotomy of the hip.* In: Chapman MW, ed.: *Operative Orthopaedics.* Philadelphia, Pa: J. B. Lippincott; 1988:649–662.

55. Opitz JL. Total joint arthroplasty. Principles and guidelines for postoperative physiatric management. *Mayo Clin Proc.* 54:602–612, 1979.

56. Aufranc OE, Harris SM, McKay SJ, Dinardo DM. Rehabilitation in revision arthroplasty. In: Turner RH, Scheller AD, eds. *Revision Hip Arthroplasty:* New York, NY: Grune and Stratton; 1982:379–396.

57. Chandler HP. Postoperative rehabilitation of the total hip patient. In: Stillwell WT, ed.: *The Art of Total Hip Arthroplasty.* New York, NY: Grune and Stratton; 1987:371–401.

58. Ecker ML, Lotke PA. Postoperative care of the total knee patient. *Orthop Clin North Am.* 20(1):55–62, 1989.

59. Insall JN. *Surgery of the Knee,* New York, NY: Churchill Livingstone; 1984:646–648.

11

Metabolic Bone Diseases and Aging

Mehrsheed Sinaki and John J. Nicholas

Skeletal tissue consists of an extracellular matrix (35% organic and 65% inorganic) and cells. The functions of bone tissue are twofold: (a) it provides the mechanical framework for the body, and (b) it is the body's major source of calcium. The skeletal system must be strong enough to withstand mechanical stress generated by weight bearing and physical activity and also dense enough to contribute to the maintenance of serum calcium concentration within a narrow range by yielding a part of its mineral content on demand (1). The most common metabolic disorder of bone is osteoporosis, and probably it is the least well understood. Paget's disease is also a common bone disorder, second in incidence to osteoporosis. Although Paget's disease of bone is generally grouped with metabolic bone disease, it is a unifocal or multifocal disease of the skeleton with unknown cause. These disorders of bone are discussed on the following pages.

Skeletal formation and resorption are coupled by coordinated actions of osteoblasts and osteoclasts in young adults. The actions of bone cells are regulated by hormones and systems as well as by local factors. Any disturbance in the coupling of formation and resorption can favor increased bone porosity or density. Bone, like other connective tissues, is affected by the process of aging. The effect of aging can extend to the point of morbidity and become pathologic.

Disorders of bone may result from diverse origin (intrinsic or extrinsic). Any factor that compromises the synthesis of calcifiable collagen can affect the endurance of bone and result in metabolic bone disease. These factors can range from disturbances of vascularity in bone and compromised nutrition of bone to changes in the mechanical loading of bone. Finally, hormonal imbalances, such as adrenal, gonadal, thyroid, pituitary, and parathyroid, are capable of producing bone disease.

Therefore, it is obvious that metabolic bone disease may be primary (due to an intrinsic factor affecting the skeleton) or secondary to external factors. It is a very simplistic approach to try to summarize these factors in one or two pages. The focus of this chapter is on care of the aged population affected by these skeletal changes.

Basic calcium phosphate salts are found deposited on the collagenous organic matrix. Bone, although a solid structure, is a metabolically active tissue. Hormones play a significant role in disturbances of bone. Parathyroid hormone can contribute to bone formation or resorption. Cortisol and other glucocorticoids have been shown to inhibit protein synthesis in vitro in several connective tissues, including bone. Therefore, they play an important role in new bone matrix synthesis. They also contribute to stabilization of lysosomal membranes, which is important in bone resorption. Thyroid hormone seems to inhibit bone cell protein synthesis in vitro. Also, in hyperthyroidism, increased metabolism contributes to an increment in bone turnover, which, with aging, favors resorption more than formation. Obviously, resorption results in bone loss. The sex hormones, both testosterone and estrogen, are known to exert metabolic influences on bone. This role is in addition to their involvement in epiphyseal closure during the early years of life. Growth hormone not only stimulates cartilage growth but also increases amino acid uptake in animal bone. Vitamin D plays two roles: (a) it affects intestinal absorption of phosphorus and calcium, and (b) in supraphysiologic levels, it can stimulate bone resorption, similar to the effect of parathyroid hormone. Calcitonin is a 32-amino-acid protein produced by thyroid C cells in higher mammals. It suppresses bone resorption through inhibition of osteoclastic activities.

OSTEOPOROSIS

Osteoporosis (increased porosity of bone) is a chronic disease that affects elderly people and is more severe in women than in men. The bone loss occurs predominantly from increased resorption disproportionate and in excess of bone formation. Osteoporosis can be primary or secondary to several disorders (Table 11.1). The types of osteoporosis are as follows: postmenopausal (type I), senile (type II), and secondary (type III) (2).

Table 11.1. Some Common Causes of Osteoporosis[a]

Hereditary, congenital: osteogenesis imperfecta, neurologic
  disturbances (myotonia congenita, Werdnig-Hoffmann disease),
  gonadal dysgenesis
Acquired (primary and secondary)
  Generalized
    Idiopathic (premenopausal women and middle-aged or young
      men; juvenile osteoporosis)
    Postmenopausal (type I)
    Senile (type II)
    Secondary (type III)
      Nutrition
        Malnutrition, anorexia nervosa
        Vitamin deficiency (C or D)
        Vitamin overuse (D or A)
        Calcium deficiency
        High sodium intake
        High caffeine intake
        High protein intake
        High phosphate intake
        Chronic alcoholism
        Sedentary life-style
      Gastrointestinal diseases (liver disease, malabsorption
        syndromes, alactasia, subtotal gastrectomy)
      Nephropathies
      Chronic obstructive pulmonary disease
      Malignancy (multiple myeloma, disseminated carcinoma)
      Immobility
      Drugs: phenytoin, barbiturates, cholestyramine, heparin
      Endocrine disorders
        Acromegaly
        Hyperthyroidism
        Cushing's syndrome (iatrogenic or endogenous)
        Hyperparathyroidism
        Diabetes mellitus (?)
        Hypogonadism
  Localized
    Inflammatory arthritis
    Fractures and immobilization in cast
    Limb dystrophies
    Muscular paralysis

[a]Modified from Sinaki M. Spinal osteoporosis. In: Sinaki M, ed. *Basic Clinical Rehabilitation Medicine*. Toronto: B. C. Decker; 1987:215–224. By permission of Mayo Foundation.

Primary osteoporosis is a major public health problem (3); an estimated 6 million persons are affected in the United States. Osteoporosis is radiographically demonstrable in the spine of about 25% of white women older than 60 years. Osteoporosis is costly and taxing on health care systems. In this country, about 1 million fractures per year occur in women after age 45 years; 70% of these are attributable to osteoporosis.

Osteoporosis consists of a heterogeneous group of syndromes in which there is reduced bone mass per unit volume, which results in increased porosity of bone and increases the likelihood of fracture (4). In osteoporosis the ratio of mineral to matrix is normal, but in osteomalacia, mineral is significantly reduced. Osteoporosis becomes clinically significant only when the bone fractures. Osteopenia is the reduction of bone mass without the occurrence of fractures. There are several types of

clinical osteoporosis. Type I occurs from age 51 years to 75 years, and the ratio of women to men is 6:1. Bone loss is mainly trabecular and fracture sites are the vertebrae (crush) and distal radius. Parathyroid function is decreased, as is calcium absorption. Type II occurs after age 70 years, and the ratio of women to men is 2:1. Bone loss is trabecular and cortical, and fracture sites are the vertebrae (multiple wedge) and hip. Parathyroid function is increased, and calcium absorption is decreased. Another form of primary osteoporosis is idiopathic osteoporosis found in premenopausal women, young or middle-aged men, or juveniles. Secondary osteoporosis (type III) results from an identifiable cause, such as early oophorectomy (in women), hypogonadism (in men), immobilization, pharmacologic doses of glucocorticoids or thyroid hormones, subtotal gastrectomy, and chronic obstructive pulmonary disease. Osteopenia and osteoporosis associated with multiple myeloma, disseminated carcinoma, or a long history of alcohol abuse are among some of the commonly missed diagnoses.

Symptoms of Osteoporosis

Osteoporosis is asymptomatic until fractures occur. Limb fractures are usually clinically evident, but some vertebral fractures, particularly the wedge fractures associated with type II (senile) osteoporosis, may not catch the physician's attention. Limb fractures aside, the osteoporotic patient who seeks medical care is usually one in whom the reduction of bone mass is so advanced that vertebral compression fractures are identifiable radiographically. Such fractures occur most frequently in the lower thoracic and upper lumbar areas, but the mid-thoracic and lower lumbar vertebrae are also often affected (5). Cervical and upper thoracic vertebrae are rarely, if ever, involved (Fig. 11.1) (6).

Vertebral fractures are often manifested by pain at the involved level of the spine. In patients with symptomatic osteoporosis, back pain is usually a major complaint and can be acute or chronic. The pain may develop gradually or occur suddenly when a person falls, lifts a heavy object, or performs some other activity. Indeed, acute pain that occurs in the absence of a previously known fracture should strongly suggest a vertebral compression fracture, especially in a patient in whom osteoporosis has previously been diagnosed. Sometimes a minor fall or even an affectionate hug may lead to fracture of a vertebra or rib. Because some vertebral fractures may not be apparent on radiographs for up to 4 weeks after the injury (7), evaluation of the serum alkaline phosphatase level or follow-up radiographs may be necessary for a firm diagnosis of fracture.

Acute Pain

An increase in the porosity of bone contributes to its susceptibility to fracture in elderly persons (8, 9). Pa-

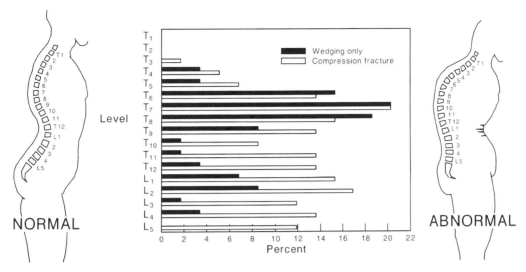

Figure 11.1 Incidence of wedging and compression fractures at various levels in radiographic evaluation of osteoporotic spine. From Sinaki M, Mikkelsen BA. Postmenopausal spinal osteoporosis: flexion versus extension exercises. *Arch Phys Med Rehabil.* 65:593–596, 1984. By permission of American Congress of Rehabilitation Medicine and the American Academy of Physical Medicine and Rehabilitation.

tients can have severe spinal osteoporosis without experiencing vertebral fractures if routine activities, such as lifting and bending, are avoided. Certainly, the susceptibility to fracture is much greater than that of persons without the disease, and it is essentially only a matter of time before exposure to even mild trauma will cause vertebral compression. Fortunately, compression rather than displacement of vertebral bones is the rule. Treatment of compression fractures must focus on relief of pain and prevention of further fractures. The fractures will heal in time, although the resulting bone deformity will remain. Development of kyphosis and scoliosis is the result of these changes.

Acute back pain is usually due to a recent vertebral fracture. It can be diminished by bedrest for 2 to 4 days (on a hard mattress with a soft covering such as synthetic sheepskin or a 2-inch foam pad), although prolonged bedrest can aggravate bone loss. Proper positioning of the patient and correct use of pillows are crucial factors in the effectiveness of bedrest. The patient may need application of proper back support to decrease pain induced by upright posture. The purpose of supporting the spine is to permit ambulation while allowing rest for the painful area of the back.

Moderate heat (10) and a gentle massage (11) of the paraspinal muscles will help decrease pain resulting from spasms. Massage should be done exclusively with gentle stroking because deep massage and heavy pressure may exacerbate the pain.

Mild analgesics may be used when needed to relieve pain. Strong analgesics with codeine should be used only in the most refractory cases, and then for only brief periods. Constipation can be especially distressing to a patient with persistent back pain. Steps should be taken to avoid this problem; if present, it should be treated.

If acute pain persists despite a trial of bedrest, a properly fitted back support is appreciated more by most patients than any other treatment measure. Full-support, rigid polypropylene braces or bivalved body jackets (Fig. 11.2) are preferred and usually give the best relief (12). Unfortunately, some patients, usually elderly persons, do not tolerate rigid back braces. These braces are obviously confining, and some of the jackets may weigh as much as 4 pounds. In these instances, a semirigid thoracolumbar support with shoulder straps is a good alternative (13) (Fig. 11.3). The shoulder straps help remind patients with kyphotic posture to avoid stooping. Rigid back braces, which are usually better tolerated by young patients, provide stronger support (13).

Sometimes severe kyphoscoliosis interferes with proper fitting of conventional back supports. Also, in the presence of diaphragmatic hernia, obesity, or emphysema, the increment of intraabdominal pressure is poorly tolerated. In such cases, a newly developed posture training support (PTS) can be used. This may be of help if the patient does not tolerate conventional back supports (14) (Fig. 11.4). For proper fitting of the PTS, the weighted pouch should fit below the shoulder blades and above the waistline of the subject. The shoulder straps contribute to shoulder extension, and the weight compensates for some of the upper body weight.

Chronic Pain

Chronic pain may be due to vertebral fractures or may result from kyphotic or scoliotic changes in the spine with inappropriate stretching of ligaments. Sometimes kyphosis causes pressure of the lower part of the rib cage over the pelvic rim and results in significant flank pain

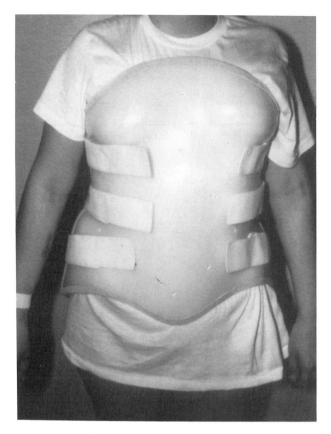

Figure 11.2. Anterior view of rigid back support (bivalved body jacket). This brace, made of polypropylene, is custom-fitted. From Sinaki M. Postmenopausal spinal osteoporosis: By permission of Mayo Foundation.

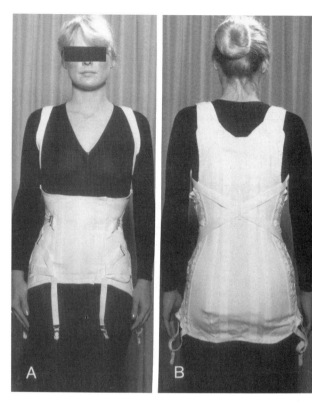

Figure 11.3. Thoracolumbar support with rigid or semirigid stays applied on each side of spine. Addition of shoulder straps further decreases kyphotic posture and reminds patient to avoid severe stooping. Proper padding can be added to shoulder straps to decrease pressure over bony prominences. A, Anterior view; B, Posterior view. From Sinaki M. Exercise and physical therapy. In: Riggs BL, Melton LJ III, eds. *Osteoporosis: Etiology, Diagnosis, and Management*. New York, NY: Raven Press; 1988:457–479. By permission of Raven Press.

and tenderness (15). In healthy posture there is sufficient space between the lower ribs and the iliac crest, and thus no contact occurs. In severe cases of osteoporosis with compression fractures and severe dorsal kyphosis and loss of height, iliocostal contact occurs (Fig. 11.5). In the case of flank pain, measures that can widen the space between the lower ribs and iliac crest are helpful. In our experience, application of a PTS has been helpful in these cases (Fig. 11.6) (16). Flank pain can be overlooked in osteoporotic patients (12). Severe kyphosis can also result in dyspnea because of reduction in functional vital capacity, and patients do not tolerate any additional abdominal pressure. Therefore, this type of chronic pain needs to be treated primarily with measures that improve posture. These include proper back extension exercises and use of a PTS. The biomechanical approach of the PTS appropriately positions weights below the inferior angles of the scapulae, counteracting the tendency to bend forward, and decreases kyphotic posturing, which is due to weakness of back extensors. The usual effective weight is 1¾ pounds. By improving the patient's posture and balance during ambulation, one can reduce the risk of falls (Fig. 11.7).

Improving the muscular support of the spine by proper strengthening exercises should be tried whenever possible. Strong back muscles contribute to good posture and skeletal support. In a recent study, the back extensor strength of osteoporotic and normal women aged 40 to 85 years was compared. The results demonstrated that the osteoporotic women had significantly lower back extensor strength than the normal women (Fig. 11.8) (17, 18). Furthermore, this decrease in strength was demonstrated to be specific to the back and not part of generalized muscle weakness (18). This finding suggests that the discrepancy in back strength between normal and osteoporotic women probably develops because of pain and discomfort or lack of proper recruitment of back muscles. The study also demonstrated that the levels of physical activity of the two groups were comparable and not significantly different, except for involvement of the younger, normal women (aged 40 to 59 years) in more sports activities (Figs. 11.9 and 11.10). This finding further indicated that one needs to improve the safety of life-style in osteoporotic women because they are as involved in the activities of daily living as normal women. Exercises that improve back strength contribute to the maintenance of good posture (19, 20). Extension exercises (21) and exercises to reduce lumbar lordosis

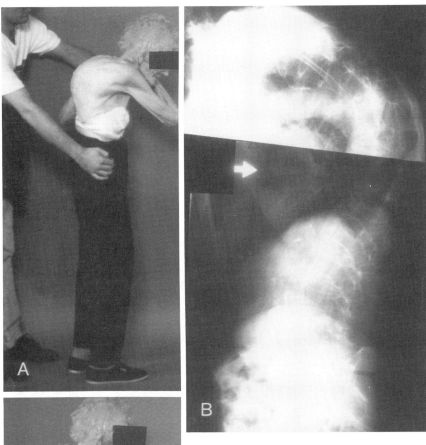

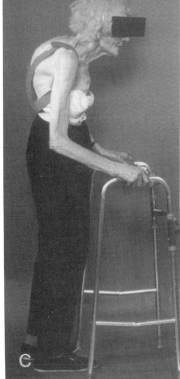

Figure 11.4.   Use of posture training support (PTS). A, Patient with severe kyphosis and poor balance secondary to postural changes. Patient had lack of tolerance for conventional bracing and so was fitted with the posture training support. **B,** Radiograph of the patient's spine. **C,** Patient was able to walk better with the PTS on. (*A* and *C*, from Sinaki M. A new back support in rehabilitation of osteoporosis program - exercise: posture training support. *In* Osteoporosis 1990. Third International Symposium on Osteoporosis, Copenhagen, Denmark. Edited by Christiansen C, Overgaard K. Ll. Kirkestraede 1, DK-1072 København K. Denmark, Osteopress ApS, 1990: 1355–1357. By permission of the publisher.)

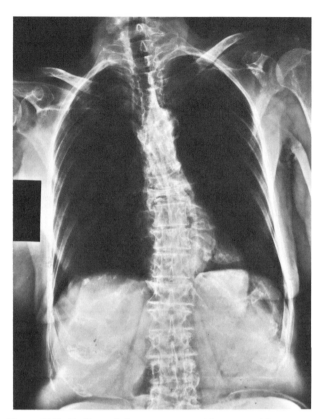

Figure 11.5   Radiograph from a 72-year-old woman with osteoporosis who had compressions of T-7, T-8, T-9, and the visualized lumbar vertebrae and anterior wedging of T-11. Radiograph demonstrates iliocostal contact in standing posture.

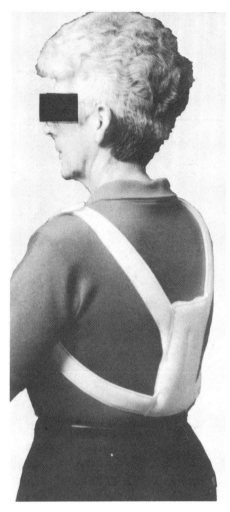

Figure 11.6.   Posture Training Support. Pouch permits weights from ¼ pound to 2 pounds, in ¼-pound increments, to be added in a gradual, progressive, balanced manner for patient tolerance and acceptance. From PTS Posturing brochure A838, 1991, Jackson, Mich: Camp International. By permission of BISSELL Healthcare Corporation.

are recommended. The exercise program should be individualized for each patient according to the severity of bone loss and the patient's ability; the program can range from back extension exercises while prone to pectoral stretching and back extension while sitting (Figs. 11.11 through 11.13). Weight-bearing exercises are helpful for maintenance of musculoskeletal health (Fig. 11.14). These exercises should be prescribed by a physician to avoid injury to the fragile skeleton.

Flexion exercises are not recommended because they can increase the vertical compression forces on the vertebral body, increase the possibility of anterior wedge fractures, and further increase the kyphosis. In a study by Sinaki and Mikkelsen (6), 59 women with postmenopausal spinal osteoporosis and back pain had been instructed in a treatment program that included back-strengthening extension exercises in 25, back-strengthening flexion exercises in 9, and combined extension and flexion exercises in 19; no therapeutic exercises were prescribed in 6. Their ages ranged from 49 years to 60 years (mean, 56 years). Follow-up ranged from 1 year to 6 years (the mean for the age groups was 1.4 years to 2 years). All the patients had spinal radiographic studies before treatment and at follow-up examinations, at which time any further wedging and compression were recorded. Additional vertebral fractures, by group, oc-

curred as follows: extension group, 16%; flexion group, 89%; extension and flexion group, 53%; and no exercise group, 67%. In comparision with the extension group, the occurrence of wedging or compression fractures was significantly higher in the flexion group and in the extension and flexion group. The authors concluded that significantly more vertebral compression fractures occur in patients with postmenopausal spinal osteoporosis who follow a back-strengthening exercise program that involves flexion of the spine than in those who perform extension exercises. Therefore, extension or isometric exercises seem to be more appropriate for patients with spinal osteoporosis (Figs. 11.11 through 11.13).

Assistive Devices

Fracture of the hip is the drastic event in osteoporosis. It mainly occurs in type II (age-related) osteo-

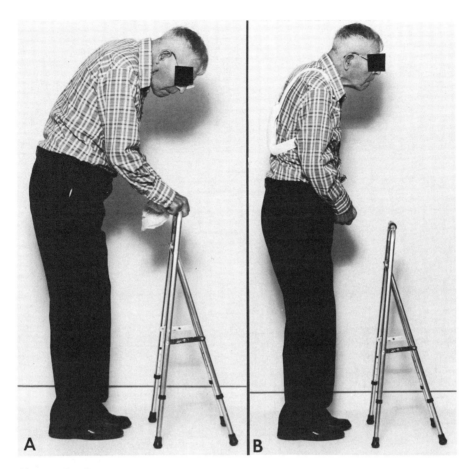

Figure 11.7. Patient with (A) and without (B) Walkane. Application of Posture Training Support enabled the patient to ambulate without the Walkane. From Sinaki M. Musculoskeletal rehabilitation in osteo-porosis. In: Riggs BL, Melton LJ. *Osteoporosis: Etiology, Diagnosis, and Management.* 2nd ed. New York, NY: Raven Press; 1993. By permission of Mayo Foundation.

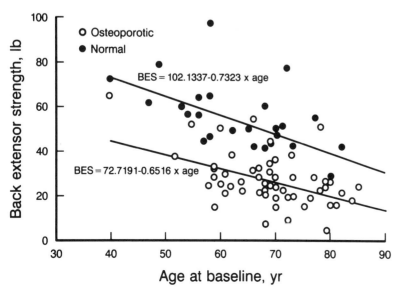

Figure 11.8 Relationship of back extensor strength (BES), in pounds, to age, for normal and osteoporotic subjects, with least-squares regression lines fitted separately to each group. Slopes are not significantly different, but intercepts are (*P*<0.001). From Sinaki M, Khosla S, Limburg PJ, Rogers JW, Murtaugh PA. Muscle strength in osteoporotic versus normal woman. *Osteoporosis Int.* 3:8–12, 1993. By permission of European Foundation for Osteoporosis.

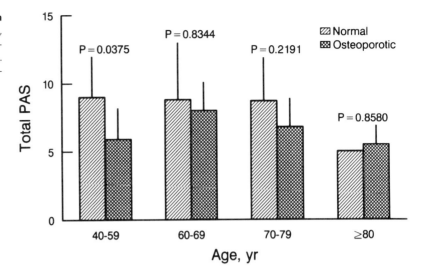

Figure 11.9. Total physical activity score (PAS) in normal and osteoporotic women. From Sinaki M, Khosla S, Limburg PJ, Rogers JW, Murtaugh PA. Muscle strength in osteoporotic versus normal women. *Osteoporosis Int.* 3:8–12, 1993. By permission of European Foundation for Osteoporosis.

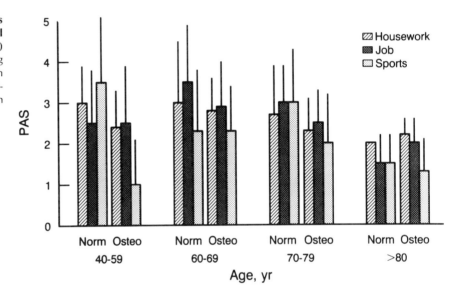

Figure 11.10. Mean scores on components of physical activity scores (PAS) in normal (Norm) and osteoporotic (Osteo) women. From Sinaki M, Khosla S, Limburg PJ, Rogers JW, Murtaugh PA. Muscle strength in osteoporotic versus normal women. *Osteoporosis Int.* 3:8–12, 1993. By permission of European Foundation for Osteoporosis.

porosis. Hip fracture is generally associated with a specific episode of trauma, usually a fall. In elderly persons, the prevalence of failing vision, muscle weakness, incoordination, and faulty posture increases the risk of falls. The use of assistive devices (canes or walkers) is of utmost importance in improving a patient's safety of gait and, in some instances, in decreasing low back pain induced by ambulatory activities.

Recreational Activities and the Osteoporotic Spine

Early instruction on the principles of proper posture may decrease the rate of worsening of the kyphosis and of falls. To avoid strenuous flexion of the spine, patients should refrain from heavy lifting and should carry any weights close to the body.

Not all types of exercise are appropriate for these patients because of the fragility of their vertebrae. Ex-

ercises that place compressive forces on the vertebrae beyond the biomechanical competence of bone, whether or not accompanied by extension strengthening exercises, tend to cause an increased number of vertebral fractures. Golfing, a favorite sport among elderly persons, can be harmful in patients with osteoporosis if unguarded strenuous bending and twisting are attempted. During the midswing while golfing, the spine is exposed to compressive forces that may exceed the ultimate biomechanical competence of vertebral bodies; therefore, compression fractures can occur. Cases of vertebral compression fractures sustained during golfing have been reported (22). Until more studies of kinematics and kinetics of the spine during the golf swing become available, application of rigid back supports is recommended for golfers who have osteoporosis of the spine and do not change their sports activities. Bowling involves similar risks. However, patients who enjoy these sports and who would feel a psychologic loss in giving them up

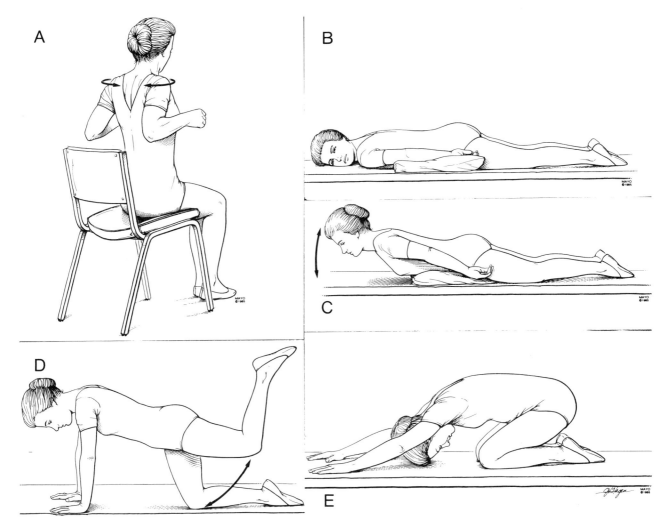

Figure 11.11. Back extension exercises. A, In sitting position. This position avoids or minimizes pain in patients with severe osteoporosis. **B** and **C,** In prone position. **D,** Exercise for improving strength in lumbar extensors and gluteus maximus muscles. **E,** In cat-stretch position. From Sinaki M. Exercise and physical therapy. In: Riggs BL, Melton LJ III, eds. *Osteoporosis: Etiology, Diagnosis, and Management.* New York, NY: Raven Press; 1988:457–459. By permission of Mayo Foundation.

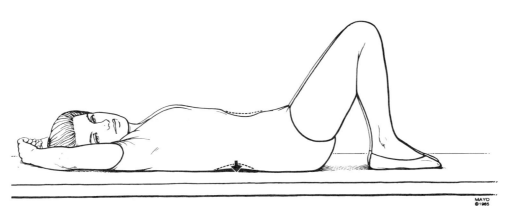

Figure 11.12. Exercise to decrease lumbar lordosis with isometric contraction of lumbar flexors. From Sinaki M. Exercise and physical therapy. In: Riggs BL, Melton LJ III, eds. *Osteoporosis: Etiology, Diagnosis, and Management.* New York, NY: Raven Press; 1988:457–459. By permission of Mayo Foundation.

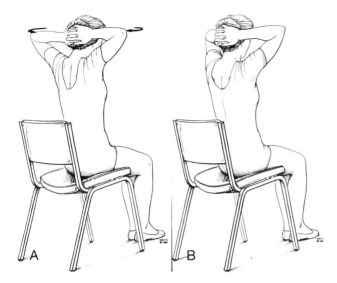

Figure 11.13. A and B, Deep-breathing exercise combined with pectoral stretching and back extension exercise. Patient sits on a chair, locks her hands behind her head, and inhales deeply while she gently extends her elbows backward. While exhaling, she returns to the starting position. This is repeated 10 to 15 times. From Sinaki M. Exercise and physical therapy. In: Riggs BL, Melton LJ III, eds. *Osteoporosis: Etiology, Diagnosis, and Management.* New York, NY: Raven Press; 1988:457–459. By permission of Mayo Foundation.

Laboratory and Radiographic Evaluation

Diagnostic evaluation for osteoporosis consists of a thorough history and physical examination. Routine radiography often includes anteroposterior and lateral thoracic views and lumbar spine films. Radiographs should be evaluated for vertebral biconcavity, or "cod fish" appearance, wedging (the anterior height of the vertebra is less than the posterior height, except for the fifth lumbar vertebra), and obvious compression fracture of the vertebral body. The examination also includes radiographs of the chest to look for lymphomas and rib fractures; complete blood cell count to rule out anemias of malignancies, especially in multiple myeloma; chemistry group tests to assess the level of alkaline phosphatase, which can increase in osteomalacia, bony metastasis, and new fracture (these tests will also demonstrate an increase in phosphorus and calcium in hyperparathyroidism); urinalysis to check for proteinuria secondary to nephrotic syndrome and low pH secondary to renal tubular acidosis causing osteopenia; 24-hour urine test to exclude hypercalciuria; determination of the erythrocyte sedimentation rate (elevated in multiple myeloma); and serum protein electrophoresis to determine changes indicative of multiple myeloma. A normal serum electrophoresis pattern excludes the presence of multiple myeloma in 90% of patients. Increased total thyroxine concentration may be a cause of osteoporosis because of increased bone turnover (24).

Type I (postmenopausal osteoporosis) is diagnosed by exclusion. Radiographs of the spine substantiate the presence of osteoporosis, but objective assessment of bone mass is not evident in conventional radiographs until at least 25% to 30% of bone mineral has been lost. Some of the optional procedures for further confirmation of the diagnosis of osteoporosis are dual-energy absorptiometry and quantitative computed tomography to determine the bone density of the lumbar spine (25) and to evaluate the risk of fracture. These procedures may also help to assess the efficacy of a therapeutic trial. Iliac

should be advised to wear an adequate back support to prevent stooping. Swimming is ineffective for improving the bone mineral density of the spine, but it is an important exercise for fitness (23). Walking is a safe, weight-bearing exercise for the fragile skeleton. Bicycling is also acceptable if the patient has a proper posture and avoids bending positions (that is, sits up straight). The cautious approach is always recommended when an exercise program is to be prescribed for a patient with a fragile skeleton. A feasible exercise program can contribute to the maintenance of skeletal health. A patient's coordination and balance should be considered before prescribing an exercise program.

Figure 11.14. Muscle strengthening and weight-bearing exercises that may decrease bone loss. (These exercises were developed for the osteopenic spine by M. Sinaki through a grant from the Retirement Research Foundation. These techniques are designed to decrease strain on the spine despite weight bearing.) **A and B,** Shoulder extensors contribute to reduction of kyphotic posturing. Shoulder extensors can be strengthened with a proper combination of weight lifting and weight-bearing exercises while balance is maintained. One knee is bent to avoid lumbar strain. *Note:* The amount of weight lifted is about 1 to 2 pounds in each hand, not to exceed 5 pounds in each hand. The amount of weight needs to be prescribed according to the patient's bone mineral density (status of osteoporosis) and the condition of the upper extremities. **C through E,** Bilateral or unilateral spine and hip weight-bearing exercise. To avoid straining the spine and to maintain balance, leaning or holding onto a steady ob-

ject for support is recommended. When weight is lifted above the head, knees should be bent slightly to avoid straining the lumbar spine. *Note:* The amount of weight lifted is about 1 to 2 pounds in each hand, not to exceed 5 pounds in each hand. The amount of weight needs to be prescribed according to the patient's bone mineral density (status of osteoporosis) and the condition of the upper extremities. **F,** In cases of limited shoulder abduction, weight lifting *only* to the shoulder level is recommended. *Note:* The amount of weight lifted is about 1 to 2 pounds in each hand, not to exceed 5 pounds in each hand. The amount of weight needs to be prescribed according to the patient's bone mineral density (status of osteoporosis) and the condition of the upper extremities. From Sinaki M. Metabolic bone disease. In: Sinaki M. *Basic Clinical Rehabilitation Medicine.* 2nd ed. Chicago, Ill: Mosby-Year Book; 1993:211–238. By permission of Mayo Foundation.

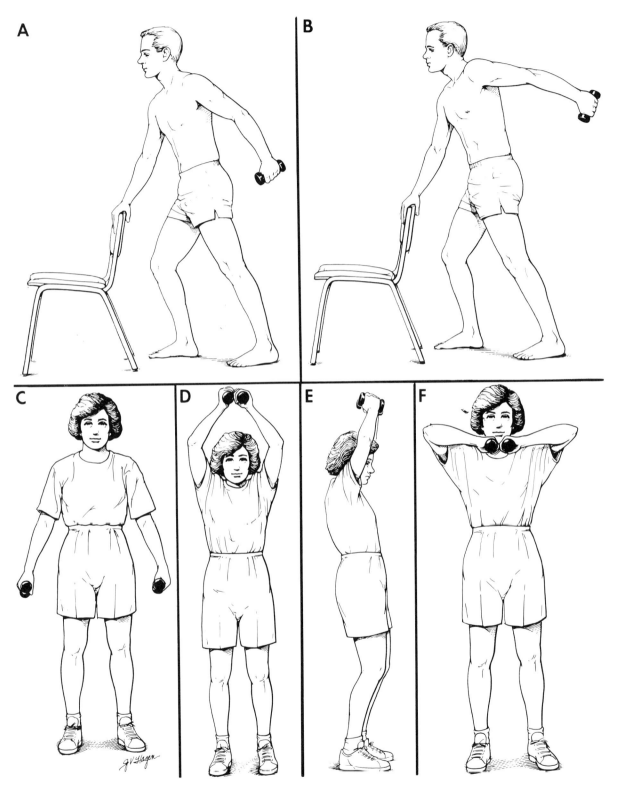

Figure 11.14

crest biopsy (after tetracycline double labeling for bone histomorphometry) to evaluate high turnover bone loss and therapeutic decisions is useful for characterizing osteoporosis but is not justified in patients who have type I disease without atypical features. Examination of bone marrow is needed to exclude multiple myeloma and metastatic malignancy (26).

Therapeutic Measures

Usually, acute pain from a new vertebral fracture is self-subsiding and takes anywhere from a few weeks to 2 or 3 months to abate (Table 11.2). Chronic pain due to postural deformity may persist. Improvement of faulty posture with feasible exercise programs or application of proper back support can help to decrease this pain (Table 11.2).

Acute pain is most often managed through implementation of sedative measures and proper positioning principles. Among the strong analgesics, codeine sulfate or its derivatives result in constipation; thus, simple analgesics are preferred if they are adequate. At this stage, physiatric management is vital. Physical therapists and occupational therapists can be of great help in providing the proper means to decrease the duration of immobility and expedite the course of recovery. Proper therapeutic exercise programs, preferably spinal extension exercises, are recommended (6, 12). Proper exercise and rehabilitative measures have the potential to build bone mass and decrease the rate of bone loss or decrease the frequency of falls.

In type I osteoporosis, the results of ongoing studies suggest that certain progestogens and anabolic agents produce effects similar to those of estrogen (27). For years, anabolic steroids and androgens have been known as potential therapeutic agents for osteoporosis (28). However, androgens are not well tolerated by women because of their masculinizing effects. More recently, Chesnut et al (29) examined the effects of stanozolol and found a small but significant increase in total body

calcium during 2 years of treatment. However, anabolic agents are poorly tolerated by women and can cause hepatic toxicity.

Approximately 10% to 20% of men with osteoporosis have partial or complete hypogonadism of various causes (30). It has been recommended that patients with low plasma testosterone levels should receive replacement therapy, such as testosterone enanthate, under the supervision of an endocrinologist.

The most commonly advocated pharmacologic treatments for involutional osteoporosis are estrogen, calcitonin, calcium, and vitamin D. These medications act by inhibiting or decreasing bone resorption.

Treatment with estrogen delays or halts bone loss and reduces fractures (31, 32). The precise mode of action of estrogen on the skeleton has been under much discussion and even today is unclear. A search for estrogen receptors in bone initially was thought to have positive results (33), but a more careful evaluation of the issue concluded that the protein-binding estrogen in bone was in fact α-fetoprotein and that true estrogen receptors were not present in bone (33, 34).

However, it was recently demonstrated that cultured human osteoblast-like cells possess the properties of target cells for estrogen. The presence of specific estrogen receptors in osteoblasts could indicate a direct effect of estrogen on these cells (35).

Estrogen and calcitonin are bone antiresorptive agents and have been approved by the Food and Drug Administration for use in osteoporosis. In women who have undergone oophorectomy and hysterectomy, a daily dose of 0.625 mg of conjugated equine estrogen (Premarin) is recommended. Transdermal estrogen (Estraderm) has also been shown to be effective as a means to prevent bone loss. Calcium may be beneficial in a small percentage of patients with high-turnover osteoporosis. In this group, diphosphonates may also be effective, but further evaluation of this approach is needed. Estrogen is more effective than calcium but has significant side effects. The most common side effects are mastodynia and fluid retention. More serious but less common ones are endometrial cancer, venous thrombosis and pulmonary embolism, aggravation of hypertension, and cholelithiasis. Calcitonin can be used to inhibit bone resorption in osteoporosis, but its effects on bone mass are limited. Osteoporosis with skeletal pain can be treated successfully with 50 to 100 international units (IU) of salmon calcitonin subcutaneously daily for 5 days a week. If bone pain is not the major factor, as in young postmenopausal women, the recommended treatment is 50 IU, 3 times weekly. Intermittent calcitonin therapy has been successful in reduction of vertebral fracture rates in some cases. Reported side effects such as nausea, anorexia, or mild gastric discomfort can occur in 8% to 10% of patients treated with salmon calcitonin; facial flushing and dermatologic hypersensitivity occur in 5%

Table 11.2. Management of Acute Pain in Patients With Osteoporosis[a]

Bedrest (less than 1 week); significant aggravation of bone loss is not likely to occur during 1 week of bedrest

Analgesics

Avoidance of constipation

Avoidance of exterional exercises

Proper positioning principles to decrease pain and avoid undue strain on spine

Application of a properly fitted and protective support may expedite the resumption of ambulatory activities

Physical therapy: mild heat and stroking massage

[a]Modified from Sinaki M. Spinal osteoporosis. In: Sinaki M, ed. *Basic Clinical Rehabilitation Medicine*. Toronto: B.C. Decker; 1987:215–224. By permission of May Foundation.

to 10%, and local pruritic reactions at injection sites occur in about 10% of patients (36).

Sodium fluoride stimulates osteoblastic activity and has been demonstrated to result in an increase in trabecular bone density of the axial skeleton but does not increase cortical bone density in the appendicular skeleton. Calcium should be administered with sodium fluoride to prevent or minimize the mineralization defect that may occur when fluoride is given alone. The new bone is well mineralized but less resilient. Recent controlled trials have demonstrated an increase in the rate of hip fractures in the treated patients (37). When the treatment group was compared with the placebo group, their bone mineral density had increased 35% (P<0.0001) in the lumbar area (predominantly cancellous bone), 12% (P<0.0001) in the femoral neck, and 10% (P<0.0001) in the femoral trochanter (sites of mixed cortical and cancellous bone), but the bone mineral density had decreased by 4% (P<0.02) in the shaft of the radius (predominantly cortical bone). The number of new vertebral fractures was similar in the treatment and placebo groups, but the number of nonvertebral fractures was higher in the treatment group (72 vs. 24; P<0.01). Therefore, it was concluded that fluoride therapy increases skeletal fragility.

One of the risk factors for osteopenia is inadequate calcium intake (38). Adequate calcium intake, assumed from Heaney and associates' data (39), is a total of 1.5 g/d of elemental calcium. A nutritional diet rich in calcium reduces the risk of osteoporosis (Table 11.3) (40).

Finally, an adequate intake of calcium and vitamin D is required to permit normal bone development and potentially to decrease excessive loss of bone tissue with advancing age. For patients with mild disease, only calcium and vitamin D supplementation need be used. For women within 15 years of menopause, and in some selected cases of older women, low-dose estrogen therapy (cyclic doses of 0.625 mg of conjugated estrogen) may be used. To decrease the risk of endometrial hyperplasia (and carcinoma), concomitant progestogen therapy (5 mg daily during the last 10 days of the cycle) is advocated.

Vitamin D plays a significant role in the absorption of calcium. The recommended daily intake of vitamin D is 400 IU. Although higher levels of supplementation increase the risk of vitamin D intoxication, elderly persons residing in nursing homes may tolerate two to three times the recommended daily allowance of vitamin D if cutaneous generation of vitamin D, mediated through exposure to the sun, is reduced.

Mechanical loading and a carefully designed exercise program play a significant role in the maintenance of skeletal health and the prevention of osteopenia secondary to immobility. Mechanical strain induces a deformation in bone tissue through altering the piezoelectric forces in the bone, which stimulates osteoblastic activity. Mechanical strain applied to in vitro bone cells results in an increase in deoxyribonucleic acid synthesis and collagenous protein synthesis (41). Rehabilitative measures have the potential to build bone mass and decrease the rate of bone loss. Implementation of proper physical therapeutic measures can decrease the risk of falls and promote safety in the ambulatory activities of daily living.

PAGET'S DISEASE OF BONE

In 1877, Sir James Paget (42) described a patient whose skull and bones of the arms and legs were clinically deformed. This man had worn several hats throughout the years, and he had needed an increasingly larger hat size. In addition, the man had lost height, and his legs had become visibly bowed. He ultimately died of osteogenic sarcoma of the left elbow. On pathologic examination, his bones were found to be thickened, and the normal bony architecture was seriously disrupted. This disease has become known as Paget's disease of bone.

Prevalence

In 1932, Schmorl (43) reported that Paget's disease of bone occurred in about 3% of 4,614 autopsy cases of patients older than 40 years. A subsequent radiologic study calculated that the disease occurred in 3.5% of patients older than 45 years (44). The disease is especially common in the British Isles and Italy, but it is rare in the Scandinavian countries.

Table 11.3. Food High in Calcium[a]

Food	Serving Size, oz	Calcium Content, mg
Milk		
Whole	8	290
Skim	8	300
Buttermilk	8	285
Yogurt		
Low-fat, plain	8	415
Low-fat, fruited	8	315
Frozen	8	200
Cheese		
Low-fat cottage	8	154
American	1	174
Cheddar	1	204
Swiss	1	272
Ice cream	8	176
Sardines (with bones)	3	372
Salmon	3	180
Shrimp	8	147
Tofu (bean curd)	4	154
Broccoli (cooked)	8	136
Turnip greens (cooked)	8	267

[a]From Sinaki M, Dale DA, Hurley DL. *Living with Osteoporosis: Guidelines for Women Before and After Diagnosis.* Toronto: B. C. Decker; 1988.

Presentation

The clinical prevalence of this disease is much lower than that determined from radiographic or autopsy results. In many instances, Paget's disease of bone is found on radiography, but it is not clinically apparent or significant. Paget's disease of bone is not clinically significant if it is in the pelvis, and it does not become involved in the pathogenesis of joint disease unless it involves the acetabulum, in which case the weight-bearing area could become a fracture site. The disease is often discovered incidentally on radiographs or when a physician investigates the reason for an increased serum alkaline phosphatase value. Rarely does a patient complain of bony deformities or an increase in hat size. Paget's disease of bone occasionally is found when a pathologic humerus or tibial fracture occurs.

Pathology

The development of Paget's disease of bone is thought to occur in three phases: an osteolytic phase, an osteoblastic phase, and a mixed phase. Initially, osteocytes increase in number and appear abnormal in size and activity, and a marked increase in bone resorption occurs. The osteolytic phase may be confused with metastatic cancer and is frequently prolonged in skull lesions. In the second phase, there is a response from the osteoblast, and the bone becomes dense. Both of these phases may be seen on bone scans. Commonly, the osteoblastic and osteolytic phases are present at the same time in adjacent parts of a bone (mixed phase). The bones are subject to fracture in both the osteolytic and the osteoblastic phases. Ultimately, Paget's disease of bone presents as a very dense bone that is less active on bone scan. Although the bone appears thicker and more dense than normal bone, it is structurally less strong and is, therefore, more subject to fracture (45).

Etiology

The cause of Paget's disease is unknown, but preliminary evidence suggests that a slow-acting virus causes increased activity of the osteoclasts. The reason that a particular site is involved and not another is not at all clear, but it is thought that the disease starts at more than one location at a time.

Laboratory Findings

The serum alkaline phosphatase and the 24-hour urinary hydroxyproline values are both elevated. Bone scans show asymmetric uptake of radionuclide. Standard radiographs reveal coarse and irregular bony trabeculae with increased density or decreased density, depending on the stage of the disease.

Clinical Findings

The clinical findings of Paget's disease depend on the site of involvement. Increased osteolysis of the skull (termed osteoporosis circumscripta cranii) may have no pathologic implications other than an increase in hat size. When the base of the skull is involved, a syndrome of adult hydrocephalus will occur with ataxia, dementia, and incontinence. Deafness is a common occurrence in patients with Paget's disease and may be due to pagetic involvement of the ossicles or deformity of the bone canal.

Occasionally, Paget's disease causes pain in bones. If Paget's disease occurs at or near the knee or hip joint, there may be advanced osteoarthritic changes. If Paget's disease occurs in the spine, the increased density of the bony vertebrae or the supporting structures may compromise the spinal cord and cause spinal stenosis with paraplegia.

Physical examination of the bones reveals an increase in size and deformity. The skin over these bones has increased warmth and tiny multiple petechiae due to vascularity.

Rarely, cancer occurs at the site of Paget's disease. If it occurs, most commonly an aggressive osteogenic sarcoma is seen. The exact incidence of this clinical finding is unknown, but it is probably less than 1% of cases (46). Metastatic carcinoma may be present at the site of Paget involvement and must be distinguished from primary osteogenic sarcoma because the treatments for these disorders are remarkably different (47). Furthermore, multiple myeloma appears to occur in Paget's disease of bone with increased frequency.

Fractures occur in the osteolytic, osteoblastic, and mixed phases of Paget's disease of bone. These fractures occur often after "trivial" trauma and appear to be pathologic. However, the fractures, when stabilized, heal rapidly (48).

Treatment

Three agents are available for the treatment of Paget's disease of bone. The first, mithramycin, is an anticancer agent that markedly and promptly diminishes the activity of the osteoclast within hours to days of its administration. The second drug, calcitonin, also diminishes osteoclastic activity but does so more slowly, requiring days to weeks for its effect to be seen. Calcitonin must be given subcutaneously and is expensive. Finally, a diphosphate may be given orally at a modest expense, but it requires weeks to months for its actions to become apparent. The diphosphate is the drug of choice simply on the basis that it may be orally administered, its cost is modest, and the side effects are fewer than the others, especially mithramycin.

The question, then, is when to treat patients with Paget's disease of bone. Some clinicians believe that Paget's disease should be symptomatic before treatment is administered. Symptoms may occur when Paget's disease is at the site of osteoarthritis or when pain from bone occurs at the site of pagetic activity. Others believe that because Paget's disease is progressive without spontaneous remission, treatment should be started promptly and continued until activity has been suppressed; prompt therapy is also needed when pagetic involvement is near a joint or has affected the base of the skull or spine.

Serial determinations of the serum alkaline phosphatase value are appropriate for monitoring treatment. Although concentrations of the enzyme diminish in a predictable fashion with treatment, a complete remission is achieved in only 50% of patients, and many patients simply have a decreased concentration. Treatment with calcitonin, for example, is often followed by a diminished enzyme value or a plateau. The disease may then develop an "escape" when the activity seems to increase, even while the same dose is administered.

The dosage of calcitonin is usually 100 MRC (Medical Research Council) units 3 times per week subcutaneously. Additional amounts have not been shown to be more effective. Diphosphonate is given orally at a dosage of 5 mg per kg of body weight every 24 hours for 6 months. If an increased dosage is used or treatment is continued for a longer period, osteomalacia will likely occur to such an extent that fractures and bone pain will increase. Series of treatments with diphosphonate are then given with a 3-month rest interval between treatments. These treatments are continued until the serum alkaline phosphatase value has been reduced by 50% or until symptoms are relieved.

In addition, when operation for a total knee or total hip arthroplasty or for spinal stenosis is being contemplated, calcitonin should be given for several weeks preoperatively to diminish the likelihood of hemorrhage from the bone at the time of the procedure. Because diphosphonate is likely to cause some osteomalacia, it is usually not given while a fracture is being treated or after joint operation. In addition, the diphosphonate is excreted through the kidneys, and its use in patients with renal failure has not been defined.

Physiatrists may hesitate to treat the occasional patient who presents with Paget's disease. However, physiatrists who are interested in the treatment of patients with musculoskeletal disease and who eventually evaluate several affected patients can become expert in the treatment of this condition. Certainly they will understand the use of canes, walkers, and crutches for patients who cannot ambulate properly before and after operation, and they can treat paraplegia. They should also treat weakness after fracture, total joint replacement, or amputation for cancer. Physiatrists should develop expertise in treating this interesting and long-recognized disease of the skeletal system.

References

1. Mazess RB, Cameron JR. Bone mineral content in normal U.S. whites. In: Mazess RBN, ed International Conference on Bone Mineral Measurement. Washington, DC: United States Department of Health, Education, and Welfare; 1973:228–237. DHEW publication NIH 75-683.
2. Yalleger JC. The pathogenesis of osteoporosis. Bone Mineral. 19:215–227, 1990.
3. Holbrook TL, Grazier K, Kelsey JL, Stauffer RN. Frequency of occurrence, impact and cost of selected musculoskeletal conditions in United States. Chicago, Ill: American Academy of Orthopaedic Surgeons; 1984.
4. Sinaki M. Spinal osteoporosis. In: Sinaki M, ed. Basic Clinical Rehabilitation Medicine. Toronto: B.C. Decker; 1987:215–224.
5. Saville PD. The syndrome of spinal osteoporosis. Clin Endocrinol Metab. 2:177–185, July 1973.
6. Sinaki M, Mikkelsen BA. Postmenopausal spinal osteoporosis: flexion versus extension exercises. Arch Phys Med Rehabil. 65:593–596, 1984.
7. Nordin BEC, Horsman A, Crilly RG, Marshall DH, Simpson M. Treatment of spinal osteoporosis in postmenopausal women. Br Med J. 280:451–454, 1980.
8. Iskrant AP, Smith RW, Jr. Osteoporosis in women 45 years and over related to subsequent fractures. Public Health Rep. 84:33–38, 1969.
9. Riggs BL, Melton LJ III. Involutional osteoporosis. N Engl J Med. 314:1676–1686, 1986.
10. Lehmann JF, De Lateur BJ. Diathermy and superficial heat and cold therapy. In: Kottke FJ, Stillwell GK, Lehmann JF, eds. Krusen's Handbook of Physical Medicine and Rehabilitation. 3rd ed. Philadelphia, Pa: W.B. Saunders; 1982:275–350.
11. Knapp ME. Massage. In: Kottke FJ, Stillwell GK, Lehmann JF, eds. Krusen's Handbook of Physical Medicine and Rehabilitation. Philadelphia, PA: W.B. Saunders; 1982:386–388.
12. Sinaki, M. Postmenopausal spinal osteoporosis: physical therapy and rehabilitation principles. Mayo Clin Proc. 57:699–703, 1982.
13. Lucas DB. Spinal bracing. In: Licht S, ed. Orthotics: Etcetera. New Haven, Conn: Elizabeth Licht, Publisher; 1966:274–305.
14. Sinaki M. New posture training back support in rehabilitation of osteoporosis program-exercise. Arch Phys Med Rehabil. 71:808, 1990. Abstract.
15. Urist MR. Orthopaedic management of osteoporosis in postmenopausal women. Clin Endocrinol Metab. 2:159–176, July 1973.
16. Kaplan RS, Sinaki M. The Posture Training Support (PTS): preliminary report on a case series of patients with symptomatic improvement of osteoporotic complications. Mayo Clin Proc. In press.
17. Sinaki M, Rogers J, Limburg P, Tiegs R, Khosla S, Murtaugh P. Comparison of back muscle strength in osteoporotic versus normal women. In: Overgaard K, Christiansen C, eds. Third International Symposium on Osteoporosis. Glostrup Hospital, Denmark: Department of Clinical Chemistry; 1990. Abstract 524.
18. Sinaki M, Khosla S, Limburg PJ, Rogers JW, Murtaugh PA. Muscle strength in osteoporotic versus normal women. Osteoporosis Int. 3:8–12, 1993.
19. Rogers JW, Sinaki M, Bergstralh EJ, Limburg PJ, Wahner HW. Correlation of bone mass, kyphosis, and back strength in healthy, active postmenopausal women. Arch Phys Med Rehabil. 71:803, 1990. Abstract.
20. Rogers J, Sinaki M, Bergstrahl E, Limburg P, Wahner H. The effect of back extensor strength, physical activity, and vertebral bone density on postural change. Arthritis Rheum. 33(Suppl):S124, 1990. Abstract.
21. Sinaki M. Exercise and physical therapy. In: Riggs BL, Melton LJ III, eds. Osteoporosis: Etiology, Diagnosis, and Management. New York, NY: Raven Press; 1988:457–479.

22. Ekin JA, Sinaki M. Vertebral compression fractures sustained during golfing: report of three cases. *Mayo Clin Proc.* 68:566–570, 1993.

23. Jacobson PC, Beaver W, Grubb SA, Taft TN, Talmage RV. Bone density in women: college athletes and older athletic women. *J Orthop Res.* 2:328–332, 1984.

24. Sinaki M. Exercise and osteoporosis. *Arch Phys Med Rehabil.* 70:220–229, 1989.

25. Wahner HW, Riggs BL. Methods and application of bone densitometry in clinical diagnosis. *Crit Rev Clin Lab Sci.* 24:217–233, 1986.

26. Riggs BL. Practical management of the patient with osteoporosis. In: Riggs BL, Melton LJ III, eds. *Osteoporosis: Etiology, Diagnosis, and Management.* New York, NY: Raven Press; 1988:481–490.

27. Lindsay R, Hart DM, Purdie D, Ferguson MM, Clark AS, Kraszewski A. Comparative effects of oestrogen and a progestogen on bone loss in postmenopausal women. *Clin Sci Mol Med.* 54:193–195, 1978.

28. Albright F. The effect of hormones on osteogenesis in man. *Recent Prog Horm Res.* 1:293–345, 1947.

29. Chesnut CH III, Ivey JL, Gruber HE, et al. Stanozolol in postmenopausal osteoporosis: therapeutic efficacy and possible mechanisms of action. *Metabolism.* 32:571–580, 1983.

30. Seeman E, Melton LJ III, O'Fallon WM, Riggs BL. Risk factors for spinal osteoporosis in men. *Am J Med.* 75:977–983, 1983.

31. Genant HK, Cann CE, Ettinger B, Gordan GS. Quantitative computed tomography of vertebral spongiosa: a sensitive method for detecting early bone loss after oophorectomy. *Ann Intern Med.* 97:699–705, 1982.

32. Christiansen C, Christensen MS, Larsen NE, Transbøl IB. Pathophysiological mechanisms of estrogen effect on bone metabolism. Dose-response relationships in early postmenopausal women. *J Clin Endocrinol Metab.* 55:1124–1130, 1982.

33. van Paassen HC, Poortman J, Borgart-Creutzburg IHC, Thijssen JHH, Duursma SA. Oestrogen binding proteins in bone cell cytosol. *Calcif Tissue Res.* 25:249–254, 1978.

34. Chen TL, Feldman D. Distinction between alpha-fetoprotein and intracellular estrogen receptors: evidence against the presence of estradiol receptors in rat bone. *Endocrinology.* 102:236–244, 1978.

35. Eriksen EF, Colvard DS, Berg NJ, et al. Evidence of estrogen receptors in normal human osteoblast-like cells. *Science.* 241:84–86, 1988.

36. Avioli LV, Gennarie C. Calcitonin therapy in osteoporotic syndromes. In: Avioli LV, ed. *The Osteoporotic Syndrome: Detection, Prevention, and Treatment.* New York, NY: Wiley-Liss, 1993:137–154.

37. Riggs BL, Hodgson SF, O'Fallon WM, et al. Effect of fluoride treatment on the fracture rate in postmenopausal women with osteoporosis. *N Engl J Med.* 322:802–809, 1990.

38. Jowsey, J. Osteoporosis: its nature and the role of diet. *Postgrad Med.* 59:75–79, 1976.

39. Heaney RP, Recker RR, Saville PD. Calcium balance and calcium requirements in middle-aged women. *Am J Clin Nutr.* 30:1603–1611, 1977.

40. Sinaki M, Dale DA, Hurley DL. *Living with Osteoporosis: Guidelines for Women Before and After Diagnosis.* Toronto: B.C. Decker; 1988.

41. Buckley MJ, Banes AJ, Levin LG, et al. Osteoblasts increase their rate of division and align in response to cyclic, mechanical tension in vitro. *Bone Mineral.* 4:225–236, 1988.

42. Paget J. On a form of chronic inflammation of bones (osteitis deformans). *Medico Trans.* 60:37–63, 1877.

43. Schmorl G. Über Ostitis deformans Paget. *Virchow's Archiv fur Pathologische Anatomie und Physiologie.* 283:694–751, 1932.

44. Pygott F. Paget's disease of bone: the radiological incidence. *Lancet.* 1:1170–1171, 1957.

45. Hamdy RC. Paget's disease of bone. In: *Endocrinology and Metabolism Series, I.* New York, NY: Praeger; 1981:22–37.

46. Poretta CA, Dahlin DC, Janes JM. Sarcoma in Paget's disease of bone. *J Bone Joint Surg [Am].* 39:1314–1329, 1957.

47. Nicholas JJ, Srodes CH, Herbert D, Hoy RJ, Peel RL, Goodman MA. Metastatic cancer in Paget's disease of bone: a case report. *Orthopedics.* 10:725–729, 1987.

48. Hamdy RC. Paget's disease of bone. In: *Endocrinology and Metabolism Series, I.* New York, NY: Praeger; 1981:47–54.

12
Rehabilitation of Fractures in the Geriatric Population

Barry D. Stein and Gerald Felsenthal

FRACTURES FROM OSTEOPOROSIS/FALLS

Fractures in the elderly are usually not from automotive or other high-velocity trauma. They are a result of "low energy" trauma such as falls in the home. These falls most commonly result in fractures in five locations: the hip, the distal shaft of the radius (Colles' fractures), the pelvis, the surgical neck of the humerus, or the ribs.

Etiology of Low-Velocity Traumatic Fractures

Investigating the reasons for a fracture in any patient is important to prevent reoccurrence. This is true whether the patient had an uncomplicated fracture with little need for additional care or a complex fracture and a personal situation requiring extensive assistance. Personal, familial, and societal health costs can be saved through prevention of future falls and fractures. There is an increase in fracture frequency with aging. This is due to two problems: increasing osteoporosis and falling with aging.

Frequency of Falls

The rise in fracture incidence with aging is not adequately explained by osteoporosis alone. A fracture results when the stress upon a given bone is greater than its strength to resist such force. About 90% of fractures of the hip, pelvis, and forearm result from a fall. There is a fatigue fracture in less than 10% (i.e., "I felt the bone snap before I fell"). Fatigue fractures may be the ones in which the osteoporosis is the most severe. In other fractures, one has to consider the problem of falls.

Many risk factors for fractures are actually risk factors for falls. These factors that increase the risk of falls can be grouped into several large categories: genetic (sex and race), age-associated factors, preexisting illnesses, life-style, medications, and the environment (Table 12.1). The clinician may uncover a variety of risk factors during a careful history and physical examination. Several formalized evaluations have been published to identify persons at high risk for falling (1, 2) Once a person has already fallen, clarification of the events surrounding the fall may provide preventive information (3–5).

Type of Fall

The causes of fractures are still not well explained if one only considers osteoporosis and the frequency of falls. Only 3%–5% of falls result in fractures. Other factors play a role in whether a fall will result in a fracture and why one type of fracture occurs as opposed to another (Figure 12.1). Contributing factors to fractures include the following (6):

Table 12.1. Some Factors Implicated in Traumatic Fractures of the Elderly

Aspects of aging	Illnesses
Primary osteoporosis	Cerebrovascular accident
Impaired balance/vision	Syncopal episodes
Alterations in gait	Hypotensive illnesses
Loss in muscle/fat "padding" at hip	Secondary osteoporosis
	Hyperthyroidism
Falls forward (Colles'/humerus) vs falls down (hip/pelvis)	Hypoparathyroidism, etc.
	Osteomalacia
Environment	Parkinson's disease
Outdoor	Dementia
Cracked walkway	Arthritis
Poor lighting	Paraparesis
Poor weather	Previous fractures
Uneven ground	Life-styles
Crime (assault and battery)	Exercise/nutrition
Indoor	Alcoholism/other abused drugs
Throw rugs	Bedrest/immobilization
Wires across path	Shoe style
Slippery tub	Medications
Poor lighting	Benzodiazepines
Stairs/railings	Tricyclic antidepressants
Pet causing a fall	Antipsychotic medications
Genetic	Corticosteroids (secondary
Sex (females > males)	osteoporosis)
Race (white > black)	Barbiturates

123

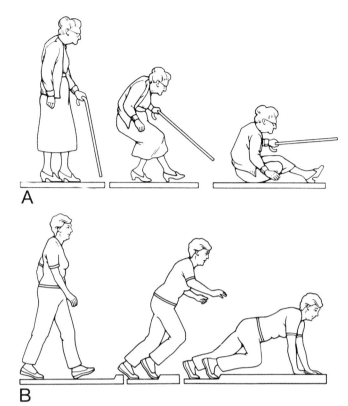

Figure 12.1. Orientation of the fall. A, When a fall occurs while a person is standing still, walking slowly, or slowly descending a step, there is little forward momentum and the principal point of impact will be near the hip. **B,** When a fall occurs during rapid walking, there is enough forward momentum for the person to land on hands or knees instead of the hip. From *Journal of Gerontology,* Medical Sciences, Vol 44, No 4, M107–111, 1989. Copyright© The Gerontological Society of America.

1. Orientation of the fall. A fall occurring when standing still, walking slowly, or transferring slowly will have little forward momentum. The point of impact will be near the hip. A fall during rapid walking has enough momentum to carry the faller onto the hands or knees instead of the hip. Gait speed slows after age 65, placing the hip at more risk.
2. Protective responses in a fall decrease with age, influencing the direction of the fall. Examples of factors leading to decreased protective response include sedation from drugs, impaired muscle function with aging (7–9), loss of protective reflexes, and dementia.
3. Local shock absorbers that surround the bone (fat and muscle) may decrease with age. The addition of local padding in a thin person, if tolerated, may reduce the risk of a fracture.
4. Bone strength (osteoporosis). Multiple studies associate bone weakness with hip fractures.

REHABILITATION OF THE PATIENT WITH A FRACTURE

Successful rehabilitation of the patient who has sustained a fracture involves:

Table 12.2. Architectural/Environmental Considerations for Successful Rehabilitation

Apartment
  Hallway length
  Elevator or stair access
  Distance from parking lot
House
  One level
  Multiple levels
  Location of living room, bathroom(s), bedroom(s), kitchen, laundry room
Apartment or House
  Width of doorways and pathways (for wheelchairs)
  Carpeting and whether it is "wall-to-wall" or "area" (consider if it has nonskid properties and curled up edges if an area rug)
  Bathroom safety grab bars/bathtub nonstick surface
  Telephone/other wires/oxygen tubing on the floor
  Amount of "clutter" in the living areas
  Nighttime indoor and outdoor lighting
  Potential slippery surfaces, including stairs
Transportation
  Public (including proximity/accessibility)
  Self (including question of resuming driving)
  Family (including proximity/accessibility)

1. Identification and treatment of pertinent surgical, medical, and psychiatric issues,
2. Clarification of patient's current and prior functional abilities,
3. Assessment of the patient's familial, social, and environmental situation (Table 12.2),
4. Initial prognostication based on helpful or hindering factors from the above information,
5. Establishment of realistic goals for the patient from the above information,
6. Formulation of therapy orders and precautions,
7. Modification of therapy and prognosis based on progress in therapy or other issues that may arise,
8. Early and continuous planning for a safe return to an out-of-hospital environment, and
9. Continuation of rehabilitation program as patient progresses to different sites of care.

The initial discussion of the rehabilitation of the patient with a fracture will focus on the patient who has sustained a hip fracture treated with operative fixation.

Hip Fractures

Fractures of the hip are generally classified by the location and the severity of the injury. Injuries of the neck or subcapital area of the femur can be classified (Figure 12.2) most easily as nondisplaced (Garden classification Type I & II) or displaced fractures (Type III & IV).

Injuries of the trochanteric region have been classified in several ways. The basic issue is recognizing stable and unstable fractures (Figure 12.3). Stable fractures do not have any involvement of the calcar femorale. This

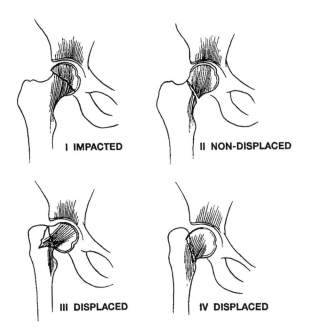

Figure 12.2. Garden classification of femoral neck fractures. It is important to recognize that Type I (impacted) and Type II are nondisplaced fractures, while Type III and Type IV are displaced fractures. It is usually difficult to differentiate Type III and Type IV fractures. From Zuckerman JD, ed. *Comprehensive Care of Orthopedic Injuries in the Elderly.* Baltimore, Md: Urban & Schwarzenberg; 1990.

posteromedial portion of the intertrochanteric and femoral neck regions is a dense cortical strut of bone that bears much of the weight of the body. Any comminution resulting in a separate calcar femorale is unstable. Conversion of this fracture to a stable situation requires specific operative techniques. Another unstable fracture is the reverse obliquity pattern. In this fracture, the medial aspect of the fracture is superior to the lateral aspect. The femoral shaft has a tendency in this injury to displace medially (10).

These fracture types have a large effect on orthopedic and rehabilitative care. For example, an unstable intertrochanteric fracture will require specific operative intervention considerations. Moreover, it will require limited weight bearing for weeks to months. This decreased weight bearing alters mobility, with additional great effect upon the activities of daily living (ADLs).

ORTHOPEDIC APPROACH

Conservative

Conservative treatment for fractures is nonoperative treatment. It is occasionally used for selected medically high risk patients (11). This occurs far less often

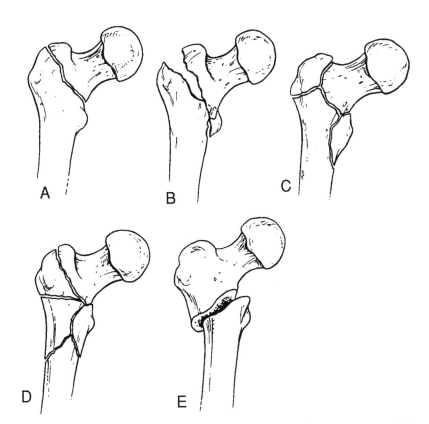

Figure 12.3. Classification of intertrochanteric fractures. (A) is a two-part fracture and is stable; (B) is also a stable pattern because the medial fragment is small and does not significantly compromise the posteromedial buttress; (C) represents an unstable fracture because of the large posteromedial fragment; (D) is an unstable intertrochanteric fracture with subtrochanteric extension; (E) is a reverse obliquity pattern and is also unstable because of the tendency for the shaft to displace medially. From Zuckerman JD, ed. *Comprehensive Care of Orthopedic Injuries in the Elderly.* Baltimore, Md: Urban & Schwarzenberg; 1990.

nowadays due to the advancement in techniques for medically stabilizing patients. Nonoperative treatment has also been done for nonambulatory, demented patients. In these patients it is felt that surgery and its risks have a minimal chance to favorably help such a patient's life-style (12). Nonoperative treatment of hip fractures involves weeks to months of bedrest, occasionally traction (13), and nonweight-bearing ambulation (as possible) for a prolonged period of time. Excellent nursing care is critical for the avoidance of many of the complications of bedrest. Malunion, pain, and higher mortality rates are complications. When the nonoperative approach is used for patients due to poor medical condition (as opposed to nonambulatory, demented patients), there can be improvement in a comprehensive rehabilitation facility. The chances of ambulation are only 55% compared to a 76% chance for those with surgical intervention (11).

Operative

Many operative techniques have been employed throughout the years for fractures of the hip. The literature in this area is extremely extensive (10) and is beyond the scope of this review.

In general, however, there are a few basic types of procedures performed for a person with a hip fracture. Nondisplaced femoral neck fractures are usually treated with multiple nails. When there is displacement of the femoral head, the risk of subsequent aseptic necrosis is quite high, and the treatment is usually a hemiarthroplasty. Stable intertrochanteric fractures are generally treated with a sliding screw and side-plate system. Unstable fractures may require medial support when the calcar femorale is involved. When the patient has known severe arthritis at the involved joint, the surgeon may elect to perform a total hip arthroplasty to try to provide a pain-free hip (14).

COMPREHENSIVE APPROACH

The comprehensive rehabilitative approach to elderly patients with a hip fracture has been steadily evolving (15). It was first attempted in the United States in the 1950s (16–18) and in the United Kingdom in 1961 (19). All too often, the hip fracture patient with great needs has not been helped to her or his potential (20,21). Rehabilitation enables improved independence (22–24).

Preoperative care

Many aspects of preoperative care can greatly influence final rehabilitation and recovery by reducing the complications of bedrest and other problems. Early use of soft mattresses, possibly even in the emergency room, may decrease the formation of skin ulceration. Initial demonstrations of techniques in deep breathing, often with the use of incentive spirometry, may speed postoperative teaching and decrease atelectasis. Increasing lower extremity venous blood flow will decrease the chance of stasis, a known risk factor for deep venous thrombosis. Techniques include calf pumping (repetitive ankle plantarflexion/dorsiflexion), quadriceps setting (isometrically "tightening" the quadriceps), and placement of antiembolism stockings preoperatively as well as postoperatively. Range of motion (ROM) and/or strengthening exercises and assistive devices may be shown to the patient. These techniques should be utilized unless contraindicated (25).

Rehabilitation Management

Many patients are able to go directly home after orthopedic treatment and continue with therapy at home or in an outpatient facility. Other patients need further inpatient comprehensive rehabilitation. In either situation, rehabilitation management begins as quickly as feasible postoperatively.

The patient should be mobilized within the first 1 to 2 days postoperatively, if possible. This is essential to prevent or reduce contractures, decubitus ulcers, skeletal and cardiac muscle weakening, disuse osteoporosis, atelectasis leading to pneumonia, deep venous thrombosis, and psychologic dependency (26). The amount of mobilization can vary with associated surgical or medical problems.

Nursing management at this stage includes encouraging the patient's own self-care, including using the trapeze in bed (if permitted). The patient should exhale while using the trapeze to prevent Valsalva maneuver. Routine coughing and deep breathing are encouraged. Instruction in skin care, monitoring of any concurrent cast or splint care, and psychologic support are vital. Additional pain management includes the use of medications. Reduction of pain through relaxation techniques has also been attempted by nursing at this stage (27).

Physical therapy management at this stage generally includes ROM and isometric exercises of appropriate muscle groups. The patient progresses to resistive exercises (with weights, manual resistance, therabands, and trapeze) (25). The physical therapist carefully integrates these exercises into a full program of transfer and gait retraining (see below). The actual mobilization out of bed usually takes place, medically permitting, on postoperative day one or two.

If bedrest has been present for a long period, a tilt table will often be helpful. Prolonged periods of bedrest will lead to a decrease in circulating blood volume and orthostatic hypotension. A tilt table can provide a controlled environment for increasing adaptability to the upright position (28).

Dislocation Prevention. Dislocation is known to occur 1% to 10% of the time after hip hemiarthroplasties.

It occurs more commonly with the posterior operative approach than the anterior approach (10). After a posterior operative approach, that portion of the hip capsule has been weakened. The prosthesis can dislocate posteriorly if the hip is moved in sufficient flexion, adduction, or internal rotation. Limits placed upon these movements are generally a maximum of 90 degrees of hip flexion, no hip adduction beyond the midline, and no internal rotation. The hip may conceivably tolerate more motion than this before any dislocation. Surgeons will passively move the hip in a generous ROM in the operating room after placement of the prosthesis. Still, the above limits for active movement are appropriate. These restrictions permit sitting, yet prevent incautious movements during the early crucial weeks of capsule healing.

If hip flexion is restricted to less than 90 degrees, recovery may be greatly affected during this period of limited motion. An upright sitting posture is prevented. The patient must slouch and have a wheelchair back that leans backwards. The use of a toilet instead of a bedpan becomes less likely if the flexion limitation is too much less than 90 degrees. Bathing and dressing may become far more limited than usual.

Restriction of these motions should be continued for at least 6 weeks and possibly as long as 3 months after a posterior approach for hemiarthroplasty. The exact timing depends upon the operative conditions and the surgeon's preference.

It is not enough to tell a person postoperatively to avoid certain motions. These motions are very natural, and a single moment of forgetfulness may result in dislocation. In addition, the patient may be in pain, receiving narcotics, depressed, schizophrenic, or delerious. Thus, there are several techniques for limiting motion. The first is the use of joint restraining devices immediately postoperatively. The most restrictive device is an abduction brace. Some physicians find this most helpful in a demented patient who is unable to learn hip motion precautions and is judged to be at a higher risk of dislocation. Another device is a long hip abduction pillow. This is a somewhat triangular foam wedge positioned between the thighs and legs. It extends across the knee joint and fastens with hook and loop ("Velcro") straps. It is sometimes used immediately postoperatively for safeguarding of hip movements when the patient is in great pain and is less able to concentrate on correct positioning. A smaller knee spreader is a foam wedge as above, but is only about 15 cm long and is located between the thighs. It too is fastened with Velcro. This has the advantage of not restricting knee movement. One primary goal in rehabilitation is to restrict only the joints that need restriction.

Knee immobilizers on the injured extremity are occasionally used to restrict hip flexion. When the knee is immobilized in extension, any hip flexion results in the more difficult "straight leg raise." This therefore tends to reduce the ease of improper hip movements. This use of knee immobilizers unnecessarily restricts movement of a second, nonoperated joint. The person's movements are restricted unnecessarily. The exception is perhaps for severe arthritis of the ipsilateral knee, but even in this case one should be cautious. It is not rehabilitatively appropriate to place a person at risk for decreased ROM in a second joint of the same limb where there is already decreased ROM in one joint (the hip). To immobilize the knee is to risk a stiff lower extremity with a greater energy expenditure in bed mobility, transfers, and ambulation (circumduction). A knee that does not bend may also result in a longer lever arm acting upon the hip.

Other equipment to prevent dislocation includes elevated toilet seats and the exclusive use of higher sitting surfaces. This is instituted to prevent excessive hip flexion. Stool softeners (such as dioctyl sodium sulfosuccinate, a detergent), often with stimulants of peristalsis (such as casanthranol) are frequently given. This is to prevent inadvertent hip flexion and dislocation while straining from postoperative constipation. Long-handled devices for washing, for donning socks and shoes, and for grasping high or low objects are supplied to the patient by the occupational therapist. Of great importance is extensive patient teaching and reminding by rehabilitative nursing, physical therapists, occupational therapists, physicians, and family regarding the above movement restrictions.

An anterior surgical approach allows flexion, adduction, and internal rotation. Since anterior supporting stuctures are weakened, the hip is unstable in extension and external rotation.

The clinical presentation of posterior dislocation includes pain, adduction, internal rotation, and shortening of the involved limb. Anterior inferior dislocations are abducted and externally rotated, and the rare anterior superior dislocation is extended and externally rotated. Standard pelvic anteroposterior roentenograms confirm the diagnosis of dislocation. Complications include a 10 % to 15% incidence of sciatic nerve injuries in posterior dislocations and neurovascular injuries in anterior superior injuries (10). A hip dislocation is an orthopedic emergency.

Weight Bearing. A controversy in orthopedics for many years has been the amount of weight that can be tolerated by a fracture after treatment. Many orthopedic surgeons are concerned about the amount of weight placed upon a freshly fractured limb with internal fixation. Even with a solid, well-impacted, anatomically acceptable anchoring provided by a nail or screw fixation, some surgeons prefer to delay significant weight bearing for many weeks. When increased amounts of weight bearing are permitted by the surgeon depends upon the surgeon's approach to weight bearing, bone fragility noted at the time of operation, stability of fixation, and appearance of the fracture/operative site on sequential x-ray films. Weight bearing is also influenced by the likelihood of the patient being able to understand and comply with the weight restriction (29). The trend over the decades has been to allow greater weight bearing on the fractured limb with internal fixation, within orthopedically stable limits.

With nail or screw fixation, hip fractures are mobilized with either immediate weight bearing (23, 30–35) or with much slower resumption of weight bearing (30). The amount of weight allowed depends on fracture stability and the preference of the surgeon. Many European and some American orthopedic surgeons advocate immediate weight bearing if the fixation is judged to be stable (see fracture type, above). Thus the majority of intertrochanteric fractures and femoral neck fractures have "as tolerated weight bearing" orders in the early postoperative period.

Other surgeons prefer 6 weeks or more of nonweight bearing or very light weight bearing for all internal fixations. The orthopedic concern is whether there will be shifting of the fixation and even nail or screw breakage during the stresses of ambulation. Any failure of fixation may require a second operation in a sometimes frail, elderly person. With this approach, clinical orthopedic and roentgenographic reevaluation occur a few weeks (up to 6 weeks) postsurgery. If there is satisfactory healing, the patient is advanced to partial weight bearing. At approximately 2 or 3 months another reevaluation occurs, and full weight bearing is usually permitted.

Obviously, these different approaches have a large impact upon the patient's rehabilitation. An aged person with questionable balance will have a greatly different recovery if immediately permitted to bear weight versus not immediately permitted to bear weight. Putting weight on the involved limb (assuming this is orthopedically appropriate) means improved balance. Many social and environmental decisions regarding the patient's future are made in the first weeks after a fracture. If there is no orthopedic contraindication concerning potential fixation failure, a more rapid weight resumption is preferable. It can help ensure less disruption in future ADL, environmental, psychologic, and social status (the question of community living versus nursing home, for example).

With hemiarthroplasties, surgeons may also restrict early weight bearing on noncemented and sometimes even cemented prostheses. The patient will then have both ROM and weight bearing precautions. This has the potential to place much strain upon the patient's medical, cognitive, social/familial, and environmental situation.

Weight Bearing Precautions.   Proper teaching of weight bearing precautions requires reinforcement from the physician, physical therapist, occupational therapist, nursing staff, and an educated family.

Nonweight Bearing: The patient supports weight on the noninvolved limbs, and the involved limb or limbs are left to dangle. A geriatric patient usually uses a nonwheeled walker. The additional weight placed on the upper extremities often exacerbates preexisting arthritic or soft-tissue problems and may cause much pain in some persons. In addition, the dangling lower extremity requires one to hop. This is more tiring to the patient than is walking, and the movement is more clumsy. Another problem is the almost universal inability to negotiate stairs with greatly restricted weight bearing; the arms in the frail elderly are rarely up to the task of supporting their body weight. Also, the trickier balance requirements of stairs are usually too hazardous with nonweight bearing for this falling-prone group of patients.

Toe-Touch or Touch-Down Weight Bearing: This phrase, used for hip or pelvic injuries, refers to the weight being placed only upon the phalanges, and perhaps the metatarsals, of the involved lower extremity. Actually, as full weight bearing could occur in this position (consider the ballerina), a very light weight placement on the limb is taught by the therapist simultaneously. The toe-touch posture creates a mnemonic for the patient to restrict weight bearing. The minimal permitted weight allows the patient to avoid the pendular effect of the nonweight bearing instruction and improves the balance. Educating the patient initially is done with the therapist's own visual observation or foot underneath for immediate feedback. A scale under the patient's foot may also be used. As in nonweight bearing, a walker instead of crutches is usually the device of choice in the elderly due to the greater stability provided by the four legs of the walker. Exacerbation of upper extremity soft tissue problems, the inability to climb stairs, and reduced endurance from an altered gait pattern are still issues with this amount of permitted weight. Some therapists find that a very light foot flat weight bearing is just as effective or more effective than the use of the toe touch approach.

Partial Weight Bearing: This is typically about 50% of the patient's body weight for lower extremity fractures. Occasionally, an older person can negotiate stairs with this permitted amount of weight.

Weight Bearing as Tolerated or Full Weight Bearing: This is helpful when there is reasonable satisfaction regarding the stability of the bony union (see fracture stability, above) and when there is satisfaction that the patient can express any distress.

Percentages: Some surgeons prefer to describe permitted weight on the limb in percentages of body weight, such as "10%," "10% to 20%," "30%," and the like. This should not be mistaken for a precise request for weight bearing accuracy to two significant digits.

Reduction of Weight: On rare occasions it may be

Table 12.3. Some Examples of Therapy Precautions

Range of motion precautions
"Cardiac" or "strict cardiac" precautions
"Pulmonary" precautions
"Poor balance" or "falling precautions"
"Impulsivity" or "patient needs 100% supervision"
Patient on anticoagulation
Potential for hypoglycemia
Impaired vision
Impaired hearing
Impaired heat sensation
Peripheral neuropathy

necessary to reduce the current weight bearing status. This may be from concern for the bony union or patient compliance problems. It also may also be deemed needed for weight unloading of the bone if avascular necrosis of the femoral head is diagnosed. In general one should try to clarify the reason for any increase in pain or new pain in the postoperative period.

For other examples of precautions that might be used to alert the rehabilitation personnel see Table 12.3.

Leg Length Discrepancy. Proper fixation with nails or screws requires impaction of the bone. This on occasion may result in limb shortening. Sufficient limb shortening may result in additional gait abnormalities. This can be corrected with an appropriate shoe lift.

Physical Therapy. Safe mobility is the prime goal. People tend to consider safe ambulation synonymous with safe mobility. However, there are other critical goals involved with achieving safe mobility in addition to ambulation. These include improved mobility in bed; transfer skills out of bed, chair, or wheelchair; sitting and standing balance skills; improved ROM; and muscle strengthening. The physical therapeutic techniques used may be modified by the presence of precautions necessitated by concommitant disease and due to the fracture and its treatment.

ROM exercises may be needed to improve or maintain joint function. Care should be taken to follow any ROM precautions. Maintainance of the patient's premorbid ROM in all uninvolved joints is desirable. The upper extremities are used for bed mobility, transfers, and weight bearing with ambulation, and maintainance of their ROM is needed.

Four types of ROM exercises are typically used: passive, active assisted, active, and resistive (36, 37). Passive ROM is helpful early when the patient's own muscle motion is not feasible (from injury). The arc of motion should be slow and painless (or minimally painful) to prevent damage. Active assisted ROM exercises involve a combination of the patient's own movements guided and often assisted by the therapist. Active muscle use without excessive strain can be achieved with this technique. If needed, this may first be done in a horizontal position, without fighting gravity. Later this can be performed against gravity. When cognitively able, the patient may be taught to use an uninjured upper extremity to help range the injured lower extremity. This helps continue exercises outside of the physical therapy gym. With improvement, the patient continues with active ROM exercises.

The use of cold modalities may help in the motion of a painful, swollen region (after clearance by the physician for any question of an orthopedic/medical problem), and heat may help ready the contracted joint for increased ranging. Heat may be contraindicated in a person with compromised vascularity or severe peripheral neuropathy (as in many diabetics) or in a confused patient. Transcutaneous electrical nerve stimulation (TENS) may often be helpful in controlling pain (38).

As the ROM improves and the pain subsides, the emphasis in the physical therapy program is shifted to the strengthening of muscles by progressive resistive exercises (39). The limb with the fracture receives a gentle course of exercises. Isometric exercises (increased muscle tension without movement) are administered at first. The patient then progresses to isotonic and/or isokinetic exercises. A skate board attached to the limb with the patient supine is one way to begin thigh abduction exercises. The other limbs receive a more vigorous workout, as they work more to support a patient's body weight during the healing period. This is true whatever the weight bearing status of the involved limb, as pain is a natural warning signal for weight reduction for those who can "weight bear as tolerated." Gradually increasing weights, attached to the limbs, are used in exercise.

Once drains are out and the wound is healing, hydrotherapy in a Hubbard tank or a heated pool (if not contraindicated) can be very therapeutic. The heat can be relaxing and analgesic, and the buoyancy can provide an easier means to start ROM activities. Standing and ambulation can also begin earlier (39). However, many elderly persons do not swim or may fear entering the water. In addition, pool facilities may not be available (40).

Ambulation may begin in the parallel bars in order to teach the patient proper balance with the indicated weight restrictions. A swing-to gait is taught. As soon as this is learned, progression to a walker occurs (39). Attention is paid to the strength and range of motion needed in the upper extremities for such ambulation. As appropriate depending on weight restrictions, strength, balance, and coordination, advancement to a four-pronged cane may be made. Often in the United States this occurs with outpatient physical therapy. Many patients do not have the strength and balance to progress beyond a walker until some point after the orthopedic surgeon permits weight bearing as tolerated, which may not occur until after the patient has been discharged from the hospital. Occasionally, an outpatient advancement to a straight cane or even to no assistive device may occur (see Prognosis).

In some facilities, a home visit by the physical and/or occupational therapist is done prior to patient discharge (41). This enables a home assessment for environmental risks for falls, as well as occasional valuable social information obtained by interviews of the patient, family, or other caregivers.

Occupational Therapy. With occupational therapy training, the patient learns how to translate gains in strength, ROM, and the like into self-care and independent living activities (42). Adaptive equipment such as long-handled shoe horns, sponges, and reachers; bathtub benches; shoes with permanently tied elastic laces; elevated toilet seats; and devices to don socks without bending over are examples of tools for independence in bathing and dressing. These devices are very helpful for those patients restricted in hip movement for 2 or 3 months after a hemiarthroplasty. Practical daily restrictions regarding ROM and weight bearing are thoroughly reviewed in the course of training with the occupational therapist. In addition, many patients without restrictions of their hip movement (i.e., no hemiarthroplasty) find these tools very useful. The pain from the fracture and operative site restricts easy hip motion during ADL, and the adaptive equipment enables dressing and bathing to occur with less time, energy, and discomfort.

The activity training with the occupational therapist is an opportunity for thorough evaluation of a particular skill. When a person dresses with the occupational therapist, for example, the activity is analyzed as it occurs. The component parts of the activity are characterized by problems that occur and their potential solutions. Components of dressing include obtaining clothes from the dresser, correctly starting underwear over the feet, getting it over the hips (with any standing needed), balance while standing for moving the clothes over the hips, and maintainance of any weight-bearing and movement restrictions with this activity.

This analysis of the elements of daily activities also allows the opportunity for education of energy conservation techniques in selected patients. This can be helpful for persons with impairing cardiac, pulmonary, and rheumatic diseases.

Rehabilitation Nursing. The rehabilitation nurse's role is multifaceted (43). The traditonal nurturing role of the nurse is combined with a goal to make the patient as independent as possible. A rehabilitation nursing program includes mobilization of the patient (44) and monitoring the bowel and bladder status as well as general oral intake of meals.

Often, the patient puts forth the best effort in the gym and is tired later in the day. What may be a minimal assist transfer to the commode in the morning occupational therapy evaluation can be a maximal assist transfer for the nursing staff at 10 o'clock in the evening. This is a natural situation in the beginning stages of recovery when there is poor endurance. If this is seen throughout the day and does not resolve with time, it can be a valuable clue to the patient's current mood, cognition, and social dynamics (e.g., secondary gain). Generally, however, the patient appreciates the continuity of therapy and nursing encouragement for progression in safe mobility and ADL's.

Nutritional Aspects. Hip fractures have been related to undernutrition. A study of hospital mortality reported differences between three groups: well nourished, thin, and very thin. The mortality in the three groups was 4.4% (normal), 8%, and 18% (very high), respectively. There was also a positive correlation between a lower core body temperature and amount of thinness (45).

The same researchers then reported an interventional study. One hundred twenty-two of the patients in the thin and very thin groups were entered into a randomized controlled supplementary feeding study. Starting within 5 days after the operation, 4.2 MJ (1000 kcal) of tube feeding per night were given. This was tolerated by 78% of the selected patients. The thin patients who received the feeding did not differ in mortality (12%). The very thin patients showed a difference in mortality when fed (8%) compared to no supplementary feedings (22%). However, this did not reach statistical significance. Of great interest is that the time to reach functional goals was statistically significantly shorter when the tube feeding were given (46).

Although tube feeding may not be appropriate in the majority of patients, it is thus clear that adequate nutrition is important in the patient's functional progress as well as medical status.

Psychologic Aspects. An epidemiologic survey of hip fracture patients (47) found that 7.5% were admitted with delirium. These patients had an increased risk of death of more than 3:1 compared to others without delirium. Persons at greater risk of delirium were older than 85 years and had at least one serious medical condition.

One study (48) found a 51% prevalance of depression early after a hip fracture using the Center for Epidemiological Studies Depression Scale (CES-D) scale. The more severe the postoperative depressive symptomatology, the poorer the 12-month recovery for ADLs. Another paper evaluated depression and dementia early after a hip fracture. Depression, as measured by the CES-D, was found in 32% of persons. Cognitive limitation, as measured by the Mini-Mental State Examination (49), was found in 43% of patients. In this survey, 12% had severe cognitive impairment (less than 17 of 30 possible points), and 31% had mild impairment (17 to 23 points). Both depression and cognitive deficits were associated with poor recovery in mobility and ADL (50). When depression and cognitive deficits occur together, patients have even greater decreases in functional abilities and the worst prognosis (51, 52). When impaired mental states are considered alone without measuring depression, the prognosis has been variously described as poor (53) and as not statistically clear (54). There is a need for further clarification of the role depression plays in recovery from hip fracture.

Fear of falling and suffering another fracture plays a role in recovery. Early after discharge home, 50% of patients remarked that fear of falling inhibited their mobility after returning home. Twelve to 15 months after discharge, 23% still reported that this fear limited their mobility (55).

Social Aspects. The social worker coordinates the transition from hospital to home or elsewhere with the patient and family. Persons with a greater number of social supports have a more complete recovery of their prefracture level of function (50, 56). To aid in this transition, it is important that caregivers be trained in caring for the patient status posthip fracture repair. If a person is returning home or to a group/boarding home, the caregivers should be knowledgeable in any special techniques needed to care for the patient (i.e., transfer skills, weight bearing or hip motion precautions, medication use and precautions, etc.). Family training sessions during inpatient rehabilitation can be valuable.

Other Medical Problems/Precautions. *Deep Venous Thrombosis.* The risk of deep venous thrombosis (DVT) of the lower extremity can be very high (45% to 70%) in orthopedic hip surgery (57). The danger of this condition is primarily a pulmonary embolus (PE), which can cause pain, pulmonary disability, and, in 10% of person, death (58). A PE can occur approximately 50% of the time with femoral vein thrombi (59, 60). Pulmonary emboli have been shown to occur with calf thrombi (61). However, a careful review of the literature concluded that clot propagation into the thigh is necessary before fatal PE (62). In addition, DVT often creates venous hypertension that can cause chronic limb edema, chronic pain, and skin ulcerations (63–65).

Approximately half of all deep venous thrombi do not show clinically (66). Fortunately, with proper prophylaxis, the absolute number of DVT is lowered. Most institutions use clinical observation as a surveillance technique for thrombotic disease. Clinical signs include unilateral swelling, edema, warmth, posterior calf or pretibial tenderness with palpation, venous prominence or cords, and erythema. A useful clinical technique is to compare circumferences of the extremities. Calf differences greater than one to two centimeters, especially with other clinical signs, can be a cause for close watching or, when appropriate, further testing. The lower extremity is commonly swollen for at least several days after a hip fracture and operative procedure. Local thigh swelling without distal calf swelling may well represent postfracture/postoperative local edema. In addition, 32% of patients in one series of patients who had an opera-

tion for fracture of the hip had ipsilateral knee effusions for up to 3 weeks (67). Therefore, the examiner may wish to look for clinical signs in addition to swelling. An increase in skin temperature and calf tenderness by simple palpation are useful findings. "Homan's" sign (pain with ankle dorsiflexion) is much less helpful (68–71). Patient complaints of pain, as well as the use of any anticoagulants or physical measures to reduce DVT, may be considered in the clinical assessment. Frequently, a high index of suspicion is helpful as only additional tests will diagnose the presence or absence of a thrombus (72). These include contrast venography (73), real time ultrasound (74), and nuclear venography (75). Recently, real time ultrasound has become a popular, accurate means of assessing the presence of femoral or popliteal DVT. It should be noted that recent literature suggests that impedance plethysmography is inaccurate for patients with a hip fracture (76, 77). For fuller discussion of these and other methods, the reader is referred to other sources (78, 79).

Interestingly, in orthopedic hip fracture patients there is an early and a late type of deep venous thrombosis. Thromboembolic disease can be found extremely early in a hospital stay. Some authors have pointed to intraoperative reasons for the early DVTs (80). However, deep vein thrombosis has even been observed before any operation. One study found that 5 of 40 (12.5%) elderly patients with hip fractures had popliteal or femoral DVTs either preoperatively or postoperatively. This study was performed using ultrasonography as part of the preoperative evaluation and then repeating it within a few days postoperatively (80). This finding has been further clarified. A certain percentage of preoperative thrombi are joined by additional postoperative thrombi. One group (81) ultrasonically demonstrated a 7% incidence of femoral or popliteal DVT preoperatively in patients with an acute hip fracture. This percentage increased during the next 10 to 14 days of hospitalization to 15% (and 19% if calf vein DVT was included). This occurred despite the patients receiving either warfarin, serial compression boots, or gradient elastic stockings (81). Another study (82) used contrast venography. It demonstrated that 15 of 176 patients (9%) had thromboembolic disease preoperatively (13 had popliteal or higher DVT; one had a pulmonary embolus, and one had a calf DVT). Postoperatively, 11% of patients developed thromboembolic disease, despite use of antiembolism stockings, low molecular weight dextran, and early mobilization. Thus, many above-knee thrombi seem resistant to the above preventive measures because of their extremely early appearance. Even with some preventive measures, there may be 10% to 20% of patients with these dangerous clots early (the first week or two) in the hospital stay, half occurring preoperatively. Therefore, even with prophylaxis, the chance of DVT, though reduced, is real.

DVT Prophylaxis. If no preventive measures are undertaken, a variety of reports show thrombus rates of 40% to 50% after a hip fracture (57). A decrease of rates to 10% to 20% occurs with preventive measures. It thus seems that many postoperative DVTs may be reduced in number. These later DVTs are likely related to the problems of bedrest. They are notable for often originating in either calf of the patient. From there, they may potentially enlarge into the thigh (62).

Physical preventive measures include preoperative and postoperative calf pumping, antiembolism stockings (above-knee if possible), and early ambulation (within the first few days postoperatively). Early ambulation improves the venous flow rate (83). Without ambulation or other prophylaxis, a general hospital population may develop calf DVT within the first week of bedrest and thigh DVT (most likely by extension from the calf veins) by the second week (84). However, ambulation alone has not been proven to decrease DVT (calf extending to thigh) (85). One study demonstrated the calf DVT already forming by one and one-half days after surgery in some persons (86). The practice of preventing DVT by early ambulation alone is insufficient. Physicians have been searching for alternate acceptable means of prevention.

Some patients are judged to be at too high of a risk to receive anticoagulants. For those persons, the use of intermittent compression devices has been promoted (87, 88). This technology is promising, but the reliance on well-functioning machinery as well as patient and staff tolerance for its 24-hour use (except during ambulation) may undermine its effectiveness. Peroneal nerve palsy has been reported following sequential pneumatic compression (89). Compression-graded stockings are effective in reducing the incidence of DVT when used correctly (90). Frequently, however, the stockings roll down and may even act in a tourniquet-like manner (91).

Several other methods have been tried for prophylaxis of DVT. Various anticoagulants have been tried and are the subject of reviews (92). These include aspirin, heparin, and warfarin. The studies are widely variable in quality and conclusions. This area is a topic of much research, and conclusions may change in the next few years. Warfarin has been called the most effective agent in preventing DVT in orthopedic patients although drawbacks with its use exist. All anticoagulants may be associated with a certain percentage of bleeding complications (hematuria, gastrointestinal (GI) bleeding, wound bleeding, etc.), which may be minimized by lower doses of these agents.

Of note is that the combined use of either anticoagulation or intermittent compression with compression stockings seems more effective than the use of only one technique (93–95). One should also keep in mind that the use of these techniques will not guarantee DVT prevention; rather, the rate of occurrence is decreased.

DVT Treatment. If a DVT is diagnosed, a decision regarding treatment option is needed. There has been some dispute regarding the treatment of isolated calf DVT, as compared to proximal DVT (62, 96). For any DVT, there may be concern that a patient's potential for falls, poor patient judgement (impulsive behavior that may lead to injury), or other medical condition contraindicates anticoagulation. In these cases, an inferior vena cava filter should be placed (97). Otherwise, anticoagulation should commence to reduce the possibility of a pulmonary embolus. One should be aware of potential complications of treatment for DVT and PE with either a filter or anticoagulation (98–100). Physical activity (exercises of the involved limb, transfers out of bed, or ambulation) is deferred for the first days of heparin anticoagulation. This is done due to the concern that the thrombus may not initially be firmly adhering to the venous wall (101, 102). Vigorous physical activity too early may place a person at risk for a pulmonary embolus. Stabilization of the thrombus may take 7 or so days (59). This may be an appropriate time for resumption of out-of-bed activity, although clinical information in this area is not available.

Skin Ulcerations (Decubitus Ulcers). Pressure over bony prominences when supine or sitting results in compression and shearing forces that reduce capillary flow. Friction, injury, and moisture (incontinence) can worsen this situation. In immobile persons, the result can be ischemia and skin ulcerations (103–105). In one prospective study of 100 consecutive patients admitted for femoral fractures, 66 developed varying degrees of ulceration. Of these 66, 18% were preoperative, 13% occurred the day of operation, and there were additional 22% during the next 3 days. The preoperative and operative pressure sores were associated with high pressure surfaces (emergency room tables, etc.). Fifty-six of the 66 patients with ulcers had milder epidermal ulceration. Another eight patients had ulcers in the dermis, and two had ulcers of the deeper subcutaneous tissue. Most patients had more than one ulcer (106). A retrospective chart review of medical complications in hip fracture patients noted a 5.8% incidence of skin ulcers (107). The smaller percentage may reflect the different data gathering methods. Possibly only the more severe cases (dermal and greater involvement) were noted.

Besides pain, complications in advanced cases of ulceration include osteomyelitis (108) and bacteremia (109). Prevention includes the use of very soft surfaces and repositioning every 2 hours (varying the position from supine to right or left 30 degree oblique positions) if orthopedically permissible (110). Treatment may become complex, involving pressure elimination, adequate nutrition, establishment of continence, and dressings such as polyurethane, hydrocolloid, or two to three times a day gentle debridement using gauze dressings moistened with saline solution ("wet to dry dressings"). A hard plastic boot is commercially available for cradling the ulcerated heel from any rubbing whatsoever (the Multipodis boot). Surgical debridement, cultures, appropriate antibiotics, and occasionally, plastic surgery may be required (111–113).

Problems of Fixation. Fixation may arise from development of osteonecrosis, problems with the type of fixation used, an inaccurate reduction, displacement after fixation, and nonunion (10). Attention to changes in pain complaints, use of radiologic techniques, and close cooperation with the orthopedic surgeon is important.

Infection. The incidence of wound infection has recently been reported to range from 2% to 10% in hip fractures when both superficial and deep wounds are considered. Older series reports ranged up to 20%, and the improved figures are likely due in part to perioperative antibiotic prophylaxis (10).

Similarly, there has been a reduced incidence of fracture-associated, pneumonia-related mortality in the past decades. This is likely due in part to the use of incentive spirometry, chest physiotherapy, and earlier patient mobilization to reduce atelectasis.

Urinary tract infection has been noted in one survey (114) to involve 14% of hip fracture patients. Infection can be more likely with bladder overdistention. This retention is probably due to anesthesia, narcotics, and the recumbent position of the patient early postoperatively. The use of an indwelling catheter for a short period can reduce overdistention. However, indwelling catheters used for more than 48 hours are associated with an increased incidence of urinary tract infection (115). The use of antibiotics and an indwelling catheter simultaneously may result in resistant urinary tract organisms. As a general approach, an initial perioperative use of an indwelling catheter should be followed by a voiding trial as early as possible. Intermittent catheterization should be considered for voiding problems beyond the immediate perioperative period. Reduction of recumbency is also important for reducing bladder retention.

Reducing all types of infection is desirable not only for the immediate, obvious benefit but also to reduce the chance of the organism spreading to the operative site and causing an osteomyelitis.

Peripheral Neuropathy. Peripheral neuropathy exists in varying amounts among the older population, often due to illnesses such as diabetes, alchoholism, chronic obstructive pulmonary disease, and/or arthritis. Impaired vision and decreased somatosensation at the ankle may contribute toward falls (116).

Peripheral neuropathy due to fractures is documented by multiple authors. Fortunately, this occurs infrequently. Recognition of this issue can help the patient.

The literature for total hip replacement has some

relevance to this topic. Total hip replacement is a potential treatment of acute femoral neck fractures when there is preexisting significant acetabular disease (rheumatoid arthritis, osteoarthritis, Paget's disease) (10). It is associated with subclinical sciatic, femoral, and obdurator nerve damage in 70% of patients, although clinically only about 1% of patients have problems (117). Electrodiagnostic studies will help determine these rare injuries.

Clinical nerve involvement can be either solely peroneal or sciatic. The latter has been documented with operative limb lengthening exceeding 4.0 cm (118) and with hemorrhaging occurring around the sciatic nerve (119). Treatment may include surgical decompression, orthotic support of any foot drop, exercises (120), and treatment of any pain. It can take up to 2 years to ascertain the total amount of recovery.

Femoral nerve injuries after a hip procedure occur similarly from retroperitoneal hemorrhaging in hemophiliac or anticoagulated patients (121, 122). A retroperitoneal bleed may also result in lumbar plexopathy (123, 124). These neuropathies from bleeding may be manifested by initial lower abdominal pain that later radiates to the lumbar and/or anterior thigh region, hypesthesia, quadriceps weakness, flexion of the thigh to reduce discomfort, and a falling hematocrit. Prompt diagnosis can be difficult, but, if suspected, a computed tomography (CT) scan may enable early diagnosis and intervention. Acute treatment includes discontinuation of anticoagulation and possible transfusion. Consideration of a vena cava filter may be appropriate in those persons anticoagulated due to a deep venous thrombisis.

Complete neurologic recovery occurs in only a third of cases treated conservatively and partial recovery in another 40%. Serial electromyographic (EMG) studies can help determine the extent of the injury and prognosis. Some authors have advocated surgical decompression in nonhemophiliac cases. In the recovering stage, quadriceps exercises are prescribed, with consideration of a knee brace and extended use of a walker due to any quadriceps weakness. Pudendal nerve palsy has very rarely occurred in thin hip fracture patients due to pressure while on the operating table (125). Acetabular injuries, a variety of pelvic fracture, may have a 5% incidence of sciatic palsy (126).

Central Nervous System Disorders. There is a known relationship between cerebrovascular accidents (CVAs) and hip fractures. Various studies show that 4% to 15% of hip fracture patients have had a prior stroke. The fracture generally occurs on the same side as the paresis. A fracture that occurs within a week after a CVA has a poor functional prognosis. If there are at least 6 months after the CVA before any fracture occurs, the functional prognosis is better (127).

The information regarding treatment and outcome of patients with Parkinsonism and subcapital hip fractures is limited. Morbidity and mortality rates are higher than in those without Parkinson's disease. A large, detailed retrospective study of the Mayo Clinic experience found a 2% rate of dislocations. Of those patients who were ambulatory prior to the fracture, 80% were able to walk afterwards (128).

Pain. A clarification of the discomfort should be made. Usually it is routine postoperative pain with associated reflex muscle contraction. However, it may be from orthopedic complications, neuropathy, muscular strain, infection, bleeding, arthritis, DVT, or other problems. Appropriate diagnosic tests may be needed in certain cases.

Assuming routine postoperative pain, injectable and oral narcotics are commonly used by surgeons for initial effective pain relief. Most patients wean themselves from these medications in a short amount of time. However, some may have been chronic narcotic users before the fracture. In these cases, clarification of the potential role of narcotic analgesics in the original fall may be illuminating.

Other means to reduce postoperative pain exist. Relaxation techniques have been shown to reduce pain and narcotic use (28). Physical measures include TENS, icing, and heat (38). Alternate medications, as appropriate, may be helpful for the patient (acetaminophen, antidepressants, injectable or oral nonsteroidal antiinflammatory agents, etc.).

Some persons may be depressed, expressing their problems through somatization with pain complaints. Anxiety, depression, and schizophrenic disorders can complicate pain problems. Since prolonged pain itself can be a cause for depression, it is appropriate to try to treat any pain before necessarily considering any psychologic component. These problems can impede rehabilitation and increase hospital length of stay, so prompt attention can be helpful.

A variety of other medical problems (129) may be present in the geriatric fracture patient. The rehabilitation physician should be aware of how the patient's medical problems impact upon and interact with the rehabilitation program (Table 12.4).

PROGNOSIS

As discussed in various sections above, there are certain problems that can seriously compromise the recovery from a hip fracture. A recent epidemiologic study confirmed that the prognosis after a hip fracture is adversely affected by increased age, a prefracture high dependency level, dementia, postsurgical delerium, depression, a poor social network, and any subsequent rehospitalization or major fall (50).

Mortality after hip fracture is 20% to 25% at 6 months to 1 year (130–132). Significant risk factors of mortality were dementia, postoperative pneumonia, malignant neoplasia, deep wound infection, age greater than 85 years, and American Society of Anesthetists's risk classification of III or IV (131,132).

In some studies, about 10% to 20% of persons after a hip fracture end up going to a nursing home (23, 133, 134). Another study distinguished between discharge after fracture to a nursing facility (5% of patients) and to supervised boarding facilities (12% of patients) (135). Other studies show a much greater rate (45%) of discharge to institutional care (50). With regard to patients who are discharged to a nursing home (136) or to a hospital for chronic care (137) studies show 66% remain institutionalized and 33% percent return home after one year.

The ambulation recovery rate is limited after a hip fracture. It must be noted that the patient's prefracture status required a walking aid for 33% to 43% of patients, and some are nonambulatory prior to the fracture (23, 133). Some report that only about 25% to 50% of patients recover to prefracture ambulatory status, and the others require a new ambulatory aid or physical assistance (138–140). However, recovery to prefracture abilities is not a static measurement. With longer recovery time, there is improved function for up to 6 to 12 months. One report (50) noted return to prefracture abilities in about 37% at 2 months, but by 6 months and after, 62% achieved their prefracture ambulatory status.

Table 12.4. **Impact of Medical Problems on Rehabilitation Program**

	Special Rehabilitation Aspect
Insulin-dependent Diabetes Mellitus	Patient often needs less insulin as mobility improves; consider frequent dose adjustments. Therapists should be notified of diagnosis.
Hypertension	Diuretics may cause incontinence (due to impaired mobility) and dehydration (with decreased postoperative oral intake). Beta-blockers may exacerbate any postoperative depression or impaired cognitive state.
Anticoagulation	Consideration of the patient's likelihood of falling may help decide regarding potential new anticoagulation versus inferior vena cava screen for DVT. Therapists should be notified re medication.
Psychiatric Problems; Sleep Disorders	Antipsychotic medications, antidepressants, benzodiazepines, barbiturates, alcohol, and other drugs of abuse can have effects upon rehabilitation for good or ill: monitor closely.
Cardiac or Pulmonary Disorders	Therapists should be notified of diagnosis for monitoring purposes.

Some patients never walk again after the injury. Two studies (133, 134) indicate that 7% to 9% of all patients with hip fracture were bedridden or wheelchair bound prior to the injury. By 1 year after the fracture, 22% to 30% of surviving patients were nonambulatory (133, 139, 141). The chance of being nonambulatory greatly increases with increasing age (139), although aggressive, empathic therapy may yield far better results than previously reported for persons greater than 90 years old (142). The walking recovery may be better for those with a femoral neck fracture compared to an intertrochanteric fracture (143).

Of those patients who walk after a hip fracture, about 50% to 85% require some form of walking aid at 1 year (23, 55, 133, 139, 143). Ten percent to 30% require a walker—the higher figure especially for those over 85 years of age (23, 54, 55). One study demonstrated that at 1 year, about 50% of patients required some type of cane—some or all of the time. Fifteen percent of persons could walk unaided. The percentage of use of each of these assistive devices is greater earlier in the recuperative year (55). Twenty-eight percent of persons after discharge required the assistance of another for ambulation in one study (144).

Many people have regained their prior ADL status by 6 months postsurgery (145). At 1 year following the injury, 60% to 90% of persons have regained prefracture status in various self-care ADL (29, 47). Fifty percent to 80% of persons by that time have reached prefracture function for various independent living skills (47).

The Swedish rapid rehabilitation program has received much attention (23, 24, 31–33, 129, 143). It was actually designed to decrease the need for intensive inpatient rehabilitation with an effective coordination of services in the first days after a hip fracture. Thus, this system is actually a rough equivalent of an early consultation to a rehabilitation service. On analysis, it is not the equivalent of a comprehensive inpatient rehabilitation service. A certain percentage of persons still seem to be transferred to facilities offering comprehensive inpatient rehabilitation (23, 143).

In one interesting study, an adaptation of the Swedish rapid rehabilitation program was applied by Jette et al (138) in the United States. No difference was noted between patients in this experimental program and those receiving standard therapy. Patients with stable fractures were allowed to weight bear as tolerated by the second day after surgery. This program was described as offering intensive rehabilitation. However, a closer inspection reveals that this version of intensive rehabilitation was different only in the provision of some family education, the existence of staff evaluations and meetings, a postdischarge (not before discharge) home visit for environmental assessment, and intermittent home telephone calls after discharge by the physical therapist for monitoring progress. This program had many of the trappings of a typical American comprehensive inpatient rehabilitation program, but lacked the core: greatly increased (i.e., typically 3 hours or more) therapy services, occupational therapists, experienced rehabilitative nursing, psychologic support, selected appropriate predischarge home evaluation, and physiatric coordination of all of these issues. In fact, 40% of the patients (with unreported functional, psychologic, and social problems) were discharged to rehabilitation facilities. The lack of increased therapy may certainly play a role, as increased amounts of therapy after a fracture are correlated with increased function (146).

Randomized controlled studies of the efficacy of comprehensive inpatient rehabilition are starting to appear (147–150). Although earlier studies were inconclusive the latest trial clearly demonstrated early improvement with comprehensive inpatient rehabilitation (150). More studies are needed.

Pelvic Fractures

Pelvic fractures have been classified in various ways. One common way describes fractures that:

1. Do not break the continuity of the pelvic ring (for example, a pubic ramus fracture),
2. Cause a single break in the pelvic ring (i.e., two ipsilateral pubic rami fractures or the symphysis pubis),
3. Cause double breaks of the pelvic ring (for example, Malgagne's double vertical fractures or dislocation of the pelvis), and
4. Fracture of the acetabulum (undisplaced or displaced).

A fracture of a single pubic ramus is initially treated with analgesia and bedrest. Early mobilization, as with hip fractures, is recommended. Weight bearing on the limb is permitted. The pain of weight bearing can be decreased by weight relief through the use of a walker, cane, or other devices. Sacral and coccygeal fractures, often from a fall onto the buttocks, are also often relieved by a brief period of bedrest. Stool softeners, sitz baths for muscle spasm, and sitting on a foam or inflatable ring often in a semireclining position are also helpful. Fractures that involve two ipsilateral pubic rami fractures or the symphysis pubis are usually treated similarly to fractures of a single pubic ramus.

Fractures that cause double breaks in the pelvic ring are usually the result of high-velocity trauma. Skeletal fixation is performed when possible for the advantages of early stabilization and thus early mobilization. The alternate treatment is prolonged bedrest.

Undisplaced acetabular fractures are sometimes treated with bedrest and sometimes traction for 1 or more weeks, followed by 2 or 3 months of nonweight bearing activity. Other patients may be treated with more immediate mobilization out of bed to avoid the complications of bedrest. Displaced acetabular fractures may be treated nonoperatively (skeletal traction for 2 or 3 months) or operatively. Degenerative arthritis and ectopic bone formation have been complications in the more severe acetabular fractures. Sciatic nerve palsy, vascular injury, and infection have occurred on occasion with acetabular surgery (126).

Colles' Fractures

Rehabilitation after fractures of the distal radius should include ROM exercises of the digits, elbow, and shoulder starting after orthopedic treatment. Weight-bearing activities and strong gripping or lifting are avoided during healing. Upon cast removal, wrist flexion and extension exercises may begin, although one should avoid excessive movement initially. Attention should be paid to attempted maintainance of forearm supination, which may be compromised with these fractures.

After a Colles' fracture, hematoma, postoperative deformity, or posttraumatic synovitis of the wrist flexor tendons can lead to carpal tunnel syndrome (CTS) (151, 152). This syndrome of pain, numbness, weakness, and paresthesias in the median nerve distribution of the hand is due to increased pressure in the carpal canal (153). Subclinical electrodiagnostic findings have been reported to occur in 52% of persons after distal radial fractures (perhaps from postfracture edema). However, clinical reports show an incidence of complaints from about zero to 6.3% (154). If there are symptoms of CTS associated with a Colles' fracture, immediate reduction and minimal early wrist flexion is recommended. If, after this, CTS symptoms do not improve in the next day or two, carpal tunnel release has been recommended to prevent permanent nerve loss (155).

Very rarely, ulnar nerve palsy has been reported to occur with Colles' fractures (156).

Humeral Fractures

Humeral fractures are minimally displaced more than 80% of the time. However, one should ascertain the stability of even minimally displaced fractures by noting whether there is bony impaction, and, if on X-ray films, the proximal portion of the humerus rotates with the distal fragment as a unit. When this occurs, then ROM exercises may begin. Pendulum exercises are then instituted and weight bearing is initially avoided. Usually at 3 to 4 weeks, a trial of active ROM program against gravity is begun. If this is tolerated, then gentle progressive strengthening exercises are begun, usually progressing from isometric exercises. Most patients regain 50% to 75% of their preinjury ROM following this fracture, usually enough to continue with their ADL (157).

Vertebral Fractures

The treatment for osteoporotic vertebral fractures is symptomatic. Initially, bedrest may help, taking care to avoid an excess. Analgesics, superficial heat (with care taken to avoid thermal injury), and muscle relaxants may all play a role in initial care. A corset may prove helpful for some persons initially, although there may be some problems with tolerance. In 3% of patients, there may be neurologic deficits associated with spinal cord compromise; CT or magnetic resonance imaging (MRI) with possible surgical consideration is then needed (158).

References

1. Nevitt MC, Cummings SR, Kidd S, et al. Risk factors for recurrent nonsynocopal falls: a prospective study. *JAMA.* 261:2663–2668, 1989.
2. Tinetti ME, Speechley M, Ginter SF. Risk factors for falls among elderly persons living in the community. *N Engl J Med.* 319:1701–1707, 1988.
3. Rubenstein LZ, Robbins AS. Falls in the elderly: a clinical perspective. *Geriatrics.* 39:67–78, 1984.
4. Sabin TA. Biologic aspects of falls and mobility limitations in the elderly. *J Am Geriatr Soc.* 30:51–58, 1982.
5. Tideiksaar R, Kay AD. What causes falls? A logical diagnostic procedure. *Geriatrics.* 41:32–50, 1986.
6. Cummings SR, Nevitt MC. A hypothesis: the causes of hip fractures. *J Gerontol.* 44:M107–111, 1989.
7. Aniansson A, Zetterberg C, Hedberg M, et al. Impaired muscle function with aging. *Clin Orthop.* 191:193–201, 1984.
8. Wheeler J, Woodward C, Ucovich RL, et al. Rising from a chair. Influence of age and chair design. *Phys Ther.* 65:22–26, 1985.
9. Young A, Stokes M, Crowe M. The size and strength of the quadriceps muscles of old and young men. *Clin Physiol.* 5:145–154, 1985.
10. Zuckerman JD, Schon LC. Hip fractures. In: Zuckerman JD, ed. *Comprehensive Care of Orthopedic Injuries in the Elderly.* Baltimore, MD: Urban & Schwarzenberg; 1990.
11. Pillar T, Gasper E, Poplingher AR, et al. Operated versus non-operated hip fractures in a geriatric rehabilitation hospital. *Int Disabil Studies.* 10:104–106, 1989.
12. Lyon LJ, Nevins MA. Management of hip fractures in nursing home patients: to treat or not to treat? *J Am Geriatr Soc.* 32:391–395, 1984.
13. Hornby R, Evans JG, Vardin V. Operative or conservative treatment for trochanteric fractures of the femur. *J Bone Joint Surg.* 71-B:619–623, 1989.
14. Stromgvist MD, Kelly I, Lidgren L. Treatment of hip fractures in rheumatoid arthritis. *Clin. Orthop.* 228:75–78, 1978.
15. Felsenthal G, Stein BD. Rehabilitation of dysmobility in the elderly: a case study of the patient with a hip fracture. In: Brody SJ, Paulson LG, eds. *Aging and Rehabilitation II: The State of the Practice.* New York, NY: Springer; 1990.
16. Cocchiarella A, Yue SH. Rehabilitation of geriatric patients with hip fracture. *J Am Geriatr Soc.* 14:1172–1176, 1966.
17. Katz S, Ford AB, Heiple KG, et al. Studies of illness in the aged: recovery after fracture of the hip. *J Gerontol.* 19:285–293, 1964.
18. Katz S, Heiple KG, Downs TD, et al. Long term course of 147 patients with fracture of the hip. *Surg Gynecol Obstet.* 124:1219–1230, 1967.
19. Clark ANG, Wainwright D. Management of the fractured neck of femur in the elderly female: a joint approach of orthopedic surgery and geriatric medicine. *Gerontol Clin.* 8:321–326, 1966.

20. Currie CT. Hip fracture in the elderly: beyond the metalwork. *Brit Med J.* 298:473–474, 1989.

21. The old woman with a broken hip. *Lancet.* 2:419–420, 1982.

22. Boyd RV, Hawthorne J, Wallace WA, et al. The Nottingham orthogeriatric unit after 1000 admissions. *Injury.* 15:193–196, 1983.

23. Ceder L, Ekelund L, Inerot S, et al. Rehabilitation after hip fracture in the elderly. *Acta Orthop Scand.* 50:681–688, 1979.

24. Thorngren M, Nilsson LT, Thorngren KG. Prognosis-determined rehabilitation of hip fractures. *Comp Geontol A.* 2:12–17, 1988.

25. Duncan BF, Fritts JA. Early rehabilitation for the bed-confined orthopaedic patient. *Contemp Orthopaedics.* 7:47–53, 1983.

26. Knapp ME. Aftercare of fractures. In: Kottke FJ, Stillwell GK, Lehmann JF, eds. *Krusen's Handbook of Pyysical Medicine and Rehabilitation.* 3rd ed. Philadelphia, Pa: W.B. Saunders, 1982.

27. Ceccio CM. Postoperative pain relief through relaxation in elderly patients with fractured hips. *Orthop Nurs.* 3:11–19, 1984.

28. Halar EM, Bell KR. Contracture and other deleterious effects of immobility. In: DeLisa JA, ed. *Rehabilitation Medicine: Principles and Practice.* 2nd ed. Philadelphia, Pa: J.B. Lippincott;1993.

29. Elabdien BSZ, Olerud S, Karlstrom G. Ender nailing of pertrochanteric fractures. Results at follow-up evaluation after one year. *Clin Orthop.* 191:53–63, 1984.

30. Ainsworth TH. Immediate full weight bearing in the treatment of hip fractures. *J Trauma.* 11:1031–1040, 1971.

31. Ceder L, Lindberg L, Odberg E. Differentiated care of hip fracture in the elderly. *Acta Orthop Scand.* 51:157–162, 1980.

32. Ceder L, Thorngren KG, Wallden B. Prognostic indicators and early home rehabilitation in elderly patients with hip fractures. *Clin Orthop.* 152:173–184, 1980.

33. Ceder L, Svensson K, Thorngren KG. Statistical prediction of rehabilitation in elderly patients with hip fractures. *Clin Orthop.* 152:185–190, 1980.

34. Hansen BA, Solgaard S. Impacted fractures of the femoral neck treated by early mobilization and weight-bearing. *Acta Orthop Scand.* 49:180–185, 1978.

35. Zuckerman JD, Zetterberg C, Kummer FJ, et al. Weight bearing following hip fractures in geriatric patients. *Top Geriatr Rehabil.* 6:34–50, 1990.

36. Joynt RL, Findley TW, Bada W, et al. Therapeutic exercise. In: DeLisa JA, ed. *Rehabilitation Medicine: Principles and Practice.* 2nd ed. Philadelphia, Pa: J.B. Lippincott; 1993.

37. Zuckerman JD, Newport ML Rehabilitation of fractures in adults. In: Goodgold J, ed. *Rehabilitation Medicine.* St. Louis, Mo: Mosby; 1988.

38. Basford JR. Physical agents. In: DeLisa JA, ed. *Rehabilitation Medicine: Principles and Practice.* 2nd ed. Philadelphia, Pa: J.B. Lippincott; 1993.

39. Moskowitz E. *Rehabilitation in Extremity Fractures.* Springfield, Ill: Charles C Thomas; 1968.

40. Means KM. Falls and fractures. In: Maloney FP, Means KM, eds. *Physical Medicine and Rehabilitation. State of the Art Reviews.* 4(1):39–48, 1990.

41. Rosenblatt DE, Campion EW, Mason M. Rehabilitation home visits. *J Am Geriatr Soc.* 34:441–447, 1986.

42. Trombly CA. *Occupational Therapy for Physical Dysfunction.* 2nd ed. Baltimore, Md: Williams & Wilkins; 1983.

43. *Rehabilitation Nursing.* Ditmar S, ed. St. Louis, Mo: Mosby; 1989.

44. Liss SE, Wylie WJ. Practical aspects of mobilizing the elderly patient following hip fracture. *Texas Med.* 74:69–73, 1978.

45. Bastow MD, Rawlings J, Allison SP. Undernutrition, hypothermia, and injury in elderly women with fractured femur: an injury response to altered metabolism? *Lancet.* 1:143–146, 1983.

46. Bastow MD, Rawlings J, Allison SP. Benefits of supplementary tube feeding after fractured neck of femur: a randomized controlled trial. *Brit Med J.* 287:1589–1592, 1983.

47. Magaziner J, Simonsick EM, Kashner M, et al. Survival experience of aged hip fracture patients. *J. Public Health.* 79:274–278, 1989.

48. Mossey JM, Mutran E, Knott K, et al. Determinants of recovery 12 months after hip fracture: the importance of psychosocial factors. *Am J Public Health.* 79:279–286, 1989.

49. Folstein MF, Folstein SE, McHugh PR. "Mini-Mental State": a practical method for grading the cognitive state of patients for the clinician. *J Psychiatr Res.* 12:189–198, 1975.

50. Magaziner J, Simonsick EM, Kahsner TM, et al. Predictors of functional recovery one year following hospital discharge for hip fracture: a prospective study. *J Gerontol.* 45:M101–107, 1990.

51. Billig N, Ahmed SW, Kenmore P, et al. Assessment of depression and cognitive impairment after hip fracture. *J Am Geriatr Soc.* 34:499–503, 1986.

52. Billig N, Ahmed SW, Kenmore PI. Hip fracture, depression, and cognitive impairment: a follow-up study. *Orthop Rev.* 17:315–320, 1988.

53. Baker BR, Duckworth T, Wilkes E. Mental state and other prognostic factors in femoral fractures of the elderly. *JR Coll Gen Pract.* 28:557–559, 1978.

54. Cheng CL, Lau S, Hui PW. Prognostic factors and prognosis for ambulation in elderly patients after hip fracture. *Am J Phys Med Rehabil.* 68:230–233, 1989.

55. Ungar DM, Warne RW. Morbidity following successful treatment of proximal femoral fractures. *Austr Fam Phys.* 15:1157–1158, 1986.

56. Cummings SR, Phillips SL, Wheat ME, et al. Recovery of function after hip fracture. The role of social supports. *J Am Geriatr Soc.* 36:801–806, 1988.

57. Consensus conference: prevention of venous thrombosis and pulmonary embolism. *JAMA.* 256:744–749, 1986.

58. Hull R, Hirsh J. Advances and controversies in the diagnosis, prevention, and treatment of venous thromboembolism. *Prog Hematol.* 12:73–123, 1981.

59. Gallus AS. Established venous thrombosis and pulmonary embolism. *Clin Haematol.* 10:583–611, 1981.

60. Kakkar VV, Howe CT, Flanc C, et al. Natural history of postoperative deep-vein thrombosis. *Lancet.* 2:230–233, 1969.

61. Bentley PG, Kakkar VV, Scully MF, et al. An objective study of alternative methods of heparin administration. *Thromb Res.* 18:177–187, 1980.

62. Philbrick JT, Becker DM. Calf deep venous thrombosis. a wolf in sheep's clothing? *Arch Intern Med.* 148:2131–2138, 1988.

63. Beninson J. Six years of pressure-gradient therapy: a general survey. *Angiology.* 12:38–45, 1961.

64. Kakkar VV, Howe CT, Laws JW, et al. Late results of treatment of deep venous thrombosis. *Brit Med J.* 1:810–811, 1969.

65. Strandness DE, Langlois Y, Cramer M, et al. Long-term sequelae of acute venous thrombosis. *JAMA.* 250:1289–1292, 1983.

66. Dalen JE, Alpert JS. Natural history of pulmonary embolism. *Prog Cardiovasc Dis.* 17:257–270, 1975.

67. Pun WK, Chow SP, Chan KC, et al. Effusions in the knee in elderly patients who were operated on for fracture of the hip. *J Bone Joint Surg.* 70–A: 117–118, 1988.

68. Cranley JJ, Canos AJ, Sull WJ. The diagnosis of deep vein thrombosis: failability of clinical symptoms and signs. *Arch Surg.* 111:34–36, 1976.

69. Fric M, Pechan J, Mikulecky M, et al. Evaluation of clinical signs and symptoms in active deep venous thrombosis of the calf. *Cor Vasa.* 27:346–352, 1985.

70. McLachlin J, Richards T, Paterson JC. An evaluation of clinical signs in the diagnosis of venous thrombosis. *Arch Surg.* 85:738–744, 1962.

71. Talbot S. The value of clinical signs of venous thrombosis. *Br J Clin Pract.* 29:221–226, 1975.

72. Camerota AJ, Katz ML, Grossi RJ, et al. The comparative value of noninvasive testing for diagnosis and surveillance of deep venous thrombosis. *J Vasc Surg.* 7:40–49, 1988.

73. Rabinkov K, Paulin S. Roentgen diagnosis of venous thrombosis in the leg. *Arch Surg.* 104:133–144, 1972.

74. Becker DM, Philbrick JT, Abbitt PL. Real-time ultrasonography for the diagnosis of lower extremity deep venous thrombosis: the wave of the future? *Arch Intern Med.* 149:1731–1734, 1989.

75. Yao JST, Henkin RE, Conn J, et al. Combined isotope venography and lung scanning: a new diagnostic approach to thromboembolism. *Arch Surg.* 107:146–151, 1973.

76. Camerota AJ, Katz ML, Grossi RJ, et al. The comparative value of noninvasive testing for diagnosis and surveillance of deep venous thrombosis. *J Vasc Surg.* 7:40–49, 1988.

77. Patterson RB, Fowl RJ, Keller JD, et al. The limitations of impedance plethysmography in the diagnosis of acute deep venous thrombosis. *J Vasc Surg.* 9:725–730, 1989.

78. Wheeler HB, Anderson F. Diagnostic approaches for deep vein thrombosis. *Chest.* 89 (suppl):407S–412S, 1986.

79. Haake DA, Berkman SA. Venous thromboembolic disease after hip surgery: risk factors, prophylaxis, and diagnosis. *Clin Orthop.* 242:212–231, 1989.

80. Froehlich JA, Dorfman GS, Cronan JJ, et al. Compression ultrasonography for the detection of deep venous thrombosis in patients who have a fracture of the hip: a prospective study. *J Bone Joint Surg.* 71-A: 249–256, 1989.

81. Dorfman GS, Froelich JA, Cronan JJ, et al. Lower-extremity venous thrombosis in patients with acute hip fractures: determination of anatomic location and time of onset with compression sonography. *AJR.* 154:851–855, 1990.

82. Roberts TS, Nelson CL, Barnes CL, et al. The preoperative prevalence and postoperative incidence of thromboembolism in patients with hip fractures treated with dextran prophylaxis. *Clin Orthop.* 255:198–203, 1990.

83. Wright HP, Osborn SB, Edmonds DG. Effect of postoperative bed rest and early ambulation on the rate of venous bloodflow. *Lancet.* 1:22–25, 1951.

84. Gibbs NM. Venous thrombosis of the lower limbs with particular reference to bed-rest. *Brit J Surg.* 45:209–236, 1957.

85. Browse NL. The prevention of venous thromboembolism by mechanical methods. In: Bergan JJ, Yao JST, eds. *Venous Problems.* Chicago, Ill: Year Book Publishers; 1978.

86. Hartsuck JM, Greenfield LJ. Postoperative thromboembolism: a clinical study with 125-I Fibrinogen and pulmonary scanning. *Arch Surg.* 107:733–739, 1973.

87. Hartman JT, Pugh JL, Smith RD, et al. Cyclic sequential compression of the lower limb in prevention of deep venous thrombosis. *J Bone Joint Surg.* 64-A:1059–1062, 1982.

88. Hull RD, Raskob GE, Gent M, et al. Effectiveness of itermittent pneumatic leg compression for preventing deep vein thrombosis after total hip replacement. *JAMA.* 263:2313–2317, 1990.

89. Pittman GR. Peroneal nerve palsy following sequential pneumatic compression. *JAMA.* 261:2201–2202, 1989.

90. Borow M, Goldson H. Postoperative venous thrombosis: evaluation of five methods of treatment. *Am J Surg.* 141:245–251, 1981.

91. Lewis CE, Antoine J, Mueller C, et al. Elastic compression in the prevention of venous stasis: a critical reevaluation. *Am J Surg.* 132:739–743, 1976.

92. Hull RD, Raskob GE. Prophylaxis of venous thromboembolic disease following hip and knee surgery. *J Bone Joint Surg.* 68-A:146–150, 1986.

93. Borow M, Goldson HJ. Prevention of postoperative deep venous thrombosis and pulmonary emboli with combined modalities. *Am Surg.* 49:599–605, 1983.

94. Colditz GA, Tuden RL, Oster G. Rates of venous thrombosis after general surgery: combined results of randomized clinical trials. *Lancet.* 2:143–146, 1986.

95. Torngren S. Low dose heparin and compression stockings in the prevention of postoperative deep venous thrombosis. *Br J Surg.* 67:482–484, 1980.

96. Mohr DN, Ryu JH, Litin SC, et al. Recent advances in the management of venous thromboembolism. *Mayo Clin Proc.* 63:281–290, 1988.

97. Jones KT, Barnes RW, Greenfield LJ. Greenfield vena caval rationale and current indications. *Ann Thorac Surg.* 42(suppl):S48–55, 1986.

98. Bach JR, Zaneuski R, Lee H. Cardiac arrythmias from a malpositioned Greenfield filter in a traumatic quadriplegic. *AM J Phys Med Rehabil.* 69:251–253, 1990.

99. Carabasi AR, Moritz MJ, Jarrell BE. Complications encountered with the use of the Greenfield filter. *Am J Surg.* 154:163–168, 1987.

100. Hirsh J. Is the dose of warfarin prescribed by American physicians unnecessarily high? *Arch Intern Med.* 147:769–771, 1987.

101. Cox JST. The maturation and canalization of thrombi. *Surg Gynecol Obstet.* 116:593–599, 1963.

102. Moser KM, Guisan M, Bartimmo EE, et al. In vivo and post mortem dissolution rates of pulmonary emboli and venous thrombi in the dog. *Circulation.* 48:170–178, 1973.

103. Bader DL, Barnhill RL, Ryan TJ. Effect of externally applied skin surface forces on tissue vasculature. *Arch Phys Med Rehabil.* 67:807–811, 1986.

104. Seiler WO, Stahelin HB. Recent findings on decubitus ulcer pathology: implications for care. *Geriatrics.* 41:47–60, 1986.

105. Shea JD. Pressure sores: classification and management. *Clin Orthop.* 112:89–100, 1975.

106. Versluysen M. How elderly patients with femoral fractures develop pressure sores in hospital. *Br Med J.* 292:1131–1313, 1986.

107. El Banna S, Raynal L, Gerebtzof A. Fractures of the hip in the elderly: therapeutic and medico-social considerations. *Arch Gerontol Geriatr.* 3:311–319, 1984.

108. Thornhill-Joynes M, Gonzales F, Stewart CA, et al. Osteomyelitis associated with pressures ulcers. *Arch Phys Med Rehabil.* 67:314–318, 1986.

109. Bryan CS, Dew CE, Reynolds KL. Bacteremia associated with decubitus ulcers. *Arch Int Med.* 143:2093–2095, 1983.

110. Seiler WO, Stahelin HB. Decubitus ulcers: preventive techniques for the elderly patient. *Geriatrics.* 40:53–60, 1985.

111. Krasner D. Utilizing the nursing process to manage heel ulcers. *Ostomy/Wound management.* 17:48–57, 1987.

112. Seiler WO, Stahelin HB. Decubitus ulcers: treatment through five therapeutic principles. *Geriatrics.* 40:30–42, 1985.

113. Witkowski JA, Parish LC. Cutaneous ulcer therapy. *Int J Dermatol.* 25:420–426, 1986.

114. Broos PLO, Van Haaften KIK, Stappaerts KH, et al. Hip fractures in the elderly. Mortality, functional results and social readaptation. *Int Surg.* 74:191–194, 1989.

115. Michelson JD, Lotke PA, Steinberg ME. Urinary-bladder management after total joint-replacement surgery. *N Engl J Med.* 319:321–326, 1988.

116. Manchester D, Woollacott M, Zederbauer-Hylton N, et al. Visual, vestibular and somatosensory contributions to balance control in the older adult. *J Gerontol.* 44:M118–127, 1989.

117. Weber ER, Daube JR, Coventry MB. Peripheral neuropathies associated with total hip arthroplasty. *J Bone Joint Surg.* 58-A:66–69, 1976.

118. Edwards BN, Tullos HS, Noble PC. Contributory factors and etiology of sciatic nerve palsy in total hip arthroplasty. *Clin Orthop.* 218:136–141, 1987.

119. Fleming RE, Michelson CB, Stinchfield FE. Sciatic paralysis: a

complication of bleeding following hip surgery. *J Bone Joint Surg.* 61-A:37–39, 1979.

120. Herbison GJ, Jaweed MM, Ditunno JF. Exercise therapies in peripheral neuropathies. *Arch Phys Med Rehabil.* 64:201–205, 1983.

121. Jackson S. Femoral neuropathy secondary to heparin induced intrapelvic hematoma: a case report and review of the literature. *Orthopedics.* 10:1049–1052, 1987.

122. Stern MB, Spiegel P. Femoral neuropathy as a complication of heparin anticoagulation therapy. *Clin Orthop.* 106:140–142, 1975.

123. Chiu WS. The syndrome of retroperitoneal hemorrhage and lumbar plexus neuropathy during anticoagulant therapy. *South Med J.* 69:595–599, 1976.

124. Emery S, Ochoa J. Lumbar plexus neuropathy resulting from retroperitoneal hemorrhage. *Muscle Nerve.* 1:330–334, 1978.

125. Hofman A, Jones RE, Schoenvogel R. Purdendal-nerve neurapraxia as a result of traction on the fracture table. *J Bone Joint Surg.* 64-A:136–138, 1982.

126. Moskovich R, Zuckerman JD. Pelvic and acetabular injuries. In: Zuckerman JD, ed. *Comprehensive Care of Orthopedic Injuries in the Elderly.* Baltimore, Md: Urban & Schwarzenberg; 1990.

127. Poplinger A-R, Pillar T. Hip fracture in stroke patients: epidemiology and rehabilitation. *Acta Orthop Scand.* 56:226–227, 1985.

128. Staehel JW, Frassica FJ, Sim FH. Prosthetic replacement of the femoral head for fracture of the femoral neck in patients who have Parkinson disease. *J Bone Joint Surg.* 70-A:565–568, 1988.

129. Cedar L, Elmqvist D, Svensson SE. Cardiovascular and neurological function in elderly patients sustaining a fracture of the neck of the femur. *J Bone Joint Surg.* 63-B:560–566, 1981.

130. Gallagher JC, Melton LJ, Riggs BL, et al. Epidemiology of fractures of the proximal femur in Rochester, Minnesota. *Clin Orthop Relat Res.* 150:163–171, 1980.

131. White BL, Fisher WD, Laurin CA. Rate of mortality for elderly patients after a fracture of the hip in the 1980s. *J Bone Joint Surg.* 69-A:1335–1340, 1987.

132. Wood DJ, Ions GK, Quinby JM, et al. Factors which influence mortality after subcapital hip fracture. *J Bone Joint Surg.* 74-B:199–202, 1992.

133. Alberts KA, Nilsson MH. Consumption versus need of institutional care after femoral neck fracture. *Scand J Rehabil Med.* 21:159–164, 1989.

134. Jensen JS, Tondevold E. Mortality after hip fractures. *Acta Orthop Scand.* 50:161–167, 1979.

135. Thomas TG, Stevens RS. Social effects of fractures of the neck of the femur. *Br Med J.* 3:456–458, 1974.

136. Keene JS, Anderson CA. Hip fractures in the elderly: discharge predictions with a functional rating scale. *JAMA.* 248:564–567, 1982.

137. Snaedal J, Thorngren M, Ceder L, et al. Outcome of patients with a nailed hip fracture requiring rehabilitation in a hospital for chronic care. *Scand J Rehab Med.* 16:171–176, 1984.

138. Jette A, Harris BA, Cleary P, et al. Functional recovery after hip fracture. *Arch Phys Med Rehabil.* 68:735–740, 1987.

139. Miller CW. Survival and ambulation following hip fracture. *J Bone Joint Surg.* 60-A:930–934, 1978.

140. Moller BN, Lucht U, Grymer F, et al. Early rehabilitation following osteosynthesis with sliding hip screw for trochanteric fractures. *Scand J Rehabil Med* 17:39–43, 1985.

141. Naden D, Denbesten L. Fractures of the neck of the femur in the aged: review of 224 consecutive cases. *J Am Geriatr Soc.* 17:198–204, 1969.

142. Kauffman TL, Albright L, Wagner C. Rehabilitation outcomes after hip fracture in persons 90 years old and older. *Arch Phys Med Rehabil.* 68:369–371, 1987.

143. Dolk T. Influence of treatment factors on the outcome after hip fractures. *Upsala J Med Sci.* 94:209–221, 1989.

144. Leung PC, Cheng YH, Ho YF, et al. Fractured proximal end of the femur in the elderly—A medico-social study. *Gerontolog.* 34:192–198, 1988.

145. Jensen JS, Tondevold E, Sorensoen PH. Social rehabilitation following hip fractures. *Acta Orthop Scand.* 50:777–785, 1979.

146. Bohannon RW, Kloter KS, Cooper JA. Outcome of patients with hip fracture treated by physical therapy in an acute care hospital. *Top Geriatr Rehabil.* 6:51–58, 1990.

147. Gilchrist WJ, Newman RJ, Hambler DL, et al. Prospective randomized study of an orthopedic geriatric inpatient service. *Brit Med J.* 297:1116–1118, 1988.

148. Kennie DC, Reid J, Richardson IR, et al. Effectiveness of geriatric rehabilitative care after fractures of the proximal femur in elderly women: A randomized controlled trial. *Brit Med J.* 297:1083–1086, 1988.

149. Reid J, Kennie DC. Geriatric rehabilitative care after fractures of the proximal femur: one year follow up of a randomized clinical trial. *Brit Med J.* 299:25–26, 1989.

150. Cameron ID, Lyle DM, Quine S. Accelerated rehabilitation after proximal femoral fracture: a randomized controlled trial. *Dis Rehabil.* 15:29–34, 1993.

151. Ambrose L, Stuchin SA. Hand and wrist injuries. In: Zuckerman JD, ed. *Comprehensive Care of Orthopedic Injuries in the Elderly.* Baltimore, Md: Urban & Schwarzenberg; 1990.

152. Lewis HH. Median nerve decompression after Colles' fracture. *J Bone Joint Surg.* 60-B:195–196, 1978.

153. Gelberman RH, Hergenroeder PT, Hargens AR, et al. The carpal tunnel syndrome: a study of carpal canal pressures. *J Bone Joint Surg.* 63-A:380–383, 1981.

154. Stark WA. Neural involvement in fractures of the distal radius. *Orthopedics.* 10:333–335, 1987.

155. Dawson DM, Hallett M, Millender LH. *Entrapment Neuropathies.* Boston, Mass: Little, Brown; 1983.

156. Shea JD, McClain EJ. Ulnar-nerve compression syndromes at and below the wrist. *J Bone Joint Surg.* 51-A:1095–1103, 1969.

157. Zuckerman JD, Buchalter JS. Shoulder injuries. In: Zuckerman JD, ed. *Comprehensive Care of Orthopedic Injuries in the Elderly.* Baltimore, Md: Urban & Schwarzenberg; 1990.

158. Schneider PL, Dzenis PE, Kahanovitz N. Spinal trauma. In: Zuckerman JD, ed. *Comprehensive Care of Orthopedic Injuries in the Elderly.* Baltimore, Md: Urban & Schwarzenberg; 1990.

13

Disorders of the Cervical and Lumbosacral Spine

Avital Fast

SPINAL DISORDERS IN THE ELDERLY

This chapter will deal primarily with disorders of the cervical and lumbar spine in the geriatric patient. Osteoporosis and compression fractures will not be reviewed since they are dealt with in Chapter 11. Significant progress has been made in the last 20 years in clarifying the pathophysiology of spinal disorders. Distinct clinical syndromes have been identified, and specific new therapeutic approaches, mostly surgical, have been adopted. The dramatic progress made in radiology, with the introduction of computerized tomography (CT) and magnetic resonance imaging (MRI), enhances our understanding of spinal pathology and allows us, in many patients, to identify the location and the specific structures leading to the patient's complaints.

It should be remembered, however, that the new imaging modalities do not solve all of our clinical problems. In many instances, false positive studies may confuse the unwary physician. In patients with unremitting pain, bone scan and occasionally bone biopsy may be necessary in order to establish the correct diagnosis. Since most elderly patients are expected to have abnormal radiologic studies, a detailed history taking and a thorough clinical examination are essential in directing the clinician toward the right diagnosis.

Disc degeneration is a common underlying process in many cervical and lumbar spine syndromes. Degeneration of the disc plays a central role in the production of spinal pain and is of paramount importance in the pathogenesis of the spondylotic spine. As we age, the disc undergoes enzymatic, biochemical, and structural changes. In the aged individual the amount of proteoglycans decreases. The disc loses its ability to retain water, dessicates, and becomes fibrotic. The discal collagen structure changes with the replacement of type II collagen by type I. As degeneration progresses, the nucleus pulposus is gradually replaced by fibrocartilage, and

the annulus fibrosus develops fissures and rents. Whereas many degenerated discs do not herniate, most herniated discs show signs of disc degeneration. Narrowing of the discs alters the load distribution in the motion segment, leading, at times, to segmental instability. As a result of excessive stresses borne by the spinal articulations, i.e., the facets, they develop osteoarthritic changes. Whereas in the lumbar spine there are only two joints connecting the vertebral bodies—the zygapophyseal joints, the cervical vertebrae have two additional joints—the joints of Luschka. These joints are located in the posterolateral aspect of the lower five cervical vertebrae. Their clinical importance lies in their proximity to the nerve root canal. Osteoarthritic spurs, hypertrophic ligamenta flava, and enlarged facet joints may narrow the intervertebral foraminae and the spinal canal, thus leading to neurologic compromise and pain.

Herniated discs, although less common in the aged population, can occur in all age groups and tend to produce symptoms by exerting tension and compression on the nerve roots or spinal cord. The physician approaching the elderly with neck or back pain should remember that there may not be a direct correlation between the severity of findings, as seen on the X-ray films, and the clinical picture. In spite of the fact that degenerative changes tend to increase with age, the prevalence of clinical symptoms does not follow the same curve. Indeed, the prevalence of back pain actually decreases beyond the fifth decade.

Frequently, one is confronted with a patient who has advanced spondylotic changes shown in the X-ray films but with minimal complaints and no changes in the neurologic examination (1). These patients are best served if left alone or treated symptomatically with analgesics.

It should be remembered that advanced osteophytes may prevent segmental instability, thus rendering the spine stable and symptomless. Many elderly patients

141

have decreased spinal range of motion. The relatively stiff spine may be normal for the elderly and does not require medical intervention.

CERVICAL SPINE

Degenerative disc disease and cervical spondylosis undoubtedly play a much more prominent role in the etiology of neck problems in the elderly than do acute disc herniations. In fact, Kelsey et al (2), in an epidemiologic study of acute proplapsed cervical discs, did not find a single patient with acute herniation in the 60 to 64 year age group.

In a study of 120 cardaveric spines, removed at routine necropsy from elderly patients, the following important observations were made: appoximately 50% of men and 30% of women in their sixth decade demonstrated a significant amount of degenerative spondylotic changes. The most frequently and most severely damaged nerve roots were those emanating from the lower cervical spine. Degeneration and scarring of nerve roots was commonly associated with abnormal discs. An additional important factor in nerve pathology, especially in the lower cervical spine, was apophyseal joint arthritis (3).

Disc degeneration is most common in the C5-6 disc followed in order of decreasing frequency by C6-7 and C4-5. The changes of spondylosis increase with age and in the cervical spine may reach a prevalence of up to 82% in the sixth decade.

The elderly patient may seek help for the following reasons: nonradiating neck pain without neurologic compromise or predominant radiculopathy in which the main complaints are pain, numbness, and weakness in the upper extremity. Cervical myelopathy, in which spinal cord compromise is the predominant feature, may present with gait dysfunction and deterioration in the functional status. Sometimes, a combination of all of the above may exist.

Although degeneration of the cervical discs and osteoarthritic changes are the most common underlying pathologic processes leading to the above clinical presentations, one should remember, especially in the elderly patient, that other pathologic processes may present in a similar fashion and should be included in the differential diagnosis of neck and arm pain (4).

Tumors may initially present with pain limited to the cervical spine. They may also mimic cervical radiculopathy with or without neural deficits. In advanced cases, tumors may compress the spinal cord and thus mimic cervical myelopathy.

Any patient with unrelenting pain, night pain, or lack of response to conservative management should undergo diagnostic work-up to rule out the existence of space-occupying lesions or infection. Erythrocyte sedimentation rate; complete blood count; serum calcium, phosphorus, uric acid, alkaline and acid phosphatase; serum protein electrophoresis; urine analysis; chest radiograms, and bone scans may help establish the correct diagnosis. Bone scans are more sensitive than radiograms and will detect tumors at an earlier stage.

Compression of the brachial plexus may be caused by lung tumors. Unrelenting upper extremity pain, simulating radiculopathy, may be the first manifestation of carcinoma of the lung. In these cases, chest radiograms or CT point towards the malignant lesion.

Thoracic outlet syndrome, especially the true neurogenic one, should also be included in the differential diagnosis. Since carpal tunnel syndrome is common in the elderly, its role in the painful and paresthetic upper extremity should be established. Electromyography, nerve conduction, and somatosensory evoked potential studies should be included as part of the work-up of cervical radiculopathy in patients with unclear diagnosis. These studies may help differentiate between peripheral causes of upper extremity pain.

Finally, other neurologic disorders that are common in the elderly must be considered. Amyotrophic lateral sclerosis may, in the first stages, present almost identically to cervical myelopathy. Complete comprehensive neurologic examination, including that of the cranial nerves and the lower extremities, may guide the physician toward the correct diagnosis.

CERVICAL RADICULOPATHY

The clinical syndrome of cervical radiculopathy may be similar in both young and elderly patients. The underlying pathologic processes that lead to the radiculopathy, however, may be different. In the majority of young patients, "soft disc"—namely, protrusion or herniation of the nucleus pulposus—is the most common cause of radiculopathy. In elderly patients, the herniating nuclear material may be transformed into a fibrous or cartilaginous mass (5). Calcification may occur in later stages leading to the formation of bony bars. In addition, in the aged cervical spine, radiculopathy or myefjloradiculopathy may be caused by osteoarthritic spurs coming from the vertebral bodies or joints of Luschka or from apophyseal arthritic changes. These changes are referred to as "hard disc" in the neurosurgical literature (6). Occasionally, the predominant pathologic processes are located in the posterior elements of the spine. In these cases, hypertrophy of the laminae may be the main reason for the patient's complaints (7).

Cervical radiculopathy may present with sensory and/or motor symptoms related to the upper extremity. The anatomy of the cervical roots and the location of the pathologic processes determine the quality of the patient's complaints. The sensory nerve roots are larger than the motor roots and are located in the upper portion of the intervertebral foramen. In this location they are located rostrally and posteriorly to the motor fibers (8).

Pathologic processes that impinge upon the upper portion of the foramen may produce sensory symptoms only. Pain and numbness in a dermatomal distribution may be the hallmark of the clinical presentation. In some patients, deformation and narrowing may be limited to the lower portion of the intervertebral foramen. In these cases, weakness and atropy of upper extremity muscles, with no concomitant sensory findings, may be the only findings. Other pathologic conditions such as amyotrophic lateral sclerosis must also be considered.

In the majority of cases, both the sensory and motor roots are compromised, and the clinical picture presents accordingly (8). The sensory findings are by far more common than the motor findings (9). Cervical radiculopathy, especially in the older population, is much more common in males. In the majority of cases, pain is a predominant complaint and is localized in the neck, upper extremity, or both (10). Upper extremity numbness and weakness may accompany the pain. Physical examination will detect sensory deficits in dermatomal distribution, weakness of muscles supplied by a certain nerve root, and limitation in the cervical range of motion. In about 30% of the patients, muscle atrophy may be found (10).

The clinical picture of cervical radiculopathy is well recognized. In most cases, awareness of this syndrome, combined with the fact that pain is a predominant early complaint, leads to timely diagnosis and proper management in many patients.

CERVICAL MYELOPATHY

Cervical spondylotic myelopathy (CSM), an entity found mostly in the elderly, is commonly underdiagnosed and thus requires an indepth discussion with attention to details. CSM is the most common cause of spinal cord dysfunction in patients over the age of 55 years (11). The normal cervical spinal canal has ample space and can accommodate significant amount of spondylotic changes. Usually, the spinal cord occupies about half of the canal space in the upper cervical spine. In the lower cervical spine, from C-4 downward, the relations change, and the spinal cord occupies larger portions of the canal. At the C5-7 level, the spinal cord takes at least 75% of the available space (11). This relationship leaves a limited amount of space to be occupied by cervical spondylotic changes. It has been determined that the critical anteroposterior diameter, below which cervical myelopathy will occur, is 13 mm. Following degenerative disc disease, secondary changes affect the vertebral bodies and the zygapophyseal joints. Osteophytic spurs develop, and the facets become hypertrophied. In addition, the ligamenta flava and the laminae may hypertropy. Intradural and extradural adhesions may

form. All the above processes may take up more than the available space and render the canal stenotic (Fig. 13.1).

The position of the cervical spine is of importance in relation to the space available for the spinal cord. During flexion of the neck, the cervical spinal canal increases in length, and the ligamenta flava are stretched. During hyperextension, the ligamenta flava buckle and tend to fold into the spinal canal. If the ligamenta flava are hypertrophied, they may compress the spinal cord during hyperextension.

The pathophysiology of CSM is complex. Direct compression and stretching of the spinal cord may lead to demyelination and axonal injury. In addition, ischemia may be caused by pressure on the blood vessels feeding and draining the spinal cord and by spasm of spinal arteries and their branches (12–14). Central bars forming between vertebral bodies or posterolateral osteophytes may compress the anterior spinal artery or its branches and render the spinal cord ischemic.

Cervical myelopathy may occur in diffuse idiopathic skeletal hyperostosis (DISH). DISH, also known as senile ankylosing hyperostosis or Forestier's disease, is commonly found in elderly males (15, 16). This disorder is distinguished by excessive ossification of ligaments and entheses. The disorder may elicit spinal pain, stiffness, dysphagia, and, occasionally, neurologic findings, e.g., myelopathy.

Cervical myelopathy may also be found in cases of ossification of the posterior longitudinal ligament (OPLL). This disorder, common in patients of Japanese origin, may be seen in Caucasians (17). It is more common in males and clinically does not become symptomatic before age 50 years. Diagnosis may be best established with cervical spine CT. Ossified posterior longitudinal ligament is most commonly found at the C-5 vertebral level. Up to 50% of patients with OPLL may have DISH. The clinical picture of CSM may be quite different from that of cervical radiculopathy. Since CSM is progressive in the majority of cases, early detection and close monitoring are of importance.

Whereas in cervical radiculopathy pain is an important clinical feature, a significant number of patients with CSM have minimal pain or no pain at all. In fact, CSM has been likened to a silent thief, quietly robbing the patient of strength and functional capacity. Commonly, one may see an elderly patient with a longstanding history of neck pain who gradually, over months or years, develops gait disturbances, hyperreflexia in the lower extremities, and a positive Babinski sign. Weakness and progressive loss of dexterity in the upper extremities may appear. The patient may notice that the upper extremities are becoming increasingly clumsy. Difficulties unbuttoning shirts and a change in handwriting may be noticed. Atrophy of the small muscles of the hands may be observed. The only complaint the pa-

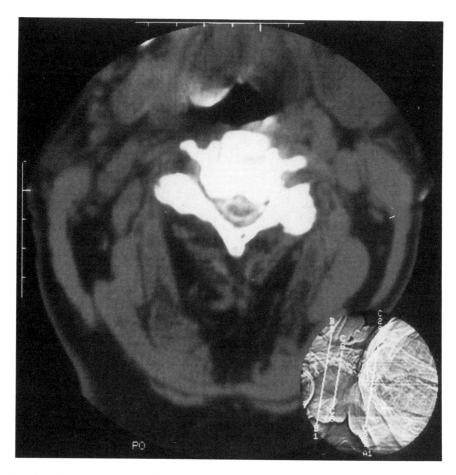

Figure 13.1. Cervical myelopathy. Spurs emanating from the uncinate processes narrow the spinal canal and mildly indent the thecal sac.

tient may verbalize is that of decline in the level of functioning and increased disability (9, 18). The sensory complaints, the functional deterioration, and the weakness may seem nonspecific to the inexperienced clinician.

The patient's gait may become unstable, and he or she may start falling. Frequent falls may become the presenting complaint in patients who, for a long time, ignored the upper extremity functional deterioration. In most patients, the sphincters are spared. Bladder incontinence, however, may occur at times. The sensory changes may involve pain, temperature, and proprioception. Touch is commonly preserved (14). Since pain is not a predominant complaint and CSM progresses gradually, many patients may seek help in relatively late stages of the disease.

It is important to emphasize that physical examination of the elderly patient, presenting with cervical radiculopathy or myelopathy, should include the lower extremities. The physician should specifically look for upper motor neuron findings, such as hyperreflexia, spasticity, and an upgoing toe.

Occasionally, CSM may develop acutely, following, what seems to be, a simple hyperextension injury of the cervical spine. The patient may sustain a whiplash injury, fall forward hitting the forehead, or be forced into hyperextension during general anesthesia. Radiologic studies usually demonstrate degenerative changes without evidence of an acute fracture. Following hyperextension, the patient develops acute myelopathy similar in findings to that described above. Occasionally, spinal cord injury may occur, and the patient may end up with a serious neurologic compromise such as quadriplegia or quadriparesis.

Among the incomplete spinal cord syndromes, central cervical cord syndrome is the most commonly observed. As the name implies, the central portion of the cervical spinal cord is most severely affected (19). Central cervical cord syndrome classically develops following hyperextension injuries of the cervical spine. The compressing forces create localized shearing stress in the cord cross-section. If the forces are limited, a root syndrome will occur. As the compressive and shearing stresses become more significant, central cord syndrome or anterior cord syndrome may result (20). The elderly patient may have, prior to the injury, a mild to moderately stenotic canal. During hyperextension, the infolding ligamenta flava further compromise the canal leading to spinal cord compression. Since the motor fibers of the upper extremities are more centrally located, patients with central cervical cord syndrome display more significant impairment of the upper extremities with relative sparing of the lower extremities, leading to what is referred to by some clinicians as the "walking quad." In addition, the patient may develop a neurogenic bladder, neurogenic bowel, varying degrees of sensory loss below the level of the lesion, and sexual dysfunction (21, 22). The predominant clinical finding in the lower extremities is that of an upper motor neuron compromise. The upper extremities, however, suffer from a lower motor neuron lesion. As a result, atrophy and areflexia are the predominant finding in the upper extremities.

Recovery in these cases occurs first in the lower extremities and bladder. The upper extremities may recover last, leaving the patient, in cases of incomplete recovery, severely disabled.

Cervical and lumbar spinal stenosis commonly coexist. In the elderly population, this combination may be rather common. Epstein et al (22) stated that up to 5% of patients with CSM may have concomitant lumbar spinal stenosis. My impression is that tandem stenosis is more common and should be actively searched for in patients presenting with stenosis in one region. In patients with tandem stenosis who require surgical decompression, there may be improvement in complaints related to the lumbar spine following decompression of the cervical stenosis. The natural history of cervical radiculopathy and cervical meylopathy should be considered before therapeutic approaches and indications for surgery are discussed.

DePalma et al (23) have reviewed the natural history of cervical disc degeneration. They followed 388 patients who failed to respond to conservative management. Surgery was advised to all the patients. Of 388 patients only 281 consented to undergo surgery. The remainder, 107 patients, were managed conservatively and served as a control group. When litigating patients were excluded from the nonoperated group, the percentage of patients rated as satisfactory following surgical or conservative intervention was about the same—62%. The satisfactory response was almost identical in the two groups. Patients with radicular symptoms did far better following surgery than those treated conservatively. Litigation adversely affected the results of conservative therapy. About one fourth of patients in both groups did not return to work (23).

In another study, two groups of patients were followed. One group consisted of patients with myelopathy. The other group consisted of patients with cervical spondylosis and radiculopathy. Patients belonging to the latter group had no further complaints or only slight intermittent symptoms in the majority of cases. However, a small subgroup had some disabling symptoms. Patients who initially presented with radiculopathy hardly ever progressed to myelopathy. The myelopathy group patients had long periods without new or worsening symptoms. Exacerbations, however, did occur at long or short intervals for many years (24).

Clark and Robinson (25) reported that in the majority of patients with CSM there may be gradual worsening with the appearance of new symptoms and signs. Whereas sensory symptoms tended to be transient, motor deficits persisted or even deteriorated with time. LaRocca (18), on the other hand, in a recent review of the natural course of CSM, concludes that at present there is not enough information in the literature to make a precise prognostication in patients presenting with CSM.

The diagnosis of cervical radiculopathy and CSM should be made clinically. Electrodiagnostic studies, including nerve conduction studies, F wave determination, H reflexes, and electromyography of paraspinal and upper extremity muscles, may help confirm the diagnosis and establish the amount of nerve compromise (26). Whereas CT and MRI studies are crucial, especially prior to surgical intervention, one should remember that there are false positive studies. With the help of an experienced radiologist, these studies, especially MRI, may help rule out other conditions that may clinically resemble cervical radiculopathy and myelopathy.

LUMBAR SPINE

Low back pain (LBP) is a common complaint observed in elderly patients. The pain may be caused by the same processes that are seen in younger patients, i.e., herniated discs or myofascial pain syndromes. In addition, degenerative processes, metabolic diseases, and especially malignant metastatic diseases and pyogenic vertebral osteomyelitis should always be considered in the diagnostic work-up. Features that should alert the clinician to the possibility of a serious disease are weight loss, fever, unremitting backache, night pain, anemia, and an elevated sedimentation rate. Patients presenting with the above features should be carefully examined. The clinician should include the abdomen and pelvis in the routine examination of the patient with back pain.

X-ray studies, CT scans, and MRI may be helpful in establishing the correct diagnosis. We should remember, however, that radiologic studies, especially in elderly patients, may demonstrate significant abnormal findings even in asymptomatic individuals. Since by age 50 years about 97% of all lumbar discs exhibit degeneration (27), caution should be exercised when interpreting radiologic studies and assessing their clinical relevance.

A study of lumbar spine MRI's in a group of 67 individuals who had never suffered from LBP or sciatica demonstrated abnormal false positive findings in 57% of the patients who were 60 years of age or older. Herniated discs, multiple degenerated discs, and spinal stenosis were commonly observed (28). Similar observations were made with CT studies. It may be concluded that abnormal radiologic studies in the younger population are more likely to be of clinical relevance. In elderly patients, however, the MRI findings may, in fact, reflect normal spine aging and may be causally unrelated to the back symptoms. In some cases, bone scans, blood tests, and, when indicated, bone biopsy, are necessary to substantiate the diagnosis.

Herniated discs, leading to significant morbidity, are much more common in the third and fourth decade than later in life. They may be, however, seen in the elderly patient. In the older age group, above 50 years, degeneration and herniation frequently occur at higher levels than those commonly seen in younger age groups. In these patients, the clinical picture may be misleading since the pain may present with atypical referral patterns.

It should be remembered, though, that spinal cord tumors may have a similar and sometimes identical clinical presentation to that of herniated discs (29, 30). Any patient who was diagnosed as suffering from herniated disc that does not respond to conservative measures or who has night backache and constitutional symptoms should be worked-up and other diagnostic entities should be considered.

SPINAL TUMORS

Although tumors of the spine are rare, they should be considered and diagnosed as early as possible. Metastatic cancer and multiple myeloma are the tumors most frequently encountered in the aged group. The patient with a herniated disc will complain of pain related to activity (worse while sitting, absent at night). The cancer patient may specifically complain of nocturnal backache. During the day, the pain may not be as severe. The nocturnal pain is caused by vascular engorgement of the tumor and increased intraosseous pressure.

Since about 50% of the bone substance has to be involved before the tumor may be detected in plain radiograms, bone scans, appropriate blood tests, and CT or MRI should be performed if the X-ray studies are negative. It should be remembered that lytic tumors such as multiple myeloma and hypernephroma do not light up the bone scan, may yield false negative studies, and remain undetected by bone scans.

Indeed up to 5% of bone scans yield false negative results. If a false negative scan is suspected, further prompt diagnostic work-up including MRI and blood tests is mandatory. Every effort should be made to detect spinal metastasis as early as possible.

Metastatic cancer is the most common malignancy, affecting the spine, particularly the thoracic and lumbar vertebrae. Five percent to 10% of cancer patients will develop neurologic complications secondary to metastatic spine disease (30).

Metastatic lesions are usually located in the vertebral bodies. The posterior elements, however, are not spared. Cancer of the lung, kidney, breast, prostate, thyroid, and gastrointestinal system tend to metastasize to the spine. These tumors commonly present with back pain, radicular pain, and weakness. In many cases, the spinal manifestations appear first, long before symptoms from the organs from which the cancer originated become manifest.

In most metastatic spine patients, the neurologic presentation is acute or subacute. There may be pain, followed shortly by sphincter paralysis or relentless, progressive paraparesis or paraplegia (30). Some patients develop acute paraplegia within the span of a few hours. In these patients, early diagnosis and aggressive management are crucial. Initially, the patient should receive a bolus of intravenous steroids (Decadron) to be followed by radiation therapy and/or surgical decompression. In order to determine the location and extent of metastatic spread, an emergency myelogram or an MRI, where available, should be obtained (31). Early aggressive approach may reverse the neurologic complications, improve the quality of life, and even prolong life by avoiding the dreaded complication of complete spinal cord damage. Delayed diagnosis and procrastination may result in irreversible neurologic catastrophy. Sixty percent to 95% of the patients who are ambulatory at the time of diagnosis will retain their functional level following therapy. Of the patients becoming paraplegic, however, only 30% will regain their ability to walk following therapeutic interventions (32).

The presence of night pain is not pathognomonic of spinal tumor since it may be seen in other entities. Paget's disease and bacterial vertebral osteomyelitis are commonly associated with night backache. Paget's disease, more commonly observed in males, occurs mostly in Caucasians. About one third of the patients afflicted with symptomatic Paget's disease complain of spine pain. In many patients, it will be difficult to differentiate between pain produced by plain osteoarthritic changes and that produced by the pagetic bone.

The clinical presentation of Paget's disease depends on its location. When the cervical and dorsal spine are affected, severe neurologic compromise, i.e., paraparesis or paraplegia may occur. Involvement of the lumbar spine may cause pain, straightening of the lumbar lordosis, facet syndrome, or frank radiculopathy via entrapment of lumbar roots. About 1% of patients with Paget's disease may develop sarcomatous changes (33).

PYOGENIC VERTEBRAL OSTEOMYELITIS

Pyogenic vertebral osteomyelits (PVO) should be considered in elderly patients presenting with LBP and fever. PVO may occur at all ages. It peaks in the elderly in the seventh decade (34). PVO may occur in immune compromised patients, diabetics, or alcoholics, following urinary tract infections, after instrumentation of the genitourinary tract, and in elderly patients who receive steroid therapy.

The infection commonly spreads into the lumbar spine. The elderly may present with back pain. Unlike mechanical or osteoarthritic pain, osteomyelitis leads to unremitting rest pain that increases with motion. The pain may be accompanied by fever. In many cases, blood analysis discloses a high sedimentation rate and frequently a high white blood count. The patient may have local tenderness and severe muscle spasm. Many patients, due to delay in diagnosis, present with progressive neurologic deterioration and even complete paralysis. In these cases, the infection spreads from the bone into the epidural space forming an epidural abscess and compromising the spinal cord.

X-ray films may help differentiate PVO from metastatic disease. In cancer, the radiologic findings are commonly limited to one vertebra and do not extend across the intervertebral disc. In PVO, the infection commonly extends through the disc to involve two adjacent vertebrae (34). The combination of back pain, local tenderness, fever and radiculopathy should trigger an immediate diagnostic and therapeutic response. Prompt early recognition and antibiotic therapy may present neurologic catastrophy and improve the quality of life.

SPINAL STENOSIS

Spinal stenosis (ST) is commonly seen in the elderly. ST causes significant morbidity and hampers the quality of life of the geriatric patient. Patients with ST may be seen first by their general practitioners, who may not be thoroughly familiar with this entity. Unfamiliarity leads to a delay in diagnosis and compromised quality of life.

The anatomy of the lumbar spine is briefly reviewed in Figure 13.2. The figure includes a lateral view and an axial view as may be seen in CT studies. With advancing years, as the discs degenerate, more stress is borne out by the posterior elements, especially the facets. With time, degenerative changes occur in the facets. They degenerate, develop osteophytes, and hypertrophy. The ligamenta flava, pedicles, and sometimes the laminae may also thicken in response to the added stress. These processes in turn lead to the gradual narrowing of the lateral recesses, encroachment of the roots in the intervertebral foraminae, and narrowing of the central spinal canal (Fig. 13.3). The above processes are seen as a normal part of aging, and, indeed, elderly individuals commonly have narrower canals than do younger ones. When degenerative changes occur in a preexisting narrow canal or when they narrow the sagittal diameter of a normal lumbar canal below 11 mm, the clinical picture of ST becomes manifest.

Initially, the patient may present with vague com-

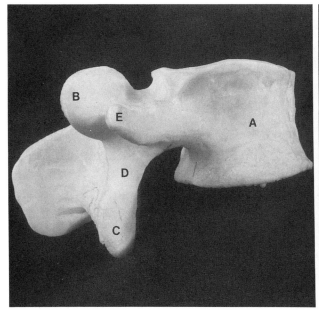

Figure 13.2A.   Lateral view of the fourth lumbar. A—vertebral body; B—superior articular facet; C—inferior articular facet; D—pars interarticularis; E—transverse process.

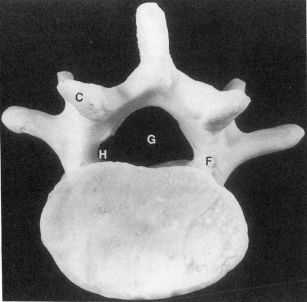

Figure 13.2B.   Axial view of some vertebra. Viewed from below. F—pedicle; G—central canal; H—lateral recess.

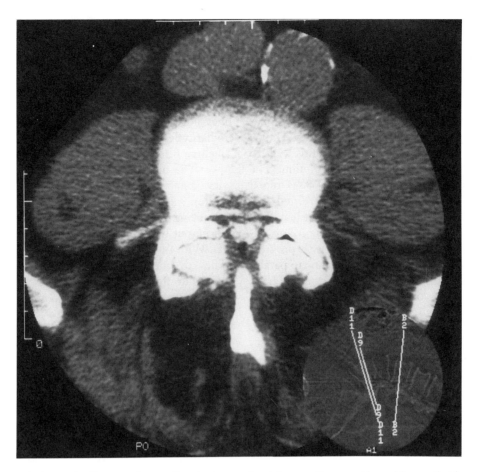

Figure 13.3. Severe spinal stenosis. The central, as well as the lateral, canal is narrowed. There is severe facet hypertrophy. There is facet degeneration as evidenced by gas that has accumulated in the right facet. There is severe narrowing of the lateral recess.

plaints. The physical examination may be completely normal. The patient, who had long-standing LBP, gradually develops symptoms related to the lower extremities. Leg cramps, intermittent claudication, or frank unilateral or bilateral sciatica may develop. The patient develops intermittent claudication in the form of tightness in the calves, tingling, paresthesias, dysesthesias, or outright pain. Stooping forward or sitting down usually relieves the symptoms.

The signs and symptoms of ST are worse in conditions that narrow the spinal canal or the intervertebral foraminae. During hyperextension, infolding of the ligamenta flava occurs, and there may be further protrusions of the discs. This leads to narrowing of the neural canal and relative closure of the foramina and thus increases the ST. This explains why the classical patient may note that it is easier to walk uphill (when the body stoops forward) as opposed to downhill (at which time the trunk tends to be hyperextended). Whereas patients with herniated discs prefer to stand rather than sit, patient with sciatica induced by spinal stenosis, are comfortable sitting (Table 13.1).

Neurogenic intermittent claudication and vascular claudication may clinically look alike. Indeed, in elderly

Table 13.1. Diagnostic Differences Between Herniated Disc and Spinal Stenosis

	Herniated Disc	Spinal Stenosis
Age	30–50 yr	>60 yr
Back pain	+	+
Sciatica	+	+
Symptoms	Usually unilateral	Frequently bilateral
Pain increases	Sitting	Walking, standing
Pain decreases	Standing, lying down	Sitting, stooping
Neurologic findings	Positive	Frequently negative
SLR[a]	Positive	Commonly negative
Natural history	Recovery in 90%	Persistent or worsening

[a] SLR = Straight leg raising test.

patients, the two conditions may coexist. It is important to examine the peripheral pulses or resort to more sophisticated studies in order to establish the role, if any, of the vasculature in symptom production.

The differences between these two conditions are summarized in Table 13.2. In many spinal stenosis patients, the physical examination may not be helpful since the patient may have a normal neurologic examination or display neurologic changes that are inconsistent. The patient may have weakness in one lower extremity that

Table 13.2.   Diagnostic Differences Between Neurogenic Claudication and Vascular Claudication

	Neurogenic Claudication	Vascular Claudication
Age	Elderly	Elderly
Back pain	+	−
Claudication	+	+
Weakness	±	−
Reflex changes	±	−
Sensory findings	±	−
SLR[a]	Usually −	−
Pain relief	Sitting, stooping	Standing
PVD[a]	−	+
Walking distance to claudication	Variable	Constant
Back X-ray studies	+	−

[a]SLR = Straight leg raising test; PVD = peripheral vascular disease.

disappears in the subsequent examination. The sensory changes may also seem inconsistent. Since in many elderly patients it is hard to obtain the knee jerks and, especially, the ankle jerks, their absence in the patient with ST may not be of diagnostic value. In many cases, the straight leg raising sign is negative even in the presence of clear leg pain-sciatica. It is, therefore, apparent that the diagnosis of spinal stenosis is based primarily on the case history. The physical examination is seldom contributory (35).

Radiologic studies, especially CT and MRI, help delineate the stenotic segment and directly demonstrate the offending structures (Fig. 13.3). Hypertrophied facets may encroach on the central and the lateral canal and produce stenosis. The ligamenta flava, especially at the level of the L-4 vertebra may become hypertrophied and thus render the canal stenotic. Stenosis affecting the lateral recess is not uncommon and, unlike central spinal stenosis, may lead, at times, to intense unrelenting leg pain. In the majority of these patients, the physical examination remains normal with a negative straight leg raising test. In some patients, inconsistent mild neurologic deficits may be found. The lateral recess is the area created by the superior articular facet posteriorly, the pedicle laterally, and the posterior boundary of the vertebral body anteriorly. As the superior articular process hypertophies, the lateral recess narrows and entrapment of the exiting root may occur. Stenosis of the lateral recess commonly affects the L-4 or the L-5 nerve roots. This area should be carefully evaluated in a patient referred for surgery, since decompression limited to the central canal will not relieve the symptoms caused by lateral entrapment.

Patients who do not respond to conservative measures should be referred for surgery. In these cases, decompression may be achieved through wide laminectomies and, when indicated, facetectomies. The conservative approach prior to surgery should include flexion exercises and a delordosing brace. This may be combined

with epidural steroid injections. Old age per se is not a contraindication for spinal stenosis surgery. On the contrary, many elderly patients, once they recover from the surgery, are expected to enjoy an improved quality of life (35). It should be explained to the patient that, although the back pain may not get better following surgery, the complaints related to the lower extremities, especially the intermittent claudication, may disappear.

Before surgery, cervical spine X-ray films should be obtained so that cervical spinal stenosis will not be overlooked. Cervical hyperextension during intubation may prove to be disastrous in a patient with cervical stenosis. In cases with tandem lesions, the cervical spine should be operated before the lumbar spine is approached.

Very commonly, one may see, especially in females, degenerative spondylolisthesis. Unlike spondylolytic spondylolisthesis, in which a break in the pars interarticularis may be demonstrated and is responsible for the slip, degenerative spondylolisthesis occurs with an intact pars. Degenerative spondylolisthesis usually occurs at the L4-5 level (spondylolytic spondylolisthesis usually occurs at L5-S1 level) and rarely progresses beyond grade one (36, 37). Staging the amount of slip can be determined on a lateral view of the lumbosacral spine. The clinician divides the upper border of the vertebra below the slip into four quarters. In grade one, the slipping vertebra progresses up to 25% of the anteroposterior diameter of the upper surface of the vertebra below, as viewed on the lateral radiogram (37). Degenerative spondylolisthesis can lead to backache, buttock, and thigh pain. The pain may be intermittent and long periods of remission are common. In cases with persistent severe pain, surgical intervention may be considered (38).

In some patients, degenerative spondylolisthesis accompanied by segmental instability may lead to lateral stenosis, affect the roots, and thus lead to symptom production.

FACET SYNDROME

The facet syndrome, still a controversial entity, may be commonly seen in elderly patients. The facet joints are true synovial joints. They are innervated by the medial branch of the posterior primary ramus. Their function in the normal spine is to control the plane of mobility, limit the rotation of the spine, and participate in weight bearing.

Under normal physiologic conditions, the facets transmit about 20% of the axial weight (39). In the aging spine, due to increasing degeneration of the intervertebral discs, more weight is borne by the facets, and they are exposed to abnormal motions and stress. The articular processes respond by developing osteoarthritic spurs; their covering cartilage degenerates, and they may become the source of pain. Occasionally, we encounter patients with radiologically proven facets arthritis in the presence of normal-looking intervertebral discs.

Hypertonic saline injections into the facet joints or in the vicinity of the facets has been shown to cause LBP that may radiate down to the buttocks (40). The facet syndrome should be included in the differential diagnosis of an elderly patient with backache and unilateral sciatica. Patients with facet syndrome frequently complain of pain located at the low back and radiating down to the buttock or thigh. The pain never crosses the midline. The patient may notice tenderness in the back, in the area overlying the facet. Muscle spasm may develop. The pain increases specifically by hyperextension of the spine.

In some patients, hamstring spasm may develop. In these patients, the straight leg raising test may be limited. In most patients with the facet syndrome, the straight leg raising test remains negative.

The diagnosis of the facet syndrome should be made after other causes for back pain have been ruled out. Fluoroscopically guided facet injections may be tried. Since each facet is innervated by posterior primary rami from adjacent spinal nerves, blocking of three facets—the involved one and the adjacent two—should be performed. If the patient does not get relief, other causes of back pain should be considered.

MANAGEMENT

Management of the elderly patient with back pain and sciatica should follow the same principles utilized in younger age groups (35). Caution should be exercised whenever nonsteroidal antiinflammatory medications are prescribed. Since these medications can affect renal function, their use in an elderly patient with compromised kidney function should be limited. Since geriatric patients commonly use a multitude of medications, the clinician who prescribes nonsteroidal antiinflammatory medications, antidepressants, and muscle relaxants should be aware of possible drug interactions between these medications and those that the patient is taking regularly for other medical conditions. One should prescribe bedrest sparingly in the elderly. It has been shown that during recumbency about 1% of the lumbar spine mineral content may be lost in one week! (41). The frail deconditioned elderly may further functionally deteriorate following an unjustified period of immobilization.

The elderly patient should be encouraged to remain as active as his physical condition permits. He or she should be advised that even mundane activities such as walking and stair climbing are beneficial.

Gradual general conditioning exercises should be prescribed, and the patient should be encouraged to stop smoking and reduce alcohol intake.

Decreased spinal motion is commonly observed in the elderly. It results from progressive osteoarthritic changes and spur formation. This should be regarded as a normal aspect of spine aging, which, in some cases, may be responsible for disappearance of symptoms that disturbed the patient for many years. In these patients, the physiatrist should not aspire to normalize the spinal range of motion. The objectives, rather, should be the toning of the abdominal and back musculature and attaining a higher level of conditioning.

The osteoporotic patient, especially in the presence of compression fractures, should perform extension exercises and refrain from flexion exercises. Osteoporotic patients should be evaluated by dual photon absorptiometry, and every effort should be made to keep their bone density above the fracture threshold. Adequate calcium and vitamin D intake combined with weight-bearing exercises and maintenance of high activity levels are recommended. In some patients, estrogen replacement should be prescribed. For the elderly woman who has already lost height due to compression fractures and presents with acute pain due to a fresh fracture support via a thoracolumbar hyperextension brace may be advocated.

The exercises of choice for the spinal stenosis patient are flexion exercises. These may be combined with a delordosating brace. Spinal stenosis patients who do not obtain pain relief, even in the absence of markedly abnormal neurologic findings, can be referred for surgical decompression. In these patients, the role played by peripheral vascular disease in symptom production should be established prior to spinal surgery.

Various physical modalities should be used concomitantly with exercises. Heat, cold, massage, and transcutaneous electrical stimulation may help alleviate the pain. I would not recommend the routine use of spinal manipulations in the elderly and would refrain from cervical manipulations in these individuals. The presence of atherosclerosis, metabolic bone disease, and, at times, undetected metastatic disease, substantially increases the risk of manipulations and may, occasionally, lead to neurologic catastrophies.

References

1. Teresi LM, Lufkin RB, Reicher MA, et al. Asymptomatic degenerative disk disease spondylosis of the cervical spine: MR imaging. *Radiology.* 164:83–88, 1987.
2. Kelsey JL, Githens PB, Walter SD, et al. An epidemiologic study of acute prolapsed cervical intervertebral disc. *J Bone Joint Surg.* 66A:907–914, 1984.
3. Holt S, Yates PO. Cervical spondylosis and nerve root lesions. *J Bone Joint Surg.* 48B:407–423, 1966.
4. Kurz LT. The differential diagnosis of cervical radiculopathy. *Semin Spine Surg.* 1:194–199, 1989.
5. Brain WR, Northfield D, Wilkinson M. The neurological manifestation of cervical spondylosis. *Brain.* 75:187–225, 1952.
6. Hunt WE. Cervical spondylosis: natural history and rare indications for surgical decompressions. *Clin Neurosurg.* 27:466–480, 1979.
7. Epstein JA, Epstein BS, Lavine LS, Carras R, Rosenthal AD.

Cervical myeloradiculopathy caused by arthritic hypertrophy of the posterior facets and lamina. *J Neurosurg.* 49:387–392, 1978.

8. Teng P. Spondylosis of the cervical spine with compression of the spinal cord and nerve roots. *J Bone Joint Surg.* 42A:392–407, 1960.

9. Lestini WF, Wiesel SW. The pathogenesis of cervical spondylosis. *Clin Orthop.* 239:69–93, 1989.

10. Gregorius FK, Estrin T, Crandall PH. Cervical spondylotic radiculopathy and myelopathy. A long term follow-up study. *Arch Neurol.* 33:618–625, 1976.

11. White AA. Symposium on cervical spondylotic myelopathy. *Spine.* 13:829–830, 1988.

12. Parke WW. Correlative anatomy of cervical spondylotic myelopathy. *Spine.* 13:831–837, 1988.

13. Gooding MR. Pathogenesis of myelopathy in cervical spondylosis. *Lancet.* 2:1180–1181, 1974.

14. Clark CR. Cervical spondylotic myelopathy: history and physical findings. *Spine.* 13:847–849, 1988.

15. Gamache FW, Voorhies RM. Hypertrophic cervical osteophytes causing dysphagia. A review. *J. Neurosurg.* 53:338–344, 1980.

16. Utsinger PD. Diffuse idiopathic skeletal hyperostosis. *Clin Rheum Dis.* 11:325–351, 1985.

17. Yu YL, Leong JCY, Fang D, Woo E, Huang CY, Lau HK. Cervical myelopathy due to ossification of the posterior longitudinal ligament. A clinical radiological and evoked potentials study in six Chinese patients. *Brain.* 111:769–783, 1988.

18. LaRocca H. Cervical spondylotic myelopathy: natural history. *Spine.* 13:854–855, 1988.

19. Stauffer ES. Diagnosis and prognosis of acute cervical spinal cord injury. *Clin Orthop.* 112:9–15, 1975.

20. Bosch A, Stauffer ES, Nickel VL. Incomplete traumatic quadriplegia. A ten year review. *JAMA.* 216:473–478, 1971.

21. Merriam WF, Taylor TKF, Ruff SJ, McPhail MJ. A reappraisal of acute traumatic central cord syndrome. *J Bone Joint Surg.* 68:708–713, 1986.

22. Epstein NE, Epstein JA, Carras R. Cervical spondylosis, stenosis and myeloradiculopathy in patients over 65: diagnostic techniques and management. *Neurol Orthop.* 6:13–23, 1988.

23. DePalma AF, Rothman RH, Levitt R, Hammond NL. The natural history of severe cervical disc degeneration. *Acta Orthop Scand.* 43:392–396, 1972.

24. Lees F, Aldren Turner JW. Natural history and prognosis of cervical spondylosis. *Br Med J.* 2:1607–1610, 1963.

25. Clark E, Robinson PK. Cervical myelopathy. A complication of cervical spondylosis. *Brain.* 79:483–510, 1956.

26. LaBan MM. Electrodiagnosis in cervical radicular and myelopathic syndromes. *Semin Spine Surg* 1:222–228, 1989.

27. Miller JAA, Schmartz C, Schultz AB. Lumbar disc degeneration: correlation with age, sex, and spine level in 600 autopsy specimens. *Spine.* 13:173–178, 1988.

28. Boden SD, Davis DO, Dina TS, Patronas NJ, Wiesel SW. Abnormal magnetic-resonance scan of the lumbar spine in asymptomatic subjects. *J Bone Joint Surg.* 72A:403–408, 1990.

29. Sim FH, Dahlin DC, Stauffer RN, Laws ER Jr. Primary bone tumors simulating lumbar disc syndrome. *Spine.* 2:65–79, 1977.

30. Constans JD, Divitiis ED, Donzelli R, Spaziante R, Meder JF, Haye C. Spinal metastases with neurological manifestation. Review of 600 cases. *J Neurosurg.* 59:111–118, 1983.

31. Portenoy RK, Lipton RB, Foley KM. Back pain in the cancer patient: an algorithm for evaluation and management. *Neurology.* 37:134–138, 1987.

32. McLain, RF, Weinstein JN. Tumors of the spine. *Semin Spine Surg.* 2:157–180, 1990.

33. Altman RD. The spine in Paget's disease of bone. *Semin Spine Surg.* 2:130–135, 1990.

34. Schwartz ST, Spiegel M, Ho G Jr. Bacterial vertebral osteomyelitis and epidural abcess. *Semin Spine Surg.* 2:95–105, 1990.

35. Fast A. Low back disorders: conservative management. *Arch Phys Med Rehabil.* 69:880–891, 1988.

36. Rosenberg NJ. Degenerative spondylolisthesis. Predisposing factors. *J Bone Joint Surg.* 57A:467–474, 1975.

37. Meyerding HW. Spondylolisthesis. *Surg Gynec Obstet.* 54:371–377, 1932.

38. Fast A, Robin GC, Floman Y. Surgical treatment of lumbar spinal stenosis in the elderly. *Arch Phys Med Rehabil.* 66:149–151, 1985.

39. Lippitt AB. The facet joint and its role in spine pain. Management with facet joint injection. *Spine.* 9:746–750, 1984.

40. Hirsch D, Ingelmark B, Miller M. The anatomical basis for low back pain. *Acta Orthop Scand.* 33:1–17, 1963.

41. Krølner B, Toft B. Vertebral bone loss: an unheeded side effect of therapeutic bed rest. *Clin Sci.* 64:537–540, 1983.

14

Management of Foot Disorders in the Elderly

Alberto Esquenazi and Elaine Thompson

The foot is one of the least appreciated and most overworked anatomic structures in the body. Feet are constantly abused by individuals walking and standing on hard surfaces and wearing ill-fitting shoes. Most individuals will suffer some form of foot or ankle pain during their life span. The ankle-foot complex provides a base of support as well as a springboard for locomotion. It can be likened to a trampoline, demonstrating a mechanism by which shock is absorbed during weight acceptance and a propulsive force is generated for mobility. The geriatric ankle-foot can be visualized as a "fatigued trampoline," which has decreased shock absorption and spring abilities as the result of disorders associated with bony disfigurement, joint pathology, muscle imbalances, and skin and toenail pathology.

The aging process, in association with other systemic conditions such as diabetes and atherosclerosis, can leave the foot insensitive, predisposed to ulceration, and with decreased healing capabilities. This can be further complicated by vision, cognition, and memory deficits.

This chapter will provide the reader with an understanding of the biomechanical causes for underlying pathology in the geriatric foot, identification of commonly seen musculoskeletal dysfunctions and neurologic abnormalities, and a discussion of preventative care and therapeutic treatment strategies for the conservative management of geriatric foot disorders.

NORMAL LOCOMOTION

It is important from the clinical standpoint to understand the events of the walking cycle so that foot disorders can be correlated to cause the effect during gait. Some basic terminology is needed to identify the components and events of the gait cycle. From the perspective of a single limb, the gait cycle has two basic components: stance phase, during which the limb is in contact with the ground, and swing phase, during which the limb is off the ground. The stance phase can be

subdivided into the following event and functional subphases: (a) initial contact, (b) loading response, (c) midstance, (d) terminal stance, and (e) preswing. The swing phase can be subdivided into the following functional subphases: (a) initial swing, (b) midswing, and (c) terminal swing (1–3).

A stride is one complete gait cycle. The stride period can be defined as the time from initial contact of one foot until the next initial contact of the same foot. The stride period becomes useful for data normalization for the purpose of comparing subjects with different stride periods. It is also useful to temporally normalize to this interval for the purpose of averaging successful strides within a subject. The stride period (100%) is the sum of the stance period (60% to 65%) and the swing period (35% to 40%). The stance-to-swing ratio has been calculated in normal subjects in their fourth decade of life, walking at their comfortable speed, and it will vary with changes in walking velocity. The stride length is equal to the left step length plus the right step length and should be equal for left and right strides. The stride can also be analyzed according to whether one or both feet are in contact with the floor. Double support is the period of time during which both feet are in contact with the ground. With increasing cadence, the double support period steadily decreases until it disappears during running. Single support is the period when only one foot is in touch with the ground and is exactly equal to the swing period of the contralateral limb (Fig. 14.1).

The step period is the time measured from an event in one foot to the subsequent occurrence of the same event in the contralateral foot. The step period is useful for measuring asymmetry between left and right sides. Step length is the distance covered in the direction of progression during one step. The cadence is the number of steps per minute. Gait velocity is the average horizontal speed of the body along the plane of progression, commonly reported in meters per second. In the geriatric population, a decrease in the walking velocity and

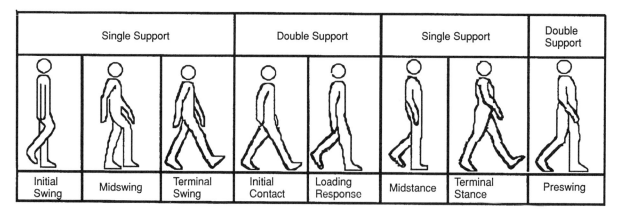

Single Support			Double Support		Single Support		Double Support
Initial Swing	Midswing	Terminal Swing	Initial Contact	Loading Response	Midstance	Terminal Stance	Preswing

Figure 14.1. Normal gait cycle.

step length and widening of the base of support are common findings.

FOOT-ANKLE ANATOMY AND BIOMECHANICS

The human foot is a rather unique and complex anatomic structure that, with its sagittal and transverse motions, provides impact absorption during stance phase, permits a stable weight-bearing base of support, and generates dynamic propulsion essential for normal locomotion. Anatomically, the foot is divided into the hindfoot, consisting of the talus and the calcaneus; the midfoot, comprising the navicula, cuneiform, and cuboid; and the forefoot, which includes the metatarsals and phalanges.

The biomechanics of the foot cannot be looked upon as an isolated entity, but only as an integral part of the biomechanics of the entire lower limb. The main function of the human gait is to achieve safe and efficient forward locomotion through a series of finely coordinated cyclical motions. A thorough understanding of the biomechanics of the ankle-foot is essential in the management of lower limb problems. Although it is frequently taken for granted, we need only to observe an individual with a gait abnormality that is the result of a foot dysfunction to realize how critical this weight-bearing structure is to locomotion. Disruption of the normal biomechanics of the lower limb may alter the gait pattern and contribute to increased energy expenditure (2, 4).

During locomotion, the ankle-foot complex needs to function both as a stable base of support and as a dynamic lever. The combination of the ankle, the subtalar, and the midtarsal joints affords the necessary control of the foot for both stability and mobility functions. The axes of motion at the ankle and subtalar joints are often described as "triplanar" in that there is not one conventionally described plane, i.e., sagittal, frontal, or transverse, that describes the joint axes position. Motion occurring at each joint can be referred to as composite.

Supination is the composite motion consisting of plantar-flexion, inversion, and adduction components. Pronation is the composite motion consisting of dorsiflexion, eversion, and abduction components.

The ankle joint axis passes approximately through the lateral and medial malleoli. This causes the joint axis to have an orientation from superior anteromedial to inferior posterolateral. The ankle joint during composite motion displays a greater degree of dorsiflexion and plantar-flexion than other component movements.

The talus is referred to as the keystone of the ankle complex as it is the common component of both the true ankle joint and the subtalar joint. The subtalar joint axis is oriented from a superior, anteromedial position to an inferior, posterolateral position. The axis position resembles most closely a sagittal axis, causing inversion and eversion to be the largest components of movement. During subtalar joint pronation, the talus drops down, causing the ankle joint to dorsiflex and the tibia to rotate medially. The pronated position of the subtalar joint also creates a more mobile forefoot due to bony configuration, ligamentous structures, and its relation to the two axes of the midtarsal joint. During subtalar joint supination, the talus moves up and out causing the ankle joint to plantarflex and the tibia to rotate laterally. Subtalar joint supination causes a rigid forefoot due to its relationship with the midtarsal joints.

The midtarsal joint (transtarsal) is comprised of two separate joints: the talo-calcaneo-navicular and the calcaneo-cuboid, each with a separate joint axis. The oblique and longitudinal axes of the midtarsal joint become parallel during subtalar joint pronation. This "unlocks" the forefoot, allowing a more pliant, flexible structure. Supination of the subtalar joint disassociates the oblique and longitudinal axes, which in turn "locks" the forefoot and provides for a rigid forefoot (5).

The action of the subtalar joint is critical during gait if the foot is to function properly. During the loading response, the subtalar joint is pronated so that the pliant foot is able to absorb the shock of increasing vertical forces. As the stance phase progresses, the subtalar joint supinates in preparation for preswing, creating a rigid lever for the purpose of propelling the body weight forward onto the contralateral limb.

The lesser four toes, with three phalanges, have both proximal interphalangeal joints (PIP) and distal interphalangeal joints (DIP). Prime movements of the interphalangeal joints (IP) are flexion and extension, with accessory movements consisting of gliding and rotating. As the hallux has only two phalanges, only one IP is formed.

The shape of the 26 bones to the foot, in combination with ligaments, muscles, and the plantar aponeurosis, forms three arches in the foot: the medial longitudinal arch located between the calcaneus and the first, second, and third metatarsal heads; the lateral longitudinal arch located between the calcaneus and the fourth and fifth metatarsal heads, and a transverse arch located posterior to the metatarsal heads. The arch support system is critical to the body's weight distribution during stance and locomotion and also serves as a tunnel of protection for tendons, nerves, and vessels located on the plantar surface of the foot.

The plantar aponeurosis is a thick band of fascia that originates from the calcaneus and blends with the skin, flexor tendon sheaths, and transverse metatarsal ligaments. During metatarsophalangeal extension and weight bearing, the plantar aponeurosis in combination with the long and short plantar ligaments and the plantar calcaneo-navicular ligament tightens preventing collapse of the longitudinal arch structure of the foot. The tarsometatarsal joints consist of articulations between the first metatarsal and medial cuneiform, the second metatarsal and all three cuneiforms, the third metatarsal and the lateral cuneiform and cuboid, and the fourth and fifth metatarsals with the cuboid. Gliding is the primary motion occurring at these joints. The metatarsal phalangeal joints permit flexion, extension, abduction, adduction, and slight rotation.

Muscular activity of the foot can be classified as either intrinsic or extrinsic. The deeply located intrinsic foot musculature both originates from and inserts in the foot. Extrinsic musculature originates proximal to the ankle and inserts in the foot. The muscles of the ankle and foot are innervated by spinal root levels L-4 through S-3 (6). The tibial and common peroneal nerve, originating from the sciatic nerve, supply innervation to the structures of the ankle-foot complex. The posterior calf muscles as well as the intrinsic foot musculature are innervated by the tibial nerve. The tibial nerve gives rise to the sensory sural nerve, innervating the lateral margin of the heel and a triangular area on the outer side of the foot. Other cutaneous branches of the tibial nerve supply the back and medial area of the heel, the plantar surface of the foot and toes, and the dorsal surface of the distal phalanges. The common peroneal nerve supplies lateral and anterior muscles of the ankle-foot complex and the dorsal muscles of the foot. The superficial peroneal nerve, a branch of the common peroneal nerve, supplies cutaneous innervation to the dorsum of the foot and proximal phalanges and a portion of the anterior surface of the leg. The lateral sural cutaneous nerve, a branch of the common peroneal, combines with the sural nerve and superficial peroneal nerve to innervate the lateral sides of the distal leg and feet and the border of the heel (7).

The blood supply to the foot and ankle complex is comprised of the anterior and posterior tibial arteries. Anterior medial and lateral malleolar branches of the anterior tibial artery disperse to the deeper structures of the anterior compartment. The dorsalis pedis artery, the distal continuation of the anterior tibial artery, branches to form the tarsal branch, the arcuate artery, and the metatarsal arteries, which supply the anterior foot and toes. The plantar arterial system comprises the medial and lateral plantar artery and is formed by the terminal branches of the posterior tibial artery.

CHARACTERISTICS OF THE GERIATRIC FOOT

The geriatric patient who has had long-standing pathologic foot biomechanics may demonstrate abnormally adapted or misshapen bones of the leg and foot in response to abnormal wear patterns. The effects of physiologic aging, often combined with a decrease in activity, lead to increased incidence of foot disorders. The skin is among the first structures to demonstrate changes with hair loss of the dorsum of the foot. The nails have a tendency to become thickened and brittle.

It has been demonstrated that both the number and size of muscle fibers decrease with age. MacLennan et al (8) have suggested that the decrease in strength is associated with an increasing proportion of skeletal muscle being replaced by fibrous tissue. The decrease in strength accompanied by the effects of static and dynamic loading, mostly on hard surfaces and with inadequate footwear throughout the years, causes the foot to have changes in morphology and, with this, changes in physiology. The foot tends to widen as the transverse arch support weakens. Abnormal bony configurations, such as hallux valgus and hammer toes, are common (9). In addition, chronic microtrauma may result in injury to the skin and acute or chronic inflammatory changes in osseous and soft tissues.

With increasing age, tensile stiffness and fracture strength decrease. It has been documented that 30% of women over 65 years of age have osteoporosis, leading to predisposition to fracture occurrence (8). Impaired proprioception may lead to trips or falls, resulting in possible ankle sprains or ankle and foot fractures. The geriatric patient with decreased light touch, pressure, pain, or temperature sensation may have increased susceptibility to soft tissue injury, infection, and gangrene, further complicated by decreased vascularization.

SKELETAL DISORDERS

Changes in the bone structure and joint surfaces can lead to faulty biomechanics of the ankle-foot complex, with deterioration of the longitudinal and transverse arches and skeletal abnormalities. Excessive pronation in the subtalar joints has been associated with a decrease in longitudinal arch support. As the forefoot "unlocks," it is less able to maintain stability during loading and causes increased pressure on the second and first metatarsal heads. The weakening of the plantar aponeurosis and foot ligaments further lessens the protection of the longitudinal arch. Excessive pronation occurs due to long-standing pathomechanics, such as excessive calcaneal varus, forefoot varus, tibial valgus, knee flexion contractures, and femoral anteversion. Poor muscle tone and obesity may increase the degree of abnormal ankle-foot pronation as well.

Transverse arch destruction has also been associated with excessive pronation. As undue stress is applied to the metatarsal heads, metatarsalgia, a burning in the ball of the foot associated with a decrease in plantar fat pad and thickening of callous, is likely. Patients with rigid pes cavus deformities of the foot or with arthritis resulting in increased weight born on the forefoot may also demonstrate metatarsalgia. It has been shown that patients with metatarsalgia have a slower than normal gait with increased lateral trunk sway and abnormally greater hip, knee, and ankle flexion (9). Increased pressure on the metatarsal heads and forefoot can lead to compression of the digital nerves, usually in the third intermetatarsal space, known as plantar (or Morton's) neuroma. Plantar neuromas and metatarsalgia are found commonly in women who have worn narrow-toed high-heeled shoes for a continued period (9).

Hallux valgus, perhaps the most common foot anomaly, is comprised of three skeletal abnormalities: lateral angulation and medial rotation of the large toe, bony enlargement of the medial side of the head of the first metatarsal bone at the metatarsophalangeal joint, and formation of a bursal sac over the point of the bony enlargement (9). Also associated with hallux valgus formation is a first metatarsal bone that is congenitally short or deviated medially. Hereditary patterns seem to exist, and the condition is often bilateral. Formation of bunions is associated primarily with middle-aged women. Some authors document that the use of pointed or ill-fitting shoes contributes to hallux valgus conditions (9). Hammer toes, the contracted position of metatarsophalangeal joint extension, combined with PIP flexion and DIP extension, has been associated with hallux valgus deformities. The hammer toe often is aggravated by muscle imbalance and encouraged by those who wear slippers. Painful dorsal keratoses are often present.

Correction of faulty biomechanics of the ankle-foot complex should begin as early as possible in the child or adult to prevent or lessen disabling foot problems commonly seen in the geriatric population.

Care must be taken in treating the geriatric patient who demonstrates abnormal pronation. Orthotic usage as prescribed for younger patients may be too rigid for the limited adaptive capabilities of this population, causing increased stress on other joint structures. The clinician must be trained in performing complete biomechanical examinations to identify areas of skeletal abnormalities that may be fixed or rigid and hence noncompliant to corrective orthotic management. The use of functional orthoses may be limited to the application of semirigid, as opposed to rigid, orthoses with little or no posting. Accommodative foot orthoses are fabricated out of soft materials and designed to control the foot posture only, not to correct it. These orthoses may prove beneficial if inflammation is caused by repetitive trauma during ambulation (10). The use of patellar-tendon-bearing orthoses to unload the ankle-foot complex may be helpful in the most severe cases.

Although several foot deformities have been associated with high-heeled, narrow-toed shoes in women, precaution must be taken prior to recommending that the geriatric patient with excessive pronation wear low-heeled shoes. By decreasing heel height, increase in pronation will occur as part of the normal biomechanics of the ankle-foot complex and further increase in pronation will be present as a result of a tight heel cord. Increase in pain and decrease in balance will be seen in these cases. Optimal toe box width and height should continue to be encouraged, with only minimal decrease in the normally worn heel height.

Additional conservative management should include range of motion, strengthening, and conditioning exercises, with emphasis throughout the lower limbs. Optimizing body weight, improving posture during standing and locomotion, and encouraging joint conservation should be additional goals.

ARTHRITIS OF THE FOOT

Various arthritides may affect the numerous small joints of the foot. Clinical presentation, radiographic findings, and pathomechanics are useful in accurately diagnosing the problem. Clinicians need to remember that arthritic problems may present as food symptomatology, but the disease is systemic. Treatment should be directed not only to the foot but also to possible systemic involvement.

Degenerative Joint Disease

Degenerative joint disease is commonly diagnosed in the elderly and middle-aged individual. History of trauma or osteochondritis is prevalent. Although all joints in the foot can be affected, the first metatarsophalangeal joint and first metatarsocuneiform joint are most commonly involved. The same degenerative process that affects the hop and knee is present in the foot and consists of biochemical changes of the articular cartilage and bony proliferation with joint distortion and destruction. Symptoms include pain and stiffness that are more severe in the morning and after prolonged standing or walking. The involved joint(s) may be warm, painful, and have evidence of joint effusion. Compensatory alterations in the gait pattern may produce pain in other areas of the foot, lower limb, and back. Radiographic changes include joint space narrowing, osteophytes and sclerotic joint margins. As the disease progresses, obliteration of the joint may also be observed (11). The common pedal manifestations are plantar fasciitis, spur formation, periostitis, tendonitis, and tenosynovitis. Conservative management includes rest, physical modalities, nonsteriodal antiinflammatory drugs (NSAIDs), strengthening exercises, appropriate footwear, and the possible use of a cane or other appropriate assistive devices. Orthotic management to accommodate foot deformities, immobilize specific joints, and redistribute forces may be used. Shoe modifications to complement the orthotic management are helpful. Local steroid injections should be used judiciously. Severe cases that do not respond to conservative management may be treated surgically.

Rheumatoid Arthritis

Rheumatoid arthritis produces foot pain in the same manner that it affects other joints in the body. The inflammatory synovial process is usually symmetric and most commonly affects the metatarsophalangeal and PIP joints. Symptoms may include pain, warmth, and swelling around the affected joints. Pain is increased by weight bearing or with motion. Hallux valgus deformity occurs in the majority of patients (11). Calluses form over deformed joints with areas of increased pressure. Achilles and posterior tibial tendonitis and plantar fasciitis are common.

Treatment is directed to decreasing pain and inflammation, preventing deformities, and restoring function. Aspirin and NSAIDs should be used as first-line medications. The use of remissive agents and systemic steroids should be reserved for the treatment of severe cases. Local steroid injections are useful. Properly fitting footwear and shoe inserts that are light and have modifications to redistribute weight, increase support, and control motion are most important. Orthoses and modified shoes may be required when deformities are severe. Rigid foot othoses should be avoided as they are not well tolerated by the rheumatoid patient. Canes and other assistive devices should be used to maintain level of function.

Seronegative Arthridities

The seronegative arthridities are Reiter's syndrome, ankylosing spondilitis, and psoriatic arthritis. Two additional types of arthritis that may affect the foot-ankle are gout and systemic lupus erythematosis. While their pathophysiology is different from that of osteoarthritis and rheumatoid arthritis, the clinical manifestations of the ankle and foot are similar and, as such, intervention should be done accordingly.

THE INSENSATE FOOT

In the United States, the overall cost of treatment of diabetic foot lesions, gangrene, and amputation are over $200,000,000 every year, excluding rehabilitation and time lost from work. The causes of tissue destruction include pressure over prolonged time, high mechanical pressure, repetitive stress, and thermal and chemical trauma (12, 13).

Ulceration of the foot is commonly the result of a combination of neuropathic changes, infection, and vascular compromise. The insensate foot can become deformed because of muscle weakness and atrophy secondary to motor nerve involvement, or toe clawing, and depression of the metatarsal heads can occur leading to fat pad atrophy with abnormal weight distribution and the development of Charcot's joint.

Autonomic nervous system dysfunction results in decreased sweating, producing "dry foot." The skin becomes cracked, scaly, fissured, and inflamed. Over time, the foot can develop an open wound that may be complicated by cellulitis, osteomyelitis, and eventually tissue destruction, possibly resulting in lower limb amputation. For treatment purposes, the insensate foot can be categorized into three general groups: (a) insensate food without ulceration, (b) insensate foot with ulceration, and (c) insensate foot with healed ulceration.

The insensate foot without ulceration requires daily foot care, including skin lubrication with an emollient, skin inspection, and observation of areas of pressure, i.e., redness, calluses. Toenails should be trimmed every 6 weeks, preferably by a professional. Proper footwear with modifications and molded semirigid orthoses for pressure redistribution should be used. Footwear should be changed frequently to avoid moisture concentration.

The insensate foot with ulceration should be treated with appropriate antibiotic coverage followed by wound débridement and care to maintain a clean and healthy ulcerative base to permit gradual healing. Lower limb elevation to control edema should be encouraged. Application of Unna boot or, preferably, a plaster of Paris total contact cast to redistribute weight bearing over the foot surface, protect against trauma, and further control edema is indicated (14–16). The cast should be changed every 1 to 2 weeks, with wound care administered at the time of cast changes. The patient should be instructed to walk with short steps in an attempt to decrease shearing forces and may benefit from the use of a cane or walker. In our experience, 30 days is the average healing time for ulcers following this treatment protocol.

The insensate foot with healed ulceration requires modifications in the weight-bearing characteristics of the foot through the use of modified shoes and orthoses that have a shear reducing liner. Ambulation should be limited in distance and with short steps. Lubrication and close monitoring of skin should be emphasized. The use of a cane or walker should be recommended to the patient when appropriate (12).

SKIN AND TOENAIL PROBLEMS

Skin Problems

One of the most common skin problems in the elderly population is dryness or xerosis. The problem is the result of a lack of hydration and lubrication accompanied by keratin dysfunction. Pruritus and heel fissures may result. The use of emollient is the recommended treatment intervention. Chronic pruritus requires differentiation from tina pedis infection or other dermatitis (17). Areas of increased stress on the foot are often clinically detectable by examining the changes in skin on the plantar and dorsal surfaces of the foot. Corns are localized, painful, hard thickening of the skin in response to continous abnormal pressure. Two types of corns can be identified: (a) hard corns, which are circumscribed, superficial lesions approximately 1 cm to 3 cm in diameter with a firm seedlike core; and (b) soft corns, which are often found on the lateral aspect of the third or fourth proximal phalanx of the toe and are soft, thick, raised calluses with either a hard core or ulcerated center (18). Calluses are a softer thickening of the skin located on the plantar surface of the foot. Pressure relief combined with the use of arch supports, orthoses, or padding may be appropriate in an attempt to decrease areas of high pressure. Medical or podiatric treatment for excessive and painful calluses and corns may include surgical excision. In cases where skin breakdown occurs, early intervention including local wound care and the use of antibiotics is important. In patients with a history of diabetes or arterial insufficiency, early use of systemic antibiotics is imperative.

Nail Problems

The most common nail problem in the elderly is onychogryposis or abnormal toenail growth (18). To a lesser extent, ingrown toenails and onychomycosis may be present. Where decreased arterial supply is present, toenail abnormalities may warrant special attention to avoid the risk of wound or skin infection. Any foot infection in an elderly patient, particularly those with arterial insufficiency and/or diabetes mellitus, carries the potential for gangrene and amputation and calls for prompt, vigorous treatment.

Proper hygiene, appropriate footwear, and adequate nutrition play a role in preventing problems associated with the skin and toenails. Due to decreased visual and sensory acuity, the geriatric patient should be encouraged to seek podiatric management for routine toenail cutting and skin care.

FOOTWEAR AND FOOT-ORTHOSES

The shoe was developed as simple protection against rough, uneven ground. The first records of footwear go back 4000 years to the Egyptians, who wore papyrus sandals; later shoes were made with leather. The high heel was introduced by Catherine de Medici as a compensation for her short stature.

To a large extent, shoe styling today is considered more important than proper fit and comfort (19). Incorrectly designed or ill-fitted footwear is the most common cause of pain and foot dysfunction. Additional factors affecting proper shoe fit include insufficient room to insert prescribed modifications and shoe collapse during weight bearing. Unless the foot is healthy and shod appropriately, pain and disability can occur. The shape, fit, and comfort of the shoe are determined by the last over which the shoe is manufactured. (The last is the wood or metal mold upon which the shoe is constructed.) Lasts vary to accommodate different shapes of the same sized feet. It is difficult to believe that there is no national standard of sizes for shoes; sizes vary from manufacturer to manufacturer and from one set of lasts to another. Some generally accepted norms in the United States and England include length increases by one third of an inch per size and width increases by one twelfth of an inch at the sole and one fourth of an inch at the upper. When fitting the painful or deformed foot, softness of materials to reduce shear and friction and the use of molded inserts to distribute pressure throughout the plantar surface are prime requirements.

Extra Depth shoes allow removal of a ¼ to ⅜ inch insole, significantly increasing the available space for deformed toes or the application of foot orthoses. For proper fit, the clinician must determine if the shoe is the appropriate size for the individual foot. The patient should be in the standing position, with the closure system applied. The length of the shoe should exceed the longest toe by at least one half inch. To determine appropriate shoe width, one quarter inch should be gathered when pinching the shoe vamp distal to the closure system. During walking, no gap or pistoning action should occur in the heel area, unless the shoe is stiff. The border of the counter should not touch the malleolae (Fig. 14.2).

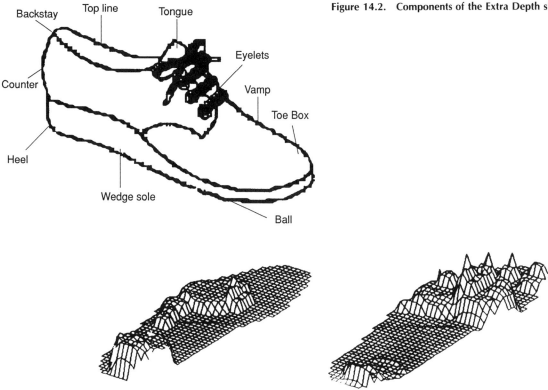

Figure 14.2.   Components of the Extra Depth shoe.

Backstay
Top line
Tongue
Eyelets
Vamp
Toe Box
Counter
Heel
Wedge sole
Ball

Figure 14.3.   Illustration of 3D forces obtained with a pedobarograph.

Orthoses can be used to immobilize and support a joint, to correct or accommodate a deformity, and to redistribute weight. As in all orthotic management, the complexity of the problem and the treatment goals will dictate the orthotic design and materials to be used. For most cases, physical examination with attention to the affected areas of the foot-ankle and observation of gait by a skillful clinician will prove effective in evaluating and understanding the symptomatology presented by a patient. The use of sophisticated technology, i.e., pedobarograph, force platform, or computerized gait analysis, is required to understand complex cases and when quantitative information of the problems and effects of intervention are necessary (Fig. 14.3).

Orthotic management of the painful/deformed foot is divided into two levels: foot orthoses (FOs) and ankle-foot orthoses (AFOs). A variety of materials and fabrication techniques are available to achieve the above mentioned objectives. Metal, leather, thermoplastics, laminated plastics, and open and closed cell foams are some examples of materials commonly utilized.

For the mild deformities, foot orthoses with arch support and Calcaneal control as provided by University of California Biomechanics Laboratory in shoe type FOs Design are used most commonly. To manage more severe cases, three types of AFOs are frequently used in our practice. They are rigid molded plastic AFOs, patellar tendon bearing AFOs (plastic, metal, or a combi-

nation) and short (lower third of calf) molded plastic AFOs. All include weight redistribution characteristics and appropriate footwear with modifications, i.e., rocker bar or bottom, cushioned heel, flair, etc. as needed (Fig. 14.4).

PHYSICAL THERAPY MANAGEMENT

The goals of physical therapy care include patient education; encouraging optimal position, mobility, and function; decreasing pain and stiffness; and preventing further dysfunction, if possible.

Postural abnormalities should be corrected without adding unusual stress to other musculoskeletal structures. Joint mobility can be encouraged with the use of modalities, joint mobilization, and soft tissue stretching techniques. Painful inflammatory conditions may benefit from the use of modalities and rest followed by gradual progressive use and therapeutic exercises. Decrease in strength and muscle imbalances can be appropriately managed with therapeutic exercises that emphasize both open and closed chain kinetic muscle function (20). General conditioning exercises should be provided as appropriate. Proprioceptive training with the use of an ankle strengthening platform may further increase range of motion in addition to improving strength, coordination, and balance.

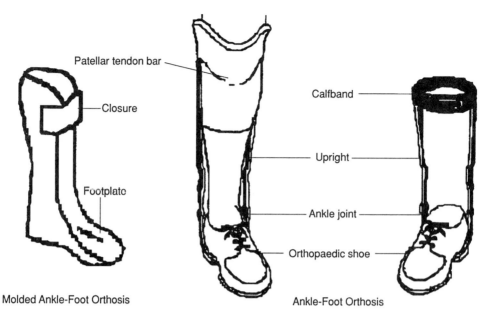

Patellar tendon bar
Closure
Footplate
Molded Ankle-Foot Orthosis

Calfband
Upright
Ankle joint
Orthopaedic shoe
Ankle-Foot Orthosis

Figure 14.4. Orthoses useful in the management of severe ankle-foot deformities.

The medical and podiatric care of wounds of the foot can be assisted by physical therapy intervention. Mechanical débridement with whirlpool can be useful; care should be taken to avoid water temperatures in excess of 94°F in those patients with arterial insufficiency. Electrical stimulation, including iontophoresis, ultrasound, phonophoresis, hyperbaric oxygen chamber, and compressive boots, have shown limited success in prompting wound closure in chronic foot ulceration in geriatric patients (5, 21, 22).

PREVENTIVE CARE

The foot is one of the most important anatomic structures of the human body. It is essential to articulate with the ground and allow ambulation, thus permitting interaction with the environment. Although the foot is a stress tolerant structure, basic preventive care is needed to prolong its functional integrity. Cumulative trauma to the foot caused by the use of narrow-toed, high-heeled, or ill-fitting shoes should be avoided. The foot should be inspected regularly, washed with soap and warm water, followed by pat drying with a towel. The skin must be kept well lubricated at all times. Excess moisture may be controlled by applying lamb's wool in between the toes along with a drying powder. White cotton socks absorb moisture better and limit allergic reactions. Trimming of toenails every 4 to 6 weeks is recommended, best if done by a professional. When cutting the nail, care should be taken to avoid cutting the skin; the nail top should be cut straight.

Integrity of the skin can be maintained by eliminating unnecessary trauma and irritation produced by ill-fitting shoes, chemical, and thermal factors. Shoes that are manufactured of light, soft, breathable materials are preferable. The toe box should have adequate space in height and width. Leather soles are preferable; when walking on slippery surfaces (e.g., snow) rubber covers should be applied. Patients should be instructed not to walk barefooted.

SUMMARY

A well-preserved, functional foot structure will permit the elderly subject to maintain a longer lasting active lifestyle. The understanding of the anatomy, physiology, and biomechanics of the foot-ankle as it relates to weight bearing and locomotion is indispensable for the diagnoses and management of related problems. Preventive care and early intervention are essential and include the use of appropriate footwear and, when needed, shoe modifications and orthotic management. In the more severe deformities, unloading of the foot with the use of upper limb support or patellar tendon bearing orthoses is indicated. In the management of open wounds, mechanical débridement, judicious use of antibiotics, and the application of total contact casting followed by correction of the foot-ankle biomechanics is the preferred therapeutic mode. The physician, podiatrist, orthotist, and physical therapist all play an important role in the preservation of the functional foot, but most important is preventive care patient education.

References

1. Bampton S. *A Guide to the Visual Examination of Pathological Gait.* Philadelphia, Pa: Temple University—Moss Rehabilitation Hospital, Rehabilitation Research and Training Center #8; 1979.
2. Inman VT, Ralston HJ, Todd F. *Human Walking.* Baltimore, Md: Williams & Wilkins; 1981.

3. Winter DA. *The Biomechanics and Motor Control of Human Gait.* Waterloo, Ontario: Waterloo University Press; 1987.

4. American Physical Rehabilitation Network. Program Outline *When the Feet Hit the Ground Everything Changes.* Toledo, Ohio; 1984.

5. McPoil TG, Brocato RS. The foot and ankle: biomechanical evaluation and treatment. In: Gould JG, ed. *Orthopaedic and Sports Physical Therapy.* 2nd ed. St.Louis, Mo: Mosby; 1990.

6. Magee DJ. *Orthopedic Physical Assessment.* Philadelphia, Pa: W.B. Saunders; 1987.

7. Truex, RC. *Human Neuroanatomy.* 6th ed. Baltimore, Md: Williams and Wilkins; 1969.

8. Payton OD, Poland JL. Aging process: implications for clinical practice. *Phys Ther.* 63:41–48, 1983.

9. Edelstein JE. Foot care for the aging. *Phys Ther.* 68:1882–1886, 1988.

10. Gartland JG. *Fundamentals of Orthopaedics.* 4th ed. Philadelphia, Pa: W.B. Saunders; 1987.

11. Mann RA. Arthritides. In: *Surgery of the Foot.* 5th ed. St Louis, Mo: Mosby; 1986.

12. Anderson JG. Treatment and prevention of plantar ulcers: a pratical approach. *Leprosy Rev.* 35:251, 1964.

13. Sims SS, Cavanagh PR, Ulbrecht JS. Risk factors in the diabetic foot: recognition and management. *Phys Ther.* 68:1887–1901, 1988.

14. Coleman WC, Brand PW, Birke JA. The total contact cast a therapy for plantar ulceration on insensitive feet. *J Am Podiatr Assoc.* 74(11):548–551, November 1984.

15. Mueller MJ, Diamond JE. Biomechanical treatment approach to diabetic plantar ulcers. *Phys Ther.* 68(12):1917–1920, 1988.

16. Nawoczenski DA, Birke JA, Graham SL, Koziatek E. The neuropathic foot—a management scheme: a case report. *Phys Ther.* 69:287–291, 1989.

17. Helfand AE. Common foot problems in the aged and rehabilitation management. In: Williams TF, ed. *Rehabilitation in the Aging.* New York, NY: Raven Press; 1984.

18. McGarvey CM. Skin and toenail problems. In: Hunt GC, ed. *Physical Therapy of the Foot and Ankle.* New York, NY: Churchill Livingstone; 1988.

19. Kaplan L. Shoes and the foot. In: Ruskin A, ed. *Current Therapy in Physiatry.* Philadelphia, Pa: W.B. Saunders; 1984.

20. Berkenblit MB, Feldman AG, Fukson OI. Adaptability of innate motor patterns and motor control mechanisms. *Behav Brain Sci.* 9:585–638, 1986.

21. Dyson M, Sauckling J. Stimulation of tissue repair by ultrasound: a survey of the mechanisms involved. *Physiotherapy.* 64:105, 1978.

22. Gault WR, Gatens PR Jr. Use of low intensity direct current in management of ischemic skin ulcers. *Phys Ther.* 56:265–269, 1976.

15

Peripheral Vascular Disease and Ischemic Skin Ulceration

John B. Redford

Of all the diseases threatening older persons, vascular disorders are certainly the most common. Occlusive arterial disease, primarily associated with arteriosclerosis, is the most prevalent. Venous thrombosis occurs slightly less frequently but is the most common vascular complication in institutions and often is succeeded by chronic venous insufficiency. Lymphedema is much less widespread in old persons; it is virtually always obstructive—secondary to lymphatic removal or neoplasm. Vasculitis and vasospastic disorders, usually associated with connective tissue diseases do occur, but, rarely, for the first time, in the elderly except for giant cell arteritis. Unfortunately, once these conditions have developed, reversal of the pathology has eluded advances in medical science—the pathogenesis can be slowed but not reversed. Prevention of complications and treatment of these diseases by physical measures in the elderly can do much to slow their inevitable course. Therefore, physical medicine, particularly through prescribed exercise regimens, plays a major role in management of vascular disease. Physiatrists are also often involved in management of the immobility or the ulcerative skin lesions induced by vascular diseases. It is essential to use physical measures to manage skin breakdown in geriatric patients. Decubitus ulcers in the elderly are extraordinarily pervasive. They not only produce high expense and morbidity but also may even lead to death. Often skin ulceration can be avoided by early attention to preventive measures widely advocated in rehabilitation medicine.

OCCLUSIVE ARTERIAL DISEASE

Occlusive arterial disease is primarily a disease of the large and medium-sized arteries in the lower extremities. Clinically, it appears as two closely related conditions, arterial embolism and atherosclerosis producing arterial insufficiency. Arterial embolism is most frequently a result of thrombus formation in the arteriosclerotic heart, seeding clots to the peripheral arteries. Arteriosclerosis first develops with fatty streaks forming in the lining of large and medium-sized arteries. This change is followed by arterial wall thickening and plaque formation; subsequently, ulceration, calcification, and thrombosis lead to occlusion. Other factors such as hypertension, excessive serum lipids, and diabetes accelerate the process. The damage primarily occurs at major arterial bifurcations. Atherosclerosis is common in the aorta and in the carotid, coronary, iliac and lower extremity arteries. As the lower limb vessels lose their perfusing ability, preexisting collateral vessels dilate to carry blood around the main vessels affected by stenosis. Because the disease progresses throughout life, arterial occlusion is most common in the elderly.

In arterial embolism, when a blood vessel is blocked suddenly, the clinical picture is usually very clear. Depending on the site and the extent of the occlusion, symptoms, and signs develop that include five features: pain, paresthesia, paralysis, pallor, and pulselessness. A cool, pale, distal limb with absent pulses is found on physical examination. Once diagnosed by arterial studies, the patient undergoes anticoagulation. Then, immediate removal of the embolus is undertaken either directly through the arterial wall or with a balloon-tipped catheter under local anesthesia aided by urokinase or streptokinase. Acute arterial thrombosis occurs less commonly and may be associated with peripheral aneurysms, but the same procedures are applied.

Unlike acute embolism and thrombosis, the usual picture of arterial insufficiency is much less dramatic. It often begins as intermittent claudication; the patient complains of pain, most commonly in the calf muscles, brought on by exercise and immediately relieved by rest. The pain can also be felt in the thigh and even in buttock muscles if the occlusion is at a higher level. The latter is usually associated with aortoiliac disease, the former with superficial femoral artery occlusion. The amount of exercise needed to bring on the condition is usually very consistent; but if unattended, the time of pain onset may become reduced because of progressive arterial occlusion and decrease in muscle perfusion.

There are a number of diseases, particularly in the elderly, that resemble intermittent claudication: musculoskeletal conditions such as arthritis of the hip and knee, neuropathic entrapment syndromes, diabetes associated with peripheral neuropathy, and, perhaps of most significance, neurospinal disorders, particularly spinal stenosis. The most distinct feature of intermittent claudication is that it is always associated with exercise and immediately relieved with rest. Although spinal stenosis may mimic these findings, its pain generally lasts longer after rest, and it may also occur in standing. To rule out intermittent claudication without resorting to more expensive technology, presence of normal peripheral pulses is usually sufficient, especially if there are clinical findings, such as reflex changes, specific limitations of joint range, or sensory and motor disturbances.

Clinical Diagnosis

Occlusive arterial disease is a condition that is almost entirely diagnosed by the history and physical examination. In history taking, it is important to learn the duration and distance of walking that elicits the muscle pain. Other symptoms are more variable but might include weakness, easy fatigue, numbness, paresthesias, and cramping of muscles. In more severe cases, pain may occur at rest or as a feeling of deadness or coldness. Symptoms are often worse when in bed at night and better when the feet are dependent. Patients may, in fact, find relief by sitting up and dangling their legs if the ischemic pain is approaching the point of becoming continuous. Skin breakdown and early gangrene sometimes may present with little pain and are often induced by trauma, exposure to cold, and even soaking the feet in hot water to relieve pain and coldness. This practice increases the metabolic demand of the tissues, subjecting them to decompensation and burns that fail to heal.

In taking the history, the clinician should seek factors contributing to arteriosclerosis: hypertension, smoking, a family history of arteriosclerosis—particularly lipid disorders—and diabetes, a condition that accounts for up to 30% of all peripheral arterial disease. The history should note whether the patient is using cardiac drugs such as propranolol and clonidine or even ergot preparations for migraine headaches because these drugs can have an adverse effect on the peripheral circulation. Important points to consider include a history of anemia, congestive heart failure, or chronic obstructive pulmonary disease, all of which may reduce the availability of oxygen to the tissues. Physical examination of the lower extremity usually confirms the degree of ischemia as related in the patient's history. In single segment disease, absent or diminished distal pulses may be noted with little skin change, but in more advanced cases, the patient exhibits decreased skin temperature and shiny, hairless, distal skin. The feet may show rubor on dependency and pallor on elevation. To evaluate for aneurysms, it is important not only to palpate the peripheral pulses but also the aorta and other major vessels. Auscultation over major vessels for the detection of bruits may be helpful.

Diabetic atherosclerosis may present a somewhat different picture; in this disease, virtually all arterial vessels are involved, including more of the medium and small-sized arteries, as well as the capillaries. In contrast to nondiabetics, diabetic patients are more likely to present with local foot infection or skin ulcers; if diabetic neuropathy accompanies the ischemia, the patient may have little or no sensation to warn of impending gangrene.

The well-known picture of the "diabetic foot" consists of peripheral neurologic loss, atrophic skin, and deformed nails attached to claw toes. Depending on underlying bony destruction and neuropathy, diabetics have thinning of plantar fat pads and calluses, combined with varying degrees of foot deformity and joint destruction.

Laboratory Diagnosis

If vascular disease is suspected, the patient should be referred to a vascular diagnostic laboratory. Particularly important are objective measurements to detect progression before clinical deterioration occurs. Initial evaluation generally includes a screening test using Doppler ultrasound techniques to obtain systolic pressures bilaterally from brachial, dorsalis pedis, and posterior tibial arteries. Ankle/arm pressure indices are reported as a ratio of ankle systolic blood pressure divided by brachialsystolic pressure. Indices equal to or greater than 1.0 are normal. Patients with intermittent claudication have indices ranging from 0.5 to 0.8; those with pain at rest usually have indices less than 0.5. Falsely high readings can occur with Doppler ultrasound when there is calcific medial sclerosis, and so the method needs skilled interpretation (1). An ultrasound technique combining real time B-mode imaging with pulsed Doppler flow detection is called duplex scanning. Vessels are located by the B-mode image, and their patency assessed; arterial flow patterns are detected by the pulsed Doppler flow component. Color flow imaging of the latter is now available. For the lower limb vessels, the system has a sensitivity of 82%, a specificity of 92%, a positive predictive value of 80%, and a negative predictive value of 93% (2).

Pulse volume recordings with measurement of arterial waveforms are helpful in assessment as well. Transcutaneous measurements of oxygen to assess skin oxygen content have also been used; they correlate with extensive occlusive disease and help determine the potential for wound healing, especially if amputation is being considered.

Arteriography is reserved for patients in whom it is critical to determine the site of the anatomic lesion prior to operative intervention. All patients who have pain at rest or expected tissue loss due to ulceration or gangrene should have arteriography. The increased risk of renal complications following contrast media infusions requires close monitoring of hydration during arteriography to protect renal function in the elderly.

Prevention and Medical Management

All patients and their families, regardless of the degree of ischemia, must be educated about the natural history of arteriosclerosis, especially the dangers of tobacco and diabetes. Smoking unequivocally increases the risk of limb loss from occlusive arterial disease as heavy smokers have a vascular reconstruction rate more than 3 times that of nonsmokers. Because diabetes increases the risk of amputation fivefold, education about diabetic control is absolutely critical. The commonly associated conditions of coronary heart disease and hypertension require effective therapy. Keeping the body warm, which helps induce distal vasodilation, and using warm socks and other means to avoid vasoconstriction on exposure to cold are strongly recommended, but the use of direct heating to the ischemic limb must be discouraged.

As the majority of amputations for ischemic limbs result from some type of trauma, protecting the foot from trauma may be the most significant preventive measure. Of particular importance is care of the feet. The patient should be instructed to inspect the feet daily and should use lanolin ointment to prevent excessive drying and fissuring of the skin. Prompt treatment of fungal infections or ingrown toe nails should be undertaken. Podiatrists who remove calluses, trim overgrown or thickened toenails, and advise about foot wear can play a major role in diabetic foot care. The patient should be instructed to wear shoes that have a wide toe box, good insole, firm shank support, and soft pliant tops. These requirements are generally met by high quality, comfortable sports shoes or special walking shoes. Shoes with extra vertical space inside, called depth-inlay shoes, are especially valuable as they allow more space for toe deformities and orthotic inserts. If the foot is deformed, custom-made shoes or foot orthoses may be necessary to prevent skin breakdown. A shoe that allows instant molding to conform with the foot and reduces the need for more expensive custom-made shoes is now available. (Extra Depth, Thermolds, P. W. Minor, Batavia, NY). All patients should be instructed in the meticulous care of the foot; formation of multidisciplinary clinics for those with dysvascular and insensitive feet have had a real impact on reducing the incidence of amputations (3). Fi-

nally, if the patient is bedridden as a result of the ischemic pain, every precaution must be made to prevent the undesirable effects of bedrest and immobility, such as hip and knee flexion contractures. These precautions would include daily range of motion exercises of the hips, knees, and ankles and use of special protective devices over the heels and bony prominences. Attempts must be made to control edema, but must prohibit use of high compression garments because compressive hose may actually increase the likelihood of skin ischemia when circulation has reached a critical stage. The head of the bed should be elevated and prolonged elevation of the ischemic extremity should be avoided.

In recent years, a number of drugs have been introduced to improve blood flow in ischemic tissues. Pentoxifylline increases the membrane flexibility of red blood cells and theoretically improves blood flow around the corners and angles in vessels. The drug has been shown to improve walking distances in double blind studies of patients with intermittent claudication (4). Therefore, it is probably worth a trial, particularly in patients whose chief complaint is intermittent claudication. The use of anticoagulants has generally not been recommended except in cases of acute thrombosis and embolism. However, low-dose aspirin therapy to reduce the chances of thrombosis in peripheral vessels is probably worth considering. There is no evidence that vasodilating drugs are effective in occlusive arterial disease if taken orally.

Untreated intermittent claudication gradually worsens, but regular exercise until the onset of symptoms followed by rest with repetition can improve exercise tolerance (5). Some have even recommended an ankle-foot orthosis that reduces the action of the calf muscle during walking to help prevent intermittent claudication, particularly if vascular surgery is not a feasible alternative (6). A controlled study of the effects of rocker-soled shoes on intermittent claudication showed that these shoes significantly increased both total distance walked as well as distance patients walked before experiencing painful calf symptoms (7). Leg exercises were once thought to increase the development of collateral circulation, but their effects are due to improved oxygen utilization in tissue. Supervised exercises are generally recommended and can include use of treadmill, bicycle, or pedalator. Unsupervised walking, particularly as a group activity, which encourages long-term continuation and practice, is better used after formal instruction for a week or two by a therapist. Patients should be encouraged to walk as quickly as possible until the pain is difficult to tolerate. They should do this several times a day, timing their walking to gradually increase exercise tolerance. Those with angina or congestive heart failure are unlikely to benefit from exercises unless their program is carefully monitored, but all others can almost be guaranteed to improve.

Surgical Treatment

Patients who have severe lower limb ischemia with pain while resting, cyanosis, dependent rubor, and ankle systolic pressures lower than 40 mm Hg are candidates for either arterial reconstruction or amputation. Severe disabling intermittent claudication or even a less severe form interfering with employment are also surgical indications. Two major treatment approaches are now available: transluminal angioplasty and direct arterial surgery. Transluminal angioplasty is mostly applicable in large peripheral vessels with short segmental stenoses. It is performed by dilating the occluded arteries by means of special catheters. It can be combined with surgical techniques that are usually reserved for larger occlusions. Arterial flow is reestablished either by thromboendarterectomy or various bypass grafts. Lately, grafts have been frequently used in the small vessels below the knee. Thus, as new materials become available, many diabetics, who previously had no chance of small vessel grafting, are now benefiting from surgical procedures.

Amputation is considered an operation of last resort. Amputation level depends on both the patient's general condition and local factors such as the extent of gangrene or ulceration, condition of adjacent skin areas, degree of infection, and severity of pain. If transmetatarsal amputation is not feasible, the next level is generally below the knee. Syme's amputations, if neuropathy is present, are generally not suitable for ischemic foot lesions. Preservation of the knee is a critical consideration, especially in the elderly. Prosthetic restoration is much more successful in below-knee than above-knee amputations. Seventy-five percent of unilateral below-knee amputees achieve independent ambulation with prosthetic training, but less than 50% of unilateral above-knee amputees are successful in prosthetic wear (8). All amputations require the same techniques used in skilled plastic surgical repair, and below-knee amputations are best performed with a long posterior flap to provide good distal padding. Above-knee amputation may be required later, but in borderline cases it is still better to try a below-knee amputation first. From surgical experience, no patients with an absent Doppler signal in the popliteal artery will heal an amputation below the knee. Immediate postoperative rigid dressings that prevent excessive edema and promote earlier healing are enabling surgeons to save many more residual limbs below the knee. However, in cases where there are significant knee contractures, i.e., 45 degrees or more, a through-knee or an above-knee amputation is a better choice. New types of prostheses have now made fitting through-knee amputations much more feasible. Because they have the advantage of some distal end-bearing, such amputations represent the best choice for prosthetic restoration if the below-knee level is not practical.

In the geriatric amputee who has prospects of walking, it is absolutely critical to be up and ambulating as quickly as possible. In most rehabilitation programs, this is feasible through the use of rigid dressings of plaster or Unna's paste bandage, which speeds up stump healing. Both require careful supervision of stump healing by a team of nurses, therapists, and physicians. Their use can be quickly succeeded by walking with temporary prostheses, which are now readily available in most rehabilitation centers (9). Even without ready-made temporary limbs, some programs recommend air splints that can be blown up enough to support some weight on the amputated side (10). No longer should a patient be forced to wait 2 to 3 months before ambulating on a prosthesis. Unfortunately, with much delay in fitting and edema control, stump contractures and other complications caused by prolonged immobility or bedrest may make prosthetic fitting impossible.

VENOUS DISORDERS

Diseases of the veins are very common in elderly people. They are of particular concern to the physiatrist because they are frequently seen in patients with various forms of paralysis. Acute deep venous thrombosis, the most common vascular problem in hospitals, may lead to pulmonary embolism—a most dreaded complication. Deep venous thrombosis is associated with muscle paralysis because the venous circulation is based partly on muscle contraction and its absence reduces the maintenance of flow. In the lower limb, this flow is against gravitational force, and this requires a series of valves that prevent backflow. When these valves become incompetent, notably in varicose vein disorders, but also in thrombotic venous disorders, stasis develops; thin venous walls become damaged, and secondary clotting with obstruction occurs at the site of the damaged valves.

Acute venous thrombosis is generally divided into two forms, superficial and deep. Superficial thrombophlebitis presents primarily in the lower leg with skin reddening, marked local tenderness along veins, and palpable thrombosed veins. It resembles acute cellulitis but can be distinguished by using Doppler ultrasound assessment. Rarely does it lead to involvement of deep veins or pulmonary emboli. Superficial thrombophlebitis usually resolves with conservative management and without any complications, although it can contribute to long-term venous stasis. Deep venous thrombosis (DVT) is a much more difficult and serious diagnosis than is superficial. The disorder seems to be directly correlated with progressive enlargement of intramuscular veins, mainly in the calf, which occurs during aging. At the present time, the incidence is probably increasing because today critically ill patients survive longer and high-risk older persons undergo more extensive surgical procedures.

The pathophysiology of DVT has been known for a century. The triad of stasis, intimal injury, and hypercoagulability was first described by Virchow. Stasis is probably the major factor; it results from surgery, paralysis, or prolonged immobilization. Over 40% of patients with hip fractures develop DVT (11) and in spinal cord injury, the incidence approaches 75% (12), which justifies the popularity of prophylactic anticoagulant therapy in such patients. Clinically, DVT is most common in immobilized patients after surgery but is also common in those with stroke, myocardial infarction, and acute paralysis, as well as persons with cancer, heart failure, and a previous history of thrombophlebitis or varicose veins. Most lethal pulmonary emboli arise in the femoral, iliac, and pelvic veins. Unfortunately, thromboses in these veins are the most difficult to detect clinically; clinical detection is accurate only about half the time.

Clinical assessment of DVT consists of examination of the lower limbs for unexplained swelling, along with palpation of muscles for tenderness by deep pressure. Usually, detection of tenderness is possible only in the calf. Deep pain in the muscles on maneuvers such as passively dorsiflexing the foot or Homan's sign is rather nonspecific. Daily circumferential measurement of the calves and thighs in patients after surgery or with recent paralysis has been advocated by some as a means to detect the onset of deep venous thrombosis. However, as in other maneuvers advocated for prevention of DVT, this does not seem to be widely practiced.

Laboratory Diagnosis

Because of the unreliable clinical signs for detecting venous thrombosis, laboratory studies are paramount. Impedance plethysmography is considered the most useful noninvasive method of detecting venous thrombosis; it is particularly helpful in assessing proximal thrombosis, although of little value in calf and popliteal veins. It is low-cost, safe, and noninvasive; it is generally felt to precede the venogram, although such an x-ray is considered the ultimate objective method for assessing acute DVT. Impedance plethysmography has been demonstrated to be sensitive and specific in over 95% of the cases (13). Although venous Doppler examination is easy to perform and most useful in diagnosing thrombosis below the knees, it needs careful interpretation and so is not widely advocated for detecting DVT. Although very accurate for detection, I-125 fibrinogen scanning has not proven useful for routine clinical use, but it has been used as a research tool to demonstrate the incidence and natural history of DVT.

Management

Because of the high incidence of DVT associated with forced immobility and other conditions of the elderly, preventive measures have been widely advocated.

If immobility is unavoidable, particularly following surgery of the hip or pelvic region, use of antithrombotic drugs and full-length supporting stockings such as TED-hose has been widely practiced. Limited information is available as to whether such stockings are really helpful. Furthermore, unless close attention is paid to keeping them in place, they may roll up at the proximal margins and actually increase venous stasis. A more physiologic approach, particularly in patients who may not be candidates for anticoagulation, is the use of intermittent pneumatic compression devices. These apply a wave of pulsatile pressure from distal to proximal regions of the lower extremity, thus simulating the pumping of venous blood toward the heart as provided by muscle action. There is good reported evidence of the preventive value of this relatively simple method, especially after surgery. Some authorities advocate that venous pumping be more widely used in hospitals (14).

Confirmed DVT is treated by systemic use of heparin administered by continuous intravenous infusion after a bolus loading dose and warfarin sodium after the first day. A daily check of heparin dosage is made by partial thromboplastin times. The heparin is usually given for 10 days, at which time oral anticoagulants are continued for at least 6 weeks for uncomplicated or isolated thrombosis. However, for DVT with suspected or confirmed pulmonary embolism, a 3-month to 6-month course is advocated. During the acute phase, the patient should be at bedrest with the lower limb elevated for at least 7 days and then gradually mobilized after the pain and swelling have subsided.

The patient, once up, should wear gradient elastic stockings and be encouraged to exercise. Some still advocate wrapping the lower limbs with elastic bandages when the patient is ambulatory, but, in our experience, most elderly patients are unable to wrap their limbs effectively, particularly since it is necessary to provide more support distally than proximally. Less expensive alternatives to bandage wraps are knitted elasticized sleeves of various weights and widths (Compresogrip—Knit-Rite, Kansas City, Mo., Elastonet—Jobst, Toledo, Ohio). These tubular supports can be doubled over the limb at the foot and ankle or layered distally to provide the gradient support needed to prevent the postphlebitic syndrome. Once the acute thrombosis has subsided, the patient should be encouraged to exercise the calves and thighs isometrically for 5 minutes at least 3 to 4 times daily to help stimulate venous return. One should also advise patients to elevate the legs whenever possible during sitting and keep them higher than the rest of the body when resting on a couch or in bed.

Chronic Venous Insufficiency

Not every patient develops postphlebitic venous insufficiency, but it is difficult if not impossible to detect which patient may eventually have this problem. Generally, patients should try the measures outlined above for at least a month or two after leaving the hospital. Then they should take the supports off and watch for leg edema occurring toward the end of the day. If no edema occurs, they probably can stop using the stockings without further concern. Patients with varicose veins or a previous history of thrombophlebitis should continue wearing supports indefinitely. Sometimes venous insufficiency develops insidiously, and blood in the deep veins is forced into the superficial venous system, especially during exercise. This results in chronic interstitial edema and rupture of small cutaneous vessels. Following this occurrence, there is a deposit of hemosiderin—stasis pigmentation—accompanied by skin atrophy with fibrosia nd obstruction of the lymphatics. With or without additional trauma, these changes may lead to loss of skin blood flow and stasis ulceration.

To prevent this unfortunate sequence of events, all patients after suspected venous thrombosis should be advised to look for any increase in dependent edema, especially toward the end of the day and report it to their physicians. If swelling is occurring, an experienced professional should measure the patient for custom-made elastic hose, especially if commercially available gradient stockings cannot be fitted or worn adequately. The prescription of such hose in elderly patients should be carefully considered as it is most difficult for the aged to apply them unaided. This is particularly true for persons with hand deformities or loss of strength in the upper limbs. Many elderly patients will not comply with wearing hose regularly unless there is a careful explanation of their use and some means provided to help them or their families put them on. One company that makes pressure gradient hose has a sock donner that operates very effectively, but only if used with the company's products (BUTLER, Med, USA, Arlington Hts Ill, 60005). Zippers have been used in some custom-made hose and can be helpful, particularly if placed behind the stocking; the foot can be placed into the hose—like slipping on a shoe—and then the rest of the stocking zipped up behind. Garter belts or some suspension must be worn at the top to avoid the rolling down of the margin, which may further aggravate the distal edema. Patients must be educated on the frequent replacement of these stockings, as they will only be effective 6 to 9 months.

If the edema is primarily below the knee, a better alternative to the stocking is a compression legging called CircAid (15). A series of pliable, nonstretchable compression bands are adjusted to conform with leg circumference in a comfortable distal to proximal pattern with a decreasing pressure gradient. The bands are locked in place by hook and loop closures using a patented closing system (See Figs. 15.1 and 15.2). The bands are easily closed, tightened, and opened making them useful for

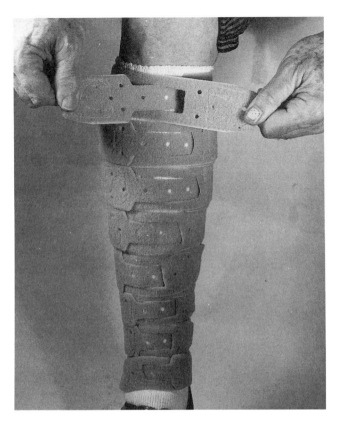

Figure 15.1. Legging orthosis in place, with the top circumferential band being adjusted. From Vernick S H, Shapiro D, Shaw F D. Legging orthosis for venous and lymphatic insufficiency. *Arch Phys Med Rehabil.* 68:459–461, 1987.

the physically handicapped person who cannot don elastic hose. The legging is superior to elastic support as it applies unyielding pressure and does not stretch out and lose its effectiveness over time. It must be applied over a tubular sock or stockinette, which helps absorb sweat. It cannot be applied over bony surfaces, and some persons may need supplemental elastic anklets and knee and thigh supports.

Additional methods of care include skin-moisturizing lotions to prevent the drying and cracking of skin that may lead to ulceration. The local massage accompanying the application of these lotions is also helpful as gentle massage may reduce local edema. Physicians should counsel patients with venous stasis on avoiding trauma to the lower limbs and encourage them to engage regularly in activities such as walking or bicycling. Surgical management should be reserved for those with severe varicose veins that are painful or cosmetically unacceptable.

LYMPHEDEMA

Lymphedema is excessive swelling of a limb after obstruction or insufficiency of the lymphatic system. The lymphatic system returns water and protein from tissue fluid spaces to the blood stream. If this protein-rich fluid

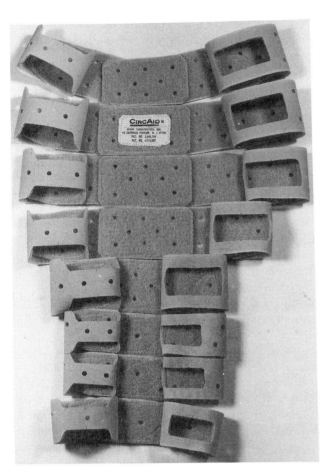

Figure 15.2. View of the rear side of the orthosis. Anchor bands, short pieces of loop tape backed with hook tape, hold band ends together. Front band ends are looped back to avoid entanglement. From Vernick SH, Shapiro D, Shaw FD. Legging orthosis for venous and lymphatic insufficiency. *Arch Phys Med Rehabil.* 68:459–461, 1987.

is not removed by the lymphatics, there is raised osmotic pressure in the tissue interspaces, and this increases the ability of the tissues to hold water. As edema fluid accumulates, tissues are stretched and further damage capillaries and small lymphatics; eventually fibrinous materials accrue and tissue fibrosis ensues. At this stage, the pitting edema, evident early in the process, ceases, and the whole limb becomes swollen and very unyielding to touch or pressure. This whole process is accelerated by trauma or infection. Patients often relate a history of surgical removal of lymph nodes followed by minimal edema until trauma or infection ensue and cause the whole limb to enlarge.

Lymph flow from the extremities is mainly by active vasomotion of the lymphatics. The musculoskeletal "muscle pump" aids flow, but excessive use of the limb after much lymphedema is present seems to actually aggravate the condition. As in chronic venous disease, dependency also worsens the lymphedema.

In elderly persons, lymphedema has two main causes: obstruction of lymph drainage either secondary to lymphatic cancer or surgical ablation of cancerous lymph nodes and an infection resulting in destroyed lymph nodes and channels. Often both may be involved in the process. Lymphedema of the upper limb is most commonly seen in elderly women secondary to removal of lymph nodes following mastectomy. In radical mastectomy, it develops in 30% to 40% of cases, although with wide adoption of less radical surgery, this form of lymphedema should be decreasing. Radiation of the lymph nodes may result in obstructive damage. In the lower limb, lymphedema is probably most often seen secondary to prostate cancer or lymphomas (16).

The diagnosis of lymphedema is generally made from the history and physical examination and rarely needs to be supplemented by laboratory tests. The patient generally complains of persistent limb swelling and heaviness that is often painless but may produce an aching discomfort, particularly in the lower extremity. With infection, the pain will be much more acute, and signs of inflammation such as tenderness, redness, and increased temperature will be apparent. The condition may come on insidiously but sometimes starts quite abruptly without any evident preceding trauma or infection.

In cases of suspected malignancy, laboratory tests include computerized tomography (CT) scan or magnetic resonance imaging (MRI) of the abdomen and pelvis for the lower limb and of the chest and shoulder for the upper. Occasionally, venography may be required for diagnosis and prognosis because venous and lymphatic obstruction may occur together.

Management

Without evidence of new malignancy or a significant infection, management of lymphedema is largely by physical methods. Use of diuretics and restriction of sodium may be somewhat helpful in the treatment of chronic lymphedema. However, results of these measures are often disappointing because removal of the excess protein from tissue fluid is the mainstay of treatment. Treatment relies on three main approaches: elevation, massage, and exercise. The patient should be encouraged to elevate the affected limb as much as possible during the day and as much as is compatible with sleep at night. The limb needs to be higher than the heart but not necessarily vertical; each session of elevation should last at least one-half hour. Although massage to mobilize fluid can be applied manually, this is somewhat time-consuming and must be done skillfully. Most therapy programs rely on pneumatically operated compression devices. These are usually applied with pressure from 50 mm Hg to 70 mm Hg from three-quarters of an hour to several hours in a series of daily sessions. The therapist measures the limb during each session to plot progress. Generally, at least 5 to 6 days are required to make significant changes in limb volume. During intervals between application of the pumping devices, the patient should be taught to exercise against an elastic support. We favor woven tubular elastic supports (Compresso-grip, Elastonet) mentioned earlier. The patients perform isometric muscle contractions with minimal joint motion under the support and should exercise at least 3 to 4 times a day for up to 5 minutes each time.

When the physical treatment seems to have accomplished as much reduction as possible—determined by circumferential measurements—the patient is provided with an elastic sleeve or stocking of the gradient type. Its length depends on the clinical presentation, but, generally full-length garments that include the hand and the foot are prescribed. Patients should be warned they might have to wear such garments for an indefinite period. Often there will be no return of the lymph channels, and edema will reoccur without wearing supports or regular pumping of the limb. The compression legging described earlier for chronic venous insufficiency has also been advocated for patients with leg lymphedema (15). Others have advocated the use of Unna's paste boots, although these have been more widely used for ulcers associated with venous insufficiency.

Intermittent pneumatic compression is applied with a sleeve comprised of either a single-chambered or multichambered system. In the latter, a series of compartments that encircle a limb are sequentially inflated from distal to proximal regions. In the average case, the multichambered system seems to have no advantage over the single-chambered, but if the edema is severe, particularly in the lower extremities, the more expensive and sophisticated multichambered varieties, such as the Wright Linear Pump, may be necessary and have proven effective (17). Pneumatic sleeve pumping must be monitored closely during the initial application because pulmonary edema may develop in high risk patients. Of course, if there is any sign of infection in the limb, massage or these pneumatic devices should not be applied.

Pneumatic compression units are available for home use. They can be rented or purchased in most major cities in the United States and used daily for patients who may choose this method of lymphedema control or even control of chronic venous insufficiency and venous ulceration. A simple to use home-based unit that uses sequential gradient compression to the legs has been marketed by Kendall Healthcare Products, Mansfield, Mass. Patients must be warned to report to their physicians increased swelling associated with any sign of infection or minor trauma to ensure complications can be treated promptly.

Long-term results with the above methods are generally quite good, but as in many chronic conditions, the patient must be educated fully to understand the condition. Patient compliance with use of the apparatus and elastic supports is best done by long-term followup and return visits to the physician who ordered the treatment.

SKIN ULCERATION

Ulceration of the skin occurs frequently in elderly persons, especially those with peripheral vascular diseases. Most ulcers are one of four types: (a) decubitus ulcers (pressure sores), (b) ischemic ulcers from occlusive vascular disease or cutaneous arteriolar disease, (c) neurotrophic ulcers, and (d) venous stasis ulcers. A mixed etiology is evident in many ulcers, for example a combination of occlusive vascular disease and pressure may cause heel ulcers in a bedridden patient. Ultimately, all ulceration is caused by death of cells from deprivation of oxygen and nutrition. Furthermore, any factor adversely affecting metabolism of cutaneous cells increases their susceptibility to death: anemia, malnutrition, diabetes, even old age, all may play a role.

Cutaneous ulceration is particularly common among elderly residents of long-term care institutions and may even become a political or legal issue in respect to sufficiency of care. Obviously, if local treatment is to be effective, management must be directed toward the whole problem. This includes: control of general infection or diabetes, correction of malnutrition, and diagnosis and treatment of anemia. In institutions, adequacy procedures, equipment for care, and ratio of trained nursing staff to residents must also be addressed.

Decubitus Ulcers

Much that has been written concerning the cause and prevention of decubitus ulcers is summarized in the following paragraphs. For excellent reviews, see Chapter 31 in DeLisa & Gans (18) or Allman (19).

Excessive pressure and compression of the skin, particularly over bony prominences, plays a primary role in ulceration; skin ischemia caused by pressure exceeding the tissue capillary pressure (13 mm Hg to 32 mm Hg) produces skin hyperemia followed by local ischemia and cell death. The exact degree of excessive pressure required is controversial, but there is a direct relationship between the duration pressure is applied and the likelihood of ischemic changes. High pressure over a large area is less damaging than localized lower pressure; low pressure for a long period of time is more damaging than high pressure for a short period. Obviously, frequent turning and use of specialized mattresses and cushions that reduce pressure are essential in prevention and management of pressure sores. A wide variety of devices are now marketed to prevent and assist in healing decubitus ulcers.

Shearing or frictional forces accompanied by stretching of blood vessels reduce pulsatile blood flow through the skin and add to the direct compression force that may be causing the skin ischemia. Frictional forces are particularly noteworthy in patients sitting in chairs or lying semireclined in bed because this may stretch the skin over the buttock or lower spine. Such stretching may be increased during poorly performed transfers from bed to chair, etc. Those attending the severely disabled should always keep this possibility in mind in frail elderly persons.

Heat causes metabolic rate to rise 10% for every degree rise in tissue temperature. Because increased temperature causes increased cellular metabolism, the effects of ischemia may be magnified if the skin is excessively warm. Seat cushions and mattresses that maintain heat and moisture have been shown to compound the problem of pressure sore development. Therefore, adequate air flow around areas of pressure and alleviation of warm, moist skin conditions are essential approaches to prevention and healing of pressure sores.

Increased interstitial fluid or edema increases the capillary-to-cell distance and reduces the rate of diffusion of oxygen and nutrients from blood vessels to the tissues. Because local edema is the initial result of pressure and friction, it compounds the ischemic problem. Needless to say, the prevention or relief of edema, often by local massage where feasible, plays a primary role in management of all skin ulcerations. Edema also may be a result of cardiac, renal, or metabolic diseases, and these conditions need primary management if ulcers are to be prevented.

Aging deprives the skin of its pliability and elasticity; an associated progressive decrease in blood flow takes place. Thus, elderly persons, particularly if thin and malnourished, are much more prone to ischemic pressure ulcers than are the young. Medical instruction for the patient, family, and all caregivers associated with the elderly must include a discussion of why older people are at risk for ulcers and the various ways to prevent them. In an old person, early recognition of the persistence of skin hyperemia, particularly over bony prominences, is perhaps the most important single factor in prevention.

Skin infection may occasionally play a primary role in the causation of decubitus ulcers. By producing local inflammation, infection increases tissue pressure, which can compromise blood flow enough to start skin breakdown. Certainly, persisting superficial infection prevents adequate healing of an ulcer even though pressure may be removed and adequate circulation and nutrition restored. Therefore, careful searches for source and type of infection, with attention to management by cleansing and antibiotics, play an important role in prevention and treatment of pressure ulceration.

Ischemic Arterial, Neurotrophic, and Venous Stasis Ulcers

Ischemic ulcers caused by occlusive arteriosclerotic disease usually start with skin trauma. Most ulcers occur on the toes or heel but may be anywhere in the distal limb. Pain, especially at night, is characteristic of ischemic ulcers. Cutaneous lesions have a pale base or a covering of black eschar with the surrounding skin appearing normal unless infection is present. Ischemic ulcers from occlusive vascular disease may require restoration of blood flow through surgical intervention and skin grafting before they will heal. Otherwise, management depends on prevention of further trauma, good control of infection, and general measures to improve blood supply to the affected areas.

Neurotrophic ulcers arise in skin deprived of sensation and subject to repeated pressure and shearing forces. In industrialized nations, by far the most common cause is diabetic neuropathy. In this disorder, painless ulcers start on the sole of the foot over major weight-bearing areas, particularly under the heel or the head of the first metatarsal. Neurotrophic ulcers nearly always have a callus surrounding them because they develop through chronic trauma and pressure, often due to poor footwear.

Treatment requires careful débridement and removal of the callus around the edge, followed by cleaning with an antiseptic solution such as povidone iodine, which must be removed by saline before applying a dressing. In care of neurotrophic and decubitus ulcers, biocclusive dressings (for example Duo-Derm, Vigilon, OpSite, and Restore) have improved ulcer care (20). They may aid in débridement, provoke formation of good granular tissue, and cause more rapid healing compared with traditional methods such as wet to dry dressings. The thickness of some of these dressings add protective padding, as well as protection from outside infection. A major advantage is that they need only be changed once or twice a week, depending on the size and stage of ulcer healing. However, their use is not advised on deep wounds or if significant wound infection is present. Erythema, purulent drainage, and a foul odor all suggest that infection must be sought and controlled, especially since osteomyelitis may underlie neurotrophic ulcers. The other main consideration in management of neurotrophic ulcers is to reduce trauma and prevent the patient from "do it yourself" cures with various lotions or salves. Great success in this regard has been reported by using careful débridement and cleansing combined with special techniques of plaster casting, but, as in all such programs, a carefully coordinated team effort is critical to achieving success (21).

Once the ulcer is either healed or nearly so, the physician should prescribe special footwear, with or without a shoe orthosis, to redistribute weight on the foot. Recently introduced special padded hosiery to protect the diabetic foot promises to aid further in preventing diabetic ulcers (SILOPAD-Softsock, Silipos, Niagara Falls, NY 14304). Proper shoes or foot orthoses are vital in preventing recurrence. Another key to prevention is instruction in foot care, as previously discussed, including avoidance of chemicals on corns and applying hot water bottles and heating pads. Dysvascular patients should inspect their feet every day and never walk barefoot. Of course, if the trophic ulcer is also associated with osteomyelitis or occlusive vascular disease, surgical intervention may be required to ensure healing.

Venous stasis ulcers usually occur distally on the medial side of the leg. They are usually painless, hurting only if infected. The ulcer presents as a shallow open wound with irregular edges and a healthy-appearing base surrounded by firm, brown-pigmented skin from longstanding venous stasis. The approach to treatment is to reduce venous pressure and edema and keep the ulcer clean and uninfected. Traditionally, this has been accomplished by cleansing the ulcer, followed by an occlusive semirigid dressing wrapped around the foot and lower leg, the Unna paste boot. This may be left in place for several weeks allowing the ulcer to heal spontaneously. It provides good pressure control to reverse the edema, as well as protection from outside infection.

In recent years, new approaches have been advocated in the treatment of stasis and other ulcers using occlusive hydrocolloid dressings. Such dressings have been shown not only to break down human fibrin clots in vivo but also to promote more new blood vessel growth than traditional adherent gauze dressings (22, 23). These dressings can be used under the Unna boot, a compression legging orthosis, or compression bandages. Recently, the introduction of adhesive compression bandages, such as Expandover (Sherwood Medical, St. Louis, Mo.) or one from ConvaTec (Squibb), promises to improve the ability to hold such dressings in place without the use of a gradient pressure stocking or the somewhat awkward and messy Unna paste dressing. A recent report from London, comparing patients who used gradient compression stockings alone with those using stockings and home pneumatic compression showed that the latter group using pressure devices healed the venous stasis much earlier than the former (24).

If the ulcer needs mechanical débridement and control of infection prior to applying the pressure dressing, mechanical treatment with hydrotherapy may be used and supplemented by enzymatic débridement. Ulcers greater than 3 cm in diameter not responding to medical control may eventually require grafting.

SUMMARY

This chapter has outlined the diagnosis and treatment of common vascular diseases affecting the elderly. Particular emphasis has been given to management of the cutaneous ulceration that may result from these disorders or from ischemia caused by local pressure. Physical treatment measures are stressed as they play an important role in prevention and management of all these conditions. Some of these measures are: *(a)* exercises to prevent the secondary effects of immobility and improve both arterial and venous circulation; *(b)* various pads, mattresses, and cushions to prevent and treat skin breakdown; *(c)* special attention to footwear and physical measures in care of the dysvascular foot; *(d)* manual massage and pneumatic compression devices; *(e)* supportive garments, including a recently introduced compression legging orthosis; *(f)* hydrotherapy for débriding and cleansing ulcers; and *(g)* recently introduced hydrocolloid dressings that aid débridement and accelerate wound healing by promoting new blood vessel growth.

References

1. Strandness DE. Diagnostic considerations in occlusive arterial disease. *Vasc Surg.* 11:271–277, 1977.
2. Kohler, TR, Nance DR, Cramer MM. Duplex scanning for the diagnosis of aortoiliac and femoropopliteal disease. *Circulation.* 76:1074–1080, 1987.
3. McAnaw MP, Troyer-Caudle J, Heath P, et al. Development of a multidisciplinary dysvascular and insensitive foot clinic. *Wounds.* 2:7–17, 1990.
4. Porter JM, Cutler BS, Lee BY, et al. Pentoxyfylline efficacy in the treatment of intermittent claudication: multicenter controlled double blind trial with objective assessment of chronic occlusive arterial disease patients. *Am Heart J.* 104:66–72, 1982.
5. Cronenwett JL, Warner KG, et al. Intermittent claudication. Current results of non-operative management. *Arch Surg.* 119:430–436, 1984.
6. Honet, JC, Strandness DE, et al. Short-leg bracing for intermittent claudication of the calf. *Arch Phys Med Rehabil.* 49:578–585, 1968.
7. Richardson JK. Rocker-soled shoes and walking distance in patients with calf claudication. *Arch Phys Med Rehabil.* 72:554–558, 1991.
8. Kegel B, Carpenter ML, Burgess EM. Functional capabilities of lower extremity amputees. *Arch Phys Med Rehabil.* 59:109–120, 1978.
9. Leonard JA, Andrews KL. Rigid removable dressings, immediate postoperative prostheses, and rehabilitation of the amputee. In: Ernst CB, Stanley JC, eds. *Current Therapy in Vascular Surgery.* Philadelphia, Pa: B. C. Decker, 1991.
10. Bonner FJ, Green RF. Pneumatic airleg prostheses: report of 200 cases. *Arch Phys Med Rehabil.* 63:383–385, 1971.
11. Merli G, Martinez J. Prophylaxis for deep vein thrombosis and pulmonary embolism in the surgical patient. *Med Clin North Am.* 71:(3)377–397, 1987.
12. Merli G, Herbison G, Ditunno J, et al. Deep vein thrombosis: prophylaxis in acute spinal cord injured patients. *Arch Phys Med Rehabil.* 69:661–664, 1988.
13. Hull R, Hirsch J, Sackett DL, et al. Combined use of leg scanning and impedance plethysmography in suspected venous thrombosis. *N Engl J Med.* 296:1497–1500, 1977.
14. Carpini JA, Scurr JH, Hasty JH. Role of compression modalities in a prophylactic program for deep vein thrombosis. *Semin Thrombosis Hemostasis.* 14 (suppl):77–87, 1988.

15. Vernick SH, Shapiro D, Shaw FD. Legging orthosis for venous and lymphatic insufficiency. *Arch Phys Med Rehabil.* 68:459–461, 1987.
16. Smith RD, Spittell JA, Schirzer A. Secondary lymphedema of the leg: its characteristics and diagnostic implications. *JAMA.* 185:80–82, 1963.
17. Kim-Sing C, Basco VE. Postmastectomy lymphedema treated with the Wright Linear Pump. *Can J Surg.* 30:368–370, 1987.
18. Donovan WH, Dinh TA, Garber SL, et al. Pressure ulcers. In: DeLisa JA, Gans BM, eds. *Rehabilitation Medicine Principles and Practice.* (2nd ed.) Philadelphia, Pa: J. B. Lippincott; 1993.
19. Allman RM. Pressure ulcers among the elderly. *N Engl J Med.* 320:850–853, 1989.
20. Sebern MD. Pressure ulcer management in home health care: efficacy and cost effectiveness of moisture vapor permeable dressing. *Arch Phys Med Rehabil.* 67:726–729, 1986.
21. Helm PA, Walker SC, Pullium G. Total contact casting in diabetic patients with neuropathic foot ulcerations. *Arch Phys Med Rehabil.* 65:691–693, 1984.
22. Van Rijswij KL, Brown D, Friedman S, et al. Multicenter chemical evaluation of a hydrocolloid dressing for leg ulcers. *Cuts.* 35:173–176, 1985.
23. Varghese MC, Bain AK, Carter DM, et al. Local environment of chronic wounds under synthetic dressings. *Arch Dermatol.* 22:52–57, 1986.
24. Smith PC, Sarin S, Hasty J, Scurr JH. Sequential gradient pneumatic compression enhances venous ulcer healing: a randomized trial. *Surgery.* 108:871–875, 1990.

16
Geriatric Stroke Rehabilitation

Susan J. Garrison

Approximately 20% of all patients who survive stroke will require comprehensive rehabilitation services, involving physical and occupational therapies and, occasionally, speech therapy. Twenty percent of those requiring rehabilitation will require assistance to ambulate. All will eventually walk independently if they live long enough after stroke for natural recovery to occur. Stroke rehabilitation therefore involves learning compensatory skills for lost muscle function, while awaiting natural recovery.

This chapter is written from the standpoint of the author's years of experience of treating hundreds of stroke patients 65 years of age and older, coupled with ongoing review of the literature. Many topics discussed as related to geriatric stroke have not been adequately researched in the literature, particularly with respect to female patients and the old, old. These are areas for further research. Many studies of interest, because they include large numbers of stroke patients, are not from the United States; while of academic interest, they do not always apply to the American geriatric population due to cultural differences and beliefs about sickness and age, differences in rehabilitation therapy, and payment issues. It is probable that more than 20% of patients over age 65 years who survive stroke will require comprehensive rehabilitation due to preexisting comorbidity with resultant activities of daily living (ADL) impairment.

STROKE REHABILITATION SETTINGS

With the advent of diagnosis-related group (DRG) exempt rehabilitation units in 1983, many acute care hospitals developed on-site comprehensive inpatient rehabilitation units. Previously, rehabilitation patients may have been admitted to various acute medical units in hospitals or to free-standing rehabilitation hospitals. There, emphasis was typically on young adult spinal cord injured or traumatic amputees. Even in the Veteran Administration Hospital (VAH) systems, few stroke patients were in their 70s, 80s, and 90s. By law, patients admitted to DRG-exempt rehabilitation units must meet certain criteria to be eligible for rehabilitation. Services include twice a day therapies such as physical therapy (PT), occupational therapy (OT), and speech therapy, if necessary. The DRG is coded as combined rehabilitation. Because the DRG code for acute cerebrovascular disease continues to decrease, there is a financial incentive for institutions to discharge these patients from acute care. Patients who do not qualify as acute stroke rehabilitation candidates may qualify for skilled nursing facility care (SNF). Others may receive therapy at home or in nursing homes until their abilities improve enough to be considered for acute rehabilitation; conversely, they deteriorate medically or surgically so that acute inpatient care may be justified. The patient, when stabilized, may then be assessed to potentially benefit from stroke rehabilitation. See Figure 16.1.

CANDIDATES FOR STROKE REHABILITATION

As in all rehabilitation, the optimum candidate for stroke rehabilitation must be capable of learning, synthesizing, and using new behaviors. Lack of verbal communication does not automatically disqualify potential candidates; patients may respond to gestures or other visual cues (1).

Previous studies summarized by Jongblood (2) indicate several factors as poor prognostic indicators for functional recovery after stroke. See Table 16.1.

Advanced age alone is not a true indicator of poor prognosis. Past studies have not included significant numbers of the very old; often discharge to "home" was utilized as a stroke rehabilitation outcome indicator (3, 4). However, "home" may not be an appropriate outcome indicator. Safety factors such as physical disability and communication impairment in those who live alone may preclude return to the home setting. More research effort is needed in this area. Functional abilities after rehabilitation, rather than placement setting, are better indicators.

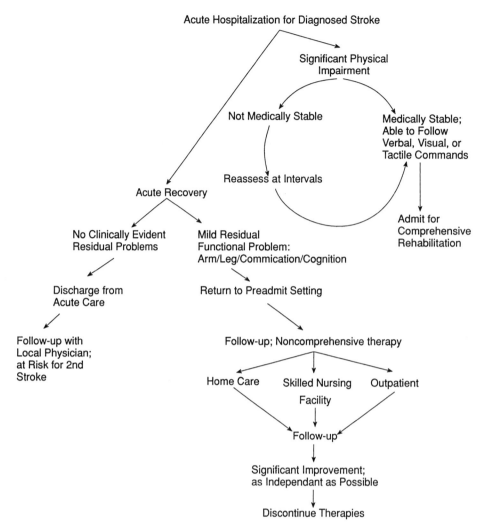

Figure 16.1. Stroke Rehabilitation Treatment.

Table 16.1. Prognostic Indicators of Poor Outcome[a]

Advanced age
Inability to understand commands
Medical/surgical instability
Previous stroke
Severe memory problems
Urinary/bowel incontinence
Visual/spatial deficits

[a]Adapted from Jongblood L. Prediction of function after stroke: a critical review. *Stroke* 17:765–776, 1986.

Under current Medicare guidelines, stroke patients are eligible for a 2-week trial of inpatient rehabilitation. The potential for progress is assessed during this time period. All patients admitted must be capable of participating in therapy sessions as determined by their needs and demonstrate increasing functional abilities. Poor motivation is not a valid reason for exclusion from rehabilitation. The causes for such labeled behavior should be sought out and addressed (5). Many factors including emotional, physical, and social concerns combine to make geriatric stroke rehabilitation a case-by-case challenge (6).

The concept of the frail elderly is significant. A subgroup of the elderly, this group utilizes a far greater share of medical resources than do other members of the population. The definition of frailty is still controversial; the need for definition is not. Winograd et al (7) developed clinical screening criteria to select hospitalized elderly at high risk for mortality, nursing home placement, and rehospitalization. Three groups of increasing frailty, Independent, Frail, and Severely Impaired, were identified. By definition, all patients with cerebrovascular accident (CVA) were defined as Frail. These groups were more predictive of nursing home utilization and mortality than were age or DRGs.

The implementation of DRGs for acute care has created financial incentive to discharge patients from acute care as soon as possible. This has resulted in earlier poststroke admissions to DRG-exempt units. Some institutions utilize hospitalwide screening teams for patients admitted with specific diagnoses, such as stroke. Appropriate candidates are followed closely throughout their acute care stays and transferred to inpatient rehabilitation as soon as medically stable (8).

OUTCOME PREDICTION

There are numerous studies of outcome following stroke rehabilitation; few have appropriately studied stroke in the aged (2, 9). Use of "return to work" as a stroke outcome indicator is invalid because the large majority of these patients have already retired. Return to home as an outcome may not be feasible due to lack of spouse or family support.

In a study of 114 stroke patients admitted to a rehabilitation center, Lehmann et al (10) found that age did not predict functional gains, but did predict that older patients were more likely to be institutionalized following hospital discharge. Kelly-Hayes et al (11) studied the living situation of stroke members of the Framingham Study. Whereas a male's level of education had no apparent impact on institutionalization following stroke, older women, married or single, with minimal education and moderate to severe impairment were at highest risk for institutionalization.

FUNCTIONAL EVALUATION

Functional outcomes are utilized today as a means of justification for rehabilitation. The most commonly used for stroke include the Barthel Index and its successor, the Functional Independence Measurement System (FIMS) (12, 13). Refer to Chapter 43 in this text for further details.

Due to the cost of rehabilitation, stroke rehabilitation should be geared toward delivery of care that assures maximal independence, gained as quickly as possible. Staged stroke rehabilitation is now indicated for specific cases. Similar to staging of inpatient rehabilitation hospitalization for spinal cord injured patients, staged stroke rehabilitation is best utilized for the geriatric stroke patient who experiences slowed lower limb muscular functional return. This patient eventually walks, though weeks to months after initial inpatient rehabilitation has occurred. Readmission to the inpatient setting allows for upgrading skills as functional muscular recovery occurs. Staged rehabilitation may also be appropriate for the patient who experiences increasing function in the dominant, previously paralyzed upper limb. Participation in intensive, twice a day therapies may allow for more independence in activities of daily living.

GERIATRIC STROKE RESEARCH

Millions of dollars are funded into stroke research for prevention and acute care-related questions. However, despite the fact that two thirds to three fourths of stroke patients are over the age of 65 years at the onset of stroke, little is devoted to that age group in stroke rehabilitation research. A task force of the National Institute of Health formulated the following stroke-specific research recommendations (14).

1. Study systems and sites for stroke rehabilitation.
2. Establish beneficial interventions for severely impaired patients, normally excluded as rehabilitation candidates.
3. Evaluate efficacy of cognitive retraining techniques.
4. Establish efficacy of modalities such as biofeedback, electrical stimulation, and neuromuscular facilitation through controlled trials.
5. Evaluate the role of assistive devices.
6. Evaluate the team process in terms of roles, communication, efficiency, and approach to patient care.

Other areas for research include the timing of rehabilitation, differences in learning of left versus right hemiplegics as well as poststroke males versus females, and the effect of caregiver role and support.

ANATOMY, ETIOLOGY, AND EPIDEMIOLOGY OF STROKE

Stroke occurs when there is a lack of blood supply to the brain. There are three types of stroke—thrombotic, embolic, and hemorrhagic. The majority of strokes are thrombotic, due to arteriosclerosis. Embolic strokes generally have a cardiac focus of origin. Hemorrhagic strokes, typically due to hypertension, account for only 10% of strokes. It is this group of strokes that has decreased in recent years, most likely as a result of better medical control of hypertension. The SHEP Cooperative Research Group (15) found that, in persons 60 years of age and older with isolated systolic hypertension, low-dose first step antihypertensive medication reduced the total stroke incidence by 36%. In addition, major cardiovascular events were significantly reduced.

Approximately two thirds to three fourths of strokes occur in the over 65-year-old age group. Incidence apparently increased in the 1980's, with over half in the age group of 75 years and older. The prevalence is increasing as this segment of the US population grows more quickly than any other. It is believed that better management of general health is allowing more patients to survive and ultimately sustain strokes (16, 17). Woo et al (18) compared risk factors for ischemic and hemorrhagic strokes in those aged 70 years and older to a younger population. They found that the risk factors differ; for those age 70 years and above, atrial fibrillation and ischemic heart disease are correlated with ischemic strokes. Hypertension and diabetes were risk factors for both groups. Hypertension was a risk for hemorrhagic stroke only in the younger patient population. Risk factors for stroke are listed in Table 16.2.

Table 16.2. Stroke Risk Factors

Major
    Age
    Cardiac impairment
    Diabetes mellitus
    Hypertension
    Previous stroke, TIAs
Minimal
    Behavioral factors
    Caffeine
    Cigarette smoking
    Obesity
    Sedentary life-style

For the purposes of this chapter, the stroke rehabilitation candidate will be considered as having experienced a middle cerebral artery infarction, with typical deficits of contralateral upper and lower limb paralysis.

The poststroke patient's diagnosis should be documented as, for example, left hemiplegia, secondary to right cerebrovascular accident, thrombotic, on specific date. Such a designation provides for a functional, etiologic, and time-related diagnosis.

Based on the patient's initial physical examination, early predictions of functional abilities can be made. Typically, poststroke patients may be areflexic for up to 48 hours. According to Twitchell (19), patients who then become hyperreflexic are likely to experience continued recovery. Those who remain flaccid without reflex or voluntary muscular recovery of the affected limb for a prolonged period of time have less chance of recovery. However, this study was not confined to patients above age 65 years, and was completed prior to the use of computed tomography (CT) scans and magnetic resonance imaging (MRIs) for diagnosis of stroke.

Many articles indicate that recovery from stroke is complete at 6 months. It is now recognized that clinically apparent recovery of muscular function and changes in tone occur for a period of at least 2 years following stroke. Physiologic recovery may require even more time. In the past, large numbers of patients simply were not routinely followed over prolonged periods in order to document clinical changes.

Unfortunately, Medicare reimbursement for poststroke rehabilitative care, both inpatient and outpatient, is linked to time of stroke onset, rather than specific diagnosis or rate of recovery. Therefore, patients who continue to make functional gains over prolonged periods may not have financial resources for continued therapy.

REHABILITATIVE CARE IMMEDIATELY POSTSTROKE

Acute hospitalization with enforced bedrest and superimposed illness can severely affect the elderly patient's strength (20), and create additional functional impairment (21). From the onset of stroke, the geriatric patient should receive careful preventive nursing and medical care. Comorbidity typically includes coronary artery disease, hypertension, peripheral artery disease (noncerebral), prior cerebrovascular disease, and diabetes mellitus. Blood pressure should be stabilized. Other potential medical problems should be documented and addressed as frequently as necessary (22). Careful positioning of paralyzed limbs minimizes skin problems; the patient may not be able to self-monitor position. Passive range of motion of affected joints is performed twice a day. As soon as possible, the patient should be sitting up out of bed with assistance. Frequent physical assessments should include documentation of muscular strength and tone of the affected extremities. Nutritional aspects, particularly with respect to possible swallowing problems, should be addressed. Communication issues such as use of language and auditory acuity are important considerations. Bladder and bowel incontinence may result from lack of communication, presence of bilateral hemispheric lesions, or from problems proceeding the stroke.

TYPICAL REHABILITATION CARE

The geriatric patient in acute rehabilitation must be physically able to tolerate twice daily sessions of PT, OT, and speech, if communication is impaired. Treatment occurs in therapy departments, where appropriate equipment such as parallel bars, standing frames, and mats are available. There is usually a kitchen facility in addition to areas for practicing ADLs such as dressing and bathing.

The patient is first taught mobility on the mat, learning to roll from side to side, to sit up, and to perform transfers from mat to wheelchair. Both static and dynamic sitting balance is practiced. Pregait activities include sit-to-stand exercises, balance, and weight shifting in the parallel bars. Left hemiplegics, due to lack of attention span, may require a quiet, isolated therapy area. Mirrors may be helpful. Right hemiplegics with communication problems will benefit from the use of gestures, tactile cues, and observation of other patients practicing skills, rather than verbal instructions (1).

Short and long-term rehabilitation goals addressing the areas of mobility, ADLs, and communication are formulated for all patients after initial evaluations are completed. The patient is expected to formulate goals as well. These goals form the basis of the team meetings, usually held weekly, to document multidisciplinary progress and formulate new goals.

Family members are encouraged to participate in therapy sessions to receive feedback on the patient's abilities as well as to learn care skills. Questions about care and activities are directed to the appropriate team member. A therapeutic home evaluation allows the patient and family to practice newly acquired skills and assess potential problem areas for further work.

Independence in mobility is addressed through bed mobility, transfers, usually standing-pivot, and ambulation with assistive devices. The patient who does not yet have enough hip strength to ambulate may be prescribed a hemiplegic wheelchair. Such a chair is typically 2 inches lower than a standard wheelchair, so that the patient may use the unaffected foot for propulsion and the unaffected arm for steering. The typical wheelchair prescription is shown in Figure 16.2.

Over time, as the patient experiences muscular recovery of the affected leg, ambulation may be possible. Assistive devices, in order of increasing independence, include hemi-walkers or pyramid canes, wide-based quadcanes, narrow-based quadcanes, and straight canes. Typically, due to poor voluntary muscular function of the affected upper limb, the gait device will be held only in the uninvolved limb. Therefore, a standard or rolling walker is not usually appropriate for a geriatric hemiplegic patient.

Return of muscular function poststroke occurs proximally to distally. The patient may have enough hip and quadriceps muscular function to stand and attempt ambulation. However, because the anterior tibialis has not yet recovered, the patient experiences foot drop. This can be corrected by the use of a plastic leg brace, known as an ankle-foot orthosis (AFO). Inexpensive off-the-shelf models are available. When more medial-lateral ankle stability is required, a custom AFO can be fabricated. If the patient experiences genu recurvatum of the affected knee, the custom AFO can be set into 5 degrees of dorsiflexion. Use of plastic orthotic devices has virtually replaced the use of short metal braces, except in specific spasticity cases (23). Lower limb orthotic devices are reimbursed by Medicare as durable medical equipment. (Refer to Chapter 14 for further information on orthotic devices.)

The affected upper limb is at risk of dependent edema, shoulder subluxation, and injury (24, 25). A sling may assist in reduction of subluxation and protection of the limb. However, it should only be worn when transferring, standing, or ambulating to prevent enhancement of increasing flexor tone. Other devices for shoulder and arm support include a wheelchair lap board with elbow pad, elevated foam pads, arm troughs, overhead slings (rarely used), and pillows. Use of overhead trapeze for bed mobility is discouraged, as it may create muscular shoulder injury in the uninvolved upper limb. The affected hand may be positioned in a resting wrist-hand orthosis (WHO) or a tone inhibitive splint, depending upon need.

Shoulder-hand syndrome, a type of reflex sympathetic dystrophy, may occur in the affected upper limb. Prevention, through careful position and vigorous passive range of motion, is the best treatment (26–28).

Transfers to bedside commode should be practiced in therapy and performed on the nursing unit. The patient should be encouraged to do as much as possible both independently and safely. Bedpans, which are difficult to use, cause skin breakdown, and reinforce the acute sick role, should be avoided. Diapers should be used only for limited time periods in situations in which incontinence may prevent completion of therapies. Timed voiding may be helpful.

Long-term use of a hospital bed at home, either manual or electric, is usually not necessary. Such a bed may impede bed to wheelchair transfers because of its height. (Refer to Chapter 38 in this text for further equipment information.)

Although bowel and bladder complaints are frequent after stroke, unilateral stroke should not neurologically affect bowel or bladder function since there is bilateral innervation. There should be no need for a bowel retraining program after stroke; however, dietary changes, lack of privacy, and lack of access to laxatives may result in constipation. Tube feedings may result in diarrhea. Fecal impaction may also cause diarrhea; manual inspection and removal of the impaction, by enemas or manually, is necessary. In all bowel problems, causes should be identified and corrected if possible; the focus should remain on functional ability and not bowel habits.

Almost all patients have an indwelling urinary catheter placed during the time of acute stroke management. Therefore, they will be candidates for urinary tract infections (UTIs). Upon admission to rehabilitation, the possibility of a UTI should be ruled out. All UTIs, even if asymptomatic, should be treated in the geriatric stroke patient unless there is a chronic urologic problem. Incontinence of urine is usually considered a problem of awareness, mobility, and communication in the poststroke geriatric patient (29–31). Use of adult diapers should be discouraged. Males can use condom catheters with leg bags, if necessary. Timed voiding immediately upon awakening, every 2 hours during the day, and immediately prior to sleeping should decrease urinary incontinence.

Lightweight hemiplegic wheelchair with removable desk arms, detachable swing away footrests.

Diagnosis - hemiplegia secondary to cerebrovascular accident.

Length of need - indefinite.

This equipment is medically necessary.

Figure 16.2. Wheelchair prescription.

Table 16.3. Characteristics of Right and Left Hemiplegics[a]

Right Hemiplegic (Left Brain Injured)	Left Hemiplegic (Right Brain Injured)
Communication impairment	Visual/motor perceptual problems; left side neglect
Learns from demonstration	Loss of visual/spatial memory
Can learn from mistakes	Overestimates his/her abilities; impulsive
May require supervision due to communication problems	Requires supervision due to lack of insight/judgment; denies disabilities

[a]From Garrison SJ. Learning after stroke: left versus right brain injury. *Top Geriatr Rehabil.* 6:45–52, 1991. With permission.

COGNITIVE ASPECTS

Left versus Right Hemiplegics

Comparisons of left and right hemiplegics' behavior is as in Table 16.3 (1). Left hemiplegic patients generally have visuospatial problems and lack insight and judgment. Safety is an issue; falls are frequent. Right hemiplegics have difficulty with communication, but can learn from visual cues and practice.

There is controversy about treating hemiplegics based on intact or impaired brain function. Shah et al (32) advocate a lateralized stroke program, in which intact functions of the affected hemisphere and the unimpaired hemisphere are used. Dombovy et al (33), however, feel that this promotes learned nonuse of the involved limbs and that more attempts should be made to access and retrain neuronal circuitry in the involved hemisphere. The best way to treat the geriatric patient would involve the most expedient method using all intact learning abilities. Patients who are illiterate, do not speak the language of the therapists, and have not been in a student situation in over 50 or 60 years may have difficulty when attempting to learn new material.

Multiinfarct Dementia

Patients who have had previous strokes or transient ischemic attacks (TIAs) account for 50% of all CVAs. When undergoing rehabilitation, these patients may demonstrate evidence of multiinfarct dementia (MID). MID is characterized by an abrupt onset with a stepwise, fluctuating course, often with sustained improvements (34). Diminished ability to learn may result from the short and long-term memory deficits common in MID patients (35). These patients must be evaluated on an individual basis with specific rehabilitation goals. Sometimes training the family or caregiver can best meet the patient's needs, rather than simply focusing on patient teaching.

Poststroke Depression

Poststroke depression is an increasingly recognized phenomenon. According to Robinson et al (36), whose studies are not confined to the over-age-65 population, the most likely candidate for poststroke depression is the left-frontotemporal impaired, at 2 to 4 months after stroke. It is likely that there is an interruption in a neuroclinical transmitter. This is true depression, differentiated from a temporary situational depressed mood over loss of health or function. The Dexamethasone Suppression Test (DST) has not been shown to be helpful in the diagnosis of poststroke depression (37). Table 16.4 lists typical general antidepressants for geriatric patients, as compiled by Bennett and Bienenfeld (38). Wade et al (39) advocate treatment with nortriptyline (Pamelor) 30 mg to 50 mg per day, which has less anticholinergic side effects than does amitriptyline (Elavil) and can be monitored by blood levels. Use of popular general antidepressants, such as fluoxetine hydrochloride (Prozac), should be avoided until appropriate geriatric trials are completed.

Other methods of treating poststroke depression include use of stimulants. Methylphenidate (Ritalin) has been evaluated as an alternative to antidepressants. Johnson et al (40), in a retrospective study of 10 geriatric stroke patients, found seven showed clinical improvement in mood and attention span while on methylphenidate. However, eight patients had a diagnosis of adjustment disorder with depressed mood; one had major depression, and one had major depression and anxiety disorder.

Although electroshock therapy (ECT) has been considered for geriatric depression, it has not been thoroughly evaluated in geriatric poststroke depression. ECT is very controversial. Loss of memory as a result of ECT may be too impairing during an acute rehabilitation experience (41).

STROKE COMPLICATIONS

Typical poststroke complications include repeat stroke, deep venous thrombosis with risk of pulmonary embolism, dysphagia with possible aspiration pneumonia, spasticity, seizures, shoulder-hand syndrome, and musculoskeletal injuries due to falls and/or use of assistive equipment. Typical comorbidity in the geriatric stroke population, such as coronary artery disease, hypertension, noncerebral peripheral artery disease, prior cerebrovascular disease, and diabetes mellitus, has already been cited. Other problems prevalent in the geriatric stroke population include decreased visual and auditory acuity, polypharmacy, poor nutritional status, osteoarthritis, impaired skin integrity, and psychiatric illness. Each problem will be discussed here in detail.

Table 16.4. Antidepressants for Treatment in Geriatric Patients[a]

Drug	Anticholinergic Side Effects	Hypotension	Sedation	Potential to Alter Cardiac Rate & Rhythm	Adult Dose (mg/d)	Geriatric Dose (mg/d)
Tertiary amines						
Amitriptyline Elavil Endep	+ + +[b]	+ +[b]	+ + + to + + + +[b]	+ + +	75–300	30–100
Imipramine Tofranil	+ + to + + +	+ +	+[b]	+ +	75–300	30–100
Doxepin Adapin Sinequan	+ + +	+ +	+ + to + + +	+ +	75–300	30–150
Trimipramine Surmontil	+ +	+ +	+ + +	+ + +	75–300	50–100
Secondary amines						
Nortriptyline Pamelor	+ +	+	+	+	50–150	30–50
Desipramine Pertofrane Norapramin	+	+ to + +	+	+	75–300	50–150
Amoxapine Asendin	+	+ +	+	+ +	200–600	25–100
Protriptyline Vivactil	+ +	+ +	+	+ +	15–60	15
Maprotiline Ludiomil	+ + to + + +	+ +	+ + to + + +	+	150–300	50–100
Atypical						
Trazodone Desyrel	+	+ +	+ +	+ to + +	200–600	50–150

[a]From Bennett JA, Bienenfeld DG. Antidepressant drug therapy for geriatric patients. *J Pract Nurs.* 39:42–51, 1989. With permission.
[b]+ + + + = very strong; + + + = strong; + + = moderate; + = mild.

General Medical

The geriatric patient is at risk for all medical complications present prior to the stroke. The medical model of diagnosis does not accurately define presentation of acute illness in the elderly. Besdine (42) has listed behavioral manifestations of disease that he terms Functional Presentations. Refer to Table 16.5

In many instances, the geriatric patient's complaints may not fit the traditional medical model. Fried et al (43) have identified four new diagnostic models: the Synergistic Morbidity, the Attribution and the Facilitating Complaint, The Causal Chain, and the Unmasking Event. Awareness and utilization of these models can help assure more timely and accurate diagnoses of medical illness in the elderly stroke patient.

Repeat Stroke

Repeat stroke is common; the body has already demonstrated its susceptibility to conditions that result in stroke. Approximately 50% of all stroke and TIAs are sustained by patients with previous stroke. Hypertension should be carefully controlled. Patients who have had embolic stroke should undergo a thorough cardiovascular examination and begin lifetime anticoagulant

Table 16.5. Besdine's Functional Presentations of Disease[a]

Nonspecific disabilities signaling onset of acute illness:
- Acute confusion
- Dizziness
- Failure to thrive
- Falling
- New onset or worsening of dementia
- Stopping eating or drinking
- Urinary incontinence
- Weight loss

[a]Adapted from Besdine RM. The educational utility of comprehensive functional assessment in the elderly. *J Am Geriatr Soc.* 31:651–656, 1983.

therapy, usually with warfarin (Coumadin). Prevention of repeat thrombotic stroke is still treated medically by aspirin. Ticlopidine (Ticlid) has proven more efficacious than aspirin only in limited subsets of stroke patients (44–46). Dipyridamole (Persantine) is probably not effective in preventing stroke (47–49).

Deep Venous Thrombosis

Deep venous thrombosis (DVT) and subsequent pulmonary embolism pose a threat to the poststroke patient. Occurring in 20% to 50% of the affected (paralyzed) extremity, the diagnosis may be missed if there is not a high degree of suspicion. Continuous use of intermittent compression units is not feasible when patients must travel to therapy departments. Use of low-dose subcutaneous heparin (5,000 units daily) has been advocated (50). Further controlled studies are needed. When DVT is diagnosed, the patient should undergo initial intravenous anticoagulation with heparin, with conversion to oral warfarin by the third day. The affected extremity should be elevated and not vigorously ranged until the clot has organized, usually at about 3 days. Patients who develop subsequent DVTs while anticoagulated may require the placement of an inferior vena cava filter. Approximately 10% of adult stroke patients with DVT subsequently experience life-threatening pulmonary embolism; however, these figures have not been confirmed in the geriatric population (51).

Dysphagia

All stroke patients should be suspected of dysphagia until proven otherwise by a bedside swallowing evaluation by a trained professional. Typically, the speech pathologist or, in some settings, the occupational therapist or rehabilitation nurse will assess the patient's ability to swallow upon command and observe for obvious difficulties in the oral stage as well as for coughing. Patients who experience difficulty on bedside swallowing evaluations are assessed by a modified barium swallow, performed under fluoroscopy with the assistance of a therapist.

Dietary modifications, including exclusion of straws, thickening liquids, and use of appropriate food textures can allow the patient to eat by mouth while decreasing the risk of aspiration and risk of pneumonia. Each patient is individual; the psychosocial dynamics of food representing love and the pleasure of eating cannot be overemphasized. Patients and families must be educated and appropriate behaviors reinforced.

Enteral feedings are indicated for patients who cannot have anything by mouth due to poor coordination of the swallowing process. Typically, a percutaneous endoscopic gastrostomy tube is placed. Everyone must be educated in the patient's need to remain NPO. As recovery of the swallowing process, documented by repeat barium swallows, occurs, facilitative feeding may be started within guidelines set by the speech/swallowing therapist. Thermal stimulation, in which an iced mirror is used at the back of the oropharynx, aids in the recovery process in specific cases.

Spasticity

Increased tone in the affected extremities may progress to spasticity. There are no antispasticity medications, including diazepam (Valium), baclofen (Lioresal), and dantrolene (Dantrium), that selectively relax only the affected muscles. Diazepam, due to its central nervous system depressant effect, should not be used in the geriatric patient following stroke. Lioresal also has a central nervous depressant effect, even though its primary site of action is at the spinal cord. Dantrolene is a calcium channel blocker of skeletal muscle; it makes all muscle groups weak (52).

In selected cases, upper extremity spasticity may be decreased by custom-fabricated tone inhibitive orthoses, positioning, and stimulation of the extensors (flexor antagonists). Lower extremity spasticity may be diminished by positioning, use of AFOs with tone inhibitive sole plates, and stimulation of the flexors (extensor antagonists) (53). Rarely, local phenol blocks may be helpful. None of the orthopedic tendon lengthening procedures have been used widely in the geriatric stroke population. Medications are not used unless the spasticity causes pain or severely limits function, such as ambulation. When prescribed, medications should be used only sparingly in selected cases with constant vigilance for adverse side effects.

Seizures

Seizures occur in approximately 10% to 15% of all poststroke patients (54), more frequently after embolic than thrombotic stroke (55). There is currently no role for seizure prophylaxis in stroke. Phenytoin (Dilantin) remains the drug of choice. Recent studies have confirmed that phenytoin at therapeutic levels has no more adverse neuropsychologic effects than carbamazepine (Tegretol) (56).

Musculoskeletal and Peripheral Nerve Injuries

Geriatric patients are at risk for injury when moving about an unfamiliar environment cluttered with wheelchairs, walkers, and bedside commodes. The stroke patient, with altered balance, possible poor communication, and/or lack of insight and judgment can be injured by falls, overzealous handling by health personnel, and overuse of adaptive equipment. Overhead trapeze bars can cause shoulder injuries; the trapeze should be avoided and the patient taught mobility using the bedside rails. Any gait assistive device can cause peripheral nerve injury, particularly carpal tunnel syndrome. A stroke patient who recovers fine motor movements of the affected fingers prior to recovery of shoulder function should be evaluated for a possible brachial plexus injury (57).

Fractures from falls usually involve the appendicular skeleton. Gait belts, when applied too tightly, may result in nondisplaced rib fractures. Any injury will prolong the rehabilitation effort.

Auditory Acuity

Auditory problems may complicate the rehabilitation effort. Uhlmann et al (58) correlated hearing impairment and cognitive dysfunction in the elderly. In some settings, speech pathologists perform auditory screening evaluations on all geriatric rehabilitation patients. Those who need further evaluation should be followed by an audiologist. Recommendations for amplification should be discussed with the patient and family. An assistive listening device (ALD) or pocket talker, which has a microphone, volume control, and ear phone, can be used to selectively amplify speech in a noisy environment.

Visual Impairment

Particularly among rehabilitation patients over age 70 years, severe visual impairment (maximal corrected visual acuity greater than 20/200 but less than 20/70) is common (59). Prescription lenses should be evaluated and corrected if indicated. Glasses must be worn for therapies when vision is poor. Cataracts may also impair rehabilitative efforts.

Visual neglect is another problem area. Wade et al (39) studied 117 consecutive acute stroke admissions, finding that over the first 3 months nearly one fourth of all patients improved in visual neglect, and probable improvement in verbal recall and attention span was found in one fifth. There is some evidence that right hemiplegics who experience visual neglect, when compared to left hemiplegics with neglect, have a poorer functional outcome (60).

Polypharmacy

Due to comorbidity, many geriatric stroke patients are on several medications. These may include antihypertensives, antiarrhythmics, and hypoglycemics. Nonsteroidal antiinflammatory, pain, sedative-hypnotic, and/or antidepressant medications may also be a part of the drug profile. The potential for adverse drug interactions is great. The more medications and dosages, the higher the chance for interaction and noncompliance, through error or missed dosages (61). Amounts of sedatives-hypnotics should be tailored for the geriatric population and used sparingly, only when necessary (62).

Nutrition

Nutritional problems, suspected by history and clinical examination, are confirmed using laboratory data and input from dieticians. Poor dentition, lack of financial resources, poor memory, depression, long-standing chronic illness, and life-long food preferences often combine to result in inadequate caloric intake. Studies indicate that 10% to 50% of patients admitted to a general acute hospital have a history of alcohol abuse (63). This too contributes to a poor nutritional state. The patient who is malnourished cannot endure physical exercise and is at risk for poor wound healing and skin breakdown. Dysphagia as a cause of malnutrition has already been addressed. Constans (64) found that short-term hospitalization of elderly patients resulted in loss of lean body mass in as little as 15 days.

Osteoarthritis

Patients who have significant degenerative joint disease of the knees often experience an increase in arthritis-related pain on the unaffected lower limb, particularly the knee. This is probably due to increased weight bearing by the nonaffected side during standing-pivot transfers and ambulation. Recognition of the problem, use of nonsteroidal antiinflammatory medications, and specific activity limitations usually decrease pain. As muscle recovery occurs, balance improves, and there is less stress on the painful knee. If muscular recovery of the stroke affected limb is prolonged, the patient may eventually require a total knee replacement due to continued pain and deformity.

Skin Integrity

The geriatric patient is at risk for skin injury due to tissue fragility. This occurs as a result of the aging process, use of medications such as steroids, poor nutrition, and lack of independence in mobility. When a patient with fragile skin is repeatedly assisted in transfer activities, bruising and skin breakdown can occur. Devices such as bedpans, poorly-fitting wheelchairs, and orthotic devices can also cause problems. Other skin problems can result from dry skin, poor circulation, and drug reactions (65). Prevention is the best treatment, along with close observation for the potential development of skin problems.

Neuropsychiatric Problems

Cushman (66) reviewed 1493 cases of stroke; she found that the 101 cases with psychiatric diagnosis had greater length of stay than average. The four categories of psychiatric illness included dementia, organic brain syndrome with psychosis, organic brain syndrome with other changes, and reactive depression. Stroke patients with psychiatric illness, regardless of discharge disposition, stayed longer than those without psychiatric illness. The data suggest that the geriatric stroke population has a greater vulnerability to psychiatric illness; further studies are needed. Poststroke depression has been discussed previously in this chapter.

Patient and Family Education and Psychosocial Aspects of Stroke

The patient and family need education regarding stroke and rehabilitation from the time the stroke occurs. Often, patients and families are in denial about the stroke and subsequently experience stages of grieving over loss of function. The patient may feel guilty because he or she has experienced a stroke. Depression as related to stroke has already been discussed in this chapter. Issues regarding caregivers with respect to the spouse and/or children may severely impair rehabilitation attempts. Children with unresolved sibling rivalries, now in their 60's and 70's, may continue to fight as adults. These family members and patients need education, social services support, and psychologic or psychiatric intervention, if necessary. If the patient has severe communication problems, family members may find themselves in disagreement over health care decisions (67).

Evans et al (68) reviewed the literature about the effects of stroke and family functioning. They summarized the following: the family can have a great influence on recovery; families who are coping poorly are less compliant with treatment; although necessary, education alone does not assist in coping with stroke-related emotional and behavioral changes; and finally, families who need support groups often are unable to participate.

The physician and health care team should educate patients and families about stroke and recovery through the use of pamphlets (69–73), books (74), and videotapes (75–77). The American Heart Association (AHA) has a nationwide toll-free number (1-800-242-8721) as a service to professionals and the lay public for information on stroke and heart disease. The National Stroke Association also has educational materials, which may be obtained using their toll-free number (1-800-STROKES). Materials should be readily available, distributed, and discussed as often as possible with the patient and family.

SUMMARY

The practice of geriatric stroke rehabilitation is difficult. Elderly patients may be severely upset that they have sustained a stroke, or they may appear to be passive about their situation. Comorbidity increases with age. These patients and their caregivers require significant attention and support. The rehabilitation team may also need support in caring for patients and their families. The geriatric stroke patient will recover—each on an individual time basis; some over prolonged periods. Rehabilitation team members and family members should receive ongoing education so that these slow gains may not be overlooked. It is no longer acceptable to deny rehabilitation simply because of age, even though the patient may only live for weeks to months following stroke rehabilitation. At this time in our society, the right to rehabilitation has been legislated. Our patients are living to older and older ages. They deserve the time and encouragement to experience natural stroke recovery based on appropriate, well-researched medical support. Providing such care is the challenge they provide to us.

References

1. Garrison SJ. Learning after stroke: left versus right brain injury. *Top Geriatr Rehabil.* 6:45–52, 1991.
2. Jongblood L. Prediction of function after stroke: a critical review. *Stroke.* 17:765–776, 1986.
3. Feigenson JS, McCarthy ML, Greenberg SD, Feigenson WD. Factors influencing outcome and length of stay in a stroke rehabilitation unit. Part 2. Comparison of 318 screened and 248 unscreened patients. *Stroke.* 8:657–662, 1977.
4. Feigenson JS, McDowell FH, Meese P, McCarthy ML, Greenberg SD. Factors influencing outcome and length of stay in a stroke rehabilitation unit. Part 1. Analysis of 248 unscreened patients—medical and functional prognostic indicators. *Stroke.* 8:651–656, 1977.
5. Hesse KA, Campion EW. Motivating the geriatric patient for rehabilitation. *J Am Geriatr Soc.* 31:586–589, 1983.
6. Goodstein RK. Overview: cerebrovascular accident and the hospitalized elderly—a multidimensional clinical problem. *Am J Psychiatry.* 140:141–147, 1983.
7. Winograd CH, Gerety MB, Chung M, Goldstein MK, Dominguez F, Vallone R. Screening for frailty: criteria and predictors of outcomes. *J Am Geriatr Soc.* 39:778–784, 1991.
8. LaBan MM, Muzljakovich D, Perrin, JC. Improving the efficiency of patient selection for continuing rehabilitation in a general hospital: the stroke option rehabilitation team. A commentary. *Am J Phys Med Rehabil.* 71:55–56, 1992.
9. Rusin MJ. Stroke rehabilitation: a geropsychological perspective. *Arch Phys Med Rehabil.* 71:914–922, 1990.
10. Lehmann JF, DeLateur BJ, Fowler RS, et al. Stroke rehabilitation: outcome and prediction. *Arch Phys Med Rehabil.* 56:383–389, 1975.
11. Kelly-Hayes M, Wolf PA, Kannel WB, Sytkowski P, D'Agostino RB, Gresham GE. Factors influencing survival and need for institutionalization following stroke: the Framingham Study. *Arch Phys Med Rehabil.* 69:415–418, 1988.
12. Granger CV, Hamilton BB, Keith RA, Zielezny M, Sherwin FS. Advances in functional assessment for medical rehabilitation. *Top Geriatr Rehabil* 1 (3):59–74, 1986.
13. Hamilton BB, Granger CV, Sherwin FS, Zielezny M, Tashman JS. A uniform national data system for medical rehabilitation. In: Fuhrer MJ, ed. *Rehabilitation Outcomes: Analysis and Measurement.* Baltimore, Md: Brookes Publishing Company; 1987:137–147.
14. Task Force on Medical Rehabilitation and Research. United States Department of Health and Human Services. Presented at the National Institute of Health Meeting; July, 1990; Washington, DC.
15. SHEP Cooperative Research Group. Prevention of stroke by antihypertensive drug treatment in older persons with isolated systolic hypertension. Final results of the Systolic Hypertension in the Elderly Program (SHEP). *JAMA.* 265:3255–3264, 1991.
16. Kuller LH. Incidence rates of stroke in the eighties: the end of the decline in stroke? *Stroke.* 20:841–843, 1989.
17. McGovern PG, Burke GL, Sprafka JM, Xue S, Folsom AR, Blackburn H. Trends in mortality, morbidity, and risk factor levels for stroke from 1960 through 1990. The Minnesota Heart Survey. *JAMA.* 268:753–759, 1992.
18. Woo J, Lau E, Kay R. Elderly subjects aged 70 years and above have different risk factors for ischemic and hemorrhagic strokes compared to younger subjects. *J Am Geriatr Soc.* 40:124–129, 1992.
19. Twitchell TE. The restoration of motor function following hemiplegia. *Brain.* 74:443–480, 1951.

20. Hoenig HM, Rubenstein LZ. Hospital-associated deconditioning and dysfunction. *J Am Geriatr Soc.* 39:220–222, 1991.
21. Hirsch CH, Sommers L, Olsen A, Mullen L, Winograd CH. The natural history of functional morbidity in hospitalized older patients. *J Am Geriatr Soc.* 38:1296–1303, 1990.
22. Goldberg G, Berger GG. Secondary prevention in stroke: a primary rehabilitation concern. *Arch Phys Med Rehabil.* 69:32–40, 1988.
23. Ofir R, Heiner S. Orthoses and ambulation in hemiplegia: ten year retrospective study. *Arch Phys Med Rehabil.* 61:216–220, 1980.
24. Calliet R. *The Shoulder in Hemiplegia.* Philadelphia, Pa: F. A. Davis; 1980.
25. Hurd MM, Farrell KH, Waylonis GW. Shoulder sling for hemiplegia: friend or foe? *Arch Phys Med Rehabil.* 55:519–522, 1974.
26. Garrison SJ, Rolak LA. Rehabilitation of the stroke patient. In: DeLisa JA, Currie D, Gans B, Leonard JA, McPhee M, eds. *Principles and Practice of Rehabilitation Medicine.* 2nd ed. Philadelphia, Pa: J. B. Lippencott; 1993.
27. Tepperman PS, Greyson ND, Hilbert L, Jimenez J, Williams JI. Reflex sympathetic dystrophy in hemiplegia. *Arch Phys Med Rehabil.* 65:442–447, 1984.
28. Davis SW, Petrillo CR, Eichberg RD, Chu DS. Shoulder-hand syndrome in a hemiplegic population: a 5-year retrospective study. *Arch Phys Med Rehabil.* 58:353–356, 1977.
29. Borrie MJ, Campbell AJ, Caradoc-Davie TH, Spears GF. Urinary incontinence after stroke: a prospective study. *Age Aging.* 15:177–181, 1986.
30. Brockelhurst JC, Andrews K, Richards B, Laycock PJ. Incidence and correlates of incontinence in stroke patients. *J Am Geriatr Soc.* 33:540–542, 1985.
31. Khan Z, Hertanu J, Yang W, Melman A, Leiter E. Predictive correlation of urodynamic dysfunction and brain injury after cerebrovascular accident. *J Urol.* 128:86–88, 1981.
32. Shah M, Avidan R, Sine RD. Self-care training: hemiplegia, lateralized stroke program, Parkinsonism, arthritis, and spinal cord dysfunction. In: Sine RD, Liss SE, Roush RE, Holcomb JD, Wilson G, eds. *Basic Rehabilitation Techniques.* Rockville, Md: Aspen Publishers; 1988.
33. Dombovy ML, Bach-y-Rita P. Clinical observations on recovery from stroke. *Adv Neurol.* 47:265–276, 1988.
34. Duthie EH Jr, Glatt SL. Understanding and treating multi-infarct dementia. *Clin Geriatr Med.* 4:749–766, 1988.
35. Schuman JE, Beattie EJ, Steed DA, Merry GM, Kraus AS. Geriatric patients with and without intellectual dysfunction: effectiveness of a standard rehabilitation program. *Arch Phys Med Rehabil.* 62:612–618, 1981.
36. Robinson RG, Jubos KL, Starr LB, Rao K, Price TR. Mood disorders in stroke patients: importance of location of lesion. *Brain.* 107:81–93, 1984.
37. Grober SE, Gordon WA, Sliwinski MJ, Hibbard MR, Aletta EG, Paddison PL. Utility of the dexamethasone suppression test in the diagnosis of post-stroke depression. *Arch Phys Med Rehabil* 72:1076–1079, 1991.
38. Bennett JA, Bienenfeld DG. Antidepressant drug therapy for geriatric patients. *J Pract Nurs.* 39:42–51, 1989.
39. Wade DT, Wood VA, Hewer RL. Recovery of cognitive function soon after stroke: a study of visual neglect, attention span and verbal recall. *J Neurol Neurosurg Psychiatry.* 51:10–13, 1988.
49. Johnson ML, Roberts MD, Ross AR, Witten CM. Methylphenidate in stroke patients with depression. *Am J Phys Med Rehabil.* 71:239–241, 1992.
41. Murray GB, Shea V, Conn MB. Electroconvulsive therapy for post-stroke depression. *J Clin Psychiatry.* 47:258–260, 1986.
42. Besdine RW. The educational utility of comprehensive functional assessment in the elderly. *J Am Geriatr Soc.* 31:651–656, 1983.
43. Fried LP, Storer DJ, King DE, Lodder D. Diagnosis of illness presentation in the elderly. *J Am Geriatr Soc.* 39:117–123, 1991.
44. Gent M, Blakely JA, Easton JD, et al. The Canadian American ticlopidine study (CATS) in thromboembolic stroke. Design, organization, and baseline results. *Stroke.* 19:1203–1210, 1988.
45. Hass WK, Easton JD, Adams HP, et al. A randomized trial comparing ticlopidine hydrochloride with aspirin for the prevention of stroke in high-risk patient. *N Engl J Med.* 321:501–507, 1989.
46. Gent M, Blakely JA, Easton JD, et al. The Canadian American ticlopidine study (CATS) in thromboembolic stroke. *Lancet.* 1(8649):1215–1220, 1989.
47. Bousser MG, Eschwege E, Haguenau M, et al. "AICLA" controlled trial of aspirin and dipyridamole in the secondary prevention of athero-thrombotic cerebral ischemia. *Stroke.* 14:5–14, 1983.
48. Canadian Cooperative Study Group. A randomized trial of aspirin and sulfinpyrazone in threatened stroke. *N Engl J Med.* 299:53–59, 1978.
49. American-Canadian Cooperative Study Group. Persantine aspirin trial in cerebral ischemia: II. End point results. *Stroke.* 16:406, 1985.
50. Hirsh J. Heparin. *N Engl J Med.* 324(22):1565–1574, 1991.
51. Warlow C, Ogston D, Douglas AS. Deep venous thrombosis of the legs after strokes. *Br Med J.* 1:1178–1183, 1976.
52. Young RR, Delwaide PJ. Drug therapy spasticity: parts I and II. *N Engl J Med.* 40:124–129, 1981.
53. Katz RT. Management of spastic hypertonia after stroke. *J Neuro Rehab.* 5:S5–S11, 1991.
54. Moskowitz E. Complications in the rehabilitation of hemiplegic patients. *Med Clin North Am.* 53:541–558, 1969.
55. Buonanno F, Toole JF. Management of patients with established ("completed") cerebral infarction. *Stroke.* 12:7–16, 1981.
56. Dodrill CB, Troupin AS. Neuropsychological effects of carbamazepine and phenytoin: a reanalysis. *Neurology.* 41:141–143, 1991.
57. Kaplan PE, Meredith J, Taft G, Betts H. Stroke and brachial plexus injury: a difficult problem. *Arch Phys Med Rehabil.* 58:15–18, 1977.
58. Uhlmann RF, Larson EB, Rees TS, Koepsell TD, Duckert LG. Relationship of hearing impairment to dementia and cognitive dysfunction in older adults. *JAMA.* 261:1916–1919, 1989.
59. Wainapel SF, Kwon YS, Fazzari PJ. Severe visual impairment on a rehabilitation unit: incidence and implications. *Arch Phys Med Rehabil.* 70:439–441, 1989.
60. Egelko S, Simon D, Riley E, Gordon W, Ruckdeschel-Hibbard M, Diller L. First year after stroke: tracking cognitive and affective deficits. *Arch Phys Med Rehabil.* 70:297–302, 1989.
61. Hussar DA. Drug interactions in the older patient. *Geriatrics.* 43:20–30, 1988.
62. Allen RM. Tranquilizers and sedative/hypnotics: appropriate use in the elderly. *Geriatrics.* 41:75–88, 1986.
63. Moore RD, Bone LR, Geller G, Mamon JA, Stokes EJ, Levine DM. Prevalence, detection, and treatment of alcoholism in hospitalized patients. *JAMA.* 261:403–407, 1989.
64. Constans T, Bacq Y, Brechot JF, Guilmot JL, Choutet P, Lamisse F. Protein-energy malnutrition in elderly medical patients. *J Am Geriatr Soc.* 40:263–268, 1992.
65. Walther RR, Harber LC. Expected skin complaints of the geriatric patient. *Geriatrics.* 39:67–80, 1984.
66. Cushman L. Secondary neuropsychiatric complications in stroke: implications for acute care. *Arch Phys Med Rehabil.* 69:877–879, 1988.
67. Molloy DW, Clarnette RM, Braun EA, Eisemann MR, Sneiderman B. Decision making in the incompetent elderly: "the daughter from California syndrome." *J Am Geriatr Soc.* 39:396–399, 1991.
68. Evans RL, Hendricks RD, Haselkorn JK, Bishop DS, Baldwin

D. The family's role in stroke rehabilitation: a review of the literature. *Am J Phys Med Rehabil.* 71:135–139, 1992.

69. *How Stroke Affects Behavior.* Dallas, Tex: American Heart Association; 1991.

70. *Proper Diet After Stroke.* Englewood, Colo: National Stroke Association; 1992.

71. *Recovering From a Stroke.* Dallas, Tex: American Heart Association; 1986.

72. *Strokes, A Guide for the Family.* Dallas, Tex: American Heart Association; 1989.

73. *Stroke: Reducing Your Risk.* Englewood, Colo: National Stroke Association; 1989.

74. Josephs A. *Stroke: An Owner's Manual: The Invaluable Guide to Life After Stroke.* Long Beach, Calif: Amadeus Press; 1992.

75. *Brain at Risk: Understanding and Preventing Stroke* (videotape). Englewood, Colo: National Stroke Association; 1990.

76. *The Healing Influence* (videotape). Santa Fe, NM: Danamar Productions; 1991.

77. *What is Aphasia* (videotape). Detroit, Mich: Lane State University Press; 1991.

17

Rehabilitation of Elderly Patients After Traumatic Brain Injury

Loren Fishman

From an epidemiologic and neuroanatomic viewpoint, traumatic brain injury (TBI) is special in the elderly. People over 74 years of age most closely approach the better-studied 15- to 29-year-old group with nearly three quarters of that group's incidence (30/10,000 vs 42/10,000) and nearly three quarters of that group's risk (1). A representative study found 15% to 16% of 2900 TBI admissions to be over 65 years of age (1). Yet, the contexts in which TBI arises are different, initiating different sequences of acute management, treatment, and outcome (Table 17.1).

EPIDEMIOLOGY AND ECONOMICS

The 15- to 29-year-old group of TBI victims is predominantly male (2), but in persons over 65 years of age, men and women are nearly equally affected (Table 17.2). Falling is the most common cause of TBI over 65 years of age (3); pedestrian accidents yield the most fatalities. Fifty percent to 60% of the mortality is associated with alcohol, especially in males (2, 4–7).

In the elderly, the severity of a traumatic event is frequently deepened by advancing medical or neurologic illness. These conditions may precipitate the event and affect its outcome, much as "risk taking" influences incidence and outcome in the young. In fact, premorbid status is most valuable as a guide in initial prognosis. See Table 17.3 (1, 8) for other factors important in predicting outcome from severe head injury.

Mortality is higher in the elderly (4, 9, 10), in spite of the fact that serious injury occurs as frequently among the young (Table 17.2). Yet, serious disability following TBI is equally likely at any age (1). The parity may be due to the fact that severely injured elderly are more likely to succumb to medical complications such as hospital-acquired pneumonia.

Table 17.2. Severity of Head Injury in Elderly and Younger Patients (n = 1020)

Category	65 Years and Over		Under 65 Years	
Severe	26	(6%)	79	(5%)
Moderate	46	(10%)	168	(11%)
Minor	377	(84%)	1324	(84%)
Total	499	(100%)	1571	(100%)
Male:female ratio	55:45		73:27	

From: Miller JD, Pentland B, Berrol S. Early evaluation and management. In: *Rehabilitation of the Adult and Child with Traumatic Brain Injury*. Philadelphia, Pa: F. A. Davis; 1990.

Table 17.3. Factors Important for Outcome From Severe Head Injury

Age
Motor response
Glasgow Coma Scale
Pupils
Eye movements
Presence of hematoma
Secondary insult
Intracranial pressure
Cerebral blood flow/metabolism
Brain electrical activity
Enzyme/chemical markers

From: Miller JD, Pentland B, Berrol S. Early evaluation and management. In: *Rehabilitation of the Adult and Child with Traumatic Brain Injury*. Philadelphia, Pa: F. A. Davis; 1990.

Table 17.1. Causes of Minor Head Injury in Elderly and in Younger Patients

Cause of Injury	65 Years and Over (n = 377)	Under 65 Years (n = 1324)
Domestic/fall	77%	34%
Vehicle occupant	5%	20%
Pedestrian	12%	8%
Assault	4%	26%
Sport/work	0%	12%

From: Miller JD, Pentland B, Berrol S. Early evaluation and management. In: *Rehabilitation of the Adult and Child with Traumatic Brain Injury*. Philadelphia, Pa: F. A. Davis; 1990.

Reemployment is not usually a goal in rehabilitation of elderly victims of TBI. Independence in activities of daily living, safe return to previous residence, and functional pursuit of social and avocational activities are core objectives in this age group.

Possibly because of these differences, there are differing views (11) on the economic consequences of TBI in the elderly. Three opinions characterize the literature:

1. Treatment of the elderly after TBI is proportionally more expensive and less successful than treatment of the young, as the elderly are proportionally more medically and functionally affected (2, 5, 12–14).
2. Both groups are the same ceteris paribus (7, 15, 16).
3. There is a parabolic relationship in which the most severely and minimally injured are equal regardless of age, but in the middle group the elderly take longer to regain "outpatient" status (17).

This chapter's premise is that enhanced understanding and skill in rehabilitating elderly TBI patients will improve clinical judgment and patient recovery, thereby reducing personal, social, and economic costs, and promoting our interests as healers, patients, and taxpayers. We will outline the pathophysics of TBI and the physiology of the aging brain, illustrating why TBI, in the elderly, is a somewhat distinct condition requiring ther-

apeutic modifications for proper care. We will focus on key aspects of acute management and on cognitive rehabilitation after TBI, which represents a true challenge: Can these often grievously injured individuals be nurtured and guided sufficiently to reenter a society that is sophisticated enough to have saved them?

PATHOPHYSICS

Woodpeckers and billygoats routinely sustain head trauma of a magnitude that would cause severe injury to the human central nervous system (18). Static pressure in humans, even enough to fracture the skull, produces no cognitive sequelae (19). The degree of neurologic injury appears to correlate well with acute acceleration and is connected more closely with the physics of head trauma than with the structural anatomy.

The diameter of the human rostral cortex is more than 10 times that of the medullary, pontine, and mesencephalic brainstem (Fig. 17.1). As volume varies with the cube of diameter, mass is correlated with volume, and assuming a relatively constant density, the ratio of the mass of the cortex to the mass of the brainstem is greater than 1,000 to 1. Tensile strength varies with the square of a linear dimension like diameter, with cross-sectional area, yielding a ratio closer to 100 to 1.

Structural Anatomy

The tentorial membrane has a stabilizing influence, holding the cerebellum in place during the forward, backward, or lateral concussive moments of head injury (Fig. 17.1). Cerebellar connections through the peduncles, the paramedian and lateral reticular nuclei, and the nucleus reticularis tegmenti pontis of Bechterow also sustain the midbrain and brainstem, while the more voluminous rostral structures move with greater freedom beyond these points of tether.

Additionally, the structure of the cervical vertebrae maximizes mobility. Following abrupt changes in speed, this "ball and chain" arrangement develops grossly disparate velocities in the more rostral versus the more caudal parts of the brain. Mass times velocity equals momentum. The mass of the freely and more rapidly moving telencephalon and diencephalon is 1000 times greater than the midbrain and medulla, while the tensile strength of the relatively stationary midbrain and medulla is 100 times less able to withstand such tensile stress (Fig. 17.1). Grossly, then, tracts of the midbrain and brainstem are more than 100,000 times as vulnerable to the tremendous forces generated by abrupt acceleration, resulting in diffuse axonal injury in them.

Functional Anatomy

The reticular formation comprises the medial two thirds of the brain stem. This region contains longitu-

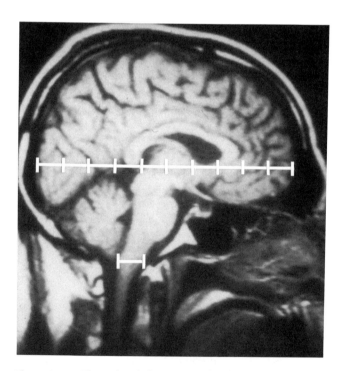

Figure 17.1. The ratio of diameters (and radii) of human rostral cortex to brainstem is greater than 10 to 1. The volumetric ratio is greater than 1000 to 1. The tentorial membrane and midbrain-cerebellar connections concentrate tensile forces and shear at the distal midbrain, pons, and medulla.

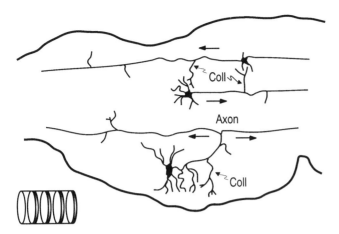

Figure 17.2. Ascending and descending fibers have multiple collateral synapses in the medullary and pontine reticular formation, (coll.) likely to modulate reception and response patterns at "higher" levels. Adapted from Scheibel ME, Scheibel AB. Structural substrates of integrative patterns in the brainstem reticular core. In: Jasper HH, Proctor LD, et al, eds. *Reticular Formation of the Brain.* Henry Ford Hospital Symposium. Boston, Mass: Little, Brown; 1958. With permission of the publisher.

dinal cells with long perpendicular branches, displaying the segmental kind of distribution common to interneurons of the spinal cord (Fig. 17.2). Facilitatory and inhibitory projections from this region are distributed throughout the cortex. Medullary, pontine, and cerebellar nuclei are critical to effective intellectual processes and smooth motor output. Breaks and disruptions here destroy the coordinating integration of cortical activity by means of the brainstem. The idea of cerebral control through brain stem influence was validated first by Morruzzi and Magoun (19) and since has been supported by investigations of Mountcastle and Powell (20), Pompeiano, (21) Ajmone (22), and others (23).

Applied Gerontology

The above describes the picture for TBI victims of any age. Once involved, older people are at risk for greater injury due to neurophysiologic and histologic developments occurring after age 50 years (1, 3, 24, 25). Calcification and thickening of the meninges increase brittleness in tissue supporting the vascular supply to the older brain (25–28), lowering its tolerance to shearing and tensile forces. Chronologically progressive and irreversible loss of posterior tract neurons (24), as well as smaller losses in other spinal tracts, and a 10% to 20% loss of cortical volume accompany a 7% to 10% actual loss of cortical neurons. This serves to increase the density of the rostral brain and widen the space in which velocity and hence momentum can grow in the relatively unchanged dimensions of the intracranial vault.

Age-related changes in the pathogenesis of TBI can be summarized as follows. Greater momentum is developed by a denser cerebrum accelerating over a greater

distance within the skull. Reduced axonal and other support below the diencephalon, especially in the more distal, less mobile brainstem, renders this region, easily the most vulnerable at any age, even more susceptible to diffuse axonal injury. Tracts traversing this locale are essential to effectively integrating more rostral brain functions. In addition, brittleness of the vascular supply and adhesions in the leptomeninges increase with age. It is not surprising then that acute and chronic subdural hematomas and other intracranial hemorrhages dominate the pathology following TBI in the elderly (3, 4, 27, 29, 30). Intracranial hemorrhage is more prevalent in the elderly even without regard to skull fracture, with which it is closely correlated in the young (31). Ocular damage is more common in elderly TBI than in any other type of central nervous system injury (32). This may be a coup-contracoup phenomenon, exacerbated by the increased momentum and brittleness of the aging brain. Still, the concept of diffuse axonal injury and its sequelae is keenly relevant in this group of patients.

ACUTE CHANGES FOLLOWING TBI IN THE ELDERLY

Overview

The physiatrist is somewhat likely to encounter acute changes, both because of the gradual development of some of the vascular and endocrine complications in the weeks following TBI and because of the possibility of additional falls—the most common cause of such injuries in the elderly—in the rehabilitation gym. By far the most serious complications in the first hour following brain injury involve cardiovascular reflexes and the airways (33).

Applied Gerontology

Cerebral function is estimated to require a little less than 40 mL of blood per min per 100 g of tissue (24). The average young adult supplies 50 mL to 60 mL per min per hundred g of cerebral tissue (24). An age-related 20% decrease between ages 30 years and 70 years, with proportionately reduced perfusion (34), exposes the older brain-injured patient to significant risks. In contrast, some authors state that glucose utilization is well-maintained in the elderly, and flexible O_2 consumption can increase arteriovenous O_2 differences to make up some of the gaps (24, 27, 34, 35).

Naturally, there may be other relevant impairments, such as dysrrhythmias, anemia, or emphysema. One study found that 40% of elderly patients presenting after TBI had undiagnosed concurrent conditions (1). Forty percent of elderly patients involved in minor TBI were significantly less mobile 6 weeks later. Over 16% were unable to return home (1). A chest radiogram, electrocardiogram, blood count, and serum glucose are sensible in every elderly TBI victim (1), along with a physical examination and at least the minimental status examination (33).

Earliest Clinical Course

Coma often begins immediately after moderate or severe head injury. The reflexes are depressed, respiration becomes arrested; a transitory bradycardia and hypotension also occur almost at once (36).

First Findings

A pupil dilating immediately after TBI, with only consensual response to light, suggests a lacerated optic nerve, which may result from fracture of the sphenoid bone. In the immediate postevent context, cervical injury including Jefferson's fracture (a burst atlas often due to force applied at the vertex of the skull), Hangman's fracture (anterior subluxation with fractured pedicles of C-2, e.g., after the chin strikes a stair or steering wheel), teardrop fractures (anterior fragment from vertebral compression, often with injured ligaments and consequent cervical spinal instability), and atlantoaxial subluxation secondary to arthritic changes in the elderly must be sought (36). Age-related changes in the oropharynx, trachea, and thorax require the most deft and circumspect intubation and cardiopulmonary resuscitation (CPR) of which a team is capable. Tracheostomy has been noted to reduce mortality 50% in patients with decerebrate rigidity (25).

While a patient is being stabilized, attention alternates between assessment of damage from the TBI and avoidance of secondary injury due to cerebral hypoxia, brain swelling, or cardiorespiratory failure. There is a linear relationship between depth of coma and brainstem reflexes. These may supplement the Glasgow Coma Scale, if observed, in descending order: Glabellar tap, oculovestibular reflex (bilateral cold irrigation), pupillary light reflex, horizontal oculovestibular reflex (unilateral irrigation), and oculocardiac reflex (bradycardia with ocular pressure) (37). In the elderly, ophthalmologic surgery, changes in the utricle and saccule, progressive supranuclear palsy and Parkinsonism, medications, and pacemakers can complicate these reliable guides to patient status.

Early Clinical Observations

Battle's sign, postauricular bogginess, and hemorrhage form the external auditory meatus suggest an underlying fracture. Immediate posttraumatic deafness, with or without vestibular signs, may be due to a petrosal fracture. "Raccoon's eyes" suggest fracture in the anterior cranial fossa and intracerebral hemorrhage.

The nasal bones are the most frequently fractured facial bones; ecchymosis of the floor of the mouth often signals mandibular fracture, the second most common facial fracture.

Superficial laceration within a sinus with fracture and torn meninges may present with cerebrospinal fluid rhinorrhea. Hygroma and dissecting aneurism can also present early (18). Evidence of these conditions suggests neurosurgical consultation.

A state of shock rarely lasts after TBI (36); persistent shock may be caused by cervical cord injury, including central cord syndrome. Prevertebral swelling may be the only sign of cervical vertebral displacement when the patient is placed in a normal position for taking films. If the cause of TBI is more violent than a fall, intraperitoneal hemorrhage or other nonneurologic sources of shock may exist. Changes of sensorium, retinal and/or conjunctival punctate hemorrhages, a petecchial axillary rash, adult respiratory distress syndrome, and urinary fat may reflect fatty emboli from fracture sites. Pulmonary edema caused by pulmonary embolism is estimated to occur in 50% of patients with severe TBI, most frequently 48 hours postinjury (36).

Later Clinical Findings

In the slightly less acute context, the following signs strongly suggest acute subdural hematoma: ipsilateral Horner's sign, Hutchinson's pupil (ipsilateral dilating pupil), hemiparesis, monoparesis, or a "hypernormal" computed tomography (CT) or magnetic resonance imaging picture (MRI), lacking the usually exaggerated sulci and abbreviated gyri in an elderly patient. Swelling and increased pressure may artifactually inflate the cerebral mantle from within, giving imaging studies a spuriously youthful appearance.

Confusion, and exaggeration of certain personality traits can intensify as weeks turn into months, as a chronic subdural hematoma enlarges from the osmotic effects of hemolyzed blood and cleaved serum proteins. Burr holes or surgical evacuation are the treatment of choice (13); again, it is reported that age *itself* is not a factor in rehabilitation outcome (37, 38).

Serial CT or MRI are useful for diagnosis and prognosis: brainstem densities indicate future difficulties with attention and arousal; poor memory often follows swelling of the temporal lobes (1). However, the patient's medical condition and surgical hardware often prohibit MRI and may vitiate the clarity of CTs.

The length of time in a coma, augmented by the depth of coma (Table 17.4) is still a fairly reliable indicator of outcome (10, 29, 37, 39). These factors sum acute and chronic injury in their synergistic effects (13, 40). An exception is acute epidural hemorrhage caused by tear of the middle meningeal artery or vein. Less frequently, a dural tear in a venous sinus can cause the

Table 17.4. Assessment of Conscious Level (Glasgow Coma Scale) [a]

	Examiner's Test	Patient's Response	Assigned Score
Eye opening	Spontaneous	Opens eyes on own	E4
	Speech	Opens eyes when asked to in a loud voice	3
	Pain	Opens eyes upon pressure	2
	Pain	Does not open eyes	1
Best motor response	Commands	Follows simple commands	M6
	Pain	Pulls examiner's hand away upon pressure	5
	Pain	Pulls a part of body away upon pressure	4
	Pain	Flexes body inappropriately to pain (decorticate posturing)	3
	Pain	Body becomes rigid in an extended position upon pressure (decerebrate posturing)	2
	Pain	Has no motor response to pressure	1
Verbal response (talking)	Speech	Carries on a conversation correctly and tells examiner where he/she is, who he/she is, and the month and year	V5
	Speech	Seems confused or disoriented	4
	Speech	Talks so examiner can understand victim but makes no sense	3
	Speech	Makes sounds that examiner cannot understand	2
	Speech	Makes no noise	1

[a] Coma Score (E + M + V) = 3 to 15.
From: Miller JD, Pentland B, Berrol S. Early evaluation and management. In: *Rehabilitation of the Adult and Child with Traumatic Brain Injury*. Philadelphia, Pa: F. A. Davis; 1990.

characteristic "lucid interval." It may be as long as several days or a week and may or *may not* be preceded by brief coma (31). This possibility calls for close observation of the elderly patient after a seemingly inconsequential fall. There is evidence that MRI can detect hemorrhages unrecognized by CT or other means (1, 41). If an epidural hemorrhage is found, surgical results are excellent at any age and alternatives are dismal (12, 25, 35, 42).

Peripheral Nerve Injury

Olfactory, optic, oculomotor, auditory, and the anterior two thirds of the trigeminal nerve are frequently injured. Facial nerve injury may not become apparent for several days to a week. The reason for this delay is unknown (36). Still, the fact that facial palsy is frequently late in onset does not preclude the possibility of a later secondary or independent cause. Blink reflex studies may be useful at onset. The palsy is frequently limited to a few weeks.

In the days following TBI, weakness of the upper extremities, more than the lower extremities, without bowel or bladder involvement may reveal central cord syndrome. Intramedullary edema between C-5 and T-1 is the most frequent cause because of the spinal cord's thickening in this region (Fig. 17.3). However, peripheral nerve injury may also cause flaccid upper extremities without effects on bowel and bladder (43). The brachial plexus is most commonly injured (43).

Intracranial Pressure and Rehabilitation

If one separates primary effects and later developments after TBI, then hypoxia in the first hours and pneumonia in the early days following hospitalization account for the greatest percentage of subsequent deaths in the elderly. Chest physical therapy must begin swiftly in the intensive care unit (ICU). Vibration and percussion, with massage and stretching of the auxiliary muscles of respiration, clear lung fields and reduce atelectasis. Postitional changes, including bed rotation, do not systematically affect intracranial pressure (ICP) (1).

Passive limb ranging in the ICU avoids contractures and reduces heterotopic ossification. It is also a powerful stimulus for spontaneous respiration. Postural drainage is valuable to reduce atelectasis, but may be more hazardous vis-a-vis ICP.

It is critical that the therapist be sensitive to ICP changes and the ominous presence of plateau waves (26 mm Hg to 60 mm Hg, lasting 1 to 10 min) and withhold therapy when they are present. Ropper (36) states that at least 50% of patients who die as a result of head injury do so solely because of uncontrolled rises in ICP.

Any of the diverse tissues making up the blood brain barrier may be the cause of increased ICP. If for any reason intracranial pressure should rise, cerebral perfusion pressure (CPP), mean blood pressure minus the intracranial pressure, can drop below 40 mm Hg to 60 mmHg a threateningly low level. Beyond the marginal cerebral blood flow in the elderly already reviewed, there

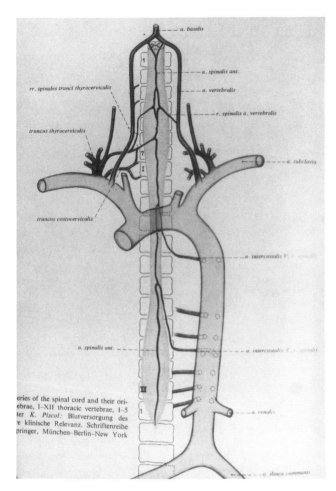

Figure 17.3. Thickening of the spinal cord occurs at C5-T1 and T10-L1, where the larger roots to the limbs are given off. The elderly cervical spine is at greater risk in TBI because of osteoarthritis, with cervical stenosis reducing bony clearance and compliance to edema still further; osteoporosis with supportive muscular weakness increasing vulnerability to fracture, and circulatory decline favoring ischemia. From Piscol K. Blutversorgung des Ruckenmarks und ihre Kleinische Relevanz. *Schriftenreihe Neurologie*, VIII. Berlin: Springer-Verlag; 1972. Copyright Springer-Verlag.

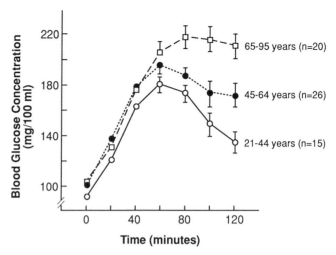

Figure 17.4. Elderly metabolic adjustment may require 4 hours . . . just in time for the next hospital meal. Reproduced, with permission, from Pozefsky T, Colkerm JL, et al. The cortisone-glucose tolerance test: the influence of age on performance. *Ann Intern Med.* 63:988–1000, 1965.

is further reduction of CPP in ventilator patients receiving positive end-expiratory pressure (PEEP).

For example, in a patient with ICP of 25 mm Hg and mean blood pressure of 100 mm Hg, the CPP, the actual effective gradient protecting the brain from ischemia, is 75 mm Hg. PEEP of 10 mm Hg lowers this closer to 65 mm Hg. If the patient is suctioned or receives painful ranging, the Cushing reflex may produce hypertensive bradycardia with mean blood pressure now near 140 mm Hg. At this precise moment, CPP rises towards 105 mm Hg. After a short time, however, greatly accelerated cerebral edema increases intracranial volume. This rapidly raises ICP, lowering CPP by the same amount. Essential measures to control the blood pressure will then disastrously reduce CPP.

Hyperventilation to reduce arterial PCO_2 from 30 mm Hg to 22.5 mm Hg is effective. The sedative gamma-hydroxybutyrate [European use (1)] reduces blood flow volume but not systolic blood pressure. In the United States, pulmonary arterial and capillary wedge pressure monitor hypovolemia in this situation. Here, prevention is more likely than cure.

Steroids are no longer universally used in cerebral edema. Their antiinsulinemic effects are heightened even in nondiabetic elderly (Fig. 17.4) and compounded by endocrine changes after TBI. One beneficial side effect of steroid-induced hyperglycemia is osmotic diuresis. Disadvantages include slowed wound healing, raised blood pressure (since greater insulin resistance raises insulin requirements), cecal hemorrhage, and ketotic or nonketotic coma. Increased levels of circulating steroids may reduce dendritic expansion after central nervous system injury (44) (Fig. 17.5).

Subacute medical care focuses on endocrine, electrolyte, and acid-base considerations (45). Recently, fludrocortisone has proven effective in the treatment of antidiuretic hormone (ADH) disturbances. Hypervolemic, hyponatremic, and hyperchloremic acidoses are common acid-base disturbances.

Cardiopulmonary Resuscitation

Excellent texts describe acute care of the traumatically brain injured (1, 34, 35). The preceding section only highlights aspects especially significant for elder TBI in the physiatric setting. The final issue regards resuscitation. On the one hand, CPR followed by surgery for acute bleeds may yield total recovery. Yet, medical pos-

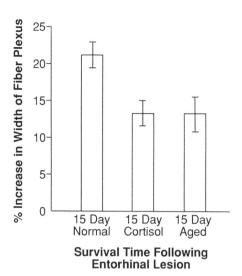

Figure 17.5. There is substantially less reactive growth with elevated blood steroid. This is curiously equal to the reduced plasticity seen in the elderly in this study. With permission of the publisher, from Cotman CW Scheff SW. Synaptic growth in aged animals. In: Cherkin A, et al, eds. *Physiology and Cell Biology of Aging.* New York, NY: Raven Press; 1979:118.

sibilities also include a long, unalterable terminal course. There is frequently no assurance of outcome in the early moments after a critical event.

Over 50% of survivors of cardiopulmonary resuscitation over 60 years of age supported the procedure on subsequent questioning. Yet, 42% were against the resuscitation. Older patients were much less positive towards the procedure after surviving a second resuscitation (34–36, 38, 41, 42, 46).

The outcome of CPR is a function of the patient's underlying disease processes and their severity and premorbid functional status. Delayed initiation or inadequate performance of CPR greatly increases the risk of brain damage in the successfully resuscitated. Safe limits of delay are reduced in the elderly for the many reasons already mentioned. Hypothermic patients and those under the influence of barbituates or alcohol can do better after delays greater than the classic 5 minutes, probably because of slowed metabolism. Individuals resuscitated after near drowning have done well after resuscitations lasting even several hours. The combination of hypothermia and excellent physical condition helps these persons. The same reasoning applies, mutatis mutandis, to the elderly.

Complications of CPR are generally mechanically associated and include rib fractures, collapsed lung, ruptured stomach, and broken teeth. While arguments can be made for or against the presence of "crash" carts in the physiatric gymnasium, older patients unquestionably deserve a staff skilled and ready to perform CPR.

APPLICATION OF PHYSICAL MEDICINE AND REHABILITATION DISCIPLINES TO THE TREATMENT OF OLDER INDIVIDUALS SUSTAINING BRAIN INJURY

In the acute and subacute phases following TBI, it is useful to distinguish lifesaving application of physical medicine and rehabilitation (PM&R) from life-improving aspects. For example, chest physical therapy prevents life-threatening pneumonia in severely injured older people, while maintaining joint mobility in the ICU may exponentially raise subsequent functional independence but is not in itself lifesaving. Well-informed physiatric judgment can mediate the interphases between Physical Therapy, Occupational Therapy, Speech Therapy, Dietary, and the life-sustaining applications of medical technology to patients. The earlier discussion of CPP and plateau waves illustrates this physiatric function.

Concerning functional aspects, perhaps the most formidable obstacle any therapist encounters in treating older victims of TBI is behavioral, presenting a parallel to what is seen in younger patients. The young may present with giddy, impulsive, Kluver-Bucy behavior (hyperphagia, hypersexuality, and dysinhibition) and inexhaustibly garbled speech. Elderly patients are more likely to become labile and childish, with "antisocial" passivity (46, 47), dependence, and grossly disruptive indecision. In rehabilitation, patient activity is generally preferable to passivity, yet inhibition of asocial behaviors is key to the orderly pursuit of societal, medical, and personal goals.

Exercises reviewed later concentrate on attention, memory, and perception, the three areas of largest deficit commonly seen after TBI (48). Work on these deficits is often called "Cognitive Rehabilitation." However, few concentrate on difficulties in the gray region where the patient's "inner life" interfaces with his or her behavior. Recently, Prigatano and Kaye, et al have begun this important work (47, 49–51).

In the elderly, behavioral difficulties may be addressed in a social and, if possible, familial context. Meaningful work on poststroke depression has been done by Hibbard et al and its efficacy assessed (52). In the post-TBI elderly, however, such behaviors do not always respond to discourse, and inclusion in a social group may presuppose exactly the level of inhibition for which treatment is sought.

Brilliant work of L'Hermitte (53, 54) examined utilization and imitation behaviors. Patients exhibiting environment-dependent behaviors generally have sustained frank damage to the tissues of the heteromodal association cortex (Fig. 17.6). However, if reticular formation structures are not intact and are unable to balance cerebral responsivity in their complex pattern of facilitation and inhibition, the same functional deficits may occur without any direct damage to the cortex itself.

Impulsivity makes up a large piece of organic and inorganic pathology in the DSM-3 classification (Tables 17.5 and 17.6). Impulsivity and childish behavior (47, 55, 56) add much to families' burden of care for the post-TBI elderly (14, 57, 58).

One treatment is pharmacologic, employing major tranquilizers, anxiolytics, lithium, and benzodiazepines (59). Monosialoganglioside GM-1 appears neurotrophic and neuritogenic (60, 61), but results of current studies with Alzheimer's disease are at best mixed. Apart from carbamazepine, which is less sedating than some antiseizure medications, currently utilized medicines may actually lead to disorientation and an iatrogenous rise in the contextually inappropriate behaviors that constitute impulsivity.

The practice of giving these medications may be viewed as the pharmacologic equivalent of the medieval bleeding of patients. This approach reduces *all* impulses through sedation and is not specific to the behaviors constituting impulsivity. What is needed is a working definition of impulsivity.

Logically, to be unimpulsive, a patient must (*a*) recognize the impulse to be inhibited, (*b*) want to inhibit it, and (*c*) be able to inhibit or resist it. Clinical contact and neuropsychologic assessment usually can determine whether, e.g., a patient with Kluver-Bucy syndrome does not *recognize* her antisocial impulses; recognizes them but does not *want* to suppress them, or recognizes them, wants to suppress them, but simply *cannot*.

Once the deficit has been identified, a host of exercises can be prescribed to "develop the inhibition muscles." If the problem is resisting an identifiable "bad impulse," the patient has to learn to selectively attend

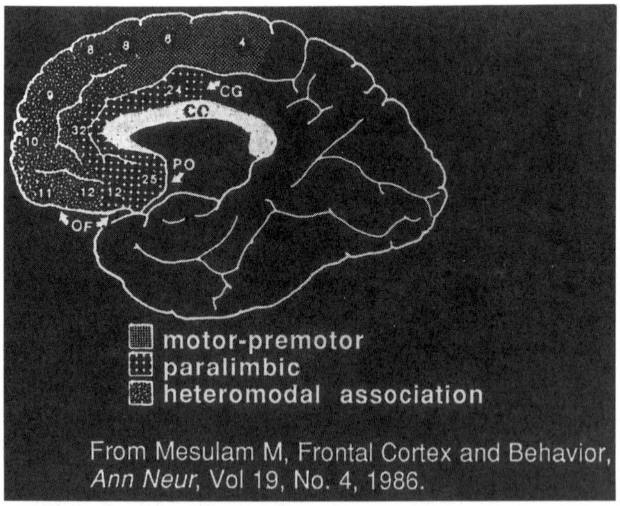

Table 17.5. Diagnostic Considerations in Pathologic Impulsivity in DSM-III Categories with Impulsivity[a] as Principal Diagnostic Feature

Disorders usually first evident in infancy, childhood, or adolescence
  Attention deficit disorder
  Oppositional disorder
  Stereotyped movement disorders (including tic disorders and
    Tourette's disorder)
  Childhood onset pervasive development disorder
Organic mental disorders
  Organic personality syndrome
  Alcohol idiosyncratic intoxication
  Substance-induced intoxication, delirium, or withdrawal
  Delirium (nonsubstance-induced)
Disorders of impulse control not elsewhere classified
  Pathologic gambling
  Kleptomania
  Pyromania
  Intermittent explosive disorder
  Isolated explosive disorder
  Atypical impulse control disorder
Personality disorders
  Histrionic
  Antisocial
  Borderline

[a]The amount of attention given impulsivity in DSM-3 is suggestive of the breadth and irrepressibility of this behavioral phenomenon.
From: Woodcock JA. A neuropsychiatric approach to impulse disorder. *Psych Clin North Am.* 9(2): 341–352, 1986.

Table 17.6. Diagnostic Considerations in Pathologic Impulsivity in DSM-III Categories with Impulsivity[a] as Common Association

Disorders usually first evident in infancy, childhood, or adolescence
  Mental retardation
  Conduct disorders
  Anorexia nervosa
  Bulimia
  Infantile autism
Organic mental disorders
  Dementia
  Organic delusional syndrome
  Organic hallucinosis
  Organic affective syndrome
Schizophrenic disorders, paranoid disorders, psychotic disorders not
  elsewhere classified
Affective disorders
Anxiety disorders
Psychosexual disorders
  Paraphilias
Personality disorders
Narcissistic disorders
Compulsive disorders

[a]The amount of attention given impulsivity in DSM-3 is suggestive of the breadth and irrepressibility of this behavioral phenomenon.
From: Woodcock JA. A neuropsychiatric approach to impulse disorder. *Psych Clin North Am.* 9(2): 341–352, 1986.

■ motor-premotor
▨ paralimbic
▧ heteromodal association

From Mesulam M, Frontal Cortex and Behavior, *Ann Neur*, Vol 19, No. 4, 1986.

Figure 17.6.   Impulsive behavior, including imitation and utilization behavior, may result from direct heteromodal cortical damage. Impulsive behavior also might be expected if lower centers facilitating and inhibiting the heteromodal cortex, e.g., in the brainstem, are dysfunctional. Reprinted, with permission of the publisher, from Mesulam M. Frontal cortex and behavior. *Ann Neurol.* 19(4):320–325, 1986.

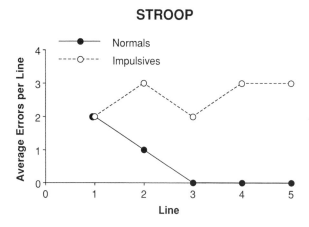

Figure 17.7. The Stroop consists of three visual presentations. In the first, the patient reads words for colors. There are five lines with a random distribution of the words "red," "blue," and "green." In the second presentation, dots of these colors are randomly distributed in the same five lines. In each of these, the patient starts at the upper left and reads across each row. In the third visual presentation, the color words are written in different colors. The patient must inhibit the urge to read the words (quite a strong urge) and instead name the colors the words are written in.

In the computerized version, each visual presentation is randomized each time it is presented. Of course an observer must determine how many mistakes are made. The figure above shows the difference between normals and impulsives, who originally make the same number of errors. It is noteworthy that normals reduce the speed of reading the words and identifying the colors in the third screen, while impulsives, continuing at the same speed, give a curve which suggests that they do not learn. From personal researches, L.M. Fishman and B. Dworetsky.

to given stimuli and more or less to ignore the impulse that has been identified as undesirable. A Stroop exercise (62) (Fig. 17.7), dichotic listening tasks in which attention must be paid to one of multiple voices or the auditory rather than the visual component of complex stimuli, or "go/no go" exercises, may be put to good use here.

If the difficulty is recognizing undesirable impulses or in patient motivation to inhibit them, then socialization and group work or cognitive rehabilitation in the sense of the work of A. T. Beck may be more to the point (63).

A logical analysis of impulsivity into these three components should be distinguished from analytical approaches such as Bracy's (64), which is helpful in other contexts (65). In this program, complex activities are broken down into "simple cognitive acts." While this analysis may be of great practical value to the stroke patient, the traumatic brain-injured patient presents a different picture: here organization, coordination, and integrative synthesis of simple mental processes are significantly impaired. To analyze and disassemble the parts of a complex activity may not benefit a traumatic brain-injured patient since it is the assemblege itself that can present the patient's greatest problem. It is as though one would take apart a bridge to see how it works.

Frank social pressure may be the ideal treatment, since social contexts are exactly where behavioral dysfunction is most destructive. Behavioral treatment programs turn the tables on the usual antisocial nature of impulsivity (66), for a target behavior is required for *inclusion* in the group. A broad scope is essential for classical behavioral management, which pervades an entire unit and all of its activities (67).

Behavioral Treatments

Our experience in using behavioral treatments for traumatic brain injury in the elderly is extrapolated from their use in younger people with traumatic brain injury and from elderly people with acquired cognitive impairments.

The vulnerability of the aging brain in which head trauma occurs requires that clinicians become less dependent on medications and more dependent on non-pharmacologic interventions such as behavioral treatments. Further, the relative lack of predictability in clinical presentation of the elderly traumatically brain-injured patient, in comparison to acquired brain injuries, means that clinicians who use behavioral treatments must become even more creative and flexible in their application, potentially over a longer trajectory in rehabilitation. Behavioral interventions are an essential, and at times the central, component of any rehabilitation program for people of any age with head trauma (67). Clinicians see the elderly both in traumatic brain injury programs (68) and in other settings where TBI is not emphasized, occult, or part of a constellation of combined neurolgic, orthopedic, and other organ systems impairments (69, 70). These other settings include general rehabilitation units, acute hospitals, nursing homes, and home care.

The environmental milieu in which behavioral treatments occur is different for traumatic brain injury rehabilitation in all age groups (67). A safe and orderly environment is created. The ultrastructured day defines the everyday life of patients. Consistency of approach among various providers is the key to communication. These approaches can become more integrated into these settings, where elderly with traumatic brain injury may be commonly seen, in the following ways: sensitivity to the degree of patient distractibility and stimulation; development of a daily individualized schedule, including intermittent rest periods, that is consensually defined among care providers and that aims to optimize meaningful engagement with the milieu; and development of an individual behavioral management plan that is utilized by all care providers to ensure interactional consistency.

Several points must be articulated to address specifically how to approach behavioral interventions in cognitively impaired elderly patients, especially those with traumatic brain injury. Understanding the detailed cognitive or neuropsychologic profile of the patient is essential. Various members of the rehabilitation team provide this information. The rehabilitation physician considers the patient metabolically and structurally (71, 72). The clinical psychologist or psychiatrist defines any related affective or thought disorders (73). This is critical in those patients demonstrating regressed, amotivational, and abulic behaviors. The various therapists define certain aspects of the neuropsychologic profile. Physical therapy provides data regarding gross motor learning. Occupational therapy provides data regarding fine motor learning and screens for strengths and deficits at various levels of cognitive hierarchy, such as memory, problem solving, and organization of intellectual and motor activities as they relate to activities of daily living. Speech therapy provides specific information regarding oral motor learning during swallowing and expressive communication work. The speech therapist provides cognitive information at various levels of the cognitive hierarchy as it relates to receptive communication (74). The neuropsychologist becomes essential, testing utilizing a formal and comprehensive battery of tests that indicate cognitive strengths and then orchestrating the definition of the neuropsychologic profile of the brain-injured elderly client (75).

This team cognitive assessment is labor intensive but necessary. There are obviously some overlaps in the division of labor, but these professionals are observing from different contexts. There is cross-validation among different examiners of specific observations relating to the cognitive profile during this assessment. The groundwork is defined, then, to create an individual behavioral treatment program. The actual translation of the cognitive profile into behavioral treatments must now occur. The rehabilitation physician and the neuropsychologist coordinate this translation (72, 74, 75).

How does this translation occur? First, goals are set that appreciate a more prolonged recovery trajectory over time. For example, global goals are broken down into short-term and even microshort-term goals. These goals are articulated in a manner that breaks down mobility, activities of daily living, cognition, and behavior into their minimally observable components. This requires ongoing goal revision from week to week. Cognitive goals that define desired skills or behaviors are set; for example, increase attention span to 5 minutes continuously; increase orientation to daily schedule using a log book with cueing; follow three-step commands; and decrease distractibility during a therapy session to 5 minutes every 15 minutes. Behavioral goals that define behaviors that must be minimized and subject to more aggressive behavioral management include the following: decrease verbal or physical aggression to two episodes per hour; decrease perseveration in conversation; and decrease urinary/fecal incontinence to once daily while awake (76, 77). The nature of these goals for elderly head trauma patients is oriented toward achieving smooth and optimal function in basic survival skills for life in the least restrictive specific environment, rather than toward achieving resumption of work and life in a variety of situations, as is the ultimate endpoint of interventions for younger patients (78, 79).

Second, a behavioral management plan must be operationalized. Behavioral management plans must not infantalize the elderly patient. The general rule is that they must reinforce desired behaviors and ignore undesired behaviors (80). This requires education and maturity by care providers. Behavioral management plans in rehabilitation settings are usually nursing centered in that the nursing staff is the most consistent among rehabilitation personnel. They spend more time with patients during the structured day. Behavioral management plans, then, define the nursing care plan. A behavioral psychologist as a consultant or a core member of the rehabilitation team becomes vital in setting up these explicit behavioral management programs for the elderly patient. The behavioral psychologist works closely with the rehabilitation team to operationalize the behavioral management plan as concretely as possible (80). Cognitive and behavioral goals and behavioral management plans, by being central components in the rehabilitation of elderly who have brain injury, become the clinical indicators of progress and outcome for concurrent traditional therapy interventions and medication interventions used to modify behavior and facilitate optimal function for the elderly head trauma patient.

There is little research on outcome of elderly brain-injured patients after rehabilitation interventions. Davis and Acton (78) present outcome data over 4 years on a small sample (N = 26) of older patients (average age = 65 years) treated at a traumatic brain injury rehabilitation unit. In comparison to younger patients (average age = 21 years), older patients had an insignificantly greater length of stay (70 versus 60 day average). Outcome among the older group was not as good as among the younger group, but was encouraging for the older group: 58% (15/26) were discharged home (versus 25/26 or over 90% for the younger group) immediately after rehabilitation, but this increased to 85% (22/26) when patients were followed over 2 years to 5 years. All of the younger patients were independent in activities of daily living, while 54% (14/26) of the older patients were independent, and another 35% (9/26) required supervision or were dependent in activities of daily living over 2-year to 5-year follow-up.

The work of the group at Jewish Memorial Hospital in Boston, Massachusetts (76, 77, 80, 81), although not specific to head trauma rehabilitation but addressing behavioral treatments in rehabilitation for elderly patients with both traumatic and acquired brain injury, demonstrates that a behavioral-neuropsychologic approach promotes functional gains and desired behaviors during actual involvement in the rehabilitation program. Sustaining optimal function and desired behaviors after discharge is more strongly correlated with stability of medical conditions, the close involvement of a family member, and home rather than institutional discharge. The integrity of the social support system to manage behavioral treatments after discharge emerges as vital in guaranteeing that the investment in rehabilitation for elderly head trauma patients is worthwhile (82). Clinicians, especially social workers, must become more creative and flexible in constructing and supporting a social network that aims either to avoid long-term institutionalization or to promote carry-over of behavioral treatments in nursing homes.

Excellent assessment instruments are available (83), such as the Duke Older Americans Resources and Service Procedures (OARS) (84), the Beaumont Lifestyle Inventory of Social Support (BLISS) (85), and the Family Help Available Scale (FHA) (86, 87).

Management of Elderly Patients' Problems Following Traumatic Brain Injury

The greatest risks elderly TBI patients face in physical therapy relate to the cervical spine. Ropper (82) defines these concerns as: (a) cord compression from vertebral dislocations, (b) proper treatment of fractures through the pedicles, facets, or vertebral bodies, and (c) instability from fractures that may cause misalignment and cord compression in the future.

With nonsurgical cervical injury, a halo-type support may be preferred, since Minerva, poster, and Philadelphia-type collars exert less predictable forces on the edentulous jaw. State-of-the-art temporomandibular joint (TMJ) studies include dynamic electrophysiologic and kinesiologic evaluation. Special maxillofacial procedures for fractures in the elderly (88) give more effective support that allows the patient to eat, speak, and participate in therapy earlier. Elderly victims of TBI often require special head and neck physical therapeutic evaluation (89–91).

THE SECOND FALL

Protecting the elderly TBI patient from a second fall is critical (3). The fall may be seen not only as a leading cause, but also as one chief effect of TBI. Despite precautions, the very goal of increased mobility often renders older TBI patients increasingly vulnerable to loss of balance or support.

Steinberg (Chapter 20), Lewis (92), and others (93–96) outline conditions that may contribute to a patient's initial propensity to fall. Other changes relate to recovery from TBI itself; Payton and Poland (97, 98) estimate a 3% loss of muscle strength for each fully immobilized day. Changes in pulmonary function, peripheral O_2 utilization, and sympathetic vascular accommodation

impair the initiation of vertical activities as well as endurance.

Applied Gerontology

A third set of factors concern acute injuries superimposed on chronic degenerative changes. In the midbrain, there is a 40% reduction in the cristae of all semicircular canals, similar changes in the maculae, sacculi, and utriculi, and severe or total losses of saccular statoconia, or otoliths (35). Reduction in vestibular end organ sensitivity and their connections along the medial longitudinal fasciculus combine with reduced neck range of motion to produce imbalance on turning (24, 25, 91, 99). New visual restrictions or extraocular muscle asymmetries further increase the need for the very head, neck, and shoulder coordination that head trauma may impair (23, 99). Vertigo, poor balance, and dizziness (100) are both major complaints of aging and major sequelae of TBI (101).

Leg length discrepancy following associated fractured hip, reduced muscle force/velocity of contraction (92), and restricted range of hip, knee, and ankle extension because of hospitalization are other consequences of TBI that strongly predispose to future falls. It can be a fine line between "fallophobia" and a rational response to the formidable array of obstacles in these situations (93, 99–104)!

Brainstem auditory evoked potentials (BSAEPs) are less clear-cut in the elderly (Fig. 17.8) and usually less

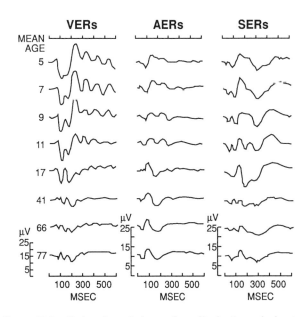

Figure 17.8. Reduced resolution and amplitudes in evoked potentials may require comparison with contralateral studies more frequently in the elderly. In TBI, with diffuse axonal injury, the contralateral may be a poor control. From Beck EC, Dustman RE, Schenkberg T. In: Ordy JM, Brizzee KR, eds. *Neurobiology of Aging.* New York, NY: Plenum; 1975:175–192. Reproduced with permission of the publisher.

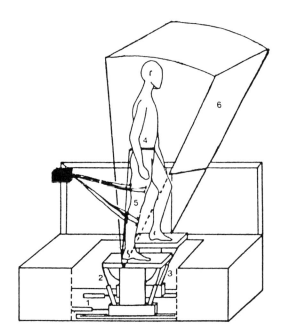

Figure 17.9. The footplates are moved anteriorly or posteriorly and rotated by hydraulic cylinders 1,2,3. Hip belt, 4, detects torso sway; surface electrodes pick up thigh, knee, and ankle extensors, and knee and ankle flexors. The visual environment, 6, can be rotated in parallel with body sway to control for visual cues. From Wollacott MH, Shumway-Cook AT, Nasher LM. Aging and posture control: changes in sensory organization and muscular coordination. *Int J Aging Hum Develop.* 23:97–114, 1986. Redrawn with permission of the publisher.

helpful than electronystagmography (ENG) (39, 99, 105) since destabilizing causes are commonly in the vestibular apparatus. Rational adaptation and use of other end organ input, e.g., vision and proprioception, can be more helpful. A systems approach may be replacing the conception of impaired reflexivity in the evaluation of poor balance (23, 105). In patient evaluation and treatment, static devices have given way to dynamic assessments (94–96). For example, in Shumway's movable platform, stabilizing force of 1.5%, 3%, and 4% of the patient's weight is delivered horizontally through a belt around the patient's midsection (95) (Fig. 17.9). The environment can be manipulated to observe the functional significance of proprioceptive and visual input. Physical therapeutic exercises for impaired oculovestibular responses, positional vertigo, and bilateral vestibular loss are fruitful applications of the systems approach (99).

Dizziness

While Meclizine may reduce vestibular function (99), case reports describe the use of small doses of scopalamine to improve balance and reduce true vertigo and dizziness after TBI. Functional gains are reported to continue after the medicine is stopped (106). While the exact mechanism is unknown, the anticholinergic medication may reduce cholinergic input from the inner ear in favor of visual, proprioceptive, cutaneous, contextual, and environmental cues. Caution is urged since clinical investigations using scopalamine to induce Alzheimer-like symptoms (106–108) show short-term memory loss and organizational deficits in some patients. After screening for tachydysrhythmias and taking urologic and general medical problems into account, a transderm patch might be used judiciously to be removed at the onset of dysfunctional side effects.

OSTEOPOROSIS

Osteoporosis places the reambulating elderly TBI patient at additional risk. Didronal may simultaneously reduce the formation of heterotropic ossification and increase bone mass. Yet Didronal is not reported to reduce the number of actual fractures. Physical therapy and dietary changes can help alleviate this problem.

Inactivity hypercalcemia profoundly affects the number and activity of osteoblasts and osteoclasts, but it does so indirectly by regulating hormonal levels that in turn affect the local osteoblasts and osteoclasts migrating from bone marrow. Fortunately, the most influential of these, parathyroid hormone, calcitonin, and 1,25 dihydoxyvitamin D3, derive from the parathyroid gland, the C cells of the thyroid gland, and the kidneys, respectively. Their control therefore bypasses the hypothalamic pituitary axis, which is frequently deranged in TBI.

Physical therapy has the dual role of increasing range of motion and producing mechanical tension in tendons. This has been noted to increase bone mass and effectively *reverse* osteoporosis (109). Functional mechanical strain has been reported to activate cell remodeling such that adequate deposition of supportive tissue occurs along the lines of force according to Wolff's law.

Working with turkeys' wings, Lanyon (109) found that 100 moderate daily stresses heightened RNA synthesis in osteocytes and that increased functional loading led to *increased* periosteal bone mass. He states that exercise that is "(1) unusual, (2) diverse (i.e., multiple unusual situations), (3) vigorous (in order to produce high strains and high strain rates), (4) repeated daily, and (5) of short duration" (109 p22) should have the greatest conservative or osteogenic effect. Simkin et al (110) showed increased bone mass, measured by Compton scattering in postmenopausal wrists, after using such an exercise pattern. Exercises of this type were more effective in reversing osteoporosis if they were *not* along a tendon's usual lines of force (109).

Deft use of appropriate range of motion parameters can fashion therapy vigorous enough to reduce the likelihood of heterotopic ossification and osteoporosis, increase range, and yet be sufficiently gentle to avoid promoting spasticity or osteoarthritis.

DIET

Apart from frank anosmia secondary to bilaterally shearing the first cranial nerve at impact, rehabilitation of the elderly TBI patient must contend with chronologic, physiologic, olfactory, and gustatory changes. In spite of regenerative capacity, mitral cells and olfactory receptors show sharply accelerated loss after ages 65 years to 70 years, sometimes bringing about a complete absence of sense of smell within a few years (111–116). There may be more profound central changes since olfactory pathways are specifically affected in Alzheimer's disease (117), and Alzheimer's disease is more common after TBI. Cognitive aspects of the entorhinal system remain largely conjectural.

Taste buds from vallate, fungiform, and foliate papillae regenerate every 7 to 10 days (116–119). However, decreased total number, particularly of the fungiform papillae (salty taste), are noted after age 40 years, with accelerated loss after 80 years. While olfactory identification appears to drop approximately 30% from age 60 years to age 90 years, gustatory threshold as tested by current perception thresholds varies by a factor of five in an almost linear fashion from age 15 years to age 90 years. There is a slight steepening at 80 years. A significant decrease in salivary volume, amylase, and amylase activity (needed for tasting sweetness) contribute to decreased perception of taste. Dentures may also contribute to this decline (119, 120).

Over 70% of the elderly are estimated to lack an effective sense of taste. This is irrelevant in the acute context, where tube feedings must supply 3000 calories (1) daily, with adequate protein to keep a positive nitrogen balance and extra calories if movement disorders raise total metabolism. But when exercise is possible, accelerated osteoporosis must be approached from the dietary standpoint of a person long deprived of sunlight, as well as one with inactivity hypercalcemia and bone loss.

The opposite influences of anterior and posterior pituitary hormones (ACTH and ADH) demand "tight control" of water metabolism to avoid dilution and hypernatremia, respectively. Besides osmotic aspects and the antiinsulinemic effects of steroids on most TBI patients, type II and type I diabetics require tight dietary regulation. Unless blood glucose is carefully controlled, triglycerides and cholesterol tend to rise as apolipoprotein B100 becomes glycosylated, destroying the liver's feedback loop to limit low density lipoproteins. High levels of insulin, the greatest hormonal promoter of adipose tissue, also dispose toward hypertension, myocardial infarction, and myopathic cardiac changes (120). Higher insulin levels are more likely in ventromedial hypothalamic damage after TBI (121).

The goals of diet include an adequately nutritious and pleasant fare that may be self-prepared and administrable. For this, the dietitian might work closely with other services, for example, occupational therapy. Deglutition is, of course, studied in speech therapy. In adaptation of the elderly individual, with cranial nerve and bony injuries, hormonal changes, cognitive deficits, and long confinement, to the demands of independent living, the dietitian is truly a central figure of the rehabilitation team.

COGNITIVE RETRAINING

One approach to the problems in rehabilitation after TBI is remediation of their neuropsychologic causes (Table 17.7). Cognitive rehabilitative use of pacing, anchoring, and self-monitoring techniques, and the establishment of quiet, action-oriented, undistracting milieux can be part of physical therapy as well as occupational therapy (76, 122, 123). In some measure these techniques are employed in speech therapy and psychologic counseling after TBI. Cognitive therapy, as developed by Beck et al, has been applied to elderly victims of poststroke depression (63), emphasizing a collaborative therapeutic relationship, with recreational therapy and vocational rehabilitation, for example. We shall discuss the cognitive aspects under "Cognitive Rehabilitation" but this is only to focus our discussion not to suggest narrow application of the techniques.

There is an element of tautology in the proposition that activities of daily living are essential to the satisfaction of universal recurrent needs. A minimum of fine and gross motor ability, a modicum of common sense and perceptual acuity, and the capacity to make rational choices appear to be the three minimum daily requirements of self-reliance at any age. This implies effective powers of observation, memory, and strategy and a sense of *gestalt*. Reasonably focal and surveillant attention must function without disabling emotional instability. In our

Table 17.7. Deficits of Cognition

Cognitive	
Linguistic	Memory[a]
Planning–Sequencing[a]	Judgment
Strategy[a]	Attention[a]
Perceptual	
Neglect[a]	Figure-ground[a]
Orientation	Spatial relations[a]
Identification-classification-gestalt[a]	
Constructional apraxia[a]	
Emotive	
Shallow lability	Self-centeredness
Irritability-euphoria	Depression
Attention[a]	Distractibility[a]
Impulsivity	Denial
W/C locking	
Kluver-Bucy	

[a]Substantial means of cognitive rehabilitation available.

form of life, effective use of tools and symbols yields "decisional capacity," the key to personal independence. Therefore cognitive rehabilitation—while important to all physical medicine and rehabilitation following traumatic brain injury—is the very core of occupational therapy (124). Little training or adaptation is possible without learning, and cognitive rehabilitation has the paradoxical task of teaching people how to learn.

"Once development was ended, the founts of growth and regeneration of the axons and dendrites dried up irrevocably. In adult centers, the nerve paths are something fixed and immutable; everything may die, nothing may be regenerated" (125).

Later in life, there are particularly severe cerebral losses of golgi Type II neurons in the third pyramidal layer (24). These are sustained chiefly in the superior temporal gyrus, precentral gyrus, and the area of the striatum. Of noncerebral structures, the cerebellum and, *uniquely* among the brainstem nuclei, the locus ceruleus degenerate somewhat after age 65 years (119). In the spinal cord, large fibers are lost, particularly in the dorsal columns (24). Most aging central nervous systems lose dendritic spines and show significantly more dendritic distortions (3, 24, 26).

Nevertheless, the mature brain actually demonstrates considerable plasticity; injury is often followed by an *increase* in dendritic fields (24, 44, 126–135) (Figs. 17.10, 17.11, 17.12). More recently, Gerald Edelmann's brilliant "Neuronal Group Selection" (130) presents a detailed technical framework for central nervous system restructuring in health and defacto rehabilitation com-patible with the "no growth" state to which Ramon y Cajal refers above.

COGNITIVE REHABILITATION

Successful efforts to enhance man's teachability date from antiquity. Still, tension exists between "aptitude tests" and efforts to improve performance on them. An aptitude test that documented improved scores on the basis of training might, eo ipso, be discounted as an effective assay of native ability. If an individual cannot learn, how can teaching help him or her? If one can learn, why not get on with the task of teaching what needs to be

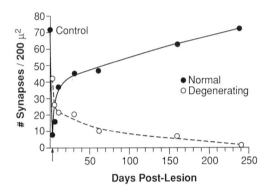

Figure 17.10. Changes in the number of degenerating (open circles) and normal synapses (closed circles) following a unilateral entorhinal lesion. From Cotman CW, Scheff SW. Compensatory synapse growth in aged animals after neuronal death. In: Strehler BL, ed. *Mechanisms of Aging and Development.* SA Lausanne, Switzerland: Elsevier Sequoia; 1978. With permission of the publisher.

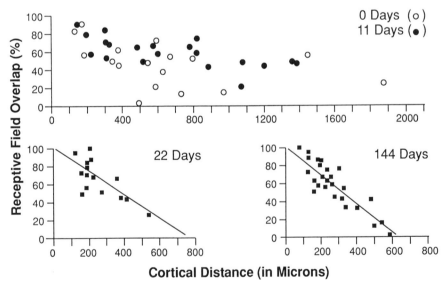

Figure 17.11. Receptive field changes of area 1 in adult monkeys' somatosensory cortices after division of the median nerve. Electrodes placed in previous receptive fields of dorsal digits 1–3, measurements at 11, 22, and 144 days. Receptive fields first expand after the lesion, then return to tighter 600 micron limit. From Merzenich MM. Progression of change following median nerve section in the cortical representation of the hand in areas 3b and 1 in adult owl and squirrel monkeys. *Neuroscience.* 10:639–665, © 1983. Copyright Wiley-Liss, a Division of John Wiley and Sons, Inc. Reprinted with permission of the publisher.

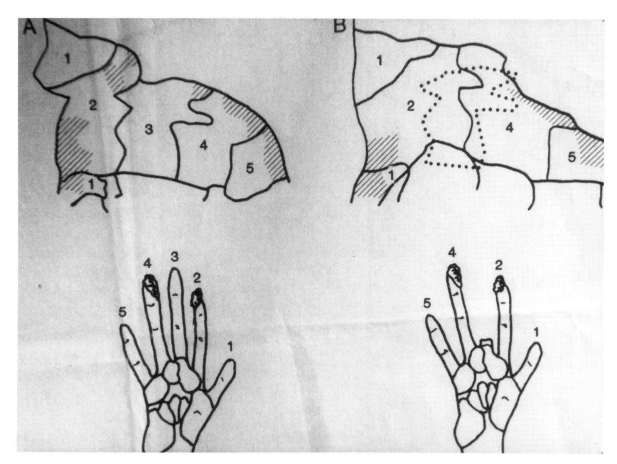

Figure 17.12. After amputation of the middle finger the somatosensory region that registered signals from it vanishes. (In **A,** area 3) The field itself changes (see **B**) to amplify representation of the remaining fingers, rededicating the area that represented the amputated third digit. Other digits' fields appear to change too. Reprinted with permission of the publisher, from Merzenich MM, Nelson RJ, Stryker MP, et al. Somatosensory cortical map changes following digit amputation in adult monkeys. *J Comp Neurol.* 224:591–605, © 1984. Copyright Wiley-Liss, a Division of John Wiley and Sons, Inc.

known? This Platonic conundrum is reincarnated in the paradox of cognitive rehabilitation.

Yet, performance on *any* type of test can be improved by practice. This may be particularly true where the "test" is independent functioning in everyday life. Cognitive rehabilitation, then, like other types of rehabilitation, improves a less-than-optimal function. As cell death within the embryo's limb buds makes for greater manipulation with the appearance of individual fingers, cell death in the central nervous system can actually enhance learning capacity. Cell death itself appears to be a powerful stimulus for new synaptic formation in adult and older mammals (Figs 17.10, 17.11, and 17.12).

Less Can Be More

As a counterargument to the theory of cephalization, loss or congenital absence of higher functional competence has been shown to markedly facilitate one type of learning (131–134). In spite of the considerable impairments imposed by cortical losses, laboratory animals and profoundly retarded children and adults have outperformed normals in associational learning tasks (131–134) (Tables 17.8 and 17.9).

Unlike representational or abstract learning, associational learning (like classical conditioning) connects stimulus to response without rational relationship between the two. Cue fading, back-chaining, and similar behavioral techniques effectively promote this type of learning. Knowledge obtained in this fashion may form the substructure upon which more intellectual types of learning and skills are based.

Pharmacological Adjuvants to Cognitive Therapy

A number of cognitive enhancers are currently being tried. Among them are methylphenidate (135), tricyclics and serotonin reuptake inhibitors (136), physostigmine and lecithin (137), gangliosides (138), Pimoline, dihydroergocristine (139), vinpocetine (140), buspirone, (−) eburnamonine (141), YM 14673 (142) and whole classes in the experimental stage. Evidence suggests that some sites of activity are in the brainstem and thalamus.

Table 17.8. Success with Behavioral Cognitive Rehabilitation

Author	Subject	Conditions	Modality	Results
Zihl, von Cramon (1980)	Human	Destriate	Nonverbal choice	+
Pöppel (1973)	Human	Destriate	Nonverbal choice	+
Weiskranz (1980)	Human	Destriate	Nonverbal choice	+
Humphrey (1974)	Monkey	Destriate	Association learning	+
Nielson (1982)	Human twins	Destriate	Forced choice	+
Oakley (1979)	Rats	Decorticate	Alleyway running	+ +
Oakley (1981)	Rats	Decorticate	Autoshaping	+ +
Zeiler (1972), Cavanaugh & Davidson (1977)	Infants/young children		Teach association	Infants outdo older children
Anderson et al (1981)	Infants/young children		Teach association	Infants outdo older children
Wilcove, Miller (1974) Rogain et al (1976)	College students/ children w/IQ<35		Autoshaping	Children outdo college students
Lowe (1989), Davey (1981)	Children	Younger/older	Operant conditioning	Younger = better
Oakley & Russell (1977)	Rats/rabbits	Destriate	Nictitating membrane	+ +
Meyer, Yutsey, Dalby & Meyer (1983)	Rats	Total cortiectomy	Relearning discrimination	+

Table 17.9. The Impaired Show Great Aptitude for Association Learning

Author	Subject	Conditions	Modality	Results
Carr (1980)	Human	Micrencephalic	Association learning	+
Sarimski (1982)	Human	Micrencephalic	Association learning	+
Skinner (1965)	Human	Micrencephalic	Fading/shaping	+
Jones & Cullen (1981)	Human	Micrencephalic	Association learning	+
Lambert (1981)	Human	Micrencephalic	Association learning	+
Quattlebaum (1972)	Human	Micrencephalic	Association learning	+
Piontokovsky (1961)	Rats	Prenatal radiation	Association learning	Superior (+ +)
Fowler et al (1962)	Rats	Prenatal radiation	Association learning	Superior (+ +)
Shibagaki et al (1981)	Rats	Prenatal radiation	Association learning	Superior (+ +)
Furchtgott et al (1976)	Rats	Prenatal radiation	Association learning	Superior (+ +)
Tamaki & Inouye (1976)	Rats	Prenatal radiation	Association learning	Superior (+ +)
Lowe, Davey (1981)	Young children	Normal	Association learning	Like nonverbal mammals
Oakley (1979)	Rats	Neodecorticated	Association learning	+ +
Lowe (1983)	Older children	Normal	Association learning	Unlike nonverbal mammals

Rational drug management includes reduction of medicines known to exert anticognitive or sedative effects, strengthen depression, or increase confusion. Lipid-soluble beta-blockers, anticholinergics, benzodiazepines, even some ACE inhibitors have been suggested in this context. The reader is referred to informative works of Nathan Cope and others (59, 143–145), for this intricate field requires a chapter or book all its own.

Using medications without cognitive rehabilitation may be comparable to an athlete attending the training table but not practice.

COMPUTERIZED COGNITIVE REHABILITATION

The computer was created by the mind of man in its own image and therefore would seem a perfect tool for accomplishing cognitive rehabilitation. A large number of excellent and diverse programs have been devised and used by Gianutsos (122), Bracy (64), Prigatano (47, 50), and others. Some (122, 146–148) have noted that there are a number of ways in which computers can help (Fig. 17.13). Still, computerized cognitive rehabilitation remains largely without reported results, and its use by the elderly may be especially controversial (7, 154, 155) (Table 17.10). Regardless of whether the therapy is delivered via computers or otherwise, it is important to distinguish *tests* from *exercises* in cognitive rehabilitation. This is a difficult distinction since both test and exercise must engage a given ability to be effective. However, since cognitive rehabilitation endeavors to increase a patient's learning, abstraction, or application of a principle in a new realm, testing within the same context and focus as the exercise begs the question of whether real cognitive rehabilitation is taking place.

The circumstances that test a given ability are clearly effective in training for it. For example, in order to run a given race better, training on that very course

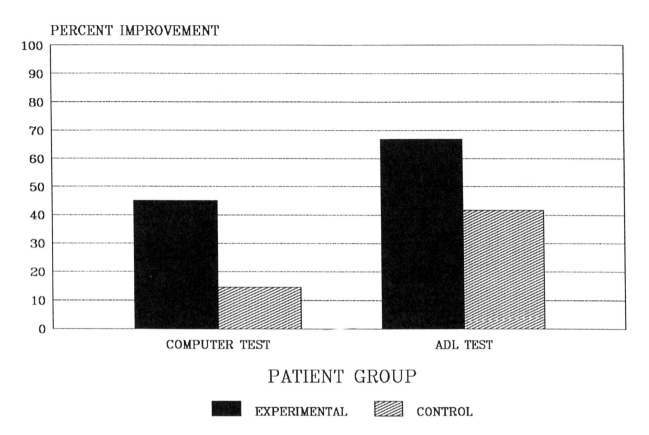

CONFERENCED PATIENTS
CONTROL VS. EXPERIMENTAL GROUPS

INITIAL LIMB RANDOMLY ASSIGNED (P < .05)

Figure 17.13. Each computer-aided occupational therapy session benefited adult inpatients as much as 2.2 occupational therapy sessions conducted without the computer. From Namerow NS. Cognitive and behavioral aspects of brain-injury rehabilitation. *Neurol Clin.* 5(4):569–583, 1987, with permission of the publlisher.

exploits the "learning effect." It is equally clear that a test sensitive to a given behavioral quality engages that quality in its proper performance. However, such practice and testing certainly cannot be used in a valid experimental context.

One study (151) used an independent, practical scale measuring speed of reacquisition of daily living skills as an index of cognitive improvement. Both treatment and control subjects were in an inpatient population, with nearly identical daily exposures and environment; patients who received computerized cognitive rehabilitation and conferencing with the rehabilitation team did impressively better than those without. Computerized cognitive rehabilitation proved a significant positive factor, provided the team continued to conference the patients (Fig. 17.13). It was critical, in other words, that the therapists used the computer as a tool and not as a substitute for their rational intervention and guidance.

Applicability of Computerized Cognitive Rehabilitation

The computer is generally applicable to patients in Level VII or Level VIII in the Rancho of Los Amigos scale (Table 17.11). A few calmer confused/appropriate or confused inappropriate, nonagitated patients can use it to advantage.

The computer may be ideal for clinical and experimental delivery of cognitive therapy. Its nonjudgmental, nonconfrontational, uniform yet randomizable presentation of multimodal stimuli, visual, auditory, verbal and nonverbal, bright, moving, even flashing colors, can be programmed to progress in difficulty along with patients' developing skill, usefully accessing patients' past strengths and weaknesses.

The computer can time, tabulate, and compare a patient's responses to his or her own earlier responses

Table 17.10. Some Studies in Cognitive Rehabilitation

Author	Conditions	Modality	Results
Prigatano et al (1984)	TBI[a]	Comprehensive program	+ (P = .001)
Lincoln (1985, 1987)	TBI	Compatible Rx	No change
Kulik et al (1980)	Students	CAI[a]	+ (50%–63%)
Weinberg (1977)	Perceptually impaired	Visual-spatial training	
Gianutsos, Klitzner (1981, 1983)	TBI, CVA[a]	Software	+
Bracy (1984)	TBI	Software	+
Rao, Bieliavskas (1983)	Brain injury	Software	+
Sunburst	Brain injury	Software	No results reported
Diller (ORM) (1974)	Brain injury	Software	
Sbordone (1984–1987)	Brain injury	Software	No results reported
Smith (1983)	Brain injury	Software	No results reported
Lambert (1985)	Brain injury	Software	Attention (no effect)
Maley (1982)	Brain injury	Software	Attention (no effect)
Skilbeck (1984)	Brain injury	Software	+
Browning (1986)	Brain injury	Video discs	No results reported
Thorkildsen (1983)	Brain injury	Video discs	No results reported
Glisky et al (1986)	Memory impaired	Domain-specific training	+
Namerow (1987)	TBI	Comprehensive computers	+
Ruff, Baser (1989)	TBI	Neuropsychologically structional vs nonstructional	Both beneficial; more benefit with neuro-psychology

[a]TBI = traumatic brain injury; CAI = computer-aided instruction; CVA = cerebrovascular accident.

Table 17.11. Rancho Los Amigos Recovery Levels

I. *NO RESPONSE:* Stimuli produce no response.

II. *GENERALIZED RESPONSE:* Inconsistent, nonpurposeful responses may be only to pain.

III. *LOCALIZED RESPONSE:* Responds with purpose. May follow simple commands; may focus attention, e.g., visually.

IV. *CONFUSED, AGITATED:* Heightened level of activity. Agitation appears related to internal confusion. Unaware of present events. Confused, disoriented, aggressive behavior.

V. *CONFUSED, INAPPROPRIATE, NONAGITATED:* Appears calm, receptive. Follows commands; does not concentrate on task; distractable; responds to external stimuli with some excitement. Does not learn. Inappropriate verbal output.

VI. *CONFUSED APPROPRIATE:* Well-directed behavior with cueing; can relearn old skills and activities of daily living (ADL); some awareness of self and others. Disabling memory deficits involving both encoding and retrieval.

VII. *AUTOMATIC APPROPRIATE:* Robot-like appropriate behavior, minimal confusion, shallow recall, poor insight, judgment, problem-solving and planning skills. Can initiate tasks but needs structure to continue.

VIII. *PURPOSEFUL APPROPRIATE:* Alert and oriented; can recall and integrate the past. Can learn new activities and can continue working independently; independent living skills; can possibly drive; low stress tolerance; impaired judgment and abstract reasoning; most people function at reduced levels in society.

and those of other patients. It is fit for research into the efficacy of cognitive rehabilitation, since the human factor, with endless nuances of empathy and countertransference, is eliminated. Nevertheless, in what follows, though a computerized mode or screen picture may accompany the text, there is no inherent reason why non-computerized delivery of the exercises should not benefit the patient. Ways in which computerized therapy may enhance rehabilitation will be discussed briefly following this section.

Rules of thumb for computerized cognitive rehabilitation of elderly patients include:

1. Hand-eye coordination is an important factor that needs to be analysed *out* when timing the purely cognitive aspect of performance (24, 151).
2. Progressive difficulty is essential.
3. Randomly ordering exercise items eliminates *undesirable* learning effects while maximizing the range of possible challenges, e.g., to improve vigilance and flexibly focal attention.
4. Progressive and entertaining visual and auditory (multimodal) rewarding is effective.
5. The patient must be informed of the correct answer when he or she fails to provide it.
6. The patient may be encouraged to use the left, numerical, symbolic side of the brain to supplement a dysfunctional right side of the brain, and vice-versa. (In Figure 17.14, superimposition of a numbered and lettered grid promotes spatial orientation as the higher functioning left brain with its symbolic abilities comes to the aid of a right brain unable to locate objects in space.)
7. Motor impersistence and poor attention span can be treated if the patient is asked to remain still while the computer or therapist "does the work" (Fig. 17.15).

There are several advantages to using the computer that are inherent in this still new technology.

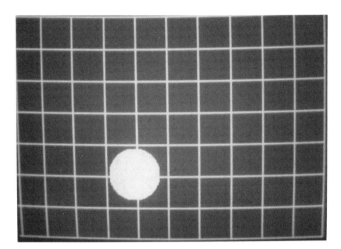

Figure 17.14. Numbering and lettering rows and columns serves, like chess notation, to improve awareness of position and memory of objects in space. An intact left hemisphere can thus aid the patient with tasks often performed with the right hemisphere.

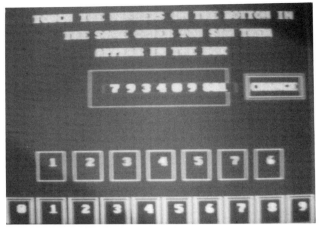

Figure 17.16. Forward or backward digit-span can be specified; timing and erasures can be recorded, as well as digit repetitions, interference from past exercises, and characteristics of fatigue.

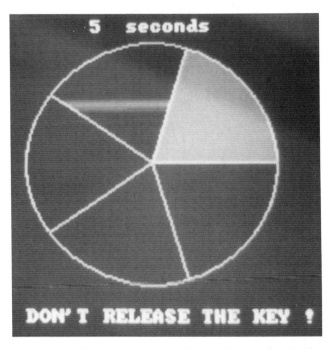

Figure 17.15. The spokes of the wheel can be increased to 30. The spaces fill up at the rate of one per second, with audiovisual rewards commensurate to the wait.

MEMORY

The computer improves on the paper and pencil version of "digit span" by recording "erasures" (Fig. 17.16). This detects perseveration, interference, low confidence, and a host of other cognitive and noncognitive difficulties that interfere with memory and for which effective treatment is available.

PERCEPTION

Computerized rehabilitation is recursive, beginning at the simplest possible discrimination of fore-

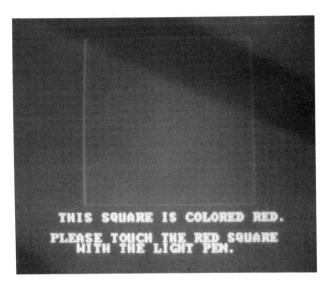

Figure 17.17. Computerized cognitive rehabilitation can begin at the simplest possible discrimination: a thing and its border . . .

ground and field and building from this to the associational-type of learning, without cognitive content, to very abstract and/or symbolic activities (Figs. 17.17 and 17.18). Graphic movement on the monitor can create perceptual exercises for hemispatial neglect and a large number of other conditions (Fig. 17.19).

ATTENTION

The computer allows for peripheral visual, i.e., nonfoveal stimulation of dorsolateral facilitatory (arousal) pathways or, e.g., heightened association and memory in foveal, inhibitory, orbital-frontal pathways (focal attention) involving the hippocampus (152, 153). These latter connections mediate stimulus-response multimodal applications of new learning, the goal of cognitive rehabilitation.

Figure 17.18. . . . to a very abstract notion, as in the command: "Touch the part of the screen that is not red, not green, not yellow."

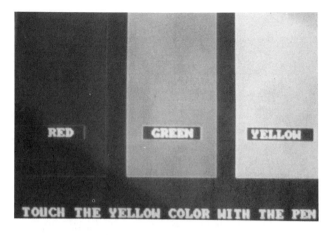

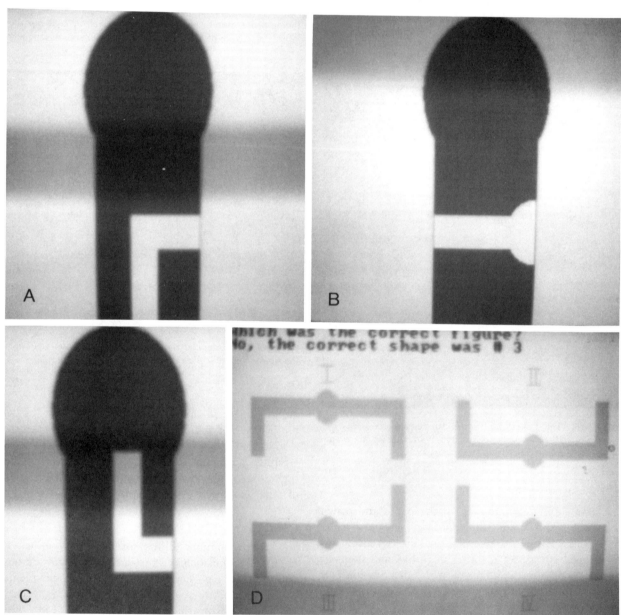

Figure 17.19. The shapes pass across the keyhole, but are never seen in their entirety. The patient must assemble them in his mind to identify the figure. At first, individuals with left neglect do worse with images coming from their left, especially if they move slowly. Impulsive people are apt to see the first half of an object and then guess. Yet, most learn, with practice.

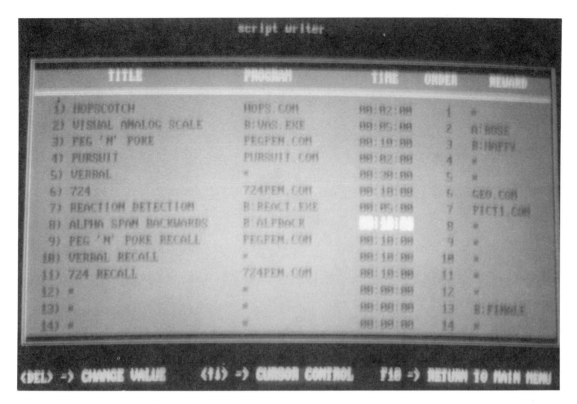

Figure 17.20. This is a prescription, which also measures the patient's response to itself, compares it with the patient's and other patients' performances, and easily measures compliance. It can be updated in person, by mail, and soon, by modem. With permission of the Arcon Group, Manhasset, New York.

Training Time

In recovery after TBI, people of all ages often regain personality and character traits long before cognitive rehabilitation is complete. Old habits, including study and work styles and "Type A" characteristics, reappear while sizeable cognitive deficits are still present. Computerized cognitive rehabilitation can proceed in the home (Fig. 17.20). Discs can present specific prescribed activities and record the patient's work, so that each task can be advanced, regressed, or revised along the relevant parameters. Discs can be mailed or brought in personally.

Patients with proper motivation can make truly astonishing gains through long hours at the computer, improving their cognitive ability with the computer's always accessible, infinitely patient, and confidential participation. William J. Lynch's recent discussion (154) of computer selection is logical and sophisticated.

Future Implications

A final advantage to computerized rehabilitation is that stimuli (e.g., presented screens) can simultaneously trigger the sweep of a brain-mapping device (Fig. 17.21). In the future, brain-mapping devices may feed back electrophysiologic data from brain processes to an expert system while the patient is working with the computer.

Cognitive rehabilitation of this type might adjust responsively to the patient's current level of function. Evidence suggests at least that electroencephalographic (EEG) output changes with patients' cognitive abilities (155), and P300 is known to rise in amplitude with the improbability of the "odd-ball" stimulus and increase latency with more difficult perceptual distinctions (156). Using electrophysiologic feedback, one might, for example, identify the best modality and exercise on which a patient can focus his or her attention at a given time. It is even possible that an expert system could locate brain circuitry immediately called into play by these manipulable parameters. Such a sensitive and immediately responsive therapy might improve cognitive and perceptual skills significantly. Any *functional* brain mapping would, in itself, provide rich information regarding the efficacy of cognitive rehabilitation programs.

Neuropsychology

More unanimously appreciated are the efforts of neuropsychologists. Albert and Moss's *Geriatric Neuropsychology* (157) describes gerontologic neuropsychologic changes, their causes, and neuroimaging, with a finely focused section on cognitive assessment. Much of the geriatrically oriented literature is devoted to Alzheimer's disease and stroke (158). Yet, despite the frustratingly diffuse cognitive sequelae after TBI, with characteristi-

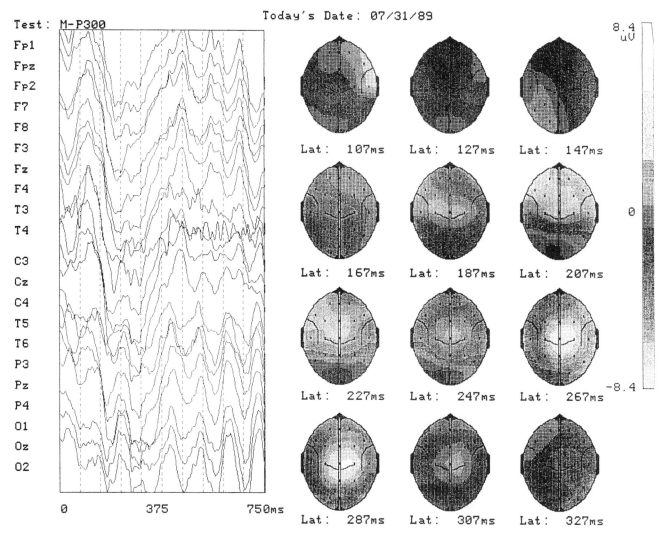

Figure 17.21. Strong positivity in the hippocampal region between 250 and 300 milliseconds denotes a perceived departure from an expected pattern. The P-300's amplitude varies inversely with the probability of the unexpected event; latency is directly related to the difficulty of distinguishing expected from unexpected stimuli. These parameters correspond well with cognitive and perceptual tasks, respectively.

cally poor relationship between test scores and patient abilities (159), neuropsychologic assessment is still the sine qua non of responsibly self-critical cognitive rehabilitation.

While testing the elderly after TBI, the neuropsychologist's casual and clinical observations of the patient may be as helpful as the test results themselves. Certainly, the combination of the two adds insight to designing treatment and subsequent evaluation. In one study (160) a combination of computerized cognitive rehabilitation and neuropsychologic evaluation rendered occupational therapy sessions 2.2 times more effective in raising scores on a Barthel-like measure of ADL than therapy given without computers and neuropsychologists (160).

Adaptation to Loss

As mentioned earlier, a domain-specific approach that has been used frequently with mentally retarded, microencephalic and decorticated mammals, can be applied to the cognitively impaired. Association learning, i.e., the type of understanding Pavlov's dog showed in salivating after constant conjunction of the bell and food, two essentially unrelated things, may occur quite readily in spite of cognitive impairment. This not abstract, non-insightful type of learning frequently is actually *superior* in the cognitively impaired. One study found young children with IQ's below 35 performing better than college graduates (132) (Tables 17.7 and 17.8).

An example of domain-specific knowledge is described by Glisky and Schachter (147). A well-defined context allows a computer to introduce a wide array of knowledge-based skill structures to higher functioning cognitively impaired individuals.

Another use of computers is as "cognitive orthotic devices" (50, 66, 150, 158). The computer becomes a type of guide, to pace and integrate such overlapping tasks as preparing a baked potato with a cheese sauce or planning an afternoon visit of grandchildren.

Autoshaping and vanishing cue techniques appear particularly successful in cognitively impaired patients. Computers can cluster temporal and spacial cues quite readily, using their summation to initiate behaviors (131–134), which then through cue-fading can become increasingly autonomous.

A more extended use of the computer is as a "prosthetic memory," where ostensibly the patients is so impaired and so dependent that he or she relinquishes a good deal of autonomy to the computer and uses it as a means of organizing thoughts and making decisions. At this time, such use of the computer appears rather fanciful, since a patient who cannot decide what information to access from the computer would appear to have just as difficult a time deciding how to access the proper advice about which information to access. Other people might best communicate directly with the computer, not its "moving part," the patient. We are thus left either with a patient acting on the basis of a computer's decision, i.e., with the computer responsible for what the patient does, or an infinitely regressive situation in which a patient, with computer, still cannot do what needs to be done (50, 150).

Summary

One benefit from occupational therapeutic interaction with elderly TBI patients is sensitive, germane development and direction of intentional actions to attain functional independence and personal goals.

SPEECH THERAPY

Communication, especially receptive skill, is critical to all therapeutic disciplines and to patient welfare. If problems with dysphagia and dysphonia and maxillofacial injuries after TBI are added, it is clear why speech therapists are prominent in TBI programs. Like occupational therapy, speech therapy's approaches to patients with CVA are often appropriate after traumatic brain injury (161, 162).

Dysphagia

Swallowing disorders may be predicted reliably from imaging studies, when bruxism, or oropharyngeal spasticity, with or without bulbar or pseudobulbar palsy appears, e.g., at Rancho Los Amigos' Level III. Later, partial paralysis or slowing of swallow reflex triggering can be studied in detail using videofluoroscopic techniques. Degree of aspiration and its causes can be studied adding different consistencies of material to this methodology (163, 164) (modified barium swallow). Appropriate food consistencies and bolus size, the contribution of advanced cervical osteoarthritis, and chewing, can be evaluated in this way.

The classic, effective method of tilting the patient's head to the side of difficulty in order to narrow or occlude the dysfunctional region of the oropharynx has also been advanced. Work on pharyngoesophageal dysphagia after lateral medullary syndrome (165) revealed that lateral rotation could aid swallow in spite of essentially flaccid pharyngeal musculature and reduce upper esophageal sphincter tone, thereby increasing the ease of bolus passage. Please see Palmer's chapter on dysphagia (Chapter 23) in this volume.

Communication Problems

The most serious speech-related losses specific to elderly TBI patients follow from the physiologic reduction of auditory capacity with increasing age (164). To these are added progressive losses in the superior temporal gyrus and parietal associational area mass (161, 162, 164, 166).

Wernicke's aphasia, but not Broca's, is significantly correlated with greater age. The inverse relationship between age and auditory comprehension is also stronger in aphasias (166). In spite of a correlation of age with various hearing and fluent aphasic abnormalities, it is felt by some that age does not greatly influence the functional linguistic quality of life of aphasics (161, 162).

Particular Speech Problems of the Elderly After TBI

Some aspects of the treatment of CVA cannot be applied to the TBI patient: performance on exam does not necessarily predict conversational skill. This is partially due to defects in prosody and partially because subtests with individual subset scoring are needed to evaluate the specific yet diffusely located impairments of speech after TBI. Here, too, clinical acumen has no substitute, both in administering the precise hybrid of tests in a battery and in noting behavioral changes. For example, a patient who performs poorly at the beginning of a session may have attentional problems, while errors late in a session may suggest limited stamina.

A personally oriented approach has greater success. A functional frame of reference for accountability is more useful than a simplistic, mechanistic view. Correct remedial therapy and compensatory strategies may be alternated with good effect.

More serious motoric deficits that impinge on linguistic expression have been a focus of engineering. An entire literature has gone beyond the Cannon Communicator (163–165). Practical analysis of expressive deficits has also led to sizeable advances in person-to-person therapy.

Although different syndromes have different timetables (166), stimulation model of response-filling, e.g., "John has a — —-(color)—-bead," can be the transition to self-cueing repetitions, and eventually competent self-initiated performance.

Anxiety reduces performance more severely in speech than in some other areas. This clinical impression may be related to the linguistically involved patient's loss of language as a problem-solving tool. The use of the right side of the brain in ostensibly symbolic tasks can have a markedly positive effect on communication, if not on speech itself.

Group Speech Therapy After TBI

The general pragmatics of speech and factors such as body language, acceptable distance from the speaker/listener in casual and unfamiliar situations, and reading of facial expressions are a few of the better-examined preconditions to linguistic behavior. Reestablishment of these preconditions is critical to the resocialization of the significantly impaired TBI patient. One advantage to group treatment of speech disorders is its resemblance to the conditions under which language is originally acquired.

All patients appear to improve in the first year after onset of aphasia (8, 161, 162, 167–170). In the second year, 40% of the patients improved (162, 170), the greatest improvement occurring with intermittent therapy (170). Swedish folk schools succeed with therapy 3 years after the onset of aphasia.

Naming tests, simple repetition, word fluency, and token tests can be used to balance skills versus expectations (171). Sarno (170) has noted that the manner of stimulus presentation is important in gaining speech therapy goals. This is particularly true in elderly victims of TBI.

The social context for speech therapy has lead to broadly diverse treatment philosophies concerning groups. After elderly TBI, these groups may have highly specific composition, or they may be as informal as a family (1, 8, 12, 46, 58, 65, 123, 124, 172, 173). Some are used for monitoring as well as treatment (174). In any event, they serve an orienting and sociologic function, promoting the development of skills essential to elderly people surviving severe TBI.

References

1. Rosenthal M, Griffith ER, Bond MR, Miller JD. *Rehabilitation of the Head Injured Adult.* Philadelphia, Pa: F.A. Davis; 1983.
2. Pentland B, Jones PA, Roy CW, Miller JD. Head injury in the elderly. *Age-Ageing.* 15(4):193–202, 1986.
3. Terry RD, ed.: *Aging and the Brain, Aging, 32.* New York, NY: Raven; 1988.
4. Kirkpatrick JB, Pearson J. Fatal cerebral injury in the elderly. *J Am Geriatr Soc.* 26(11):489–497, 1978.
5. Roy CW, Pentland B, Miller JD. The causes and consequences of minor head injury in the elderly. *Injury.* 17(4):220–223, 1986.
6. Ruff FM, Marshall LF, Klauber MR, et al.: Alcohol abuse and neurological outcome of the severely head injured. *J Head Trauma Rehabil.* 5(3):21–31, 1990.
7. Wilson BA, Baddeley AD, Cockburn JM. How do old dogs learn new tricks: teaching a technological skill to brain injured people. 25(1):115–119, 1989.
8. Lundgren CC, Perschino EL. Cognitive Group: a treatment program for head-injured adults. *Am J Occup Ther.* 40(6):397–401, 1986.
9. Braakman R. Systematic selection of prognostic features in patients with severe head injury. *Neurosurg.* 68:362, 1980.
10. Jennett B, Teasdale G, Braakman R, et al. Prognosis of patients with severe head injury. *Neurosurg.* 4:283, 1979.
11. Davis DS, Acton P. Treatment of the elderly brain-injured patient. Experience in a traumatic brain injury unit. *J Am Geriatr Soc.* 36(3):225–229, 1988.
12. Cole JR, Cope DN, Cervelli L. Rehabilitation of the severely brain-injured patient: a community-based, low-cost model program. *Arch Phys Med Rehabil.* 66(1):38–40, 1985.
13. Hernesniemi J. Outcome following head injuries in the aged. *Acta Neurochir, Vienna.* 49(1–2):67–79, 1979. Read in abstract.
14. McMordie WR, Barker SL. The financial trauma of head injury. *Brain-Inj.* 2(4):357–364, 1988.
15. Najenson T, Groswasser Z, Mendelson L, Hackett P. Rehabilitation outcome of brain damaged patients after severe head injury. *Int Rehabil Med.* 2(1):17–22, 1980.
16. Rao N, Jellinek HM, Harberg JK, Fryback DG. The art of medicine: subjective measures as predictors of outcome in stroke and traumatic brain injury. *Arch Phys Med Rehabil.* 69(3 Pt 1):179–182, 1988.
17. Saywell RM Jr, Woods JR, Rappaport SA, Allen TL. The value of age and severity as predictors of cost in geriatric head trauma patients. *J Am Geriatr Soc.* 37(7):625–630, 1989.
18. Thorn GW, Adams RD, Braunwald E, et al. *Harrison's Principles of Internal Medicine.* 8th ed. New York, NY: McGraw Hill; 1977.
19. Moruzzi G, Magoun HW. Brain stem reticular formation and activation of the EEG. *Electroencephalogr Clin Neurophysiol.* 1:455–473, 1949.
20. Mountcastle VB, Powell TPS. Neural mechanisms subserving cutaneous sensibility, with special reference to the role of afferent inhibition in sensory perception and discrimination. *Bull Johns Hopkins Hosp.* 105:201–232, 1959.
21. Pompeiano O. Vestibulospinal relations: vestibular influences on gamma motoneurons and primary afferents. In: *Basic Aspects of Central Vestibular Mechanisms. Progress in Brain Research*, XXXVII. Brodal A, Pompeiano O, eds. Amsterdam: Elsevier; 1972:197–232.
22. Ajmone Marsan C. The thalamus. Data on its functional anatomy and on some aspects of thalamocortical integration. *Arch Ital Biol.* 103:847–882, 1965.
23. Engberg A. Vestibular stimulation after head injury: effect on reaction times and motor speech parameters. *Arch Phys Med Rehab.* 70(13):893, 1989.

24. Kenney RA, Fry HD. *Physiology of Aging - A Synopsis.* 2nd ed. Chicago, Ill: Year Book Medical Publishers; 1989.

25. Graham DI, Adams JH, Doyle D. Ischaemic brain damage in fatal non-missile head injuries. *J Neurol Sci.* 39:213, 1978.

26. Terry RD. Physical changes of the aging brain. In: Behnkey JA, Finch CE, Moment GB, eds. *Biology of Aging.* New York, NY: Plenum Press; 1978.

27. Amacher AL, Bybee DE. Toleration of head injury by the elderly. *Neurosurg.* 20(6):954–958, 1987.

28. Brizze KR, Ordy JM, Knox C, Jirge SK. Morphology and aging in the brain. In: Maletta GJ, Pirozzolo FJ, eds. *The Aging Nervous System.* New York, NY: Praeger; 1980.

29. Ohno K, Suzuki R, Masaoka H, et al. [A clinical study on head injuries in the aged]. *No Shinkei Geka.* 15(6):607–611, 1987.

30. Pedachenko GG, Shapovalov IuV. [Disruption of sodium-potassium metabolism in the acute period of craniocerebral injuries in the aged]. *Zh Vopr Neirokhir.* (6):40–44, 1983.

31. Sibata S, Mori K. [Elderly patients with traumatic intracerebral hematoma who talk and deteriorate]. *No Shinkei Geka.* 17(2):177–180, 1989.

32. White MF Jr, Morris R, Feist RM, et al. Eye injury: prevalence and prognosis by setting. *South Med J.* 82(2):151–158, 1989.

33. Greer M. Emergency evaluation of head injuries in the elderly. *Geriatrics.* 34(10):73–84, 1979.

34. Cooper PR, ed. *Head Injury.* 2nd ed. Baltimore, Md: Williams & Wilkins; 1987.

35. Behnke JA, Finch CE, Moment GB, ed. *The Biology of Aging.* New York, NY: Plenum Press; 1978.

36. Ropper AH. Trauma of the head and spinal cord. In: Braunwald E, Isselbacher KJ, Peterdorf RG, et al. *Harrison's Principles of Internal Medicine.* 9th ed. New York, NY: McGraw Hill; 1987.

37. Born JD, Albert A, Hans P, et al. The relative prognostic value of best motor response and brain stem reflexes in patients with severe head injury. *Neurosurg.* 16:595, 1985.

38. Miller JD. Prediction of outcome after injury—a critical review. In: Vigouroux R, ed. *Advances in Neurotraumatology, I.* Berlin: Springer-Verlag; 1986: 229.

39. Shin DY, Ehrenberg B, White J, Bach J, DeLisa JA. Evoked potential assessment: utility in prognosis of chronic head injury. *Arch Phys Med Rehabil.* 70:189–193, 1989.

40. Bakay L, Glassauer FE. *Head Injury.* Boston, Mass: Little, Brown; 1980.

41. Povlishock JT, Becker DP, Cheng CLY, et al. Axonal changes in minor head injury. *J Neuropathol Exp Neurol.* 42:225, 1983.

42. Povlishock JT, ed. *Central Nervous System Trauma: Status Report.* Washington, DC: NINCDS, NIH; 1985:139.

43. Cosgrove JL, Vargo M, Reidy ME. A prospective study of peripheral nerve lesions occurring in traumatic brain-injured patients. *Am J Phys Med Rehabil.* 2(1):15–23, 1989.

44. Cotman CW, Scheff SW. Synaptic growth in aged animals. In: Cherkin A, Finch CE, Kharasch N, Makinodan T, Scott FL, Strehler B, eds. *Physiology and Cell Biology of Aging, Aging,* VIII. New York, NY: Raven; 1979.

45. Ishikawa SE, Saito T, Kaneko K, Okada K, Kusuya T. Hyponatremia responsive to fludrocortisone acetate in elderly patients after head injury. *An Intern Med.* 106(2):187–191, 1987.

46. Corrigan JD, Arnett JA, Houck LJ, Jackson LRD. Reality orientation for brain injured patients: group treatment and monitoring of recovery. *Arch Phys Med Rehabil.* 66(9):626–630, 1985.

47. Prigatano GP, Altman IM. Impaired awareness of behavioral limitations after traumatic brain injury. *Arch Phys Med Rehab.* 71:1058–1064, 1990.

48. Kaye K, Grigsby J, Robbins LJ, Korzun B. Prediction of independent functioning and behavior problems in geriatric patients. *J Am Geriatr Soc.* 38:1304–1310, 1990.

49. Ommaya AK, Gennarelli TA. Cerebral concussion and traumatic unconsciousness: correlation of experimental and clinical observations on blunt head injuries. *Brain.* 97:633, 1974.

50. Wood RL. Attention disorders in brain injury rehabilitation. *Neurosurgery.* 21(6):327, 1988.

51. Prigatano GP. Recovery and cognitive retraining after craniocerebral trauma. *J Learn Disabil.* 20(10):603, 1987.

52. Hibbard MR, Grober SE, Gordon WA, et al. Cognition therapy and the treatment of post stroke depression. *Top Geriatr Rehabil.* 5(3):43–55, 1990.

53. Lhermitte F, Pillon B, Sercaru M. Human autonomy and the frontal lobes. Part I: Imitation and utilization behavior: a neuropsychological study of 75 patients. *Ann Neurol.* 19(4):326–334, 1986.

54. Lhermitte F. Human autonomy and the frontal lobes. Part II: Patient behavior in complex and social situations: the "Environmental Dependency Syndrome." *Ann Neurol.* 19(4):335–343, 1986.

55. Brooks DN, Aughton ME. Psychological consequences of blunt head injury. *Int Rehabil Med.* 1(4):160–165, 1979.

56. Wilson JA, Pentland B, Currie CT, Miller JD. The functional effects of head injury in the elderly. *Brain-Inj.* 1(2):183–188, 1987.

57. Hacki JM, Benzer A, Putz G, et al. How much reintegration can be achieved in patients after severe craniocerebral injury? *Anaesthesist.* 35(3):171–176, 1986.

58. Quine S, Pierce HP, Lyle DM. Relatives as lay-therapists for the severely head-injured. *Brain-Inj.* 2(2):139–149, 1988.

59. Weinberg RM, Auerbach SH, Moore S. Pharmacologic treatment of cognitive deficits: a case study. *Brain-Inj.* 1(1):57–59, 1987.

60. Finger S, Stein DG. *Brain Damage and Recovery: Research and Clinical Perspectives.* Orlando, Fla: Academic Press; 1982.

61. Ala T, Romero S, Knight F, et al. GM-1 treatment of Alzheimer's disease. *Arch Neonl.* 47:1126–1130, 1990.

62. Comalli PE Jr, Wapner S, Werner H. Interference effects of Stroop color-word test in childhood, adulthood, and aging. *J Genet Psychol.* 100:47–53, 1962.

63. Beck AT, Rush AJ, Shaw BF, Emery G. *Cognitive Therapy of Depression.* New York, NY: Guilford Press; 1979.

64. Bracy O. Computer based cognitive rehabilitation. *Cognitive Rehabil.* 1(1):7, 1983.

65. Bernal G, Jacobson LI, Lopez GN. Case histories and shorter communications. Do the effects of behavior modification programs endure? *Behav Res Ther.* 13:61–64, 1975.

66. Giles GM, Wilson JC. The use of behavioral techniques in functional skills training after severe brain injury. *Am J Occup Ther.* 42:658–665, 1988.

67. Howard ME. Behavioral management in the acute care rehabilitation setting. *J Head Trauma Rehabil.* 3(3):14–22, 1988.

68. Davis CS, Acton P. Experience of the elderly-brain injured patient. Experience in a traumatic brain injury unit. *J Am Geriatr Soc.* 36(3):225–229, 1987.

69. DeMaria EJ, Kenney DR, Merriam MA, Casanova LA, Gann DS. Survival in trauma after geriatric patients. *Ann Surg.* 206(6):738–743, 1987.

70. Kauder DR, Schwab CW. Comorbidity in geriatric patients. In: Maull K, Cleveland HC, Strauch G, Walforth C, eds. *Advances in Trauma.* St. Louis, Mo: Mosby; 1990:215–230.

71. Lehman LB. Head trauma in the elderly. *Postgrad Med.* 83(7):140–147, 1988.

72. Long DF. Issues in behavioral neurology and brain injury. In: Ellis DW, Christensen AL. *Neuropsychological Treatment After Brain Injury.* Boston, Mass: Kluwer; 1989:39–90.

73. Silber JM, Hales RE, Yudofsky SC. Psychopharmacology of depression in neurologic disorders. *J Clin Psych.* 51(suppl):33–39, 1990.

74. Sandel ME. Interventions in the inpatient setting. In: Ellis DW,

Christensen AL, eds. *Neuropsychological Treatment After Brain Injury.* Boston, Mass: Kluwer; 1989:157–181.

75. Christensen AL: The neuropsychological investigation as a therapeutic and rehabilitative technique. In: Ellis DW, Christensen AL, eds. *Neuropsychological Treatment After Brain Injury.* Boston, Mass: Kluwer; 1989:125–127.

76. Foley AM, Shahrokhi K, Robinson KM. A behavioral neuropsychological approach strategy for the difficult geriatric patient. *Arch Phys Med Rehabil.* 70:114–117, 1989.

77. Robinson KM, Marcus P, Gepford P. Geriatric rehabilitation in a chronic hospital; meeting the clinical and administrative challenge of providing rehabilitation services to elderly people with severe disability. Presented at 18th Annual Conference, American Hospital Association, Rehabilitation Section; December, 1988; Hollywood, Fl.

78. Davis CS, Acton P. Experience of the elderly-brain injured patient. Experience in a traumatic brain injury unit. *J Am Geriatr Soc.* 36(3):225–229, 1987.

79. O'Donohue WT, Fisher TE, Krasner L. Behavior therapy and the elderly: a conceptual and ethical analysis. *Int J Aging & Human Devel.* 23(1):1–15, 1986.

80. Lightfoot OB, Shahrokhi K, White S, Wilking S, Sessions C, Nelles S. Behavioral neuropsychiatry in a chronic disease rehabilitation hospital #1. Presented at Third Congress of the International Psychogeriatric Association; August 1987; Chicago, Ill.

81. To A, Lightfoot OB, Shahrokhi K, Sessions C, White S. Long-term follow-up of behaviorally disordered geriatric patients. Presented at American Association for Geriatric Psychiatry; February 1990; San Diego, California.

82. Ropper AH. Trauma of the head and spinal cord. In: Braunwald E, Isselbacher KJ, Petersdorf RG, Wilson JD, Martin JB, Fauci AS, eds. *Harrison's Principles of Internal Medicine.* 11th ed. New York, NY: McGraw-Hill; 1987.

83. Brown LJ, Potter JF, Foster BG. Caregiver burden should be evaluated during geriatric assessment. *J Am Geriatr Soc.* 38:455–460, 1990.

84. Fillenbaum GC. *Multidimensional Functional Assessment of Older Adults: The Duke Older Americans Resources and Service Procedures.* Hillsdale, NJ: Lawrence Erlbaum; 1988.

85. Tamler MS, Perrin JCS. Beaumont lifestyle inventory of social support: can it predict disposition prior to an inpatient rehabilitation admission? *Am J Phys Med Rehabil.* 71:149–155, 1992.

86. Miller IW, Bishop DS, Epstein NB, Keitner GI. The McMaster family assessment device: reliability and validity. *J Marital Fam Ther.* 11(4):345–355, 1985.

87. Kabacoff RI, Miller IW, Bishop DS, Epstein NB, Keitner F. A psychometric study of the McMaster family assessment device in psychiatric, medical, and nonclinical samples. *J Fam Psychol.* 3(4)177–186, 1990.

88. Vero D. Long-standing bilateral dislocation of the mandible in the elderly. *Int J Oral Surg.* 10(suppl 1):313–317, 1981.

89. Martin AD, Brown E. The effects of physical activity on the human skeleton. Evaluating and treating head and neck dysfunction in the older person. *Top Geriatr Rehabil.* 4(2):2, 1989.

90. Paris SV. Cervical symptoms of forward head posture. *Top Geriatr Rehabil.* 5(4):11–19, 1990.

91. Amacher AL, Bybee DE. Toleration of head injury in the elderly. *Neurosurg.* 20(6):954–958, 1987.

92. Lewis CB. *Aging: The Health Care Challenge.* Philadelphia, Pa: F.A. Davis; 1985.

93. Tideiksaar R, Kay AD. What causes falls? A logical diagnostic procedure. *Geriatrics.* 41(12), 1986.

94. Wolfson LI, Whipple R, Amerman P, Kleinberg A. Stressing the postural response: a quantitative method for testing balance. *J Am Geriatr Soc.* 34:845–850, 1986.

95. Woollacott MH. Changes in posture and voluntary control in

the elderly, research findings and rehabilitation. *Top Geriatr Rehabil.* 5(2):1–11, 1990.

96. Woollacott MH, Shumway-Couk AT, Nashner LM. Aging and posture control: changes in sensory organization and muscular coordination. *Int J Aging Hum Devel.* 23:97–114, 1986.

97. Payton OD, Poland JL. Aging process: implications for clinical practice. *Phys Ther.* 63(1):41–48, 1983.

98. Brody SJ, Pawlson LG, eds. *Aging and Rehabilitation II—The State of the Practice.* New York, NY: Springer; 1988.

99. Herdman SJ. Treatment of vestibular disorders: traumatically brain-injured patients. *J Head Trauma Rehabil.* 5(4):63–76, 1990.

100. Morimatso M, Hirai S, Etu F, Yoshikawo M. [Vertigo and dizziness in the elderly]. *Jpn J Geriatr.* 12:405–413, 1975. Cited by Corso JF. *Aging Sensory Systems and Perception.* New York, NY: Praeger; 1981.

101. Christiansen J, Juhl E, eds. [The prevention of falls in later life]. *Danish Med Bull.* 34(suppl 4):1024, 1987.

102. Gryfe CI, Amies A, Ashley MJ. A longitudinal study of falls in an elderly population: I. Incidence and morbidity. *Age-Ageing.* 6:201–210, 1977.

103. Kalchthaler T, Bascon RA, Quintos V. Falls in the institutionalized elderly. *J Am Geriatr Soc.* 26(9), 1978.

104. Murphy, J, and Isaacs, B: The post-fall syndrome. *Gerontologist.* 28:265–270, 1982.

105. Werner RA, Vanderzant CW. Multimodal evoked potential testing in acute mild closed head injury. *Arch Phys Med Rehabil.* 72:31–34, 1991.

106. Goldberg E, Gerstman LJ, Mattis S, Hughes JE, Sirio CA, Bilder RM Jr. Selective effects of cholinergic treatment on verbal memory in posttraumatic amnesia. *J Clin Neuropsychol.* 4(3):219–234, 1982.

107. Brody EM, Kleban MH, Moss MS, Kleban F. Predictors of falls among women with Alzheimer's disease. *J Am Geriatr Soc.* 32(12):877–882, 1984.

108. Graves AB, White E, Koespell TD, et al. The association between head trauma and Alzheimer's disease. *Am J Epidemiol.* 131(3):491–501, 1990.

109. Lanyon LE. Strain-related bone modeling and remodeling. Evaluating and treating head and neck dysfunction in the older person. *Top Geriatr Rehabil.* 4(2):13–24, 1989.

110. Simkin A, Ayalon J, Leichton J. Increased trabecular bone density due to bone loading exercise in postmenopausal osteoporotic women. *Calcif Tissue Int.* 40:59–63, 1987.

111. Bhatnagark KR, Baron G, et al. The number of mitral cells in volume in the aging human olfactory bulb: a quantitative morphological study. *Anat.* 218:73–87, 1987.

112. McBride MR, Mistrette CM. Taste responses from the chorda tympani nerve in young and old fisher. *J Gerontol.* 41:306–314, 1986.

113. Myslinski NR. The effects of aging on oral-facial nerve and muscle. Evaluating and treating head and neck dysfunction in the older person. *Top Geriatr Rehabil.* 5, 1990. p 31–38.

114. Nakashima T, Kimmelman P, Snow J. Structure of human fetal and adult olfactory neuroepithelium. *Arch Otolaryngol.* 110:641–646, 1984.

115. Doty RL, Shaman P, Appelbaum SL, et al. Smell identification changes with age. *Science.* 226:1441–1443, 1984.

116. Cherkin A, Finch CE, Kharasch N, Makinodan T, Scott FL, Strehler B, eds. *Physiology and Cell Biology of Aging, Aging,* VIII. New York, NY: Raven; 1979.

117. Servy M. Olfaction in Alzheimer's disease. *Prog Neuropsychopharmacol Bio Psychiatr.* 10:579–586, 1986.

118. Corso JF. *Aging Sensory Systems and Perception.* New York, NY: Praeger; 1981.

119. Ordy JM, Brizzee KR, Beavers TL. Sensory function and short-

term memory. In: Maletta GJ, Pirozzolo FJ, eds. *The Aging Nervous System*. New York, NY: Praeger; 1980.

120. Bernstein D. *Lectures on Diabetic Diet*. Bronx, NY: AECOM; 11 April 1990.

121. Bray GA, Gallagher T. Manifestations of hypothalamic obesity in man: a comprehensive investigation of eight patients and a review of the literature. *Medicine*. 54:301, 1975.

122. Gianutsos R, Grynbaum BB. Helping brain-injured people to contend with hidden cognitive deficits. *Int Rehabil Med*. 5(1):37–40, 1983.

123. Harrington DE, Levandowski DH. Efficacy of an educationally-based cognitive retraining programme for traumatically head-injured as measured by LNNB pre- and post-test scores. *Brain-Inj*. 1(1):65–72, 1987.

124. Carter LT, Oliveira DO, Duponte J, Lynch SV. The relationship of cognitive skills performance to activities of daily living in stroke patients. *Am J Occup Ther*. 42(7):449–455, 1988.

125. Ramón y Cajal S. May, RM trans. *Degeneration and Regeneration of the Nervous System*. London: Oxford University Press; 1928.

126. Landry P, Deschênes M. Intracortical arborizations and receptive fields of identified ventrobasal thalamocortical afferents to the primary somatic sensory cortex in the cat. *J Comp Neurol*. 199:345–371, 1981.

127. Merzenich MM, Jenkins WM, Middlebrooks JC. Observations and hypotheses on special organizational feature of the central auditory nervous system. In: Edelman GM, Gall WE, Cowan WM, eds. *Dynamic Aspects of Neocortical Function*. New York, NY: Wiley; 1984:397–424.

128. Merzenich MM, Kaas JH, Wall JT, Nelson RJ, Sur M, Felleman DJ. Topographic reorganization of somatosensory cortical areas 3b and 1 in adult monkeys following restricted deafferentation. *Neuroscience*. 8:33–55, 1983.

129. Merzenich MM, Nelson RJ, Stryker MC, Schoppman A, Zook M. Somatosensory cortical map changes following digit amputation in adult monkeys. *J Comp Neurol*. 224:591–605, 1984.

130. Edelman GM. *Neural Darwinism*. New York, NY: Basic Books; 1987.

131. Oakley DA, Russell IS. Manipulandum identification in operant behavior in neodecorticate rabbits. *Psych Behav*. 21:943–950, 1977.

132. Goldstein LH, Oakley DA. Expected and actual behavioral capacity after diffuse reduction in cerebral cortex: A review and suggestions for rehabilitative techniques with the mentally handicapped and head injured. *Brit J Clin Psychol*. 24:13–24, 1985.

133. Oakley DA. Instrumental reversal learning and subsequent fixed ratio performance on simple and go/nogo schedules in neodecorticate rabbits. *Physiol Psychol*. 7:29–42, 1979.

134. Oakley DA. Learning with food reward and shock avoidance in neodecorticate rats. *Exp Neurol*. 63:627–642, 1979.

135. Weinberg RM, Auerbach SH, Moore S. Pharmacologic treatment of cognitive deficits: a case study. *Brain-Inj*. 1(1):57–59, 1987.

136. Song F, Freemantle N, Sheldon TA, et al. Selective serotonin reuptake inhibitors: meta-analysis of efficacy and acceptability. *Brit J Med*. 306:683–687, 1993.

137. Goldberg E, Gerstman LJ, Mattis S, Hughes JE, Sirio CA, Bilder RM. Selective effects of cholinergic treatment on verbal memory in posttraumatic amnesia. *J Clin Neuropsychol*. 4(3):219–234, 1982.

138. Gabel BA, Dunbar GL, Stein DG. Gangliosides minimize behavioral deficits and enhance structural repair after brain injury. *J Neurosci Res*. 12(2–3):429–443, 1984.

139. Fioravanti M, Buckley AE, Agnoli A. A multidimensional approach to the assessment of clinical validity in a study on CCVD

treatment: dihydroergocristine versus placebo. *Arch Gerontol Geriatr*. 6(1):83–93, 1987.

140. Balestreri R, Fontana L, Astengo F. A double-blind placebo controlled evaluation of the safety and efficacy of vinpocetine in the treatment of patients with chronic vascular senile cerebral dysfunction. *J Am Geriatr Soc*. 35(5):425–430, 1987.

141. Facciolla D, Ruocco A, Rossi A, Serra C, Bulfalino L, Cavrini P. [Clinical and electrophysiologic changes produced by (−) eburnamonine in acute and post-acute stages of head injuries]. *Riv Neurol*. 53(1):15–33, 1983.

142. Yamamoto M, Shimizu M. Effects of a new TRH analogue, YM-14673 on a passive avoidance test as a possible criterion of improvement in cognitive disturbance in rodents. *Naunyn Schmiedebergs Arch Pharmacol*. 338(3):262–267, 1988. Read in Abstract.

143. Larson EB, Walter AK, Buchner D, Reifler BV. Adverse drug reactions associated with global cognitive impairment in elderly persons. *Ann Intern Med*. 107:169–173, 1987.

144. Cope DN, ed. Neuropharmacology. *J Head Trauma Rehabil*. 2(4),34–42 1987.

145. Cope DN. The pharmacology of attention and memory. *J Head Trauma Rehabil*. 1(3):34, 1986.

146. Weinberg J, Diller L, Gordon WA, et al. Visual scanning training effect on reading-related tasks in acquired right brain damage. *Arch Phys Med Rehabil*. 58(11):479–486, 1977.

147. Glisky EL, Schacter DL, Tulving E. Computer learning by memory-impaired patients: acquisition and retention of complex knowledge. *Neuropsychologia*. 24(3):313–328, 1986.

148. Kurlychek RT, Levin W. Computers in the cognitive rehabilitation of brain-injured persons. *Crit Rev Med Inform*. 1(3):241–257, 1987.

149. Lincoln NB, Whiting SE, Cockburn J, Bhavnani G. An evaluation of perceptual retraining. *Int Rehabil Med*. 7(3):99–101, 1985.

150. Namerow NS. Cognitive and behavioral aspects of brain-injury rehabilitation. *Neurol Clin*. 5(4):569–583, 1987.

151. Fishman LM. Computerized treatment of impulsivity. *Arch Phys Med Rehabil*. 69:709–710, 1988.

152. Auerbach SH. Neuroanatomical correlates of attention and memory disorders in traumatic brain injury: an application of neurobehavioral subtypes. *J Head Trauma Rehabil*. 1(3):1–12, 1986.

153. Bear DM. Hemispheric specialization and the neurology of emotion. *Arch Neurol*. 40:195, 1983.

154. Lynch WJ. Selecting a computer for rehabilitation. *J Head Trauma Rehabil*. 5(4)101–103, 1990.

155. Williamson PC, Mersky H, Morrison S, et al. Quantitative electroencephalographic correlates of cognitive decline in normal elderly subjects. *Arch Neurol*. 47:1185–1188, 1990.

156. Picton TW. The P-300 wave of the human event-related potential. *J Clin Neurophysiol*. 9(4):456–479, 1992.

157. Albert MS, Moss MB. *Geriatric Neuropsychology*. New York, NY: Guilford Press; 1988.

158. Kirsch NL, Levine SP, Fallon-Krueger M, Jaros LA. The microcomputer as an orthotic device for patients with cognitive limitations. Presented at American Congress of Rehabilitation; 1984; Boston, Mass.

159. Cicerone KD, Wood JC. Planning disorder after closed head injury: a case study. *Arch Phys Med Rehabil*. 68(2):111–115, 1987.

160. Fishman LM, Tabaddor K, Hillman G, et al. The ghost and the machine. *Top Geriatr Rehabil*. 5(3):56–65, 1990.

161. Sarno MT. Verbal impairment after closed head injury. Report of a replication study. *J Nerv Ment Dis*. 172(8):475–479, 1984.

162. Sarno MT. Language and speech defects. *Scand J Rehabil Med*. 17(suppl):55–64, 1988.

163. Logemann JA. *Evaluation and Treatment of Swallowing Disorders*. San Diego, Calif: College-Hill Press; 1983.

164. Adamovitch BB. Treatment of communication and swallowing disorders. In: Rosenthal M, Griffith ER, Bond MR, Miller JD, eds. *Rehabilitation of the Head Injured Adult.* Philadelphia, Pa: F.A. Davis; 1983.

165. Logemann JA, Kahrilas PJ, Kobara M, Vakil NB. Benefit of head rotation on pharyngoesophageal dysphagia. *Arch Phys Med Rehabil.* 70:767–771, 1989.

166. Schechter I, Schejter J, Abarbanel M, Groswasser Z, Solzi P. Age and aphasic syndromes. *Scand J Rehabil Med.* 12(suppl):60–63, 1985.

167. Levine SP, Kirsch NL, Perlman OZ, Cole TM. Engineering therapy: an approach to treatment of a patient with severe cognitive and physical handicaps. *Arch Phys Med Rehabil.* 65(11):737–739, 1984.

168. Groher ME. Speech and language assessment. In: Rosenthal M, Griffith ER, Bond MR, Miller JD, eds. *Rehabilitation of the Head Injured Adult.* Philadelphia, Pa: F.A. Davis; 1983.

169. Coleman CL, Cook AM, Meyers LS. Assessing non-oral clients for assistive communication devices. *J Speech Hear Dis.* 45:515, 1980.

170. Sarno MT. Speech therapy. Lecture at New York Academy of Medicine; April 3, 1990; New York, NY.

171. Dahlberg C, Weintraub A, Howard S. *Language Disturbances in Traumatic Brain Injury.*

172. Menninger K, Mayman M. Episodic dyscontrol: a third order of stress adaptation. *Bull Menninger Clin.* 20(4):153, 1956.

173. Mysiw WJ, Corrigan JD, Hunt M, Cavin D, Fish T. Vocational evaluation of traumatic brain injury patients using the functional assessment inventory. *Brain-Inj.* 3(1):27–34, 1989.

174. Jackson RD, Mysico WJ, Corrigan JD. Orientation group monitoring system—an indicator for reversible impairments in cognition during post traumatic amnesia. *Arch Phys Med Rehabil.* 70(1):33–36, 1989.

18
Degenerative Central Nervous System Diseases

S. Sheela Jain and Joel A. DeLisa

Degenerative central nervous system (CNS) disorders are often of unknown etiology, are mainly treated symptomatically, and may have a progressive course. In caring for these patients one has to not only address the immediate functional needs, but also plan for addressing more significant impairments. In prescribing equipment for these individuals, one has to be aware of the patient's and significant other's tolerance for gadgets and recognize financial constraints. In this chapter we will only deal with adult motor neuron disease and Parkinsonism, but the principles apply to other CNS degenerative diseases as well.

MOTOR NEURON DISEASE

Motor neuron disease (MND) refers to a heterogeneous group of diseases that are characterized by disorders of motor neurons in the cerebral cortex, brainstem, and/or spinal cord and are associated, to varying degrees, with weakness, atrophy, and long-tract motor signs (1).

Generalized Description

Diseases of the motor neuron may be diffuse or focal. The majority are diffuse systemic degenerations of unknown etiology selectively destroying upper and lower motor neurons (UMN and LMN) (Table 18.1) (1). Amyotrophic lateral sclerosis (ALS) is the most common disorder affecting the motor neuron. It involves both UMN and LMN.

Characteristically, there is a combination of UMN and LMN signs that spread to almost all muscles of the body except possibly the extraocular muscles and sphincters. ALS may be categorized into four subtypes based on the combination of UMN and LMN involvement of the bulbar and spinal motor neurons. The subtypes are (1): (*a*) LMN-bulbar: progressive bulbar palsy, (*b*) LMN-spinal: progressive muscular atrophy, (*c*) UMN-

bulbar: progressive pseudobulbar palsy, and (*d*) UMN-spinal: primary lateral sclerosis.

Involvement of the UMN produces weakness without atrophy, usually asymmetrical, in either the proximal or distal limb muscles or the bulbar muscles (1, 2). Reflexes are hyperactive, and pathologic reflexes are present. Spasticity commonly occurs at different levels; there may be spastic gait or spastic dysarthria with bulbar palsy. Muscle cramps are frequent and are often what prompts the patient to seek medical assistance.

LMN damage produces clinical abnormalities. Loss of anterior horn cells (AHC) and their peripheral axons results in the loss of muscle-fiber innervation. The weakness is usually painless. The nerve terminals of intact motor units will reinnervate these muscle fibers, and, if they can keep pace with the loss of AHC, weakness and atrophy will not occur. Up to one third of the motor neurons innervating a muscle may be lost before clinical signs of weakness or atrophy are found. The denervated muscle becomes weak, flaccid, and atrophic, the typical signs of LMN disease.

Pathologically, there are degenerative changes and atrophy in motor neurons throughout the neuraxis, including reduction of the large motor neurons in the cervical and lumbar spinal cord. Peripherally, there is a marked reduction in the number of large myelinated fibers in the ventral roots. The data indicate that ALS is predominantly a neuronopathy, with quantitatively similar axonal degeneration at both proximal and distal levels.

In ALS, one finds both UMN and LMN manifestations. The illness is insidious in onset. Classically, the first involvement is often the intrinsic hand muscles, but it may start in the bulbar or distal muscles of the lower extremities. The disease usually starts distally and may be asymmetrical and symmetrical. Ultimately, muscle weakness and wasting becomes bilateral and widespread. Fasciculations tend to be prominent and are usually as-

Table 18.1. Some of the Suggested Etiological Factors in ALS

Abiotrophy: premature aging of motorneurons
Axonal transport: orthograde, retrograde ("suicide")
Biochemical factors: decreased RNA and protein synthesis
Calcium metabolism: hyperparathyroidism, West Pacific foci
Circulating endogenous neurotoxins: directed at perikaryon,
 terminal sprouts
Endemic factors: hexosaminidase A, DNA repair enzymes, thiamine
 pyrophosphatase
Genetic factors: familial ALS
Heavy metals: lead, mercury
Immunologic factors
Injuries, fractures, animal skins, etc.
Neuronal receptors: androgens, thyrotropin-releasing hormone
Paraneoplastic factors: lymphoma, paraproteinemia
Viruses: polio, postpolio syndromes

Table 18.2. Classification of Motor Neuron Disorders

Infants
 Infantile muscular atrophy (Werdnig-Hoffmann)
Childhood/adolescence
 Juvenile muscular atrophy (Wohlfart-Kugelberg-Welander)
 Juvenile progressive bulbar palsy
 Progressive bulbar palsy of childhood (Fazio-Londe)
Adults
 Adult progressive bulbar palsy
 Amyotrophic lateral sclerosis
 Hereditary spastic paraplegia
 Primary lateral sclerosis (Erb)
 Progressive bulbar-spinal muscular atrophy (Magee)
 Progressive muscular atrophy or spinal muscular atrophy (SMA)
 Pseudobulbar palsy
 Upper limb SMA (Aran-Duchenne)

sociated with an increase in tone, hyperreflexia, and extensor plantar responses.

Epidemiology

ALS occurs almost as frequently as multiple sclerosis, with an incidence rate ranging from 0.4 to 1.8 per 100,000 population and a prevalence rate of 2.5 to 7.0 per 100,000 (1, 3). These rates occur fairly uniformly throughout the world except in Guam and the Kiji peninsula, where they are much higher. The disease is 95% sporadic, 5% being hereditary and mainly autosomal dominant (4). In the hereditary form, there is good penetrance, but the expression can vary within the same family. Most cases of inherited ALS are due to a genetic defect on the long arm of chromosome 21. This gene generates the enzyme responsible for destroying free radicals. For sporadic ALS, the mean age of onset is about 55 years, and the male:female ratio is 2:1.

In one large series, ALS presented with upper extremity involvement 41%, lower extremity involvement 40%, and bulbar involvement 19% (5). Bulbar involvement is usually found in cranial nerves V, VII, IX, X, and XII. The initial symptoms may present with respiratory involvement including the diaphragm. The location of the symptoms depends upon the part of the nervous system affected first and usually involves all four extremities within 1 year of onset. This type of onset suggests that ALS actually encompasses several different diseases that may have separate causal agents.

The mean duration of ALS is 2 to 6 years, with death usually due to respiratory failure and/or pneumonia, depending on whether the patient chooses some type of ventilatory support. The 5-year survival rate is approximately 40%, with 10% of the patients surviving beyond 10 years. Some patients have lived as long as 20 years after the initial onset of ALS. There may be considerable variability in the course of the disease, with plateaus and possibly even reversals. Patients with the

Table 18.3. Other Forms of Motor Neuron Disorders (MND)

Degenerative disorders
 Friedreich's ataxia
 HMSN type II
 Scapuloperoneal syndrome
 Shy-Drager Syndrome
Infectious disorders, all of which may demonstrate multifocal
 anterior horn cell destruction
 Coxsackie virus
 Herpes zoster
 Jakob-Creutzfeldt disease
 Poliomyelitis
MND associated with diabetes mellitus
 Diabetic amyotrophy
 Possible relationship to hypoglycemia
MND associated with juvenile asthma
MND associated with structural lesions
 Syringomyelia or syringobulbia
 Cervical spondylosis
Paraneoplastic syndrome
Postradiation therapy neuronopathy
Toxic motor neuronopathies
 Dapsone
 Disulfiram

worst prognosis are those with bulbar symptoms and those who are diagnosed after the age of 50 years.

Classifications

In general, classification is based on the patient's age at onset and the associated clinical findings. Some of the motor neuron disorders based on time of onset are noted in Table 18.2 (1). Other less common forms of MND are listed in Table 18.3 (1).

The diagnosis is based on the clinical picture and is supported by electrodiagnostic abnormalities, normal cerebral spinal fluid, a neurogenic picture on muscle biopsy, and absence of radiographic abnormalities indicative of spinal cord compression. Increases in serum creatinine phosphokinase (CPK) are common in ALS and correlate with muscle weakness and atrophy.

Differential Diagnosis

Given the grave prognosis of ALS, the diagnosis should be made only when other causes that might produce a similar clinical picture have been ruled out. This includes cervical spondylosis, tumors, anomalies of the foramen magnum and upper cord, CNS syphilis, syringomyelia, heavy metal intoxications (such as lead and mercury), diabetic amyotrophy, hyperparathyroidism, late effects of polio, postradiation myelitis, and paraproteinemias.

Weakness

ALS also presents itself as stiffness, clumsiness, atrophy, and/or fasciculations. Exercise early in the disease is used to prevent disuse weakness and to strengthen unaffected muscles (6). Later, energy conservation and work simplification should be stressed (2, 7, 8). Many physicians believe that fatigue may increase weakness, and thus, Progressive Resistive Exercises (PREs) are not recommended. Although there are no studies with respect to ALS to support this statement, experience with polio patients substantiates this concern. Contractures are also to be avoided. Cramps can be a problem and may respond to treatment with calcium supplements such as quinine 180 mg to 300 mg daily or Dilantin 100 mg to 200 mg daily.

Some patients with a defect of the neuromuscular junction have responded to an anticholinesterase drug such as Mestinon. This dosage must be titrated carefully and used with a specific functional goal in mind. The fasciculations tend mianly to be distal in origin, and their presence and severity does not appear to be related to the course of the disease. Treatments consist of rest, caffeine avoidance, and Valium, if indicated.

The extent of spasticity depends on whether UMN or LMN symptoms are prevalent. Valium and Dantrium are usually ineffective, and although Lioresal is considered the drug of choice, the authors have not found it to be particularly helpful.

Ambulation difficulties are due to weakness of the lower extremities, as well as the trunk and upper extremities. The painless foot drop responds to an insert ankle-foot orthosis with the ankle in the neutral position (2).

Activities of Daily Living

Adaptive equipment can be provided to aid in self-care activities. The types of equipment prescribed will depend on what the patient desires to do for him or herself. The prescription should be tempered by financial resources, gadget tolerance, and the value as perceived by the patient (2, 9).

Dysphagia

One of the treatment goals is to maintain nutrition and hydration (10). Adequate fluid is essential to maintain good urinary output and to avoid urinary tract infections, as well as loosen pulmonary secretions (2). Because of the progressive weakness and spasticity of bulbar muscles in some ALS patients, dysphagia is a common component.

With respect to swallowing, there may be problems with chewing, reflex swallowing, aspiration, and/or malnutrition (11). One of the most common early symptoms is that the patient will complain of choking on saliva while reclining or on postnasal congestions. The initial swallowing problems are with liquids and, later, solids. Some techniques to providing safer swallowing are: stimulate the receptors using taste, temperature, or texture and if bulbar symtpoms are present, take the food in the upright position with the neck flexed (2). Custards, casseroles, and other foods that hold together in a bolus are recommended, while pureed foods, sticky foods such as white bread, or foods that produce thick mucus such as chocolate or uncooked milk products should be avoided. Pills can be placed in jelly or custard and be swallowed as a single bolus (2).

Thick secretions can be liquified by dissolving a papase tablet under the tongue 10 minutes before meals or by swabbing the tongue with a small amount of meat tenderizer made from papaya and wiping the secretions (2). An aspirator is also helpful. A cricopharyngeal myotomy may be helpful for a patient who has a good productive cough and adequate tongue and pharyngeal strength to propel the bolus into the esophagus. This is a rare patient in our experience.

Sialorrhea

Drooling occurs due to the lower lip or other facial weakness and/or swallowing problems. A person secretes about 0.5 to 2 cc of saliva each minute. Anticholinergic drugs such as atropine and scopolamine have been disappointing for long-term treatment of this disorder. A transtympanic neurectomy that interrupts the parasympathetic innervation of the submaxillary, sublingual, and parotid glands will reduce the volume of saliva at rest and the patient's response to parasympathetic stimulation (2, 8, 12). A combined unilateral transtympanic neurectomy and parotid duct ligation takes about 2 to 3 hours to perform and may provide control for up to 6 months. If the patient has intact palative salivary glands, then the loss of taste on the anterior tongue will not be a problem.

When the patient is not able to handle liquids or when there is a high risk of aspiration, an alternative method of intake is essential. If the gag reflex is diminished, the patient may pass an orogastric tube to meet the hydration and nutrient needs. A cervical esophagostomy is an alternative solution, but most people prefer a percutaneous gastrostomy.

Dysarthria

The destruction of speech is due to paresis and spasticity of the lips, tongue, palate, and larynx due to the involvement of cranial nerves V, VII, IX, X, and XII, and the respiratory muscles (13). One often finds a mixed spastic-flaccid dysarthria with slowness of articulation, hypernasality, and strained voice quality with UMN lesions and a stridulous or breathing sound with LMN lesions. There are also problems with articulation due to decreased strength of the tongue, lips, cheeks, and mandibular muscles. To counter these problems the patient should be taught energy conservation using short phrases and key words (2), and may communicate using writing, gesturing, or an alphabet/word board. The patient may also benefit from an augmented communication device. Criteria for prescribing such a device are:

1. Speech is unintelligible for effective communication.
2. The patient has no ability to use the hands for written communication.
3. The patient has no ability to learn to use other alternative devices.
4. The patient will accept a machine, as opposed to other means, such as a signal system.

Respiratory Failure

Atrophy of the respiratory muscles results in restrictive pulmonary syndrome. Pulmonary diffusion capacity may be diminished because of chronic microatelectasis and the inability to manage airway secretions. Acute obstructive episodes may occur as a result of mucus plugging. Inspiratory muscle weakness results in dyspnea, hypoventilation, and chronic ventilatory insufficiency. Motor dysfunction of the pharynx, glottis, and larynx produces aspiration, while weakness of the larynx, glottis and expiratory muscles produces an impaired cough. The most common respiratory problems are hypoventilation and impaired clearance of secretions, which lead to infection and acute respiratory failure (14–18).

The respiratory muscles most affected vary with the distribution of the disease (16). The diaphragm is usually affected, while the upper and midthoracic spinal segments are relatively spared. Respiratory evaluation should consist of a screening function test to rule out the presence of a significant obstructive component, which may be present in patients with premorbid pulmonary disease. Typically the presence of decreased lung volumes, i.e., vital capacity, in the presence of normal forced expiratory flows, is sufficient to rule out a significant obstructive component and establish the diagnosis of restrictive pulmonary syndrome.

In the presence of symptoms of hypoventilation or a decrease in vital capacity to less than about 1000 mL, nocturnal oxygen saturation and/or end-tidal carbon dioxide monitoring should be performed (14). Significant decreases in oxygen saturation or elevations in carbon dioxide tension indicate the need for nocturnal ventilatory aid. Although most of these patients will eventually require a tracheostomy for ventilatory support, this should be contingent on the family's commitment to maintain the patient in the home environment and the availability of 24-hour access to technical support. Noninvasive methods of ventilatory aids may be effective so long as oropharyngeal muscle strength is adequate. The pneumobelt may be especially useful for these patients because this device assists ventilation, and the forced expiration may aid in the mobilization of secretions. Oxygen therapy, which depresses the ventilatory drive, should be avoided.

Secretions can be aided by suctioning, postural change, and chest physiotherapy, including manual assisted coughing. Vigorous postural drainage and percussion are not well tolerated, and the positions available for drainage are often limited to half lying and half side-lying. Gentle shaking or vibration often gives some relief with removal of secretions. Aggressive chest physiotherapy does not usually result in lasting improvement in ventilatory function and may lead to excessive tiredness and a decrease in respiratory excursions. These techniques should be carried out frequently for short periods. Manual assisted coughing is effective but may be effort intensive. A forced mechanical exsufflation device is very effective and simple to use.

One of the major decisions in dealing with these patients is whether to use a total ventilatory support with a tracheostomy or to use a noninvasive ventilation system (Chapter 22). The following issues need to be addressed when making this decision:

1. Technical support—is it available 24 hours per day?
2. Primary caregivers—will there be more than one?
3. Both the patient and the support system must agree on the type of support.
4. Bioethical decisions—these are of particular importance with irreversible pathology.
5. Living Will—this should be written before respiratory failure develops.
6. Patient has the option of discontinuing the support.

Psychologic Aspects of Care

Psychologically these patients are no different than other seriously ill persons (2). Situational reactive depression is comon. The progressive disability, increasing dependence, difficulties in communication, and the reaction of people around them all contribute to the mood disturbances. In the authors' experience, antidepressants such as the tricyclics are not usually needed or particularly helpful (2). Rather, one needs to counsel the patient and care provider regarding the management of the progressive losses and eventual outcome. The patient should have the opportunity to express feelings, concerns, and frustrations (2). Attention must be given to planning for heavy personal care on a 24-hour basis, as well as discussing issues such as feeding, communication, ventilator decision, death, and dying (2). Hope should always be present and new treatment modes discussed. Suicide among this population is very uncommon (2).

Treatment

The etiology is unknown and selection of experimental compounds is based on assumed etiologies or pathologic observations. Current medications such as attentuated cobra venom, plasmaphoresis, ganglioside therapy, and interferon have not altered the course of the disease. Thyrotropin-releasing hormone (TRH), when given in high intravenous doses, will temporarily improve muscle strength and function, (1, 19, 20). However, it is not a cure.

PARKINSON'S DISEASE

Parkinson's disease (PD) is a chronic, slowly progressive, degenerative neurologic disorder of the CNS, which was first described by James Parkinson in 1817 (21). It is characterized by the presence of resting tremor, bradykinesia, rigidity, and loss of postural reflexes.

Parkinsonism can be categorized into three etiological groups (Table 17.4):

1. Idiopathic Parkinsonism: Idiopathic Parkinsonism is the most common form of PD, but its cause remains unknown. It has been suggested that the disease represents selective acceleration of the normal aging

Table 18.4. Classification of Common Forms of Parkinsonism

Primary or idiopathic Parkinsonism (Parkinson's disease)
Secondary or acquired Parkinsonism
  Infections: postencephalitic
  Toxins: manganese, carbon monoxide, carbon disulfide, synthetic
    drug 1-methyl-4 Phenyl-1,2,3,6 tetrahydropyridine (MPTP)
  Drugs: antipsychotic, reserpine
  Hypoparathyroidism
  Vascular (atherosclerotic)
Parkinsonism-plus, in which additional neurologic signs are present
  Striatonigral degeneration
  Progressive supranuclear palsy
  Shy-Drager syndrome
  Normal pressure hydrocephalus
  Alzheimer's disease
  Wilson's disease
  Huntington's disease

process. This is because the symptoms mirror those associated with advanced age. These symptoms include flexed posture, shuffling gait, and slowing of the reaction time and speed of movement. However, only a small number of elderly suffer from PD, and its incidence declines after age 80 years.

2. Secondary Parkinsonism: There are numerous disorders where Parkinsonism may be the predominant or less dominant feature. This includes brain tumors that affect basal ganglia function, encephalitis, and cerebrovascular disease. Secondary Parkinsonism may also arise as a result of poisoning with manganese or carbon monoxide, surgical removal of the parathyroid, or may be drug-induced by the toxicity of neuroleptic drugs, such as reserpine, butyrophenomes, or phenothiazines. Drug-induced, postencephalitis, and vascular Parkinsonism are the three most common types of secondary Parkinson's disease and are discussed below.

  a. Drug-Induced Parkinsonism: Reserpine depletes the storage of dopamine in the dominergic nerve terminals in the striatum and hence in high doses may result in Parkinsonism. Antipsychotic drugs such as butyrophenomes and phenothiazines can block postsynaptic dopamine receptors in the striatum and thus produce severe extrapyramidal symptoms that resemble idiopathic Parkinsonism. Levodopa is not able to reverse this complication because dopamine receptors are blocked and occupied by the antipsychotic medication. If the toxic drug is withdrawn, symptoms may clear over several weeks or months. However, oral anticholinergic drugs have been found to be effective in treating this form of Parkinsonism.

  b. Postencephalitic Parkinsonism: PD was first noted in 1919 in many patients who suffered from encephalitis lethargica (VonEconomo's encephalitis) during World War I and in patients who had suffered from viral encephalitis. Clinically, it progresses more slowly and is more sensitive to levodopa therapy than is idiopathic PD.

  c. Vascular Parkinsonism: Arteriosclerotic or vascular Parkinsonism may occur in middle age as well as old age. It may follow a stroke, but is more commonly seen as a complication of multiple small infarctions involving striatum. Diagnosis is made using a computed tomography (CT) scan and magnetic resonance imaging (MRI). Gait disturbance and loss of postural reflexes are present, while tremor and bradykinesia are rare. AntiParkinson's drugs have little benefit in treating this type of PD.

3. Parkinsonism-Plus: These are multisystem degenerative diseases with signs of Parkinsonism and other neurologic deficits (Table 18.4). They are beyond the scope of this chapter and will not be discussed.

Epidemiology

Primary or idiopathic PD affects 1% of the population over 50 years of age in the United States (22). In 1968, there were over one million victims, varying in age from 35 years to 80 years. It has a prevalence rate of 1.5 per 1,000 in North America and Europe, and an estimated incidence rate of 20.5 per 100,000 per year (23). Males and females are effected equally. PD ranks behind cerebrovascular diseases and arthritides as the third most common chronic disease of late adulthood (24). Preliminary investigations have suggested increased risk associated with the rural environment and well water consumption (25).

Course and Prognosis

The incidence of PD increases with age, reaching a maximum at age 75 years and declining after that. The age of onset is the fifth and sixth decade. The onset is so insidious that flagrant signs may not become apparent until much later in life. Patients with early tremor progress more slowly, though the average duration is approximately 14 years. The mortality rate is 1.5 to 2.5 times higher than among controls. Death is usually due to pneumonia or cardiovascular disease.

Pathology

Much remains to be learned about the pathophysiology of Parkinsonism. It has long been known to be a disorder of the extrapyramidal system with most changes being present in the substantia nigra. There is cell loss and degeneration of a group of pigmented neurons that produce the neurotransmitter dopamine. Lewy bodies (concentric hyaline eosinophilic cytoplasmic inclusions) are seen microscopically in the substantia nigra and locus ceruleus neurons. It is believed that a loss of dopamine in basal ganglia may cause an imbalance between this and other neurotransmitters such as acetylcholine, glutamate, aspartate, and gamma-aminobutyric acid. It has recently been shown that many different dopamine receptors in the basal ganglia may undergo pathologic changes and that dopamine may not be the only neurotransmitter affected in Parkinsonism (26).

Clinical Manifestations

Tremor is the most common symptom. The dopaminergic pathway of the substantia nigra exerts a tonic modulatory influence by inhibiting the cholinergic striatal interneurons. Loss of inhibitory input may cause excessive striatal excitatory output, which facilitates oscillatory loops in the thalamocortical system, resulting in Parkinson's tremor. Initially, the tremor is the pill-rolling type, with flexion and extension of the index finger

and thumb into the palm. This may then spread to the rest of the fingers, hands, forearm, and even more proximally to the trunk, neck, and ankles. The tremor is rhythmic, four to eight beats per minute, and is most pronounced at rest. Electromyographic (EMG) tracings show rhythmic alternating bursts in agonistic and antagonistic muscles. It is suppressed by activity and sleep and is aggravated by fatigue or stress. This differentiates it from intention tremors, which occur during activity. When the disease has advanced, Parkinson's tremor can also be present during activity.

Rigidity appears in two forms: plastic or lead-pipe and cogwheel. Plastic or lead-pipe rigidity is seen when resistance is present uniformly throughout the passive range of motion (ROM) of the limb. Attempted passive ROM results in cogwheel rigidity, when the resistance is intermittent, producing a series of jerks. Both of these varieties involve flexor and extensor limb muscles. Patients often find it difficult to ambulate due to stiffness and heaviness in the legs. Their gait is very stereotyped with poverty of motion, mostly due to insufficient extension at the hip, knee, and ankle and lack of reciprocal movements of the upper extremities. Rising from a chair or bed may be difficult or impossible. Patients may also have difficulty initiating movements. For example, when starting to walk they may feel as if their feet are stuck to the floor, but once started, the step length may increase, and the patients may lean forward and walk faster to avoid falling forward. The gait is described as a "festinating" gait. It is said that Parkinson's patients walk as if they are trying to catch up with their center of gravity. When negotiating a turn, patients take short frequent steps, twisting around rather than walking. Loss of postural reflexes can cause the patients to become unable to maintain standing balance, and they may fall from a push forward or backward. Repetitive movements are performed slowly with progressively reduced amplitude. Postural deformities appear: the head is flexed forward; the trunk is stooped and may be tilted to one side; hands may develop ulnar deviation with flexion at metacarpophalangeal joints and extension at interphalangeal joints; arms may be adducted and elbows flexed.

Akinesia, hypokinesia, and bradykinesia are terms used interchangeably, to mean slowness of voluntary movement. Patients are less mobile, and their movements are slow and deliberate as if they are making an effort to initiate the movement. Programming and execution of movement have been studied by Sheridan et al and confirmed to be slow (27). In the beginning stages of the disease, the patient walks slowly, and the reciprocal swing of the upper extremity is lost. As the disease progresses, gait becomes shuffled with very small steps, and hand dexterity is lost. Many patients are unable to button their clothes, tie their shoe laces, etc. Micrographia, where the writing becomes smaller and is cramped and unintelligible develops, and the patient gradually becomes dependent in the activities of daily living.

Cranial nerve dysfunction may result in difficulty with chewing, swallowing, and blinking. This is due to bradykinesia of the muscles supplied by the ocular, facial, and glossopharyngeal nerves. The postencephalitic Parkinson patient may exhibit an oculogyric crisis in which the eyes move and remain in an uncontrolled position, mostly upward and outward. Voice quality changes occur with speech becoming very low volume, monotonous, and unintelligible. Akinesia also leads to a blank or mask-like face with paucity or lack of expression. Infrequent blinking and reduction in ocular movement may result in a staring appearance, which causes the patient to appear intellectually impaired or depressed.

Autonomic nervous system dysfunction is also evident. Patients may have increased salivation or sialorrhea. A decreased rate of swallowing may lead to pooling of saliva and drooling. Increased perspiration and seborrhea with oily skin, bladder incontinence, and heat intolerance are also present. Decreased peristalsis may result in constipation. Respiration may become shallow, and symptomatic postural hypotension may be present.

Sensory symptoms such as generalized or localized warmth, coldness, or numbness may be present. A subjective feeling of motor restlessness may be seen when the patient is not able to sit or lie still.

Adhesive capsulitis of the shoulder is a common symptom of the disease. Riley et al (28) found a significantly higher incidence of both history of shoulder complaints and a frozen shoulder (diagnosed by history of spontaneous onset of painful and progressively severe restriction of shoulder joint mobility lasting for a variable period and followed by a gradual resolution with or without medical intervention and with no evidence of intrinsic shoulder pathology) in patients with PD. Those developing frozen shoulder had initial disease symptoms indicative of akinesia twice as frequently as those with a tremor. In 8% of the patients studied, frozen shoulder was the first symptom of the disease, occurring 0 to 2 years prior to the onset of more commonly recognized features. It had no effect on the severity or the prognosis of the disease.

Perceptual motor and visuospatial deficits were found during neuropsychologic studies (29). The deficits are believed to be due to the disease affecting the basal ganglia structures that are necessary for voluntary movements that require sequencing or planning and not related to the motor deficit.

Emotional and personality changes occur in the later stages of PD. Patients become less assertive, more passive, dependent, and indecisive. Depression is common and is found in approximately 40% of the patients. Sleep disturbance and dementia may be seen in advanced stages of the disease.

Diagnosis

PD is a clinical diagnosis and usually recognized by physicians during physical evaluation. The patient may have mask-like face, resting tremor, rigidity, paucity of movement, difficulty getting out of chair, and/or typical shuffling gait. However, the patient initially may only have mild symptoms of tremors, clumsiness, fatigue, and difficulty in walking on one side only, and symptoms may gradually extend to the other side.

Management

There is no known cure for Parkinson's disease. Management of the disease includes lifetime care with the goals of treatment being to maximize the patient's functional abilities and minimize disability. The three methods of treatment, pharmacologic, rehabilitative, and neurosurgical, are discussed below.

PHARMACOLOGIC TREATMENT

Drug therapy is needed when the symptoms become annoying and restrict normal activity and has been found to improve the quantity and quality of life for idiopathic Parkinsonism patients (30). Before L-dopa was discovered, patients with Parkinsonism had a mortality rate that was three times higher than the current rate. It has decreased to 1.5 times higher after the introduction of L-dopa (31). However, problems are also seen secondary to L-dopa and other dopamine agonists (32). Optimal symptomatic relief is obtained by using a number of pharmacologic strategies and "as needed" dosing to reduce adverse effects (33). The drugs used in the treatment of PD include carbidopa-levodopa, bromocryptine, amantadine, and anticholinergic agents.

Levodopa is the drug of choice for the treatment of idiopathic Parkinson's because of its ability to correct the abnormalities of recruitment and firing pattern of motor units (34). However, postencephalitic Parkinson's patients only tolerate levodopa in very small doses and are more prone to develop side effects. The treatment should be started with very small doses, with gradual weekly increases to achieve maximum benefit with minimal or no side effects. A combination of carbidopa and levodopa will help reduce the gastrointestinal and cardiovascular side effects of levodopa, as the dose can be markedly reduced.

Because levodopa therapy is associated with disabling long-term complications and may speed the loss of cells, therapy is not started when the disease is mild and symptoms do not cause any disability. When the symptoms become annoying and cause restriction of activities, then the lowest dose required to obtain the needed relief in disability is started. No effort should be made to abolish all signs of PD. About 65% of patients report loss of efficacy of the drug after 5 to 10 years of therapy, probably due to progression of the disease. The relief from each dose may also become effective for shorter periods ("wearing-off"), resulting in disability fluctuation during the day. These fluctuations may cause akinesia or freezing for prolonged periods ("on-off" phenomenon). Stopping the medication ("drug holiday") may make the patient responsive gain to L-Dopa in 5 to 10 days. The different pharmacologic agents, their indications, usual dosage, and side effects are noted in Table 18.5

Patients with PD require careful adjustments of medication so care must be taken to note the time of onset and extent of relief provided by each medication. Duration of symptomatic relief should also be noted, as well as athetoid movements and the time and relationship to dose administration. Careful charting of precise times of medication administration is essential for the physician to adjust each patient's regime.

REHABILITATION

Rehabilitation of a patient with PD will not stop the downhill course of the disease but will add quality to the patient's life. The interdisciplinary team approach will provide maximum benefit to the patient. However, there have been very few efforts at this approach due to the progressive degenerative nature of the disease. The treatment strategy will depend upon the individual patient's needs and will be dictated by the specific deficits that predominate an individual illness. Lasting goals cannot be achieved, and the patient's performance may vary on a day-to-day basis or within a few hours, depending on the blood levels of the medication. These factors must be kept in mind by the entire team when developing a treatment program.

The long-term benefit of physical therapy has been controversial. Gibberd (35) showed that a short course of physical therapy did not improve function in patients whose medical regimen was stable. However, his study was limited because the therapy was done in the hospital and the patients did not exercise at home.

Several studies have shown that PD patients may benefit from continued therapy. Stefaniwsky and Bilowit (36) found that movement initiation and speed were improved in Parkinson's patients after training with sensory cues for 3 weeks. Szekely (37) used exercises suggested by the American Parkinson's Disease Association in a 13-week program of both professionally supervised and unsupervised home exercise and documented significant improvement in gait but not in posture, stance, or time taken to write a signature.

Long latency stretch responses are known to be abnormal in PD (38). Palmer (39) compared slow stretching exercises recommended by the Parkinson Foundation to an upper body karate training program

asnd found similar outcomes. The majority of the patients improved in gait, tremor, grip strength, and motor coordination of tasks requiring fine control.

Schenkman et al (40) have suggested a model for multisystem evaluation and treatment and individuals with Parkinson's. This model demonstrates that many of the impairments, e.g., rigidity and postural instability, of patients with PD may have contributions from both a CNS and a non-CNS nature. Since the disabilities of PD, e.g., difficulty with mobility, dementia, and depression, are the outcomes of the total impact of impairments, they occur both as a direct result of the degenerative process and as a result of sequelae indirectly affecting musculoskeletal and cardiopulmonary systems. The rehabilitation team may not be able to correct the direct CNS pathology but can teach compensatory mechanisms to reduce potential sequelae.

Patients have to struggle against rigidity and bradykinesia, which may result in frustration and fatigue. Thus, the patient may need frequent rest periods. However, these should be monitored, as prolonged rest periods may result in increased rigidity. In the early stages there may be no disability, but as the disease progresses the patient may become stiff, immobile, lose joint range, and develop contractures and disuse atrophy. These disabilities result from rigidity, bradykinesia, tremors, and the loss of postural reflexes and can be minimized by a properly designed physical therapy exercise and activity program.

Decreased Rigidity

Relaxation of axial and limb musculature are important to increase flexibility and decrease rigidity (41). Slow rhythmic rotational movements beginning with very small ROM exercises are used to achieve relaxation. Rotation is lost early in the disease; therefore passive rotation should be started and progressed to active rotation. Biofeedback, contract-relax, and neuromuscular facilitation techniques as described by Voss (42) can be used to accomplish active rotation. Patients should lie supine or on the side and start self-relaxation exercises from this supported position, then gradually be taught self-relaxation exercises in sitting and standing positions.

Increased Flexibility

Patients should be given exercises for rotation of each segment of the spine. The therapy is directed toward increasing lumbar, thoracic, and cervical extension so that the stooped posture can be corrected. Straight leg raises and knee bend exercises can be included, and patients may use an exercise bike and a pulley to achieve reciprocal motion and maintain mobility of arms and legs.

Table 18.5. Medications in the Treatment of Parkinsonism

Medication	Usual Dose	Indications	Side Effects
Neurotransmitter replacement			
L-Dopa (levodopa)	100 mg 2 times/d; (1.5–6 g)	Can reverse cardinal symptoms of Parkinsonism; sustained effectiveness (not used alone); less effective for tremor	Acute side effects can be nausea, hypotension, sedation, hallucination, frequent development of dyskinesia, and "on-off phenomenon" with chronic use
Carbidopa with levodopa L-Dopa with carboxylase inhibitors (Sinemet)	10/100 mg, 25/100 mg, 40/200 mg, 25/250 mg 3 times/d and the dose should be adjusted	Can reverse cardinal symptoms of Parkinsonism; less side effects; may have longer duration of dose by dose effects; effective for tremor and dystonia	May have increased evidence of dyskinesia and on-off symptoms when compared to L-Dopa alone; postural hypotension, confusion may occur
Anticholinergics (commonly used)			
Trihexyphenidyl (Artane)	2 mg 3 times/d (6–20 mg)	Effective for tremor, dystonia, rigidity; long-term side effects lacking; limited usefulness for bradykinesia and imbalance	Side effects may be confusion, impairment to vision and memory, urinary retention, dry mouth
Benztropine mesylate (Cogentin)	1–2 mg 3 times/d (1–10 mg)	May be useful in patients with sialorrhea	
Procyclidine (Kemadrin)	2 mg 3 times/d (7.5–30 mg)	Good for neuroleptic-induced Parkinson's	
Receptor Agonists			
Amantadine (Symmetral)	100 mg 2 times/d	Effective for all Parkinson's symptoms; long-term side effects lacking; less effective than L-Dopa alone; useful in combination; good for neuroleptic-induced Parkinson's when unable to tolerate anticholinergics; often has limited period (3–6 months) of efficacy	Dry mouth, nausea, vomiting, dose-related side effects present. Blurring of vision, leg edema, mental impairment, livedo reticularis are other side effects
Bromocriptine mesylate (Parlodel)	1.25 mg 2 times/d, increased in small (2.5 mg) increments (20–30 mg)	Effective for all Parkinsonism symptoms; less effective as single drug therapy than L-Dopa; greater and more selective effectiveness than L-Dopa; lack of on-off effects and dyskinesia with long-term therapy	Side effects include hypotension, nausea, confusion (usually dose-related), anorexia, vomiting, nausea, erythromelalgia; expensive
Permax (Pergolide)	1–5 mg	More potent than Parlodel	Similar to L-Dopa
Monoamine oxidase B inhibitor			
Deprenyl (Selegiline)	5–10 mg	Extends dose effects of L-Dopa. May retard the progression of PD	May increase dose-related L-Dopa side effects

Gait and Posture

To stabilize gait, the feet should be kept 10 to 12 inches apart to broaden the base of support when walking, especially when turning or changing direction. The therapist must remember that patients tend to lose their balance each time they perform an activity that moves the center of gravity outside the base of support. To counter this, balance activities should follow weight shifting activities in each position. Patients should be taught to vigorously swing their arms while walking to improve balance and decrease fatigue caused by a rigid shuffling gait. The therapist should gradually shift the patient's center of gravity and try to elicit normal righting reflexes.

Some patients may markedly improve their walking by carrying a hockey stick or a cane with a 6" projection made of leather or cardboard. The "sill" will help the patient take the first step. Patients should be taught to dorsiflex their toes if they feel their feet are stuck to the floor. High "step gait" is practiced by walking over boxes or other obstacles placed irregularly on the floor.

The hips and knees tend to remain flexed, and the patient has a stooped posture due to rigidity and proprioceptive deficits. They should work on stretching the hip and knee extensors, abductors, hamstrings, and gastrocnemius muscles. Shoulder extensors, abductor and internal rotators, elbow extensors, forearm supinators, and finger-hand extensors should also be stretched. Postural reeducation is extremely important, as it helps the patient maintain flexibility and range of motion.

Upper Extremity

There is a tendency for the patient to develop flexion at the metacarpophalangeal (MCP) joints and extension at the interphalangeal (IP) joints, resulting in reduced hand function. To counter this, patients should have exercises for the hands. One such exercise is to have the fingers fully abducted and extended at the MCP and IP joints and have the patients close and open their fists. The forearms should be fully supinated and pronated, and the shoulder should retain full ROM to counter adhesive capsulitis. Preston (43) has described radial compression neuropathy in patients with advanced Parkinsonism. The site of nerve injury was the upper part of the arm where the radial nerve pierces the intermuscular septum. A combination of bradykinesia and improper position in a bed or wheelchair may lead to nerve compression at this site. Preventive methods should include frequent position changes and avoidance of sleeping in wheelchairs. If radial neuropathy develops, a wrist splint should be used to prevent fixed wrist flexion deformity.

The inability to rise from the sitting position can be decreased by placing the patient's feet directly under the center of gravity and rocking the body forward and backward in the chair. If the rear legs of the chairs are raised, or front legs shortened, by about 2 inches to 4 inches, it will help the patient rise from the sitting position.

Respiratory

Benson (44) suggested that rhythmic relaxed breathing is an essential component of the relaxation response. Relaxed rotation of the upper extremity and neck and deep breathing can help increase chest expansion and be used to increase vital capacity. This will help prevent musculoskeletal limitations that contribute to the high incidence of pulmonary complication in patients with PD.

Swallowing Difficulty

Dysphagia and a variety of other swallowing abnormalities can occur in Parkinson's disease. Subjective discomfort, difficulty in handling pills, and high incidence of bronchopulmonary pneumonia are some of the complications commonly found. Patients may complain of coughing when eating, food sticking in their throat, and difficulty swallowing pills. Logemann (45) has suggested that there is abnormal lingual control of swallowing, as lingual festination may prevent the bolus from passing into the pharynx. Reduced pharyngeal peristalsis may also occur, as well as delayed swallowing reflex and repetitive and involuntary reflux from vallecula and piriform sinuses into the oral cavity (46). Patients may not swallow pills, which are then retained in the vallecula for long periods of time. This may result in erratic absorption of medication and thereby interfere with the clinical efficacy of oral medication. They may also have swallowing difficulties without having any other symptoms of the disease and may suffer from silent aspirations.

The clinical severity of the disease does not correlate well with the swallowing abnormalities, as these can occur in both early and late stages of the disease. It is recommended that patients with complaints of dysphagia or with a history of pneumonitis have a modified barium swallow evaluation, as they may be unable to identify the specific nature of their dysfunction. Treatment strategies can help prevent these silent aspirations and decrease morbidity. If the patients are found to have an abnormal barium swallow, the speech therapist can teach the patient mechanical modification of swallowing, for example, supraglottal swallow. This will help protect the airway and, hence, prevent aspiration. Anticholinergic medications can also impair swallowing. In some patients, levodopa treatment can improve swallowing but increasing the dose will not provide additional benefit.

Facial exercises such as a look of surprise, grimacing, frowning, blowing, smiling, puckering, etc., are extremely important to try to fight some of the masked facies and can be used to improve breathing patterns. Tongue exercises to improve its mobility by sticking the tongue out, moving it from corner to corner of the lips, and moving it within the mouth, are also useful.

Self-Care

Adaptive equipment, such as eating and kitchen utensils and comb and hairbrush with built-up handles, may be provided, and an electric toothbrush should be used to ensure proper hygiene. A plate guard to avoid spillage, Velcro closures or zippers in place of buttons, grab bars near bathtubs and toilets, and bathtub seat and raised toilet seat may help the patient in activities of daily living. Stairways should have strong railing, preferably on both sides, for safety.

Nutrition

Nutrition is likely to be neglected by the patient, as tremor interferes with self-feeding. The treatment team can help the patient in feeding activities and should discourage incoordinated chewing efforts. The patient should be allowed to feed himself, if possible, under supervision. Poor swallowing and excessive salivation may require careful attention. A soft, high-residue, low-protein, and high or low calorie diet is normally indicated. Fluids are not tolerated well by these patients, but it is necessary to maintain adequate intake.

Psychotherapy

Patients undergo personality changes and many suffer from depression due to the slow progression of the disease and the resulting dependency on others. Psychosocial support and counseling for the family is an integral part of the treatment plan as the family members taking care of the patient may become overwhelmed and depressed. Antidepressant medication may be prescribed for the patient when indicated.

It has been suggested that Parkinson's patients do better in a group rehabilitation setting (47). These patients have a clearer understanding of the disease, which can then help them become less fearful and improve their quality of life. Patients can socialize, communicate, and become concerned and involved with others rather than becoming self-centered. Home exercise is an integral part of the treatment plan and should be taught as soon as possible to ensure ongoing intervention.

Family involvement is extremely important due to the chronic progressive nature of the disease. If the family understands the disease and its effect on the patient, they will be better able to cope with its progressive nature and thus will be able to participate in the patient's management and clinical care in a beneficial manner.

NEUROSURGICAL TREATMENT

Before the advent of levodopa, management of tremor and rigidity could be achieved by surgical destruction of the ventrolateral nucleus of the thalamus. Stereotactic techniques utilizing heating or freezing were found to help reduce tremor and rigidity, but had no effect on bradykinesia, loss of balance, or dysarthria. Computed tomography-based stereotaxis and microelectrode recording techniques are now used for precise localization and placement of the surgical lesion (48). While thalamotomy results in complete abolition of the resting tremor in the contralateral upper extremity, it is rarely indicated in medically intractable Parkinson's tremor.

Recently, autograft transplantation of adrenal medulla into the striatum of patients with advanced PD has been attempted (48) in an effort to reverse the Parkinsonism.

Preclinical Parkinson's Disease

Most investigators now believe that a presymptomatic period exists in all PD patients, and the emphasis of further research should be to identify patients in this period and thereby attempt disease prevention. Deprenyl is considered neuroprotective by slowing the progress of the disease. Presymptomatic diagnostic criteria can be clinical symptoms, biochemical markers, and imaging. Biochemical markers being studied include abnormalities of autooxidation of DA (49), DA neuron antibody, and decreased cerebrospinal fluid (CSF) growth promoting activity (50). Adhesive capsulitis occurring up to 2 years before symptoms of PD is considered a preclinical symptom by Riley (28). Until the etiologic factors responsible for PD are identified and a specific diagnostic test developed, subjective clinical evaluation is the only way to diagnose PD.

SUMMARY

The variability in the distribution of muscle weakness and the progressive nature of the condition means that the rehabilitation techniques and the treatment plan have to be modified to the needs of the individual patient. There is no effective drug treatment available for long-term management, and thus, the most common form of management is symptomatic and supportive.

References

1. DeLisa J. Electrodiagnosis in motor neuron disorders. *Phys Med Rehab.* 3:701–712, 1989.
2. DeLisa JA, Mikulic MA, Miller RM, Melnick RR. Amyotrophic lateral sclerosis: comprehensive management. *Am Fam Physician.* 19(3):137–142, 1979.
3. Mulder DW. *The Diagnosis and Treatment of Amyotrophic Lateral Sclerosis.* Boston, Mass.: Houghton Mifflin; 1980:1–397.
4. Horton WA, Eldridge R, Brody JA. Familial motor neuron disease. *Neurology.* 26:460–465, 1976.
5. Rosen AD. Amyotrophic lateral sclerosis: clinical features and prognosis. *Arch Neurol.* 35:638–642, 1978.
6. Andres PL, Hedlund W, Finison L, et al. Quantitative motor assessment in amyotrophic lateral sclerosis. *Neurology.* 36:937–941, 1986.
7. Gauthier L, Dalziel S, Gauthier S. The benefits of group occupational therapy for patients with Parkinson's disease. *Am J Occup. Ther.* 41:360, 1987.
8. Smith RA, Norris FH. Symptomatic care of patients with amyotrophic lateral sclerosis. *JAMA.* 234:715–717, 1975.
9. Sinaki M, Mulder DW. Rehabilitation techniques for patients with amyotrophic lateral sclerosis. *Mayo Clin Proc.* 53:173–178, 1978.
10. Slowie LA, Paige MS, Antel JP. Nutritional considerations in the management of patients with amyotrophic lateral sclerosis (ALS). *J Am Diet Assoc.* 83:44–47, 1983.
11. Robbins J. Swallowing in ALS and motor neuron disorders. *Neurol Clin.* 5:213–229, 1987.
12. Parisier SC, Butzer A, Binder WJ, et al. Tympanic neurectomy and chorda tympanectomy for the control of drooling. *Arch Otolaryngol.* 104:273–277, 1978.
13. Hillel AD, Miller R. Bulbar amyotrophic lateral sclerosis: patterns of progression and clinical management. *Head & Neck.* 11:51–59, 1989.
14. Bach JR, Alba AS. Management of chronic alveolar hypoventilation by nasal ventilation. *Chest.* 97:52–57, 1990.

15. Braun SR. Respiratory systems in amyotrophic lateral sclerosis. *Neurol Clin.* 5:9–31, 1987.
16. Serisier DE, Mastaglia FL, Gibson GJ. Respiratory muscle function and ventilatory control. I: In patients with motor neuron disease. II. In patients with myotrophic dystrophy. *J Med NS.* 51:205–226, 1982.
17. Sivak ED, Gipson WT, Hanson MR. Long-term management of respiratory failure in amyotrophic lateral sclerosis. *Ann Neurol.* 12:18–23, 1982.
18. Moss AH, Casey P, Stocking CB, Roos RP, Brooks BR, Siegler M. Home ventilation for amyotrophic lateral sclerosis patients: outcomes, costs, and family and physician attitudes. *Neurology.* 43:438–443, 1993.
19. Mitsumoto H, Salgado ED, Negroski D, et al. Amyotrophic lateral sclerosis: effects of acute intravenous and chronic subcutaneous administration of thyrotropin-releasing hormone in controlled trials. *Neurology.* 36:152–159, 1986.
20. Tyler HR. Double-blind study of modified neurotoxin in motor neuron disease. *Neurology.* 29:77–81, 1979.
21. Parkinson J. *An Essay on the Shaking Palsy.* London: Sherwood, Neely and Jones; 1817.
22. Duvoisin R. *Parkinson's Disease, a Guide for Patient and Family.* New York, NY: Raven; 1978.
23. Rajput AH, Offord KP, Beard CM, Kurland LT. Epidemiology of Parkinsonism: incidence, classification and mortality. *Ann Neurol.* 16:278–282, 1984.
24. Elliot FA. *Clinical Neurology.* Philadelphia, Pa; W.B. Saunders; 1970.
25. Schoenberg BS. Environmental risk factors for Parkinson's disease: the epidemiologic evidence. *Can J Neurol Sci.* 14:407–413, 1987.
26. Lieberman A. Dopamine agonists. *New Perspectives Trends Clin Neurol.* 4(3):1–19, 1988.
27. Sheridan MR, Flowers KA, Hurell J. Programming and execution of movement in Parkinson's disease. *Brain.* 110:1247–1271, 1987.
28. Riley D, Lang AE, Blair RDG, et al. Frozen shoulder and other shoulder disturbances in Parkinson's disease. *J Neurol Neurosurg Psychiatry.* 52:63–66, 1989.
29. Stern Y, Mayeux R, Rosen J, Ilson J. Perceptual motor dysfunction in Parkinson's disease: a deficit in sequential and predictive voluntary movement. *J Neurol Neurosurg Psychiatry.* 46:145–151, 1983.
30. Hoehn MM, Yahr MD. Parkinsonism: onset, progression and mortality. *Neurology.* 17:427–442, 1967.
31. Yahr MD. Evaluation of long-term therapy in Parkinson's disease: mortality and therapeutic efficacy. In: Birmayer W, Horn Y, Kiewicz O, eds. *Advances in Parkinsonism.* Basle: Editions Roche; 1976.
32. Lesser RP, Fahn S, Snider SR, et al. Analysis of the clinical problems in Parkinsonism and the complications of long term levodopa therapy. *Neurology.* 29:1253–1260, 1979.
33. Levitt PA. New perspectives in the treatment of Parkinson's disease. *Clin Neuropharmacol.* 9 (suppl 1):S37–S46, 1986.
34. Milner-Brown HS, Fisher MA, Weiner WJ. Electrical properties in motor unites in Parkinsonism and a possible relationship with bradykinesia. *J Neurol Neurosurg Psychiatry.* 42:35–41, 1979.
35. Gibberd FB, Page NGR, Spencer KM, et al. Controlled trial of physiotherapy and occupational therapy for Parkinson's disease. *Br Med J.* 282:1196, 1981.
36. Stefaniwsky L, Bilowit DS. Parkinsonism: facilitation of motion by sensory stimulation. *Arch Phys Med Rehabil.* 54:75–77, 90, 1973.
37. Szekely BC, Kosonovich NN, Sheppard W. Adjunctive treatment in Parkinson's disease: physical therapy and comprehensive group therapy. *Rehabil Lit.* 43:72–76, 1982.
38. Mortimer JA, Webster DD. Evidence for a quantitative association between EMG stretch responses and Parkinsonian rigidity. *Brain Res.* 162:169–173, 1979.
39. Palmer SS, Mortimer JA, Webster DD, et al. Exercise therapy and Parkinson's disease. *Arch Phys Med Rehabil.* 67:741–745, 1986.
40. Schenkman M, Butler RB. A model for multisystem treatment of individuals with Parkinson's disease. *Phys Ther.* 69:932–943, 1989.
41. Schenkman M, Donovan J, Tsubota J, et al. Management of individuals with Parkinson's disease: rationale and case studies. *Phys Ther.* 69:944–955, 1989.
42. Voss DE, Ionta MK, Myers BJ. *Proprioceptive Neuromuscular Facilitation: Patterns and Techniques.* 3rd ed. Philadelphia, Pa: Harper and Row; 1985.
43. Preston DN, Grimes JD. Radial compression in advanced Parkinson's disease. *Arch Neurol.* 42:695–696, 1985.
44. Benson H. *The Relaxation Response.* New York, NY: Avon Books; 1975.
45. Logemann JA, Blonsky ER, Boshes B. Lingual control in Parkinson's disease. *Trans Am Neurol Assoc.* 98:276–278, 1973.
46. Bushmann M, Dobmeyer SM, Leeker L, Perlmutter JS. Swallowing abnormalities and their response to treatment in Parkinson's disease. *Neurology.* 39:1309–1314, 1989.
47. Davis JC. Team management of Parkinson's disease. *Am J Occup Ther.* 31(5):300–308, 1977.
48. Kelly PJ, Ahlskog JE, Van Heerden JA, et al. Adrenal medullary autograft transplantation into the striatum of patients with Parkinson's disease. *Mayo Clin Proc.* 64:282–290, 1989.
49. Carlssou A, Forstedt B. Catechol metabolites in the cerebrospinal fluid as possible markers in the early diagnosis of Parkinson's disease. *Neurology.* 41(5 suppl 2):50–51, 1991.
50. Carvey PM, McRae A, Lint J, et al. The potential use of a dopamine neuron antibody in a straital derived neurotropic factor as diagnostic markers in Parkinson's disease. *Neurology.* 41 (5 suppl 2):53–58, 1991.

19

Peripheral Nervous/Muscular System

Daniel Dumitru, Arthur Gershkoff, and Nicolas E. Walsh

PERIPHERAL NERVOUS SYSTEM

Peripheral neuropathic diseases commonly occur in the elderly (65 years or older) and cause considerable functional impairment reducing their quality of life. The major issues in rehabilitation involve reversing, minimizing, or compensating for weakness, sensory loss, or pain. The older patient often suffers from diseases of other organ systems, which compound the disability from these ailments and impede rehabilitation. For example, osteoarthritis of the knees or ankles may interfere with ambulatory training in a patient recovering from acute inflammatory demyelinating polyneuropathy (Guillain-Barré syndrome). Similarly, mild neuropathy by itself may present no functional limitation; however, combined with a total knee arthroplasty or lower extremity fracture, it can prolong the rehabilitation process.

Histologic and Physiologic Changes in the Aging Peripheral Nervous System

Changes in morphology occur with aging in the cell bodies of sensory ganglia, dorsal roots, peripheral axons, and the distal neural receptors. Increased lipofuscin deposits are seen in ganglion cells. Schwann cells show evidence of paranodal or segmental demyelination and remyelination. Axonal loss appears in nerve roots and distal nerves. It is felt by some that many of these changes could be explained by repetitive minor trauma. The number of Meissner corpuscles in the fingers and toes decreases, and encapsulated receptors show age-related changes in the structure of their terminals. Autonomic nerves and sympathetic ganglia also reveal changes with aging, including depletion of cells, marked increase in neuronal pigmentation, and vacuolation of cell bodies (1).

Loss of vibratory sense, as measured by an increase in vibratory perception threshold (VPT), is well-documented to occur with aging, with up to 82% of elderly persons demonstrating decreased vibratory sense in the distal lower extremities (2). A wide variety of causes

have been suggested: atherosclerosis of spinal cord vessels, peripheral nerve ischemia, myelin changes, nutritional deficiency, nerve root trauma, and diminished numbers of sensory receptors in the elderly (1). None have been proven definitively to cause the altered VPT. Proprioception and light touch, as measured by von Frey hair perception testing or finger touch-pressure threshold, also diminish with age, but this is reported less frequently on clinical exam than is vibratory loss. Pain perception may also decrease.

Other changes in the neurologic examination that occur with aging include: loss of ankle deep tendon reflexes (up to 70%), reduced pupillary light reflex, reduced meiotic component of the near visual reflex, restriction in upward gaze (20%), and cogwheel visual tracking (31%). To what extent changes in peripheral nerves contribute to these alterations is unclear. Many of these findings may reflect otherwise subclinical central nervous system disease (3).

Inflammatory Demyelinating Polyneuropathies

Acute inflammatory demyelinating polyneuropathy (AIDP) or Guillain-Barré syndrome is an acute-onset, progressive motor paralysis caused by autoimmune-induced demyelination. The incidence is 1 to 2 per 100,000 and possibly higher in the elderly. The prognosis for functional recovery is usually good. However, severe cases associated with Wallerian degeneration suggest a more prolonged disease course and a greater likelihood of incomplete recovery, especially for the elderly (4). In about half of patients, paralysis compromises the ability to swallow, speak, and breathe normally. One fifth of all patients require intubation and ventilatory assistance (5).

In addition to motor nerves, sensory nerves are also involved with demyelination, and paresthesias are common. A true disabling sensory loss in the hands and feet, however, usually does not occur. Pain that is severe, deep, and aching and associated with elevated creatine phosphokinase occurs frequently and probably reflects a muscular rather than axonal origin. Occasionally, a severe burning and shooting type of pain involving primarily the lower extremities may occur. The muscular pain usually responds to steroids, while the more severe neurologic pain may require narcotics (6).

Plasmapheresis is thought to reduce the severity of demyelination and axonal damage in AIDP if started immediately, but its value in the elderly is controversial (4, 7). Other agents have been used with variable success. Early rehabilitation involves passive range of motion to paretic limbs to prevent contractures, repositioning for comfort and to prevent skin breakdown, cautious strengthening with active assisted and active range of motion, joint protection of the lower extremities to prevent overstretching of soft tissues, and splinting of the upper extremities. A deep water tank can permit active exercises and even ambulation before muscles have achieved antigravity strength. As strength improves, the water level can be lowered. Eventually, mobility training can be moved to the parallel bars and advanced to the use of other assistive devices (8).

It is important to avoid overfatiguing recovering muscles, as this may aggravate weakness or even cause a relapse (9). Early mobilization must be done cautiously; a significant percentage of patients have autonomic instability and are at risk for postural hypotension. With these measures, patients are protected from complications and are likely to make optimal use of the neurologic recovery usually associated with AIDP.

Chronic inflammatory demyelinating polyneuropathy (CIDP) occurs much less frequently than AIDP, but is more likely to leave the patient with significant functional impairment. There are two forms, a relapsing type affecting younger individuals and a chronic progressive type that affects primarily middle-aged and elderly persons (10). When approaching these patients, it is important to set goals that are realistic in light of the fluctuating course of the disease. As in AIDP, it is critical to avoid overfatiguing muscles.

Drug-related and Toxic Neuropathies

Urinary tract compromise is common in older individuals, and care must be taken when medication is prescribed. With chronic use, the urinary tract bacterial suppressant nitrofurantoin can cause a distal neuropathy. Symptoms usually commence within 45 days of starting the drug and include tingling dysesthesias of the toes, feet, and fingers (11). More severe cases can progress to paresis associated with axonal damage (12).

Other drugs used in the elderly have been noted to cause neuropathy. The antidysrhythmic agent amiodarone can cause a chronic demyelinating neuropathy. The rheumatic gold formulations, antimicrobials isoniazid and metronidazole, as well as the neoplastic thera-

peutic agents cisplatin and vincristine, can cause chronic axonal damage, sometimes to a severe degree. Withdrawal of the medication is essential to limit neurologic damage (13). Phenytoin is reported to cause peripheral neuropathy in 7% to 30% of chronic users, with the elderly particularly affected (14). Ironically, pyridoxine, which is used to prevent peripheral (and central) nervous system toxicity from isoniazid and to reduce symptoms from neuropathy in carpal tunnel syndrome and diabetes, can cause a painful peripheral neuropathy if administered in megadoses of 500 mg per day or more (15).

Nutritional Deficiencies and Alcoholic Neuropathy

A variety of nutritional deficiencies affecting the elderly are associated with painful sensorimotor polyneuropathies. While individual vitamin deficiencies such as beriberi (Vitamin B_1), pellagra (niacin), and pyridoxine (Vitamin B_6) do occur, they are unusual in this country and are often associated with malabsorption syndromes. The most common neuropathy of this class is alcoholic neuropathy. This neuropathy typically presents with burning feet, occasionally in conjunction with distal weakness and paresthesias. Cramping may occur and is more common in milder cases (16). Abstinence from alcohol, restoration of a balanced diet, and B-vitamin supplementation usually lead to symptomatic improvement. Mentholated salves and lotions can reduce the pain and burning sensations (11).

Associated with pernicious anemia, vitamin B_{12} deficiency is often found in the elderly and usually results from malabsorption caused by autoimmune-induced gastric atrophy, partial or total gastrectomy, or pancreatic insufficiency. Intrinsic factor becomes deficient, leading to malabsorption of oral vitamin B_{12} in the terminal ileum. Up to 75% of patients with deficient blood levels will develop peripheral neuropathy, the symptoms of which may be severe. These include paresthesias, stocking-glove loss of sensation, and distal muscle wasting. Infrequently, paresthesias may be dysesthetic. Orthostatic hypotension, impotence and impaired urination may also occur (17).

Vitamin B_{12} deficiency causes functional disability primarily from myelopathy, the symptoms of which often overshadow those from neuropathy. The severe posterior column demyelination is responsible for significant loss of position sense in the lower extremities. If untreated, the disease may progress to involve the corticospinal and spinothalamic tracts. Reflexes may be increased or diminished, depending upon the extent of corticospinal tract and peripheral nerve involvement. Megaloblastic anemia may lead to a tragic misdiagnosis of isolated folate deficiency; treatment of the latter without also correcting B_{12} deficiency may reverse the megaloblastosis, but will not prevent the central and peripheral nervous system disease from progressing. Vitamin B_{12} replacement usually resolves the neurologic manifestations if neuropathic symptoms predominate or if myelopathic symptoms are of less than 3 months duration. Rehabilitation issues usually center around gait impairment, which may be severe, as a result of ataxia, weakness, and spasticity (18).

Postherpetic Neuralgia

Herpes zoster is largely a disease of the elderly. The incidence varies from 1/1000 to 3/1000 in persons under age 50 years to 5/1000 to 10/1000 in octogenarians. Predisposing factors are lymphoproliferative disorders or treatment with corticosteroids, radiation, or cytotoxic agents producing an immunocompromised status. A characteristic vesicular rash with a red base erupts in a dermatomal distribution. Sensory nerves are affected almost universally, with resulting burning, neuralgic pain, hyperesthesias, and focal sensory loss. Transient clinical weakness from motor pathway dysfunction occurs rarely; however, in combination with pain, it can cause functional disability. The frequency of motor involvement is tripled when herpes zoster is associated with malignancy, which is more likely to occur in the elderly (10). Severe pain always occurs during the vesicular eruption and then gradually declines as the skin lesions heal (19, 20). The thoracic dermatomes are the most frequently affected, but any dermatome can be involved. Presentation on the nose suggests spread of herpes zoster to the eye, necessitating emergency ophthalmologic evaluation.

Pain that persists after healing of the skin lesions is termed postherpetic neuralgia (PHN), and older persons are at a greater risk for developing this complication. Of patients who contract herpes zoster, only about 10% to 15% of those under 45 years of age experience PHN lasting longer than one month, while greater than 50% of persons over 60 years of age suffer from PHN of this duration (20). Thus, PHN ranks as a major cause of persistent neuropathic pain in the elderly.

A variety of agents administered at the start of the acute eruption have been shown to reduce the severity or persistence of PHN, including oral steroids, amantidine, vidarabine, interferon, levodopa, and adenosine monophosphate (20, 21). Acyclovir may accelerate healing of the eruption, but does not affect the development of PHN. It is recommended that immunocompetent patients more than 50 years old be treated with corticosteroids and an antiviral agent (usually acyclovir) (19). Topical compresses with Burow's solution or calamine lotion and vaseline-impregnated bandages promote clearing of cutaneous lesions.

Salicylates, nonsteroidals, and narcotics may be useful for acute pain, but do not affect the development of PHN. Narcotics should be used cautiously as they tend to become less effective and problematic if pain becomes chronic. Sympathetic blocks are reportedly useful for severe, acute pain (19, 20). For chronic treatment, tricyclic antidepressants have been proven effective in reducing PHN. Transcutaneous electrical nerve stimulation is worth trying (19). Physical and occupational therapy can reverse deconditioning, contractures, or mobility and self-care deficits patients develop secondary to the pain.

Diabetic Neuropathy

Diabetes is one of the most common causes of neuropathy in the elderly. The actual incidence of neuropathy increases from 7.5% at the time diabetes is diagnosed, to about 50% after the disease has been present 25 years (10). The longer the disease is present and the poorer the control, the greater the likelihood that clinical signs and symptoms of neuropathy will develop (22). The most common diabetic neuropathy is symmetric distal polyneuropathy, which typically progresses slowly over many years. This commonly manifests with sensory symptoms that are minimally bothersome but can occasionally be quite severe. Patients experience burning, tightness, paresthesias, and aching distal pain. Lancinating pain may also be present and can be triggered by sensory stimuli. Five percent to 10% of diabetics may experience severe sensory loss, which can be associated with ulceration or Charcot joints, both occurring as a result of repetitive minor trauma. In advanced cases, distal motor weakness may be severe, leading to a dropped foot and intrinsic-minus (clawfoot) deformities.

Autonomic involvement in symmetric distal neuropathy can involve many systems. Symptoms occur in approximately 30% of all diabetics. Patients can have impaired sensation of bladder fullness, leading to overdistention and urinary retention. Sexual impotence is common in males, but often has other contributing factors. Constipation and diarrhea occur frequently. In diabetic gastroparesis, gastric emptying and peristalsis are slowed, causing depressed appetite and dyspepsia. Gustatory sweating, excessive truncal sweating, or anhydrosis may occur. Impaired cardiovascular reflexes are thought responsible for silent myocardial infarction, hypoglycemic unawareness, and occasionally in advanced cases, symptomatic postural hypotension (23).

Proximal diabetic neuropathy may be symmetric or asymmetric (24–26). The term diabetic amyotrophy has been used to describe both groups. There is definite overlap in these clinical syndromes, both of which usually affect the elderly (10). Symmetric proximal neuropathy is usually slow in onset, over weeks to months, and is thought to have a metabolic origin. The syndrome encompasses most cases of diabetic polyradiculopathy, which starts unilaterally in 75% of cases but eventually involves bilateral pelvifemoral weakness and wasting. Pain is a prominent early symptom that usually improves significantly.

In addition to entrapment neuropathies, asymmetric diabetic neuropathies include focal and multifocal syndromes that are thought to be caused by vascular lesions (24). These typically present with a sudden onset of pain, followed by weakness that progresses rapidly over several days. Mononeuritis multiplex usually involves the lumbar plexus. There can also be a focal lumbar radiculopathy or acute femoral neuropathy, which have similar presentations. Other nerves and plexuses can also be involved. Diabetic ophthalmoplegia is the most common cranial neuropathy of diabetes. Pupillary responses are spared, but severe pain develops around the eye in 50% of patients, in addition to diplopia and ptosis. Third nerve palsies are most frequent, followed by sixth nerve palsies.

It is generally accepted that reversal of nerve damage from diabetic neuropathy is difficult, if not impossible. However, various substances have been explored to limit or slow damage; some may reduce sensory symptoms and allow a patient to recover at least partial strength and function. Close control of blood sugar with insulin and strict diet is considered foremost among these. Nonsteroidal drugs and vitamin B_6 and B_{12} supplements have been documented as helpful in controlling painful symptoms, possibly through metabolic mechanisms (27, 28). Initially promising, an aldose reductase inhibitor, such as sorbinil, has been removed from clinical trials because of a high rate of side effects, including fatalities (29).

For adjunctive pain relief of both lancinating and burning pain, a large body of controlled studies supports the use of amitriptyline and other tricyclic antidepressants in treating neuropathic symptoms (30–32). Analgesic effectiveness is similar in depressed and nondepressed patients. In at least one study (31), there was no relationship between analgesia and improvement in mood. The antiepileptics carbamazepine and phenytoin and the antidysrhythmic mexiletine have also reduced pain (33–35).

Entrapment Neuropathies

These are common syndromes that cause varying degrees of impairment in the elderly. Nerves and nerve roots can become compressed mechanically by bones or soft tissues and typically cause pain, sensory loss, and weakness in their characteristic distributions. Usually pain radiates distally, but it can radiate proximally as well. The latter can confuse the diagnostic process. The importance of early recognition and intervention, before irreversible axonal damage occurs, cannot be overemphasized.

Carpal tunnel syndrome is extremely common and causes paresthesias, numbness, and occasionally a burning pain in the fingers and hands. Proximal arm pain, even into the shoulder and neck, worse at night, frequently occurs. Patients often complain of dropping objects. Wrist splints are usually helpful in controlling mild motor and sensory symptoms; one inexpensive type is an elastisized wrist gauntlet with hook and loop closures and a bendable metal voler insert. The splint needs to be custom-fitted so that the wrist is dorsiflexed in a comfortable position. Avoidance of activities stressful to the wrist may be necessary. Steroid injections into the carpal tunnel may be helpful, but must be given carefully to avoid inadvertant injection into the median nerve, which itself can cause nerve damage and scarring (36). Pyridoxine in modest doses (50 mg to 100 mg per day) may improve symptoms. If symptoms are anything more than mildly annoying, then surgical release of the transverse carpal ligament should be considered, as it is curative in more than 90% of patients, as long as no axonal damage has occurred.

Rheumatic Diseases: Rheumatoid Arthritis and Polyarteritis

Both rheumatoid arthritis and polyarteritis cause symmetric neuropathies and asymmetric mononeuropathies. The former tend to develop subacutely over weeks to months, while the latter tend to develop more acutely. The symmetrical neuropathies can be very mild or subclinical, but can also start with severe burning pain and progress to significant weakness. Approximately 50% of patients with polyarteritis and 1% to 2% of patients with rheumatoid arthritis have clinical peripheral nerve involvement. Rheumatoid arthritis patients with neuropathy typically have suffered from their disease for more than 10 years. Differentiating rheumatoid neuropathy from polyarteritis neuropathy rests with the associated clinical findings, which include predominate severe arthritis in the former and characteristic skin lesions, renal disease, and other evidence of widespread vasculitis in the latter. High-dose steroids and immunosuppressant agents usually control the vasculitis of polyarteritis and may allow the neuropathy to improve (37).

Rheumatoid arthritis can also cause single or multiple mononeuropathies, particularly over pressure areas such as the carpal or cubital tunnels. Joint deformity or swelling may contribute significantly to the problem. Management includes relief of pressure, careful splinting, and control of the inflammatory arthritis.

Carcinomatous Neuropathies

Carcinomatous neuropathy involves a number of disease processes (38). The most common type is a diffuse chronic sensorimotor neuropathy. Less common are acute onset and chronic relapsing varieties, both of which are thought to have an inflammatory demyelinating origin. The motor weakness and sensory loss may be mild or severe.

Predominate sensory neuropathy occurs less frequently overall; but women are far more likely to be affected than men. In contrast, men and women are affected more equally by a sensorimotor neuropathy. The onset is usually subacute and involves numbness, dysesthesias, and parasthesias of the extremities starting distally and spreading proximally. Gait dysfunction may result from sensory ataxia or from true motor weakness. The latter occurs only in the late stages of this neuropathy. A variety of humoral, metabolic, and nutritional factors may contribute to this neuropathy. Often it is difficult to know what specifically causes the neuropathy and associated debility. Treatment of the neoplasm and normalization of nutritional and metabolic abnormalities are equally important. Both sensorimotor and sensory neuropathies can present clinically months or even years prior to manifestation of the tumor, confounding diagnosis and treatment. Fluctuations of the neuropathic symptoms may or may not correlate with tumor size, debilitation, or antineoplastic therapy. Carcinoma can also cause focal neuropathies through local infiltration or compression of nerves and plexuses. Shrinkage of the tumor by radiation, surgical debulking, or chemotherapy can help control symptoms.

Rehabilitation of these patients must encompass: (a) cautious strengthening of muscles weakened from neuropathy, (b) reversal of deconditioning caused by immobility during and following medical and surgical treatment, (c) control of symptoms from antineoplastic therapies, (d) avoidance of pathologic fractures from metastatic bone disease and osteoporosis, and (e) overcoming depression and pain associated with both the tumor and neuropathy. Complicated and severely debilitated patients may require multidisciplinary treatment to regain lost function. Comprehensive inpatient rehabilitation is justifiable only for patients with the stamina to tolerate an intensive interdisciplinary therapy program.

Paraproteinemic Neuropathies

Clinical neuropathy occurs in 13% of patients over 50 years of age with multiple myeloma. Like carcinomatous neuropathy, it often precedes the diagnosis of the neoplastic process by months or years. It may be acute, subacute, relapsing, or chronic, but is usually progressive and nonpainful, with disability caused primarily by motor weakness. In the most severe cases, patients can advance to complete quadriplegia. Benign monoclonal gammopathy occurs in about 3% of the general population and increases with age. It is associated with a severely demyelinating neuropathy that can also produce axonal loss in severe cases. The neuropathy associated with IgG gammopathy is usually chronic and progressive. IgM gammopathy occurs much less frequently, but a higher percentage of patients have peripheral nerve involvement that usually starts with paresthesias and numbness in the hands followed by similar symptoms in the feet. There is associated tremor, ataxia, and Raynaud's phenomenon. Steroids, immunosuppressants, and plasmapheresis have limited the neuropathic symptoms (39).

Of considerable interest has been the discovery of IgM antibodies that bind to myelin and myelin-associated glycoproteins (MAG). This marker is present in approximately half of patients with IgM neuropathy, and weakness is a prominent additional symptom. Response to chemotherapy, steroids, and plasmapheresis, alone or in combination, is variable, even though all should theoretically reduce anti-MAG antibodies in the body (40).

MUSCULAR/NEUROMUSCULAR JUNCTION DISORDERS

The common decline in neuromuscular performance with advancing age is often multifactorial. It may result from age-related factors as well as concomitant disease processes. Factors that impact upon muscle performance include changes in the cardiopulmonary and musculoskeletal functions and nutrition, as well as alterations in the neural and endocrine systems. Disease processes leading to changes in neuromuscular function are often indistinguishable from those caused by normal aging. In addition, physical activity also frequently decreases with age; it is often difficult to separate the effects of aging on the neuromuscular system from those of disuse.

Histologic and Physiologic Changes of the Normal Aging Neuromuscular System

A large and diverse group, the elderly differ physiologically from the young and from each other depending on whether they are healthy or ill, active or sedentary. Certain neuromuscular findings are observed in the elderly although their cause and effect are not always known or agreed upon. The muscular system changes that are associated with aging include: altered neuromuscular junction, reduced muscle mass, shift in fiber type distribution, decreased cell metabolism, and a decline in muscle function.

Neuromuscular junction changes with normal aging include an increased number of preterminal axons entering an endplate and increased length of the motor endplate. The endplate composition is altered to include a larger number of smaller conglomerates of acetylcholine receptors as well as perijunctional acetylcholine receptors (41). Metabolically impaired neuromuscular junctions have been suggested as the cause for alterations in the synthesis and release of the transmitter acetylcholine. This can eventually result in complete denervation and atrophy of muscle fibers prior to the loss of spinal motor neurons.

Muscle atrophy is a common feature of aging. Multiple factors have been suggested for this decrease in muscle mass, including age-related loss of anterior horn cells and disuse atrophy due to alteration of activity. There is clear evidence for the loss of motor units in older subjects. Individuals over 60 years of age have approximately half the number of motor units of subjects under 60 years of age (42).

Disuse, cachexia, and aging are all associated with selective atrophy of type 2 muscle fibers (43, 44). The preferential atrophy of type 2 muscle fibers secondary to disuse has been established. Muscle biopsies in the aged patient show type 2 atrophy with type 2B fibers selectively involved. A cross-sectional study (45) suggested that the loss of type 2 fibers with aging is partly due to a slow loss of alpha motor neurons innervating the type 2 fibers. However, this cross-sectional study did not determine whether this loss of type 2 fibers was due to the aging process, decreased physical activity, or a combination of the two. Research on the effects of aging on the total number and size of fibers, as well as the proportion of type 1 and type 2 fibers, have yielded differing results (45–48).

Age may alter the metabolism and function of muscle fibers such that excitability thresholds increase and membrane resistance decreases. The level of intracellular sodium increases while potassium decreases. Shifts in the ion balance of muscle fibers are related to changes in their membrane permeability and altered function of the sodium potassium pump (49).

Loss of muscle function with aging is probably due to decrease in fiber number as well as size. This is accompanied by a decline in strength with a 20% to 30% loss between the ages of 60 years and 90 years (43). Significant decrements in maximum power output (work rate) have been reported (45% decrease between the ages 50 years and 80 years). There is also a reduction in myofascial tissue elasticity and extensibility, making it more susceptible to injury following minor trauma (50).

Exercise and the Elderly

A longitudinal study evaluating the muscle function of aging men and women noted a decrease in muscle strength with age. This was thought to be the result of a changed activity pattern with a lack of fast and forceful movements in daily living. Other studies have shown a decrease in maximum isometric torque in men and women between the ages of 60 years and 70 years due to altered daily activity (51). These and similar studies suggest physical activity may prevent disability due to decreased muscle strength and function.

Investigators studying how physical training influences muscle morphology and strength in different age groups concluded that age-related muscle fiber atrophy was diminished following training, as evidenced by increased fiber size. Muscle strength was found to be lower in elderly patients throughout the study, suggesting that strength decline in old age is not primarily due to muscle fiber atrophy (52). The effects of a 12-week endurance training program at 70% peak O_2 consumption in elderly and young healthy individuals showed that the elderly had more adipose tissue and less muscle mass than the young. The initial peak VO_2 was lower in the elderly, but the absolute increase of 5.5 mL to 6 mL per kilogram per minute after training was similar for both groups. Muscle biopsies showed that before training muscle glycogen stores were 61% higher in the young and that glycogen utilization per joule during submaximal exercise was higher in the elderly. Glycogen stores and muscle O_2 consumption increased significantly in response to training only in the elderly. The absolute changes that training produced in peak VO_2 were similar in both age groups, but the muscle oxidative capacity was 128% greater in the elderly. This suggests that peripheral factors play an important role in the elderly's exercise endurance (53). Multiple studies have shown that endurance type training leads to enhanced capacity for aerobic metabolism in the elderly (54). Grimby suggests that part of the observed reduction in muscle mass with age is the result of inactivity as well as a loss of motor units. Muscle changes appear to be quantitative rather than qualitative until the age of 70 years. A reduction in the size of type 2 fibers was noted in the quadriceps but not other muscles, presumably due to differences in activity pattern and motor unit recruitment. Limitations in aerobic capacity may result from reduced muscle mass as well as impaired circulatory and respiratory systems (55).

Aerobic capacity can be shown to increase along with static and dynamic muscle strength utilizing 12-week programs of dynamic and static exercises. The fiber composition revealed a significantly higher proportion of type 2 fibers after training, as well as enzymatic evidence of training with significant increases in enzymes such as muscle myokinase and lactate dehydrogenase. Several studies have shown that aerobic capacity and muscle strength are improved with training in 70-year-old individuals (56). Other research has suggested that inactivity, concomitant disease, and advancing age give the greatest correlation with muscle wasting (57).

Men over 65 years of age who participate in regular walking exercise regimes show greater muscle strength in the triceps surae. Muscle strength correlates positively with the rate of walking and distance walked. These results raise the possibility that more and faster walking may help maintain calf muscle strength and independent life-style in old age (58). In the elderly, the loss of strength in proportion to body weight often results in low safety margins for activities such as stepping up or down a stair (59). Researchers have noted gains in lean body mass and skeletal muscle function following training programs in older adults. This indicates that loss of skeletal muscle with age is reversible and possibly preventable with exercise (60–64). Studies suggest that, although some decline in physiologic functions can be attributed primarily to aging, more important factors include inactivity and clinical or subclinical disease. Moderate rhythmic and dynamic exercises performed at an intensity greater than 50% of VO_2max for 15 minutes to 60 minutes daily in multiple sessions are recommended to enhance general well-being and fitness (65–68).

Polymyositis/Dermatomyositis

Polymyositis is a diffuse inflammatory myopathy of unknown cause producing symmetrical weakness of voluntary striated muscle of the shoulder and pelvic girdles. Polymyositis and dermatomyositis (PM-DM) occur from infancy to late adult life with a peak incidence in the 5th to 6th decades. There is an approximate 2 to 1 predominance of females afflicted with reported incidence rates varying from 0.1 to 0.9 per 100,000 (69). The disease may progress to involve muscles of the neck and diaphragm. In dermatomyositis, inflammatory cutaneous changes accompany the weakness and muscle pain.

Polymyositis often begins insidiously over a 2 to 3 week period with the primary complaints being muscle weakness and tenderness, as well as joint pain. Proximal muscle weakness of the shoulder and pelvic girdles occurs in 75% to 100% of patients. Other common symptoms include neck flexor weakness (65%), dysphagia (50%), and pain or tenderness (50% to 75%). Approximately 10% of the patients with DM-PM have distal muscle weakness. In PM-DM, an erythematous rash appears on the face and upper extremities in 25% of the cases. Classical dermatomyositis occurs in approximately 30% of the patients with PM-DM. A characteristic heliotropic rash occurs on the eyelids, accompanied by periorbital edema in these patients. Connective tissue disorders and neoplasms are associated with PM-DM in approximately one quarter of all cases (69).

High-dose corticosteroid therapy is recommended for treatment of PM-DM. Prednisone may be administered at 60 mg to 80 mg per day in divided doses for several weeks, with a gradual reduction (5 mgs every 2 to 3 weeks) to a maintenance dose of 5 mg to 15 mg of prednisone per day. In most cases, steriod therapy is maintained at this lower level indefinitely (70). The muscle weakness and atrophy observed in PM-DM may be compounded by a steroid myopathy. High-dose steroids may produce iatrogenic problems, including vertebral compression fractures in the thorax and lumbar spine (71). Immunosuppressive therapy (methotrexate and azathioprine) has been utilized by some centers when there has been an inadequate response to prednisone or to allow reduction in the dosage of prednisone.

Rehabilitation intervention includes range of motion to prevent contractures and modalities to relieve painful muscle spasm during the acute phase. In the remittive phase, active exercises are utilized for muscle strengthening, activities of daily living to improve function, and conditioning training to increase endurance. Psychologic support is necessary to improve coping skills for PM-DM patients. Long-term recreational exercise programs should be instituted to maintain strength and endurance.

Polymyalgia Rheumatica

Polymyalgia rheumatica (PMR) is a connective tissue disorder characterized by diffuse nonarticular pain, aching, and stiffness, usually occurring in the proximal musculature about the neck and shoulder girdle. Polymyalgia rheumatica affects people during their middle age to late adult life, peaking during the 8th decade with no sexual predominance (70). As a connective tissue disorder, PMR is closely related to cranial arteritis and rheumatoid arthritis. In PMR, myositis does not occur. Impaired usage of the limbs results from pain and stiffness rather than from muscle weakness.

Polymyalgia rheumatica is a chronic, self-limiting disease with a median duration of 11 months (72). Serious complications of this disease include arterial insufficiency, coronary occlusion, cerebral vascular accident, and blindness. Patients often present with pain and stiffness of the back, shoulder, and neck, which are usually more severe in the morning. They may also complain of severe throbbing headaches involving the temporal and occipital regions. Forty percent of patients with temporal arteritis also develop PMR, and approximately 16% of patients with PMR have active temporal arteritis (73).

Small doses of corticosteroid drugs have been shown to effectively reduce inflammation and speed recovery. Prednisone, less than 10 mg per day usually minimizes symptoms within 4 days. Long-term steroid therapy is often utilized until the disease remits (70). Nonsteriodal antiinflammatory drugs are also effective in less severe cases, when duration of treatment and dosage are individualized (72).

Rehabilitation management of these patients routinely involves multiple modalities, including heat or cold, for muscle pain. Psychologic support programs can help patients cope with this disease process. In the acute phase, the rehabilitation is directed towards maintaining range of motion and muscle strength. In the chronic phase, patients often require reconditioning and strengthening programs.

Myasthenia Gravis

Myasthenia gravis is an autoimmune disorder of neuromuscular transmission, involving destruction of the postsynaptic acetylcholine receptors at the neuromuscular junction. Often associated with thymic tumor in the elderly, it may occur at any age with a peak incidence for females in the third decade and the peak incidence for males in the 7th decade of life. The reported incidence rates vary from 0.2 to 0.5 per year per 100,000 (74). Myasthenia gravis is characterized by chronic fatigueability and weakness of muscles, especially in the face and throat. The onset of symptoms is often gradual with ptosis, diplopia, and weakness of the facial muscles. This disease may involve the extraocular muscles selectively or be generalized in muscular involvement. Muscle usage typically aggravates the symptoms.

Myasthenia gravis is currently treated with anticholinesterase medications, alternate day prednisone therapy, other immunosuppressants, or plasmapheresis. Aminoglycoside administration can reduce the number of acetylcholine quanta released; therefore, aminoglycosides should be avoided or used cautiously in patients with myasthenia gravis. Chlorpromazine, quinine, quinidine, procainamide, and beta-blockers may amplify the neuromuscular transmission defect (74).

Rehabilitation in these patients needs to selectively stage therapy at the high points of muscle strength during the day and to incorporate a metered approach in all physical activities. Exercise, meals, and activities should be planned during the energy peaks following utilization of medication. Energy conservation is essential in these patients, who have periodic remissions, exacerbations, and day-to-day fluctuations. Strenuous exercise, stress, infection, and needless exposure to hot or cold weather should be avoided.

Myasthenic Syndromes

Myasthenic syndromes are genetic or acquired disorders of neuromuscular transmission, associated with abnormal weakness and fatigue not due to myasthenia gravis. The elderly may acquire a deficiency of pseudocholinesterase due to liver disease, the use of monoamine oxidase inhibitors, or exposure to organophosphate compounds. This does not normally manifest unless the patient is given a depolarizing relaxant drug such as succinylcholine.

Nutritional, metabolic, and toxic myasthenic-like symptoms may also develop in the elderly. Patients receiving beta-blocking agents have had clinical syndromes resembling myasthenia gravis, which may result from a neuromuscular depressant effect or an immunologic complication of the medication (75). A small number of patients have developed myasthenic syndrome while taking D-penicillamine. These symptoms resolve with medication withdrawal.

Lambert-Eaton myasthenic syndrome (LEMS), with or without neoplasm, is associated with a malignant tumor in two thirds of the cases, occurring primarily in men over 40 years of age and with 80% of the tumors being a small cell carcinoma of the lung (76). This form of myasthenic syndrome has also been linked with carcinoma of the bronchus, breast, stomach, prostate, and other organs. The remaining one third have nonneoplastic Lambert-Eaton myasthenic syndrome, which may present at any age.

Muscle weakness and fatigue are the most common symptoms. Lower extremities are more severely affected than upper extremities and the proximal muscles more than distal. Some patients complain of muscle pain, peripheral paresthesias, or symptoms involving cranial muscles. In the majority of patients, autonomic nervous system abnormalities are manifest with dryness of the mouth, impotence, and hydrosis. During maximal voluntary muscle contraction, strength reduces initially, increases after a few seconds, and then diminishes with continued exertion.

Rehabilitation efforts must selectively stage therapy at the high points of muscle strength during the day and use a titrated approach in all physical activities. Energy conservation is essential in these patients who have periodic remissions, exacerbations, and day-to-day fluctuations. As with myesthenia gravis, strenuous exercise, stress, infection, and needless exposure to hot or cold weather are to be avoided.

Rhabdomyolysis

Rhabdomyolysis involves necrosis of the muscle fiber in response to multiple clinical circumstances. In the elderly, acute rhabdomyolysis may occur secondary to heat stroke, muscle ischemia, crush injury, and generalized anoxia. High temperatures secondary to fever accompanying bacterial and viral infections and malignant hyperthermia also result in rhabdomyolysis. Drugs and toxins associated with rhabdomyolysis include: heroin, methadone, amphetamine, barbiturates, diazepam, meprobamate, isoniazid, amphotericin B, alcohol, phencyclidine, clofibrate, emetine, azathioprine, aminocaproic acid, and 5'-azacytidine. In addition to trauma and pharmacologic exposure, metabolic derangements such as severe hypernatremia, diabetic ketoacidosis, and hyperosmolar coma have been associated with rhabdomyolysis (77).

The clinical presentation often includes severe muscle pain, tenderness, and weakness of the limb; swelling of the effected muscles may require fasciotomy. Acute oliguric renal failure may result from severe myoglobinuria. Management of the situation requires removal of the precipitating event and control of the immediate sequelae. Rehabilitation after the acute episode involves increasing muscle strength and endurance as well as activities of daily living, depending upon the muscle groups involved.

ELECTROPHYSIOLOGIC ASPECTS OF AGING

It is relatively easy to assess the dynamic functional integrity of both the peripheral and central nervous systems through specific electrophysiologic techniques. By artificially inducing action potentials in a peripheral nerve, neural propagation can be evaluated peripherally and/or centrally. If a mixed nerve (motor and sensory fibers) in a limb is activated, one may consider initially the propagating action potential to travel distally. This distal propagation can terminate in a number of muscles or the nerves supplying some cutaneous aspect of the extremity. By placing surface or subcutaneous electrodes in a muscle or along the cutaneous course of the nerve, one may calculate the velocity with which the action potential propagates.

For example, if the recording electrode is placed on the median innervated thenar muscles and the median nerve is stimulated at the antecubital fossa and wrist, a compound muscle action potential can be recorded with each stimulation. The more proximal stimulus will take longer to activate the muscle than will the distal stimulus, and these latencies can be accurately documented. Subtracting the wrist from the elbow latency yields a time of travel between the two activation points for the fastest conducting fibers. Dividing the interstimulus distance by the time difference results in a nerve conduction velocity (NCV). This speed of propagation is usually expressed in meters/second (m/s). In this instance, a motor conduction velocity is obtained. Comparing the obtained value with a previously established normative data base establishes whether the nerve under investigation is normal or subject to pathology. The distal time segment is typically not included in motor velocity measurements (hence subtracting it from the proximal time) because of the uncertainty of the time delay across the neuromuscular junction (78). Also, it is possible to record from the median innervated digits, resulting in a sensory nerve conduction velocity; this may be accomplished with either stimulation site (wrist or elbow in the above example). Subtraction of the distal segment is unnecessary as a neuromuscular junction is not involved in the sensory fibers. The amplitude of the evoked muscle or sensory response conveys an approximation of the number of axons activated. A drop in the amplitude implies axonal loss or a less synchronous arrival of the individual nerve action potentials.

A needle electrode may be inserted directly into a skeletal muscle to evaluate its electrophysiologic status (electromyography or EMG). Aside from the endplate region, a normal muscle is electrically silent at rest. If spontaneous activity is present, this typically heralds some form of disease process. With voluntary activation, the individual motor unit characteristics may also be assessed. Alterations in the morphology of motor unit action potentials (MUAPs) may suggest possible pathologic processes affecting the patient.

The central nervous system may also be evaluated through peripheral nerve excitation. Instead of recording from distal sites, one may place surface electrodes along the proximal course of the nerve such as Erb's point, the cervical spine, and, finally, overlying the cerebral cortex. Somatosensory evoked potentials (SEPs) can be used to determine the integrity of the entire somatosensory pathway from the peripheral aspects of the extremity to the somatosensory cortex. Brainstem auditory evoked responses (BAERs) consist of a series of auditory clicks that the patient hears, with the ensuing electrical potentials produced along the auditory pathway recorded. Lesions affecting the eighth nerve or its central extensions can be evaluated for possible pathologic involvement. Finally, the visual pathway may be investigated with a series of checkerboard pattern reversals, with the resulting neural impulses measured. The electrophysiologic examination is a dynamic study of the nervous system and compliments the static anatomic depictions of neural integrity such as the magnetic resonance imager (MRI) or computerized tomographic scans (CT). To appreciate the electrophysiologic alterations with age, it is first necessary to consider the normal anatomic changes of the aging nervous system.

Neuromuscular Alterations Pertinent to Electrophysiology

The density of large myelinated fibers in the distal portions of the sural nerve increases rapidly from birth to 3 years of age, reaching a stable adult value by 3 years. A maximum fiber density of 6480/mm^2 is achieved by the third decade. The large fiber density progressively declines to 54% (3480/mm^2) of the second decade by 90 years of age (79). After 60 years of age, stenosis of the vasa nervorum is rather pronounced (79, 80). One may conclude, therefore, that only about half of the large sensory myelinated fibers innervating the distal portions of the lower extremities survive the aging process. Of additional interest is the relationship between the distances separating the nodes of Ranvier (internodal length) and diameter of myelinated fibers. Below the age of 65 years, there is a linear correlation of internodal length and diameter. At all ages above 65 years, there is less of a linear correlation and increased scatter of values, suggesting a shortening of the internodal length (81, 82). A lessening of the internodal length can result from demyelination and remyelination (83). This process is ongoing with age and does not affect all of the large myelinated fibers equally. The above findings have been documented in multiple peripheral nerves of both the upper and lower extremities.

Histochemical studies of limb muscles from elderly individuals without evidence of neuromuscular disease revealed: fiber size variation, hyaline or granular degeneration, loss of striations, clumps of pyknotic nuclei, increased fat and connective tissue, and, most significantly, neurogenic fiber type grouping (84). The fiber type grouping is more pronounced in the lower than upper extremities and distally more so than proximally. The etiology of fiber type grouping was presumed secondary to degeneration and regeneration of the peripheral nervous system, with secondary reorganization of the muscle fibers belonging to individual motor units.

In addition to age-related changes of the peripheral nervous system, the central nervous system also demonstrates alterations associated with aging. The most conspicuous changes were noted in the posterior columns (85, 86). A progressive loss of large myelinated fibers proportional to the decreasing numbers of posterior spinal nerve root fibers was noted (87). A loss of fibers was also noted in the peripheral and central projections of the acoustic nerve. Degeneration of the eighth nerve extensions was observed in the pathways through the brainstem into the white matter of the cerebrum (88). The optic nerve displays similar changes to those previously noted for both peripheral and central nerves (89). The optic nerve is invested by oligodendroglia, and myelination is usually complete by 4 years. It is small at birth and reaches adult size by 12 to 15 years. This nerve contains a maximum of approximately one million axons in the mid-thirties. Optic nerve axonal density demonstrates a progressive decrease with age that becomes rather obvious by 60 years.

Nerve Conduction Studies

One may consider either motor or sensory responses with respect to nerve conduction studies. A number of parameters can be evaluated when investigating electrophysiologic aspects of the peripheral nervous system. The evoked response's amplitude, duration, latency, and conduction velocity can be easily quantified.

Several generalizations can be made regarding peripheral evoked sensory nerve actions potentials (SNAPs). The conduction velocity demonstrates a consistent decline approximating 1 m/s to 2 m/s per decade (90–94). The SNAP's duration is about 10% to 15%, and 20% longer in the 40 to 60 and 70 to 88 year-old individuals than in the 18 to 25 year-old persons, respectively. Compared to the 18 to 25 year-old group, the SNAP's amplitude is one half and one third, respectively, for the 40 to 60 and 70 to 88 year-old groups (91). The distal sensory latencies revealed a similar prolongation with age.

The results of aging on conduction velocity have been examined in a number of upper and lower extremity nerves (Table 19.1). Motor nerve conduction velocities reveal similar changes to those of the sensory nerves. The newborn's motor nerve conduction velocities are about half of adult values, which are reached by 3 to 5 years of age (95). After the age of 50 years, the conduction velocity of the fastest motor fibers progressively declines, approximating 1 m/s to 2 m/s per decade (96–99). There is a concurrent increase in the distal motor latency and decrease in the motor response's amplitude with advancing age.

The above nerve conduction study findings may be explained to some degree by considering the histologic changes associated with aging of the peripheral nervous system. The maximal adult nerve conduction velocities are achieved coincidentally when myelination of the large fibers is completed in the 5-year-old child (95, 100). The subsequent reduction in sensory and motor conduction velocity and amplitude, with increases in the distal latency and response duration, correlates well with advancing age. The aging nervous system demonstrates loss of large fibers and evidence suggestive of progressive demyelination and remyelination, particularly after the sixth decade (81–83). Large fiber loss, combined with segmental demyelination/remyelination, has been suggested as a cause for a slowing of the conduction velocities. Additionally, the evoked response's amplitude decline may result from a loss of fibers. Buchthal (91) has postulated that the primary cause of the noted electrophysiologic changes directly stems from an alteration in the nerve's membranous properties to sustain the appropriate current density necessary for maximum conduction velocities.

Needle Electromyographic Findings

Standard concentric needle evaluations of motor unit action potentials clearly reveal a relationship between the potential's duration and individual's age. From 1 to 85 years there is a progressive increase in the MUAP's mean duration of 5.7 ms (1 to 4 years) to 10 ms (85 years) (101, 102). The MUAP's duration relates to (a) differences in the arrival times of the nerve impulse to the individual single muscle fiber's endplates, (b) length of the region within which the endplates of the motor unit are situated, (c) propagation velocity of the different muscle fibers, and (d) length over which the single muscle fiber action potential propagates. In light of these histologic changes of denervation/reinnervation with subsequent remodeling of the motor unit, one may postulate various reasons for increasing MUAP duration with age.

The subclinical loss of a few motor fibers will render all of the muscle fibers innervated by that nerve to be denervated. As a result, neighboring motor units, through the process of peripheral sprouting, may rein-

Table 19.1. NCV[a] Changes with Age

Nerve Study	Age Range (years)	Mean NCV (30 years)	NCV Drop m/s/dec
Median (m)[97]	10–80	59	0.7
Median (s)[97]	10–80	68	0.7
Median (s)[91]	18–88	65	1.6
Ulnar (m)[99]	3.5–82	58	2.2
Ulnar (m)[97]	10–80	59	0.8
Ulnar (m)[98]	20–90	58	1.3
Ulnar (s)[97]	10–80	65	1.1
Ulnar (s)[91]	18–89	64	1.4
Musc. (m)[94]	15–74	68	2.0
Musc. (s)[94]	15–74	66	2.0
Peroneal (m)[96]	15–74	50	1.1
Peroneal (m)[97]	10–80	49	0.8
Peroneal (s)[90]	15–65	56	1.0
Tibial (m)[97]	10–80	45	0.5
Sural (s)[90]	15–65	57	1.0

[a]Median and ulnar nerve motor (m) and sensory (s) values apply to the wrist to elbow segment. Peroneal, tibial, and sural nerves represent the distance between the popliteal fossa and ankle. Musc. refers to the musculocutaneous nerve elbow to axilla segment. The mean nerve conduction velocity (NCV) is given for 30 years of age for the study quoted to serve as a reference point. The mean drop in meters/second/decade (m/s/dec) is provided as determined in the study noted.

nervate those orphaned single muscle fibers prior to regrowth of the original axon. The sprouted motor unit will now contain more muscle fibers than it "normally" should. Interesting characteristics of the newly innervated muscle fibers will have specific effects upon the waveform's morphology, representing the remodeled motor unit (103). Initially, the newly formed peripheral nerve sprouts may be less than optimally myelinated. This will result in a somewhat slower conduction velocity. The result is less synchronicity of the summated electrical activity contributing to the MUAP, with a possible increase in the number of phases and/or duration of the recorded potential. The added muscle fibers will also increase the spatial extent of the endplate zone, contributing to the total potential's duration. The conduction velocity of recently innervated muscle fibers may also be slower than their nondenervated counterparts again leading to less synchronous potential summation and possible increases in MUAP duration. An increase in neuromuscular junction jitter (time of neuromuscular junction transmission delay) and blocking (failure of neuromuscular transmission) has been demonstrated in individuals older than 60 years, supporting the contention of recently formed neuromuscular junctions from a reinnervating process (104). Single-fiber electromyographic investigations have also documented increased fiber density of the aged population, adding further support to peripheral sprouting secondary to drop-out of motor fibers with aging (104).

As the peripheral sprouts mature and the terminal neural conduction velocity increases with diminished jitter and blocking, an increase in the electrical summation of the MUAP can be expected to occur to some extent.

The improved temporal summation of electrical activity should result in an increase in the MUAP's amplitude in older individuals. Macroelectromyography has indeed documented the expected increase in the amplitude of the MUAP with aging (Table 19.2) (103). Motor unit counting techniques have also shown a reduction in the total number of motor units, but an increase in the size of those remaining in people of advanced age (105). The electrophysiologic findings support the histologic data in substantiating the alterations of the peripheral neuromuscular system with aging.

Somatosensory Evoked Potentials

Somatosensory evoked potentials are commonly recorded following stimulation of the peripheral nervous system through the median or tibial nerves. Evaluating the effects of aging upon SEPs is rather complex; the latency is dependent upon height as well as peripheral and central action potential transit. Elderly individuals are usually somewhat shorter than younger individuals. Also, the peripheral nervous system conduction slowing must be differentiated from possible central nervous system conduction changes.

A number of SEP alterations have been documented with advancing age, giving appropriate consideration to peripheral nerve conduction's slowing and diminishing stature. Cortical SEP onset latency increased by 0.015 ms/m per year and 0.08 ms/m per year for the median and tibial nerves, respectively (106). These changes reflect slowing in both the peripheral and central conduction pathways. Central conduction time (transit between the cervical spine and somatosensory cortex),

Table 19.2. Electrophysiologic Alterations in Aging Muscle

Age (years)	MU[a] Count (105)	Mean Fiber Density (104)	% Increased Jitter (104)[a] (μs)	% Increased Blocking (104)	Macro EMG Amplitude (103) (μV)[a]
10–19	280	1.50	0.33	0.33	132
20–29	268	1.38	0.0	0.0	158
30–39	252	1.47	0.0	0.0	159
40–49	240	1.48	0.33	0.0	207
50–59	227	1.51	0.6	1.0	190
60–69	<100	1.55	1.6	1.3	207
70–79	<100	1.78	2.81	0.3	351
80–89	<100	2.32	—	—	—

[a]Macro EMG of tibialis anterior muscle expressed in microvolts (μV) and jitter measured in microseconds (μs). Motor unit (MU) count represents an estimate of the number of motor units in the median nerve innervated thenar muscles.

however, revealed a rather constant interval between 10 and 49 years, but increased abruptly by 0.3 ms (5.6%) beyond the fifth decade and remained constant again up to 79 years (107). Peripheral slowing of the SEP response can be explained by the above noted changes in loss of myelinated fibers, increased internodal length, and possible alterations in the axonal membrane's ability to sustain the appropriate current density. The increase in central conduction time may stem from slowing of posterior column conduction, loss of larger fibers, increased synaptic delay, or other as yet unknown factors.

The recorded SEP amplitude reveals rather interesting changes with age. In stimulating the median nerve at the wrist, a cervical spine potential at C-2 can be recorded (N 14) in addition to the cortical potential (N 20) (107). The amplitude of N 14 remained essentially unchanged between 10 and 39 years. It then decreased about 0.004 microvolts/year progressively in persons 40 years and beyond. The N 20 amplitude, however, decreased between 10 and 39 years and then increased 0.005 microvolts/year. The amplitude ratio, N 20/N 14 initially diminished and then increased after the age of 40 years. A number of explanations have been postulated to explain this finding in the cortical N 20 amplitude, but none have been substantiated experimentally; the true cause remains unknown.

Brainstem Auditory Evoked Potentials

Brainstem auditory evoked potentials are routinely utilized to assess hearing loss or to detect retrocochlear lesions and brainstem dysfunction. The BAER is a series of seven (I-VII) positive cortically recorded far-field potentials. Their respective sites of origin are postulated to be: I (auditory nerve), II (cochlear nucleus), III (superior olivary complex), IV (midbrain/lateral lemniscus), V (inferior colliculus), VI (medial geniculate body), and VII (auditory radiation from thalamus to cortex) (108). Although the sites of origin appear well identified, much work is needed to clearly identify the actual neural generators of these far-field potentials.

As individuals age, there is a progressive increase in the latency of all the evoked peaks. The greatest latency delay is in the first peak. This is most likely due to the alterations noted previously for peripheral nerves. One may also measure the interpeak latency to assess the slowing of conduction in more central pathways. Studies investigating the interpeak latency values reveal that throughout life only a small amount of slowing occurs in the central nervous system pathways with respect to the auditory system (108, 109). Elderly persons typically incur a high frequency hearing loss, and this prolongs the BAER latencies. This time delay has been attributed to a shift in the responses originating in the basal portion of the cochlea to the more apical aspect (110).

Visual Evoked Potentials

A positive cortically recorded potential peak occurring at approximately 100 ms (P100) results when the eye observes a reversing checkerboard pattern. This waveform is referred to as the pattern visual evoked potential (PVEP). The PVEP demonstrates a progressive increase in the P100 latency with advancing age of 7% to 13% (109). This increase depends upon the check size and luminance of the pattern observed. A small check size reveals almost a twice as large prolongation in the P100 latency (2.6 ms/decade) as compared to a large check size (1.4 ms/decade) with advancing age (111). At low levels of luminance, the P100 latency increases after the fourth decade, approximating 1.4 ms/decade. At high levels of luminance, only a small increase in the P100 latency is observed (0.7 ms/decade) (112). These occurrences may result from the differential effects of the aging process on the various spatial frequency processing abilities of the human visual system.

References

1. Schaumburg HH, Spencer PS, Ochoa J. The aging human peripheral nervous system. In: Katzman R., Terry RD, eds. *The Neurology of Aging.* Philadelphia, Pa: FA. Davis; 1983:111–122.
2. Klawans HL, Tufo HM, Ostfeld AM, Shekelle RB, Kilbridge JA.

Neurologic examination in an elderly population. *Dis Nerv Syst.* 32:274–279, 1971.

3. Jenkyn LR, Reeves AG. Neurologic signs in uncomplicated aging (senescence). *Semin Neurol.* 1:21–30, 1981.

4. McKhann GM, Griffin JW, Cornblath DR, et al. Plasmapheresis and Guillain-Barré syndrome: analysis of prognostic factors and the effect of plasmapheresis. *Ann Neurol.* 23:347–353, 1988.

5. Grob D. Common disorders of muscles in the aged. In: Reichel W, ed. *Clinical Aspects of Aging.* Baltimore, Md: Williams & Wilkins; 1989:296–313.

6. Ropper AH, Shahani BT. Pain in Guillain-Barré syndrome. *Arch Neurol.* 41:511–514, 1984.

7. Gruener G, Bosch EP, Strauss RG, et al. Prediction of early beneficial response to plasma exchange in Guillain-Barré syndrome. *Arch Neurol.* 44:295–298, 1987.

8. Gashi F, Kenrick MM. Guillain-Barré syndrome: review of the literature, case presentation, and physiatric management. *South Med J.* 68:1524–1528, 1975.

9. Pease WD, Johnson EW. Rehabilitation management of diseases of the motor unit. In: Kottke FJ, Lehmann JF, eds. *Krusen's Handbook of Physical Medicine and Rehabilitation.* 4th ed. Philadelphia, Pa: W. B. Saunders; 1990:754–764.

10. Thomas PK. Peripheral neuropathy in late life. In: Assal JPH, Liniger C., eds. *Peripheral Neuropathies 1988: What is Significantly New?* Padova: Liviana Press; 1989:183–196.

11. Panis W, Aronoff GM. Painful peripheral neuropathies. In: Aronoff GM, ed. *Evaluation and Treatment of Chronic Pain.* Baltimore, Md: Urban & Schwarzenberg; 1985:75–82.

12. Toole JF, Parrish ML. Nitrofurantoin polyneuropathy. *Neurology.* 23:554–559, 1973.

13. Hughes RAC. Chronic polyneuropathy of undetermined cause. In: Matthews WB, ed. *Handbook of Clinical Neurology, Vol. 7(51): Neuropathies.* New York, NY: Elsevier Science Publishers; 1987:529–541.

14. Woodbury DM, Fingl E. Drugs effective in the therapy of the epilepsies. In: Goodman LS, Gilman A, eds. *The Pharmacological Basis of Therapeutics.* 5th ed. New York, NY: MacMillan; 1975:201–226.

15. Hallett M, Tandon D, Berardelli A. Treatment of peripheral neuropathies. *J Neurol Neurosurg Psychiatry.* 48:1193–1207, 1985.

16. Behse F, Buchthal F. Alcoholic neuropathy: clinical, electrophysiological, and biopsy findings. *Ann Neurol.* 2:95–110, 1977.

17. Sluga E, Donis J. Deficiency neuropathies. In: Matthews WB, ed. *Handbook of Clinical Neurology, Vol. 7(51): Neuropathies.* New York, NY: Elsevier Science Publishers; 1987:321–354.

18. Pathy MSJ. The central nervous system – clinical presentation and management of neurological disorders in old age. In: Brocklehurst JC, ed. *Textbook of Geriatric Medicine and Gerontology.* 3rd ed. New York, NY: Churchill Livingstone; 1985:391–426.

19. Porteroy RK: Pain. In: Abrams WB, Beskow R, eds. *The Merck Manual of Geriatrics.* Rahway, NJ: Merck Sharpe & Dohme Research Laboratories; 1990:105–128.

20. Watson PN, Evans RJ. Postherpetic neuralgia: a review. *Arch Neurol.* 43:836–840, 1986.

21. Sklar SH, Blue WT, Alexander EJ, Bodian CA. Herpes zoster: the treatment and prevention of neuralgia with adenosine monophosphate. *JAMA.* 253:1427–1430, 1985.

22. Clements RS, Bell DSH. Complications of diabetes: prevalence, detection, current treatment, and prognosis. *Am J Med.* 79(suppl 5A):2–7, 1985.

23. Cohen JA, Gross KF. Autonomic neuropathy: clinical presentation and differential diagnosis. *Geriatrics.* 45:33–42, 1990.

24. Asbury AK. Focal and multifocal neuropathies of diabetes. In: Dyck PJ, Thomas PK, Asbury AK, et al, eds.: *Diabetic Neuropathy.* Philadelphia, Pa: W. B. Saunders; 1987:45–55.

25. Bastron JA, Thomas JE. Diabetic polyradiculopathy: clinical and electromyographic findings in 105 patients. *Mayo Clin Proc.* 56:725–732, 1981.

26. Chokroverty S, Reyes MG, Rubino FA, et al. The syndrome of diabetic amyotrophy. *Ann Neurol.* 2:181–194, 1977.

27. Cohen KL, Harris S. Efficacy and safety of nonsteroidal anti-inflammatory drugs in the therapy of diabetic neuropathy. *Arch Intern Med.* 147:1442–1444, 1987.

28. LeQuesner PM. Trophic factors and vitamin therapy. In: Dyck PJ, Thomas PK, Asbury AK, et al, eds.: *Diabetic Neuropathy.* Philadelphia, Pa: W. B. Saunders; 1987:194–198.

29. Martyn CN, Reid W, Young RF, et al. Six month treatment with sorbinil in asymptomatic diabetic neuropathy: failure to improve abnormal nerve function. *Diabetes.* 36:987–990, 1987.

30. Kvinesdal B, Molin J, Froland A, Gram LF. Imipramine treatment of painful diabetic neuropathy. *JAMA.* 251:1727–1730, 1984.

31. Max MB, Culnane M, Schafer SC, et al. Amitriptyline relieves diabetic neuropathy pain in patients with normal or depressed mood. *Neurology.* 37:589–596, 1987.

32. Turkington RW. Depression masquerading as diabetic neuropathy. *JAMA.* 243:1147–1150, 1980.

33. Rull J. A., Quibera R, Gonzalez-Millan H, et al. Symptomatic treatment of peripheral diabetic neuropathy with carbamazepine: double blind crossover trial. *Diabetologia.* 5:215–218, 1969.

34. Chadda VS, Mathur MS. Double blind study of the effects of diphenylhydantoin sodium on diabetic neuropathy. *J Assoc Phys Ind.* 26:403–406, 1978.

35. Dejgard A, Peterson P, Kastrup J. Mexiletine for treatment of chronic painful diabetic neuropathy. *Lancet.* 1:9–11, 1988.

36. Stewart JD. *Focal Peripheral Neuropathy.* New York, NY: Elsevier; 1987.

37. Conn DL, Dyck PJ. Angiopathic neuropathy in connective tissue diseases. In: Dyck PJ, Thomas PK, Lambert EH, Bunge R, eds.: *Peripheral Neuropathy.* Philadelphia, Pa: W. B. Saunders; 1984:2027–2043.

38. McLeod JG. Carcinomatous neuropathy. In: Dyck PJ, Thomas PK, Lambert EH, Bunge R, eds.: *Peripheral Neuropathy.* Philadelphia, Pa: W. B. Saunders; 1984:2180–2191.

39. McLeod JG, Pollard JD. Peripheral neuropathy associated with paraproteinemia. In: Matthews WB, ed.: *Handbook of Clinical Neurology, Vol. 7(51): Neuropathies.* New York, NY: Elsevier Science Publishers; 1987:429–444.

40. Latov N, Hays AP, Sherman WH. Peripheral neuropathy and anti-MAG antibodies. *CRC Crit Rev Neurobiol.* 3(4):301–332, 1988.

41. Oda K. Age changes of motor innovation and acetylcholine receptor distribution on normal skeletal muscle fibers. *J Neurol Sci.* 66:327–328, 1984.

42. Brown WF, Strong MJ, Snow R. Methods of estimating numbers of motor units in biceps-brachialis muscles and losses of motor units with aging. *Muscle Nerve.* 11:423–432, 1988.

43. Teravainen H, Calne DB. Motor system in normal aging and Parkinson's disease. In: Katzman R, Terry R, eds. *The Neurology of Aging.* Philadelphia, Pa: FA Davis; 1983:85–109.

44. Tomonaga M. Histochemical and ultrastructural changes in senile human muscle. *J Am Gerontol Soc.* 3:125–131, 1977.

45. Larsson B, Rentstrom P, Svardsudd K, et al. Health and aging characteristics of highly physically active 65 year old men. *Int J Sports Med.* 5:336–340, 1984.

46. Lexel J, Henriksson-Larsen K, Winblad B, et al. Distribution of different fiber types in human skeletal muscles: effects of aging studied in whole muscle cross sections. *Muscle Nerve.* 6:588–595, 1983.

47. Grimby G, Aniansson A, Zetterberg C, et al. Is there a change in relative muscle fiber composition with age? *Clin Physiol.* 4:189–194, 1984.

48. Essen GB, Borges O. Histochemical and metabolic characteristics of human skeleton muscle in relation to age. *Acta Physiol Scand.* 126:107–114, 1986.

49. Frolkis VV, Martynenko OA, Zamostayan VP. Aging of the neuromuscular apparatus. *Gerontol.* 22:244–279, 1976.

50. Baker PCH. The aging neuromuscular system. *Sem Neurology.* 9:50–59, 1989.

51. Borges O. Isometric and isokinetic knee extension and flexion torque in men and women age 20–70. *Scand J Rehab Med.* 2:45–53, 1989.

52. Larsson L. Physical training effects on muscle morphology in sedentary males at different ages. *Med Sci Sports Exerc.* 14:203–206, 1982.

53. Meredith CN, Frontera WR, Fisher EC, et al. Peripheral effects of endurance training in young and old subjects. *J Appl Physiol.* 66:2844–2849, 1989.

54. Suominen H, Heikkinen E, Parkatti T. The effect of eight weeks physical training on muscle and connective tissue of the vastus lateralis in 69 year old men and women. *J Gerontol.* 32:33–37, 1977.

55. Grimby G. Physical activities and effects of muscle training in the elderly. *Ann Clin Res.* 20:62–66, 1988.

56. Aniansson A, Grimby G, Rundgren A, Savanbrog A, et al. Physical training in old men. *Ageing.* 9:186–187, 1980.

57. Carter AB. The Neurological Aspects of Aging. In: Rossman I, ed. *Clinical Geriatrics.* Philadelphia, Pa: Lippincott; 1986:326–351.

58. Bassey EJ, Bendall MJ, Pearson M. Muscle strength in the triceps surae: an objectively measured customary walking activity in men and women over 65 years of age. *Clin Sci.* 74:85–89, 1989.

59. Pearson MB, Bassey EJ, Bendall MJ. Muscle strength and anthropometric indicies in elderly men and women. *Age-Ageing.* 14:49–54, 1985.

60. Gorman KM, Posner JD. Benefits of exercise in old age. *Clin Geriatr Med.* 4:181–192, 1988.

61. Farrar RP, Martin TP, Araies CM. The interaction of aging and endurance exercise upon the mitochondrial function of skeletal muscle. *J Gerontol.* 36:642–647, 1981.

62. Grimby G. Physical activity in muscle training in elderly. *Acta Med Scand.* 711 (suppl):233–237, 1986.

63. Engel WK. Selective and non-selective susceptibility of muscle fiber types. *Arch Neurol.* 22:97–117, 1970.

64. Sydney KH, Sheppard RJ, Harrison JE. Endurance training and body composition of the elderly. *Am J Clin Nutrition.* 30:326–333, 1977.

65. American College of Sports Medicine. *Guidelines for Graded Exercise Testing and Exercise Prescription.* Philadelphia, Pa: Lea & Febiger; 1980.

66. Landin RJ, Linnemeier TJ, Rothbaum DA, et al. Exercise testing and training of the elderly patient. In: Wenger NK, ed. *Cardiovascular Clinics, Exercise and the Heart.* Philadelphia, Pa: F.A. Davis; 1985:201–218.

67. Mahler DA, Cunningham LN, Curfman GD. Aging and exercise performance. *Clin Geriatr Med.* 2:433–452, 1986.

68. Smith EL, Gilligan C. Physical activity prescription for the older adult. *Phys Sports Med.* 11:91–101, 1983.

69. Banker BQ, Engel AG. The polymyositis and dermatomyositis syndromes. In: Engel AG, Banker BQ, eds. *Myology: Basic and Clinical.* New York, NY: McGraw Hill; 1986:1385–1422.

70. Currie S. Inflammatory myopathies. In: Walton J, ed.: *Disorders of Voluntary Muscle.* Edinburgh: Churchill Livingstone; 1981:525–567.

71. Hicks JE, Gerber LH. Rehabilitation of the patient with arthritis and connective tissue disease. In: DeLisa JA. *Rehabilitation Medicine: Principles and Practice.* Philadelphia, Pa: J. B. Lippincott; 1989:765–794.

72. Banker BQ. Other inflammatory myopathies. In: Engel AG, Banker BQ, eds. *Myology: Basic and Clinical.* New York, NY: McGraw-Hill; 1986:1501–1524.

73. Chuang T-Y, Hunder CG, Ilstrup DM, et al. Polymalgia rheumatica: a ten year epidemiologic and clinical study. *Ann Intern Med.* 97:672–680, 1982.

74. Engel AG. Myasthenia gravis. In: Engel AG, Banker BQ, eds. *Myology: Basic and Clinical.* New York, NY: McGraw-Hill; 1986:1925–1954.

75. Simpson JA. Myasthenia gravis and myasthenic syndromes. In: Walton J, ed. *Disorders of the Voluntary Muscle.* Edinburgh: Churchill-Livingstone; 1986:585–624.

76. Lambert TH, Lennon VA. Neuromuscular transmission in nude mice bearing oat cell tumors from the Lambert-Eaton myasthenic syndrome. *Muscle Nerve.* 5:S39–S45, 1982.

77. Mastaglin FL, Argov Z. Drug-induced neuromuscular disorders in man. In: Walton J, ed. *Disorders of Voluntary Muscle.* Edinburgh: Churchill Livingstone; 1981:873–906.

78. Thomas PK, Sears TA, Gilliat, RW. The range of conduction velocity in normal motor nerve fibres of the small muscles of the hand and foot. *J Neurol Neurosurg Psychiatry.* 22:175–181, 1959.

79. Tohgi H, Tsukagoshi H, Tolyokura Y. Quantitative changes with age in normal sural nerves. *Acta Neuropath [Berl].* 38:213–220, 1977.

80. Cottrell L. Histologic variations with age in apparently normal peripheral nerve trunks. *Arch Neurol Psychiatry.* 43:1138–1150, 1940.

81. Arnold N, Harriman GF. The incidence of abnormality in control human peripheral nerves studied by single axon dissection. *J Neurol Neurosurg Psychiatry.* 33:55–61, 1970.

82. Lascelles RG, Thomas PK. Changes due to age in internodal length in the sural nerve in man. *J Neurol Neurosurg Psychiatry.* 29:40–44, 1966.

83. Vizoso AD, Young JZ. Internode length and fibre diameter in developing and regenerating nerves. *J Anat [Lond].* 82:110–134, 1948.

84. Jennekens FGI, Tomlinson BE, Walton JN. Histochemical aspects of five limb muscles in old age: an autopsy study. *J Neurol Sci.* 14:259–276, 1971.

85. Morrison RL, Cobb S, Bauer W. The effect of advancing age upon the human spinal cord. Cambridge, Mass: Harvard University Press; 1959.

86. Ohnishi A, O'Brien PC, Okazaki H, et al. Morphometry of myelinated fibers of fasciculus gracilus of man. *J Neurol Sci.* 27:163–172, 1976.

87. Corbin KB, Gardner ED. Decrease in number of myelinated fibers in human spinal roots with age. *Anat Rec.* 68:63–74, 1937.

88. Hansen CC, Reske-Nielsen E. Pathological studies in presbycusis. *Arch Otolaryngol.* 82:115–132, 1965.

89. Dolman CL, McCormick AQ, Drance SM. Aging of the optic nerve. *Arch Opthalmol.* 98:2053–2058, 1980.

90. Behse F, Buchthal F. Normal sensory conduction in the nerves of the leg in man. *J Neurol Neurosurg Psychiatry.* 34:404–414, 1971.

91. Buchthal F, Rosenfalck A. Evoked action potentials and conduction velocity in human sensory nerves. *Brain Res.* 3:1–122, 1966.

92. Downie AW, Newell DJ. Sensory nerve conduction in patients with diabetes mellitus and control. *Neurology.* 11:876–882, 1961.

93. Martinez AC, Barrio M, Perec Conde MC, et al. Electrophysiological aspects of sensory conduction velocity in healthy adults. *J Neurol Neurosurg Psychiatry.* 41:1097–1101, 1978.

94. Trojaborg W. Motor and sensory conduction in the musculocutaneous nerve. *J Neurol Neurosurg Psychiatry.* 39:890–899, 1976.

95. Baer RD, Johnson E. W. Motor nerve conduction velocities in normal children. *Arch Phys Med Rehabil.* 46:698–704, 1965.

96. Gregersen G. Diabetic neuropathy: influence of age, sex, metabolic control, and duration of diabetes on motor conduction velocity. *Neurology.* 17:972–980, 1967.

97. Mayer RF. Nerve conduction studies in man. *Neurology.* 13:1021–1039, 1963.

98. Norris AH, Shock NW, Wagman IH. Age changes in the max-

imum conduction velocity of motor fibers of human ulnar nerves. *J Appl Physiol.* 5:589–593, 1953.

99. Wagman IH, Lesse H. Maximum conduction velocities of motor fibers of ulnar nerves in human subjects of various ages. *J Neurophysiol.* 15:235–244, 1952.

100. Wagner AL, Buchtal F. Motor and sensory conduction in infancy and childhood: reappraisal. *Develop Med Child Neurol.* 14:189–216, 1972.

101. Buchthal F, Rosenfalck P. Action potential parameters in different human muscles. *Acta Psychiatr Neurol Scand.* 30:125–131, 1955.

102. Sacco G, Buchthal F, Rosenfalck P. Motor unit potentials at different ages. *Arch Neurol.* 6:366–373, 1962.

103. Stalberg E, Fawcett PRW. Macro EMG in healthy subjects of different ages. *J Neurol Neurosurg Psychiatry.* 45:870–878, 1982.

104. Stalberg E, Thiele B. Motor unit fibre density in the extensor digitorum communis muscle. *J Neurol Neurosurg Psychiatry.* 38:874–880, 1975.

105. Brown WF. Functional compensation of human motor units in health and disease. *J Neurol Sci.* 20:199–209, 1973.

106. Dorfman LJ, Bosley TM. Age-related changes in peripheral and central nerve conduction in man. *Neurology.* 29:38–44, 1979.

107. Hume AL, Cant BR, Cowan JC. Central somatosensory conduction time from 10 to 79 years. *Electroenceph Clin Neurophysiol.* 54:49–54, 1982.

108. Rowe MJ. Normal variability of the brain-stem auditory evoked response in young and old adult subjects. *Electroenceph Clin Neurophysiol.* 44:459–470, 1978.

109. Allison T, Wood CC, Goff WR. Brainstem auditory, pattern-reversal visual, and short-latency somatosensory evoked potentials: latencies in relation to age, sex, and brain and body size. *Electroenceph Clin Neurophysiol.* 55:619–636, 1983.

110. Yamada O, Kodera K, Yagi T. Cochlear processes affecting wave V latency of the auditory evoked brain-stem response. *Acta Audiol.* 8:67–70, 1979.

111. Sokol S, Moskowitz A, Towle VL. Age-related changes in the latency of the visual evoked potential: influence of check size. *Electroenceph Clin Neurophysiol.* 51:559–562, 1981.

112. Shaw NA, Cant BR. Age-dependent changes in the latency of the pattern visual evoked potential. *Electroenceph Clin Neurophsyiol.* 48:237–241, 1980.

20
Disorders of Mobility, Balance, and Gait

Franz U. Steinberg

MOBILITY

Disabilities of the elderly are most frequently caused by disorders that restrict the aging persons' ability to move about at will, with ease, and without pain. These disorders may be due to abnormalities of joints and connective tissue structures or to neuromuscular lesions. Injury to bones, another frequent cause of loss of mobility, is discussed in Chapter 12.

Contractures

Connective tissue is the main constituent of tendons and ligaments. These structures are composed of strands of collagen fibers interspersed with some elastic fibers. Tendons connect muscle to bone. Within the muscle, collagen fibers are small filaments, attached to the muscle fibers. The collagen fibers merge and eventually fuse into the tendon. In the tendon, the connective tissue fibers run in parallel, which gives the tendon a marked tensile strength. Ligaments connect bone to bone. The connective tissue fibers in ligaments are not as strictly arranged in parallel as they are in tendons. They contain more elastic fibers than do tendons. Loose areolar connective tissue fills the spaces between organs. Connective tissue fibers are imbedded in an amorphous ground substance.

Range of motion is reduced when ligaments and tendons tighten and can no longer be fully extended. Joint capsules, which are composed of fairly dense connective tissue, may also contract, and this process associated with lesions of bone and cartilage may deprive a joint of mobility. When a part of the body is immobilized for a period of time, tendons and ligaments will contract, and loose areolar connective tissue may be replaced by dense scar tissue, reducing the mobility of peripheral joints and of the spine. The most common causes of the formation of dense motion-restricting tissue are immobilization, inflammation, trauma, and reduced arterial circulation.

Under normal conditions, the upright posture of the body is maintained by ligaments that restrict abnormal motions of hip and knee joints. The hip joints can be flexed anteriorly only. Extension in standing position is limited to 160 degrees to 175 degrees. Furthermore, in order to keep the hip extended without muscular activity, the line that runs from the center of gravity of head, arms, and trunk (HAT) to the supporting foot must be kept posterior to the hip joint. The knee flexes only posteriorly since anterior flexion is prevented by tendons and ligaments. Therefore, the center of gravity must be kept anterior to the knee joint. A healthy person, therefore, can maintain a standing position without muscular effort by locking hips and knees against supporting ligaments. The only muscle activity in quiet standing is alternating contractions of soleus and anterior tibial muscles, which maintain balance (1). The mechanism of maintaining stance without muscular effort is imperiled if hips or knees develop flexion contractures. This is a common occurrence in elderly persons who spend much of the day sitting and walk very little. In order to keep hips or knees from collapsing, extensor muscles must then be activated. Standing then becomes rapidly fatiguing.

Walking is made even more difficult if one or both hips have an extension deficit. As one leg moves forward, the other leg must hold the weight of the upper part of the body over the supporting foot. This requires an active contraction of the hip extensors since the center of gravity is now anterior to the hip joint. If the hip extensors are weak, other mechanisms must compensate for the inadequate muscle action. The lumbar spine must be extended as much as possible, and the knee may be flexed. Both of these mechanisms will bring the center of gravity closer to the hip, thereby reducing the need for muscular support. However, other symptoms will become apparent. The lumbar spine may be arthritic, and excessive extension may cause back pain. The knee when bearing weight in a flexed position needs to be supported by quadriceps action. The pressure of the contracting muscle, added to the pressure of weight bearing, puts a significant load on the articular structures and will cause knee pain (2). The patient may complain that his or her back and knee hurt when walking. Only a careful examination will show that the source of pain is a hip flexion contracture.

Hip flexion contractures are frequently overlooked; hip range of motion is difficult to measure because the joint is imbedded in deep layers of soft and movable tissue. Furthermore, hip range of motion defects may be masked by the simultaneous rotation of the bony pelvis. The Thomas test (flexion of the opposite hip and knee) may uncover the extension deficit. A method to measure hip range of motion has been described by Mundale et al (3).

The development of contractures can be prevented by gentle stretching exercises. Patients who have been immobilized for whatever reason are particularly vulnerable, and active or passive range of motion exercises should be used routinely unless there is a specific contraindication. As pointed out before, limbs with impaired arterial circulation are particularly susceptible to developing joint or soft tissue contractures. Once contractures have appeared, stretching by a physical therapist should be done, preferably twice a day. Caution must be observed if the contracted joint is inflamed. Stretching may be uncomfortable; if the pain lasts for several hours after therapy, the stretch has been too vigorous, and the technique will need to be revised. Tightened muscles are not as vulnerable as joints, but care must be taken that osteoporotic bones are not inadvertently fractured by overly energetic manipulations. In general, stretching may be more effective and less traumatic if a gentler prolonged stretch is used. Hip joints can be stretched by a pulley system with the patient lying prone and with the opposite hip flexed. A knee can be stretched with the patient prone and a weight applied to the leg above the ankle. Stretching of upper extremity contractures has to be done with special care. Shoulder contractures are best treated with Codman's pendulum exercises. The patient stands with the hips flexed. The arm hangs down by gravity and is gently moved in all directions. As the condition improves, the patient may be made to exercise while holding a weight in the hand. In hemiplegic patients, the shoulder of a paralyzed upper extremity must be handled with particular caution. As long as the shoulder girdle muscles are flaccid, overly energetic abduction of the arm may stretch the joint capsule and lead to a subluxation of the joint. At a later phase, the shoulder may become contracted in adduction and internal rotation. Very vigorous stretching may enhance muscle spasticity and cause chronic pain. Caldwell et al (4) recommend that, if the arm is paralyzed and if no return of motor function can be expected, the shoulder not be abducted past 45 degrees in order to avoid pain. Elbows, wrists, and hands can be splinted to avoid contractures and to provide a gentle and long-term stretch.

Bennett (5) in a classical paper entitled "Uses and Abuses of Certain Tools of Physical Medicine" warned against stretching an extremity if the segmental muscles are excessively weak or paralyzed. Bennett had been working with poliomyelitis patients, and his dictum should be remembered: "Mobility without underlying strength to support mobility may be far more dangerous than loss of mobility" (5 p1114). For instance, a contracted knee joint with little mobility can carry the body weight even if the regional muscles are paralyzed. Once the joint is stretched so that some mobility is restored, it will collapse with weight bearing.

Muscle Activity

Extremity movements depend on the simultaneous contraction of several muscles each of which has a specific function to perform. A muscle may be the prime mover or agonist. Another muscle or group of muscles may serve as synergists. The main function of a synergist is to make the movement more forceful, but it may also compensate for unwanted actions of the agonist. For instance, the musculus tibialis anterior is the prime mover for ankle dorsiflexion. However, it also inverts the ankle, and this is an unwanted component. The musculi peroneus longus and brevis are ankle evertors, and their action simultaneous with the musculus tibialis anterior makes the ankle dorsiflex in a line parallel to the axis of the leg. An antagonist muscle has a function opposite to the agonist; it may remain inactive during the contraction of the prime mover, or it may contract weakly in order to modify the force of the motion. Finally, muscles can act as stabilizers. Their contraction immobilizes the proximal section of a limb while the distal section is made to move by the agonist. As an example, the rhomboids and trapezius muscles stabilize the scapula during the flexion or rotation of the humerus. Most skeletal muscles can perform any of the four functions and serve as agonist, synergist, antagonist, or stabilizer depending on what motion is wanted. The maximal force of a muscle is directly related to its cross-sectional area where the muscle belly is the widest. From various experimental studies the absolute muscle strength is estimated as 3.6 kg/cm^2 of the cross-sectional area (6).

Muscles lose strength with aging. This loss is associated with a decrease in the size and number of muscle fibers, especially of the fast-twitch Type II fibers. The muscle enzyme activity is also diminished (7). In spite of these changes, the muscle strength can be improved by a program of therapeutic exercise; this suggests that the changes in muscle function and structure may be due to inactivity and disuse rather than to aging. A gross enlargement of muscle size with exercise was not noted originally. However, more recently, Frontera and associates (8) noted evidence of muscle hypertrophy following exercise by measuring the size of thigh muscles by magnetic resonance imaging (MRI).

Peripheral Neuropathy

Disorders of the peripheral and central nervous system are frequent causes of the decline of mobility. Peripheral neuropathy in the elderly may be due to infections, metabolic or nutritional disorders, and exposure to heavy metals or certain drugs such as vincristine. The functional impairment of peripheral nerves may also be due to nerve root lesions or an encroachment on the proximal portion of the nerve. In many cases the cause remains undetermined. Weakness is accompanied by atrophy. Sensory loss, or distortion of sensation with or without pain, is almost always associated with a motor defect.

Prognosis and medical treatment depend upon the cause. Physical therapy needs to be applied with caution. Heat treatment should be avoided if sensation is affected. Strengthening exercises may not be effective. If applied too vigorously, they can cause severe muscle fatigue or permanent overuse damage (5). In any case, exercises have to be carefully planned and executed. All too often they will strengthen the opposing normal muscles, thereby increasing the muscular imbalance. As an example, if the finger extensors are affected and weak, squeezing a rubber ball will strengthen the finger flexors and further impair the hand function.

Central Nervous System Dysfunction

The loss of mobility due to central upper motor neuron lesions is common in the elderly. Strokes are the most frequent causes, but other cerebral lesions can present the same or similar neurologic picture. Assessment and management of these disorders are difficult because of the complexity of the upper motor neuron function, which will be summarized in the subsequent paragraphs.

Movements are initiated through two mechanisms. Contractions of individual muscles arise from the large Betz cells in the motor cortex of the cerebral hemispheres, and the impulses are transmitted through the pyramidal corticospinal tracts to the spinal cord. The terminal portions of these tracts form synapses with the anterior horn cells of the spinal cord, which send nerve fibers to connect with muscle fibers. However, many corticospinal tract fibers terminate at small interneurons, and the stimuli reach the anterior horn cells only after a series of interneuron synapses. The interneurons receive impulses from other neurons; this will modify the ensuing muscular contraction. This is the basic mechanism of finely tuned skilled movements such as making a drawing or working with a sensitive instrument. These movements are under complete voluntary control. The impulse transmission from brain to muscle is slow because the corticospinal tracts can carry only a few volitional impulses at any one time. This can be demonstrated by our inability to contract voluntarily more

than three or four individual muscles at different parts of the body at the same time.

All other activities of our daily lives are performed by coordinated multimuscular movements. The only volitional aspect is the intent and the initiation of the activity. The individual movements necessary to execute the task are automatic. These activities are under the control of the extrapyramidal sensory-motor system. Most of the activities originate in the large premotor cortical area, located immediately anterior to the motor cortical centers of the cerebral hemispheres. Impulses are transmitted to the basal ganglia (putamen and caudate nucleus) and from there through the reticular formation of the brainstem to the spinal cord.

The toning down of unduly prolonged and intensive impulses is achieved by the inhibitory effect of the basal ganglia on the reticular formation and by a negative feedback to the cortical motor area. Destruction of the basal ganglia causes muscular rigidity and an inability to perform coordinated skilled movements. Another function of the basal ganglia is to achieve and control the contraction of trunk and proximal extremity muscles in preparation of skilled movements of hands or feet. In this way, the distal parts of extremities can perform skilled movements against a stabilized trunk and proximal extremity.

The cerebellum is another part of the extrapyramidal system. Through various tracts the cerebellar hemispheres receive impulses from the cerebral cortex, the basal ganglia, the brainstem, and the nuclei of the reticular formation. The cerebellum also receives impulses directly from peripheral nerves via the spinal cord, apprising it of changes in the position of the trunk and part of the extremities. Efferent impulses go from the central lobe of the cerebellum, the vermis, to different parts of the body. These impulses correct abnormal positions and help to keep the body upright and in balance. All of these functions take place on a subconscious level. Most of our everyday activities are consciously planned but are carried out automatically. This is true for such simple tasks as getting up from a chair, moving about, ascending and descending steps, getting dressed, etc. Even very complicated tasks are carried out automatically. The finger movements of playing the piano or of typing, once learned and repeated many times, become automatic.

The entire integrative process of coordinated mobility is based on the function of hundreds of neurons and hundreds of synapses; most details remain unknown, and most of the explanations are speculative. Much has been learned from animal studies, but animal brains are not good models of what takes place in the human brain. All of the automatically performed activities have been learned. Many activities are learned early in life, so early that we cannot remember when we acquired them. We can recall learning some more complicated activities such as riding a bicycle or driving an automobile. We remember our early awkward attempts, how every motion had to be painstakingly planned, and we realize how these activities have become so automatic that we no longer give them a thought.

Each movement pattern is performed by muscles that contract in a certain sequence and with a power suitable to the task. It is assumed that as activities are done over and over again the proprioceptive pattern forms an engram in the cerebral sensory cortex. When the learned activity is to be used, the engram can be retrieved from the sensory cortex, and movements will be performed in the same sequential pattern. It is assumed that activities that must be performed very rapidly are stored in the motor cortex itself and that connections are established from there to the premotor cortex, the basal ganglia, and the cerebellum. A lesion in any of these parts of the brain can destroy the person's ability to rapidly perform skilled and coordinated movements.

It is difficult to visualize how so many neuronal processes can produce the well coordinated skilled movements that we perform every day. Physiology texts have presented concepts explaining these most complicated functions. For more details these references should be consulted (9–12).

Motor and sensory functions are disrupted in various ways by lesions of the central nervous system. Injuries to the spinal cord block both stimulating and inhibitory impulses at the site of the lesion. If the injury has caused a complete disruption of the cord, no voluntary movements will be possible below the level of the lesion. But reflex muscle contractions occur, and since no inhibitory signals can be received from above, these contractions will be violent spasms. They can be so forceful that the patient is thrown out of the wheelchair. Spasms of the lower extremities are predominantly located in the extensor muscles, and patients may have great difficulties with self-care activities such as dressing and putting on socks and shoes. Positioning in bed or chair in a way that will protect the skin from breaking down may be most difficult. Therapeutic intervention may be attempted if the spasticity disrupts the patient's life-style or presents further hazards to health and safety. Effective oral medications are diazepam (Valium), baclofen (Lioresal), or dantrolene (Dantrium). All three drugs have significant side effects. All three are sedative; diazepam can be habit-forming, and dantrolene may cause an elevation of liver enzymes. In recent years the administration of baclofen by an intrathecal pump has been quite effective in cases of intractable spasticity, but reports of further experiences need to be awaited. Dilute solutions of phenol applied intrathecally or by nerve blocks have been effective in relieving excessive spasticity. It is important to realize that lower extremity spasticity can be helpful to paraplegic patients. Many patients learn to elicit extensor spasm that last long enough

to use the muscle contraction for standing transfers or for positioning themselves in bed. However, caution needs to be exercised since extensor spasticity tends to give way suddenly causing a fall. On the other hand, patients with completely flaccid lower extremities will be quite helpless. They cannot change their position in bed because their flaccid legs are dead weight.

Strokes and other Cerebral Lesions

In aged individuals, dysfunctions of the central nervous system are most frequently caused by strokes. The neurologic deficits vary considerably depending on the location of the lesion, but the most common strokes in the aged are infarcts in the motor, sensory, or premotor areas. The resulting hemiparesis is flaccid during the initial phase. This is succeeded by a second phase in which the muscles regain tone, but voluntary movements will still be difficult or impossible. Later the pattern changes to a spastic paralysis; in the upper extremity the flexor muscles are usually affected, in the lower extremity spastic paralyses of the extensors are more common. As in spinal cord lesions, the spasticity is due to the failure of inhibitory signals to be transmitted to lower centers.

Voluntary activity as it returns is usually in synergies. In the upper extremity, an effort to flex the elbow is accompanied by an external rotation of the shoulder, abduction of the shoulder up to 90 degrees, retraction of the shoulder girdle, supination of the forearm, and flexion of wrist and fingers. The common synergy of the lower extremity is extensor in type. Extension of hip or knee are accompanied by abduction and internal rotation of the hip, plantar flexion, inversion of the ankle, and plantar flexion of the toes except that the big toe might extend. Extension synergies of the upper extremity and flexion synergies of the lower extremities are rare. In the lower extremity, a flexion synergy is particularly disturbing since hip and knee are pulled into flexion as the patient attempts to put weight on the leg.

The synergies are the same whether the precipitating motion, elbow flexion of the arm or hip-knee extension of the leg, is voluntary or by reflex. These synergistic movements obviously are not part of the correct engram of elbow flexion and knee extension. They are ordinarily suppressed by the inhibitory effect of basal ganglia as described before. In strokes, the inhibitory impulses are not functioning, at least not until further recovery has taken place. In many cases the synergies remain permanent. In this case, the upper extremity will not regain a useful skilled function.

Over the last three decades, various exercise programs under the generic name of facilitation techniques have been developed, designed to improve skills by stimulating peripheral nerves or muscles (13). Knott (14) described a method called proprioceptive neuromuscular facilitation using muscle stretch, traction, and compression of joints and giving maximum resistance to the affected muscles in order to facilitate active movements. Rood (15) used sensory stimulation by brushing or stroking certain skin areas to facilitate the contraction of the underlying muscle and simultaneously inhibiting the antagonist. Bobath (16) advocated the patient's early use of the involved extremity while the therapist suppressed the spastic synergy pattern by special techniques. In contrast, Brunnstrom (17) facilitated the development of synergies in the early phases of recovery; at a later phase she taught the patient to suppress unwanted spastic synergistic components and concentrate on contracting only those muscles that would be part of the desired movement pattern.

Each of these methods has had its devoted disciples. Clinical experience has shown that no technique is superior to the others and that the facilitation techniques actually have a great deal in common (18). Stern (19) divided a group of stroke patients into two subgroups. One received conventional stroke physical therapy, the other had one of the facilitation methods added to the conventional therapy. Stern concluded that the outcome was not improved by adding facilitation to the conventional therapy. Many therapists now use facilitation techniques by incorporating them into the routine therapeutic program.

BALANCE

Vestibular System

The forces that preserve body balance allow man to maintain an upright position against gravity. The mechanisms functioning to keep our body balance under control are complex. Unfortunately, they begin to fail with advancing age, and falls become more frequent causes of morbidity and mortality.

The vestibular apparatus, the labyrinth of the inner ear, is the main site of balance control. The labyrinth contains two chambers, the utricle and the saccule, and three semicircular canals, which are arranged at ninety degree angles to each other. The utricle and the saccule perceive shifts of the position of the head, either in forward, backward, or lateral directions. The semicircular canals perceive early rotational displacements of the head.

The utricle, saccule, and semicircular canals send impulses caused by the shift of the position of the head through the vestibular nerve to the vestibular nucleus in the brainstem. From there the signals are transmitted to the cerebellum and through reticular nuclei down the spinal cord. In the cord, antigravity muscles are by reflex alternatingly stimulated or inhibited until the loss of balance has been corrected.

It is noteworthy that the utricle and saccule are stimulated only by movement of the head either forward, backward, or laterally, and they respond only to linear acceleration. The semicircular canals perceive rotation of the head when it is first initiated and transmit impulses early enough to prevent a loss of body balance. For details, physiology texts should be consulted (9).

Disorders of Balance and Falls

Disorders of body balance in the elderly are common causes of falls. They contribute greatly to the morbidity of aged individuals, and many studies have been conducted with the goal of designing preventive measures.

Chronic disorders of the vestibular system are not common in the elderly. Usually they are associated with vertigo, and inner ear deafness may be present. The diagnosis can be confirmed by the caloric test. The ear is irrigated with cold water. If the vestibular nerve is intact, nystagmus will develop to one side and past pointing by the hand of the other side. If the vestibular nerve is not functioning at all, nystagmus will not develop. Normal body posture and locomotion, in addition to labyrinthine function, depend also on visual function and proprioception. Persons with labyrinthine dysfunction walk unsteadily with uneven step length and a tendency to deviate laterally. A blind or blindfolded person can walk quite well though cautiously. A loss of proprioception due to posterior column lesions, cerebellar lesions, or combined system disease will cause marked unsteadiness especially when the patient is made to stand with the eyes closed (Romberg test). The gait will be unsteady and ataxic unless the patient is able to correct it by visual cues. Only a minority of persons with precarious body balance exhibit the distinct neurologic or sensory disorders of poor equilibrium.

There are many other possible causes for loss of balance and subsequent falls than a failure of the three basic mechanisms responsible for maintaining body equilibrium: vestibular dysfunction, visual problems, and poor proprioception. Regardless of cause, the patient will show an unstable standing balance and characteristic gait deviations.

Disorders of the static balance can be measured by determining the body sway while the individual stands still with eyes open or closed. Lord and associates (20, 21) have extensively studied the significance of increased sway and have come to important conclusions. Increased sway when standing on a firm surface was associated with poor tactile sensation and a poor joint position sense but not with abnormal vestibular function or vision. Increased body sway when standing on a compliant surface such as foam rubber with eyes open was associated with poor visual acuity since standing on an unstable surface makes the sensory input ineffective, and the individual must now rely on the eyes to maintain a steady balance. If the eyes cannot provide this compensatory mechanism, the sway is increased. An increase in reaction time and weakness of knee and ankle muscles are additional factors responsible for an abnormally increased sway. Lord's population was comprised of 95 residents of a home for the aged in Sydney, Australia. His findings should be valuable to those who do sway studies on elderly subjects.

Another study on postural sway was reported by Era and Heikkinen (22). They tested 300 men in three age groups, 31–35 years, 51–55 years, and 71–75 years of age. Sway while standing was increased with advancing age. However, the recovery of balance after having disturbed it intentionally was the same in all age groups. The functioning of the postural control system was correlated with the vibratory perception at the ankles, grip strength, and aerobic and anaerobic capacity. It is noteworthy that in the youngest age group the postural control system was poorer in those who had a great deal of occupational exposure to noise.

Many investigators have designed balance testing methods based on every day activities. Tinetti and her coworkers (23, 24) have developed a number of such tests and have used them to construct a Fall Risk Index. They observed the patient when getting up from a standard chair without using the hands and measured the time that it took to come to standing. They determined the time it took a patient to turn 360 degrees. They made patients bend down to pick an object off the floor and to reach to a high shelf. They tested them for standing on one leg for 5 seconds without losing their balance. The reaction to a light push on the sternum was observed. Gait deviations were noted and recorded.

Duncan et al (25) used individuals' functional reach to determine how far the center of gravity could be moved away from the supporting feet without losing balance. Hsieh-Ching et al (26) tested adults of different ages by having them step over obstacles. Older persons used a slower crossing speed, shorter step length, and a shorter obstacle-heel strike distance.

Impaired balance may also be due to weakness of the lower extremities. Weakness of the hip extensors, knee extensors, and ankle muscles will cause an unsteady gait pattern. Weakness of the ankle dorsiflexors causes a foot drop, and the patient will easily stumble over very minor obstacles. Weakness of the hip abductor muscles, the musculus gluteus medius, the musculus gluteus minimus, and the musculus tensor fasciae latae contributes significantly to a decrease of standing or walking balance. The distal function of these muscles is to abduct the lower extremity at the hip joint against a stabilized trunk. However, for attaining a secure balance during walking or one-legged stance, the reverse action of the hip abductors is essential. If the supporting leg is firmly planted on the ground, the abductor muscles hold the trunk securely over the supporting leg. If the hip abductors are weak, the body weight is shifted over the supporting leg in order to decrease the length of the lever arm. If the muscle weakness is extreme and if the proprioception is decreased, the patient will not be able to compensate by shifting the weight toward the supporting leg and will fall toward the unsupported side as that foot is lifted off the ground (Trendelenburg sign).

A study done with women aged 65 years and above measured muscle strength of knee extensors and hip abductors using an isokinetic dynamometer (Cybex). The results were compared with data obtained from young women. Peak torque, work, and power were significantly lower in the older women at a level of $P < 0.001$. The endurance was not diminished in the older age group. The speed of developing an effective force was assessed by measuring the work performed in the first eighth of a second. This function was also decreased in older women at $P < 0.001$ (27). These findings have important functional implications. The failure to rapidly recruit an adequate force for restoring a lost equilibrium predisposes elderly persons to falling. Slowing of the reaction time has also been noted by various investigators as a predisposing factor to serious falls. Nevitt et al (28) studied 325 community-dwelling elderly persons who had fallen once during the preceding year. Fifty-eight percent of the participants had fallen again since the original fall that had made them eligible to participate in the study. Many participants suffered very minor injuries. Only 6% had major injuries, but those who did showed a considerable slowing in the trail making and other timed tests. The subjects had been followed by telephone or mail every week for an entire year. It can be assumed, therefore, that all data obtained were up-to-date and reliable.

A recent study by Means (29) has shown that the postural balance of persons subject to falls can be appreciably improved by a rehabilitation program. Means tested a number of fallers and a corresponding number of nonfallers on an obstacle course that he had designed. This consisted of walking on a hard surface, on foam rubber, on sand, on Astroturf, and on a shag carpet. The subjects walked up and down a ramp 8 feet for 1-foot rise, 8 steps 3 inches in height, etc. One test was to approach a door, open it, step through, and close it. The subjects were tested on sitting down and rising from an armless chair. Most of the tests were timed. As expected nonfallers did better than fallers at $P < 0.0001$. The fallers were retested after a suitable rehabilitation program, and they improved in a significant number of tests.

The rehabilitation of a patient with impaired balance consists of exercises to improve coordination and muscle strength. If the patient is severely impaired, the initial exercise must be simple before the patient is made to progress to the next phase. Gait training should start with simple weight shifts when standing in parallel bars and continue to single steps. Some patients will do better if they are first taught to walk sideways. In the advanced stage, walking backward or in tandem gait will help to enhance the patient's skills. Frenkel's exercises designed to improve proprioception will be very helpful. Patients also need to be taught how to prevent the loss of balance. They should learn to pick an object off the floor by stepping close to it and supporting themselves on a solid structure with one hand. Some movements need to be carefully planned such as turning around in a full circle, while keeping both feet on the ground. Reaching for an object on a high shelf should be done cautiously, preferably by supporting oneself with one hand and without extending the neck too far. The physician or therapist should have the patient do some of these maneuvers as tests and then advise the patient how to do them correctly.

The physician should inquire about medication. Benzodiazepines, phenothiazines, barbiturates, antidepressants, and alcohol impair body balance and lead to falls. Proper shoes are important. The use of a cane or other support should be recommended if the physician believes that it will be helpful to provide good stability.

Patients who tend to lose their balance when getting up from a chair should be checked for orthostatic hypotension (see Chapter 9).

GAIT

The inability to walk deprives an aged person of independence, and it often is the beginning of a social decline. For this reason, early impairments of walking need to be assessed carefully, and corrective actions need to be initiated as soon as possible.

Normal Gait

The rhythmic alternating movements of the legs translate the body mass from one point to the other with a minimum of energy cost. The center of gravity of the body is located anterior to the second sacral segment. During walking, this center describes a smooth sinusoidal curve with an excursion of 2 inches or less. It follows a similar side-to-side curve with an excursion of 1¾ inches. If the legs were rigid poles with monoaxial hip joints, the excursions both in the up and down and in the lateral directions would be much greater and the energy cost much higher. In the normal human being, however, the hip is a three-dimensional joint, and knee, ankle, and feet contribute to keep the movements of the center of gravity to a minimum. Biomechanical research has identified six factors that are essential for keeping the center of gravity on its sinusoidal path. These six determinants of gait consist of rotation of the pelvis, pelvic tilt, knee flexion, ankle rotation, pivoting of the ankle, and lateral movements of the center of gravity (30). The six determinants take place at defined points of the gait cycle.

The gait cycle begins with the stance phase, the heel of a foot touching the ground. Heel strike is followed by the foot flat and then by the push-off of the toes, lifting the foot off the ground for the swing phase. The period from the heel strike of one foot to the heel strike of the other foot is called step length or gait cycle. Stride length is the period from the heel strike of one foot until the same heel strikes the ground again. Cadence is the number of steps taken in a given period of time. The foot is in contact with the ground for approximately 60% of the gait cycle. In ordinary walking, there is a brief period when both feet are on the ground at the same time. The length of this period of double support is variable. It is longer with slow walking and shorter with fast gait. There is no period of double support while running.

The velocity of walking varies greatly from person to person. Each person has his or her own self-selected walking speed that feels most comfortable. This free or self-selected speed for the healthy adult varies from 75m/min to 80m/min. At this speed the energy cost of walking determined per distance walked is at a minimum. At higher as well as slower speeds the energy cost is greater. (Fig. 20.1.) Anybody who has been forced to accompany a person who walks very slowly will testify that this abnormal slow gait is very tiring. The speed of walking for healthy older persons has been determined by a number of investigations. Imms and Edholm (31) have developed an equation relating age to the self-selected walking speed (v):

$$V = 1.669 - 0.1119 \times age.$$

It will serve as an approximate guide.

Even in fit elderly persons the gait pattern changes with progressing age. Murray and coworkers (32, 33) studied these changes in the 1960s with interrupted-light

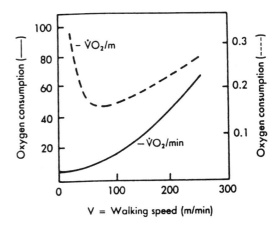

Figure 20.1. Oxygen consumption during normal walking, given in milliliters per kilogram of body weight. Left ordinate, Vo₂/min; right ordinate, Vo₂/m. Reproduced, with permission, from Levin ME, O'Neal LW, eds. *The Diabetic Foot.* 4th ed. St Louis, Mo: C.V. Mosby; 1988.

photography. Healthy young persons spend about 60% of the gait cycle in the stance and 40% in the swing phase. Murray found that as men age, more and more time of the gait cycle is given to the stance phase and less to swing. She also noted that the period of double support became longer with aging. The stride dimensions became shorter and wider. Older men also show a progressive shortening of lower limb excursions during swing phase. Steinberg et al (34) studied the hip joint excursions in elderly men without obvious gait impairments and found that the period of hip excursion was one fourth of the excursion time of younger controls. The time from hip flexion to extension was greatly prolonged in older individuals but not the time to return from hip extension to flexion.

These changes do not denote a true pathology of gait. Rather, they are compensatory mechanisms to make walking safer for the elderly when joints have become less flexible and muscles have become weaker.

These movement patterns as described serve to protect the elderly person from losing his or her balance, but they also increase the energy cost of walking. Many smaller steps are more uneconomical of energy consumption than fewer larger steps. A younger person extends the back at the beginning of stance phase in order to keep the center of gravity behind the hip joint of the supporting leg. In many elderly persons, the low back is stiff and cannot be fully extended. The person must now use the hip extensor muscles to keep the hip from collapsing into flexion and that increases the energy cost. Furthermore, a healthy person selects the speed of walking at which the energy expenditure is at a minimum. The elderly person with arthritic lower extremity joints will need to select a slower speed than the one at point of minimal energy cost. (Fig. 20.1.) Walking becomes more of an effort even though the speed is slower.

Abnormal Gait in Old Age

The gait patterns characteristic for the elderly are not truly functional disabilities. However, if they become more pronounced, they are increasingly disabling.

Most older persons walk with a shorter and wider stride. As time goes on the steps may become shorter and shorter, and the progress from one place to the next becomes less and less efficient. This senile gait has been described many times. It was first noted by Pétren who called it "Marche à petit pas." The patient walks with the head forward, the upper dorsal spine flexed, the lumbar spine flattened. Hips and knees no longer become fully extended. The steps are small, and the feet shuffle on the ground. This is accompanied by gross rowing movements of the arms. When the patient needs to turn or encounters a true or imagined obstacle, such as a change in the color of the floor covering, the steps become even smaller, and the movements become inef-

fectual. He or she gropes for support and does not do well with cane or walker.

Several observers have associated this gait with a normal pressure hydrocephalus. Accompanying symptoms are dementia and urinary incontinence (35). Some patients have been improved by shunting the hydrocephalic ventricles. But shunting has not been a panacea. Physical therapy may give some help if the patient is well motivated. This should consist of coordination exercises and gait training. Walking is an automatic activity. Patients often do better when left to use their small-step automatic gait. When asked to put one foot in front of the other, they usually become flustered and are unable to follow through. Parkinson's disease shows a similar small-step gait. However, the arms are usually held rigid on the sides. A patient with Parkinson's disease has a tendency to accelerate the gait and at times will not be able to stop until running into a wall. The diagnosis is made by neurologic examination. The muscles are rigid, and a typical tremor will be present.

With cerebellar lesions, the gait is broad-based and staggering if both hemispheres are involved. In unilateral cerebellar lesions, the patient may stagger to the affected side. The trunk may also bend to the affected side. Other cerebellar signs such as ataxia and past-pointing will usually be present.

Apraxia of gait may be due to frontal or parietal lobe lesions. Sensory abnormalities may be present as well. The volitional movements to initiate gait are impaired. The patient may stand for a long time, unable to move. Eventually he or she may walk quite well with a shuffling gait until a real or imaginary obstacle forces him or her to stop again. Other volitional leg movements such as tapping the toe or heel, will also be impaired. Abstract movements such as kicking an imaginary ball will be impossible, while there may be no difficulty kicking a real ball. This condition has been investigated and described by Meyer and Barron (36).

Gait disorders caused by strokes are of course quite common. Symptoms and signs depend on the location of the lesion. Most frequently, the flexor muscles are weak or paralyzed while the extensors recover earlier and may become spastic. The typical hemiplegic gait shows a circumduction of the leg for clearing the ground. The heel-to-toe pattern during stance phase is absent, and the entire foot is set down all at once. A steppage gait may compensate for an absent or weak ankle dorsiflexion.

The neurologic deficits in strokes are very variable, and a careful assessment needs to precede the rehabilitation program. Contractures of the external rotator muscles of the hip are fairly common. They can be prevented by proper positioning of the patient during the acute early phase. Contractures of the heel cord are a frequent complication especially if the plantar flexors of the ankle are spastic. Suitable physical therapy applied early can do much to prevent these complications. In addition to exercises, an ankle brace might help to correct the contracture. In some cases, surgical correction may have to be done at a later date.

Whether or not a stroke patient will be able to walk cannot be predicted from a neurologic examination alone. It may not be possible to elicit a voluntary motion of the affected leg, yet in a functional weight-bearing position sufficient antigravity muscle activity may be recruited by reflex action to support the body weight on the affected leg. In order to assess a patient's ability to walk, he or she must be placed into a standing position in parallel bars. The ankle muscles are usually the last to recover function. A below-knee brace will substitute for active function. If the dorsiflexors of the ankle are the only weak muscles and the plantar flexors are not spastic, a lightweight plastic brace might suffice. Weak knee extensor action can be supplemented by a metal brace with double upright bars and the ankle locked in 10 degrees of plantar flexion (37). Above-knee braces are not useful in strokes.

Musculoskeletal impairments are frequent impediments to walking. Arthritic changes of the hip joints can be exquisitely painful. An obese patient must lose weight to obtain relief. Denham (38) has shown that the loss of 1 pound of weight reduces the pressure on the hip joint by 3 pounds. Blount (39) has shown that the use of a cane in the opposite hand will relieve the pressure on the diseased hip joint by as much as 60 pounds. His ingenious calculations can be reviewed in Blount's paper entitled "Don't Throw Away the Cane." The shortening of one leg, often the complication of femoral neck or shaft fracture, can cause back pain and affect the other leg. Walking on a shortened leg causes flexion of the lumbar spine to that side. This in turn will place the vertebral facet joints into a weight-bearing position and subject them to trauma and arthritic changes. A flexion contracture of the knee will effect an unduly high pressure on the joint with resulting painful degenerative changes.

Finally, infections, circulatory deficits, or any other lesions of the feet will cause an abnormal gait and often painful limp. The older the patient, the more causes of gait abnormalities will have to be considered; a thorough diagnostic exploration will be mandatory to keep the patient walking and independent.

References

1. Kottke FJ. Therapeutic exercise to maintain mobility. In: Kottke FJ, Lehmann JF, eds. *Krusen's Handbook of Physical Medicine and Rehabilitation.* 4th ed. Philadelphia, Pa: W.B. Saunders; 1990:440.
2. Perry JJ. Normal and pathologic gait. In: *Atlas of Orthotics.* 2nd ed. St. Louis, Mo: C.V. Mosby; 1985:91–92.
3. Mundale MO, Hislop HJ, Rabideau RJ, Kottke FJ. Evaluation of extension of the hip. *Arch Phys Med.* 37:75–80, 1956.
4. Caldwell CB, Wilson DJ, Brown RM. Evaluation and treatment of the upper extremity in the hemiplegic stroke patient. *Clin Orthop.* 63:69–93, 1969.
5. Bennett RL. Use and abuse of certain tools of physical medicine. *Arch Phys Med Rehab.* 41:485–496, 1960.
6. De Lateur BJ, Lehmann JF. Therapeutic exercise to develop strength and endurance. In: Kottke FJ, Lehmann JF, eds. *Krusen's Handbook of Physical Medicine and Rehabilitation.* 4th ed. Philadelphia, Pa: W.B. Saunders; 1990:484.
7. Larsson L, Sjodin B, Karlsson J. Histochemical and biochemical changes in human skeletal muscle with age in sedentary males, age 22–65 years. *Acta Physiol Scand.* 103:31–39, 1978.
8. Frontera WR, Meredith CN, O'Reilly KP, et al. Strength conditioning in older men: skeletal muscle hypertrophy and improved function. *J Appl Physiol.* 64:1038–1044, 1988.
9. Guyton AC. The central nervous system. In: *Human Physiology and Mechanisms of Disease.* Philadelphia, Pa: W.B. Saunders; 1987:400–414.
10. Kottke FJ. Neurophysiologic therapy for stroke. In: Licht S, ed. *Stroke and Its Rehabilitation.* Baltimore, Md: Waverly Press; 1975.
11. Kottke FJ. From reflex to skill: the training of coordination. *Arch Phys Med Rehabil.* 61:551–561, 1980.
12. Kottke FJ. Therapeutic exercise to develop neuromuscular coordination. In: Kottke FJ, Lehmann JF, eds. *Krusen's Handbook of Physical Medicine and Rehabilitation.* 4th ed. Philadelphia, Pa: W.B. Saunders; 1990, 452–479.
13. Harris FA. Facilitation techniques and technological adjuncts in therapeutic exercise. In: Basmajian JV, ed. 4th ed. *Therapeutic Exercise.* Baltimore, Md: Williams & Wilkins; 1984, 110–178.
14. Knott M, Voss DE. *Proprioceptive Neuromuscular Facilitation.* 2nd ed. New York, NY: Harper & Row; 1968.
15. Stockmeyer SA. An interpretation of the approach of Rood to the treatment of neuromuscular dysfunction. *Am J Phys Med.* 46:900–956, 1967.
16. Bobath B. *Adult Hemiplegia: Evaluation and Treatment.* 2nd ed. London: William Heinemann Medical Books, Ltd; 1978.
17. Brunnstrom S. *Movement Therapy in Hemiplegia: A Neurological Approach.* New York, NY: Harper & Row; 1970.
18. Flanagan EM. Methods of facilitation and inhibition of motor activity. *Am J Phys Med.* 46:1006–1011, 1967.
19. Stern PH, McDowell F, Miller JM, et al. The effects of facilitation exercise techniques in stroke rehabilitation. *Arch Phys Med Rehabil.* 51:526–531, 1970.
20. Lord SR, Clark RD, Webster IW. Postural stability and associated physiological factors in a population of aged persons. *J Gerontol.* 46:M69–76, 1991.
21. Lord SR, Clark RD, Webster IW. Physiological factors associated with falls in an elderly population. *J Am Geriatr Soc.* 39:1194–1200, 1991.
22. Era P, Heikkinen E. Postural sway during standing and unexpected disturbance of balance in random samples of men of different ages. *J Gerontol.* 40:287–295, 1985.
23. Tinetti ME, Williams TF, Mayewski R. Fall risk index for elderly patients based on a number of chronic disabilities. *Am J Med.* 80:429–434, 1986.
24. Tinetti ME. Performance-oriented assessment of mobility problems in elderly patients. *J Am Geriatr Soc.* 34:119–126, 1986.
25. Duncan PW, Weiner DK, Chandler J, Studenski S. Functional reach: a new clinical measure of balance. *J Gerontol.* 45:M192–197, 1990.
26. Hsieh-Ching Chen, Ashton-Miller JA, Alexander NB, Schultz AB. Stepping over obstacles: gait patterns of healthy young and old adults. *J Gerontol.* 46:M196–203, 1991.
27. Steinberg FU, Schuessler P. Weakness of lower extremity muscles in the elderly: functional implications. American Geriatrics Society, Annual Meeting; Final Program; 1986; Chicago, Ill: S 38. Abstract.
28. Nevitt MC, Cummings SR, Hudes ES. Risk factors for injurious

falls: a prospective study. *J Gerontol.* 46:M164–170, 1991.

29. Means KM. Functional obstacle course performance in elderly subjects; a pilot study. Official Program, American Academy of Physical Medicine and Rehabilitation; 1992:160. Abstract.

30. Ragnarsson KT. In: DeLisa; ed. *Rehabilitation Medicine.* New York, NY: J.B. Lippincott; 1988:312–313.

31. Imms FJ, Edholm OG. Studies of gait and mobility in the elderly. *Age Ageing.* 10:147–156, 1981.

32. Murray MP, Kory RC, Clarkson BH. Walking patterns in healthy old men. *J Gerontol.* 24:169–178, 1969.

33. Murray MP, Kory RC, Sepic SB. Walking patterns of normal women. *Arch Phys Med Rehabil.* 51:637–650, 1970.

34. Steinberg FU, Roettger RF, Baker KE. Gait abnormality of old age: decrease of active hip motion. *Arch Phys Med Rehabil.* 59:538, 1978. Abstract.

35. Messert B, Wannamaker BB. Reappraisal of the adult occult hydrocephalus syndrome. *Neurology.* 24:224–231, 1974.

36. Meyer JS, Barron DW. Apraxia of gait: a clinico-physiological study. *Brain.* 83 II:261–284, 1960.

37. Lehmann JF. Biomechanics of ankle-foot orthoses: prescription and design. *Arch Phys Med Rehabil.* 60:200–207, 1979.

38. Denham RA. Hip mechanics. *J Bone Joint Surg.* 41-B:550–557, 1959.

39. Blount WP. Don't throw away the cane. *J Bone Joint Surg.* 38-A:695–708, 1956.

21

Heart Disease and Cardiac Rehabilitation in the Elderly Patient

J. Michael Anderson

SCOPE OF THE PROBLEM

Cardiovascular disease remains the number one killer in America. In 1987, heart and blood pressure diseases killed nearly one million Americans, almost as many as cancer, accidents, pneumonia, influenza, and all other causes of death combined. Almost one in two Americans will die of cardiovascular disease. More than one in four Americans currently suffer from some form of cardiovascular disease (1). Morphologic classification of 1000 consecutive autopsy cases studying heart disease in the aged revealed the prevalence of heart diseases to be 65.7%, with an incidence of 1.02 heart diseases per heart and 1.6 heart diseases per diseased heart (2) (Table 21.1).

AGING HEART AND HEART DISEASE

Basic principles governing the evaluation and treatment of older persons with heart disease are often overlooked. Older individuals who present with congestive heart failure and tachycardia are usually given a diagnosis of atherosclerotic heart disease unless a predisposing history of another form of cardiac pathology had been established earlier in life. This is despite the precept that there is no cardiac condition peculiar to older persons and none from which they are exempt. Basic principles that should govern evaluation and treatment of older persons with heart disease include: (a) the differential diagnostic possibilities should not be limited by the age factor; (b) as in other areas of medicine, age may modify the individual's response to disease; (c) nonetheless, age is only one consideration in developing an optimal therapeutic regimen, which should be individualized in every case; and (d) the elderly patients with a cardiac problem and their physicians must set and accept realistic goals as to what can be accomplished in the management of that problem (3).

Heart diseases in the aged can be thought of as falling into two main groups. The first group of diseases occurs specifically in the elderly and is summarized as degenerative heart diseases, including specific forms of valvular diseases and conduction disturbances that are associated with degeneration of the myocardium and connective tissues of the heart. The second group of heart diseases have continued from younger age (Table 21.2).

STRUCTURAL, ANATOMIC, AND FUNCTIONAL CHANGES WITH AGING

Many studies of the aging cardiovascular system are tainted by the inclusion of an unintentional bias: a failure to exclude patients with cardiovascular disease from the study population. Often when a disease-free older population is studied, changes traditionally attributed to aging, rather than to disease processes, are challenged. The exclusion of diseased individuals from studies of the elderly is difficult, particularly as the disease process may be totally asymptomatic. This is particularly true with

Table 21.1. Incidence of Heart Diseases in the Aged (in 1,000 cases)[a]

Type	Number of Cases
Normal	343
Coronary sclerosis	428
Myocardial infarction	137
Hypertrophy	237
Valvular heart disease	120
Conduction disturbance	96
Cor pulmonale	41
Pericarditis	39
Congenital heart disease	28
Aortic rupture	11
Others	22
Heart diseases	1,022
Diseased heart	657
Heart diseases per one heart	1.6

[a]From Sugiuva M, Hiraoka K, Ohkawa S, Shimoda H. A clinicopathological study on the heart diseases in the aged: the morphological classification of the 1,000 consecutive autopsy cases. *Jpn Heart J.* 16(5):528, 1975.

Table 21.2. Heart Diseases in Old Age[a]

Heart diseases from younger age
  Congenital heart disease
  Hypertensive heart disease
  Ischemic heart disease
  Rheumatic valvular disease
  Syphilitic aortic regurgitation
  Mitral regurgitation
    Papillary muscle dysfunction
    Ruptured chordae tendineae (due to endocarditis)
  Cor pulmonale
  Conduction disturbance (inflammatory, ischemic)
Heart diseases specific for aged
  Mitral regurgitation
    Ring calcification
    Ring dilatation
    Ruptured chordae tendineae (due to degeneration)
    Nodular sclerosis
  Calcified aortic stenosis
  Degenerative aortic regurgitation
  Conduction disturbance (chronic)

[a]From Sugiuva M, Hiraoka K, Ohkawa S, Shimoda H. A clinicopathological study on the heart diseases in the aged: the morphological classification of the 1,000 consecutive autopsy cases. *Jpn Heart J.* 16(5):535, 1975.

ischemic heart disease in the elderly, which is present in approximately 50% of those over 60 years of age dying from other causes. Not only is it difficult to dissociate cardiovascular disease from aging, but it is also hard to sort out age-determined manifestations of cardiovascular disease, age-related progression of disease processes, and the influence of the aging cardiac substrate upon which disease may be superimposed (4).

Morphologically, unless there is an underlying etiologic factor responsible for heart disease, the heart of the older person will remain normal or decrease in size in association with body size. The heart tends to reduce in mass relatively less than other anatomic structures with aging. The endocardium diffusely thickens with age, primarily with increases in fibrosis and collagen fibers, a process which is more pronounced in the left ventricle and atrium. The heart valves also become more fibrotic with age, thickening and increasing in rigidity. The mitral and aortic valves are typically more involved than are the tricuspid and pulmonic valves. Calcium depositions in the valve leaflets and cusps are sometimes more marked at the annulus, and they can produce rings in the mitral and/or the aortic valves. As a rule these morphologic changes are not severe enough to produce significant hemodynamic changes, although occasionally significant aortic stenosis or aortic or mitral insufficiency can occur, predisposing the patient to other sequellae, including cerebral vascular accidents, left atrial enlargement, and secondary atrial fibrillation.

Arterial walls develop increased intrinsic stiffness with age, reflecting an increase of the connective tissue components with aging. There is also an age-associated dilation of the aorta. These two changes tend to offset

each other so that the increased vascular load on the ventricle associated with the stiffer, more resistant structure is lessened by the larger inner dimension of the aorta, which needs less change in diameter to accommodate the stroke volume.

The most important facets of cardiovascular aging have been summarized as follows (4):

1. After neonatal development, the number of myocardial cells in the heart does not increase.
2. Left ventricular myocardial hypertrophy occurs in response to increased arterial vascular stiffness and dropout of myocytes.
3. When myocardial hypertrophy occurs, it is out of proportion to capillary and vascular growth.
4. The ability of the myocardium to generate tension is well maintained.
5. There is a selective decrease in beta-adrenoceptor-mediated inotropic, chronotropic, and vasodilating cardiovascular responses with aging.
6. Increased pericardial and myocardial stiffness and delayed relaxation during aging may limit left ventricular filling during stress.

Other minor physiologic changes in cardiovascular function are fairly widespread. Although the mean heart rate may fall little with age, the inherent rhythmicity of the sinoatrial node will change and increasing irregularities in cardiac rhythm develop with exercise and activity (5, 6). These changes are associated with fibrosis of branching portions of the atrioventricular (AV) bundle and the bilateral bundle branches associated with degeneration of the central fibrous body and fibrosis of the summit of the ventricular septum. Changes in vasomotor tone and vagal tone are also responsible for some of these manifestations.

RESPONSE OF THE CARDIOVASCULAR SYSTEM TO EXERCISE AND ACTIVITY

The maximum heart rate during exercise declines with age (Table 21.3). Peripheral vascular resistance increases in older people, primarily associated with increased atherosclerosis and a more rigid arterial system. Systolic blood pressure is usually increased more than diastolic pressure. These changes in blood pressure and heart rate in response to exercise tend to offset each other such that the calculated cardiac work does not reflect an age effect on workload of the heart. A decline in cardiac output appears to occur with age and is believed primarily to be due to a reduction in stroke volume. The cardiac index may decrease by 0.8% per year with aging. Older subjects have greater difficulty increasing cardiac output during maximal exertion as well. The left ventricular ejection fraction at peak exercise is lower in older individuals, and the magnitude of change

Table 21.3. Maximum Heart Rate Predicted by Age and Conditioning[a]

Age (years)	20	25	30	35	40	45	50	55	60	65	70	75	80	85	90
Unconditioned	197	195	193	191	189	187	184	182	180	178	176	174	172	170	168
90%	177	175	173	172	170	168	166	164	162	160	158	157	155	153	155
75%	148	146	144	143	142	140	128	137	135	134	132	131	129	128	126
60%	118	117	115	114	113	112	110	109	108	107	106	104	103	102	101
Conditioned	190	188	186	184	182	180	177	175	173	171	169	167	165	163	161
90%	171	169	167	166	164	162	159	158	156	154	152	150	149	147	145
75%	143	141	140	138	137	135	133	131	130	128	127	125	124	122	121
60%	114	113	112	110	109	108	106	105	104	103	101	100	99	98	97

[a]From American College of Sports Medicine. *Guidelines for Exercise Testing and Prescription.* 3rd ed. Philadelphia, Pa: Lea & Febiger; 1986: 170.

from resting values to exercise value is inversely related to age (7). Unlike in younger people where higher filling pressures indicate lower cardiac output, in "normal" older people the higher filling pressures are associated with higher cardiac output. This is believed to be primarily due to stiffness of the myocardium, which is usually seen in the elderly and is supported by demonstration of pressure patterns on cardiac catherization that resemble those of cardiac constriction.

Most of the age-related changes in the myocardial function appear relatively small when compared to the decline in oxygen consumption. Cardiovascular rehabilitation of the aged patient is based upon the capability of the aging heart to increase its output and its systolic pressures and its capability for hypertrophy (6), as well as for improving function in both the neuromuscular and musculoskeletal systems.

Physicians working with the cardiovascular systems of older individuals must always recall that the normal physiologic changes in the cardiovascular system with aging frequently impair the patient's ability to make the prompt and sudden adjustments necessary to maintain cardiac output at all times and under all conditions. The aged individual is more vulnerable to development of transitory episodes of heart failure, as well as syncope and falls that may result from a sudden discrepancy between cardiac output and that necessary to maintain adequate cerebral flow (7). An individual's capacity for exercise depends upon a number of physiologic factors, which, after the age of 65 years, may play a more important role in a person's ability to interact to the environment than does the chronologic age (8). There is a general reduction in physiologic function in man with a functional decline in capacity at a rate of about 0.75% per year after 30 years. This loss will vary from individual to individual and from organ to organ within an individual. Work capacity and capability of performing exercise or activity clearly follows this general trend. Various contributing factors include decline in muscular strength and muscle mass; decrease in the basal metabolic rate; generalized dehydration, with decreased water in individual cells; increase in body fat; cardiovascular

system changes (as described above); decrease in respiratory function, including reduction in vital capacity with concomitant increase in residual lung volume; changes within the nervous system, including reduction in the number of cells within the central nervous system and alterations in peripheral nerve function, with slowed nerve conduction velocity; and finally, alterations in the skeletal system, including loss of bone density and joint changes generally attributed to osteoarthritis (8). A sedentary life-style may be a contributing factor.

Aging in the skeletal muscle results in functional denervation due to changes in the neuromuscular junction. The distinct fiber types present in muscle mass of younger individuals tend to develop into a more homogeneous fiber composition in the elderly, with an increased loss in the fast twitch type 2 fibers. This results in approximately 50% reduction in senile muscle masses compared with normal adult muscle. Some age-mediated changes in oxidative metabolism are also manifest at old age. Functionally, advancing age is accompanied by a loss of strength, both isometric and dynamic, to a greater degree than in the loss of speed or motion. The ability to continue specific tasks decreases, but the relative work capacity does not appear to significantly change (9). Histologic and morphologic changes also occur in cartilage, ligament, and tendon, which result in decreased flexibility occurring with advancing age. The latter changes appear to be more closely related to concomitant degenerative diseases rather than to the biologic aging process itself (10).

PRESCRIBING EXERCISE FOR THE ELDERLY PATIENT

The multiple changes in the cardiovascular, respiratory, musculoskeletal, and central and peripheral nervous systems, as well as other adverse changes brought on by coexisting disease processes, must all be considered when developing physical activity and exercise programs for the elderly. Relatively few articles are written about physical conditioning in the aging adult. These articles generally recommend application of exercise guidelines, similar in terms of both frequency and duration, to those employed with younger individuals. Recommendations include appropriate warmup and cool-down exercises, each varying from 5 to 15 minutes in duration, with an interposed dynamic phase of exercise of aerobic activity, which is individually prescribed to fit the capabilities of each individual patient (11–18). The American College of Sports Medicine's guidelines recommend exercise testing in elderly individuals with two or more risk factors, with symptoms, or with known

cardiac disease (Table 21.4) (14). Although maximal testing is not uniformly recommended for elderly individuals, a low-level exercise test or submaximal test is often used for the purpose of functional assessment and exercise prescription (13).

There is a general consensus as to the intensity, frequency, and duration of exercise activity in both healthy adults and cardiac patients (Table 21.5). Elderly cardiac patients participating in exercise therapy have essentially the same safety in performing exercise activity as do the

Table 21.4.   Guidelines for Exercise Testing and Participation[a]

	Apparently Healthy		Higher Risk[b]		
	Younger ≤40 years (men) ≤50 years (women)	Older	No symptoms	Symptoms	With Disease[c]
Medical exam and diagnostic exercise test recommended prior to:					
Moderate exercise[d]	No[f]	No	No	Yes	Yes
Vigorous exercise[e]	No	Yes[g]	Yes	Yes	Yes
Physician supervision recommended during exercise test:					
Sub-maximal testing	No	No	No	Yes	Yes
Maximal testing	No	Yes	Yes	Yes	Yes

[a]From American College of Sports Medicine. *Guidelines for Exercise Testing and Prescription.* 4th ed. Philadelphia, Pa: Lea & Febiger; 1991.
[b]Persons with two or more risk factors or symptoms.
[c]Persons with known cardiac, pulmonary, or metabolic disease.
[d]Moderate exercise (exercise intensity 40 to 60% $\dot{V}O_2$max)—Exercise intensity well within the individual's current capacity and can be comfortably sustained for a prolonged period of time, i.e., 60 minutes, slow progression, and generally non-competitive.
[e]Vigorous exercise (exercise intensity > 60% $\dot{V}O_2$max)—Exercise intense enough to represent a substantial challenge and which would ordinarily result in fatigue within 20 minutes.
[f]The "no" responses in this table mean that an item is "not necessary". The "no" response does not mean that the item should not be done.
[g]A "yes" response means that an item is recommended.

Table 21.5.   Guidelines for Exercise Prescription for Healthy Adults and Cardiac Patients[a]

	Frequency	Intensity	Duration	Mode
Healthy adult	3–5 times/wk	60%–80% $\dot{V}O_2$	15–60 min	Aerobic activities, weights, games
Angina	3–5 times/wk	70%–85% anginal threshold	15–60 min	Walk, jog, bike
MI/CABG[b]				
Phase I	2–3 times/d	HR rest—20	5–20 min	Range of motion, ambulation stairs
Phase II	3–4 times/d	HR rest—20 or 50%–70% $\dot{V}O_2$	15–60 min 30–60 min	Range of motion, walk, Range of motion, walk, bike, arm ergometry
Phase III	3–4 times/wk	50%–80% $\dot{V}O_2$	30–60 min	Range of motion, walk, jog, bike, swim, games, weights
PTCA[b]	Same as Phase III			
Transplants (outpatients)	3–4 times/wk	RPE[b] 12–14	15–60 min	Range of motion, walk, bike, arm ergometry
Fixed HR[b] pacemaker	3–4 times/wk	60–80T systolic blood pressure range	15–60 min	Walk, jog, bike, swim, games

[a]From Ward A, Malloy P, Rippe J. Exercise prescription guidelines for normal and cardiac populations. *Cardiol Clin.* 5(2):204.
[b]MI/CABG = myocardial infarction/coronary artery bypass grafting; PTCA = percutaneous transluminal coronary angioplasty; HR = heart rate; RPE = rate perceived exertion.

younger patients. Additionally, attendance ratio is slightly higher in the elderly patients (17).

Guidelines for the exercise prescription in elderly cardiac patients call for lower training intensities than those utilized in younger patients. This is necessitated by the decreased functional capacity noted on exercise testing. The lower functional capacity has been attributed to multiple factors, including an increasingly sedentary life-style, associated medical problems, and superimposed musculoskeletal and neuromuscular problems.

Intensity of exercise prescription has often been based upon estimated peak oxygen uptake values or measured maximal heart rates (MHR). Most facilities do not have the capability to measure oxygen uptake directly, and estimates of oxygen uptake have not been well corroborated in elderly patients. Estimates of O_2 uptake are usually based upon the MHR results obtained from exercise tests; hence, direct use of MHR values to prescribe exercise intensity appears appropriate.

EXERCISE TESTING OF THE ELDERLY CARDIAC PATIENT

The exercise tests performed in the elderly cardiac population are not diagnostic, but rather are performed to establish appropriate parameters for exercise prescription. Because of this, every effort should be made to ensure that the conditions for the exercise test simulate as closely as possible the conditions that will be experienced during the actual participation in the exercise portion of the cardiac rehabilitation program (CRP). Unlike diagnostic exercise tests where cardiac medications usually are withheld so as to reduce the likelihood of having false positive or negative tests, the patients should be asked to continue all of their usual medications. Additionally, it is helpful to perform the test in a time frame that most closely coincides with the proposed time for exercise so that the effects of medication on the heart rate, blood pressure, and electrocardiographic and symptom responses will be as closely simulated as possible. This will result in more accurate prescription and a reduced likelihood of encountering difficulties that could ensue if a patient was tested during the time medication was having a peak or trough effect. Significant exercise alterations in heart rate response, hemodynamic alterations, electrocardiographic changes, or other untoward responses to activity, such as occurrence of angina or other cardiovascular symptoms, should be maximally reduced by following this procedure.

The type of exercise activity to be performed by the patient should be considered when selecting an exercise test protocol. The patient often experiences significantly higher heart rates using an upper extremity ergometer or stationary cycle. Musculoskeletal, peripheral vascular, pulmonary, or neuromuscular conditions often preclude exercising to peak heart rate values. The elderly patient may be more functionally limited by musculoskeletal or neurovascular deficits than by cardiovascular dysfunction. It is therefore helpful to test individuals upon the equipment and with the exercises with which they will be trained. CRPs should be familiar with and utilize protocols for testing using exercise equipment in addition to the usual, standard treadmill tests.

Graded exercise testing in the patient over 65 years of age does not appear to have an increased rate of medical complications (19, 20). As a rule, exercise testing during the first 3 to 6 weeks postmyocardial infarction (MI) utilizes a submaximal test (21). Subjective maximal exercise testing can be safely performed after this time and typically shows a relatively low aerobic work capacity, averaging about 3 metabolic equivalents; maximal heart rates are significantly reduced below those normally predicted for age, and a relatively lower increase in the pressure-rate product from rest to maximal exercise is achieved. In addition to exercise prescription, the exercise test is also helpful in identifying major risk groups (22), one of which is the presence of associated ventricular dysrhythmias. Some early studies showed that occurrence of an acute MI after age 70 years was associated with considerably higher long-term mortality than is found in younger patients. Other studies suggest, however, that exercise testing does result in effective long-term risk stratification in the older patients, with survival in low risk elderly patients comparable to that found in 50 to 59-year-old postinfarction patients. The presence of ventricular dysrhythmias resulted in marked diminution of life expectancy as compared with the nondysrhythmia group (23).

SPECIAL CONSIDERATIONS IN EXERCISE PRESCRIPTION WITH THE ELDERLY

Use of Beta-Blocking Medications

A dose-related relationship exists between the amount of beta-blocking medication and the resulting reduction in heart rate (24). The beta-blockers depress the heart rate response both at rest and during exercise. Despite this, the method of calculating exercise prescription based upon heart rate response remains the same whether or not the patient is utilizing a beta-blocker. Although the heart rate response is lower in individuals using these medications, the rate perceived exertion (RPE) and VO_2max are similar to those in individuals not using this medication.

Simultaneous use of the heart rate response and RPE are helpful parameters for exercise prescription in elderly patients using varying dosages of beta-blocking medication. Once the patient has mastered RPE monitoring, it is particularly useful to adjust exercise prescriptions in the elderly patients whose dosages of beta-blockers have been altered. During the period of medication adjustment, the patients should exercise to their assigned RPE rather than to the target heart rate. Once the dosage of the beta-blocking agent has been stabilized, the heart rate response at the RPE level assigned is usually an excellent reflection of the new target heart rate. This technique often precludes the necessity of performing a repeat exercise test in order to reestablish appropriate target heart rate values. These values can be corroborated at subsequent followup exercise tests performed for reestablishing the accuracy of the prescription, as well as for monitoring progress in improved functional capacity, according to protocols established by the CRP.

The Patient with Angina

For those patients who experience angina prior to reaching their maximal capacity, a heart rate response of 5 to 10 beats per minute below angina threshold is an appropriate upper limit target heart rate (23).

Aerobic training reduces the resting heart rate and double product of heart rate times systolic blood pressure at any given level of submaximal exercise (25) and has the effect of raising the angina threshold (26). Nitrates are useful for their vasodilatory effects on the general vasculature, as well as on the larger coronary arteries themselves. Occasionally, intermediate or long-acting oral nitrates may be indicated prior to initiation of exercise activity to enable the patient to exercise to a higher level (27). This procedure should not be performed unless the patient has first been thoroughly evaluated with continuous electrocardiographic (ECG) monitoring and frequent blood pressure and pulse determinations to ensure that no untoward hemodynamic or electrographic abnormalities are noted with the higher level of exercises, which can occur prior to onset of angina after use of the medication. The risk of the hypotension and syncope associated with the medication, with the increased potential risk of falling, is also a significant concern in the elderly population. Nonetheless, in some elderly patients with a very low tolerance to work activity because of early onset of angina, this strategy has proven effective in allowing participation in an exercise program and has resulted in significant improvement in function with a resulting rise in the angina threshold, thereby permitting them to be much more functional in their normal activities.

Patients found to have silent myocardial ischemia, manifested by horizontal ST segment depression of greater than 1 mm or upsloping ST segment depression of greater than 2 mm, should also be provided with an upper limit of the target heart rate response of 5 to 10 beats below the threshold level.

Cardiomyopathy

A small number of patients with various forms of cardiomyopathy may be referred to a cardiac rehabilitation program. These patients are typically exercised at significantly lower levels, with the initial intensity prescribed being 60% to 65% of that safely achieved on the graded exercise test. Although studies on patients with cardiomyopathy who have engaged in regular exercise programs are not available, anecdotal experiences reveal that these patients do benefit significantly, with increasing functional capacity resulting from their participation in a CRP.

Transient appearance of Q waves may occur during exercise in patients with hypertrophic cardiomyopathy. These Q waves appear related to anomalous activation of the septum, as the hypertrophic myocardium of the interventricular septum may have electrophysiologic properties different from those of normal myocardium. This does not appear to be a rate-dependent change. These noninfarctional Q waves may be more commonly seen in the resting electrocardiograms of patients with hypertensive cardiomyopathy (28).

Pacemakers and Exercise

In a group of patients over age 65 years with complete heart block, significant differences appeared to exist between these elderly patients who were paced with ventricular demand pacing (VVI) as compared with physiologic stimulation (DDD) pacemakers. There was an overall improvement in work capacity of both groups of paced individuals as compared with their functional capacity prior to insertion of pacemakers. There was a further small difference in exercise tolerance between the two groups, with those patients provided with physiologic stimulation having small but statistically significant greater increases in cumulative load and total exercise time, as well as increase in oxygen consumption (29).

Recent changes in the rate adaptive algorithm used in QT driven pacemakers has improved the speed of response of the rate-modulated pacemakers to physical exercise (30). With older models, the initial response of the pacing rate following onset of exercise was reported to be relatively slow. The improved rate responsive algorithm allows for faster rate response at onset of exercise and a smoother, more physiologic transition to the upper rate limit.

Development of heart block and sinus node dysfunction, the most common reason for permanent pacemaker implantation, appears to be related to a progressive loss of pacemaker cells in the SA node, as well as fibrous tissue replacement of the conduction fibers, as documented earlier. At present there appears to be significantly less reluctance to implant pacemakers in the elderly because of recent advances in pacemaker technology and surgical techniques that have made initial transvenous implantation relatively simple (31). If the heart is paced at a constant rate, cardiac output can only increase by a change in stroke volume, caused by increased contractility or by Starling mechanisms brought about by enhanced venous return (32). Because of the lack of heart rate responsiveness to exercise during ventricular demand pacing, use of target heart rate as a primary means of monitoring exercise activity is inappropriate. Paced individuals should be carefully followed with both perceived exertion and frequent blood pressure evaluations to ensure adequacy and safety of exercise activity and to prevent untoward hemodynamic events.

Exercise After Insertion of AICD

Patients who have been found to be at risk for sudden cardiac death and who could not be managed medically may be referred to a CRP after having had an automatic implantable cardioverter-defibrillator (AICD) inserted. Patients with the AICD are able to participate in CRPs and demonstrate improvement in functional capacity (33). It is important when prescribing exercise for these individuals to assess the heart rate cutoff of the AICD, rather than to attempt to establish a target heart rate based upon the maximum heart rate achieved during the graded exercise test, as the AICD has a preprogrammed heart rate cutoff point above which it will deliver a shock if it senses a wide QRS tachydysrhythmia. This heart rate should not be approached during exercise activity, particularly in patients with interventricular conduction defects. In selected patients, beta-blockers may be needed to limit the heart rate response during exercise in order to prevent the AICD from discharging. The monitoring for these patients, while participating in a CRP, is otherwise unchanged from the general population of elderly CRP participants.

MONITORING THE ELDERLY PATIENT DURING EXERCISE

Eighty-seven percent of respondents to a recent group of AMA DATTA panelists felt that telemetry electrocardiographic monitoring was essential to the safety and efficacy of a prescribed regimen of exercise in coronary rehabilitation. However, this report also noted there had been no controlled studies comparing the safety of exercise training conducted with on-site medical supervision, with and without continuous ECG monitoring. Although the majority of DATTA panelists considered the telemetry ECG monitoring to be an essential com-

ponent of a prescribed exercise regimen, the details of its application varied widely. The primary use of the monitoring was during the initial phase of the exercise program to determine the maximum exercise target heart rate range on an exercise treadmill and to monitor the patients during the initial 2 or 3 weeks after MI or cardiac surgery. Otherwise, continuous ECG monitoring was recommended for high risk patients, including those with severely depressed left ventricular function, complex ventricular dysrhythmias during rest, ventricular dysrhythmias appearing or increasing with exercise, decreases in systolic blood pressure with exercise; survivors of sudden cardiac arrest, and those with severe coronary artery disease and marked exercise-induced ischemia (34). This report also indicated that patients unable to self-monitor heart rate and those with MI complicated by congestive heart failure (CHF), cardiogenic shock, and/or serious ventricular dysrhythmias should also be monitored. Our program considers an acute MI complicated by CHF, cardiogenic shock and/or serious ventricular dysrhythmia to be a contraindication to participation in active exercise and does not treat this population. Patients having difficulty self-monitoring heart rate response usually have been able to safely master perceived exertion ratings, which do correlate well with both heart rate responses and oxygen consumption, and by using RPE they frequently have obviated the need for continuous ECG telemetry monitoring in this subgroup.

All elderly patients should record resting heart rate, perceived exertion ratings, and blood pressures upon entry to the exercise area, at the end of warmup exercises, every 5 to 10 minutes during the active participation in their aerobic exercise/activity, and at the end of their cooldown exercises. ECGs are obtained any time a patient experiences a significant change in regularity of heart rate or if any untoward cardiac signs or symptoms are noted. Baseline ECGs are taken for review and inclusion in the medical records on a monthly basis. Monthly ECGs are also required by current Medicare guidelines. Patients who have recently had their cardiac medications or dosages altered may also benefit from continuous ECG monitoring until they have been shown to have no untoward electrocardiographic or hemodynamic problems with their new medication regimen.

EDUCATION OF THE ELDERLY HEART PATIENT

Cardiac rehabilitation programs typically stress exercise to a greater degree than other program components. The structure and nature of the CRP tend to focus on provision of supervised exercise and activity. The exercise component is also the most widely studied parameter of CRPs. However, the educational component with its capability of altering other modifiable risk factors is the most important aspect of a CRP. Dietary instructions to reduce obesity, control hyperlipidemia, alter salt ingestion, and to treat other specific problems of the individual patient are very important. Smoking cessation and stress management are other recommended topics for the educational component of the CRP (35). Earlier reports from the American Heart Association indicated that changes in these modifiable risk factors are of greater importance in reducing long-term morbidity and mortality than is participation in the exercise portion of the CRP.

Few studies have been reported upon the efficacy of educational interventions in the cardiac patient, and even less material is available dealing with application of educational techniques in the elderly population. A behaviorally oriented educational program utilizing a problem-solving system applied to particular behaviors identified by elderly heart patients was shown to be particularly effective (36). Although long-term follow-up and substantiation of data in larger populations have not yet been reported, the preliminary results showed an excellent response of the elderly patients to the educational component of their cardiac program.

Participation in a structured exercise/activity program also appears to have a synergistic effect with the educational portion of the program for modification of risk factors. For example, smoking cessation after MI occurred at a greater rate among patients concomitantly participating in a training group as compared with a nontraining group of patients (37). Studies of compliance with cardiac rehabilitation in the elderly patient also revealed that lack of adequate information was a significant factor in those patients who were noncompliant (38). Other factors negatively impacting compliance included lack of motivation, associated diseases, an extreme low exercise tolerance, and socioeconomic problems.

Other studies have shown that elderly patients who show evidence of psychologic impairment and disability within 3 months after a MI are more likely to have increased problems with attitudes of passive hopelessness and resignation to a life of dependency and incapacity at 3 years follow-up (39). These results suggest that early intervention and education may be crucial to reduction of disability among the elderly cardiac patients. Another study revealed that, although the greatest benefit in cardiac rehabilitation in elderly patients was improvement in physical function, significant benefits were also noted in the social and emotional function. This study emphasized that older adults want to and can learn to perform new activities, that the adjustment of the individual elderly patient to aspects of cardiac disease is not necessarily more problematic than that of younger people, that teaching of the older person is worth the time and effort involved, and, finally, that, rather than perceiving health problems and age related deficits in the elderly as

barriers to adjustment and the ability to learn, these problems can be perceived as handicaps that can be overcome (40).

REIMBURSEMENT FOR CARDIAC REHABILITATION

Reimbursement for cardiac rehabilitation for the elderly is often less of a problem than it is for the individual younger than 65 years of age. Medicare presently allows for reimbursement of cardiac rehabilitation programs, but this is administered by different intermediaries on a state by state or regional basis. Implementation of Medicare guidelines may vary from state to state, depending upon requirements established by the intermediaries. Most guidelines call for exercise programs that include specific types of exercise that are individually prescribed for each patient. The patients must have a "clear medical need" and be referred by their attending physician. Determination of a clear medical need usually consists of documenting the diagnosis of acute MI within the preceding 12 months, coronary bypass surgery, and/or having stable angina pectoris.

At present, CRPs may be provided either through an outpatient department of a hospital or by any physician-directed clinic. Medicare reimbursement for the program, however, is usually subject to such limits as: requiring that a physician be on the premises and available to perform medical duties at all such times the facility is open; having immediately available all necessary cardiopulmonary emergency diagnostic and therapeutic lifesaving equipment such as oxygen, cardiopulmonary resuscitation equipment or defibrillation equipment; conducting the program in an area set aside for exclusive use of the program while in session, and having the program staffed by personnel who are trained in both basic and advanced life support techniques and exercise therapy for coronary disease. Any services of nonphysician personnel are usually required to be furnished under direct supervision of the physician, i.e., the physician must be in the exercise program area and immediately available and accessible for an emergency at all times the exercise program is being conducted (41). In some states, the physician is no longer required to be physically present in the exercise room itself.

FUTURE DIRECTIONS IN CARDIAC REHABILITATION

There appears to be an emerging consensus that cardiac rehabilitation programs, as currently structured, may need modification in the 1990's (42–45). The consensus indicates that patients can safely and effectively improve both function and/or reduce the symptoms of their cardiovascular disease through participation in a CRP. Benefits are generally attributed to both the reduction of risk factors associated with atherosclerotic and hypertensive cardiovascular disease, as well as with alterations in physiologic function associated with the exercise portion of the CRP.

Changes to occur during this next decade of cardiac rehabilitation are in the approach to and prescription of cardiac rehabilitation. The typical 12-week program, developed primarily because Medicare guidelines have reimbursed for 12 weeks in most states, will no longer be an acceptable standard. Instead, patients will be stratified depending upon risk factors, and duration of nonmaintenance portions of the CRP will be adjusted to each individual patient's need, as is currently done with the intensity of exercise activity. Low risk cardiac patients may need programs as short as 2 to 3 weeks to be instructed in appropriate exercise techniques and provided with counseling regarding disease prevention. Intermediate risk cardiac patients may need a 6 to 8 week program with a greater degree of monitoring. High risk cardiac patients may need 12 to 36 or more weeks of CRP participation, with much more intense monitoring including continuous ECG monitoring. Stratification of patients into various risk categories may be done by functional capacity at time of initial exercise test, presence or absence of significant dysrhythmias, presence or absence of ischemia on exercise stress testing, cardiac function as measured by ejection fraction, cardiac symptoms, ability to self-monitor, and any complications of the underlying disease processes.

As Medicare intermediaries and reimbursement guarantors become aware of these new position reports and suggestions emanating from the American College of Physicians and the American College of Cardiology, it is likely that implementation of such risk stratification alterations in the duration of the elderly patient's participation in the CRP will most likely follow. The driving force will be the potential for cost containment through reduction of duration of CRP participation. The impact of such changes on the elderly patients has yet to be determined. Age may become a factor in prescribing the duration of the nonmaintenance portion of the CRP, as some increase in program length may be needed to train the elderly patient, given the decreased rate of new learning and increased difficulty of mastering the self-monitoring techniques noted above. Alteration in program structure will also necessitate revising the educational component of most CRPs. The luxury of providing education related to secondary disease prevention and risk factor modification over a 12-week time period may be lost. Further, current absence of a mechanism for revenue generation for the educational portion of the CRP will make it more difficult to increase the educational components of the elderly cardiac patient's anticipated program. Patient and family education may be the greatest challenges to face the physician working with the elderly cardiac patient in the 1990's.

Acknowledgments. Special thanks to Doctors Romulo Baltazar and Marc Effron for manuscript review and to Judy Lubao for her secretarial assistance.

References

1. American Heart Association: *1990 Heart and Stroke Facts.* Dallas, Tex: AHA; 1989.
2. Sugiuva M, Hiraoka K, Ohkawa S, Shimoda H. A clinicopathological study on the heart diseases in the aged: the morphological classification of the 1,000 consecutive autopsy cases. *Jpn Heart J.* 16(5):526–536, 1975.
3. Lewis KB. Heart disease in the elderly. *Hospital Practice.* 11(2):99–106, 1976.
4. Weisfeldt ML, Lakatta EG, Gerstenblith G. Aging and cardiac disease. In: Braunwald E, ed. *Heart Disease.* Philadelphia, Pa: W.B. Saunders; 1988.
5. Burch GE. Fundamentals of clinical cardiology: interesting aspects of geriatric cardiology. *Am Heart J.* 89(1):99–114, 1975.
6. Caird FJ, Ball JLC, Williams BO. The cardiovascular system. In: Brocklehurst JC, ed. *Textbook of Geriatric Medicine and Gerontology.* 3rd ed. New York, NY: Churchill Livingston; 1985.
7. Beard OW. Age related physiological changes in the cardiovascular system. In: Cape RDT, Coe RM, Rossman I, eds. *Fundamentals of Geriatric Medicine.* New York, NY: Raven; 1983.
8. Smith EL, Serfuss RC, eds. *Exercise and Aging: The Scientific Basis.* Minneapolis, Minn: Enslow Publishers; 1981.
9. Fitts RH. Aging in skeletal muscle. In: *Exercise and Aging: The Scientific Basis.* Minneapolis, Minn: Enslow Publishers; 1981.
10. Adrian MJ. Flexibility in the aging adults. In: *Exercise and Aging: The Scientific Basis.* Minneapolis, Minn: Enslow Publishers; 1981
11. Marsiglio A, Holm K. Physical conditioning in the aging adult. *Nurse Practitioner.* 13(9):33–41, 1988.
12. Morrissey MJ, Baldwin J. Exercise and chronic heart disease. *Geriatr Nurs.* 8(3):138–140, 1987.
13. Greenland P. Cardiac fitness and rehabilitation in the elderly. *J Am Geriatr Soc.* 30(9):607–611, 1982.
14. American College of Sports Medicine. *Guidelines for Exercise Testing and Prescription.* 4th ed. Philadelphia, Pa: Lea & Febiger; 1991.
15. Sloane PD. How to maintain the health of the independent elderly. *Geriatrics.* 39(10):93–104, 1989.
16. American Running and Fitness Association. Aging and exercise. *J Geriatr Psychiatry Neurol.* 1(3):176–177, 1988.
17. Williams MA, Esterbrocks DJ, Sketch MH. Guidelines for exercise therapy of the elderly after myocardial infarction. *Eur Heart J.* 5(suppl E):121–123, 1984.
18. Anderson JM. Rehabilitating elderly cardiac patients. In: Rehabilitation Medicine—Adding Life to Years [Special Issue]. *West J Med.* 154:573–578, 1991.
19. Newman KP, Phillips JH. Graded exercise testing for diagnosis of coronary artery disease in elderly patients. *South Med J.* 84(4):430–432, 1988.
20. Glover DR, Robinson CS, Murray RG. Diagnostic exercise testing in 104 patients over 65 years of age. *Eur Heart J.* 5(suppl E):59–61, 1984.
21. Podczeck A, Frohner K, Foderler G, Meisl K, Unger G, Steinbach K. Exercise test in patients over 65 years of age after the first myocardial infarction. *Eur Heart J.* 5(suppl E):89–92, 1984.
22. Callahan P, Froelicher VF. Exercise test for identification of the high risk patient. *Chest.* 92(4):741–744, 1987.
23. Sannamaki KI. Early postmyocardial infarction exercise testing in subjects 70 years or more of age. Functional and prognostic evaluation. *Eur Heart J.* 5(suppl E):93–96, 1984.
24. Pollock ML, Pells AE III. Exercise prescription for the cardiac patient: an update. *Clin Sports Med.* 3(2):425–442, 1984.
25. Todd IC, Ballantyne D. Editorial Review. Cardiac adaptations

of training: relevance to angina pectoris. *Int J Cardiol.* 10:91–97, 1986.

26. Laslett L, Paumer L, Amsterdam EA. Exercise training in coronary artery disease. *Cardiol Clin.* 5(2):211–221, 1987.

27. Turi Z, Cohn PF. How medical therapy of angina pectoris differs in patients over 65. *Geriatrics.* 35(12):26–34, 1980.

28. Zalman F, Goldberger AL, Shabetai R. Transient Q waves during exercise in hypertropic cardiomyopathy. *Am J Cardiol.* 56:491–492, 1985.

29. Jordaens L, DeBacker G, Clement D. Physiologic pacing in the elderly. Effects on exercise capacity and exercise-induced arrhythmias. *Jpn Heart J.* 29(1):35–44, 1988.

30. Heijer PD, Nagelkerke D, Perrins EJ, ct al. Improved rate responsive algorithm in QT driven pacemakers: evaluation of initial response to exercise. *Pace.* 12:805–811, 1989.

31. Cobler JL, Akiyama T, Murphy GW. Permanent pacemakers in centenarians. *J Am Geriatr Soc.* 37(8):753–756, 1989.

32. Pehrsson SK, Hjemdahl P, Nordlander R, Astrom H. A comparison of sympatheoadrenal activity and cardiac performance at rest and during exercise in patients with ventricular demand or atrial synchronous pacing. *Br Heart J.* 60:212–220, 1988.

33. Menard-Rothe K, Callahan CM. Cardiac rehabilitation and the automatic implantable defibrillator patient: is it appropriate? *J Cardiopulmonary Rehabil.* 6:400–408, 1986.

34. Cole HM, ed. Diagnostic and Therapeutic Technology Assessment (DATTA): coronary rehabilitation services. *JAMA.* 258(14):1959–1961, 1987.

35. Sivarajan ES, Newton KM, Almes MJ, Kempf TM, Mansfield LW, Bruce RA. Limited effects of outpatient teaching and counseling after myocardial infarction: a controlled study. *Heart Lung.* 12(1):65–73, 1983.

36. Clark NM, Rakowski W, Wheeler JRC, Ostrander LD, Oden S, Keteyian S. Development of self-management education for elderly heart patients. *Gerontologist.* 28(4):491–494, 1988.

37. Taylor CB, Houston-Miller N, Haskell WL, Debusk RF. Smoking cessation after acute myocardial infarction: the effects of exercise training. *Addictive Behav.* 13:331–335, 1988.

38. Gori P, Pivotti F, Mase N, Zucconi V, Scardi S. Compliance with cardiac rehabilitation in the elderly. *Eur Heart J.* 5(suppl E):109–111, 1984.

39. Pathy MS, Peach H. Disability among the elderly after myocardial infarction: a 3-year follow-up. *J Royal College Physicians London.* 14(4):221–223, 1980.

40. Packa DR, Branyon ME, Kinney MR, Khan SH, Kelley R, Miers LJ. Quality of life of elderly patients enrolled in cardiac rehabilitation. *JCVN.* 3(2):33–42, 1989.

41. Blue Cross Blue Shield of Maryland. *Medicare Report: Cardiac Rehabilitation Programs.* December, 1989:1, 6, 7.

42. Health and Public Policy Committee, American College of Physicians. Position paper: cardiac rehabilitation services. *Ann Intern Med.* 109(8):671–673, 1988.

43. Greenland P, Chu JS. Efficacy of cardiac rehabilitation services with emphasis on patients after myocardial infarction. *Ann Intern Med.* 109(8):650–663, 1988.

44. Parmley WW. President's Page: Position report on cardiac rehabilitation. *J Am Coll Cardiol.* 7(2):451–453, 1986.

45. Wenger NK. Rehabilitation of the coronary patient in 1989. *Arch Intern Med.* 149:1504–1506, 1989.

22

Pulmonary Assessment and Management of the Aging and Older Patient

John R. Bach

Pulmonary management of the aging and older patient involves the use of many of the classical approaches of pulmonary rehabilitation. These include psychosocial and nutrition counseling, patient education, therapeutic exercise, the use of respiratory muscle aids, facilitation of the performance of activities of daily living (ADLs), etc. Although it is generally recognized that patients with chronic obstructive pulmonary disease (COPD) can benefit from pulmonary rehabilitation (1–3), the use of physiatric or physical medicine and rehabilitation (PM&R) principles for geriatric patients with respiratory muscle weakness or anyone with restrictive pulmonary syndromes or sleep disordered breathing has been largely ignored. Further, there is evidence that the latter two conditions are both underdiagnosed and undertreated in geriatric or chronically disabled individuals (4). Indeed, pulmonary dysfunction accompanies many chronic neuromuscular, musculoskeletal, and central nervous system conditions and is a direct consequence of many generalized disorders that lead the geriatric patient to a rehabilitation specialist. It is also a frequent cause of morbidity and mortality in this population.

Recent developments in the use of physical medicine respiratory muscle aids have been shown to decrease the risk of pulmonary complications, hospitalizations, and the need for invasive interventions such as endotracheal intubation and bronchoscopy. The inspiratory muscle aids include the use of noninvasive intermittent positive pressure ventilation (IPPV). This is the delivery of IPPV via a mouthpiece or nasal or oral-nasal interfaces. These techniques and the construction and use of custom patient-ventilator interfaces for delivery of IPPV, continuous positive airway pressure (CPAP), and bilevel positive airway pressure (Bi-PAP) are two new developments that deserve wider recognition and clinical application. Another is the recent release of a mechanical insufflator-exsufflator (In-Exsufflator, J. H. Emerson Co., Cambridge, Mass), an expiratory muscle aid that is extremely valuable in simulating effective coughing, particularly for individuals without indwelling endotracheal tubes. Likewise, for individuals with documented hypoxia during exercise, oxygen administration may improve exercise tolerance. Oxygen therapy may also facilitate ADLs and, for patients with COPD, prolong life.

Some patients may benefit from a combination of approaches. For example, the elderly hemiplegic patient may have decreased functional ability on the basis of unrecognized and potentially treatable respiratory impairment. Limited diaphragm and chest wall mobility may cause paradoxial diaphragm movement, decreased vital capacity (VC), reduced forced expiratory volumes, higher minute ventilation and oxygen consumption, as well as decreased PaO_2 and oxyhemoglobin saturation (SaO_2), particularly during mild exercise. Hypoxia may be exacerbated by the presence of concomitant COPD. Thus, weakness, ventilation/perfusion abnormality, and respiratory muscle dysfunction may contribute to a generally decreased level of functioning. However, when cooperative, these patients may benefit from a combination of PM&R techniques and the administration of supplemental oxygen. Likewise, information from the National Spinal Cord Injury Statistical Center (5) shows that pulmonary complications are the most frequent cause of death for up to 11 years postinjury. In a multicenter study of tracheostomized tetraplegics dependent on phrenic nerve pacemakers for electrophrenic respiratory (EPR) or tracheostomy IPPV, survival percentages at 1, 3, 5, and 7 years postinjury were 86%, 70%, 63%, and 59%, respectively (6). The majority of the deaths of these patients treated by these invasive techniques were associated with the inadequacy of the techniques themselves (7). Greater use of the noninvasive PM&R approaches can only improve these statistics (8, 9).

RESTRICTIVE PULMONARY SYNDROMES: EVALUATION

Pathophysiology

By contrast to individuals with intrinsic pulmonary disease or COPD who tend to have regional ventilation perfusion disturbances, individuals with paralytic/restrictive conditions tend to have global alveolar hypoventilation. In these patients the VC is directly related to respiratory muscle strength (10). VC normally plateaus at 19 years of age then decreases 1.0% to 1.2% per year thereafter. Maximum voluntary ventilation decreases by 0.8% per year after age 30 years (11). The rate of loss of pulmonary volumes increases, however, for patients with global alveolar hypoventilation, including disorders of the chest wall, neuromuscular disease, or any conditions leading to immobility or respiratory muscle weakness. The rate of loss of VC is most dramatic for patients with neuromuscular diseases such as amyotrophic lateral sclerosis or Duchenne muscular dystrophy. Following their plateau between ages 10 to 14 years, the latter lose about 250 mL of VC per year until the rate of loss tails off after falling below 300 mL to 400 mL (12, 13). Other patients susceptible to late-onset ventilatory failure include postpoliomyelitis patients who lose VC at a rate of 1.8% per year (14) and traumatic quadriplegics (9). This occurs because of the effects of aging, fatigue, and/or recrudescence of disease on residual respiratory muscle strength, lung compliance, and pulmonary function. Patients with severe back deformity or sleep disordered breathing can also develop severe restrictive pulmonary syndromes. Diminished pulmonary volumes may increase spontaneously in conditions such as Guillain-Barré syndrome and multiple sclerosis.

The loss of pulmonary volumes leads to acute or insidious ventilatory insufficiency. In the latter case, symptoms (15) may be minimal as gradual resetting of respiratory control centers accommodates to chronic alveolar hypoventilation (CAH). Hypercapnia is likely when the VC falls below 55% of predicted normal (10). Hypoxia, hypercapnia, and decrease in VC are exacerbated when intrinsic lung disease, kyphoscoliosis, sleep disordered breathing, or obesity complicate respiratory muscle weakness from any cause. Both dynamic and static pulmonary compliance can be diminished (16). The shallow breathing pattern, with loss of the ability to take occasional deep inspirations (sighs), contribute to loss of compliance. In tetraplegic patients, loss of compliance may be exacerbated by chest wall spasticity and fibrotic changes in intercostal muscles (17). Elderly residents of nursing facilities often receive multiple medications that can reduce the ventilatory response to hypercapnia, permit the development of microscopic atelectasis, and with it the loss of pulmonary compliance. In a recent study of nursing facility residents, including some elderly, inactive individuals with uncomplicated medical histories, mean VC was less than 40% of predicted normal (4). In many cases, the restrictive pulmonary syndrome was sufficiently severe to warrant the use of regular maximal insufflations, which, among other benefits, familiarize the patient with mouthpiece IPPV for more prolonged use when needed. CAH may also complicate usually mild generalized neuromuscular conditions such as Charcot-Marie-Tooth disease, facio-scapulo-humeral muscular dystrophy, and myotonic dystrophy and be exacerbated by acute complicating medical conditions.

Patients with expiratory muscle weakness have difficulty clearing secretions especially following general anesthesia and during upper respiratory tract infections (URIs). Chronic mucus plugging can lead to ventilation/perfusion imbalance, chronic microatelectasis, frequent pneumonias, pulmonary scarring, further loss of lung compliance, cor pulmonale, and eventually, cardiopulmonary arrest. Risk is heightened in the presence of weak oropharyngeal musculature. Mucus plugs can also cause sudden hypoxia and respiratory failure. Patients with neuromuscular disease may have varying degrees of cardiomyopathy and may be particularly susceptible to hypoxia-triggered dysrhythmia and cardiac decompensation. With proper treatment using the techniques described in this chapter, intubation can be eliminated, mucus plugs prevented or quickly cleared, and the risk of life-threatening pneumonias minimized for many.

Pulmonary Function

The symptoms of CAH most typically include fatigue, daytime somnolence, and, for patients able to ambulate, dyspnea (15). There is often a history of frequent hospitalization for respiratory impairment. Signs, particularly those of cor pulmonale, are present only in advanced stages and do not occur in properly managed patients (15).

Baseline pulmonary function testing may demonstrate the presence of intrinsic lung disease, which, if severe and accompanied by PaO_2 less than or equal to 60 mm Hg in the presence of $PaCO_2$ less than or equal to 40 mm Hg, indicates the need for supplemental oxygen therapy. If a primarily restrictive pulmonary syndrome is diagnosed, regular evaluation of VC with a portable spirometer is sufficient for monitoring patient progress and response to treatment. For many young patients for whom there is no reason to suspect intrinsic or obstructive pulmonary dysfunction, such as those with typical Duchenne muscular dystrophy, pulmonary function studies other than routine VC monitoring are unnecessary. The VC should be measured in the sitting position, supine position, and with other positional changes or while using thoraco-lumbar orthoses when applicable.

The maximum insufflation capacity (MIC) is useful for determining the potential for assisting ventilation by noninvasive means as opposed to tracheostomy IPPV. The MIC is a measure of the maximum volume of air that can be held by an individual. It is obtained by the air stacking of mechanical insufflations and is always greater than or equal to the VC. Weak oral muscles can be splinted during these insufflations by delivering the air via a Bennett lip seal (Puritan-Bennett, Boulder, Colo) held firmly over the mouth. The MIC is a function of pulmonary compliance and the strength of oropharyngeal and laryngeal muscles. An MIC of at least 500 mL is necessary to achieve useful exsufflation flows during attempts at manually-assisted coughing (18). This is necessary to prevent mucus plugging, atelectasis, and pneumonia during URIs. An MIC of less than 500 mL may be considered an indication for tracheostomy. In patients with intact bulbar musculature, the MIC should approach the predicted inspiratory capacity.

Any patient with less than 40% of predicted normal supine VC should undergo SaO_2 monitoring during sleep. Patients for whom the diagnosis of CAH is unclear on the basis of VC, nocturnal oximetry, and wake blood gases should also undergo noninvasive $PaCO_2$ monitoring. The capnograph, which can be used to measure end-tidal pCO_2, and pulse oximeter must be capable of collating and printing the data (15, 19). These studies are most conveniently performed on an ambulatory basis.

Sleep Disordered Breathing and Nocturnal Alveolar Hypoventilation

Any symptomatic patient with greater than 70% of predicted normal VC, mean SaO_2 less than 95% for at least 1 hour during sleep with multiple transient desaturations below 90%, and normal end-tidal pCO_2 is a candidate for ambulatory polysomnography to evaluate for the presence of sleep disordered breathing (20). This condition can develop into or exacerbate CAH. It may also complicate COPD.

Sleep disordered breathing refers to the occurrence of apneas and hypopneas, which may be centrally derived or result from upper airway obstruction. Carskadon and Dement (21) found that 37.5% of all subjects over the age of 62 years have apneas or hypopneas. The obstructive sleep apena syndrome (OSAS) in which the apneas and hypopneas are primarily obstructive in nature has only recently been recognized as a common entity with potentially serious cardiovascular and neuropsychiatric sequelae (22). Obstruction is most commonly due to hypopharyngeal collapse from a transluminal pressure gradient across the airway caused by the action of the inspiratory muscles and the failure of activation of the airway dilator muscles, which are normally reflexly activated at the onset of inspiration. Overt

OSAS occurs in at least 3% of the general population, but its incidence increases with age, in males and in the presence of exogenous androgens, obesity, brain stem lesions, hypothyroidism, lymphoma, nasal obstruction, hypertrophied tonsils, lingual or laryngeal cysts, micrognathia, retrognathia, macroglossia, or nasal obstruction (23). It occurs in the majority of patients with ventilatory insufficiency using negative pressure body ventilators (20, 24) or EPR. It also appears to be more prevalent in patients with generalized neuromuscular diseases.

The diagnosis of OSAS is characterized by the appearance of 10 or more obstructive apneas plus hypopneas per hour during sleep (25). An apnea has been defined as a cessation of airflow lasting at least 10 seconds. A hypopnea is defined as a decrease in tidal volume to one-third or less of the baseline value of the immediately preceding breaths that persists for greater than 10 seconds (25). Virtually every apnea and hypopnea is associated with a 4% or greater oxyhemoglobin desaturation ($dSaO_2$) or 4% $dSaO_2$ (25). Since the potential complications of OSAS appear to derive predominantly from hypoxia, SaO_2 monitoring is particularly important for the screening of this disorder. A typical sawtooth pattern of $dSaO_2$ is observed (20, 26). George et al (25) demonstrated that the number of $dSaO_2$ of greater than 3% that last for at least 10 seconds and have a particular slope predicts the total number of polysomnographically derived apneas and hypopneas with 98% sensitivity and with very few false positives and false negatives. Thus, whether quantified by computer or counted manually, the quantitation of $dSaO_2$s is useful for the screening of OSAS and monitoring the efficacy of treatment.

Obstructive apneas are often accompanied by central apneas. Indeed, there may be an etiologic association between them. It is conceivable that, for some patients with severe OSAS, central apneas result at least in part from central nervous system desensitivity to hypoxia. This desensitivity also occurs in the presence of the chronic respiratory muscle dysfunction, which may accompany any paralytic/restrictive condition as well as OSAS. CAH, therefore, may result from OSAS (27), as well as from neuromuscular, restrictive (15, 28, 29), or intrinsic pulmonary disease (30).

The diagnosis of CAH is established by the presence of chronic hypercapnia. Without the use of noninvasive pCO_2 monitoring, continuous mean nocturnal SaO_2 less than 95% for 1 hour or more in a symptomatic patient with supine VC less than 40% of predicted is sufficient to establish the diagnosis. With CAH, nocturnal hypoventilation is usually more severe than during the daytime. The pattern of nocturnal SaO_2 is often relatively smooth in CAH patients without sleep disordered breathing. The insidiously progressive hypercapnia that can occur in these patients and the resulting compensatory metabolic alkalosis results in elevated bicarbonate levels that depress the ventilatory response to hypoxia and hypercapnia. CAH can be associated with symptoms, decreases in tidal volumes, and dSaO$_2$ as severe as seen in pure OSAS, even without the presence of back deformity, muscular weakness, or obesity (15).

The untoward cardiovascular effects of OSAS result primarily from hypoxia (22, 31) and include pulmonary hypertension, right ventricular volume overload, decreased cardiac output, sudden episodes of right ventrical hypotension, and life-threatening dysrhythmias (31, 32). There is an increased incidence of systemic hypertension (31) and angina (33). CAH has the same complications as OSAS with the additional danger of respiratory arrest from severe hypercapnia and increased risk for pulmonary complications during otherwise benign URIs.

RESTRICTIVE PULMONARY SYNDROMES: MANAGEMENT

Sleep Disordered Breathing

Although the mechanism of action is unclear, in obese patients with OSAS, a weight reduction of 10% to 25% can significantly improve or completely resolve OSAS in most cases (23). Unfortunately, weight loss is very infrequently long-term.

CPAP is effective for the majority of patients. The mechanisms by which it is effective are unclear; however, one is its pneumatic splinting effect to maintain an open airway. CPAP of 5 cm H$_2$O to 15 cm H$_2$O is usually adequate. Independently varying the inspiratory and expiratory pressures, i.e., using bilevel positive airway pressure, can improve effectiveness and comfort. The Bi-PAP ventilator (Respironics Inc, Monroeville, Pa) has been designed for this. For many obesity/hypoventilation patients or patients with a combined paralytic/restrictive ventilatory insufficiency and concurrent OSAS, CPAP or Bi-PAP may be ineffective. Assisted ventilation by noninvasive IPPV at higher than typical Bi-PAP pressures can both ventilate the patient and maintain upper airway patency.

A recent study indicated that 43 of 125 patients could not tolerate long-term CPAP largely because of discomfort from the CPAP mask itself (34). CPAP is usually delivered via commercially available CPAP masks. These masks are inexpensive, but often poorly tolerated. For these patients, a commercially available kit is available for custom molding of a nasal interface (SEFAM mask, Lifecare Inc, Lafayette, Colo). Such interfaces are comfortable and effective at higher pressures. However, they are expensive ($785), delicate, and require refabrication every 6 weeks to 5 months. A transparent, custom-molded, low profile acrylic nasal interface is also available. It costs $500 and is comfortable, cosmetic, and

very durable, but is currently available only in New Jersey (Fig. 22.1) (35).

A more convenient long-term solution, effective for many OSAS patients, is the use of an orthodontic splint that brings the mandible and tongue forward (Fig. 22.2) (36, 37). This can be effective and is the commonly preferred treatment for many patients.

Nasopharyngeal tubes are effective but not tolerated by the majority of patients. There are no clear roles for oxygen or pharmacotherapeutic agents in the management of OSAS (23). Surgical options, including tra-

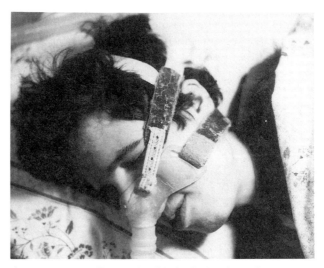

Figure 22.1. Ventilator-assisted individual with Duchenne muscular dystrophy using an acrylic custom-fabricated nasal interface for IPPV. This patient is dependent on nasal IPPV 24 hours per day.

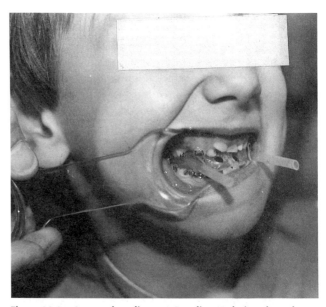

Figure 22.2. Intraoral appliance ("Equalizer") designed to advance the mandible and distract it vertically from the maxilla. Its advancement of the tongue and splinting of the uvula and pharyngeal musculature are effective in treating obstructive sleep apneas. (Courtesy of John J. Haze, D.D.S., Montville, NJ.)

cheostomy and the less frequently effective uvulopala-topharyngoplasty, and mandibular advancement procedures should be used as a last resort (38–40).

Global Alveolar Hypoventilation

REHABILITATION TECHNIQUES

The fundamental management goals include maintenance of normal ventilation 24 hours a day, prevention of chest tightness, and effective clearance of airway secretions particularly during URIs. Early diagnosis and introduction of these goals are important.

Counseling is needed to explain: the importance of maintaining normal ventilation 24 hours per day; the inspiratory muscle aids that can accomplish this; the need to avoid supplemental oxygen therapy except during episodes of acute pulmonary disease when PaO_2 may not exceed 60 mm Hg in the presence of normal ventilation (15); the need to avoid sedatives, obesity, heavy meals, extremes of temperature, humidity, excessive fatigue, crowded areas or exposure to respiratory tract pathogens; the need for appropriate influenza and bacterial vaccinations and early medical attention during URIs; the value of pursuing personal goals and encouraging self-directed activities and decision-making, as well as maximizing the level of functioning and daily activities.

The basic rehabilitation techniques include the use of lung expansion techniques, which should be performed at least twice a day to approach the predicted inspiratory capacity. Air stacking of mechanical insufflations (41) or glossopharyngeal breathing (GPB) (42, 43) should be used for this. The earlier and more aggressively that this is introduced, the better may be the ultimate effect on dynamic and possibly static lung compliance. This is important because decreased pulmonary compliance increases the work of breathing and exacerbates CAH. A positive pressure blower (Zephyr, Lifecare Inc, Layfayette, Colo), intermittent positive pressure breathing (IPPB) machine, or portable ventilator is most useful for delivering the maximal mechanical insufflations.

Respiratory muscle exercise should be used for conditions for which it has been shown to be useful (41, 44). Strengthening of accessory respiratory muscles may improve both inspiratory endurance and increase expiratory thrust when insertions are fixed during contraction.

Manually and/or mechanically-assisted coughing should be used as necessary (18, 45–47). When peak cough expiratory flows are less than 5 liters a second, unassisted coughing is inadequate. Manually-assisted coughing can be provided by first delivering a maximal inspiration or insufflation. An assistant then delivers a manual thrust to the anterior chest wall and epigastrium as the patient initiates his or her expulsive effort. Mechanically-assisted expulsion of airway secretions, which

is less labor intensive and more effective, can be achieved with mechanical insufflation-exsufflation devices (45–47) or exsufflation-biased oscillation devices (48).

Other rehabilitation specialists should also be involved in patient management. Occupational therapists can train the patient in the use of energy-saving devices and techniques, environmental control systems, and robotics, when appropriate (49). Physical therapists can train the patient and caregivers in range of motion and other exercises to optimize the patient's musculoskeletal condition and in chest therapy, postural drainage, and manually-assisted coughing. Orthotic aids should be used to maintain ambulation and erect body posture. Speech pathologists should be called upon as appropriate for the management of dysphagia and dysarthria and for augmentative communication if needed.

Oximetry biofeedback can assist the patient with CAH in maintaining more normal daytime ventilation. The patient should be instructed to keep his or her SaO_2 at 95% or greater throughout daytime hours by supplementing his or her breathing with mouthpiece IPPV (Fig. 22.3) (9, 14, 50). The oximeter can effectively gauge ventilation provided that supplemental oxygen therapy is avoided. Continuous SaO_2 monitoring is also particularly useful during URIs when sudden $dSaO_2$ is usually an indication of acute mucus plugging and chronic $dSaO_2$ an indication of atelectasis or pneumonia.

Respiratory muscle rest or inspiratory muscle assistance with the use of body ventilators or noninvasive

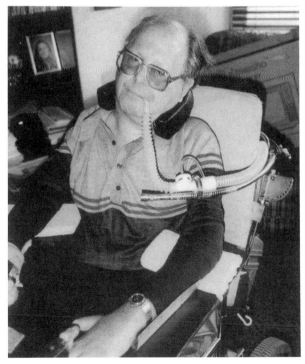

Figure 22.3. An individual supported by noninvasive methods of ventilatory support since 1955 and using mouth IPPV around the clock since 1982.

IPPV should be used to reset respiratory control centers and maintain normal arterial blood gases (see below) (15, 51–55).

GPB should be taught to patients with less than 1200 mL of VC and adequate oropharyngeal muscle strength for functional swallowing and speech. GPB is the use of the tongue and pharyngeal muscles to add to a maximal inspiratory effort by projecting boluses of air past the vocal cords into the lungs. One breath consists of 6 to 30 boluses (gulps) of 30 mL to 150 mL each. Effective GPB permits a patient to sustain ventilation for hours despite having little or no VC. It also normalizes speech production and permits the patient to take a deeper "breath" for shouting and coughing. Progress with GPB should be monitored by regularly measuring the volume of air per gulp and the number of gulps per breath.

Ventilator weaning can be facilitated by using mouthpiece IPPV and by use of manually or mechanically assisted coughing (8, 48). Conversion from tracheostomy IPPV to the safer noninvasive means of long-term ventilatory support is indicated for patients with adequate MIC (8, 9).

INSPIRATORY MUSCLE AID

Patients with CAH require various regimens of inspiratory muscle assistance. They almost invariably and appropriately refuse elective tracheostomy for IPPV. Many patients with supine VC less than 30% of predicted require at least nocturnal ventilatory support (15). Patients with less than 12% of predicted VC often require aid around the clock (15). Acute ventilatory failure and emergency tracheostomy can also be avoided by appropriate use of respiratory muscle aids. The patient must be cooperative, without substance abuse problems or a seizure disorder, which can decrease the efficacy of many noninvasive techniques, particularly during sleep.

Inspiratory muscle aid can be provided by body ventilators, devices that act directly on the body, or by noninvasive IPPV. Negative pressure body ventilators create negative pressure on the chest and/or abdomen causing air to flow into the lungs through the nose and mouth. They include the Rocking Bed (56), Iron Lung (57), Porta Lung (Fig. 22.4), Pneumowrap (Fig. 22.5), and Chest Shell (Fig. 22.6) (58–60). These devices are not feasible or are inadequate in the sitting position. Except for the Iron Lung and Porta Lung, they are generally not useful in the presence of scoliosis or extreme obesity. It may take 10 minutes or more for a personal care attendant to place a patient in a wrap ventilator (Pneumosuit, Pneumowrap). Sleeping with a significant other may not be possible. Travel with the heavier and bulkier body ventilators is inconvenient if not impossible. In addition, these devices are associated with obstructive sleep apneas in the majority of patients using

them (20). It is for these reasons that noninvasive IPPV is the method of choice for long-term ventilatory support for the majority of patients. Negative pressure body ventilators continue to be useful, however, for temporary assistance for some patients during URIs (14, 50), for use during tracheostomy site closure (8, 9), and for patients who prefer them to noninvasive IPPV.

The intermittent abdominal pressure ventilator (IAPV) consists of an inflatable bladder in an abdominal belt (Fig. 22.7). The bladder is cyclically inflated by a positive pressure ventilator. This pushes the abdominal contents up against the diaphragm and ventilates the patient. The IAPV generally augments the patient's tidal volume by 200 mL to 400 mL, but much greater volumes are often possible (61). The IAPV is not effective

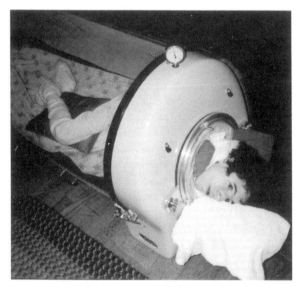

Figure 22.4.   Use of the Porta-Lung during a respiratory tract infection for a patient who otherwise uses 24-hour nasal IPPV.

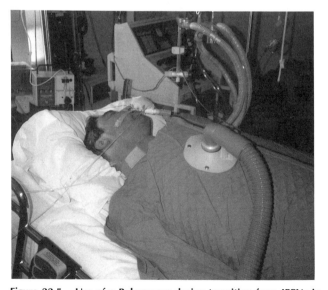

Figure 22.5.   Use of a Pulmowrap during transition from IPPV via nasotracheal intubation.

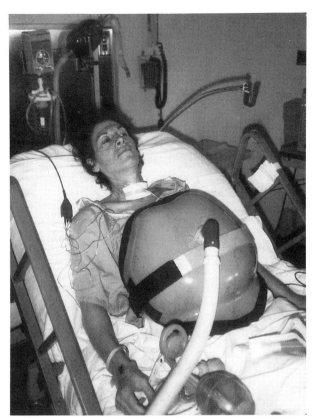

Figure 22.6. Use of a Chest Shell Ventilator during tracheostomy closure and conversion to 24-hour mouthpiece IPPV.

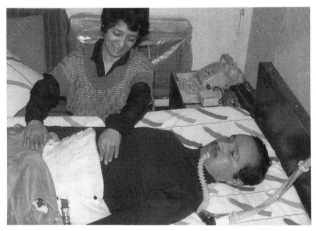

Figure 22.7. Use of mouthpiece IPPV during placement of the IAPV. The patient has used the IAPV successfully when sitting despite having no measurable vital capacity since 1955.

in the presence of scoliosis or extremes of body weight. It is effective only at greater than 30 degrees from the horizontal and is best in the sitting position at 75 degrees to 85 degrees. It is the method of choice for daytime ventilatory support for most patients with less than 1 hour of free time off the ventilator because it is cosmetic, practical, effective, and ideal for concurrent GPB and wheelchair use (61).

Recently, noninvasive IPPV has been recognized as an effective alternative to tracheostomy IPPV, EPR, and body ventilator use. IPPV can be delivered through the mouth (14, 50, 62) (Fig. 22.3), nose (15, 54, 55), or mouth and nose (19). For all three methods, custom-molded interfaces can enhance comfort and efficacy (35). These interfaces may also be useful in the management of OSAS (Fig. 22.1). Mouthpiece IPPV is also an excellent alternative method for ventilator weaning (8, 9).

THE COPD PATIENT: EVALUATION

COPD ranks as the fifth leading cause of death in the United States. It affects 10% to 40% of all Americans, including 17,000,000 reported cases, with the incidence having doubled since 1970. Fifty percent of patients have activity limitations, and 25% are bed-disabled (63). COPD is the fourth largest cause of major activity limitation. The forced expiratory volume in one second (FEV_1) decreases by 60 mL per year in COPD patients. This rate is twice that of normals. Exertional dyspnea occurs when the FEV_1 is less than 1500 mL. With the aging of the general population, a significant increase in the prevalence and severity of COPD is projected for the years to come.

The results to be expected from a comprehensive rehabilitation program include reduction in dyspnea, increased maximum oxygen consumption and exercise tolerance, and fewer hospitalizations from respiratory impairment. The significant improvement in quality of life which may be expected from continued adherence to rehabilitation principles is all the more significant because the time course in mild to moderate emphysema and chronic bronchitis without a major reversible component may be 20 to 40 years.

Pathophysiology

The chronic obstructive pulmonary diseases include chronic bronchitis, emphysema, asthma, and cystic fibrosis. These conditions usually have significant elements of both airway obstruction and parenchymal lung disease. The gas exchange surface of the lung, which under normal circumstances is effective to a 20-fold range of metabolic demand and maintains normal arterial blood gases, is greatly reduced in patients with intrinsic lung disease. Gas exchange is dependent on ventilation, perfusion, and diffusion, all of which are commonly affected. COPD is characterized by hyperinflation, oxygenation impairment, hypercapnia, airflow limitation, and decreased exercise and ambulation capacity.

Oxygen and carbon dioxide diffusion across the respiratory exchange membrane of the lung is a function of the gas partial pressures and the respiratory exchange membrane area and inversely related to membrane thickness (5). Exchange normally takes place in one third of the pulmonary capillary blood transit time. With decreased diffusion or increased blood flow, arterial PaO_2

is lower than alveolar PaO_2. PaO_2 levels fall before there is an observed rise in $PaCO_2$ because of the greater rate of diffusion of CO_2. Thus, hypoxia in the presence of normal ventilation or hyperventilation ($PaCO_2$ less than 43 mm Hg) is characteristic of intrinsic lung disease. Such patients may go into overt respiratory failure during acute pulmonary infections. As for CAH patients, pulmonary vascular resistance increases in the presence of generalized or local pulmonary tissue hypoxia, especially in the presence of acidosis. Widespread regional alveolar hypoventilation can lead to severe pulmonary artery hypertension with right ventricular failure.

Peripheral chemoreceptors in the aortic and carotid bodies sense PaO_2, $PaCO_2$, and pH. Central receptors on the surface of the medulla respond to hydrogen ion levels in the cerebrospinal fluid (5). Response to $PaCO_2$ is reduced by drugs or heavy mechanical loads such as in the presence of scoliosis or airway obstruction. The chemoreceptors gradually reset as the patient's breaths become increasingly shallow to decrease the work of breathing. This occurs at the expense of increasing dead space ventilation, hypercapnia, and a resulting metabolic alkalosis.

Deep breathing increases the work to overcome the elastic forces of the lung and chest wall and, like shallow breathing, is inefficient. However, since the flow through a partially obstructed channel is inversely related to the fourth power of the radius of that channel, and slower, deeper breaths require less flow than rapid shallow breaths, the former breathing pattern is particularly beneficial for patients with COPD, although the latter pattern is more commonly seen in these anxious and often struggling patients.

Patient Evaluation and Selection

Any motivated patient with symptomatic COPD, adequate medical and neuromusculoskeletal status to permit active participation, and who has quit smoking, is a candidate for pulmonary rehabilitation. Active patients who are still able to walk several blocks but who have noted yearly decreases in exercise tolerance are ideal candidates.

Space limitations prevent a thorough presentation of the principles of evaluation and rehabilitation of COPD patients. The reader is referred to the cited references as well as standard text books devoted to this topic (1, 3, 64).

A general medical evaluation should be undertaken and coincident conditions such as obesity and hypertension should be treated. Severe cor pulmonale, congestive heart failure, uncontrolled dysrhythmias, serious coronary artery disease, and uncontrolled angina are contraindications for a comprehensive pulmonary rehabilitation program, which necessarily includes therapeutic exercise.

Symptoms most commonly include shortness of breath, cough, and wheezing. Precipitating and relieving factors including exercise, allergies, occupational history, and emotional factors should be considered. The history of previous pulmonary diseases, hospitalizations, medications, smoking, drinking, and dietary habits should also be addressed.

The general physical examination should include respiratory rate and depth; observation for the use of scalene, sternocleidomastoid and other accessory muscles; auscultation of the lungs, and assessment for signs of cardiac dysfunction.

Laboratory, radiologic studies, and sleep blood gas monitoring should be ordered as indicated by the patient's symptoms and medical condition. Pulmonary function studies provide an indication of prognosis but are not generally felt to be alterable by rehabilitation efforts.

We recommend that clinical exercise testing be performed both before and after the program to determine the degree of functional impairment and to document patient progress. Prior to energy cost studies, an arterial blood gas should be performed to help determine the possible need for the use of supplemental oxygen (PaO_2 less than 60 mm Hg) or nocturnal pCO_2 monitoring (pCO_2 greater than 45 mm Hg). Consistently elevated pCO_2 of 50 mm Hg or greater during sleep is an indication for an attempt at nocturnal inspiratory muscle assistance as discussed previously (51–53).

Clinical exercise testing, whether by using a treadmill, stationary bicycle, or upper extremity ergometer, should include the following: vital signs, electrocardiography, oxygen consumption, carbon dioxide production, the respiratory quotient, the ventilatory equivalent, minute ventilation, and metabolic rate. The respiratory quotient is the ratio of the carbon dioxide produced divided by the oxygen consumed. The ventilatory equivalent is equal to the volume of air breathed for 1 liter of oxygen consumed. A metabolic equivalent (MET) is the resting metabolic rate per kilogram of body weight (i.e., 1 MET = 3.5 mL O_2/kg/min). Useful measures of cardiac function include the oxygen pulse, a measure of the mL of oxygen consumed per heart beat. A clinical exercise test should advance until oxygen consumption fails to increase, maximum allowable heart rate for age is reached, or electrocardiographic changes, chest pain, severe dyspnea, or fatigue occur. In general, a goal of attaining a minute ventilation of 35 times the patient's FEV_1 is reasonable. Clinical exercise testing permits the clinician to determine whether the primary disability is pulmonary, cardiac dysfunction, or exercise induced bronchospasm (65).

Management

The patient should be educated as to the reasons for cessation of smoking. These include decreasing the rate of loss of FEV$_1$. Likewise, the patient should be counseled to avoid atmospheric or vocational pollutants and other aggravating factors such as pollen, aerosols, excessive humidity, stress, large meals, people with respiratory infections, etc. Influenza and pneumococcal vaccinations are recommended. High altitude travel may require supplemental oxygen therapy. Good nutrition should be maintained and dehydration avoided.

Medical therapy involves optimal pharmacologic management of reversible bronchospasm when present including the use of xanthine derivatives, adrenergics, and aerosolized medications. Greater than 20% improvement in FEV$_1$ is significant with bronchodilator use, but many pulmonologists use bronchodilators with little objective evidence of benefit. Other medications such as expectorants, mucolytics, corticosteroids, antibiotics, and disodium cromoglycate should be used along with humidification and bronchial toilet as warranted to prepare the patient for optimum participation in the therapeutic exercise program. During URIs, early medical attention is important including the use of broad spectrum antibiotics and glucocorticoids.

Oxygen therapy should be used if the PaO$_2$ is less than 60 mm Hg. This can be delivered up to 24 hours per day. It decreases reactive pulmonary hypertension and polycythemia, improves cognitive function, and may decrease the number of hospitalizations. Transtracheal oxygen delivery avoids waste around the nose and mouth, avoids the "dead space" of the nasopharynx, and prevents discomfort and drying associated with nasal cannulas and face masks (1).

Training in the techniques of chest percussion, postural drainage, assisted coughing, and proper use of nebulizers and ventilatory equipment is often needed. Without proper training, the medication delivered by handheld nebulizers is too often deposited uselessly on the tongue.

The physical treatment modalities include the use of therapeutic exercise. This may be limited by pain in the performing muscles of unconditioned individuals. Reconditioning exercises may include walking, stair climbing, calisthenics, bicycling, and pool activities. The patient should be placed on and made responsible for a progressive program. We recommend the purchase of a stationary bicycle for the patient's home and its use twice a day. A daily 12-minute walk is recommended. A daily log should be kept of time and distance walked and bicycled. In general, the pulse should increase at least 20% to 30% and return to baseline 5 to 10 minutes after stopping exercise. Increased endurance for exercise may occur independently of changes in ventilatory muscles endurance.

Breathing exercises should be used with the goals of modifying the breathing pattern, strengthening respiratory muscles, and improving the cough mechanism. Pursed lip and diaphragmatic breathing decrease the re-

spiratory rate and coordinate the breathing pattern. Pursed lip breathing may also equalize pleural and bronchial pressure thus preventing collapse of smaller bronchi. Diaphragm resistive exercises or, more conveniently, inspiratory resistive exercises performed by inhaling through a variable diameter orifice may be used. A daily log of orifice diameter and time periods of use should also be kept. Specific ventilatory muscle training may produce a significant increase inventilatory muscle endurance (66).

Air shifting techniques should be taught. Air shifting involves a deep inspiration that is held with the glottis closed for 5 seconds. The air, thus, shifts to lesser ventilated areas of the lung and may help to prevent microatelectasis. The subsequent expiration should be via pursed lips. This technique may be most beneficial when performed several times per hour.

Relaxation exercises such as Jacobson exercises and biofeedback may be used to decrease tension and anxiety (1). Pursed-lip breathing also aids in relaxation.

Interspersing periods of respiratory muscle rest with exercise of specific respiratory muscle groups in a principle of pulmonary rehabilitation. Rest can be achieved by overnight assisted ventilation by use of a body ventilator (3) or by periods of mouth or nasal IPPV (11–14). Improved daytime gases, increased VC, decreased fatigue, and increased well-being having been reported in such programs (10, 13–15). Mechanical ventilation should be used when the pCO$_2$ exceeds 50 mm Hg or when pO$_2$ fails to improve beyond 40 mm Hg despite inhalation of 100% oxygen. The use of expiratory muscle and mucociliary clearance aids may also be very useful in this population and merit further study (48).

SUMMARY

Pulmonary disorders may be divided into conditions in which difficulties with either blood oxygenation or with pulmonary ventilation predominate. For patients with primarily a blood oxygenation impairment, life can be prolonged by oxygen therapy and the quality of life can be enhanced by a well-designed pulmonary rehabilitation program including therapeutic exercise. For patients with primarily impaired pulmonary ventilation, oxygen therapy should be avoided. Inspiratory and expiratory muscle aids can assist or support alveolar ventilation and eliminate airway secretions without resort to tracheal intubation or bronchoscopy. Oximetry biofeedback can facilitate their use.

References

1. Make B, ed. *Clinics in Chest Medicine: Pulmonary Rehabilitation.* Philadelphia, Pa: W.B. Saunders; 1986.
2. Rondinelli RD, Hill NS. Rehabilitation of the patient with pulmonary disease. In: Delisa J, ed. *Rehabilitation Medicine: Principles and Practice.* New York, NY: McGraw Hill; 1988.

3. Haas F, Axen K, Pineda H, eds. *Pulmonary Therapy Rehabilitation.* ed 2. Baltimore, Md: Williams & Wilkins; 1991.

4. Wang TG, Bach JR. Pulmonary dysfunction of residents of chronic nursing facilities. Taiwan Rehabilitation Journal. (Submitted for publication).

5. Young JS, Burns PE, Bowen AM, McCuthen R. *Spinal Cord Injury Statistics: Experience of the Regional Spinal Cord Injury Systems.* Phoenix, Ariz: Good Samaritan Medical Center; 1982.

6. Whiteneck GG, Carter RE, Hall K, Menter RR, Wilkerson MA, Wilmot CB. Collaborative study of high quadriplegia. *Arch Phys Med Rehabil.* 66:575, 1985. Abstract.

7. Bach JR, O'Connor K. Electrophrenic ventilation: a different perspective. *J Am Paraplegia Soc.* 14:9–17, 1991.

8. Bach JR, Alba AS. Noninvasive options for ventilatory support of the traumatic high level quadriplegic. *Chest.* 98:613–619, 1990.

9. Bach JR. New approaches in the rehabilitation of the traumatic high level quadriplegic. *Am J Phys Med Rehabil.* 70:13–20, 1991.

10. Braun NMT, Arora NS, Rochester DF. Respiratory muscle and pulmonary function in polymyositis and other proximal myopathies. *Thorax.* 38:616–623, 1983.

11. Burri PH. Development and regeneration of the lung. In: Fishman AP, ed. *Pulmonary Diseases and Disorders.* 2nd ed. New York, NY: McGraw-Hill; 1988.

12. Rideau Y, Jankowski LW, Grellit J. Respiratory function in muscular dystrophies. *Muscle Nerve.* 4:151–164, 1981.

13. Bach J, Alba A, Pilkington LA, Lee M. Long term rehabilitation in advanced state of childhood onset, rapidly progressive muscular dystrophy. *Arch Phys Med Rehabil.* 62:328–331, 1981.

14. Bach JR, Alba AS, Bohatiuk G, Saporito L, Lee M. Mouth intermittent positive pressure ventilation in the management of postpolio respiratory insufficiency. *Chest.* 91:859–864, 1987.

15. Bach JR, Alba AS. Management of chronic alveolar hypoventilation by nasal ventilation. *Chest.* 97:52–57, 1990.

16. Estenne M, De Troyer A. The effects of tetraplegia on chest wall statics. *Am Rev Respir Dis.* 134:121–124, 1986.

17. De Troyer A, Heilporn A. Respiratory mechanics in quadriplegia: the respiratory function of the intercostal muscles. *Am Rev Respir Dis.* 122:591–600, 1980.

18. Sorter S, McKenzie M. *Toward Independence: Assisted Cough.* Dallas, Tex: BioSciencee Communications of Dallas, Inc; 1986.

19. Bach JR, Alba AS, Shin D. Noninvasive airway pressure assisted ventilation in the management of respiratory insufficiency due to poliomyelitis. *Am J Phys Med Rehabil.* 68:264–271, 1987.

20. Bach JR, Penek J. Obstructive sleep apnea complicating negative pressure ventilatory support in patients with chronic paralytic/restrictive ventilatory dysfunction. *Chest.* 99:1386–1393, 1991.

21. Carskadon M, Dement W. Respiration during sleep in the aged human. *J Gerontol.* 36:420–425, 1981.

22. Bradley TD, Phillipson EA. Pathogenesis and pathophysiology of the obstructive sleep apnea syndrome. *Med Clin North Am.* 69:1169–1185, 1985.

23. Lombard R Jr, Zwillich CW. Medical therapy of obstructive sleep apnea. *Med Clin North Am.* 69:1317–1335, 1985.

24. Levy RD, Bradley TD, Newman SL, Macklem PT, Martin JG. Negative pressure ventilation: effects on ventilation during sleep in normal subjects. *Chest.* 65:95–99, 1989.

25. George CF, Millar TW, Kryger MH. Identification and quantification of apneas by computer-based analysis of oxygen saturation. *Am Rev Respir Dis.* 137:1238–1240, 1988.

26. Fletcher EC, Costarangos C, Miller T. The rate of fall of arterial oxyhemoglobin saturation in obstructive sleep apnea. *Chest.* 96:717–722, 1989.

27. Rapoport DM, Garay SM, Epstein H. Goldring RM. Hypercapnia in the obstructive sleep apnea syndrome: a reevaluation of the "Pickwickian syndrome". *Chest.* 89:627–635, 1986.

28. Midgren B. Oxygen desaturation during sleep as a function of

the underlying respiratory disease. *Am Rev Respir Dis.* 141:43–46, 1990.

29. Smith PEM, Calverley PMA, Edwards RHT. Hypoxemia during sleep in Duchenne muscular dystrophy. *Am Rev Respir Dis.* 137:884–888, 1988.

30. Tirapur VG, Mir MA. Nocturnal hypoxemia and associated electrocardiographic changes in patients with chronic obstructive airways disease. *N Engl J Med.* 306:125–130, 1982.

31. Parish JM, Shepard JW. Cardiovascular effects of sleep disorders. *Chest.* 97:1220–1226, 1990.

32. Ancoli-Israel S, Klauber MR, Kripke DF, Parker L, Cobarrubias M. Sleep apnea in female patients in a nursing home: increased risk of mortality. *Chest.* 96:1054–1058, 1989.

33. Barach AL, Steiner A, Eckman M, Molomut N. The physiologic action of oxygen and carbon dioxide on the coronary circulation, as shown by blood gas and electrocardiographic studies. *Am Heart J.* 22:13–34, 1941.

34. Waldhorn RE, Herrick TW, Nguyen MC, O'Donnell AE, Sodero J, Potolicchio SJ. Long-term compliance with nasal continuous positive airway pressure therapy of obstructive sleep apnea. *Chest.* 97:33–38, 1990.

35. McDermott I, Bach JR, Parker C, Sorter S. Custom-fabricated interfaces for intermittent positive pressure ventilation. *Int J Prosthodont.* 2:224–233, 1989.

36. Bonham PE, Currier GF, Orr WC, Othman J, Nanda RS. The effect of a modified functional appliance on obstructive sleep apnea. *Am J Orthod Detofac Orthop.* 94:384–392, 1988.

37. Clark GT, Nakano M. Dental appliances for the treatment of obstructive sleep apnea. *J Am Dent Assoc.* 118:611–619, 1989.

38. Katsantonis GP, Walsh JK, Schweitzer PK, Friedman WH. Further evaluation of uvulopalatopharyngoplasty in the treatment of obstructive sleep apnea syndrome. *Otolaryngol Head Neck Surg.* 93:224–250, 1985.

39. Thawley SE. Surgical treatment of obstructive sleep apnea. *Med Clin North Am.* 69:1337–1358, 1985.

40. Riley RW, Powell NB, Guilleminault C, Mino-Murcia G. Maxillary, mandibular, and hyoid advancement: an alternative to tracheostomy in obstructive sleep apnea syndrome. *Otolaryngol Head Neck Surg.* 94:584–588, 1986.

41. O'Donohue W. Maximum volume IPPB for the management of pulmonary atelectasis. *Chest.* 76:683–687, 1976.

42. Dail C, Rogers M, Guess V, Adkins HV. *Glossopharyngeal Breathing Manual.* Downey, Calif: Professional Staff Association of Rancho Los Amigos Hospital, Inc; 1979.

43. Dail CW, Affeldt JE. *Glossopharyngeal Breathing* [videotape]. Los Angeles, Calif: Department of Visual Education, College of Medical Evangelists; 1954.

44. Huldtgren AC, Fugl-Meyer AR, Jonasson E, Bake B. Ventilatory dysfunction and respiratory rehabilitation in post-traumatic quadriplegia. *Eur J Respir Dis.* 61:347–356, 1980.

45. Barach AL, Beck GJ, Smith H. Mechanical production of expiratory flow rates surpassing the capacity of human coughing. *Am J Med Sci.* 226:241–248, 1953.

46. Bickerman HA, Itkin S. Exsufflation with negative pressure. *Arch Intern Med.* 93:698–703, 1954.

47. The OEM Cof-flator Portable Cough Machine. St. Louis, Mo: Shampaine Industries.

48. Bach JR. Update and perspectives on noninvasive respiratory muscle aids: part 2 — the expiratory muscle aids. *Chest.* In press.

49. Bach JR, Zeelenberg A, Winter C. Wheelchair mounted robot manipulators: long term use by patients with Duchenne muscular dystrophy. *Am J Phys Med Rehabil.* 69:59–69, 1990.

50. Bach J, O'Brien J, Krotenberg R, Alba A. Respiratory management of patients with Duchenne muscular dystrophy. *Arch Phys Med Rehabil.* 66:524–527, 1985.

51. Braun NMT, Marino WD. Effect of daily intermittent rest of

respiratory muscles in patients with severe chronic airflow limitation. *Chest.* 85:59s, 1984.

52. Cropp A, DiMarco AF. Effects of intermittent negative pressure ventilation on respiratory muscle function in patients with severe chronic obstructive disease. *Am Rev Respir Dis.* 135:1056–1061, 1987.

53. Ambrosino N, Montagni T, Negri A, Brega S, Fracchia C, Rampulla C. Negative pressure ventilation induces long term improvement of exercise tolerance of COPD patients. *Eur Resp J.* 2:263s, 1989. Abstract.

54. Ellis ER, Bye PTP, Bruderer JW, Sullivan CE. Treatment of respiratory failure during sleep in patients with neuromuscular disease, positive-pressure ventilation through a nose mask. *Am Rev Respir Dis.* 135:148–152, 1987.

55. Kerby GR, Mayer LS, Pingleton SK. Nocturnal positive pressure ventilation via nasal mask. *Am Rev Respir Dis.* 135: 738–740, 1987.

56 Goldstein RS, Molotiu N, Skrastins R, Long S, Contreras M. Assisting ventilation in respiratory failure by negative pressure ventilation and by rocking bed. *Chest.* 92:470–474, 1987.

57. Drinker PA, McKhann CF. The iron lung. *JAMA.* 255:1476–1480, 1986.

58. Kinnear W, Petch M, Taylor G, Shneerson J. Assisted ventilation using cuirass respirators. *Eur Respir J.* 1:198–302, 1988.

59. Splaingard ML, Frates RC, Jefferson LS, Rosen CL, Harrison, GM. Home negative pressure ventilation: report of 20 years of experience in patients with neuromuscular disease. *Arch Phys Med Rehabil.* 66:239–242, 1985.

60. Bach, JR. A historical perspective on the use of noninvasive ventilatory support alternatives. In: Kutscher AH, ed. *The Ventilator: Psychosocial and Medical Aspects; Muscular Dystrophy, Amyotrophic Lateral Sclerosis, and Other Diseases.* New York, NY: Foundation of Thanatology; In press.

61. Bach JR, Alba AS. Total ventilatory support by the intermittent abdominal pressure ventilator. *Chest.* 99:630–636, 1991.

62. Curran FJ, Colbert AP. Ventilator management in Duchenne muscular dystrophy and postpoliomyelitis syndrome: twelve years' experience. *Arch Phys Med Rehabil.* 70:180–185, 1989.

63. Higgins ITT. Epidemiology of bronchitis and emphysema. In: Fishman AP, ed. *Pulmonary Diseases and Disorders.* 2nd ed. New York, NY: McGraw-Hill; 1988.

64. Hodgkin JE, Zorn EG, Connors GL. *Pulmonary Rehabilitation: Guidelines to Success.* Boston, Mass: Butterworth; 1984.

65. Jones NL, Campbell EJM. *Clinical Exercise Testing.* Philadelphia, Pa: W.B. Saunders; 1982.

66. Dimarco AF, Kelling JS, Dimarco MS, Jacobs I, Shields R, Altose MD. The effects of inspiratory resistive training on respiratory muscle function in patients with muscular dystrophy. *Muscle Nerve.* 8:284–290, 1985.

23

Rehabilitation of Swallowing Disorders in the Elderly

Jeffrey B. Palmer and Ann S. DuChane

Impairments of swallowing are common in the elderly and cause significant morbidity and mortality. They may result from stroke, nervous system disorders, connective tissue diseases, cancer, or other illnesses common in elderly individuals (1–3). In this chapter, we will briefly review the physiology of normal and abnormal swallowing, present basic principles in rehabilitation of swallowing disorders, and discuss several specific disorders in more detail. We will focus on disorders of the oral and pharyngeal stages of swallowing since these are the most amenable to rehabilitative management.

A number of concepts underlie the rehabilitation of swallowing impairments. Rehabilitation requires accurate appraisal of pathophysiology, diagnosis, and prognosis. However, it is usually not possible to reduce the underlying physiologic impairment. Instead, we focus on reducing disability through therapeutic and compensatory strategies. The guiding principle is to maintain adequate alimentation and hydration while establishing the circumstances of safe, efficient swallowing. The ultimate goal is to reduce handicap, allowing the patient to resume essential premorbid social roles. A basic rule of rehabilitation is that the best exercise for an activity is generally the activity itself. Thus, the core of the rehabilitation program is establishing a safe program of therapeutic feeding (4).

NORMAL SWALLOWING

Swallowing is a complex act, involving the coordinated activity of more than 25 muscles (Fig. 23.1) (5, 6). It occurs in relation to several processes, such as feeding, mastication, respiration, and digestion. Food is first placed in the mouth. The oral preparatory stage precedes the swallow. During this stage, food particles are reduced to a smaller size, and food consistency is altered by mixing with saliva. The food is propelled to the posterior oral cavity, where a bolus is formed between the tongue and the hard palate. Liquids boluses are generally held in the oral cavity until the time of swallow onset, but solid foods are handled differently (7). A small preswallow bolus of chewed solid food may be transported through the faucial pillars and into the oropharynx several seconds before swallow onset, while chewing continues. When the food is ready for swallowing, the anterior tongue contacts the roof of the mouth. The area of contact rapidly moves posteriorly, propelling the bolus into the pharynx. This propulsion constitutes the oral stage of swallowing (7).

Next, there is a complex, rapid, nearly synchronous series of events called the pharyngeal stage of swallowing (Fig. 23.2) (5, 6). The soft palate rises and contacts the posterior and lateral pharyngeal walls, which bulge inward. The hyoid bone and larynx are pulled upward and forward toward the chin (laryngeal elevation). This opens the pharyngoesophageal (PE) segment by pulling the cricoid cartilage (with the attached anterior pharyngeal wall) away from the posterior pharyngeal wall. At the same time, the cricopharyngeus muscle relaxes for about one-half second, allowing the PE segment to open (Fig. 23.3). This muscle holds the PE segment closed between swallows. The hypopharynx (inferior portion of the pharynx) rises with the larynx, shortening the pharynx. The tongue pushes posteriorly and downward into the pharynx, propelling the bolus through the pharynx and into the esophagus. The pharyngeal walls contract around the bolus with a wave of sequential contraction that begins at the level of the palate and sweeps downward. This produces a stripping action that empties the pharynx of residue. The pharyngoesophageal segment closes, and the oral, pharyngeal, and laryngeal structures return to their reference positions. After entering the esophagus, the bolus is propelled downward by a peristaltic wave. (In the upright position, this is strongly assisted by gravity.) The gastroesophageal sphincter relaxes, and the bolus is finally propelled into the stomach.

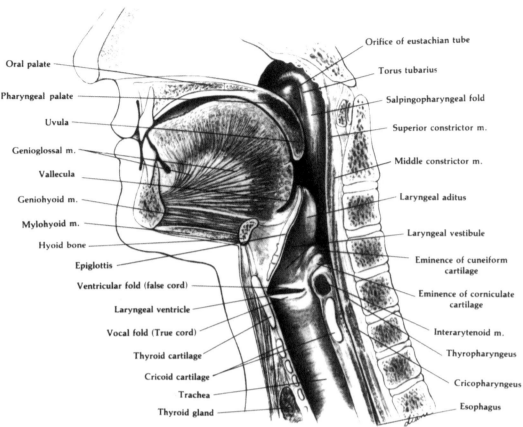

Figure 23.1.   The anatomy of the pharynx. Sagittal view of the principle anatomic landmarks of mouth, pharynx, and upper esophagus, as well as related structures of upper airway. From Donner MW, Bosma JF, Robertson DL. Anatomy and physiology of the pharynx. *Gastrointest Radiol.* 10:196–212, 1985.

Gastroesophageal reflux is prevented by the gastroesophageal sphincter, which is closed between swallows. Regurgitation from the esophagus to the pharynx is prevented by the cricopharyngeus muscle, which contracts continuously between swallows. This also prevents air from entering the esophagus during inhalation. Cricopharyngeus muscle relaxation during swallowing permits the PE segment to open. However, the active mechanism of opening is upward and anterior displacement of the larynx (5).

Several mechanisms protect the trachea from contamination by food during swallowing. Respiration ceases with the onset of swallow. The larynx is pulled forward, under the base of the tongue. The epiglottis folds over the larynx, deflecting the bolus into lateral food channels. The larynx closes tightly at the level of the glottis (vocal folds) and laryngeal vestibule (supraglottic portion of the larynx). If a small portion of the bolus is misdirected into the larynx, it is immediately ejected by reflex laryngeal closure or coughing.

Neuroanatomy

The neuroanatomy pertinent to swallowing is intricate (6). Sensation in the oral cavity (other than taste) is carried by the trigeminal nerve. Pharyngeal and laryngeal sensation are carried by the glossopharyngeal and vagus nerves. Afferent projections of these three nerves converge on the nucleus solitarius. A neural center for swallowing is thought to lie adjacent to this nucleus in the reticular formation of the brainstem.

Lower motor neurons (LMNs) for the muscles of mastication travel in the trigeminal nerve and originate in its motor nucleus. Intrinsic muscles of the tongue are supplied by LMNs of the hypoglossal nucleus and nerve. The intrinsic muscles of the larynx, pharynx, and upper esophagus are supplied by LMNs that originate in the ipsilateral nucleus ambiguous and travel (primarily) in the vagus nerve. The lower esophagus is innervated by parasympathetic pathways originating in the dorsal motor nucleus of the vagus nerve. Whereas the LMNs of swallowing are all ipsilateral to the muscles, the upper motor neurons (UMNs) lie on both sides of the brain.

Swallowing involves both smooth and skeletal muscles. The oral cavity, pharynx, and larynx contain striated muscle only. The esophagus contains skeletal muscle in its upper third and smooth muscle below. Skeletal muscle requires input from the central nervous system, but the smooth muscle portion of the esophagus may function autonomously.

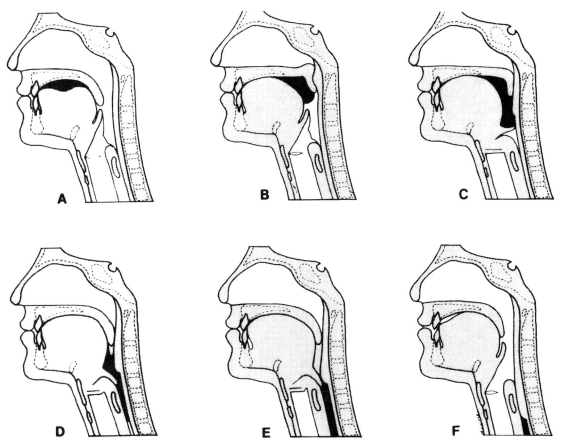

Figure 23.2 The normal swallow as seen from the lateral view. The airway is shown in white; bony structures are shown in dashed line. **A.** Bolus is held in the oral cavity with the surrounding laryngeal structures and airway at rest. **B.** Bolus is conveyed into the oropharynx. The larynx and pharynx have begun elevating in preparation for swallow. The velum has made contact with the pharyngeal wall, sealing the nasopharynx. **C.** Bolus is descending in advance of the descending wave of pharyngeal constriction. The epiglottis is now horizontal and is outlined within the bolus, with the bolus descending into the hypopharynx. The larynx has reached its maximum elevation. **D.** Bolus continues through the hypopharynx, through the open pharyngoesophageal (PE) segment, into the esophagus, with the peristaltic wave descending behind it. The nasopharynx begins to open, and the opening progresses in a descending sequence. **E.** The wave of pharyngeal contraction has obliterated the oropharyngeal cavity and moved into the hypopharynx, with the bolus descending further through the open PE segment into the esophagus. The nasopharyngeal airway continues to open in a cephalocaudal fashion. **F.** Bolus has disappeared into the esophagus. All structures have returned to the open position; the normal contours of the airway are again visible, although the larynx has not yet completed the descent to its original resting position. From Donner MW, Bosma JF, Robertson DL: Anatomy and physiology of the pharynx. *Gastrointest Radiol.* 10:196–212, 1985.

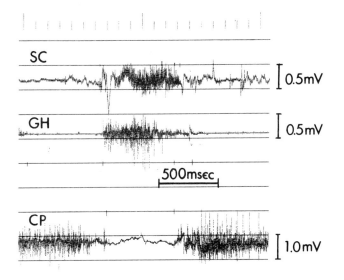

Figure 23.3 Myoelectric activity during a water swallow, simultaneously recorded in the superior pharyngeal constrictor (SC), geniohyoid (GH), and cricopharyngeus (CP) muscles, using hooked wire electrodes. From Palmer JB, Tanaka E, Siebens AA. Electromyography of the pharyngeal musculature: technical considerations. *Arch Phys Med Rehabil.* 70:283–287, 1989.

Neurophysiology

Central nervous system control varies among the stages of swallowing (6). The oral preparatory stage is under voluntary control, the pharyngeal stage is semiautomatic, and the esophageal phase is involuntary. The motions of these oral, pharyngeal, laryngeal, and esophageal structures are produced by complex interactions of various brainstem reflexes and rhythm generators.

The initiation of pharyngeal swallowing is poorly understood. Receptive fields for elicitation of reflex swallowing in animal preparations involve three cranial nerves (trigeminal, glossopharyngeal, and vagus) and a variety of receptors. Swallowing is normally initiated while the bolus is located in the oral cavity and/or oropharynx. Receptors in the oral cavity assess the physical characteristics of the food to determine whether it is appropriate for swallowing. Initiation of swallowing is intimately related to control of jaw motion. Swallow onset occurs while the upper and lower teeth are close together, but not necessarily in contact (7).

The neural control of pharyngeal swallowing is complex. Two alternative explanations have been proposed. The first postulates that swallowing is controlled by a central pattern generator, and swallowing occurs when this pattern generator responds to stimuli. According to this hypothesis, every swallow must be identical in terms of motor activity since the pattern is fixed by neuronal circuitry. This hypothesis is supported by data showing that the sequence of muscle activity during swallowing is highly reproducible under a variety of conditions.

The second hypothesis postulates that swallowing is controlled by a chain of reflexes. The motions produced by each reflex in the chain produce afferent activity in the nervous system. This afferent activity then elicits the next reflex in the chain. Thus, each event depends on the outcome of the prior event in the chain. There is variability in each reflex, so substantial variability in the overall pattern of swallowing exists. This hypothesis is supported by data showing variability in the strength and duration of contraction of particular muscles among different swallows in the same subject. Although data support the existence of a central pattern generator, recent reports show that peripheral sensory input and volition can modify the swallow (6, 8).

PATHOPHYSIOLOGY OF SWALLOWING DYSFUNCTION

Swallowing has two basic purposes. The first, and most obvious, is transport of food from the oral cavity to the stomach. The second is protection of the airway. It clears the pharynx and prevents inappropriate material from entering the larynx, trachea, and lungs. Disorders of swallowing, regardless of etiology, may jeopardize airway integrity, cause failure of transport, or both. Analyzing the mechanisms of food transport and airway protection is critical to the evaluation of every patient.

Specific Abnormalities of Swallowing

ORAL STAGE

Oral stage abnormalities include the inability to prepare food for swallowing (by forming a swallow-safe bolus), inability to transfer food to the oropharynx, and inability to retain food in the oral cavity before swallowing. Tongue control is essential to oral function. Weakness or incoordination of the tongue may cause retention of food in the buccal recesses, failure of oral transport, or uncontrolled movement of food into the oropharynx under the influence of gravity. Furthermore, a spastic tongue may obstruct oral transport.

Normal swallowing requires coordination of oral food transport with pharyngeal swallowing and respiration. If the onset of swallowing is delayed, serious problems may result. Swallow onset occurs promptly when liquid enters the pharynx in normal individuals. Delayed onset of swallowing creates a risk for aspiration; liquid may flow into the larynx under the influence of gravity. Solid food may be inhaled and obstruct the airway with potentially lethal consequences Delayed onset of swallowing is a common abnormality (3, 9).

VELOPHARYNGEAL CLOSURE

Velopharyngeal dysfunction results from inadequate apposition of the velum to the posterior and lateral pharyngeal walls. Patients may experience regurgitation of liquids into the nasal cavity. The incompetent velopharyngeal seal also forms an escape valve, impairing pressure generation within the pharynx, limiting bolus propulsion into the esophagus.

LARYNGEAL PROTECTION

Aspiration is defined as passage of food through the vocal folds. Aspiration of microscopic quantities is a physiologic event, but with larger quantities it is uncommon in normal individuals (10). Aspiration can occur before, during, or after swallowing. Before the swallow, it is commonly caused by delayed swallow, with prolonged exposure of the pharynx to food before swallowing. Aspiration during the swallow may occur if laryngeal closure is delayed or incomplete. Following the swallow, food retained in the pharynx may enter the larynx under the influence of gravity. Another mechanism for aspiration is inhalation of food. It may occur before or after the swallow.

The clinical consequences of aspiration are highly variable (11). Some patients sustain serious illness (such as aspiration pneumonia) in response to aspiration, while others suffer no ill effects. The risk of illness due to aspiration depends on several factors. One factor is the depth of aspiration, that is, whether the material merely enters the subglottic portion of the larynx or actually passes down into the distal airways and lung. A second factor is the nature of the aspirated material. Aspiration of solid food may be disastrous if it obstructs the airway. Acids are much more harmful to the lung than are alkali, so stomach contents are particularly hazardous. A third factor is the amount of material aspirated; a tiny amount is usually well tolerated. Finally, the response to aspiration is critical (12, 13). Sequelae are unlikely if prompt, effective coughing clears the larynx and trachea. However, airway protection reflexes are often impaired in dysphagic individuals. Aspiration that fails to elicit coughing (so-called "silent" aspiration) often leads to respiratory sequelae.

PHARYNGEAL TRANSPORT

Normal subjects occasionally retain small amounts of food in the pharyngeal recesses after swallowing. Excessive retention of food in the pharynx after swallowing may be produced by obstruction of the foodway or by weakness or incoordination of pharyngeal contraction. Pharyngeal paresis may be caused by a reduction in tongue driving force or weakness of pharyngeal constrictor muscles (5). Unilateral constrictor palsy usually results from LMN dysfunction subsequent to lesions of the nucleus ambiguus or vagus nerve.

The opening of the pharyngoesophageal segment is a complex process. The larynx moves anteriorly, dilating the segment, and the cricopharyngeus muscle relaxes. Functional narrowing of the pharyngoesophageal segment may be caused by a reduction in anterior motion of the larynx during swallow or by the presence of a posterior pharyngeal "bar" defect that impinges on the lumen. The physiologic basis for this bar defect has been presumed to be sustained contraction (failure of relaxation) of the cricopharyngeus muscle during swallowing. Indeed, this is the basis for performing a cricopharyngeal myotomy. During this procedure, the cricopharyngeus muscle is disrupted to reduce the resistance of the pharyngeal outflow tract. However, dyssynergy of the cricopharyngeus muscle has never been verified with electromyography. The pathophysiology of the posterior pharyngeal bar remains unclear (5, 14).

ESOPHAGEAL FUNCTION

Esophageal disorders are quite common in the elderly (15, 16). The esophagus has two critical functions: transport of food from the pharynx to the stomach and prevention of gastroesophageal reflux and regurgitation. Impairment of esophageal transport may be caused by anatomical obstruction, derangement of esophageal peristalsis, or dysfunction of the gastroesophageal sphincter. Patients may experience pain, difficulty swallowing, or regurgitation of food from the esophagus back into the pharynx.

Gastroesophageal reflux disease may have serious sequelae. Ulceration and scarring of the esophageal mucosa by stomach acid may cause strictures with resultant esophageal obstruction. If refluxed material is regurgitated into the pharynx, it may be aspirated. Serious respiratory complications may ensue since the larynx and lungs are highly sensitive to acid. Patients with reflux disease may complain of pain, difficulty swallowing, hoarseness, and regurgitation of sour or partially digested material.

Effects of Aging

Differentiating the effects of normal aging from the effects of disease is a major problem. When an elderly patient complains of difficulty with feeding and swallowing, the etiology may be a current illness, the cumulative effects of numerous past illnesses, or the effects of normal aging.

Several studies have examined the effects of aging on oral function in healthy adults. Motor performance of the lips and tongue decreases with age on a variety of tasks (17). Older subjects differ from younger subjects in masticatory function, even with normal dentition. Older subjects chew their food for a longer time and for a greater number of chewing strokes before swallowing. However, food particles are eventually reduced to a size that subjects feel they can swallow safely. This "swallow-safe" particle size does not vary with age (18). Subtle abnormalities of hyoid motion have been shown with ultrasonography. The duration of hyoid motion during swallowing increases with age. Older subjects often make multiple gestures of the tongue and hyoid bone prior to swallowing (19, 20).

Tracy and colleagues (21) recently studied differences in pharyngeal swallowing among different aged adults. Increasing bolus volume reduced the oral transit time of the head of the bolus, presumably because the head of the bolus was positioned closer to the pharynx prior to swallowing. The duration of opening of the pharyngoesophageal segment was longer for higher volumes. These effects were seen in subjects of all ages. The latency from entry of the bolus into the pharynx until the onset of laryngeal elevation increased with age. This finding was recently confirmed by Robbins et al (22). The effect of aging on the strength of pharyngeal contraction (measured manometrically) remains controversial.

Esophageal function also changes with age. Sliding hiatal hernia is more common in the elderly. Whether gastroesophageal acid reflux increases with age is uncertain; studies conflict in this regard. The amplitude of esophageal peristaltic contractions decreases with age (15, 16).

Oral, pharyngeal, and esophageal function change subtly with age in healthy adults. However, the clinical significance of these changes is unknown. It remains unclear whether these changes cause or contribute to disability. Physiologic test data (such as videofluorographic or manometric data) should be interpreted cautiously in elderly patients. Norms developed with younger populations may not apply to older individuals.

PRINCIPLES OF PATIENT EVALUATION

Medical History

The case history must be carefully scrutinized since the evidence for abnormal swallowing may be subtle. Gradual changes in diet or eating habits may mask early physiologic or organic changes (16). Data suggestive of impaired swallowing include: complaints of choking, coughing, or discomfort with swallowing; alterations in diet; history of pneumonia or respiratory complications; history of surgery, especially of the head and neck; and unexplained weight loss or dehydration.

Certain medications may impair oral, pharyngeal, or esophageal function. These include many psychotropic medications. Neuroleptic medications (phenothiazines and butyrophenones) or metoclopramide may produce irreversible involuntary movement disorders of the orofacial muscles. Benzodiazepines may produce or worsen incoordination of oropharyngeal swallowing (23). Tricyclic antidepressants have anticholinergic effects, which inhibit esophageal motility and reduce salivary flow. The medication history should be reviewed carefully in dysphagic individuals since medications may produce or exacerbate impairments of swallowing.

Psychosocial factors may have a significant impact on swallowing, especially for elderly individuals. An individual living alone may be unable to obtain supervision during meals. For a nursing home resident, prescribing a special diet may be unrealistic. Swallowing must be considered in the context of feeding. Feeding dependency is an enormous problem for the elderly (24). Problems with feeding may be difficult to differentiate from impairments of swallowing, per se.

Physical Examination

A careful examination is critical to patient evaluation. The upper aerodigestive tract is examined as a series of functional components that prepare the food, form a bolus, propel it from the lips to the esophagus, and protect the larynx. The tongue is tested for bulk, tone, and active range of motion (ROM). The velum is examined for position and symmetry at rest and during motion. The neck is palpated, and the larynx is mobilized manually. Laryngeal elevation is assessed during swallowing. Other components of the swallowing mechanism are similarly assessed.

Communication and cognitive function are frequently abnormal in dysphagic patients and should be assessed carefully (25). Speech is examined for dysphonia or dysarthria. Language, hearing, and cognitive abilities must be understood in order for clinicians to provide appropriate instructions. Severely impaired patients may be unable to learn compensatory maneuvers for safe swallowing. Physical findings must be interpreted cautiously. One must try to differentiate changes attributable to normal aging from those caused by disease. Normative data for many speech assessment tasks are lacking for elderly individuals.

The comprehensive examination includes observing the patient eating and drinking. Behaviors that should be noted include drooling, slow rate of eating, residual food in the mouth after swallowing, frequent throat clearing, change in voice quality, and posturing of the head and neck with swallowing. The method of feeding (e.g., cup or straw), position of the patient, and need for supervision should be noted.

The purpose of the physical examination is to assess components of the swallowing mechanism, to characterize the nature and severity of the swallowing deficit, to assess the patient's ability to perform compensatory maneuvers, and to determine whether a videofluorographic swallowing study is necessary. The examination can not prove the presence or absence of aspiration (26).

Radiologic Evaluation

Radiography has a critical role in evaluation of normal and abnormal swallowing (1–4, 9, 27–29). The videofluorographic swallowing study (VFSS) is a safe, effective procedure for evaluating foodway function. Videofluorography is generally preferred over cineradiography as it provides a lower radiation dose and the capacity for immediate playback. The VFSS provides precise pathophysiologic data for accurate diagnosis and rehabilitation. The objective of the VFSS is to obtain high quality images of swallowing to evaluate the mechanism of swallowing. In patients with oral and pharyngeal swallowing dysfunction, it also demonstrates the circumstances that result in safe and unsafe swallowing (4, 29–31) The VFSS should be performed by a team of individuals who understand the functional anatomy of swallowing, are experienced with the procedure, and are familiar with the patient. Ideally, the team includes the attending physician and speech-language pathologist (29).

During the VFSS, the patient is seated comfortably with adequate support and eats a variety of radiopaque solid and liquid foods. Images are recorded in lateral and posterior-anterior projections. Abnormalities of structure and function are noted with particular attention to the mechanisms of oral and pharyngeal food transport and of laryngeal protection. The esophagus is screened routinely in the upright position to exclude gross dysfunction. If esophageal pathology is suspected, further imaging is performed with the patient recumbent.

The rehabilitation approach to videofluorography is to have the patient eat various radio-opacified foods, using appropriate modifications, towards the goal of establishing a safe and efficient method of eating. An empirical approach is used to identify variables associated with safe and unsafe swallowing. Variables commonly analyzed include physical consistency of food, posture of the patient (especially position of the head and neck), and the means for presenting the food. These variables are altered systematically during the VFSS, and the effects on swallowing are observed (29–31).

The physical consistency of the food is a critical variable (32). Many patients experience aspiration or failure of bolus transport with foods of some consistencies but not others. Liquids are categorized as thin (e.g., water, clear juices), thick (e.g., nectar) or ultrathick (e.g., custard). For most patients, thick liquids are easier to control than thin liquids and produce less aspiration. Solid foods are categorized as formable (easily formed into a bolus), particulate, multitextured, and crunchy. As the complexity of the texture increases, the difficulty of controlling the bolus increases (Table 23.1) (29).

Dynamic imaging is currently the sine qua non of diagnostic tests. Only dynamic imaging can show the swallowing mechanism at work in real time. However, static imaging has an important role in evaluation of swallowing disorders. Plain radiographs provide much better image resolution and clarity than do video images. Static imaging reveals subtle abnormalities of structure that may not be visible on the dynamic recording. Plain radiographs are also much less expensive than videofluorography and can often be obtained at the bedside. Indications for a VFSS in a patient with symptoms of swallowing dysfunction include frequent choking episodes, difficulty managing secretions, wet-hoarse voice quality, respiratory complications, and unexplained weight loss. Relative contraindications include inability to cooperate with the examination and severe respiratory dysfunction.

Other Studies

ENDOSCOPY

Endoscopy is useful for visualizing the larynx, pharynx, and esophagus. It is essential for detecting and identifying mucosal lesions and is also helpful in evaluating motor and sensory function.

MANOMETRY

Manometry (pressure recording) is valuable for evaluating the strength and coordination of esophageal peristalsis and function of the lower esophageal sphincter. More recently, manometry has been used for eval-

Table 23.1. Characteristics of Solids and Liquids

Characteristic	Liquids	Solids
Ease of deformation	High	Low
Tendency to flow	High	Low
Tendency to leak	High	Low
Passage through narrow passages	Easy	Difficult
Need for mastication	Little	Much
Risk of aspiration[a]	High[b]	Low
Risk of laryngeal obstruction[a]	Low	High
Risk of pharyngeal retention[a]	Low	High

[a] These characteristics are greatly simplified to provide a frame of reference. They are not true in every case.
[b] The risk of laryngeal penetration is usually lower for thick than for thin liquids.

uating motor activity of the pharynx and pharyngoesophageal segment. Combining manometry with simultaneous videofluorography reveals the specific events associated with pharyngeal pressure waves (33).

ELECTROMYOGRAPHY

Electromyography is useful for detecting LMN dysfunction of the muscles of swallowing and differentiating LMN from UMN dysfunction. This is useful for rehabilitation since neuromuscular reeducation and strengthening techniques differ for the two types of dysfunction. Electromyography is also useful for detecting myopathy (34, 35)

RADIONUCLIDE SCINTIGRAPHY

Radionuclide scintigraphy is highly sensitive for detecting aspiration. It may also be useful for assessing pulmonary clearance mechanisms following glottic penetration (13).

PRINCIPLES OF TREATMENT

The aim of treatment is to provide adequate alimentation and hydration while establishing and maintaining conditions for safe swallowing, toward the long-term goal of resuming premorbid roles in society. Therapy is individualized on the basis of the holistic interdisciplinary evaluation. The efficacy of this approach is supported by clinical experience, including published reports. However, no controlled, prospective study of dysphagia rehabilitation has been reported. We will present basic principles of rehabilitative treatment. Pharmacologic and surgical therapies are beyond the scope of this chapter.

Therapeutic Feeding

A basic premise is that the best therapy for a swallowing disorder is swallowing itself. Whenever possible, oral feeding should be maintained. The diet prescription is based on the VFSS findings. For example, if a patient aspirated thin (but not thick) liquids, liquids should be thickened to a safe consistency. If tongue dysfunction prevents oral transport of particulate solid foods, then the solid food prescription should be limited to single texture, formable solids. Educating the patient and caregivers regarding the diet prescription and techniques for food preparation is an important part of this aspect of therapy.

Another important aspect of treatment is teaching physical maneuvers to facilitate safe swallowing. For many patients, swallowing with the neck flexed or rotated reduces laryngeal penetration or improves pharyngeal transport (36, 37). Some patients may recline, stand, or wear nose plugs to facilitate swallow. In addition, the bolus volume (38), method of presenting the food (e.g., spoon or cup), rate of eating, and need for supervision may be included in the prescription for safe swallowing (Table 23.2) (29). Patients with impaired opening of the pharyngoesophageal sphincter may learn to augment its opening volitionally. Voluntarily contracting the suprahyoid muscles (the Mendelsohn maneuver) pulls the hyoid and larynx forward, maintaining laryngeal elevation. This increases the extent and duration of sphincter opening (39).

Therapeutic Exercise

Some patients benefit from exercises to improve the flexibility, strength, and coordination of specific components of the swallowing mechanism. The variety of therapeutic exercises and maneuvers is great. Examples include range of motion or manual resistive exercises for the tongue, lips and/or jaw; object manipulation to improve tongue dexterity; or phonation exercises to increase vocal fold adduction. These exercises supplement, but do not replace, therapeutic feeding.

Pharyngeal Bypass

Patients with severe dysphagia or behavioral and cognitive deficits may be unable to maintain adequate nutrition and hydration via oral feeding. Irrespective of therapeutic feeding, nutritional needs must then be provided via a route that bypasses the pharynx (e.g., naso-gastric, gastrostomy, or jejunostomy tube feeding). The ability to eat and the socialization surrounding eating are important for quality of life. Some patients who receive a pharyngeal bypass can take some food by mouth for hedonic or social reasons. It is important to understand how the patient swallows in order to balance nutritional, health, and psychosocial needs. Whether tube feeding prevents aspiration is controversial (40).

Nasogastric tube feeding is useful for time-limited pharyngeal bypass in patients with acute illnesses. Prolonged nasogastric intubation is often uncomfortable and cosmetically unacceptable. Whether the presence of a nasogastric tube interferes with recovery of swallowing function remains conjectural.

Gastrostomy tube feeding is more acceptable for long-term pharyngeal bypass. Bolus feeding is preferred, as this method simulates normal ingestion. Gastroesophageal reflux disease is a relative contraindication to gastrostomy feeding in dysphagic patients. The tube-fed material may pass through the gastroesophageal sphincter, putting the patient at risk for regurgitation and subsequent aspiration of stomach contents. Radiographic or scintigraphic tube studies may detect aspiration subsequent to tube feedings (29). The risk of aspiration may be minimized by maintaining the upright position after feeding.

Jejunostomy tube feeding is preferred for patients with severe gastroesophageal reflux disease. Since the tube terminates in the jejunum, the pyloric sphincter helps to prevent reflux. However, bolus tube feeding is not possible with this method. Instead, the liquid diet must be infused slowly over a period of hours. This is quite unlike the normal rhythm of ingestion and may interfere with activities.

PHYSIOLOGIC DISORDERS

Physiologic disorders may affect swallowing and feeding by altering cognition, sensation, strength, or coordination. The pathophysiology varies depending on the part of the nervous system or musculoskeletal system affected. The site of the lesion (in the cerebrum, brainstem motor nuclei, cranial nerves, muscle, or connective tissue) is important for understanding the effects on the swallowing mechanism. The rehabilitation approach depends greatly on pathophysiology; it is less influenced by etiologic diagnosis.

Neurogenic disorders may alter sensation or motor activity essential to normal feeding and swallowing. UMN dysfunction often affects the strength and coordination of mastication and swallowing. These effects may be unilateral in the orofacial muscles, but are bilateral in the larynx and pharynx. LMN disorders produce weakness ipsilateral to the site of dysfunction. Myopathies produce symmetrical weakness of the muscles of swallowing, with no direct effect on sensation. How-

Table 23.2. Therapeutic and Compensatory Techniques

Head and neck position	Upright, flexed, extended, rotated
Trunk posture	Upright, reclined
Feeding devices	Spoon, cup, straw, glossectomy spoon, syringe, fork
Bolus volume	Small (<5 cc), moderate (5–15 cc), large (>15 cc)
Respiratory maneuvers	Coughing, throat clearing, supraglottic swallow
Clearance maneuvers	Double swallow, clearing liquid swallow, Mendelsohn maneuver

ever, chronic presence of saliva or other contaminants in the foodway or airway may produce accommodation of receptors in the mucosa. This effect may cause a secondary alteration of sensory performance in patients with motor dysfunction, with reduction in airway protective reflexes. We will discuss briefly several specific disorders.

Neurogenic Oral and Pharyngeal Dysfunction

STROKE

Dysphagia is a common problem after stroke; the incidence may be as high as 50% (41). Certain specific abnormalities of oral and pharyngeal swallowing occur commonly in stroke patients. Acute stroke may impair brainstem responses critical to airway protection, putting the patient at high risk for silent laryngeal penetration. This risk gradually abates in most patients. However, some continue to have significant impairments of swallowing (42).

Stroke may damage both UMN and LMN related to swallowing (43). UMN dysfunction may impair volitional control of mastication and oral food transport, as well as initiation of pharyngeal swallowing. It may also interfere with coordination and timing or oral and pharyngeal muscle activity, leading to entry of food into the pharynx long before initiation of swallowing. This is a major cause of laryngeal penetration and aspiration (44). UMN impairments of swallowing may be produced by unilateral or bilateral lesions of the cerebral cortex, diencephalon, or brainstem (45). Patients with lesions of the cerebellum or pons may exhibit impaired swallowing in association with movement disorders, including ataxia or palatal myoclonus (46).

Infarction of the medulla presents unique problems. Damage to the nucleus ambiguus (as in the lateral medullary syndrome) produces weakness of ipsilateral palatal, pharyngeal, and laryngeal muscles. The ipsilateral hemipharynx may become flaccid, resulting in failure of transport function (37). Similarly, infarction of the medial medulla may damage the hypoglossal nucleus, producing ipsilateral tongue weakness. The rehabilitation approach may be highly effective for restoring safe and efficient swallowing in stroke patients.

PARKINSON'S DISEASE

Individuals with Parkinson's disease typically exhibit abnormalities of the oral and pharyngeal stages of swallowing. Robbins (47) found that all her subjects with Parkinson's disease demonstrated abnormalities of swallowing on videofluorography, but only a portion complained of difficulty swallowing. Oral transport was characterized by repetitive tongue pumping. Onset of pharyngeal swallowing was delayed after the entry of food. Retention in the oral cavity and pharynx after swallow

lead to multiple swallows for a single bolus. Two subjects had glottic penetration of liquids during or after the swallow. Bradykinesia and rigidity appear to underlie the oral and pharyngeal motility disorders.

MOTOR NEURON DISEASE (MND)

Impaired swallowing is a frequent, disabling aspect of MND. Early in the disease course, patients may complain of choking, difficulty chewing, or food sticking in the foodway. Robbins (48) reported oral and pharyngeal stage abnormalities in MND. Patients with signs of pseudobulbar (UMN) dysfunction had difficulty with solid substances, whereas the patients with bulbar (LMN) signs had greater difficulty with liquids. Oral deficits were related to reduced force, coordination, and range of tongue movement. Bulbar patients demonstrated poor laryngeal elevation and glottic penetration before, during, and after swallowing. Logemann (3) reported finding poor lingual control and reduced pharyngal peristalsis early in the disease, with delayed pharyngeal swallowing response noted later. Ultimately, many patients require pharyngeal bypass as cranial motor nuclei become severely involved.

DEMENTIA

Impairments of feeding and swallowing are seen frequently in demented individuals. Many are dependent for feeding (23). Some dementing illnesses (e.g., Parkinson's disease, multiple cerebral infarctions) may directly affect the swallowing mechanism. The effect of Alzheimer's disease on the swallowing mechanism is unknown, but volitional aspects of eating are often affected by dementia. Demented patients may have difficulty recognizing and appropriately bringing food to the mouth. Impulsive patients may overload their mouths with food, putting themselves at risk for choking and aspiration. Alterations in orofacial reflexes (e.g., exaggerated snout, tongue thrusting, or biting reflexes) have a profound effect on oral function. Rehabilitation is difficult because of the limited ability to learn therapeutic and compensatory techniques (29).

POSTOPERATIVE CRANIAL NERVE DYSFUNCTION

Impaired swallowing may follow surgical procedures affecting the brain or cranial nerves. The pathophysiology is similar to that described for stroke. Patients are often dysphagic initially, but most recover quickly. The precise effects on swallowing depend on the site of injury. Injury of the cerebrum may impair cognition and UMN function. Brainstem or peripheral cranial nerve injury may produce LMN dysfunction with ipsilateral weakness (35). Surgery adjacent to the brainstem may cause severe dysphagia due to injury of multiple cranial nerves. Many of these patients benefit from a multidisciplinary rehabilitation approach; however, some never regain functional swallowing.

Connective Tissue Disease

INFLAMMATORY MUSCLE DISEASE

Inflammatory diseases of striated muscle (polymyositis and dermatomyositis) cause weakness of the pharyngeal musculature. About 20% of patients complain of dysphagia (49). In our experience, VFSSs in these patients may show apparent incoordination of the muscles of swallowing, although the physiologic basis for this is unclear. The dysphagia usually improves markedly with pharmacotherapy for the underlying disorder. In severe end-stage disease, it may not. These patients often benefit from a multidisciplinary rehabilitation approach, including a VFSS.

SCLERODERMA (SYSTEMIC SCLEROSIS)

In contrast to inflammatory muscle diseases, scleroderma affects smooth muscle of the foodway (50). Esophageal dysfunction develops early in the majority of patients with scleroderma and constitutes the most common manifestation of internal organ involvement. Manometry shows reduced propulsive force of the lower esophagus in about 90% of patients. Esophageal peristalsis may be diminished or absent, and dilation of the lower esophagus eventually occurs. Food is often retained in the lower esophagus. Gastroesophageal reflux is common and may lead to peptic esophagitis, ulceration, and strictures.

Patients complain of difficulty swallowing due to the esophageal dysfunction. They may avoid foods that cause dysphagia and take care to masticate thoroughly before swallowing. The dysphagia is usually worse for solids than liquids. Therapy for gastroesophageal reflux is essential to prevent its complications. If strictures are present, therapeutic dilation may be necessary periodically.

ESOPHAGEAL DISORDERS

Esophageal dysfunction is common in the elderly and may coexist with oral and pharyngeal stage deficits. Esophageal disorders may present with symptoms similar to those of pharyngeal abnormalities. These disorders are often chronic and may have serious sequelae (15).

Esophageal disorders commonly present with dysphagia, chest pain, and heartburn. A thorough evaluation is necessary since esophageal dysfunction may have many causes, including both structural and functional disorders. Dysphagia for solids only suggests a mechanical obstruction. Dysphagia for solids and liquids suggests a motility disorder. Intermittent dysphagia may be due to esophageal spasm. Progressive dysphagia with

heartburn suggests scleroderma. Progressive dysphagia without heartburn may be caused by achalasia. This disease causes loss of esophageal contractility and stenosis of the lower esophageal sphincter. Progressive obstruction of the esophagus may be caused by esophageal cancer, a disease with high morbidity and mortality. Gastroesophageal reflux disease is common, but whether it is more common in the elderly is unclear. The potential for complications of reflux is great in elderly patients. Treatment for esophageal dysfunction is complex, including behavioral, pharmacologic, and surgical therapies (15).

STRUCTURAL DISORDERS

A number of structural disorders cause swallowing impairment. These may mimic physiologic disorders since their effects (failure of transport or airway protection) are similar. A high index of suspicion is necessary to avoid misdiagnosis. Transport functions are commonly disrupted by structural disorders. Obstruction of the foodway by a mass or stricture may prevent bolus transport via a direct mechanical effect. Surgical excision of foodway structures may impair or prevent bolus propulsion. Stiffness or fixation of foodway structures (due to fibrosis or infiltration) may also impair bolus transport by altering muscle contractility. Airway protection may be compromised by fixation or surgical alteration of the larynx, tongue, or suprahyoid muscles. Foodway obstruction may secondarily affect airway protection if a large bolus accumulates adjacent to the laryngeal aditus (opening).

Cervical Spine Disorders

Disorders of the axial skeleton may impair swallowing. Osteophytes of the cervical spine may impinge on the pharyngeal foodway, obstructing transport (51). Excessive cervical lordosis may impair airway protection by impeding laryngeal elevation. Critical foodway structures may be damaged in cervical spine injuries. Prevertebral or retropharyngeal hemorrhage may obstruct the foodway. Rehabilitation strategies, such as modification of diet or posture, are frequently effective, and surgical treatment is rarely necessary.

Webs and Strictures

These soft tissue structures are usually asymptomatic unless they obstruct the foodway. A web is a membranous narrowing of the foodway covered entirely by mucosa (52). Webs are most commonly seen in the pharyngoesophageal segment and may be associated with iron deficiency anemia (Plummer-Vinson syndrome). Pharyngeal strictures are usually due to ingestion of caustic substances such as lye. These lesions may be notoriously difficult to treat. Esophageal strictures are caused by mucosal injury, usually induced by chronic acid reflux or medication. Obstructing lesions are usually treated by esophageal dilation. Removing the source of mucosal irritation is essential to preventing progression or recurrence (15).

Diverticula

Diverticula may occur in the pharynx or esophagus. The Zenker diverticulum is relatively common. This is a posterior diverticulum of the hypopharynx just above the cricopharyngeus muscle. Its etiology is uncertain, but it is thought to be a pulsion diverticulum that occurs at a weak point in the pharyngeal constrictor muscles (53). Food collects in the diverticulum and may suddenly reenter the unprepared pharynx sometime later. This can cause complaints of regurgitation and choking and may lead to aspiration. Some diverticula become very large and obstruct the foodway by external compression. Zenker diverticula may require surgical treatment, such as excision of the diverticulum. This operation usually includes cricopharyngeal myotomy, which is thought to reduce pharyngeal outflow tract resistance.

Cancer of the Oral Cavity, Larynx, and Pharynx

Malignant tumors of the oral cavity, larynx, and pharynx are quite common but rarely cause dysphagia. Therapy generally includes surgical excision, radiation, or both. Surgical techniques vary greatly, depending on the size and location of the tumor. The effects on swallowing depend on what structures are deleted, how the wounds are closed, and what reconstruction is performed (if any). These procedures may cause serious impairments of swallowing and speech (3, 54). Restoration of communicative and ingestive function is a formidable challenge. We will discuss briefly several of the more common situations.

ORAL CAVITY

Treatment for cancers of the oral cavity often includes partial or total glossectomy and mandibulectomy. The tongue is critical for mastication, oral food transport, and swallowing. Partial glossectomy may greatly reduce the mobility and strength of the tongue, making it ineffective for bolus transport and control in the oral cavity. The pharyngeal stage of swallowing may be affected to a lesser degree. Limiting the diet to soft food is often necessary. The oral cavity may be bypassed with devices that present food directly to the pharynx. These include a syringe with a short plastic tube (for liquids and semisolids) and a glossectomy spoon (for soft solids). The latter incorporates a piston-like mechanism to push the food off the end of the spoon, directly into the oropharynx. Intraoral prosthetics are sometimes helpful for reshaping the oral contour following an excision (55). These provide a smaller oral cavity, more manageable for the mobility-impaired tongue.

PHARYNX

Cancer of the pharynx often necessitates removal or disruption of many structures important to swallowing (3, 54). These include the base of the tongue, palate, faucial pillars, hyoid bone, epiglottis, larynx, and pharyngeal constrictors. The pharyngeal stage of swallowing may be severely impaired, with failure of both pharyngeal transport and laryngeal protection. Oral food transport may also be affected, due to a loss of tongue mobility. Bolus formation and control may be impaired. Stasis in the pharyngeal recesses is common.

LARYNX

Supraglottic laryngectomy is often performed for cancer of the supraglottic region, including tumors of the false vocal folds, epiglottis, or valleculae. This procedure deletes portions of the larynx above the vocal folds, including the epiglottis, laryngeal vestibule, false vocal folds, and a portion of the tongue. These structures are important to laryngeal protection during swallowing. However, most patients can learn to swallow safely by voluntarily closing the glottis prior to swallowing (the so-called "supraglottic swallow" maneuver). Cough reflexes remain intact. If food penetrates the glottis, it is subsequently ejected by spontaneous coughing. Pharyngeal transport functions are also hampered by these procedures. Patients often need multidisciplinary rehabilitation.

Total laryngectomy isolates the airway from the foodway. A permanent tracheostomy is performed for ventilation; the larynx is excised, and the pharynx is closed anteriorly. The nasal and oral cavities and the pharynx are excluded from the airway, and the ability to phonate is lost. Thus, there is no risk of food penetrating the airway. Pharyngeal transport may be impaired, depending on what has been done to the constrictor muscles and tongue.

RADIATION THERAPY

Radiation therapy of the oral cavity and pharynx often produces a decrease in saliva. The saliva also becomes more viscous and tenacious, reducing its effectiveness as a lubricant. Mucous membranes become swollen and tender, and sores may develop. Fibrosis of irradiated tissue occasionally follows long after the radiation. This may limit the mobility of foodway structures and lead to aspiration.

Tracheostomy

The effects of tracheostomy on swallowing are complex. It may make swallowing more difficult by hampering laryngeal elevation and by reducing the sensitivity of the trachea and larynx to foreign material. It drastically reduces the effectiveness of cough for clearing the larynx by providing an escape valve through the trachea. Providing a unidirectional tracheostomy valve may have beneficial effects on swallowing. Air is inspired, but not expired, through the tracheostomy. With each expiration, air flows through the larynx, washing contaminants into the pharynx. This helps restore sensitivity of laryngeal receptors (56).

Acknowledgments. Eiichi Tanaka, M.D. and Keith Kuhlemeier, PH.D. provided helpful comments on the manuscript. We thank Arthur Siebens, M.D. and Patricia Linden, M.A. for their guidance and support. This work was supported in part by Clinical Investigator Development Award #DC00024 from the National Institute on Deafness and other Communication Disorders.

References

1. Gelfand DW, Richter JE. *Dysphagia: Diagnosis and Treatment.* New York, NY: Igaku-Shoin; 1989.
2. Groher ME, ed. *Dysphagia: Diagnosis and Management.* Boston, Mass: Butterworth; 1984.
3. Logemann JA. Evaluation and treatment of swallowing disorders. San Diego, Calif: College-Hill Press; 1983.
4. Siebens AA. Rehabilitation for swallowing impairment. In: Kottke FJ, Lehmann JF, eds. *Krusen's Handbook of Physical Medicine and Rehabilitation.* 4th ed. Philadelphia, Pa.: W.B. Saunders; 1990.
5. Dodds WJ, Stewart ET, Logemann JA. Physiology and radiology of the normal oral and pharyngeal phases of swallowing. *AJR.* 154:953–963, 1990.
6. Miller AJ. Deglutition. *Physiol Rev.* 62:129–184, 1982.
7. Palmer JB, Rudin NJ, Lara G, Crompton AW. Coordination of mastication and swallowing. *Dysphagia.* 7:187–200, 1992.
8. Kahrilas PJ, Logemann JA, Krugler C, Flanagan E. Volitional augmentation of upper esophageal sphincter opening during swallowing. *Am J Physiol.* 260(Gastrointest Liver Physiol 23):G450–G456, 1991.
9. Dodds WJ, Stewart ET, Logemann JA. Radiologic assessment of the abnormal oral and pharyngeal phases of swallowing. *AJR.* 154:965–974, 1990.
10. Ekberg O, Nylander G. Cineradiography of the pharyngeal stage of deglutition in 150 individuals without dysphagia. *Br J Radiol.* 55:253–257, 1982.
11. Feinberg MJ, Knebl J, Tully J, Segall L. Aspiration and the elderly. *Dysphagia.* 5:61–74, 1990.
12. Horner J, Massey EW. Silent aspiration following stroke. *Neurology.* 38:317–319, 1988.
13. Silver KHC, Van Nostrand D, Kuhlemeier KV, Siebens AA. Scintigraphy for detection and semi-quantification of subglottic aspiration. *Arch Phys Med Rehabil.* 72:902–910, 1991.
14. Goyal RK. Disorders of the cricopharyngeus muscle. *Otolaryngol Clin North Am.* 17:115–130, 1984.
15. Castell DO. Esophageal disorders in the elderly. *Gastroenterol Clin North Am.* 19:235–254, 1990.
16. Sheth N, Diner WC. Swallowing problems in the elderly. *Dysphagia.* 2:209–215, 1988.
17. Baum BJ, Bodner L. Aging and oral motor function: evidence for altered performance among older persons. *J Dent Res.* 62:2–6, 1983.
18. Feldman RS, Kapur KK, Alman JE, Chauncey HH. Aging and mastication: changes in performance and in the swallowing threshold with natural dentition. *J Am Geriatr Soc* 28:97–103, 1980.
19. Sonies BC, Parent L, Morrish K, Baum B. Durational aspects of the oralpharyngeal phase of swallow in normal adults. *Dysphagia.* 3:1–10, 1988.
20. Sonies BC, Ship JA, Baum BJ. Relationship between saliva production and oropharyngeal swallow in healthy, different-aged adults. *Dysphagia.* 4:85–89, 1989.
21. Tracy JF, Logemann JA, Kahrilas PJ, Jacob P, Kobara M, Krugler C. Preliminary observations on the effects of age on oropharyngeal deglutition. *Dysphagia.* 4:90–94, 1989.
22. Robbins J, Hamilton JW, Lof GL, Kempster GB. Oropharyngeal swallowing in normal adults of different ages. *Gastroenterology.* 103:823–829, 1992.
23. Wyllie E, Wyllie R, Cruse RP, Rothner AD, Erenberg G. The mechanism of nitrazepam-induced drooling and aspiration. *N Engl J Med.* 314:35–38, 1986.
24. Siebens H, Trupe E, Siebens A, et al. Correlates and consequences of eating dependency in institutionalized elderly. *J Am Geriatr Soc.* 34:192–198, 1986.
25. Martin BJW, Corlew MM. The incidence of communications disorders in dysphagic patients. *J Speech Hearing Disorders.* 55:28–32, 1990.
26. Linden P, Siebens AA. Dysphagia: predicting laryngeal penetration. *Arch Phys Med Rehabil.* 64:281–284, 1983.
27. Jones B, Donner MW, eds. *Radiology of Normal and Abnormal Swallowing.* New York, NY: Springer-Verlag; 1990.
28. Logemann JA. *Manual for the Videofluorographic Study of Swallowing.* Boston, Mass: College-Hill Press; 1986.
29. Palmer JB, DuChane AS, Donner MW. The role of radiology in rehabilitation of swallowing. In: Jones B, Donner MW, eds. *Normal and Abnormal Swallowing : Imaging in Diagnosis and Therapy.* New York, NY: Springer-Verlag; 1990.
30. Linden P. Videofluoroscopy in the rehabilitation of swallowing dysfunction. *Dysphagia.* 3:189–191, 1989.
31. Siebens AA, Linden PL. Dynamic imaging for swallowing reeducation. *Gastrointest Radiol.* 10:251–253, 1985.
32. Coster S, Schwarz W. Rheology and the swallow-safe bolus. *Dysphagia.* 1:113–118, 1987.
33. McConnel FMS, Cerenko D, Hersh T, Weil LJ. Evaluation of pharyngeal dysphagia with manofluorography. *Dysphagia.* 2:187–195, 1988.
34. Palmer JB. Electromyography of the muscles of oropharyngeal swallowing: basic concepts: *Dysphagia.* 3:192–198, 1989.
35. Palmer JB, Holloway AM, Tanaka E. Detecting lower motor neuron dysfunction of the pharynx and larynx with electromyography. *Arch Phys Med Rehabil.* 72:237–242, 1991
36. Ekberg O. Posture of the head and pharyngeal swallow. *Acta Radiol Diagn.* 27:691–696, 1986.
37. Logemann JA, Kahrilas PJ, Kobara M, et al. The benefit of head rotation on pharyngoesophageal dysphagia. *Arch Phys Med Rehabil.* 70:767–771, 1989.
38. Ekberg O, Olsson R, Sundgren-Borgstrom P. Relation of bolus size to pharyngeal swallow. *Dysphagia.* 3:69–72, 1988.
39. Logemann JA, Kahrilas PJ. Relearning to swallow post stroke-application of maneuvers and indirect biofeedback. *Neurology.* 40:1136–1138, 1990.
40. Hassett JM, Sunby C, Flint LM. No elimination of aspiration pneumonia in neurologically disabled patients with feeding gastrostomy. *Surg Gynecol Obstet.* 167:383–388, 1988.
41. Gordon C, Hewer RL, Wade DT. Dysphagia in acute stroke. *Br Med J.* 295:411–414, 1987.
42. Horner J, Massey EW, Riski JE, et al. Aspiration following stroke: clinical correlates and outcome. *Neurology.* 38:1359–1362, 1988.
43. Palmer JB, DuChane AS. Rehabilitation of swallowing disorders due to stroke. *Phys Med Rehabil Clin North Am.* 2:529–546, 1991.
44. Veis SL, Logemann JA. Swallowing disorders in persons with cerebrovascular accident. *Arch Phys Med Rehabil.* 66:372–375, 1985.
45. Robbins JA, Levine RL. Swallowing after unilateral stroke of the cerebral cortex: preliminary experience. *Dysphagia.* 3:11–17, 1988.

46. Palmer JB, Tippett DC, Wolf JS. Synchronous positive and negative myoclonus due to pontine hemorrhage. *Muscle Nerve.* 13:124–132, 1991.

47. Robbins J, Logemann JA, Kirshner HS. Swallowing and speech production in Parkinson's disease. *Ann Neurol.* 19:283–287, 1986.

48. Robbins J. Swallowing in ALS and motor neuron disorders. *Neurol Clin.* 5:213–228, 1987.

49. Bradley WG. Inflammatory diseases of muscle. In: Kelly WN, Harris ED, Ruddy S, Sledge CB: *Textbook of Rheumatology.* Philadelphia, Pa: W.B. Saunders; 1981.

50. Fulp SR, Castell DO. Scleroderma esophagus. *Dysphagia.* 5:204–210, 1990.

51. Parker MD. Dysphagia due to cervical osteophytes: a controversial entity revisited. *Dysphagia.* 3:157–160, 1989.

52. Katz PO, Bohlman ME. Benign esophageal disease. In: Gelfand DW, Richter JE: *Dysphagia: Diagnosis and Treatment.* New York, NY: Igaku-Shoin; 1989.

53. Hannig C, Wuttge-Hannig A, Feussner H. Motor dysfunction of the upper esophageal sphincter in posterior hypopharyngeal diverticula: results of a motility study by high-speed cineradiography. In: Siewert JR, Holscher AH, eds. *Diseases of the Esophagus.* New York, NY: Springer-Verlag; 1987.

54. Logemann JA, Bytell DE. Swallowing disorders in three types of head and neck cancer surgical patients. *Cancer.* 44:1095–1105, 1990.

55. Logemann JA, Kahrilas PJ, Hurst P, Davis J, Krugler C. Effects of intraoral prosthetics on swallowing in patients with cancer. *Dysphagia.* 4:118–120, 1989.

56. Tippett DC, Siebens AA. Using ventilators for speaking and swallowing. *Dysphagia.* 6:94–99, 1991.

24

Evaluation of Cognition in the Elderly Rehabilitation Patient

Claudia H. Kawas

Certain cognitive skills are necessary if a patient is to participate successfully in a treatment program. Nowhere is this more important than in the rehabilitation environment. Numerous studies, however, suggest that clinicians often have difficulty recognizing cognitive disturbances in their patients. Williamson et al (1) found that only 13% of demented subjects were recognized as such by the physicians in charge of their care. Other, more recent studies (2–4) on inpatient services have found that one third to one half of cognitively impaired patients went unidentified by clinical staff. Since the likelihood of cognitive impairment increases dramatically in the older patient, evaluation of the cognitive abilities of geriatric patients is crucial to designing successful rehabilitative programs. The clinician caring for the older patient must have an understanding of the cognitive changes that occur in normal aging and age-related diseases in order to detect and circumvent these problems.

CHANGES OF NORMAL AGING

Age-related declines of cognitive functioning have been given a variety of terms in the literature. In 1962, Kral coined the phrase "benign senescent forgetfulness." He described this as "the inability of the subject to recall relatively unimportant data and parts of an experience, like a name, a place, or a date, whereas the experience . . . . can be recalled" (5p257). The forgotten information was often remote, could frequently be recalled on another occasion, and did not seriously impair functional abilities. The example was given of a woman who could remember attending, some years before, the wedding of her son in a New England city, but was sometimes unable to recall the name of the specific city. While this type of memory loss is familiar to all of us, the example is difficult to generalize to the clinical setting.

More recently, Crook and associates (6) developed the concept of "age-associated memory impairments" in

persons over 50 years of age who have complaints of memory loss. Operationally, it is defined as memory test performance that is at least one standard deviation below the mean established for young adults on a standardized test of secondary memory. This conceptualization of age-related memory loss is problematic because of the inclusion of such a wide variety of individuals with memory loss, many of whom may be depressed, delirious, or in the process of developing clinical dementia. The authors acknowledge this problem but offer no solution for potential discrimination of "organic" losses from "normal" declines.

Many of the declines of "normal" aging have been derived from cross-sectional studies comparing young individuals to older subjects (7, 8). Studies of this type cannot control for a variety of cohort effects and other factors that may strongly influence the results. Ideally, the cognitive changes of aging should be measured using the same subjects over the lifespan. A study of this type, the Baltimore Longitudinal Study of Aging (BLSA) (9) is a prospective investigation of normal aging that has been conducted for over 30 years. The effort has included almost 1,800 subjects and is now a part of the Gerontology Research Center, National Institute on Aging. The goal of the BLSA is to trace the true effects of aging as distinguished from disease, socioeconomic disadvantage, and other processes. The BLSA has documented age-related declines in a variety of psychologic and physiologic domains. It has also been noted that some functions, particularly in the realm of cognition, improve with age (Table 24.1).

Overall, the BLSA has demonstrated that declines of cognitive function are a part of the normal aging process, but probably start later in life than previously thought, may be smaller in magnitude, and may include fewer functions (9). Of prime importance, these changes have not significantly impaired social functioning in BLSA participants. Simple strategies adopted by the subjects have easily overcome these minor losses in daily life. They

Table 24.1. Cognitive Changes in Aging—Baltimore Longitudinal Study of Aging[a]

Measures Showing Decline over Time	Measures Stable or Increasing over Time
Benton Visual Retention Test	Wais Vocabulary
Concept Problem Solving	Digit Span Forward
Paired Associate Learning	Memory for Text

[a]Adapted From Shock NW, Greulich RC, Costa PT, et al. *Normal Human Aging: The Baltimore Longitudinal Study of Aging*. US Department of Health and Human Services, Baltimore City Hospitals; 1984.

include note writing, fewer instructions over more time, and "guided encoding," which is the process of making associations with the information to be remembered, as in mnemonics.

ELDERLY PATIENTS IN THE REHABILITATIVE ENVIRONMENT

Unfortunately most patients in need of rehabilitative services cannot be expected to be normal. Medical illnesses, multiple medications, reactive grief, and numerous other factors are likely to impair cognitive functioning. In particular, dementia, delirium, and depression or a combination of these are exceptionally frequent in the elderly patient. Failure to recognize these problems is common and will sabotage rehabilitation efforts.

Dementia

DEFINITIONS AND PREVALENCE

The definition of dementia (compatible with DSM III-R criteria) is a loss of cognitive abilities of sufficient severity to interfere with social or occupational functioning with loss of memory and at least one other area of cognition (language, calculations, attention, apraxias, and agnosias) in an alert patient (10).

The prevalence of dementia in community samples has been reported between 6.6 and 15.8 per 100 for those over 65 years of age (11). A recently published survey in East Boston reported 47% of those over the age of 85 years to be suffering from probable Alzheimer's disease (12). Regardless of the exact percentages, it is clear that dementia is one of the leading obstacles to healthy aging (13) and will adversely affect rehabilitative efforts.

The most common causes of dementia are Alzheimer's disease (AD) (65%), multiinfarct dementia (MID) (10%–15%), and mixed dementia (AD and MID) 15%–20%). Other etiologies include medical illnesses such as B₁₂ deficiency, thyroid disease, and syphilis. Medications, such as the benzodiazipines and beta-blockers, have been reported to produce dementia. In addition, depression has been associated with a reversible dementia, frequently termed pseudodementia. These are the most frequent causes of dementia although over 100 causes

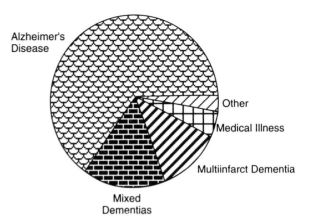

Figure 24.1. Causes of Dementia.

have been described (14). The goal of the rehabilitative staff is not to specifically diagnose a dementia but to detect its presence and the need for further workup (Fig. 24.1).

INITIAL SCREENING

Screening procedures can be very brief but still provide considerable information about the patient's cognitive status. The Mini-Mental State Examination (MMSE) (15) has been used extensively as a screening tool. Originally designed as "a practical method for grading the cognitive state of patients for the clinician," it generally requires only 5 minutes and can be administered by lay personnel with very little training. It has demonstrated high test-retest reliability (.89) and interrater reliability (0.82) (15, 16). To some extent, sensitivity and specificity of the MMSE depend on the characteristics of the population being screened. Among hospital patients, the MMSE was 87% sensitive and 82% specific in detecting dementia and delirium (cut off score 23/24) (17). False positives were most likely in patients with low education levels (Fig. 24.2).

The Blessed Information-Memory-Concentration (IMC) test (18) is also useful as a screening instrument. In clinicopathologic studies, it has shown correlation with numbers of senile plaques detected in the cerebral cortex. Although it contains many items similar to the MMSE, it does not include items that test language (reading/writing) or motor skills—an advantage when evaluating patients with limited sight or extremity paralysis. Error scores of greater than 10 are consistent with a diagnosis of dementia, but scores of 5 to 10 errors suggest possible early dementia as reported by Katzman and colleagues (19).

Instruments such as the Mini-Mental and the Blessed can be used to screen for cognitive impairment. They also provide a way of measuring improvement or decline over time. They do not, however, provide specific diagnoses. When cognitive impairment is suspected, further clinical and psychometric evaluation is necessary to identify the etiology. Table 24.2 shows the

Figure 24.2. Mini-Mental State.[a]

I. ORIENTATION (Ask the following questions)		

What is today's date?	Date (e.g., Jan. 21)	☐
What is the year?	Year	☐
What is the month?	Month	☐
What day is today?	Day (e.g., Monday)	☐
Can you also tell me what season it is?	Season	☐
Can you also tell me the name of this hospital (clinic)?	Hospital (Clinic)	☐
What floor are we on?	Floor	☐
What town or city are we in?	Town or City	☐
What county are we in?	County	☐
What state are we in?	State	☐

II. IMMEDIATE RECALL		

Ask the subject if you may test his/her memory. Then say "ball," "flag," "tree" clearly and slowly, about one second for each. After you have said all 3, ask him/her to repeat them. This first repetition determines his/her score (0-3), but keep saying them until he/she can repeat all 3, up to 6 tries. If he/she does not eventually learn all 3, recall cannot be meaningfully tested.

"Ball"	☐
"Flag"	☐
"Tree"	☐
Number of Trials: _____	

III. ATTENTION AND CALCULATION		

Ask the subject to begin with 100 and count backwards by 7. Stop after 5 subtractions (93, 86, 79, 72, 65). Score the total number of correct answers.

If the subject cannot or will not perform "the count backwards test" task, ask him/her to spell the word "world" backwards. The score is the number of letters in correct order. For example, dlrow is 5, dlorw is 3.

"93"	☐
"86"	☐
"79"	☐
"72"	☐
"65"	☐
D	☐
L	☐
R	☐
O	☐
W	☐

IV. RECALL		

Ask the subject to recall the 3 words you previously asked him/her to remember. Score 0-3.

"Ball"	☐
"Flag"	☐
"Tree"	☐

V. LANGUAGE		

NAMING
Show the subject a wrist watch and ask him/her what it is. Repeat for pencil.

Watch	☐
Pencil	☐

REPETITION
Ask the subject to repeat, "No ifs, ands, or buts."

Repetition	☐

3-STAGE COMMAND
Give the subject a piece of plain blank paper and say, "Take the paper in your right hand, fold it in half and put it on the floor."

Takes paper in right hand	☐
Folds paper in half	☐
Puts paper on floor	☐

READING
On a blank piece of paper print this sentence "Close your eyes," in letters large enough for the subject to see clearly. Ask him/her to read it and do what it says. Score correct only if he/she actually closes his/her eyes.

Closes Eyes	☐

WRITING
Give the subject a blank piece of paper and ask him/her to write a sentence. It is to be written spontaneously. It must contain a subject and a verb and be sensible. Correct grammar and punctuation are not necessary.

Writes Sentence	☐

COPYING
On a clean piece of paper, draw intersecting pentagons, each side about 1 inch, and ask subject to copy it exactly as it is. All 10 angles must be present and two must intersect to score one point. Tremor and rotation are ignored.

Draws Pentagons	☐

e.g.

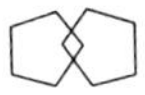

DERIVING TOTAL SCORE		

Sum the number of correct replies to the test items. If item "world spelled backward" was used then add the number of correct letters given in proper sequence (one to five). The maximum score is 30 for this test.

TOTAL SCORE ☐

[a]Reprinted with permission from Folstein MF, Folstein SE, McHugh PR. Mini-Mental State. A practical method for grading the cognitive state of patients for the clinician. *J Psychiatr Res.* 12:189–198, 1975.

Table 24.2. Work-up for the Differential Diagnosis of Dementia[a]

By the examiner
    History
    Mental status examination
    Physical examination
    Neurologic examination
Special tests[b]
    CT scan or MRI
    Chest X-ray
    ECG
    EEG
    Blood
        CBC, metabolic screen, thyroid profile,
            B_{12} level, VDRL, FTA-abs
Psychometric Evaluation

[a]Modified from Wells CE. *Dementia.* 2nd ed. Philadelphia, Pa: F. A. Davis; 1978.
[b]CT = computed tomography; MRI = magnetic resonance imaging; ECG = electrocardiogram; EEG = electroencephalogram; CDC = complete blood count; VDRL = Venereal Disease Reference Laboratory.

Table 24.3. Geriatric Depression Scale (GDS) Sensitivity and Specificity[a]

	Cut-off Scores		
	9	11	14
Sensitivity	90%	84%	80%
Specificity	80%	95%	100%

[a]From Brink TL, Yesavage JA, Lum O, Heersema PH, Adey M, Rose TL. Screening tests for geriatric depression. *Clin Gerontol.* 1:37–43, 1982.

major components for a work-up of dementia. It is not within the scope of this chapter to elaborate on the diagnostic criteria for different dementias. For further information on this topic, see Katzman et al, 1988 (20). It should be emphasized that the detection of dementia and the diagnosis of its etiology are very dependent on history. Seeking information from family and friends regarding the patient's functional abilities provides the basis for diagnosis to a greater extent than any psychometric, laboratory, or radiologic procedures.

Depression

DEFINITIONS AND PREVALENCE

The essential feature of a major depressive episode, as defined by the DSM III-R, is depressed mood or loss of interest or pleasure in most activities for a period of at least 2 weeks. The symptoms represent a change from previous functioning and are relatively persistent; that is, they occur for most of the day, nearly every day. Associated symptoms include appetite disturbance, change in weight, sleep disturbance, psychomotor agitation or retardation, decreased energy, feelings of worthlessness, inappropriate guilt, difficulty thinking or concentrating, and recurrent thoughts of death or suicide (10).

The reported prevalence of depressive symptomatology in the elderly ranges from 5% to 65% in hospital and community populations (21). Despite these variations, it is generally agreed that depression is more prevalent in older persons than in any other age group (22). Furthermore, it is well recognized that depression can be associated with reversible dementia. Termed pseudodementia (23) or the dementia associated with depression (16), characteristic symptoms include lack of motivation and drive, difficulty with verbal elaboration, poor memory retrieval, and improved performance with

encouragement (24). It is easy to understand the potential impact of these symptoms on rehabilitative efforts. Successful treatment of depression can be very effective in improving rehabilitative outcome, making recognition of the problem imperative.

Depression in the elderly may not have the classic vegetative signs of weight loss, sleep disorder, or changes in libido. Even when present, these signs may be attributed to the patient's age or medical illness. Although nothing can replace the clinical examination by an experienced psychiatrist, numerous instruments have been developed to assess depressive symptomotology in populations.

INITIAL SCREENING

There are two varieties of depression scales: examiner-rating and self-rating. Overall, the former is considered superior but requires a trained interviewer and extensive time. The prototype examiner-rating scale is the Hamilton Scale (25), which takes up to an hour to administer. This is an excellent instrument if time allows. Self-rating scales such as the Zung Scale (26) and the Beck Scale (27) have been widely used but can be misleading in the elderly. Age-related illnesses such as arthritis can result in high "somatic complaint" scores, making elders with good mental health appear depressed on the screening instrument. The Geriatric Depression Scale (GDS) (28) was designed to specifically evaluate the common manifestations of depression in later life. It consists of a 30-item questionnaire answerable with yes/no responses. Correlation with the Zung and Hamilton Scales is high, but superiority has been reported in elderly populations with the GDS. Cut-off scores for different sensitivities/specificities are shown in Table 24.3 and Figure 24.3.

DEPRESSION AND STROKE

A particular situation deserving of attention is the recently appreciated relationship between depression and stroke. Although any individual faced with medical disability (e.g., hip fracture, loss of limb, etc.) is likely to feel depression, stroke is an illness affecting the organ that is responsible for our affective state. Depression has not been clearly localized, but recent studies point to certain areas of the brain as being more closely associated with the development of depression and cognitive

Figure 24.3. Geriatric Depression Scale.[a]

1. Are you basically satisfied with your life?	yes/no
2. Have you dropped many of your activities and interests?	yes/no
3. Do you feel that your life is empty?	yes/no
4. Do you often get bored?	yes/no
5. Are you hopeful about the future?	yes/no
6. Are you bothered by thoughts you can't get out of your head?	yes/no
7. Are you in good spirits most of the time?	yes/no
8. Are you afraid that something bad is going to happen to you?	yes/no
9. Do you feel happy most of the time?	yes/no
10. Do you often feel helpless?	yes/no
11. Do you often get restless and fidgety?	yes/no
12. Do you prefer to stay at home, rather than going out and doing new things?	yes/no
13. Do you frequently worry about the future?	yes/no
14. Do you feel you have more problems with memory than most?	yes/no
15. Do you think it is wonderful to be alive now?	yes/no
16. Do you often feel downhearted and blue?	yes/no
17. Do you feel pretty worthless the way you are now?	yes/no
18. Do you worry a lot about the past?	yes/no
19. Do you find life very exciting?	yes/no
20. Is it hard for you to get started on new projects?	yes/no
21. Do you feel full of energy?	yes/no
22. Do you feel that your situation is hopeless?	yes/no
23. Do you think that most people are better off than you are?	yes/no
24. Do you frequently get upset over little things?	yes/no
25. Do you frequently feel like crying?	yes/no
26. Do you have trouble concentrating?	yes/no
27. Do you enjoy getting up in the morning?	yes/no
28. Do you prefer to avoid social gatherings?	yes/no
29. Is it easy for you to make decisions?	yes/no
30. Is your mind as clear as it used to be?	yes/no

[a] Reprinted with permission from Brink TL, Yesavage JA, Lum O, Heersema PH, Adey M. Rose TL. Screening tests for geriatric depression. *Clin Gerontol.* 1:37–43, 1982.

impairment. Robinson and colleagues (24) have reported that stroke patients with left frontal brain injury are more severely depressed than are those with lesions in other areas (29, 30). In addition, they have demonstrated a relationship between depression and severity of intellectual impairment that depended on the laterality of the lesion. Depression associated with right hemisphere injury produced no cognitive impairment. In patients with a single left hemisphere lesion, over 50% had significant intellectual impairment. The degree of intellectual impairment was associated with the severity of depression; all patients with major depression had cognitive impairment, as compared with 40% of the nondepressed patients. Moreover, during the course of a 6-month follow-up, there was improvement in MMSE scores in nondepressed patients, while depressed patients showed either no change or a slight decline (31). Treatment of poststroke depression with tricyclic anti-

depressants has been shown to improve rehabilitative outcome and should be considered in patients, particularly after left hemisphere cerebrovascular accidents.

Delirium

DEFINITIONS AND PREVALENCE

The DSM III-R (10) defines delirium as reduced ability to maintain attention to external stimuli and to appropriately shift attention to new external stimuli. Disorganized thinking, as manifested by rambling, irrelevant, or incoherent speech is usually present. The syndrome also involves a reduced level of consciousness, sensory misperceptions, disturbances of the sleep-wake cycle, disorientation to time, place, or person, and memory impairment. The onset is relatively rapid, and the course typically fluctuates.

While most clinicians associate fluctuating level of consciousness with the diagnosis of delirium, their interpretation of this is often limited. Patients who frequently sleep when left unstimulated or those who have fluctuating or poor attention are likely to be exhibiting symptoms of delirium.

The prevalence of delirium in hospitalized patients is unclear, but the elderly patient is particularly vulnerable to this problem. Medications, fevers, hypoxia, relatively mild infections, and organ failure may all contribute to delirium and cognitive impairment in the elderly.

SCREENING AND EVALUATION

The screening instruments for dementia (MMSE and Blessed IMC Test) can be useful for detection of the patient with delirium. In addition, the electroencephalogram (EEG) often shows characteristic changes and can be useful for the diagnosis. The primary clue for this problem is often contained in the patient history. The course of most dementias is gradual decline after an insidious onset. Relatively abrupt or subacute changes in mental status or sleep/wake cycles are suggestive of a toxic-metabolic etiology and should be regarded with suspicion. History should be reviewed with special attention to recent changes in medications. Laboratory studies, including complete blood count (CBC) (infection/anemia), hepatic and renal functions, arterial blood gases, glucose, electrolytes, and other serum chemistries should all be obtained.

MANAGEMENT OF COGNITIVE IMPAIRMENTS

Elderly patients frequently suffer multiple illnesses. Cognitive impairments in elderly patients are also often the result of multiple etiologies. Emphasis should be placed on discovering treatable diseases. One third of demented patients are also suffering from depression (32). Treatment of the latter can significantly improve the patient's cognitive status and general well-being. Reduction or elimination of medications, particularly those with psychotropic activity, can improve the patient's ability to participate in treatment programs. Recognition of the cognitive impairments that cannot be reversed allows the therapist to modify treatment strategies accordingly. An awareness of the cognitive changes of normal and pathologic aging is the key to devising optimal treatment for the elderly patient.

SUMMARY

The elderly are the leading consumers of health care, and the physical medicine team must be aware of the special needs of this group of patients. Cognitive impairment is more common in the elderly patient than in any other age group. Recognition of a patient's intellectual abilities is essential for devising appropriate treatment strategies. Screening for dementia, depression, and delirium should be a part of each patient's evaluation in order to provide optimal care. The routine evaluation of cognitive abilities when assessing elderly patients would greatly improve the quality and outcome of rehabilitative care.

References

1. Williamson J, Stokoe IH, Gray S, et al. Old people at home: their unreported needs. *Lancet.* 1:1117–1120, 1964.
2. Knights EB, Folstein MF. Unsuspected emotional and cognitive disturbance in medical patients. *Ann Intern Med.* 87:723–724, 1977.
3. DePaulo JR, Folstein MF. Psychiatric disturbances in neurological patients: detection, recognition, and hospital course. *Ann Neurol.* 4:225–228, 1978.
4. Roca RP, Klein LE, Vogelsang G. Inaccuracy in diagnosing dementia among medical inpatients. *Clin Res.* 30:305A, 1982.
5. Kral VA: Senescent forgetfulness: benign and malignant. *Can Med Assoc J.* 86:257–260, 1962.
6. Crook T, Bartus RT, Ferris SH, Whitehouse P, Cohen GD, Gershon S. Age-associated memory impairment: proposed criteria and measures of clinical change. Report of a National Institute of Mental Health Work Group. *Dev Neuropsychol.* 2:261–276, 1986.
7. Botwinick J. *Aging and Behavior.* 3rd ed. New York, NY: Springer; 1984.
8. Poon LW, Fozard JL, Cermak LS, Arenberg D, Thompson LW, eds. *New Directions in Memory and Aging.* Hillsdale, NJ: Lawrence Erlbaum Associates; 1980.
9. Shock NW, Greulich RC, Costa PT, et al. *Normal Human Aging: The Baltimore Longitudinal Study of Aging.* US Department of Health and Human Services, Baltimore City Hospitals; 1984.
10. *Diagnostic and Statistical Manual of Mental Disorders.* Ed 3-R. Washington DC: American Psychiatric Association; 1987.
11. Zhang D, Katzman R, Salmon D, et al. The prevalence of dementia and Alzheimer's disease in Shanghai, China: impact of age, gender, and education. *Ann Neurol.* 27:428–437, 1989.
12. Evans DA, Funkenstein HH, Albert MS, et al. Prevalence of Alzheimer's disease in a community population of older persons. *JAMA.* 262:2551–2556, 1989.
13. Katzman R. The prevalence and malignancy of Alzheimer's disease. *Arch Neurol.* 33:217–218, 1976.
14. Wells CE: *Dementia.* 2nd ed. Philadelphia, Pa: F. A. Davis; 1978.
15. Folstein MF, Folstein SE, and McHugh PR. Mini-Mental State. A practical method for grading the cognitive state of patients for the clinician. *J Psychiatr Res.* 12:189–198, 1975.
16. Folstein MF, McHugh PR. Psychopathology of dementia: implications for neuropathology. In: Katzman R, ed. *Congenital Acquired Cognitive Disorders.* New York, NY: Raven Press; 1979.
17. Anthony JC, LeResche L, Niaz U, Von Korff MR, Folstein MF. Limits of the 'Mini-Mental State' as a screening test for dementia and delirium among hospital patients. *Psychol Med.* 12:397–408, 1982.
18. Blessed GT, Roth BE. The association between quantitative measures of dementia and senile change in the cerebral grey matter of elderly subjects. *Br J Psychiatry.* 114:797–811, 1968.
19. Katzman R, Aronson M, Fuld P, et al. Development of dementing illnesses in an 80 year old volunteer cohort. *Ann Neurol.* 25:317–324, 1989.
20. Katzman R, Hasker B, Bernstein N. *Advances in the Diagnosis of Dementia: Accuracy of Diagnosis and Consequences of Misdiagnosis of Disorders Causing Dementia.* New York, NY: Raven Press; 1988.
21. Blazer D. The diagnosis of depression in the elderly. *J Geriatr Soc.* 25:52–58, 1980.
22. Gurland BJ. The comparative frequency of depression in various adult age groups. *J Gerontol.* 31:283–292, 1976.
23. Caine ED. Pseudo-dementia. *Arch Gen Psychiatry.* 38:1359–1364, 1981.
24. Robinson RC, Bolla K. Depression influences intellectual impairment in stroke patients. *Br J Psychiatry.* 148:541–547, 1986.
25. Hamilton MA. A rating scale for depression. *J Neurol, Neurosurg Psychiatry.* 23:56–62, 1960.
26. Zung WWK. A self-rating depression scale. *Arch Gen Psychiatry.* 12:63–70, 1965.
27. Beck AT, Ward CH, Mendelson M, Mock J, Erbaugh J. Inventory for measuring depression. *Arch Gen Psychiatry.* 4:561–571, 1961.
28. Brink TL, Yesavage JA, Lum O, Heersema PH, Adey M, Rose TL. Screening tests for geriatric depression. *Clin Gerontol.* 1:37–43, 1982.
29. Kubos KL, Starr LB, Rao K, Price TR. Mood disorders in stroke patients: importance of location of lesion. 107:81–93, 1984.
30. Lipsey JR, Rao K, Price TR. A two year longitudinal study of post-stroke mood disorders: Dynamic changes in associated variables over the first 6 months of follow-up. *Stroke.* 15:510–517, 1985.
31. Price TR. Depression influences intellectual impairment in stroke patients. *Br J Psychiatry.* 148:541–547, 1986.
32. Jarvik T, Trader D. Treatment of behavioral and mood changes. In: Aronson MK, ed. *Understanding Alzheimer's Disease.* New York, NY: Scribner, 1988.

25
Urologic Disorders

Inder Perkash and Gerald W. Friedland

Urologic problems in the elderly are common and important; they are costly and sometimes disabling. Elderly patients with urologic problems will classically present with one or more of the following symptoms: *(a)* frequency, including nocturia, *(b)* incontinence, *(c)* hematuria, and *(d)* retention.

FREQUENCY

Frequency is the most common presenting symptom in the elderly with urologic problems. It can be a symptom during the day and the night or particularly troublesome when it occurs at night, in which case it is called nocturia. The most common causes are local pathology, physiologic factors, medication, and metabolic changes.

Pathology in the Lower Urinary Tract

The most common local cause of frequency in men is an enlarged prostate, especially enlarged periurethral glands (formerly called median lobe enlargement).

Enlargement of the periurethral glands (Fig. 25.1) causes frequency because as those glands enlarge they may irritate nerve endings at the posterior bladder neck. If we introduce a urodynamics catheter into the bladder under sonographic control while doing transrectal sonography and if we happen to irritate the posterior bladder neck with the catheter tip, the bladder contracts; the bladder neck opens, and the periurethral striated sphincter relaxes. During normal voiding, as the bolus distends the bladder neck, this stimulates the nerve endings at the bladder neck, resulting in further bladder contraction and urethral relaxation. Any enlargement of the periurethral glands at the posterior bladder neck, therefore, would tend to duplicate these conditions since the same nerve endings are being stimulated. This may lead to an unstable bladder.

Another local cause of frequency in elderly men is urinary tract infection (UTI), especially in patients with retention, bladder cancer, and bladder stones.

In elderly women, UTI is the most important local cause of frequency since there is a lower biological resistance to infection with fecal organisms in the perineum and urethra as women age. This is due in part to the fact that the vaginal pH becomes more alkaline and there is a lower secretion of antibodies into the vaginal fluid (1, 2). Bladder cancer is also an important cause of frequency in elderly women. Finally, uninhibited bladder contractions are common in older women; as many as half of all older women have an unstable bladder to some degree.

Physiologic Factors

Physiologic factors can also be important in frequency problems; if so, they commonly result in nocturia. Common causes include excessive fluid intake at the end of the day, especially caffeine-containing drinks since caffeine is a diuretic. Another problem may be reabsorption of edema fluid from the lower extremities when the patient lies down at night. The elderly, particularly those with incipient cardiac failure, tend to pool more fluid in their lower extremities than do younger people. This can be a particular problem in elderly people who are confined to a wheelchair since their legs are lower than the rest of the body the whole day long. The elderly in wheelchairs tend to keep their legs inactive for longer periods of time as well. Because their leg muscles contract weakly and infrequently, these muscles may not pump blood and interstitial fluid pooling in their lower extremities back into the general circulation as effectively as might be desired.

Excessive tension may also cause physiologic problems leading to frequency. Many of the elderly are very tense; theirs is a real struggle for existence, which they may face with deteriorating mental and physical abilities, loss of status, and financial difficulties. This tension means that there is an excess secretion of norepinephrine, which causes vasoconstriction of the renal arterioles. This in turn results in decreased perfusion through the kidneys. This reduces the glomerular filtration rate;

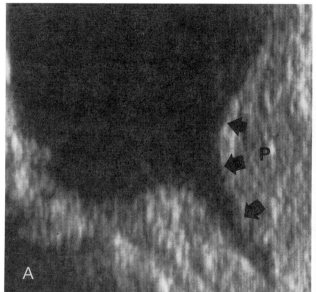
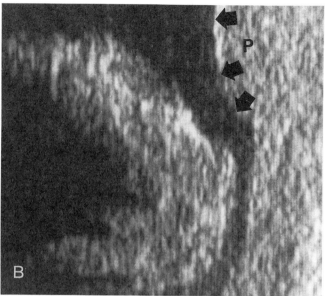

Figure 25.1. Sonographic voiding cystourethrogram performed after a sphincterotomy. A is a magnified view of the bladder neck; **B** is a view of the prostatic and proximal bulbous urethra. A slightly enlarged prostate **P** protrudes into the bladder neck posteriorly (arrows).

the kidneys themselves will filter less fluid, meaning that such people will retain fluid. When they fall asleep, they do relax; norepinephrine production declines; the renal arterioles relax, and the patient has a diuresis.

Medication-Induced Frequency

Frequency, and particularly nocturia, can be medication-induced, particularly if the patient is on diuretics.

Metabolic Causes

The patient may have an unsuspected and untreated diabetes mellitus; less commonly, the patient may have diabetes insipidus.

Investigation

The first step is to culture the urine to check for infection and to test the patient for diabetes mellitus. It is also vital to obtain three consecutive urine specimens for exfoliative cell cytology to help screen for bladder cancer. Transrectal sonography (Fig. 25.2) may also be done in men to detect median lobe (periurethral gland) enlargement (Fig. 25.1), and cystoscopy may be done to rule out bladder cancer in either sex.

Management

Fluid intake at the end of the day should be controlled and patients advised to get their legs and feet up at times during the day and to move and exercise their legs. Psychotherapy and medications are available for tension, and any infections, cancers, periurethral gland hyperplasia, stones, or diabetes mellitus or insipidus

should be treated appropriately. Patients with an enlarged prostate and with symptoms, but in whom the prostate is still relatively small, can be treated with alpha-adrenergic blockers. If this is insufficient, the patient should have a transurethral resection of the prostate.

INCONTINENCE

Incontinence is defined as the involuntary loss of urine (3). It may be transient (acute), regular (also known as established or chronic incontinence), or functional (3).

Transient Incontinence

Transient incontinence is due to reversible factors. Common causes include diabetes mellitus, acute UTI, severe constipation with fecal impaction, and acute illnesses such as coma, stroke, pneumonia, myocardial infarction, or electrolyte imbalance. Transient incontinence may also be drug-induced; cardiovascular drugs like alpha and beta-blockers, diuretics, sedatives, analgesics, hypnotic drugs, anticholinergics, drugs for treating Parkinsonism, anticonvulsants, and antihistamines may all cause transient incontinence. If the patient is taking psychotropic drugs such as Thorazine, Mellaril, Haldol, and lithium, urinary symptoms can result, usually acute retention. Some patients, however, can develop acute retention with overflow incontinence, which is then a form of transient incontinence. Older patients who are psychotic may insert foreign bodies into the bladder thereby causing acute incontinence.

Regular Incontinence

Regular incontinence is occurring when a patient has two or more episodes per month and is socially embarrassed. Throughout life, this condition is more common in women than it is in men; between the ages of 15 and 44 years, the prevalence of regular incontinence in women is 7%, in men 1%; between the ages of 45 and 64 years, it is 12% in women, 2% in men and over the age of 65 years, it is 16% in women, 15% in men (4, 5).

About 25% of the elderly who are homebound have regular incontinence, as compared to 3% of those who are fully mobile.

The total direct cost of regular incontinence is enormous, about 10.3 billion dollars each year. This includes about 7 billion dollars direct cost to the community and an additional 3.3 billion dollars in costs to nursing homes (6–9). Treating patients with regular incontinence and keeping them relatively continent, however, costs significantly more than these direct costs, so some do not consider treatment cost-effective. However, we continue to treat people with regular incontinence in order to improve their quality of life.

There are a number of different causes for regular incontinence, including urge, stress, mixed, continuous, postvoid, and reflex incontinence (3).

URGE INCONTINENCE

Urge incontinence occurs when a patient has a strong urge to void but cannot get to the bathroom in time and so is incontinent (10–13). It may have two causes, either motor or sensory.

The characteristic feature of motor urge incontinence is that, if the patient is asked to cough, the person is not immediately incontinent, as would be the case in stress incontinence, but is incontinent 10 to 15 seconds after the cough (14) due to triggering of uncontrolled bladder contractions (unstable bladder). These patients can also lose urine when sitting, lying, or sleeping, which is not the case with patients with stress incontinence.

According to studies by Resnick and his colleagues, motor urge incontinence is the most common cause of incontinence in the elderly (3). Resnick's group found that the most common cause for motor urge incontinence in the elderly, and indeed of any form of incontinence in the elderly, is detrusor hyperreflexia, which may occur after a stroke, with Alzheimer's disease (Figs. 25.3 and 25.4), Parkinson's disease, or after a head injury. A hyperreflexic bladder is one that can contract involuntarily when there is a smaller volume of urine in the bladder (15). The patient has a normal peak voiding flow rate, no postvoid residual urine, and has voluntary control over the anal sphincters. Such patients are very frequently institutionalized because of problems with incontinence.

Another important cause of motor urge incontinence is benign prostatic hyperplasia, especially when it is due to enlargement of the periurethral glands. Benign prostatic hyperplasia can cause motor urge incontinence for precisely the reasons discussed previously under frequency.

In many patients, in whom the cause is unknown, motor urge incontinence may be called "primary motor urge incontinence".

Sensory urge incontinence is most commonly due to bladder lesions; infections, carcinoma in situ, carcinoma, irradiation cystitis, and interstitial cystitis are the

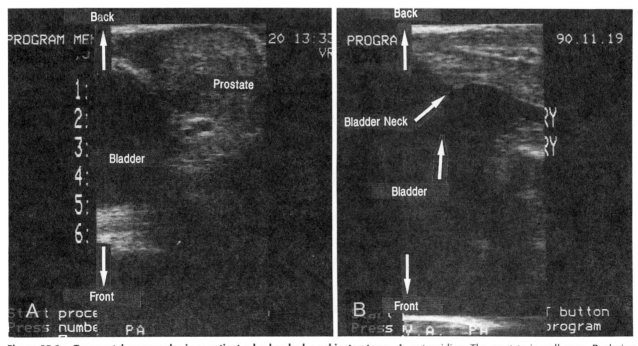

Figure 25.2. Transrectal sonography in a patient who has had a sphincterotomy. A, not voiding. The prostate is well seen. **B,** during voiding. The bladder neck and urethra open widely.

most common causes, although occasionally other lesions, such as tuberculosis, may occur.

STRESS INCONTINENCE

Stress incontinence occurs when an increase in the intraabdominal pressure causes an increase in the bladder pressure, which in turn causes voiding despite the fact that the detrusor does not contract (14). In stress incontinence, persons are incontinent the moment this rise in pressure occurs (14).

In elderly women, stress incontinence is common. The basic cause is an excessive descent of the pelvic floor, the bladder, and the bladder neck when the intraabdominal pressure rises; the secondary phenomenon is that the angle between the base of the bladder and the urethra and that between the urethra and the sagittal plane change. Stress incontinence in women can also be due to radiation-induced fibrosis involving the urethra and pelvic floor, or it may be due to a flaccid urethra, which can be one aspect of the general atony occurring as a result of the aging process.

In elderly men, the most important cause of stress incontinence is injury to the periurethral striated sphincter, the most important cause of which, in turn, is an injury after prostatectomy. The injury may also be due to external trauma.

MIXED INCONTINENCE

Mixed incontinence is a combination of stress and urge incontinence. In women, stress incontinence commonly develops first, followed by urge incontinence; in men, the reverse is true.

CONTINUOUS INCONTINENCE

Continuous incontinence is by definition a continuous, uncontrolled dribble. This form of incontinence is common in elderly men and is usually due to bladder outlet obstruction caused by an enlarged prostate. There is chronic retention not previously recognized so that urine then overflows (overflow incontinence) and continuous incontinence results. It may, however, not be an overflow phenomenon but arise because the periurethral striated sphincter was severely injured during prostatic surgery.

Continuous incontinence may also be an overflow phenomenon in elderly women with infrequent voiding syndrome. It may also be a result of diabetes mellitis. It may, however, not be an overflow phenomenon but arise because of vesicovaginal or urethrovaginal fistulae or because the patient has a very rigid (noncompliant) or flaccid periurethral striated sphincter that does not close. This can be due to previous surgical procedures or radiation-induced fibrosis. The distinguishing feature of continuous incontinence due to a fistula or a rigid

sphincter is that the person dribbles more in the upright position than otherwise.

POSTVOID INCONTINENCE

Patients with postvoid incontinence continue to dribble significantly after voiding has ceased. This is characteristic of urethral diverticula.

REFLEX INCONTINENCE

Reflex incontinence occurs without stress and without warning; the person simply voids suddenly and involuntarily. It can be caused by an upper motor neuron spinal cord lesion or a large or diffuse cerebral lesion.

Functional Incontinence

Functional incontinence occurs in patients who have completely normal lower urinary tracts but who also have severe, even overwhelming, cognitive impairment such that they can no longer recognize that the bladder is full. They then become incontinent. It may also occur in patients who are immobilized and who therefore cannot get to the toilet on time.

The Impact of Incontinence in the Elderly

From the elderly patient's point of view, incontinence of any variety may cause severe psychologic effects. These include embarrassment, anxiety, loss of confidence and self-esteem, and the feeling of being helpless and dependent. The result can be severe depression; in fact, 25% of elderly patients with incontinence have stated that they find life intolerable because of that incontinence.

There are also sexual problems, as can be imagined; when a person may smell of stale urine or void at any time, the sexual partner is not likely to be as interested.

There are also consequent social effects. The behavior of incontinent elderly persons is altered; they do not wish to leave home as often; they may not want to go to work, and their leisurely activities are curtailed. If the incontinence is severe, especially if it is associated with fecal incontinence, the incontinent person may need to be institutionalized.

There are associated medical effects, including skin maceration, rashes, pressure sores, skin infections, and the like.

The consequence is clearly that the effects of incontinence in the elderly are much more severe than we often realize.

Evaluation of the Patient

HISTORY AND PHYSICAL EXAMINATION

A very complete history will be necessary, covering all the symptoms discussed above, to locate possible causes of incontinence. A complete physical examination is also required. Both should be initiated by asking all elderly patients whether they are incontinent. It may be difficult for these patients to volunteer this information themselves; many elderly patients are never asked whether they are incontinent or not, nor do they receive special investigation for incontinence.

DIAGNOSTIC IMAGING, URODYNAMIC STUDIES, AND OTHER SPECIAL INVESTIGATIONS

With respect to diagnostic imaging and other studies, the following considerations should apply.

Urge Incontinence

Patients with motor urge incontinence should have complete urodynamic studies (16). If possible, simultaneous urodynamic studies and transrectal sonography can be very useful because such studies will show the actual functional anatomy and, in men, any prostatic enlargement, especially enlarged periurethral glands (16).

Patients with sensory urge incontinence should be cystoscoped to rule out bladder cancer.

Stress Incontinence

The only medical devices needed to establish the diagnosis of stress incontinence in women is a urethral catheter, a 50 mL syringe, and a bottle of water. It will be unnecessary in most cases to cystoscope and urethroscope the patient, perform urodynamic studies, voiding cystourethrograms (radiologic or sonographic), or chain cystograms (17).

The only exceptions are patients with mixed incontinence, patients with previously unsuccessful operations for stress incontinence, or those with rigid sphincters due to previous surgery or radiation (17). These patients should have chain cystograms (18, 19) or sonographic voiding cystourethrograms (20).

It has been found on the chain cystogram, in which a chain is placed in the bladder and upright lateral radiographs obtained during straining, that the actual angle between the base of the bladder and the urethra, or between the urethra and the vertical plane, is useless (17). After successful surgery, the actual urethrovesical junction should be several centimeters higher than a line between the bottom of the fifth sacral vertebra and the bottom of the symphysis pubis. A better choice, however, is the sonographic voiding cystourethrogram, which can be done transrectally or preferably transvaginally (20). Using a linear array transducer, which yields a true sagittal image, the relation between the urethrovesical junction and the symphysis pubis can be shown accurately and easily.

In men, the usual examination is a radiologic cystogram in the upright position. To determine whether or not the periurethral striated sphincter is functional, we ask the patient to void and then to stop voiding in midstream.

If this is successful, the periurethral striated sphincter is functional. We then wait until the urethra drains of contrast material, clamp the end of the urethra with a zipser clamp or rubber band to obstruct it, and then ask the patient to cough. If the distal urethra fills with contrast material during coughing, the patient has stress incontinence.

Mixed Incontinence

Mixed incontinence should be investigated as for urge and stress incontinence (see above).

Continuous Incontinence

A good physical examination should show whether a patient has a distended bladder, which overflows causing continuous incontinence. It is also possible to do transrectal sonography to see if there are enlarged periurethral glands; and the patient should be tested for diabetes mellitus.

A rigid sphincter in women can be demonstrated by having the woman stand in the upright position to see if the dribbling becomes worse. To check for fistulae, a cystogram with the patient in the upright lateral position will be helpful; as the patient strains, the examiner should check for dribble into the vagina. An alternative procedure if the results are ambiguous is to inject methylene blue into the bladder and place three large cotton balls into the vagina; depending on which cotton balls turns blue and where, the investigator will be able to determine that a fistula exists and at what level the fistula communicates with the vagina.

Postvoid Incontinence

In women, the history will suggest the diagnosis, and it may be possible, on physical examination, to milk the mass and express urine from the diverticulum. Neither the physical exam nor cystoscopy are very sensitive for this diagnosis; a more sensitive examination is the retrograde urethrogram using a Davis double balloon catheter. Transrectal and transvaginal sonography are also available but much less sensitive than the retrograde urethrogram.

In men, the voiding cystourethrogram is by far the best method to check for an anterior urethral diverticulum. It is also possible to place a sonographic transducer directly over the urethra, although this examination is currently not as sensitive as the voiding cystourethrogram.

Reflex Incontinence

Patients with reflex incontinence will require full urodynamic studies, preferably with a simultaneous imaging technique. We have found that transrectal sonography is the best associated technique for this purpose.

Patients with severe diffuse cerebral disease such as advanced Alzheimer's disease have no electrical activity in the periurethral striated sphincters and cannot adequately contract their periurethral striated sphincters when asked to do so, as the various neural pathways between the brain and the spinal cord are disturbed.

Treatment

Treatment may be general or specific.

GENERAL TREATMENT

General treatment would include taking care of the skin and other affected areas, as well as treating any urinary infections and underlying diseases, such as diabetes mellitus and other diseases discussed above.

SPECIFIC TREATMENT

Urge Incontinence

Specific treatments for motor urge incontinence may include muscle relaxants, such as flavoxate; anticholinergics (Fig. 25.3 and 25.4), such as propantheline or oxybutynin; and imipramine, which has both anticholinergic and alpha-agonist effects on the bladder neck (3).

Specific treatments for sensory urge incontinence include specific treatment for the underlying diseases listed above (3).

Stress Incontinence

For women with stress incontinence, specific treatments might include asking the patient to lose weight to reduce the abdominal pressure pushing the uterus downward and a specific Kegal regimen to strengthen the muscles of the pelvic floor. A pessary may be helpful in correcting uterine prolapse. Oral or vaginal estrogen and oral imipramine have also been shown to be helpful (3).

If these general approaches are not effective, full urodynamic evaluation is in order. If surgery is contemplated, the current procedure of choice is the Stamey-Pereyra procedure (14). For the treatment of postprostatectomy stress incontinence, artificial sphincters can be inserted in carefully selected cases (21–24).

Mixed Incontinence

For mixed incontinence, a combination of treatments for motor urge incontinence and stress incontinence will be indicated. For the treatment of the motor urge incontinence component, due either to a suprasacral spinal cord lesion or a brain lesion such as multiple sclerosis, anticholinergics can be very helpful.

Continuous Incontinence

Men with continuous incontinence (overflow) due to obstruction because of an enlarged prostate will require either prostatectomy or the currently popular transurethral balloon dilation of the prostatic urethra (25–32), although the success rate of the latter procedure is not established (33). Temporary relief can also be obtained by implanting a self-retaining and dilating stent (34). Medical treatment can successfully reduce the ob-

Figure 25.3. Uninhibited contractions in a patient with Alzheimer's disease, resulting in urge incontinence. After 220 mL of water was introduced into the bladder, the patient had a strong urge to void. The cystometrogram (CMG) demonstrates that the bladder pressure rose precipitously to 50 cm of water. The patient, however, held urine; the electromyogram (EMG) therefore demonstrated increased activity in the sphincter. The patient was not incontinent at this point. More fluid was introduced into the bladder; the bladder pressure rose to 80 cm of water, and the patient had a strong urge to void. The patient was initially able to hold urine (electrical activity in the sphincter increased), but the sphincter then suddenly relaxed (no electrical activity in the sphincter), and the patient was incontinent. The patient was successfully treated with anticholinergic medications.

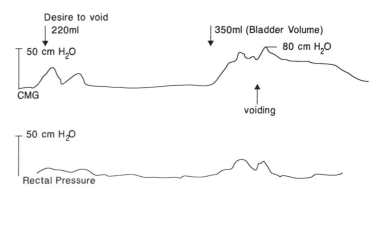

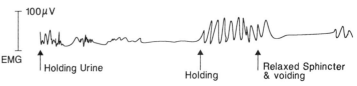

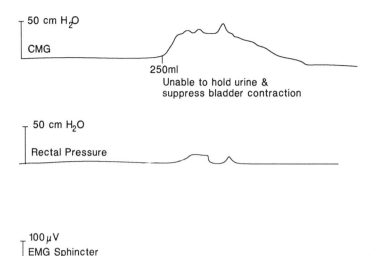

50 cm H$_2$O

CMG

250ml
Unable to hold urine &
suppress bladder contraction

50 cm H$_2$O

Rectal Pressure

100 μV
EMG Sphincter

Figure 25.4. Patient with advanced Alzheimer's disease. When 250 mL of water was introduced into the bladder, the patient had a strong urge to void. Weak electrical activity was recorded in the striated sphincter, and the patient was unable to hold urine or suppress bladder contraction. The patient was successfully treated with anticholinergic medications.

struction and relieve overflow incontinence. For those patients with prostatic hyperplasia in which the gland is still fairly small, alpha-blockers can be effective; those patients with larger glands can be treated hormonally.

For continuous incontinence in women due to fistulae or rigid sphincters, surgical treatment will be required.

Postvoid Incontinence

For postvoid incontinence, the treatment of choice is the surgical removal of the diverticulum.

Reflex Incontinence

Imipramine and anticholinergic drugs are the treatment of choice for reflex incontinence.

HEMATURIA

Hematuria is blood in the urine, which may be either gross or microscopic. It is a serious symptom in the elderly and is often due to surgical hematuria (hematuria without albuminuria or casts).

The first requirement in cases of hematuria is a good history, a good physical examination, and a urinalysis. With the results in hand, important causes can be considered, the most important of which is transitional cell carcinoma of the bladder. Other important causes include transitional cell carcinoma of the renal pelvis or ureter or renal cell carcinoma. Hematuria may also be due to a renal infarct; so it is always important to examine the patient for atrial fibrillation, which can send emboli to the kidneys. Such patients usually have severe pain. Renal, ureteral, or bladder calculi may also cause bleeding, although many patients with calculi will also feel pain. In men, hematuria may be due to benign prostatic hyperplasia. Some men with benign prostatic hyperplasia have urethral varices, which can bleed.

Elderly patients may also have medical hematuria.

Such patients may have a great deal of pain due to arthritis, in which case they may take large doses of analgesics leading to papillary necrosis, which also can cause bleeding. Papillary necrosis may also be due to diabetes mellitus or sickle cell disease. In diabetic patients, papillary necrosis is commonly associated with a urinary infection.

Investigation of Surgical Hematuria

The two most important initial investigations of surgical hematuria are cystoscopy and an intravenous urogram. Cystoscopy, urethroscopy, and even ureteroscopy may be required since cancer of the bladder is the most likely cause of painless gross hematuria in the elderly. Furthermore, if the patient is bleeding from the upper urinary tracts, cystoscopy will allow the examiner to see from which ureter the bleeding arises; the examiner can then ureteroscope the appropriate side.

The intravenous urogram, however, will detect only half of all bladder cancers and is, by itself, a poor test for bladder cancer, yet another reason why cystoscopy is so important here. The intravenous urogram with a good nephrogram and tomograms is, however, a sensitive test for kidney masses and can show areas of infarction, stones, and filling defects in the upper urinary tracts that may be due to transitional cell cancers. It is also very useful for showing some medical causes of hematuria such as papillary necrosis.

If a patient does have a kidney mass on an intravenous urogram with all the features of a renal cyst, ultrasound will be the next cost-effective examination choice, particularly since renal cysts occur in half of all elderly people. If all the typical appearances of a cyst are not present on an intravenous urogram, the next best examination will be computed tomography.

The problems of staging cancers are beyond the scope of this discussion.

Treatment of Hematuria

Treatment of surgical hematuria is the appropriate surgical treatment. For patients with analgesic nephropathy the point will be to get the patient to stop taking analgesics.

Various patients may also have radiation and chemotherapy in the event of cancer; both of which are also beyond the scope of this discussion.

RETENTION

The most common causes of retention in elderly men are benign prostatic hyperplasia and cancer of the prostrate. Such patients usually require surgery to relieve the obstruction. Medical treatment includes alphablockers, hormonal therapy, and/or intermittent catheterization.

Urinary retention in elderly women is rare. Most cases are due to obstruction caused by urethral stenosis.

In both sexes, spinal cord lesions may cause retention of urine due to detrusor-sphincter dyssynergia. Most of these patients can be managed with intermittent catheterization.

References

1. Stamey TA, Timothy MM. Studies of introital colonization in women with recurrent urinary infections. I. The role of vaginal pH. *J Urol.* 114:261, 1975.
2. Stamey TA, Howell JJ. Studies of introital colonization in women with recurrent urinary infections. IV. The role of local vaginal antibodies. *J Urol.* 115:413, 1976.
3. Resnick M, Yalla SV. Management of urinary incontinence in the elderly. *N Engl J Med.* 313:800–805, 1985.
4. Thomas TM, Flymat KR, Blannin J, Meade TW. Prevalence of urinary incontinence. *Br Med J.* 281:1243–1245, 1980.
5. Yarnell JWG, Leger AS. The prevalence, severity and factors associated with urinary incontinence in a random sampling of the elderly. *Age Aging.* 8:81–85, 1979.
6. Brazda JF. *Washington Report, The Nation's Health.* 13(3), 1983.
7. Jewett MAS, Fernie GR, Holliday PJ, Pim ME. Urinary dysfunction in a geriatric long-term care population: prevalence and patterns. *J Am Geriatr Soc.* 29:211–214, 1981
8. Ouslander JG, Kane RL, Abrass IB. Urinary incontinence in elderly nursing home patients. *JAMA.* 248:1194–1198, 1982.
9. Warshaw GA, Moore JT, Friedman SW, et al. Functional disability in the hospitalized elderly. *JAMA.* 248:847–850, 1982.
10. Brocklehurst JC, Dillane JB. Studies of the female bladder in old age. II. Cystometrograms in 100 incontinent women. *Gerontol Clin [Basel].* 8:306–319, 1966.
11. Brocklehurst JC. The aging bladder. *Br J Hosp Med.* 35:8–10, 1986.
12. Castelden CM, Duffin HM, Asher MJ. Clinical and urodynamic studies in 100 elderly incontinent patients. *Br Med J.* 282:1103–1105, 1981.
13. Fossberg E, Sander S, Beisland HO. Urinary incontinence in the elderly: a pilot study. *Scand J Urol Nephrol.* 60 (suppl):51–93, 1981.
14. Schaeffer AJ, Stamey TA. Endoscopic suspension of vesical neck for urinary incontinence. *Urology.* 23:484–494, 1984.
15. Hald T, Bates P, Bradley WE. *The Standardization of Terminology of Lower Urinary Tract Function.* Glasgow: International Continence Society; 1984:1–34.
16. Perkash I, Friedland GW. Principles of modern urodynamic studies. *Invest Radiol.* 22:279–289, 1987.
17. Shortliffe LMD, Stamey TA. Urinary incontinence in the female. Stress urinary incontinence. In: Walsh PC, Gittes RF, Perlmutter AA, Stamey TA, eds. *Campbell's Urology.* Philadelphia, Pa: W.B. Saunders; 1986:2680–2717.
18. Rubesin SE, Pollack HM, Banner MP. Simplified chain cystourethrography. *Radiology.* 145:199–200, 1982.
19. Yoshioka S, Ochi K, Takeuchi M. Simple method for chain cystography. *Urology.* 28:527–528, 1986.
20. Quinn MJ, Beynon J, Mortsesen NJ, et al. Transvaginal endosonography: a new method to study the lower urinary tract in urinary stress incontinence. *Br J Urol.* 62:414–418, 1988.
21. Scott FB, Bradley WE, Timm GW. Treatment of urinary incontinence by an implantable prosthetic sphincter. *Urology.* 1:252–259, 1973.
22. Kaufmann JJ. Treatment of postprostatectomy incontinence using a silicone-gel prosthesis. *Br J Urol.* 45:646–653, 1973.
23. Brown J, Borales P. Artificial urinary sphincter 800. *Urology.* 23:479–483, 1984.
24. Davies C, Evans C, Richards DG, Stephenson TP. The radiological appearance of artificial urinary sphincters. *Clin Radiol.* 36:95–99, 1985.
25. Castaneda F, Reddy P, Wasserman N, et al. Benign prostatic hypertrophy: retrograde transurethral dilation of the prostatic urethra in humans—Works-in-Progress. *Radiology.* 163:649–654, 1987.
26. Castaneda F, Reddy P, Hulbert J, et al. Retrograde prostatic urethroplasty with balloon catheter. *Semin Intervent Radiol.* 4:115–121, 1987.
27. Reddy PK, Wasserman N, Castaneda F, Castaneda-Zuniga WR. Transurethral balloon dilatation of prostate for prostatism: preliminary report of nonsurgical technique. *J Endourol.* 1:269–273, 1987.
28. Reddy PK, Wasserman N, Castaneda F, Castaneda-Zuniga WR. Balloon dilatation of the prostate for the treatment of benign hyperplasia. *Urol Clin North Am.* 15:529–535, 1988.
29. Gonzales JA, Devendra GL, Bolong DT. Prostatic urethroplasty—results at William Beaumont Hospital. *Semin Intervent Radiol.* 6:57–60, 1989.
30. Herrera MA, McCullough D, Harrison L, Link KM. Prostatic urethroplasty—results at Bowman Gray School of Medicine. *Semin Intervent Radiol.* 6:61–64, 1989.
31. Gill KP, Abel P, Jager HR, Williams G, Allison DJ. Prostatic urethroplasty—results at the Royal Post-graduate Medical School. *Semin Intervent Radiol.* 6:65–71, 1989.
32. Isorna S, Maynar M, Belon JL, et al. Prostatic urethroplasty results—Spanish experience. *Semin Intervent Radiol.* 6:72–78, 1989.
33. Friedland GW. The urethra—imaging and intervention in the 1990s. *Clin Radiol.* 42:157–160, 1990.
34. Yachia D, Lask D, Robinson S. Self-retaining intraurethral stent: an alternative to long-term indwelling catheters or surgery in the treatment of prostatism. *AJR.* 154:111–113, 1990.

26

Rehabilitation Management of Pain in the Elderly

Marcel A. Reischer and Henry A. Spindler

The evaluation and management of pain in the elderly is a significant and challenging problem in rehabilitation medicine. At some time, the majority of the elderly population will seek medical care because of various pains. Musculoskeletal pain is the most common (1, 2). The problem is even greater in the nursing home population with 71% (3) to 83% (4) having a pain problem and over half the patients experiencing pain on a daily basis. The incidence of pain tends to increase with age and time, and in a recent study, pain increased significantly over the final year of life with 66% of patients feeling pain "all of the time" one month prior to death (5). It is interesting to note that despite these statistics, the elderly have a tendency to underreport the severity and frequency of their pain, suggesting that pain may be an even greater problem than has been thought (1).

In evaluating any patient with pain, it is critical to differentiate pain behavior from the pain itself. This is especially true in the elderly. Decreased socialization, bedrest, increasing dependence, and outbursts of anger, may all be behavioral responses to the patient's pain. Similarly, attempts at unrealistically increased levels of independence may also be learned behavior to this.

Concepts of operant conditioning will often determine the patient's behavioral response to an episode of pain. Reinforced, these will increase in frequency. For example, if bedrest helps the patient reduce pain and also increases family involvement, the patient may learn that decreasing one's level of independence can lead to both pain reduction and other secondary gains. On the other hand, there is evidence that the elderly do not complain of pain as often because of the assumption that pain is a normal consequence of aging. This may necessitate acting out behavior by the patient, including loud and disruptive outbursts and excessive complaining. Again, this behavior may be successful in drawing the necessary attention and care to the patient, as well as providing further secondary gains in terms of family involvement. Consequently, these pain behaviors may continue even after the acute causes of pain have subsided. This may not be a conscious attempt by the patient to feign disability, but an unconscious learned behavior. The elderly may actually be taught to limit independence and "act their age" by well-meaning and caring family and physicians. Conversely, they may be taught to be mean, loud, angry, and difficult in the same fashion.

Behavioral treatment using principals of extinction may be appropriate and necessary in management, but it is critical for all involved in the care of these patients to appreciate the behavioral responses to pain.

PATHOPHYSIOLOGY

An explosion in understanding of basic physiologic mechanisms of both acute and chronic pain has occurred in the past 20 years. Concepts of gait control, endogenous opiate receptors and mediators, and other specific neurotransmitters are familiar to all now (6). Concurrently, our knowledge of the natural processes of aging has increased. Progressive decrease in sensory function including eyesight (presbyopia), hearing (presbycusis), and two-point discrimination, touch threshold, and vibrotactile threshold occur, and all worsen with age (7).

Paradoxically, however, no consensus exists on specific changes in pain perception. Age-associated changes in pain sensation have been studied both experimentally and clinically for many years. Studies using a variety of methods to induce pain in normal volunteers have given mixed results and were recently summarized by Ferrell (8). His review of the literature from 1940 to the present documented studies showing higher threshold change with aging, lower threshold change with aging, and no change in the threshold to pain with aging. The well-known clinical experience of older patients having painless myocardial infarctions and intraabdominal catastrophes is accepted. It is not clear, however, whether these clinical observations represent a distinct age-related change in pain perception (9, 10). Due to differences in methodology and subject selection, consensus still does not exist regarding the presence of age-associated changes in pain perception. One cannot automatically assume that most elderly patients experience less pain, therefore, and aggressive evaluation and treatment may preclude needless suffering and decreased quality of life in this population (11).

EVALUATION

The evaluation of the elderly patient with pain proceeds along the same general guidelines as evaluation of any patient with pain. A careful history must be taken; a thorough physical examination must be performed; appropriate ancillary studies including laboratory evaluations, radiographic and other imaging techniques must be ordered and evaluated; a diagnosis must be made after a differential diagnosis has been considered and specific treatment plans must be formulated and followed.

Several general rules regarding the management of the elderly patient with pain pertain. Many elderly patients assume that pain is an inevitable consequence of aging and will not complain. It is always necessary to specifically ask patients about the presence of pain. It is always necessary to take the patient seriously and to believe the patient. Never underestimate the potential effects of acute or chronic pain on a patient's general quality of life; it can be much more devastating than in the younger patient. It is critical to achieve an accurate diagnosis, and to merely write-off one's pain as a normal consequence of aging is wrong. It is important to treat patients aggressively and compassionately using a multidisciplinary, multilevel approach to treatment including both physical and medicinal measures. It is important to note the specific side effects and toxicities, as well as drug interaction, in the elderly patient. Be aware that both anxiety and depression can occur and interfere with the treatment response at any point in the course. Although it is important to make a definite diagnosis, do not delay treatment until the diagnosis is made. Indeed, treatment can help facilitate making the diagnosis.

History

The history must be taken from the patient carefully. A thorough general medical history is essential, of course. Patients may be seen for functional deterioration, and only careful, persistent questioning will elicit any story of pain. Questions should be kept short and direct. Some patients will ramble in an attempt to help the doctor, and it is important for all to keep focused.

Often it is useful to supplement the patient's history with information given by a relative or significant other (friend, housekeeper, social worker, landlord, or neighbor) for the full extent of disability to be appreci-

ated. When getting a history from a third party, one must be aware of the possibility of hidden agendas. Reports of significant deterioration of function around the time of a planned family vacation may be intended to justify hospital or nursing home admission, not to treat any reversible dysfunction, but to provide guilt-free, but expensive, domiciliary care. On the other hand, the extent of functional loss may be minimized by a family member unwilling to recognize the deterioration in this once strong, proud, and independent person.

A thorough social history is imperative. Loneliness, helplessness, acute stress, and anxiety may all be the consequences of pain and may only be identified through family interview. These issues can be easily addressed by making the patient and family aware that these feelings can increase the patient's perception of pain. Loneliness and social isolation can lead to the expression of pain as an attention focus in the operant conditioning mode, discussed previously. There are some clinical clues that we have found useful in helping to determine whether the patient's social response is one of learned behavior or a natural response to the patient's condition. It is important to learn about the patient's access to caring relationships, satisfaction and dependence, and needs and ability to care for oneself prior to the onset of this deterioration. Does the patient still live alone or has someone moved in? What does the patient do when the family is there and what does the patient not do? It is important to identify what would get done and who would do it if no one else were there. It is important to get clarification of the family's response to the patient when he or she is in pain and what the family's response is to the patient when there is no pain. How is the patient sleeping? Does the patient complain throughout the day of intractable pain, but is able to sleep through the night without difficulty? All of these provide clues to the patient's pain behavior and provide direction for management.

Obviously, dementia and cognitive deficits significantly hinder the giving of an accurate history. Both pain and the medication used to treat it, however, can mimic dementia and, indeed, should be considered in the differential diagnosis of reversible dementia. Making the patient and family aware that the pain itself can be causing these intellectual deficits and that with appropriate management of the pain these deficits may subside can facilitate keeping the patient functional in an independent living situation rather than in a protected environment. Similarly, depression can be a cause of reversible dementia and may also be secondary to pain, so thoughtful evaluation is essential. Just as pain may present as cognitive loss and dementia, dementia and cognitive deficits may present as patients with pain (12).

Hearing loss may also interfere with the patient's ability to respond appropriately to questions. Obviously, this makes taking history even more difficult. In the patient with impaired hearing, background noise, such as from hospital equipment or a busy ward or physical therapy department, may aggravate the hearing loss and lead to further impairment of the patient's concentration.

In the noncommunicative patient, the history must be obtained from someone other than the patient. A history of changing moods, levels of agitation, or self-care deterioration, such as the onset of incontinence, may be the only way to surmise that pain is present.

Cultural issues may also enter into the taking of an accurate history. The elderly may find it difficult or embarrassing to explain problems to the health professional who is significantly younger ("you remind me of my grandchild"). We find this particularly true when an elderly male patient speaks to a young female. These issues must be appreciated, especially if the history obtained from the patient is substantially different from that given by other family members or assessment of the patient's functional status does not jive with the patient's assessment of his own functional status. This may also explain some interobserver differences in the assessment of the same patient's status, both clinically and in the research mode.

There are other problems in taking a pain history of the geriatric patient. It has been shown that the elderly do not perceive pain to the same extent that younger patients do (13). This is true even if nondemented patients. Many elderly patients often anticipate pain as a natural consequence of growing old and will not volunteer information regarding pain while being evaluated for functional deterioration. Pain is often not even mentioned by the patient unless specifically inquired about. Attempts at listing specific precipitating cause for the pain should be made. There is a tendency by both patient and professional to ascribe pain in the elderly to chronic degenerative conditions such as osteoarthritis. Although this is, indeed, a common cause of musculoskeletal pain in the elderly, generally speaking, the radiographic abnormalities predate the clinical complaints by many years. Accordingly, the question to be answered by all involved in care is: if this is indeed osteoarthritis, why has it just become symptomatic, why has it just worsened? In our experience, there are two common answers to this question. A history of trauma should be sought. Relatively trivial trauma, particularly in the elderly, can result, for example, in internal derangement of the knee with damage to the cruciate ligaments and menisci.

The other common precipitating factor in our experience has been immobility. We have found that patients who have been immobilized for relatively short periods of time, for any number of reasons including even brief hospitalization for what is otherwise considered a relatively trivial medical illness, will subsequently develop musculoskeletal pain. These brief periods of immobility in the elderly may result in enough cardiovascular and muscular deconditioning to significantly affect the patient's ability to ambulate, endurance, and most specifically the muscular protective effect about their weight-bearing joints and axial structures. It is important to emphasize that weak and tight muscles lead to pain. The converse of this is that strengthening those weak muscles will often improve pain (14, 15). In some patients, hip and knee flexion contractures can develop following these short periods of immobilization. These contractures can result in significant pain several weeks later as a result of excessive strain to joint surfaces and soft tissues. Recognition of these two factors, trauma and immobilization, can result in successful goal-directed treatment, improvement in functional status, and decrease in pain.

Obviously, other concomitant causes of worsening pain should always be considered as well. Crystal deposition disease in the joints, bursitis, referred pain from other structures, or herniated discs with or without radiculopathy may cause worsening symptoms in a joint, and the history should try to elicit information suggesting these conditions as well.

Some patients will purposely avoid telling physicians about painful symptoms, fearing that the pain represents a serious illness such as cancer. These patients feel that if they do not describe the symptoms they perceive as being secondary to a malignancy, they will not get that malignancy. Others fear that surgery will be necessary, and they will require more care than appears to be available to them in their social setting. Some fear the loss of independence and control that illness represents to them. All of these patients tax the clinical skill and expertise of the physician.

Primary neuromuscular disorders may present as musculoskeletal pains. Myasthenia gravis may present as low back pain because of the muscular weakness involved (16). Postpolio syndrome, as well as myopathies and neuropathies, may present with pain of a musculoskeletal nature because of associated weakness in supporting structures. In patients with persistent symptoms, a history of these conditions should be obtained and a work-up undertaken.

Physical Examination

There are special issues involved with the physical examination of the elderly patient as well. A thorough examination, particularly of the neurologic and musculoskeletal systems, is important. The elderly are particularly vulnerable to degenerative changes, postural imbalances, gait disturbances, inadequate exercise, muscular weakness and immobility, and all of these predispose to soft tissue pain syndromes. A relative lack of exercise leads to increasing obesity and poor body mechanics, leading to further stresses on abnormal joint surfaces and weak supporting structures. Again, the relatively brief immobility can significantly aggravate what had heretofore been a trivial incidental finding.

There is a normal decrease in flexibility of the musculoskeletal system that occurs with aging. Accordingly, some tightness of the hamstrings, heel cords, and back extensors can be expected as a normal concomitant of aging. Similarly, there is limitation of motion of the subtalar joints. There is also limitation of the knee and finger joints normally (17–21). These limitations, however, should be symmetrical. Asymmetric limitation of motion is a significant finding regardless of the patient's age. Similarly, although there is almost universal degeneration of articular cartilage as one ages and some osteoarthritic deformity, as well as radiographic abnormalities, can be expected, asymmetric abnormalities are not the rule in the normal elderly. In general, these normal deteriorations do not result in abnormal asymmetric tenderness about the joint unless there is some complication.

Some of these normal restrictions of motion, however, can have clinical importance. We have found in particular the presence of heel cord tightness in the elderly female to be a common normal finding. This has recently been confirmed (22). The gastrocsoleus complex is a two-joint muscle. Extending the knee may cause further relative shortening of the heel cord complex and, in extreme cases, plantar flexion of the foot and ankle. Flexion of the knee relieves this and allows dorsiflexion of the foot and ankle. In our opinion, the cause of this heel cord tightening is likely long-time wear of high-heeled shoes with resultant shortening of the heel cord and posterior calf structures. A common scenario has a patient hospitalized for a medical problem, and, while recovering in the hospital, the patient starts to ambulate using just the hospital-supplied low-heeled slippers, rather than the higher heeled shoes that the patient has grown accustomed to. These hospital slippers, of course, do not accommodate for the heel cord contracture that has developed over the years as the patient's own shoes generally do. The natural tendency for the patient to fall backward will be overcome by flexing the knee, relaxing the heel cord, and thus being able to put the foot flat underneath the patient. This, however, results in the patient walking with the knees in excess flexion, resulting in increased forces and stress on the knee joint, excessive flexion of the hips, and abnormal spinal postures, leading to increased stresses and strains in those areas. This leads further to fatigue, both as a result of the pain on walking, as well as the excessive muscle contraction. This can lead to significant pain at multiple sites, and without careful physical examination and the knowledge of the pathomechanics involved, the underlying cause of the problem (the tight heel cords) may be overlooked.

Many elderly patients show what in younger people would be considered abnormal physical signs on neurologic examination. These abnormal neurologic signs may be found in about 80% of patients over the age of 70 years. These include irregular pupillary outline; loss of tone in the facial, neck and spinal musculature; loss of ankle jerks; loss of appreciation of the vibratory sensation at the ankle, and some loss of position sense in the toes. There is also a general decrease in muscle bulk with wasting of the small muscles in the hands being the most common. There may be some sluggishness of the pupillary light reflex, as well as of accommodation. These abnormalities generally do not have clinical significance, however. They are rarely associated with symptoms, and their importance is in not ascribing these as manifestations of significant organic disease. These changes appear to be independent of the presence of any mechanical difficulty associated with cervical spondylosis or other significant neurologic illness. These also appear to be independent of any specific disuse, and, indeed, strength is often maintained surprisingly well despite the wasting on physical examination.

There is also progressive restriction of upward gaze with increasing age. In the patient with cervical spondylosis this can be clinically significant. Compensation for this limitation of upward gaze may be achieved by increasing lordosis and extension of the neck, leading to foraminal narrowing, facet compression, and alterations in balance (as a result of vestibular feedback from the innervation of the facet joints) and may lead to dizziness and falls. It may also lead to increasing pain symptoms as a result of radicular compression because of further foraminal narrowing.

Certainly, disuse is an important factor in muscular weakening that may be seen in the elderly. Care, however, should be taken in ascribing disuse as a cause of the previously described normal changes with aging. Patients with disuse atrophy are typically weak. If the disuse is secondary to some joint dysfunction, it may be greater about that joint than elsewhere. Similarly, multiple contractures and postural abnormalities are more likely to be associated with disuse atrophy than with normal aging (23).

The elderly often show evidence of peripheral vascular disease affecting the blood flow to various nervous structures as well as to the limbs. Although true ischemic neuropathy and myelopathy are not common, they may be seen and certainly should be considered. It is important to examine the patient for differences of limb temperature, which could suggest the presence of vascular insufficiency or inflammation. The vascular insufficiency may have implications as the etiology of the patient's pain. It may also be a significant limiting factor in what can be done for the patient, both surgically (as it limits healing) or nonsurgically (with various heating modalities contraindicated in the presence of vascular insufficiency). Fifteen percent of the elderly population will have orthostatic hypotension, and when evaluating the patient functionally, gait disturbances may be secondary to that rather than to musculoskeletal abnormality.

Various formal scales, such as the Tinetti Gait Evaluation Scale and the Katz Activity of Daily Living Scale, may be useful in the full functional assessment of the patient. In the clinical setting, we have found that observing the patient's normal activities of daily living, such as ambulation and psychosocial functions, may correlate better with the actual level of functional deterioration. Indeed, it has been suggested that these activities of daily living may, in fact, correlate better with the presence and severity of pain than any of the formal assessment scales (2, 3).

Obviously, a thorough general physical examination can give important information regarding specific pain complaints. Neoplastic disease can cause pain locally, from metastatic disease as well as secondary trigger points. Atherosclerotic heart disease may be associated with shoulder-hand syndrome, frozen shoulder, or myofascial trigger points in various areas of the chest. Irritability of the diaphragm, both from the lung above and the hepatic structures below, can result in shoulder pain. A thorough knowledge of referred pain patterns, both from visceral structures as well as neurologic and musculoskeletal structures, is essential in doing a thorough evaluation of the patient with pain. Referred pain sites are often tender and may be confused with local pathology (24). Patients may have pain referred to one area from another one that is not painful. For example, hip disease may present as knee pain without any symptoms referable directly to the hip joint itself. Similarly, cervical radiculopathies may present as shoulder pain or elbow pain without any significant cervical symptoms. Also, referred pain patterns can vary; patients with cervical spine disease may present initially with shoulder pain and may subsequently develop elbow pain with continuing nerve root compression.

Palpation about joints for areas of localized tenderness including trigger points may also help differentiate worsening degenerative joint disease from much more easily treated trigger points, bursitis, or tendinitis (25). A localized injection will often result in immediate and long-lasting relief in that situation, obviating the need for expensive and potentially dangerous medications or surgery. Careful palpation about bony prominences, including the greater trochanter, can help establish these sites as sources of continuing discomfort for the patient (26). Palpation of the pes anserinus and the subacromial region can also help make the diagnosis of easily treatable conditions. Thorough palpation in the elderly patient with trunk pain can suggest the presence of broken ribs and/or metastatic disease.

General observation of the patient's demeanor can also give clues to the nature of the patient's complaints. Typically, acute pain is associated with some level of autonomic hyperactivity including tachycardia, diaphoresis, and increasing general anxiety levels. Chronic pain usually has no autonomic symptoms associated with it. Accordingly, the patient who is complaining of chronic pain, but who is showing some evidence of autonomic hyperactivity, may in fact be experiencing an acute exacerbation of an underlying condition.

The elderly will often have decreased vision and hearing, gait instability, and fear, which limit their ability to be distracted from the pain that they are experiencing. Appropriate attention to these other conditions, such as treatment of cataracts or a new hearing aid, may actually result in improvement in the patient's pain.

Ancillary Studies

There are special considerations in the laboratory and radiographic evaluation of the geriatric population. Roentgenograms will almost universally show some osteoporosis. Less often recognized is coexistent osteomalacia. The osteomalacia may result from malabsorption due to inadequate diet, medication interactions, or from surgery or other medical causes. Care must be taken in the elderly patients in ascribing musculoskeletal symptoms only to osteoporosis. In our experience, trauma of some sort, which often results in a fracture, is the first symptomatic incident in the patient's history of osteoporosis. Typically, the initial fracture is in the low thoracic and high lumbar spine (T-11 through L-1). If initial fractures are seen elsewhere, then consideration should be given to pathologic fractures of the spine and osteoporosis secondary to other conditions such as myeloma, thyroid disease, or metastatic disease.

In addition, radiographic evidence of degenerative joint disease is almost a universal finding in multiple areas, particularly the weight-bearing joints and the spine. Again, care must be taken in ascribing the patient's symptoms to the osteoarthritic abnormalities, particularly if they are symmetrical, and the pain is not symmetrical. There is poor correlation between the severity of radiographic abnormalities, the severity of osteodegenerative disease, and the severity of the patient's symptoms (27). Roentgenograms are helpful to rule out metastases and fracture, as well as bone diseases such as Paget's disease. However, in the patient with new onset of joint pain, when the x-ray film shows only chronic changes, we typically initiate further investigation to determine the cause of the symptoms. Again, decreased muscular protective effect about the joints, bursitis, and internal derangement, aseptic necrosis or crystal-induced synovitis are common causes and should be worked up with joint taps and imaging studies. One should not simply ascribe symptoms to osteoarthritis.

The newer imaging studies, including magnetic resonance imaging (MRI) and computerized axial tomography (CAT) scans, have provided a useful noninvasive tool for the evaluation of a patient's complaints. For example, the diagnosis of spinal stenosis was rarely made prior to the routine use of CAT scans. As noted by Fast elsewhere in this book, spinal stenosis is now recognized to be an important and common cause of back pain in the elderly. Similarly, MRI has proven to be a useful noninvasive tool in evaluation of joint anatomy of the knee and shoulder, as well as other structures. It is becoming the technique of choice for the evaluation of aseptic necrosis of the femoral head. Radioisotope scintigraphy continues to be useful in evaluation of metastatic disease and fractures, as well as aiding in the diagnosis of reflex sympathetic dystrophies. (Fig. 26.1).

Electrodiagnostic evaluations including particularly electromyography and nerve conductions studies can provide significant help in achieving a diagnosis. They are indispensible in determining the site of nerve entrapments and in evaluating neuromuscular disorders that may be contributing to the patient's pain and dysfunction. In the patient with wide-spread degenerative disease of the spine for example, electrodiagnostic evaluation may identify the specific nerve roots that are compressed and may provide valuable assistance in planning a surgical approach. Similarly, identifying coexisting nerve entrapment syndromes in the periphery, such as carpal tunnel syndrome, ulnar neuropathy, or tarsal tunnel syndrome, may obviate the need for spinal surgery, particularly if these conditions can be treated successfully. The electrodiagnostic evaluation provides a physiologic correlate to the abnormalities seen on imaging studies and can be very useful in this patient population.

Laboratory studies that are of particular value in determining the cause of pain in the elderly include erythrocyte sedimentation rate, prostate specific antigen, acid phosphatase and alkaline phosphatase, calcium and phosphorus levels, and serum protein electrophoresis, as well as thyroid function tests. Certainly a general screening, including complete blood count (CBC), electrolytes (both disorders of potassium and sodium metabolism can be associated with pain), chemical profile, and liver, muscle, and kidney function tests, provides useful information. In the chronic patient in particular, we have found a low serum albumin to be helpful in evaluating the level of chronic debility secondary to the pain dysfunction.

There are difficulties, however, in both laboratory and imaging techniques that are peculiar to the elderly. Patients with severe contracture may not be able to fit into the MRI machine. Patients with kyphosis may not be able to tolerate some of the positions necessary for adequate imaging. Confused and agitated patients may make studies technically impossible. Absence of veins may make it particularly difficult to obtain adequate blood specimens for analysis. Although each of these problems can be addressed, one needs to be aware of their existence so that time and effort are not wasted.

Diagnosis

The differential diagnosis of pain in the elderly patient is long. A number of specific pain syndromes are known to affect the geriatric population disproportionately, including peripheral vascular disease; herpes zoster, with or without postherpetic neuralgia; temporal arteritis; polymyalgia rheumatica, and trigeminal neuralgia. There are, however, three disorders in particular that have to be considered in any elderly patient who presents with acute or chronic pain. These are: malignant disease, degenerative joint disease, and depression.

It is important to differentiate malignant from nonmalignant pain. Likewise, it is important to evaluate how much of the patient's complaints are, in fact, fear of malignant pain. In some patients this may manifest as trying to hide facts, and in some cases, it may manifest in an excessively detailed history. Clinically, night pain is an important symptom to elicit. Although night pain may be secondary to nonmalignant conditions such as frozen shoulder, referred pain from a cervical or lum-

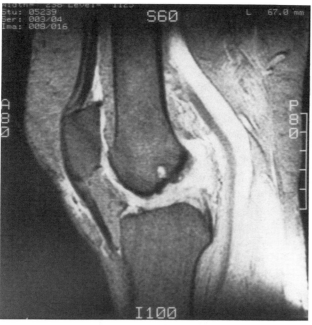

Figure 26.1. Magnetic resonance imaging study of a 78-year-old female with persistent knee pain 9 months after motor vehicle accident. The patient had been functional with occasional knee stiffness in the morning lasting less than 10 minutes, less than once a week. Following the accident, she developed continuing, progressive pain and swelling, leading to significant decrease in her level of activity. Modalities through physical therapy, including ultrasound, hot packs, and electrical stimulation, provided her no relief. The above MRI shows, in addition to some degenerative changes, the absence of the anterior cruciate ligament. Changing the therapy program to a strengthening exercise program with emphasis on the hamstrings, resulted in substantial improvement in her symptoms.

bosacral radiculopathy, pes anserinus, or trochanteric bursitis, the development of night pain is worrisome and suggests the possibility of malignant disease. Patients with known Paget's disease who experience a change in symptoms with increasing pain may be undergoing sarcomatous degeneration of their underlying disorder. On the other hand, the Paget's may be undergoing nonmalignant enlargement, and compression of a nerve may be the cause of the worsening pain (28). Asking about systemic symptoms such as a recent change in appetite, weight change, and other similar symptoms that may be associated is necessary and useful. Certainly an aggressive work-up is warranted whenever there is the possibility of malignant disease present.

A particularly important cause of malignant pain in the elderly is stomach and pancreatic cancer. These will cause pain generally referred to the thoracolumbar region, initially with minimal physical examination abnormality. Subsequently, patients may have trigger points in the involved musculature.

Depression is a common occurrence in patients with these malignancies, and one must guard against ascribing all of the patient's symptoms to depression and proceed with full evaluation of the pain. In our experience, many patients who come to us for evaluation of pain are specifically concerned about the presence of cancer, and we directly confront this issue with the patient. We have seen a number of patients whose symptoms were largely secondary to concern over the presence of disease, and when we assured them none was present, these patients required no further treatment and were able to resume normal functional life-style. When in the midst of a work-up it becomes apparent that the patient does not have malignant disease, we will often advise the patient that there is no evidence of cancer, but that further testing will be necessary to determine the exact nature of the patient's pain. In our experience, patients have been quite grateful for this.

Degenerative joint disease has already been mentioned as a cause of pain. It is important to evaluate adjacent structures including muscular function, trigger points, joint stability, neurologic function, and associated disorders such as crystal deposition disease and referred pain before ascribing the patient's symptoms purely to osteoarthritis. Again, weak muscles lead to painful joints and improvement in the patient's strength and advising the patient that improvement in strength will lead to improvement in function will often help the patient to participate more actively in the rehabilitation program (29). In particular, if careful examination about the joints can elicit the presence of local tenderness such as bursitis, marked improvement symptomatically and functionally can be expected.

Depression is common in the elderly and is commonly associated with chronic pain. The overwhelming majority of the elderly, however, have organic pathology causing pain with psychologic disturbance being a much less prominent etiology (30). Typically depressed patients tend to report both more intense pain complaints and a greater number of localized pain complaints. Pain may be generalized, in a single area, or at multiple contiguous areas. Although joint pain per se generally does not correlate with the presence of depression, depression may make this pain more intense and more disabling. Depression is both a consequence and an aggravator of chronic pain syndrome occurring in up to 90% of all patients with chronic pain syndrome. Studies have shown hypochondriacal, hysterical, and depressive symptomatologies that have reverted to normal with the treatment of the underlying chronic pain disorder. Although patients with primary depression may complain of chronic headaches, backaches, and other symptomatology, depression must be considered a diagnosis of exclusion, and ascribing the chronic pain disorder to depression alone may be simplistic (31).

Although these three, malignant disease, degenerative joint disease, and depression, must be considered in all geriatric patients with pain, there are several other conditions that are often present resulting in significant pain and disability. Myofascial pain syndromes consist of localized soft tissue pain generation associated with a trigger point and characteristic pain referral patterns. The predisposing conditions for myofascial dysfunction are very common in the elderly and include areas of previous trauma, overuse, poor body mechanics, postural imbalance, muscular weakness, a sedentary life-style, inactivity, and cold. They tend to be associated with both anxiety and depression. They may be manifestations of occult neoplasm, hypothyroidism, or electrolyte imbalance, as well as arthritis, disc disease, and various neuropathies and radiculopathies. They are both a cause and a result of sleep disturbance. All of these conditions tend to be somewhat more common in the elderly population and predispose to the development of these trigger points. The characteristic referral patterns of these trigger points can mimic very closely structural disease, and trigger points may be confused with sciatica or cervical radiculopathy. Trigger points tend to become self-perpetuating and chronic. They lead to reflex muscle spasm and splinting which, in turn, leads to increased tightness and weakness which, in turn, leads to increased trigger points, leading to further spasm and splinting. This vicious cycle may be interrupted using trigger point injections, as well as an aggressive stretching and strengthening program.

Again, these trigger points may coexist with other disorders. This is true in general in dealing with the elderly pain patient. One should not think that one has found the ultimate source of the patient's complaints until the work-up has been completed. Multiple etiologies of pain can coexist in the same patient. Indeed, multiple etiologies of pain increase the susceptibility and the sensitivity to pain in other areas from other sources. Visceral structures may cause somatic pain, and that somatic pain may manifest as trigger points. Aortic aneurysms may present as low back pain with radiation into the left hip and leg; gastric and pancreatic carcinomas even without lumbosacral plexus involvement can result in trigger points in the paravertebral area, and atherosclerotic heart disease can result in trigger points in the serratus anterior and pectoralis major presenting a complicated clinical picture.

Another type of pain that appears to be particularly common in the elderly is deafferentation pain (32). In this condition, unlike somatic pain, the dysesthesias occur because of neural damage, which leads to both a sensory loss and, paradoxically, to pain. This results in a sensory imbalance that produce poorly understood pain syndromes. These include postherpetic neuralgia (33), phantom pain, reflex sympathetic dystrophy, and the pain of brachial plexus involvement. Thalamic pain syndromes and the pain associated with paraplegia are probably similar syndromes. Patients with deafferentation pain find that normally nonpainful stimuli, such as touch, pressure, movement, and changes in ambient temperature, can significantly trigger the pain. There is often an initial element of somatic pain associated with this such as radiculopathy or herpes zoster infection and gradually the deafferentation pain will take over. It is critical to differentiate between somatic pain and deafferentation pain because the treatment modalities available and the results to be expected are significantly different. Surgery is generally not appropriate in patients with deafferentation pain. In deafferentation, sensory cell bodies in the dorsal ganglia may die, leaving second order neurons with less synaptic input. This may create an imbalance in which remaining influences have greater input into this second order pain neuron and may excite this neuron. These aberrant impulses then can be transmitted and processed centrally. It is because of this that some centrally active medications such as the tricyclics may be helpful in this situation. Certainly there does tend to be an element of peripheral involvement, however, in these deafferentation syndromes as manifested by the fact that some patients will still respond to transcutaneous electrical nerve stimulation (TENS) units, as well as some physical therapy.

Phantom sensations are a common occurrence in patients following the removal of an appendage. Phantom pain is much less common and can be quite disabling. We have found that reassuring the patient prior to the amputation that they may experience some phantom sensation will minimize the level of dysfunction. Although phantom pain is most commonly thought of as occurring with limb amputations, in fact, it can occur following the removal of any appendage. We find that particularly following mastectomies occurrence of phantom pain may be a cause of significant postsurgical pain,

and it often helps to recognize this and advise the patients of the issues involved.

Treatment

There are issues unique to the treatment of pain in the geriatric patient as well. The goals of pain treatment ultimately are to maintain and improve mobility and function. Without recognizing the effect that the patient's pain has on his or her total life-style and well-being, one cannot adequately treat the geriatric patient's pain. As mentioned earlier, clearly the concepts of operant conditioning of pain behavior are a major issue and must be overcome for a successful result in the total management of the patient's dysfunction.

It is important to formulate a distinct treatment plan and communicate this plan to the patient. The patient will ultimately be responsible for compliance with the medication and exercise regimen, and it is important to include the patient in other significant decision-making processes. It is critical to keep medication regimens simple and consistent. It is important to recognize functional decline, treat it, and prevent further decline. It is crucial to have the patient understand that curtailing physical activity and rest may help some of the patient's symptoms, but may actually, in the long run, result in worsening of the underlying condition if not appropriately combined with exercise. In general, it is important to take the patient's pain seriously and treat it aggressively.

Foley (38) has stated that the cornerstone of treatment of pain in the elderly is medication. Principals of medicinal treatment have been reviewed elsewhere in this book. There are substantial pitfalls to the use of medication, however. The typical geriatric patient is on a number of medicines per day (34). The metabolism of drugs in the elderly is altered substantially. Changes in body composition significantly affect tissue distribution of various medications. Alterations in hepatic function and renal clearance can interfere with the metabolism of drugs. Drug interactions can be a real problem in these patients with altered metabolism. Adding another medication may produce significant toxicity and unforeseen problems. Indeed, patients not on prescribed medications often take over-the-counter medications and typically neglect to mention this to the physician (35). It is important to get a history regarding other medications including specific over-the-counter pain medications whenever considering prescribing for the elderly. Over-the-counter medications often interact with the medications that are typically used in treating pain in the elderly. Nonsteroidal antiinflammatory drugs (NSAIDs) have become the mainstay of medicinal treatment. NSAIDs may not be as safe in the elderly, however, as they are in the younger population. There is evidence that the incidence of gastrointestinal (GI) bleeding is higher in the geriatric population. This class of medication will often produce salt retention, resulting in hypertension, edema, and occasionally heart failure. Renal insufficiency may develop as well. The use of alcohol with NSAIDs significantly increases the risk of GI bleeds and must be specifically warned against.

Narcotic analgesics can be used in the elderly, but must be used with caution. The elderly respond to narcotics as if given four times the dose given to young adults. This is true orally, parenterally, and even intrathecally. Peak levels are higher, and the half life is prolonged. This may lead to significant respiratory depression, confusion, or somnolence. Agitation may be a symptom of pain in the elderly, and in the noncommunicative patient it may be the only indication of the presence of pain. Paradoxically, narcotic analgesics may lead to increased agitation suggesting erroneously that a higher dose of narcotic may be necessary for control of the patient's pain. In fact, the agitation may be produced by the narcotic itself.

Constipation is a particularly troubling side effect in the elderly and should be anticipated and prevented with concomitant stool softeners, laxatives, and dietary manipulations, rather than trying to treat the problem after it develops. Nausea is another troubling side effect of narcotic analgesics and may be prevented by taking anticholinergic medications such as antihistamines and phenothiazines. The elderly are, however, increasingly sensitive to the side effects of delirium and movement disorders seen with these medications, and the patient may actually prefer the nausea.

Concern has been raised about the risks of addiction resulting from narcotic treatment of pain (36). In fact, however, addiction is rare in elderly patients treated with narcotic analgesics (37). Although there are numerous problems associated with narcotic use, if otherwise clinically indicated, we feel that fear of addiction is not a reason to withhold this medication, which would continue the patient's suffering.

Tolerance is a common physiologic problem that occurs in patients on narcotic analgesia. This tolerance leads to decreased duration of effective analgesia resulting in requests for higher doses spaced more closely together. This need not indicate worsening of the underlying condition. It should be noted that the tolerance to the respiratory depressive effects of the medication may not necessarily correlate with the tolerance to the analgesic effect, and the patient should be watched for development of respiratory depression with increasing doses of narcotics.

Other medications that have been used in the elderly with some measure of success include centrally acting medication such as the tricyclics. These act by enhancing neurotransmitter effect of various central pathways. This class of medication may provide improved sleep pattern and relieve pain (sleep disturbance is a cause of musculoskeletal pain) at much lower doses than are necessary for their antidepressant effect. Many of these drugs have anticholinergic side effects including glaucoma and urinary retention, and these can be particularly insidious in the elderly. Dysrhythmias may develop as well.

The elderly may be more sensitive to the neurologic side effects of other medications including carbamazepine and the benzodiazepines. Sedation, ataxia, dizziness, nausea, and vomiting appear to occur more often in this age group (38). Recently, topically applied capsaicin has shown some promise in the elderly in combating some chronic pain syndromes including those secondary to peripheral neuropathy and postherpetic neuralgia. Initiation of treatment will sometimes, however, cause a flare-up of the pain, and there is often poor compliance with the medication. It may also increase local metabolic demand with a rash and as a result may lead to some tissue compromise in patients with vascular insufficiency.

Local injections can be remarkably effective in alleviating the patient's pain as well. Intraarticular steroid injection will lead to marked decrease in pain and improved mobility. It may enable the patient to participate more fully with an exercise program. Trigger point injections using, in our experience, local anesthetics can provide significant relief of soft tissue pain syndrome in elderly patients and enable the patients to proceed with their lives with minimal loss of function. Although sometimes providing only temporary relief, these injections are also useful in at least helping patients resume their normal sleep pattern. Even the period of temporary relief can help the patient believe there is some hope that the ultimate outcome of treatment can be successful and result in pain relief.

Although all of these medicinal approaches can provide significant help, it is our feeling that physical measures should be the cornerstone of treatment of musculoskeletal pain in the elderly. Therapeutic modalities including superficial and deep heating, cooling, electrical stimulation, and exercise can provide substantial relief and aid in reversing the cause of the deterioration of function. Specific exercises to correct tightness and weakness that have occurred following a period of immobilization are often remarkably effective in providing pain relief and preventing recurrences of the pain. In the elderly, however, it may take significantly longer to achieve the desired effect of the exercise program than it takes in younger patients. This is important from the perspective of third party review agents who must appreciate that these patients may not rehabilitate as quickly as a younger patient.

The patient should generally exercise to a quota and not to his or her pain threshold. For example, if it is clear that a patient can walk 25 feet before pain begins, then an exercise program of walking 20 feet three to four times a day is appropriate. The distance can be increased slowly so that the patient experiences exercise and rest, rather than exercise, pain, and rest. Time and consistent increases are the keys to success.

Therapeutic heating and cooling modalities may improve tissue extensibility, decrease inflammation, and allow the patient to exercise more effectively and with less pain. Trigger point injections can help the patient to stretch and strengthen the involved structures to greater therapeutic effect.

Other modalities that have been effective in treatment for the elderly include massage, manipulation (39), infrared (40) and laser treatment (34), and a home TENS unit. We have found the TENS unit particularly useful in elderly patients since it is something that can be done at home. Also strength training, using both isotonic and isokinetic equipment, has been shown to be helpful for pain (14, 15). Cervical and lumbosacral traction can be helpful for both radiculopathies, as well as helping in stretching soft tissue structures (41).

There are significant problems, however, with the physical medicine approach in the elderly as well. It has been shown that temperature perception in the elderly is decreased (42). Accordingly, the elderly patient may not be able to tell when heating modalities are, in fact, too hot, and these patients are particularly susceptible to burns if not watched carefully. Indeed, in a recent study of the nursing home population, hot packs left at the bedside were often not used by the patients because they did not feel hot enough (3)! Heating modalities can result in significant increases in cardiovascular demand and cardiac output and result in symptomatic aggravation of the patient's coronary artery disease. Increasing metabolic demand by local heating of an extremity in a patient with vascular compromise can precipitate gangrene and, certainly in those patients who develop burns, may precipitate catastrophic limb loss. Patients with dysproteinemia may have complications from local cold treatments including tissue necrosis and gangrene. Artificial joints, metal sutures, postoperative clips, or pacemakers may be preferentially heated using some of the diathermy modalities, resulting in damage to local tissue and at times catastrophic results. Cervical traction can lead to strokes, and, indeed, a carotid bruit has been suggested as a contraindication for cervical traction (43). Also, cervical traction can lead to progressive quadriparesis because of spinal cord compression by spondylitic bars or epidural masses.

In our experience, the elderly may have some difficulty managing proper placement of TENS electrodes. This is particularly true if they have to be placed on the low back or thoracic and interscapular region. There is also the potential of the TENS unit to interfere with the function of demand pacemakers and automatic defibrillators. Our policy is not to use a TENS unit at all in patients with an automatic defibrillator and to not use it near a demand pacemaker.

Early experience with TENS units indicated a good initial response following which patients would tend to accommodate to the electrical stimulation parameters and become resistant to the therapeutic effects. Changes in the circuitry have significantly decreased the incidence of the accommodation reaction. Today, if a patient experiences initial relief with a TENS unit, continues to use it, and subsequently becomes resistant to its effect, depression is a much more likely diagnosis than accommodation to the electrical stimulation parameters.

Physical modalities are typically administered by therapists in various clinic settings, although some modalities and exercises can be continued in a home program. An important consideration in the elderly is transportation and, therefore, access to treatment. Patients simply may not have the ability to get out three to five times a week at an appointed time. This is sometimes mistaken as lack of cooperation and poor motivation by those caring for the patients and may be ascribed to depression. It is important to appreciate the fact that the elderly often no longer drive themselves and have to rely on others, needing favors from friends, family, or public transportation, to get where they have to go. Accordingly, significant flexibility in scheduling these patients is paramount. Attendance at group exercise programs at a senior citizen center should be encouraged, and home visits and home care should be considered, but we feel that, if possible, initiation of treatment in a more formal setting can be helpful. In addition to the direct effects of treatment, just getting out and socializing may have significant therapeutic benefit.

At times, a home visit from an occupational therapist may identify significant impediments to the patient's functional independence. Assistive devices, such as raised toilet seats, door knob extensors, splints, and other well-known devices and aids can significantly impact on the patient's ability to maintain functional independence at home and avoid costly, painful, and inconvenient treatment.

Other assistive devices including shoes, braces, and canes, can be very important. Good shoes that accommodate for contractures of the heel cords, as well as for the abnormalities and deformities of the toes, can increase a patient's ability to ambulate to the extent that they can then do their own shopping. We have found lower extremity braces to be somewhat less useful in the elderly patient because they are generally not well accepted. Those patients with some ankle instability have been more accepting of a high top tennis shoe than to a standard orthosis. These orthoses are often cosmetically and philosophically not acceptable to patients. Back braces are often poorly tolerated because of respiratory impairment and worsening hiatal hernia symptoms engendered by abdominal binding.

Many patients will have significant emotional difficulty accepting a cane or a walker, despite the fact that it has become very obvious to them that their current level of ambulation is not functional. Patients will at times practice with a friend's cane and not be taught how to use the cane properly or have it appropriately measured. Generally speaking, of course, a cane should be held on the side opposite the most impaired lower extremity. Typically, it is at about the level of the greater trochanter for best support. It should be noted, however, that with progressively increasing kyphosis the cane may be more functional if it is somewhat shorter so that it may provide maximum support when the elbow is flexed to about 30 degrees.

There are, of course, complications to these assistive devices as well. The risk of carpal tunnel syndrome and ulnar compression at Guyon's tunnel is increased in patients who use a cane regularly. Again, the need to use a cane or other assistive device may precipitate depression in the patient, and this should be looked for, particularly in a patient who has started to use a cane, has had some measure of success with it, and has given it up and lapsed back into functional decline. Interestingly, our experience with upper extremity braces, particularly for carpal tunnel syndrome and for arthritis of the first carpometacarpal joint, has been that patients are more tolerant of these and have used them more successfully than those for the back or lower extremity.

Paradoxically, the successful treatment of pain can often precipitate other problems. Patients whose ambulation has been hindered by pain may now walk more quickly once the pain has been alleviated. Consequently, there is some risk for unmasking significant peripheral vascular disease or angina. Patients who successfully have joint replacement operations may develop functional leg length discrepancy with resulting myofascial, sacroiliac, and lumbosacral pain problems. All of these problems can be anticipated, and the patient and his or her family should be made aware of their possible development. The patient should be seen on a regular basis in follow-up to evaluate the results and side effects of treatment. The program should be changed as dictated by the patient's response.

Surgical treatment is also available for these pain syndromes. Joint replacement surgery particularly of the hip and, to a lesser extent, the knee (44, 45) can be extraordinarily effective in improving pain and function. Particularly in an otherwise healthy patient with severe hip disease, surgical total hip replacement may actually be the most conservative treatment available to the patient. Similarly, surgical treatment of various nerve entrapments may provide remarkable relief and improvement in pain and functional status.

Nerve blocks may be helpful for some patients. Certainly those patients with reflex sympathetic dystrophy may benefit from sympathetic nerve block. Neuroablative procedures, however, including dorsal route entry zone (DREZ) procedures and cutting the spinothalamic tracts should be reserved for patients with end-stage malignant disease. Local blocks of the lumbosacral plexus and sympathetic fibers can help the patient with carcinomatous invasion of those structures.

Hypnosis and biofeedback can both be helpful in treating pain. In the patient who is cognitively intact, the relaxation and anxiety reduction that can be learned can help provide significant relief (28).

One final thought prior to discussing specific regional pain syndromes. A patient may have multiple etiologies of pain in a particular area. A chronically painful area due to a particular disorder will have a lower threshold for other sources of pain than will the contralateral extremity. Incoming nociceptive fibers open the gates by inhibiting the inhibitory neurons in the substantia gelatinosa. Therefore, a strong nociceptive influence will be assured of perception. In addition, a focus of chronic pain may promote the perception of other pains elsewhere (43). Accordingly, the elderly patient with multiple foci of pain may become severely limited and disabled by conditions that would not ordinarily be considered to be this disabling. In an otherwise healthy patient, a carpal tunnel syndrome or epicondylitis may just be a nuisance. In the elderly patient with chronic cervical radiculopathies, myofascial dysfunction, and rotator cuff deterioration, it may precipitate a major functional breakdown.

COMMON PAIN SYNDROMES

Upper Extremity

The most common site of upper extremity pain that we encounter in our practice is the shoulder. Recent studies have suggested that at least a quarter of the elderly may have shoulder pain (46, 47). Many patients will accept this pain and disability without complaint despite the fact that in most cases the cause is a soft tissue lesion that is amenable to nonoperative treatment. In a recent study (48), 98 out of 138 patients complaining of shoulder pain were found to have soft tissue lesions responsive to conservative local treatment. In those patients where no intrinsic shoulder problem could be found, cervical spondylosis with referred pain was felt to be the most common cause. True osteoarthritis of the glenohumeral joint is a rare cause of shoulder pain in the general population. Arthritis of the acromioclavicular joint is not uncommon, however, and may lead to some minimal restriction of motion as well.

The clinical evaluation of these patients is often

able to differentiate an intrinsic shoulder lesion from that secondary to referred pain. Pain with movement of the shoulder is typically associated with an intrinsic shoulder problem. The classical painful arc in the midrange of abduction is found with rotator cuff tendinitis and impingement syndromes. Pain radiating down the arm and unrelated to shoulder movement is usually referred from the neck. Tenderness at the acromioclavicular joint is important to note in arthritis of that joint. Limitation of motion is the sine qua non of a frozen shoulder, but coexistent lesions, both within the shoulder and from referred sources, must be evaluated as well. Patients with frozen shoulder are typically worse at night, often awakening because of the pain. Local metastases and apical carcinoma of the lung may also cause shoulder pain and may also awaken the patient at night, but are often associated with neurologic weakness and distal dysesthesias.

It should be noted that many of these conditions may coexist. A common scenario that we have seen in our practice is a patient with a cervical radiculopathy involving C-5 and/or C-6 leading to weakness in the rotator cuff musculature and inefficient abduction resulting in impingement of the rotator cuff. This may be a situation where neither the chronic radiculopathy nor the rotator cuff lesion alone is severe enough to cause major disability, but the combination of the two can result in major functional decline.

The clinical picture of rotator cuff tears in the elderly can be very insidious, and these patients may be unaware of any worsening of motion despite the tear. Chronic tears can be indistinguishable from tendinitis without rupture. Severe muscle wasting may develop in time, and electrodiagnostic evaluation can be very helpful in differentiating this disuse atrophy from atrophy due to neurogenic causes involving the cervical nerve root or the suprascapular nerve.

Shoulder pain may occur secondary to a general medical condition, such as following myocardial infarction or diaphragmatic irritation. Patients may develop reflex sympathetic dystrophy and/or shoulder-hand syndromes and may develop frozen shoulders following mastectomy or other surgeries. Sympathetic nerve blocks may be helpful both diagnostically as well as therapeutically in this situation.

Other treatment options for soft tissue lesions about the shoulder include local steroid injection for chronic tendinitis and bursitis. Some patients with rotator cuff tears will respond as well symptomatically. Arthroscopic decompression and repair is available for patients with severe dysfunction and weakness. Again, it is important to fully evaluate the musculature about the rotator cuff prior to surgery, and electrodiagnostic studies can be very helpful in this regard.

Physical therapy, including deep heating modalities such as ultrasound, with an active range of motion and strengthening exercise program is particularly useful in situations where there is significant limitation of motion and weakness. A prolonged course of treatment may be necessary. We have found treatment for cervical spondylosis to be particularly helpful in some patients who, despite documented intrinsic shoulder lesions, have not responded to therapy just directed to that area. Treating the chronic radiculopathy that is coexisting may significantly relieve symptoms.

Because of the risks of anesthesia associated with age, as well as osteoporosis, manipulation under anesthesia should be considered a last resort when treating the elderly patient with a frozen shoulder.

Elbow pain is also a common problem in the elderly. In our practice the most common cause of elbow pain in this group is referred pain from cervical radiculopathy, most commonly C-7. Two other important causes are medial and lateral epicondylitis. Lateral epicondylitis typically occurs following a prolonged period of relative immobilization. For example, after a long winter of minimal upper extremity activity, a patient will go out in the early spring and start to prepare the garden for planting. Because of the grasping and pulling involved, patients may develop very significant tendinitis of the lateral epicondylar musculature. It should be noted that gardening, particularly when the patient is on the hands and knees, may lead to the neck being hyperextended and can precipitate an acute cervical radiculopathy as well. Local injections and physical therapy including ice and/or deep heating modalities, electrical stimulation, and stretching and strengthening of the involved musculature can be remarkably effective for this problem. In our experience, simply giving these patients an oral antiinflammatory agent is not adequate, and those patients often develop a chronic epicondylitis. Again, consideration should be given to evaluation and treatment of possible cervical radiculopathy, particularly if the patient's symptoms are resistant to initial treatment.

Medial epicondylitis appears most frequently in the elderly following excessive activities involving resisted wrist flexion. The most common of these activities is bringing a large load of groceries into the home. Carrying the bags under the arms with excessive resisted wrist flexion will precipitate this condition. Patients may develop ulnar neuropathy as part of this syndrome as well. Local injections and physical therapy with particular emphasis on modalities, stretching and strengthening appropriate musculature can result in a rapid return to normal activities. Patients with resistant symptoms should be evaluated for ulnar neuropathies, as well as cervical radiculopathies. Less common but still significant causes of persistent symptoms include median nerve compression in the area of the pronator teres muscle and, rarely, carpal tunnel syndrome.

Carpal tunnel syndrome is the most common cause of wrist and hand pain that we see in the elderly. It is not at all unusual for patients to be referred for evaluation of muscular wasting in the hand and to find that they have been told for many years that they have been suffering from arthritis or poor circulation. Patients who have already developed significant atrophy may no longer be good surgical candidates, and any patient with persistent upper extremity symptoms and certainly specific symptoms in the wrist and hand including numbness, weakness, clumsiness, and pain, should be considered to have carpal tunnel syndrome until proven otherwise. These patients should all be evaluated electrodiagnostically.

Ulnar neuropathy at the elbow can also present with wrist and hand pain, as well as numbness and weakness. Electrodiagnostic evaluation for ulnar nerve slowing at the wrist and elbow should always be part of the electrodiagnostic evaluation of the patient with upper extremity symptoms. It should be noted that weakness engendered by nerve entrapments in the upper extremities, including median, ulnar, or radial, may lead to relative overuse of other muscles and may be an important precipitant in the development of medial and/or lateral epicondylitis, as well as tendinitis about the wrist and hand. Patients with persistent symptoms unresponsive to therapy should always be evaluated for these conditions, as well as other conditions causing weakness and incoordination of upper extremity function. Another important cause of hand disability that we have seen in the elderly population is arthritis of the first carpometacarpal joint. This often coexists with carpal tunnel syndrome. Some patients, however, will have the arthritic problem alone without the carpal tunnel syndrome. Wasting of the thenar eminence musculature secondary to splinting from the pain, as well as weakness of the thenar musculature because of the pain, will compound this confusion. Typically, a sensory examination is normal in patients with the arthritic condition. Electrodiagnostic evaluation will exclude nerve entrapments in this situation. Treatment for the arthritic condition can include local injections, systemic antiinflammatories, or orthopedic procedures including joint fusion or joint replacement.

Another common cause of wrist and hand pain in the elderly is deQuervain's stenosing tenosynovitis. This has been historically referred to as "washer woman's hand," which suggests the offending action. Excessive grasping and twisting will result in tendinitis of the extensors and long abductors of the thumb. Patients may complain of numbness associated with this condition because of the coexistent entrapment of the superficial radial nerve at the wrist. Sometimes the swelling at the wrist results in a coexistent carpal tunnel syndrome. Local injection can be very helpful, but care must be exercised to avoid hitting the superficial radial nerve. Likewise, surgery can injure that nerve although it can be quite effective. Splinting can provide significant

functional improvement, but one must be certain that there is immobilization of the appropriate joints involved. The commercially available cock-up splints do not generally provide significant immobilization of the appropriate joints although opponens splints do.

Finally, another important cause of hand pain is systemic arthritis. Despite the deformities noted in osteoarthritis, these deformities rarely affect function, and they may even be painless. Flexor tenosynovitis in the hand may cause referred pain in the palm and may cause referred pain to the interphalangeal (IP) joints of the hand. This can be a difficult diagnosis, particularly in the stage before a trigger finger develops. Once the triggering becomes obvious, however, the diagnosis is clear, and local injection and splinting may obviate the need for surgery.

Lower Extremity

Osteoarthritis of the hip is a common cause of pain in the lower extremity. Although typically pain is felt in the groin, patients may actually have pain referred to the knee with no hip symptoms whatsoever. In patients with chronic stable osteoarthritis of the hip joint to develop sudden worsening, consideration should be given to the possibility of trochanteric bursitis. Local injection can be remarkably effective. A lumbosacral radiculopathy may cause similar worsening. Indeed, chronic radiculopathy of the L-5 and S-1 nerve roots may lead to significant weakening of the hip abductor musculature causing relative overuse of those muscles and leading directly to the development of a trochanteric bursitis. Treatment of both the radiculopathy as well as the bursitis may be necessary. Although there may be radiographic evidence of osteoarthritis of the hip, treatment of these other conditions can return the patient to a relatively pain-free and functional state.

Significant care must be taken in evaluating the patient with hip pain. In the patient with severe osteoporosis, pelvic fractures can develop and may not have been seen on initial radiographic evaluation. Scintigraphic techniques may be the only ones useful in evaluating the elderly osteoporotic patient for possible pelvic fractures. Patients with a history of a fall or other trauma with continuing pain and a negative work-up should be considered for this.

Careful physical examination of the hip is obviously crucial. Painful limitation of range of motion, as well as a tender hip joint (the hip joint is found deep to the femoral vessels; a common mistake is assuming that the greater trochanter is in fact the hip joint) point to a diagnosis of specific hip joint dysfunction. In patients with negative x-ray films, consideration should be given to an MRI for the evaluation of possible aseptic necrosis.

Other important diagnoses to consider in the patient with hip pain include referred pain from radiculo-pathy and referred pain from retroperitoneal disorders. The pain of an aortic aneurism may be felt in the back and radiate into the left hip and occasionally down the left leg. Intrapelvic disease, both benign and malignant, may be referred to the hip area as well. Nonsurgical treatment of hip disorders can be quite helpful. The use of a cane (held in the hand opposite the painful hip), attempts at weight loss (for every 10 pounds of weight loss, 30 pounds of force are removed from the hip joint) can be helpful. Physical therapy including strengthening the surrounding muscles, stretching the joint capsule, and providing deep heating to the joint through ultra-sound, as well as the judicious use of medication can also be quite helpful. Treating associated conditions such as lumbosacral radiculopathy and other causes for mus-cular weakness, as well as myofascial dysfunction, can also be helpful.

In patients in whom the diagnosis of osteoarthritis of the hip is secure, consideration should be given to joint replacement surgery. The functional results fol-lowing this surgery may be spectacular with patients often able to return to a normal, active life 4 to 6 weeks after the surgery. In a patient who is otherwise in good med-ical condition, total hip replacement may actually be the more conservative treatment for osteoarthritis of the hip in the elderly patient (47).

Knee pain is also a common problem in the el-derly patient. The clinical diagnosis of osteoarthritis should be reserved for patients whose pain is associated with limitation of motion. Typically, initially there is a lack of normal extension. Subsequently the patients will develop limitations in flexion. Physical examination may who some tenderness and enlargement and thickening of the synovial tissues, and there may be a moderate increase in synovial fluid. The patellofemoral articula-tion may be the site of maximum damage, but it should be noted that asymptomatic crepitation in this joint is not uncommon.

The structures of the knee, particularly if there has been some degeneration, are particularly sensitive to further damage by trauma. This trauma may be quite trivial and not noted by the patient. Ask specifically about difficulty getting out of a cab, a slight trip over the side-walk, or a missed step, as these may precipitate the de-velopment of meniscal tears and/or ligamentous strains. Bursitis is a common problem, particularly given the fact that there are well over 30 bursae present about the knee. It may result in significant swelling and pain. There is typically point tenderness in the area of the bursa, and these may respond to local injections. Care must be taken, however, to avoid injecting a tendon directly, as this may weaken the tendon and result in rupture.

Probably the most common cause of deterioration of knee function in our experience has been the devel-opment of quadriceps weakness, most typically follow-ing a period of immobilization such as a brief hospitali-zation. Patients may also reflexly inhibit muscular function as a result of some knee pain. Accordingly, one estab-lishes a vicious cycle of pain, immobility, and weakness, leading to further pain, further immobility, and further weakness. In patients who are functionally marginal, even a small period of immobilization can make a significant functional difference. The clinician must be alert to this problem, and a strengthening program, together with modalities, may be particularly helpful in reversing the muscular wasting. As mentioned, other physiotherapy modalities including ultrasound and electrical stimula-tion may provide these patients with some benefit when combined with a strengthening program. Weight reduc-tion and intraarticular steroids can also be helpful, as can some NSAIDs. Bracing is often considered for these patients. We have not had a lot of success with braces, as the elderly find it difficult to don and doff them, ap-ply them snugly enough to give meaningful support, or tolerate them cosmetically.

If conservative treatment fails in the presence of significant knee pain, surgery is available (45). The re-sults of knee replacement surgery are not as dramatic as those of hip replacement surgery, but can still provide improvement in function and decrease in pain in many patients. Ligamentous function must be intact. Osteot-omy of the tibia can be considered when there is uni-compartmental disease. Arthroscopic surgery for men-iscal tears can provide remarkable benefit, although we have seen somewhat less success with the use of this technique in the treatment of patellofemoral disorders in the elderly patient. Chronic cruciate tears should probably not be repaired in this population. Referred pain to the knee from high lumbar radiculopathies, lum-bosacral plexus lesions, nerve entrapments, and injuries about the knee should be evaluated and treated appro-priately.

Foot and ankle pain are a common cause of dis-ability and dysfunction in the elderly. Although the foot takes a significant beating in normal activities such as walking, osteoarthritis is in fact uncommon with the possible exception of the midtarsal region. Many of the foot problems seen in the elderly are due more to the process of senescence, and these problems in turn may lead to a cascade of other symptomatic entities. The subcutaneous tissue of the foot is normally minimal with the exception of the plantar fat pad. This pad acts as a resilient buffer against the constant pounding of the metatarsal heads and the os calcis against the ground. These fat pads atrophy in the elderly. Painful callouses then develop under the metatarsal heads. Atrophy of the heel pad may cause pain under the calcaneus. Altered gait mechanics as a result may lead to tendinitis of the intrinsic and extrinsic foot muscles, presenting a com-plicated picture which may, in turn, lead to nerve en-trapments such as tarsal tunnel syndrome, further complicating the clinical picture. As with all pain problems, a full, careful history and physical examination must be undertaken. True osteoarthritis is rare in the ankle despite the obvious wear and tear of weight bearing. Particularly in obese women, however, a general synovial thickening may develop about the ankle, which can result in pain. It is differentiated from stasis edema by its lack of pitting. With increasing age, the subtalar joint gradually loses motion, and some narrowing of the joint space may be noted radiographically. The subtalar joint itself would generally not be symptomatic, but will transmit increased forces to the midtarsal joints, and osteoarthritic change may be noted there. Osteoporosis is not an issue in the typical patient with foot pain.

As a result of deformities and poor fitting shoes, in addition to weakness and deconditioning, painful tenosynovitis about the foot and ankle is common. It is most frequently seen in the tibialis posterior tendon with flexor hallucis longus tendinitis and achilles tendinitis being somewhat less common. These typically have local tenderness, but referred pain as well as coexistent nerve entrapments may occur, and these should be evaluated. Local steroid injections, systemic antiinflammatories, and shoe modifications, as well as physical therapeutic modalities and strengthening and stretching exercises can be helpful.

As a result of the posture assumed by most women when wearing high-heeled shoes, excessive stresses are placed on the anterior metatarsals. Accordingly, metatarsalgia is a common problem. Patients often complain of pain, as well as local burning. Peripheral neuropathy, radiculopathy, or nerve entrapments must be considered. Interdigital neuroma may also develop and is common in this population. A clinical clue to its presence is when the pain only occurs with walking and generally does not involve a lot of proximal radiation. Occasional tingling and numbness may be present, but the pain is the predominant complaint. Local injection and appropriate shoe modifications are the treatment of choice. As with all foot surgery in the geriatric population, there is a significant risk of skin sloughing and other complications due to associated vascular insufficiency.

Tendinitis of the achilles tendon may be seen in the elderly. Spontaneous rupture of the tendon typically occurs while the patient is in some unusual exertion, such as running for a bus. Again, conservative treatment will generally result in functional improvement with the need for surgical repair most unusual in this population.

Finally, the most common cause of foot pain in the elderly male is the plantar heel spur syndrome. Although the high-heeled shoes tend to increase the incidence of metatarsalgia in females, they tend to decrease the incidence of symptomatic heel abnormalities. This syndrome is typically associated with tightness of the plantar fascia, and the normal atrophy that one sees in the heel pad with aging may significantly aggravate the

symptoms and impact on the ability to treat the patient successfully. Patients with this condition often have a coexistent tenosynovitis in the flexor hallucis longus. Consideration should be given to the presence of a tarsal tunnel syndrome as well. Pain from a pure plantar heel spur syndrome is typically most severe on the initiation of weight bearing, especially upon arising in the morning. Patients in whom the tenosynovitis of the flexor hallucis longus is the predominant problem will generally not have pain on initiation of weight bearing, but will have symptoms with walking. Local injections, a heel lift, cut-outs, and other orthotics may be helpful in relieving symptoms. Interestingly, a spur may not be present radiographically. Physical therapy with modalities including whirlpool and ultrasound, as well as stretching exercises to the tight plantar fascia and improving strength of the flexor hallucis longus muscle, may be helpful.

SUMMARY

The evaluation and care of the elderly patient in pain is a difficult and challenging problem, but a problem of increasing importance. The goal of treatment and rehabilitation of the elderly patient in pain is to maintain and improve function by decreasing that pain. The unique physiology and pathophysiology in the elderly require a careful, thorough, and thoughtful evaluation process. In particular, a history of even minor trauma and immobilization must be sought, as these can precipitate major deteriorations in functional status. Particular care must be taken in following the effects of treatment and understanding and appreciating the multiple psychosocial issues and behavioral issues involved in the pain management of these patients. Consideration of issues such as transportation and socialization must be taken into account when evaluating and prescribing for these patients. Particular care must be taken in following the effects of treatment. To simply ascribe pain in the elderly to arthritis and to merely prescribe medication without giving thought to the full impact that the pain may have on the patient's function is a disservice. An aggressive multidisciplinary approach may ultimately help the patient to continue or resume a productive and functional existence.

References

1. Crook J, Rideout E, Growne G. The prevalence of pain complaints in a general population. *Pain.* 18:299–314, 1984.
2. Lavsky-Shulan M, Wallace RB, Kohout FJ, et al. Prevalence and functional correlates of low back pain in the elderly; the Iowa 65 Plus Rural Health Survey. *J Am Geriatr Soc.* 33:23–28, 1985.
3. Ferrell BA, Ferrell BR, Osterweil D. Pain in the nursing home. *J Am Geriatr Soc.* 38:409–414, 1990.
4. Roy R, Michel TA. Survey of chronic pain in an elderly population. *J Can Fam Phys.* 32:513–516, 1986.
5. Moss MS, Lawton MP, Glicksman A. The roll of pain in the last year of life of an older person. *J Gerontol Psychol Sci.* 46(2):51–57, 1991.

6. Bonica JJ. *The Management of Pain.* 2nd ed. Philadelphia, PA: Lea & Febiger; 1990.

7. Hinchcliff R. Aging and sensory threshold. *J Gerontol.* 17:45, 1962.

8. Ferrell BA. Pain management in elderly people. *J Am Geriatr Soc.* 39:64–73, 1991.

9. Bayer AJ, Chada JS, Farag RR, et al. Changing presentations of myocardial infarctions with increasing age. *J Am Geriatr Soc.* 34:263–266, 1986.

10. Bender JS. Approach to the acute abdomen. *Med Clin North Am.* 73(6):1413–1422, 1989.

11. Harkins SW, Kwentus J, Price DD. Pain in the elderly. In: Benedetti C, ed. *Advances in Pain Research and Therapy, VII.* New York, NY: Raven Press; 1984.

12. Anderson JM, Kaplan MS, Felsenthal G. Brain injury obscured by chronic pain: a preliminary report. *Arch Phys Med Rehabil.* 71:703–708, 1990.

13. Ferrell BA, Ferrell BR. Assessment of chronic pain in the elderly. *Geriatr Med Today.* 8(5):123–134, 1989.

14. Lexell J, Robertson E, Stenstrom E. Effects of strength training in elderly women. *J Am Geriatr Soc.* 40:190–191, 1992.

15. Fisher NM, Pendergast DR, Gresham GE, et al. Muscle rehabilitation: its effect on muscular and functional performance of patients with knee osteoarthritis. *Arch Phys Med Rehabil.* 72:367–374, 1991.

16. Wood DW, Turner RJ. The prevalence of physical disability in southwestern Ontario. *Can J Public Health.* 76:262–265, 1985.

17. Jette AM, Bottomley JM. The graying of America. Opportunities for physical therapy. *J Phys Ther.* 67:1537–1542, 1987.

18. Wright V. Stiffness, a review of its measurement and physiological importance. *J Physiotherapy.* 59:107–111, 1973.

19. Barnett CH, Cobbold AF. Effects of age on the mobility of human finger joints. *Ann Rheum Dis.* 27:175–177, 1968.

20. Such CH, Unsworth A, Wright V, et al. Quantitative study of stiffness in the knee joint. *Ann Rheum Dis.* 34:286–291, 1975.

21. Vandervoort AA, Chesworth BM, Cunningham DA, et al. Age and sex effects on mobility of the human ankle. *J Gerontol Med Sci.* 47:M17–21, 1992.

22. Carter AB. The neurologic aspects of aging. In: Rossman I. *Clinical Geriatrics.* 3rd ed., Philadelphia, PA: Lippincott; 1986.

23. Kellgren JG. On the distribution of pain arising from deep somatic structures with charts of segmental pain areas. *Clin Sci.* 4:35–46, 1939.

24. Reynolds MD. Myofascial trigger point syndrome and the practice of rheumatology. *Arch Phys Med Rehabil.* 62:111–114, 1981.

25. Swezey RL. Pseudo radiculopathy in subacute trochanteric bursitis of the subgluteus maximus bursa. *Arch Phys Med Rehabil.* 57:387–390, 1976.

26. Bayless TM. Malabsorption in the elderly. *Hosp Prac.* 14:57–63, 1979.

27. Portenoy RK, Sarkash A. Optimal control of non-malignant pain in the elderly. *Geriatrics.* 43:29–47, 1988.

28. Chen JR, Rhee RS, Wallach S, et al. Neurologic disturbances in Paget's disease of bone; response to calcitonin. *Neurology.* 29:448–457, 1979.

29. Parmele PA, Katz IR, Laughton MP. The relation of pain to depression among institutionalized aged. *J Gerontol Psychol Sci.* 46:P15–21, 1991.

30. Newton PA. Chronic pain. In: Cassel CK, Sorensen LB, Reisenberg DE, Walsh JR, eds. *Geriatric Medicine.* 2nd ed. New York, NY: Springer Verlag; 1989.

31. Watson CPN. Postherpetic neuralgia. *Neurol Clin.* 7:231–248, 1989.

32. Osserman KE, Genkins G. Studies on myasthenia gravis: review of a twenty year experience in over twelve hundred patients. *Mount Sinai Gen Med.* 38:497–537, 1971.

33. Foley KM. Pain management in the elderly. In: Hazzard WR, Andres R, Bierman EL, et al. *Principals of Geriatric Medicine and Gerontology.* 2nd ed. New York, NY: McGraw Hill; 1990.

34. Felsenthal G, Cohen BS, Hilton EB, Panagos AV, Aiken BM. The physiatrist as primary physician for patients on an inpatient rehabilitation unit. *Arch Phys Med Rehabil.* 65:375–378, 1984.

35. Chrischilles EA, Lenke JH, Wallace RB. Prevalence and characteristics of multiple analgesic drug use in an elderly study group. *J Am Geriatr Soc.* 39:979–984, 1990.

36. Long DM. Management of pain in the elderly. In: Hazzard WR, Andres R, Bierman EL, et al. *Principals of Geriatric Medicine and Gerontology.* 1st ed. New York, NY: McGraw Hill; 1985.

37. Porter J, Jick H. Addiction rare in patients treated with narcotics. *N Engl J Med.* 302:123, 1980.

38. Debner R. Topical capsaicin therapy for neuropathic pain. *Pain.* 47:247–248, 1991.

39. Cassidy JD, Kirkaldy-Willis WH. *Manipulation, Managing Low Back Pain.* 2nd ed. In: Kirkaldy-Willis WH, ed. New York, NY: Churchill Livingstone; 1988.

40. Stelian J, Gili Habot B. Improvement of pain and disability in elderly patients with degenerative osteoarthritis of the knee treated with narrow band light therapy. *J Am Geriatr Soc.* 40:23–26, 1992.

41. Laban MM, Meerschaert JR, Johnstone K. Carotid bruits: their significance in the cervical radicular syndrome. *Arch Phys Med Rehabil.* 58:491–494, 1977.

42. Sherman ED, Robillard E. Sensitivity to pain and relationship to aging. *J Am Geriatr Soc.* 12:1037–1044, 1964.

43. Marlow RM, Olson RE. Changes in pain perception after treatment for chronic pain. *Pain.* 11:65–72, 1981.

44. Harris WH, Sledge CB. Total hip and total knee replacement (part 1). *N Engl J Med.* 323:725–731, 1990.

45. Harris WH, Sledge CB. Total hip and total knee replacement (part 2). *N Engl J Med.* 323:801–807, 1990.

46. Chard M, Hazelman R, Hazelman BL. Shoulder disorders in the elderly (A community study). *Br J Rheumatol.* 28(Supplement 2):21, 1989.

47. Chakravarty KK, Webley M. Disorders of the shoulder; an often unrecognized cause of disability in elderly people. *Br Med J.* 300:848–849, 1990.

48. O'Reilly D, Bernstein RM. Shoulder pain in the elderly. *Br Med J.* 301:503–504, 1990.

27

Sexual Function in the Elderly

Fae H. Garden

The aging and elderly population is especially vulnerable to sexual dysfunction. An interplay of psychogenic and organic factors including effects of multiple medications, chronic illness, and the loss of friends or spouses contributes to this problem. Physicians and other health professionals who work with older patients are often guided in their treatment approach by a number of myths concerning geriatric sexuality. These myths are compounded when the patient in question also happens to be disabled. Woodward and Rollin (1) have described 10 commonly held beliefs about sexuality and disability in the older population. Perhaps the most widely held of these beliefs is that older disabled people are not interested in sex and that older disabled people should learn to adjust to a life of celibacy, especially after 60 years of age (1).

Although the literature concerning sexuality and aging is occasionally contradictory, it is generally accepted that sexual interest and activity does not automatically diminish with advancing age and may, in fact, continue almost indefinitely (2). Pfeiffer (3) noted that many elderly persons regularly engaged in sexual activity but that the percentage declined significantly with age. In persons aged 78 years or older, only 20% regularly participated in sexual activity. Despite this, sexual interest was reported by over 40% of persons in this age group. Older men reported greater sexual activity and interest and activity than did older women. The frequency of sexual activity among persons aged 60 to 90 years was reported to vary from once a month to three times a week. Labby (4) has noted that the earlier sexual activity began in adulthood, the more likely it was to continue into old age. This statement may be influenced by a relative lack of male partners among the aged population. Pfeiffer and Davis (5) have noted that the ratio of women to men is 130 to 100 for those between the ages of 65 and 74 years. For those 75 years and older, the ratio increases to 178 to 100.

Elderly persons who live in nursing homes often find that this environment inhibits their sexuality. Although the reason most frequently given by residents in a nursing home for not being sexually active is lack of a partner (6), the home is usually not set up for couples to have sexual relationships. Staff members are often not trained in human sexuality. Many homes have single, hospital style beds and require that doors be unlocked at all times. Family members may support the sexless environment of nursing homes because of an inability to accept their parents' sexuality (7). Other reasons for not being sexually active in a nursing home include poor health, lost interest, and inability to perform (6). Some patients will use masturbation as a sexual outlet. Masturbation by female patients may be one of the most common reasons that physicians are asked to transfer patients out of a nursing home (8). Male nursing home residents are frequently asked to undress in the presence of others and must refrain from displaying any sexual excitement (7). All of this can have a damaging effect on an elderly person's self-esteem and interpersonal relationships.

The denial of sexuality by American nursing homes is in direct contrast to those of the Netherlands. In the Netherlands, the nearly 200,000 residents of retirement and nursing homes are permitted to use the services of prostitutes. This practice has led to extensive campaigning in the television and print media to encourage the elderly to use condoms to protect themselves from sexually transmitted diseases.

CHANGES IN THE MALE SEXUAL RESPONSE WITH AGING

Masters and Johnson are credited with making the first direct observations of age changes in the physiologic response. The phases of excitement, plateau, orgism, and resolution are variably affected in a given individual as a result of aging. There appears to be a steady decline in the duration as well as the intensity of each phase (9).

A reduced speed of sexual arousal is often the first change noted by aging men (9). Testosterone, the primary hormone associated with sexual desire, is usually produced at all ages, but production decreases gradually after the age of 20 years. An accelerated decline in testosterone levels occurs after the sixth decade (10). Plasma testosterone normally rises during coitus (11), and this response may be blunted in older individuals. Androgen replacement, used to treat sexual dysfunction including decreased sexual desire, in older men has met with limited success. Changes that do occur in men receiving this treatment are often attributed to either a placebo effect or an improvement in the patient's sense of well-being (10).

Diminished libido may also be due to alterations in the sensations of vision, hearing, and smell. The sensitivity of the glans penis in detecting the difference between vibration and static touch decreases with age (12). Illness of an acute or chronic nature has a more profound effect on the speed of sexual arousal in an older person than one would expect to find in a younger individual (9).

Men who notice a decrease in their sexual desire are often influenced by negative social attitudes toward sexuality in the elderly. Many of these men were raised during a time when sex education and open sexual expression were considered immoral. They may have concerns that their continued sexual desires could label them as "dirty old men." It is the role of the counselor to help allay these fears and educate the patient about the natural changes in sexuality with aging. Bringing the partner into the discussion is essential to foster the idea of continued closeness and intimacy.

In addition to difficulties with libido, erectile changes in aging men are common and a source of great concern. Many older men take up to 10 minutes to achieve full penile engorgement. The change in penile length is less marked, and the fully erect penis may be less rigid compared with the patient's younger years. Loss of collagen tissue as well as progressive arteriosclerosis is partially responsible for this phenomenon. The usual darkening of the glans penis may not be as noticeable, and elevation of the testicles is less obvious (9). A change in coital position may be necessary due to a reduced angle of the erect penis. Cardiopulmonary changes inherent to the aging process may result in an excessively increased respiratory rate, tachycardia, and blood pressure elevation.

Erectile dysfunction in the elderly may result from psychologic as well as physiologic problems. The presence of nocturnal or morning erections can be useful in differentiating between these two etiologies. Monitoring with penile plethysmography may be useful in some cases. The duration of erection during sleep decreases steadily with aging. While an adolescent may spend 3 hours erect during an average evening of sleep, by age 65 years a healthy male will have erections during 20% of his sleep time (13). When impotence is due to physiologic processes such as diabetes, treatment options should be identified and discussed. Some alternatives include surgically implanted penile prostheses, external impotence management devices, and injectable and oral medications.

The sensation associated with ejaculation is frequently reported by older patients to be less intense. As the contractile strength of the prostate decreases with aging, so does the amount and viscosity of the ejaculate. Decreases of up to 50% of previous ejaculate volume have been noted by some men (9). The postejeculation refractory period becomes significantly prolonged, sometimes lasting for days to weeks in men over the age of seventy years (10). This phenomenon is a normal part of the aging process and should be explained to patients in straightforward terms.

Elderly men who engage in sexual activity may have questions about their reproductive capability. Testicular biopsies have demonstrated active spermatogenesis in 50% of men over the age of 70 years (13). Degenerative changes in the seminiferous tubules and germ cells are also evident.

CHANGES IN THE FEMALE SEXUAL RESPONSE WITH AGING

A woman in the United States can expect to live approximately 29 years past the age of menopause (14). Since women live longer than men, they may spend the last few years without a male partner. The onset of menopause and its associated hormone deprivation is directly related to problems in female sexual interest and performance. In a group of women age 50 years and over, 79% of postmenopausal women noted a decrease in sexual interest (15). This finding has been disputed by others (4) who indicate that a woman's interest in sex often intensifies after menopause, especially when she has the feeling that sexuality activity is acceptable and can be continued in later life. Androgens, primarily produced in the adrenal glands, are not adversely affected by menopause. The sexual stimulating properties of testosterone may play a large role in postmenopausal libido once estrogen and progesterone levels have dropped (9). The freedom from risk of pregnancy and the absence of children in the house may help to encourage continuation of sexual activity past menopause (4). Women are more likely than men to cease sexual activity or substitute masturbation for intercourse after the loss of their long-term sex partner (4).

A decrease in coital frequency has been associated with low serum estrogen levels (15). In one study (16), a serum estradiol level of 35 pg/mL or lower was found to be a critical value that predicted dwindling intercourse frequency. Most of the women who had intercourse at least once a week had estradiol levels above this value.

Vaginal dryness and resultant insertion dysparenuria are common problems cited by postmenopausal women. Vaginal lubrication is a primary function of the Bartholin glands which lose some of their effectiveness with aging. Estrogen deficiency leads to thinning and brittleness of the vaginal tissues. Women who use antihistamines and decongestants will experience mucous membrane dryness from these medications. Vaginal expansion during sexual arousal is decreased and contributes to the problem of uncomfortable intercourse.

The development of urinary stress incontinence can have a profoundly adverse effect on the woman and her partner. Decreases in muscle strength and bulk as well as limitations in movement caused by osteoarthritis and osteoporosis contribute to the development of sexual dysfunction.

Orgastic capability may decrease in some postmenopausal females. Estrogen-deficient women may experience the uterine contractions during orgasm as being painful (14).

When it has been determined that estrogen deficiency has resulted in these sexual problems and when no medical contraindications exist, estrogen replacement therapy is often instituted. Estrogen replacement, either oral or topical, retards atrophic changes in the genitals and stimulates vaginal secretions. The addition of androgens to postmenopausal hormonal replacement therapy is controversial. Sexual arousal is enhanced and sexual fantasies are increased when postmenopausal women are given androgens (17).

Bachman (15) has suggested that the use of oil based or water-based lubricants, such as K-Y Jelly, just before intercourse is helpful in women with astrophic vaginitis. An over-the-counter moisturizing gel in a tampon applicator called Replens is marked by Columbia Laboratories Inc. and can be inserted into the vagina three times a week. Through the use of water-filled polymers that adhere to the vaginal cells, a layer of moisture is maintained, which may improve comfort during intercourse. Regular performance of Kegel exercises will help to improve vaginal tone and strengthen pelvic muscles. Planning sexual activity for times when the patient is less fatigued can enhance interest and enjoyment.

EFFECTS OF PHYSICAL ILLNESS

Chronic illness accounts for much of the decline in sexual function with aging (18). In the elderly, diseases of the genitourinary tract and reproductive system have the greatest effect on sexual function. These are followed by endocrine disease, cardiovascular disease, and respiratory disease (19).

Benign Prostatic Hypertrophy

This condition is developed by nearly half of older men, and many fear that surgical treatment will impair sexual function (19). Transurethral resection of the prostate (TURP) may result in retrograde ejaculation of semen into the bladder due to external sphincter damage. While this will interfere with fertility, it does not adversely affect physical sensation or erection. In most cases, impotence associated with TURP is psychologic in origin (19). Other surgical approaches to the prostate that require an open incision are associated with an increased incidence of sexual dysfunction. The suprapubic and retropubic prostatectomies result in impotence in up to 20% of patients, while the perineal approach is associated with up to a 50% impotence rate (20).

Hysterectomy

Because of the myth that this operation results in a "loss of femininity," women may develop postoperative problems with their sexual identity. The surgery does result in shortening of the vagina and eliminates uterine contractions during orgasm. If the patient's preoperative sexual relationships were enjoyable, these changes should not cause many problems (20).

Diabetes Mellitus

Sexual dysfunction is a common complication of diabetes mellitus. Nearly 50% of diabetic men have been found to be impotent secondary to the disease (20). This is unrelated to the age of onset, severity of illness, or medication control (10). The exact pathophysiology of erectile dysfunction in diabetic men has not been clearly defined. In many cases, organic causes are mixed with significant psychologic overlay. One sex clinic has claimed that some diabetic patients with secondary impotence of up to 7 years were cured within 2 to 7 weeks of therapy (21). A careful sexual history with particular attention to the onset of impotence, occurrence of nocturnal erections, masturbation, and alcohol intake should be obtained. Measurements of vascular dilatation during rapid eye movement (REM) sleep by nocturnal penile plethysmography is useful in differentiating psychologic from organic impotence (22). The use of surgically implanted rigid or inflatable penile prostheses are helpful in cases of proven organic impotence. Patients may be offered one of a number of commercially available external impotence management devices in cases where surgery is not acceptable (23). Patient and spouse may differ in their acceptance of these devices, and both should be included in the decision-making process prior to prescription.

Diabetic neuropathy can result in the development of retrograde ejaculation. Patients may complain of having a "dry orgasm" followed by the passage of cloudy urine. Reassurance from the physician that this is a physiologic rather than a psychologic problem may be helpful.

The etiology and prevalence of sexual dysfunction in diabetic females is unclear. Early studies (24) indicated that 35% of diabetic women had orgasmic dysfunction compared with controls. In contrast to male diabetics, there was a strong correlation between sexual dysfunction and duration of the disease. Later studies (25, 26) have disputed these findings and have suggested that diabetic women show little impairment in their sexual response. The sexual response of Type I (insulin-dependent) diabetics has been studied (27). Libido and orgasmic problems as well as impaired vaginal lubrication were related to elevated blood sugar levels. Furthermore, when a woman developed diabetes after entering into a relationship, her sexual response was more likely to become impaired.

Primary Hypothyroidism

This endocrinopathy, more common in women, is manifested by lethargy, depressed motor and intellectual function, and cold intolerance. It frequently results in diminished libido and potency. While thyroxine therapy may eliminate many symptoms, sexual function can remain impaired (9).

Cardiovascular Disease

Many older men with cardiovascular disease have some apprehension about sexual intercourse (19). Decreased libido and intercourse frequency have been reported in up to two thirds of heart attack survivors. Impotence, frequently of a permanent nature, has been reported in 10% of men who have suffered a myocardial infarction (28). The fear of death during coitus is frequently cited by patients and their partners as the reason for their reluctance to resume sexual activity. Sexual intercourse rarely precipitates cardiac death (19). Instances of reported death during sex usually occur with a new partner or during an extramarital affair. With an accustomed partner, heart rates in postmyocardial infarction males rarely exceed 125 beats per minute (29). In patients without complicating symptoms of angina or congestive heart failure, sexual intercourse can typically resume within 6 weeks of an acute coronary event. When angina does accompany intercourse, physicians may recommend a dose of sublingual nitroglycerine 15 to 30 minutes before commencing sexual activity.

Hypertension

Both male and female hypertensive patients are at risk of developing sudden cardiac or cerebrovascular problems. Medical control of severe hypertension lowers but does not eliminate this risk. Drug therapy of hypertension, however, is often complicated by sexual dysfunction. Table 27.1 lists some of the commonly prescribed antihypertensive medications that have been

Table 27.1. Antihypertensive Agents Frequently Associated with Sexual Dysfunction [a]

Sympatholytics
  Methyldopa (Aldomet)
  Reserpine (Serpasil)
  Clonidine (Catapres)
Alpha-adrenergic blockers
  Phentolamine (Regitine)
  Phenoxybenzamine (Dibenzyline)
Beta-adrenergic blockers
  Propranolol (Inderal)
Diuretics
  Hydrochlorothiazide (Esidrix)
  Spironolactone (Aldactazide)
Vasodilators
  Hydralazine (Apresoline)
Norepinephrine depletion
  Guanethidine (Ismelin)

[a] The effect on sexual function of most of these drugs is dose-related or associated with chronic usage.

associated with adverse effects on sexual function. The ACE-inhibitors, such as Captopril, are among the least likely class of antihypertensives to cause erectile impairment (30).

Degenerative Joint Disease

Pain and stiffness caused by this disorder can have an adverse effect on sexual function. Timing analgesic administration to coincide with likely times of sexual intimacy can be helpful (9). Frequently, couples must be counseled to adopt changes in their usual sexual position to facilitate comfortable intercourse.

Stroke

The available data indicates that stroke patients maintain prestroke sexual desire but commonly experience sexual dysfunction including erectile and orgasmic problems (31, 32). Less than half of male subjects who were capable of achieving an erection prestroke maintained this ability poststroke. Successful ejaculation was preserved in an even smaller number of subjects (31). Vaginal lubrication in poststroke females is frequently inadequate and may result in painful coitus (32). A main predictor of the frequency of intercourse poststroke is the level of dependency on the spouse for activities of daily living and self-care (33). Overprotection by a spouse can lead to the patient assuming a dependent role, resulting in loss of the former sexual relationship. The fear of precipitating another stroke during sexual intercourse causes many couples to cease all poststroke sexual activity. Formerly used sexual positions may become uncomfortable or impractical due to the presence of hemiplegia, sensory loss, visual deficits, or spasticity.

Mental Illness

Depression, anxiety, and psychoneurosis are common psychologic illnesses in the elderly population. The presence of chronic illness or social isolation combined with depression can result in feelings of apathy and hopelessness. In this setting, it is not uncommon to find patients suffering from a loss of sexual interest. Psychotherapy and psychotropic drugs may improve the depression, but libido does not always return (9).

Confusion, a nonspecific symptom in many older persons, has also been associated with the loss of sexual response. Individuals suffering from cortical disinhibition, on the other hand, may display an increased sexual drive and occasional inappropriate attempts at sexual outlet (9). Hypersexuality may also be part of the manic phase of a manic depressive disorder.

DRUG-INDUCED SEXUAL DYSFUNCTION

Many of the drugs commonly prescribed to the elderly can result in sexual dysfunction by pharmacologically altering neurotransmission, hormonal function, or vascular flow.

In addition to the antihypertensive medications, psychoactive agents such as tranquilizers and antidepressants often have significant sexual side effects. In some cases, sexual problems may have even underlined the depression and anxiety for which these drugs were prescribed. Decreased libido, impotence, and ejaculatory difficulty have been reported with use of major tranquilizers (34). Thioridazine (Mellaril), because of its alpha-adrenergic receptor antagonism, is a strong inhibitor of ejaculation. It is also known to cause vaginal dryness. Chlorpromazine (Thorazine) is associated with a dose-related loss of libido and impotence (30). Among the antidepressants, Trazodone (Desyrel) use may result in priapism. The sedative and anticholinergic properties of these drugs can lead to decreased libido and impotence (34).

Imipramine (Tofranil) and amitriptyline (Elavil) can cause painful ejaculation (35). The minor tranquilizers, especially benzodiazephines such as diazepam (Valium) reduce libido by their depressive effect on the limbic system, septal region, and brainstem reticular formation (34).

Other prescription drugs that have been linked to sexual dysfunction are listed in Table 27.2.

Controlled studies have shown that chronic and/or excessive alcohol intake results in increased time to obtain an erection, increased time to ejaculation, and decreased orgasmic pleasure. These problems were noted to positively correlate with blood alcohol levels (34).

Nicotine, by its vasoconstrictive action, can adversely affect potency (34). The presence of atherosclerotic peripheral vascular disease often magnifies the problem.

Table 27.2. Other Drugs Associated with Sexual Dysfunction

Antihistamines
  Diphenhydramine (Benadryl)
  Dimenhydrinate (Dramamine)
  Hydroxyzine (Vistaril, Atarax)
  Promethazine (Phenergan)
  Meclizine (Antivert)
  Cimetidine (Tagamet)
Antiemetics
  Metoclopramide (Reglan)
Antiparkinson agents
  Benztropine (Cogentin)
  Trihexyphenidyl (Artane)
Muscle relaxants
  Cyclobenzaprine (Flexeril)
Antispasmodics
  Dantrolene sodium (Dantrium)
  Baclofen (Lioresal)
Miscellaneous
  Disopyramide (Norpace)
  Alcohol
  Nicotine
  Estrogens
  Lithium carbonate

COUNSELING THE ELDERLY PATIENT

When asked about their need for sexual counseling, nearly half of the subjects on a rehabilitation medicine service wanted to discuss sexual problems with a hospital staff member prior to discharge. Most of these patients expressed a preference for a like sexed physician as the person with whom they would be most willing to discuss sexual concerns (36). Unfortunately, few physicians incorporate a sexual history and physical into their routine examination. In many cases, this reflects a doctor's lack of comfort with discussing sexuality issues. Many elderly persons were raised in an environment where sexuality was not openly discussed. They are often reluctant to mention their sexual problems without a doctor's prompting. In an effort to circumvent this stalemate, Bray (10) has suggested that the person who is to provide sexual education and counseling services for the aged should be a person comfortable with sexuality issues. In many centers, this person may be a nurse, social worker, or therapist. A thorough knowledge of the effects of aging on sexuality is essential to providing effective services.

An accurate and detailed sexual history and physical examination is an essential step in identifying potentially reversible causes of sexual dysfunction. Once this has been completed, appropriate counseling can be integrated into the rehabilitation process. One popular method for providing sexual counseling is the PLISSIT model. This model allows counselors to provide four different levels of intensity when addressing a patient's sexual concerns. The levels include *Permission, Limited*

Information, Specific Suggestions, and Intensive Therapy.

Permission

Many geriatric patients will benefit from a general discussion of sexual concerns and reassurance that continuation of sexual activity is permissible. The counselor should refrain from making value judgements about a patient's sexual behavior. If the counselor identifies the possibility for an adverse outcome as a result of these behaviors, he or she is obligated to bring these concerns to the patient's attention (10). Open discussions of sexual issues will reassure the patient that the changes he or she is experiencing are part of the normal aging process.

Limited Information

Some patients will require more than verbal reassurance in order to accept changes in their sexuality. Counselors should have a supply of educational materials in the form of books, pamphlets, and videotapes that can be used to provide information in laymens terms about sex and the aging process. Patients should be given the opportunity to discuss what they have read or watched.

Specific Suggestions

At this level of counseling, patients are given assistance to improve their sexual problems. This assistance may be in the form of prescribing vaginal lubricants or suggesting variations on the patients's usual coital positions. Geriatric males with premenopausal female partners should be advised about the need for birth control if prevention of pregnancy is desired.

Specific sexual difficulties usually can be identified in the sex history. Patients and their partners can use the suggested strategies to adapt their sexual behavior to the changes occurring with aging.

Intensive Therapy

Certified sex therapists are probably the most qualified to provide assistance at this level. The therapy is time intensive and requires the provider to have a thorough understanding of human behavior. Sex therapy should be considered when the first three levels of the PLISSIT model have not been successful.

SUMMARY

Sexual functioning, as with all other phenomena of aging, is of concern to rehabilitation professionals. Sexual responsiveness can be adversely affected by poor health, anxiety, and social myths. In the absence of these factors, an older individual may reasonably expect that his or her sexual activity and enjoyment will be lifelong. Many older persons will seek help from the medical community when sexual problems arise. For this reason, members of the rehabilitation team who are comfortable in discussing sexual issues with patients should be identified and trained. This will, in turn, help the geriatric patient understand the normal changes with aging so that the patient does not fear losing his or her sexuality. The sexual concerns of an increasingly aging population should be treated as a major part of geriatric rehabilitation programs.

References

1. Woodard WS, Rollin SA. Sexuality and the elderly: obstacles and options. *J. Rehab.* 47:64–68, 1981.
2. Kofoed L, Bloom JD. Geriatric sexual dysfunction. *J Am Ger Soc.* 30:437–440, 1982.
3. Pfeiffer E, Verwoerdt A, Wang H. Sexual behavior in aged men and women. I. Observations on 254 community volunteers. *Arch Gen Psychiatry.* 19:753–758, 1968.
4. Labby DH. Aging's effects on sexual function. *Postgrad Med* 78:32–43, 1985.
5. Pfeiffer E, Davis GC. Determinants of sexual behavior in middle and old age. *J Am Geriatr Soc.* 20:151–158, 1972.
6. Wasow M, Loeb MB. Sexuality in nursing homes. In: Solnick RL, ed. *Sexuality and Aging.* Ethel Perry Andrus Gerontology Center, University of Southern California Press; 1978.
7. Driver JD, Detrich D. Elders and sexuality. *J Nurs Care.* 15:8–11, 1982.
8. Kassel V. Long term care institutions. In: Weg R. ed. *Sexuality in Later Years.* New York, NY: Academic Press; 1983.
9. Felstein I. Sexual function in the elderly. *Clin Obstet Gynecol.* 7:401–420, 1980.
10. Bray GP. Sexuality in the aging. In: Williams TF, ed. *Rehabilitation in the Aging.* New York, NY: Raven Press; 1984.
11. Fox CA. Recent research in human coital physiology. *Br J Sex Med.* 42:32–34, 1978.
12. Newman HF. Vibratory sensitivity of the penis. *Fertil Steril.* 21:791–793, 1970.
13. Riehle RA, Vaughan ED. Genitourinary disease in the elderly. *Med Clin North Am.* 67:445–461, 1983.
14. Steege JF. Sexual function in the aging woman. *Clin Obstet Gynecal.* 29:462–469, 1986.
15. Bachman GA. Sexual dysfunction in postmenopausal women: the role of medical management. *Geriatrics.* 43:79–83, 1988.
16. Cutler W, Garcia S, McCoy N. Perimenopausal sexuality. *Arch Sex Behav.* 16:225–234, 1987.
17. Sherwin B, Gelfand M. The role of androgen in the maintenance of sexual functioning in oophorectomized women. *Psychosom Med.* 49:397–409, 1987.
18. Mulligan T, Retchin SM, Chinchilli VM, Bettinger CB. The role of aging and chronic disease in sexual dysfunction. *J Am Geriatrics.* 36:520–524. 1988.
19. Dagon EM. Problems and prospects with sexuality and aging. *Wis Med J.* 80:37–39, 1981.
20. Spennrath S. Understanding the sexual needs of the older patient. *AUAA J.* Apr/June:10–17, 1983.
21. Renshaw DC. Sexual problems in old age and disability. *Psychosomatics.* 22:975–985, 1981.
22. Karacan I, Williams RL, Thornby JI. Sleep-related tumescence as a function of age. *Am J Psychiatry.* 132:932–937, 1975.
23. Zasler ND. Managing erectile dysfunction with external devices. *Practical Diabetology.* 8:1–9, 1989.

24. Kolodny RC. Sexual dysfunction in diabetic females. *Diabetes.* 20:557–559, 1971.

25. Ellenberg M. Sexual aspects of the female diabetic. *Mt Sinai J Med.* 44:495–500, 1977.

26. Schreiner-Engel P, Schiavi RC, Victorisz D. Diabetes and female sexuality: a comparative study of women in relationships. *J Sex Marital Ther.* 11:165–175, 1985.

27. Bahen-Auger N, Wilson M, Assalian P. Sexual response of the type I diabetic woman. *Med Asp Hum Sex.* 94–100, 1988.

28. Mackey FG. Sexuality and heart disease. In: Comfort A, ed. *Sexual Consequences of Disability.* Philadelphia, Pa: F. Stickley; 1978.

29. Hellerstein HK, Friedman EH. Sexual activity and the postcoronary patient. *Arch Inter Med.* 125:987–999, 1970.

30. Sexual problems in the elderly: the use and abuse of medications. A Geriatrics panel discussion. *Geriatrics.* 44:61–71, 1989.

31. Bray GD. Sexual functioning in stroke survivors. *Arch Phys Med Rehabil.* 62:286–288, 1981.

32. Monga TN, Lawson JS. Sexual dysfunction in stroke patients. *Arch Phys Med Rehabil.* 67:19–22, 1986.

33. Sjogren K, Danber JE. Sexuality after stroke with hemiplegia. *Scand J Rehabil Med.* 15:55–61, 1983.

34. Van Arsdalen KN, Wein AJ. Drug-induced sexual dysfunction in older men. *Geriatrics.* 39:63–70, 1984.

35. Drugs that cause sexual dysfunction. *Med Lett Drugs Ther.* 25:73, 1979.

36. Sadoughi W, Lashner M, Fine HL. Sexual adjustment in a chronically ill and physically disabled population: a pilot study. *Arch Phys Med Rehabil.* 52:311–317, 1971.

28

Visual Impairments

Stanley F. Wainapel

*"Moses was a hundred and twenty years old
when he died; his eye was not dim
nor his natural force abated."*
—Deuteronomy, 34:7

The above quote notwithstanding, many contemporary adults who reach even two thirds the age of the biblical patriarch do so with vision dimmed or absent altogether. Visual impairment is one of the most common and most disabling accompaniments of the aging process. The 1979 National Health Interview Survey, conducted by the National Center for Health Statistics (NCHS) (1), reported that 12.0% of men and 11.8% of women aged 65 years or older had some degree of visual impairment, making this the seventh most prevalent chronic condition among males and the eighth most prevalent among females in this age group. More recent NCHS data (Table 28.1) indicate that this figure may be as high as 12.8% and that over 2,000,000 noninstitutionalized older Americans are unable to read ordinary newspaper print because of a vision problem. By age 85 years, one person in four will have this degree of vision limitation (2).

But these numbers do not tell the whole story. Vision is one of the three major factors contributing to stable upright posture (3)—vestibular function and proprioception are the other two—and, as a consequence, it has a crucial role in balance, mobility, and falls (4–6). Hip fractures, one of the most serious sequelae of falls in the elderly, have been shown to be much more frequent in individuals with monocular or binocular vision problems (7). Moreover, the aging eye often coexists with an aging cardiovascular and/or neuromuscular system, giving rise to such doubly challenging problems as the blind amputee (8, 9) and the blind stroke patient (10). One recent survey of 271 consecutive admissions to a general inpatient Rehabilitation Medicine unit (11) included 19 (7.0%) in whom blindness or severe visual impairment were significant secondary disabilities.

Clearly, then, both the geriatrician and physiatrist can expect to frequently confront the functional problems associated with vision loss in their patients. Unfortunately, however, the subject of vision rehabilitation (as opposed to the medical-surgical management of geriatric eye diseases) has been generally overlooked in the literature of both these specialties (12). This relative neglect is particularly ironic because more than two thirds of the legally blind population are over 55 years old (13).

One reason for this omission is the historic separation of vision care services from other medical rehabilitation services. The vision rehabilitation system has existed in parallel with Rehabilitation Medicine and Geriatrics, rarely exchanging knowledge or techniques with these specialties. To some extent this tradition of insularity from the medical mainstream was justifiable and perhaps even provided a stronger sense of identity. The main clients of the vision care system were young, usually totally blind, and often employable, as in the case of the veterans of World Wars I and II who provided the impetus for modern vision rehabilitation. Additionally, there was little, if anything, that Ophthalmology could offer these cases of traumatic blindness. Over the past half-century, new professions have evolved to meet the needs of such individuals—the Orientation and Mobility (O & M) Instructor, the Rehabilitation Teacher—and the vocational focus of treatment has been of enormous benefit to its clients.

But much has changed that makes one now question the value of the continued separation of medical and vision rehabilitation systems. Dramatic new gains in ophthalmologic technology have radically improved the outlook for patients who previously had no hope of regaining or preserving their vision. A corollary of these developments is a change in the ratio of partially sighted to blind individuals that now approaches four to one

Table 28.1. Prevalence of Visual Impairment in the Elderly[a]

	Age			
	65 and Over	65–74	75–84	85 and Over
Estimated population in thousands	26,290	16,227	8,073	1,990
Percentage of persons reporting visual problems				
A. Blindness in one or both eyes	4.2	2.7	5.7	11.7
B. In one eye	3.2	2.2	4.4	6.9
C. In both eyes	1.0	.5	1.3	4.8
D. Any other trouble seeing	10.2	7.9	12.3	21.4
Disabilities reported by respondents with some vision in one or both eyes: Inability to see well enough, even when wearing glasses or contact lenses, to . . .				
E. Recognize the features of people if they are within two or three feet	2.3	1.7	2.9	5.5
F. Watch TV 8 to 12 feet away	2.9	2.0	3.7	8.2
G. Read newspaper print	6.6	4.0	8.5	20.5
H. Step off a curb or down a step	4.2	2.5	5.4	13.6
I. Recognize a friend walking on the other side of the street	7.7	4.4	10.2	25.6
Composite measures of visual impairment				
J. Severe visual impairment: Blind in both eyes or inability to read newsprint even with glasses	7.8	4.7	9.9	25.0
K. Visual impairment: Blindness in one or both eyes or any other trouble seeing	12.8	9.5	16.0	26.8

[a]Visual Impairment Among Elderly Americans (Table 1) by R. A. Nelson (*Journal of Visual Impairment and Blindness*, Vol. 81 No. 7) is reproduced with kind permission from the American Foundation for the Blind and is © 1987 from the American Foundation for the Blind, 15 West 16th Street, New York, N.Y. 10011.

(14). Most important of all, perhaps, has been the aging of the population, which has altered the type of person requiring vision rehabilitation services. That person is now likely to be older (the average age of patients consulting an ophthalmologist is 64 years) (15), less often employable or seeking employment, and more often partially sighted than totally blind. This person is almost more likely to have impairments other than visual ones that require medical, surgical, and/or rehabilitative technologies that heretofore were not utilized (or needed) by the vision rehabilitation system. This change in focus has not yet been incorporated into agencies for the blind and visually impaired, so that the older individuals who account for as much as 64% of their clientele (16) currently exist in a no-man's-land between the jurisdictional territories of Rehabilitation Medicine, Geriatrics, and Vision Rehabilitation and are therefore a notably underserved population.

This chapter attempts to present a fusion of these three disciplines' management of visual impairment in the elderly, and it is hoped that it will encourage a con-

certed effort by them to forge a more unified approach to these patients.

CLASSIFICATION AND CONSEQUENCES OF VISUAL IMPAIRMENT

Visual function and dysfunction are usually classified in terms of central acuity and peripheral fields. Acuity measurements are based on the standard Snellen eye chart, with optimal acuity rated at 20/20 and reduced vision indicated by a higher number in the denominator. Central (acuity) deficits are described as diffuse or discreet (scotomas). Visual fields are measured by manual or computerized perimetry in which a round object or light is moved through all four visual quadrants. Peripheral (field) deficits are described as concentric (loss of peripheral vision with retained central function, producing "tunnel vision") or central (loss of central vision with preservation of peripheral function, the typical presentation in macular degeneration). A third type of field deficit is the hemianopsias or quadrant losses associated with brain injury; these are classified as homonymous (identical areas of each eye), bitemporal (lateral fields of each eye), or binasal (medial fields of each eye).

When central acuity is 20/200 or less despite maximal corrective lenses, or if peripheral visual fields are reduced to 20 degrees or less in the better eye, an individual meets the criteria for *legal blindness*, a term first defined in 1935 by the Social Security Act. A legally blind person is eligible for a number of financial benefits and can receive rehabilitative services provided by state agencies for the blind and visually handicapped. Excluded from these entitlements is the much larger population of people with *low vision*, a term that is often defined as corrected visual acuity between 20/70 (the acuity below which one cannot read ordinary newspaper print) and 20/200. Over 2,00,000 Americans of geriatric age have low vision, but only about 250,000 of them are totally blind (2).

The World Health Organization has suggested a more specific classification of low vision as follows (15):

Moderate low vision—corrected acuity between 20/70 and 20/160 in the better eye.
Severe low vision—corrected acuity between 20/200 and 20/400, or visual field of 20 degrees or less, in the better eye.

As a rule, central vision losses have their greatest impact on reading and object/person identification, while peripheral visual losses affect mobility. However, the functional consequences of either deficit can be far more pervasive than this generalization would suggest, and a number of authors have drawn attention to the physical, social, and psychologic consequences. Appollonio et al (17) evaluated 1,201 community-based elderly Italians (aged 70 to 75 years) to ascertain the effects of visual and/or hearing impairments on their basic activities of daily living (ADL), instrumental ADL (IADL), and social interaction/satisfaction. They documented that those with visual impairment alone were significantly less independent in ADL and IADL and were particularly likely to have low levels of social satisfaction as measured by the SELF scale of Linn (18). Branch et al (19) found fewer physical limitations in their Massachusetts-based study of elderly persons with declining vision (only some significant IADL deficits), but their data highlighted this group's social isolation, emotional dysfunction (low morale, depression), and lower self-perception of general health status. Gillman et al (20) corroborated the negative effect of vision loss on the morale, perceived health, and general sense of well-being in a group of 486 elderly (age 60+years) residents of public housing projects in New York City. These three representative studies, each within a distinct geographic and cultural context, are a convincing demonstration of the global nature of the functional losses associated with visual impairment in the elderly.

One final illustration is found in an analysis of data from the Framingham Eye Study by Felson et al (7), who studied 2,633 subjects over a 10-year period during which 110 subjects sustained hip fractures. While the incidence of hip fracture was 3.0% in subjects with good vision (acuity 20/30 or better), it rose to 8.5% in those with moderately impaired vision (acuity 20/30 to 20/80 in at least one eye), and reached 11.3% in those with poor vision (acuity 20/100 or less in either eye). Adjusted relative risk for hip fracture rose from 1.54 in subjects with moderate visual impairment to 2.17 in those with poor vision. The greatest incidence and relative risk values occurred in subjects with varying degrees of impairment in each eye, which suggests that preserved stereoscopic vision may play an important role in preventing fracture-producing falls (Table 28.2).

Table 28.2. Incidence of Hip Fractures among Older Persons with Varying Degrees of Visual Impairment[a]

Visual Acuity	Cumulative Incidence Rate of Hip Fracture (%)	Unadjusted RR (95% CI)[b]	Multivariate Adjusted RR (95% CI)[b]
Good vision both eyes	63/2131 (3.0%)	1.00	1.00
Any impaired vision in either eye	47/502 (9.4%)	3.28 (2.25–4.79)	1.73 (1.13–2.65)
Moderately impaired vision in at least one eye	29/342 (8.5%)	2.95 (1.90–4.58)	1.54 (0.95–2.49)
Good eye—Moderate eye	19/215 (8.8%)	3.08 (1.84–5.15)	1.94 (1.13–3.32)
Moderate eye—Moderate eye	10/127 (7.9%)	2.73 (1.40–5.32)	1.11 (0.55–2.24)
Poor vision in at least one eye	18/160 (11.3%)	4.01[c] (1.61–6.78)	2.17[c] (1.24–3.80)
Good eye—Poor eye	5/89 (5.6%)	1.92 (0.77–4.78)	1.50 (0.60–3.75)
Moderate eye—Poor eye	9/44 (20.5%)	7.78 (3.87–15.64)	2.82 (1.33–5.96)
Poor eye—Poor eye	4/27 (14.8%)	5.49 (2.00–15.07)	2.46 (0.87–6.99)

[a]Reprinted with permission from the American Geriatrics Society, Impaired vision and hip fracture: the Framingham Eye Study, by Felson DT et al, JOURNAL OF THE AMERICAN GERIATRICS SOCIETY, Vol. 37, No. 6, pp. 495–500, 1989.
[b]Results of Cox models with unadjusted model testing vision as sole predictor of hip fracture and multivariate model adjusted for age, sex, Metropolitan Relative Weight, alcohol use, and, in women, estrogen use.
[c]Test for linear trend (good—good; moderate impairment in at least one eye; poor vision in at least one eye), $P < .01$.

PHYSIOLOGY OF THE AGING EYE

The eye undergoes numerous morphologic and functional changes as an individual ages. Some of the morphologic changes, such as the deposition of fatty material in the conjunctiva and the margin of the cornea to produce pinguecula and arcus senilis (21), are entirely benign. Other changes can have potentially significant functional consequences. Loss of retroorbital fat causes the eye to become more deeply recessed; when this occurs in combination with ptosis of the upper lid (due to loss of elastic tissue), the elderly person may experience a partial or total occlusion of the upper visual fields (22). Loss of corneal sensitivity may reduce awareness of acute injuries or infections (21). The enlargement of the lens produces a shallower anterior chamber, which places older persons at greater risk of developing acute angle-closure glaucoma when the pupil is dilated (21).

One of the most significant morphologic changes of the aging eye is a progressive decline in pupillary size to a minimum diameter by age 60 years. Additionally, there is an impaired ability to increase pupillary diameter for adaptation to changes in environmental illumination. The amount of light that reaches the retina of a 60-year-old is only one third as much as would reach it at age 20 years, given the same level of lighting (22). Thus, older persons need much more illumination for optimal reading and indoor mobility, a fact that needs to be kept in mind by hospitals, nursing homes, and doctors' offices when planning these environments.

The physiologic and functional changes of vision associated with aging are summarized in Table 28.3. One of the best-known and most characteristic is presbyopia, the loss of accommodation ability for near vision. A child can see objects clearly even when they are only 3 inches away from the eye, but by age 60 years or older, this near vision limit has extended to 3 feet, a distance in excess of that of the outstretched arms, so that normal reading becomes difficult or impossible without special reading glasses (21).

The gradual decline of visual acuity with age has been recognized since 1864 when it was first reported by Donders (13). Nevertheless, as is the case with other impairments, it is remarkable how many older individuals continue to have excellent vision. Although the average visual acuity of an 80-year-old is between 20/30 and 20/40, data from the Framingham Eye Study indicate that 70% of the 80-year-olds in that population had 20/20 vision, and only 15% had acuities of 20/50 or lower (23).

The distinction between normal and pathologic aging of the eye is not a clear one. For example, between ages 20 and 80 years, the anteroposterior diameter of the lens increases by 50% (22), and this is associated with the development of microopacities that do not affect acuity but can produce optical glare. When do these opacities become a cataract? And at what level of vision impairment does the cataract become pathologic? It is clear, however, that four eye disorders account for about 98% of cases of visual loss in persons over 70 years of age: cataract, age-related macular degeneration (AMD), glaucoma, and diabetic retinopathy (23). Their characteristic symptoms are summarized in Table 28.4, and their current management is briefly outlined in the next section.

COMMON EYE DISEASES IN THE ELDERLY

Of the four major causes of geriatric vision impairment, cataract is by far the most prevalent. Cataracts severe enough to reduce visual acuity to 20/30 or worse occur in 18% of persons aged 65 to 74 years and in 46% of persons aged 75 to 84 years (23). It has an insidious onset, with gradual clouding of central vision, heightened glare, and yellowed vision. When it has progressed sufficiently to produce visual and functional difficulties, the primary therapeutic approach is surgical. Cataract extraction is currently the most common operation performed on Medicare recipients (24). There are two main surgical techniques: (a) intracapsular extraction, with removal of the entire lens and its capsule; or (b) extracapsular extraction, in which the cataractous lens material and a portion of the capsule are removed, leaving the posterior capsule intact to receive an implanted plastic intraocular lens.

After intracapsular extraction, the patient's loss of refractive power can be treated with special glasses or contact lenses. The eyeglasses required are thick and heavy; they provide good central vision, but interfere with peripheral vision and produce optical distortion by increasing the apparent size of objects by 25% (25). The

Table 28.3. Physiologic Changes in the Aging Eye[a]

Functional Change	Physiologic Change
Visual acuity	Morphologic change in choroid, pigment epithelium, or retina
	Decreased function of rods, cones, or other neural elements
Extraocular motion	Difficulty in gazing upward and maintaining convergence
Intraocular pressure	Increased pressure
Refractive power	Increased hyperopia and myopia
	Presbyopia
	Increased lens size
	Nuclear sclerosis (lens)
	Ciliary muscle atrophy
Tear secretion	Decreased tearing
	Decreased lacrimal gland function
	Decreased goblet cell secretion
Corneal function	Loss of endothelial integrity
	Posterior surface pigmentation

[a]From Kane RL, Ouslander JG, Abrass IB. *Essentials of Clinical Geriatrics.* 2nd ed. © 1989, McGraw-Hill Information Services Company, New York, NY. This material is reproduced with permission of McGraw-Hill, Inc.

Table 28.4. Clinical Characteristics of Common Ophthalmologic Problems in the Elderly[a]

Signs and Symptoms	Cataract	Open-angle Glaucoma	Angle-closure Glaucoma	Macular Degeneration	Temporal Arteritis	Diabetic Retinopathy
Pain			×		×	
Red eye			×			
Fixed pupil			×			
Retinal vessel changes					×	×
Retinal exudates				×		×
Optic disc changes		×			×	
Sudden visual loss			×		×	
Loss of peripheral vision		×				
Glare intolerance	×					
Elevated intraocular pressure		×	×			
Loss of visual acuity	×			×		×

[a] From Kane RL, Ouslander JG, Abrass IB. *Essentials of Clinical Geriatrics.* 2nd ed. © 1989, McGraw-Hill Information Services Company, New York, NY. This material is reproduced with permission of McGraw-Hill, Inc.

adverse effect of these glasses on peripheral vision would be particularly serious in the presence of concomitant AMD, which has been shown to be more common among elderly individuals with lens opacities (26). Contact lenses, especially extended-wear models that do not require daily changing, can be used by most persons with adequate hand coordination, do not impair peripheral vision, and cause only 6% increase in apparent object size.

By far the best optical solution for the great majority (probably over 95%) of patients with cataracts is the combination of extracapsular lens extraction with implantation of an intraocular lens. The implanted lens produces only a 1% increase in apparent object size, and it permits good central and peripheral vision (25). A further beneficial effect of such a procedure is the associated improvements in physical and mental function in addition to the expected improvement in vision. Applegate et al (24) retrospectively reviewed 293 patients aged 70 years or older who underwent cataract extraction/intraocular lens implantation over a 15-month period and found that (a) mean visual acuity improved from 20/100 to 20/40 in the operated eye 4 months after surgery, (b) mental status improved significantly by 1 year postoperatively (though not quite significantly at 4 months), and (c) timed manual performance activities had improved significantly by 4 months after surgery. These gains in nonvisual areas would argue for the value of cataract surgery even in patients with some mental deficits (they might be partly related to sensory deprivation) and for its performance prior to starting an intensive rehabilitation program in elderly patients with superimposed neuromuscular disabilities.

Although cataracts are the most common cause of visual impairment in the elderly, AMD is the most frequent cause of *severe* visual impairment in this group. Some degree of AMD is present in more than 30% of individuals over the age of 65 years (13); it has a particularly high prevalence among elderly females (27). The macula is the portion of the retina responsible for detail vision, and AMD produces a gradual loss of central acu-

ity with preservation of peripheral vision. The older person who develops this disorder will be able to utilize his (or more likely her) retained peripheral fields to walk down a street, but will probably be unable to identify a street sign or the face of a person standing nearby. Reading a book or newspaper would be extremely difficult, if not impossible.

There are two main forms of AMD: (a) the "dry" or nonexudative type, which may be relatively benign or can produce well-defined areas of chorioretinal atrophy that impair vision; and (b) "wet" or exudative AMD, in which damage to retinal pigment epithelium and choriocapillaris results in the exudation of protein and fluid under the pigment epithelium. Exudative AMD may progress to a hemorrhagic stage characterized by the growth of small and fragile blood vessels (neovascularization), which often produce blood leaks. This is the variant with the worst prognosis for preserving any central vision (21).

AMD is a particularly discouraging disease because, of the four discussed here, it is the only one for which effective medical and surgical measures are still lacking. Although certain localized exudative lesions may be amenable to laser photocoagulation, most patients will find specialized vision rehabilitation services their only option. Fortunately, however, they are unlikely to lose their peripheral vision and can therefore remain relatively mobile.

Glaucoma produces the opposite field deficit from that associated with AMD: a gradual but progressive loss of peripheral vision that leads to "tunnel vision" and, if untreated, to total blindness. Open-angle glaucoma, the more common type, results from impaired flow of aqueous humor from the anterior to the posterior chamber of the eye with a resultant increase in intraocular pressure that can, over an extended period, damage the optic nerve. The insidious nature of open-angle glaucoma is its greatest danger; it produces no pain, and visual loss is so gradual that it goes unnoticed until a late stage has been reached. Regular measurement of intraocular pressure is therefore an essential part of the evaluation of every older patient regardless of the presence or absence of any subjective visual symptoms.

Angle-closure (narrow-angle) glaucoma is fortunately a much rarer disease, but when it does occur it represents a genuine ophthalmologic emergency. The sudden rise of intraocular pressure produces severe pain and rapidly progressive loss of vision that will be permanent unless promptly treated by the surgical creation of a free passage between the anterior and posterior chamber. This is now most frequently accomplished by a laser iridectomy.

Open-angle glaucoma can be satisfactorily controlled by the use of eyedrops that constrict the pupil (miotics), such as pilocarpine, which help to keep the intraocular pressure at an acceptable level. Pilocarpine has several disadvantages: it decreases contrast sensitivity, increases glare sensitivity, reduces night vision, and produces a sense of darkening vision lasting 20 to 60 minutes after using the eyedrops (28). Beta-blocking agents such as timolol (Timoptic) are also used locally, but they can produce systemic effects (e.g., on asthma or blood pressure) in susceptible individuals (21). Carbonic anhydrase inhibitors such as oral acetazolamide (Diamox) are sometimes used in cases that are difficult to control with eyedrops alone.

Diabetic retinopathy, the most common cause of blindness in younger adults, is also a significant cause of vision impairment among the elderly. In the 75 to 85-year age group, 30% of diabetics have some degree of retinopathy (13). Patients with less severe forms of so-called background retinopathy may have relatively little visual loss, although the retinal edema and ischemic changes near the macula can produce some central vision loss without peripheral defects. However, proliferative diabetic retinopathy can lead to multiple vitreous hemorrhages from small, fragile new vessels (neovascularization). If untreated, proliferative retinopathy and its attendant vitreous hemorrhages can rapidly lead to retinal detachment and irreversible total blindness. Fortunately, the development of laser surgery has provided an effective method for combatting this dreaded and previously untreatable situation. Laser photocoagulation can seal microhemorrhages before they produce major vision loss. Additional surgical techniques that have been brought to bear on the diabetic eye are vitrectomy (removal of blood and fibrous tissue from the vitreous by suction, replacing them with a saline infusion) and scleral buckling (reattachment of a retina that has been detached by vitreous hemorrhages) (13).

DOUBLE DISABILITIES: COMBINED VISUAL AND NEUROMUSCULAR IMPAIRMENTS

One of the challenges posed by geriatric patients is the fact that their impairments—and associated disa-

bilities—rarely occur in an isolated fashion. The degenerative processes that affect all body organs and systems make it no surprise that one often has to simultaneously address multiple impairments. Vision loss is no exception; it often coexists with other disorders and adds an extra degree of difficulty to their rehabilitation.

The patient with diabetic retinopathy, mentioned above, is a case in point. The effects of diabetes on peripheral nerve and peripheral vascular systems are such that a number of visually impaired or blind diabetics will also have a peripheral polyneuropathy or require eventual lower extremity amputation. The loss of proprioception resulting from neuropathy would further compromise the postural stability of a blind patient, who would have vestibular function as the only remaining intact mechanism for stable, upright stance (3). Furthermore, loss of two-point discrimination in the fingers could make it impossible for a blind individual to use the tactile language of Braille. The situation of the elderly blind amputee is less pessimistic. Altner et al (8) reported that eight out of twelve blind amputees seen in their program became ambulatory with a prosthesis. Two other blind diabetics with below-knee amputations were discussed by Fisher (9); both became functional ambulators.

The patient with cerebral infarction may experience visual problems such as homonymous hemianopsia, visual neglect, or dysperception of verticality as a direct result of the stroke. Additionally, some of these patients may have had previous visual loss from other causes. Wainapel (10) retrospectively reviewed 220 consecutive stroke admissions to a general rehabilitation unit over a 2-year period. There were nine admissions (4.1%) involving seven patients who were blind or severely visually impaired prior to their cerebral infarction. These patients were relatively old (age range 71 to 84 years, mean age 76.1), and all had a long experience of prior visual loss (range 5 to 47 years, mean duration 14.7 years). Cataract, glaucoma, and diabetic retinopathy were the causes of visual loss in all but one of the cases studied. Six of the seven patients could perform their ADL and ambulate with supervision or minimal assist by the time they were discharged, after a mean length of stay of 54 days. Four were able to return home, with two requiring nursing home placement, and one going to an Adult Home that required him to be ambulatory.

More recently, a retrospective review of 191 consecutive rehabilitation medicine admissions revealed 13 patients (6.8%) in whom blindness or severe visual impairment was a significant secondary disability. (11) Again, the patients were quite elderly (their mean age of 79.7 years was about 10 years older than the mean age of all 191 patients) and had experienced their visual losses prior to their current admission. The most common admitting diagnoses among these visually impaired patients were stroke (4), lower extremity amputation (2), and back pain (2). Etiologies of visual loss were macular degeneration (5), cataract (4), glaucoma (3), and diabetic retinopathy (2)—a few patients had more than one visual diagnosis. Eight of the 11 admissions resulted in the patient's discharge home ambulatory with a walker or cane, and mean length of stay (33.1 days) was actually slightly shorter than that for the 191 patients as a whole. On the basis of its prevalence among admitted patients, visual impairment or blindness constituted the fourth most frequent disability diagnosis in this unselected group of rehabilitation inpatients.

The successful outcomes documented by the above studies are gratifying evidence that doubly disabled elderly patients still have considerable rehabilitation potential, a fact that should be borne in mind when evaluating such patients for admission to rehabilitation or geriatric units. One of the keys to this success may be the time sequence of visual loss preceding neuromuscular disability by a rather long period. Visual loss—often of gradual onset—occurred at a comparatively younger age, allowing the patient to learn compensatory strategies. Moreover, these patients usually had the opportunity to experience a rehabilitation process (in this case vision rehabilitation) and could later utilize a similar approach when dealing with the medical rehabilitation system.

Could visual loss actually have been helpful to some of these patients? This may be true in the case of the patient who suffers a stroke affecting the right parietal area. Such patients can often manifest severe visual-perceptual deficits that result in a poor functional outcome in physical and occupational therapy activities. These problems were notable for their relative absence in three left hemiparetic patients who were blind (10). In fact, the only patient with any significant signs of dysperception was the one who had the greatest amount of residual vision. It is hypothesized that the prolonged and profound visual deprivation in these patients may have protected them from the disabling visual-perceptual sequelae usually associated with right brain damage.

Patients such as those described above require the professional skills and techniques typified by the medical rehabilitation model of care. But an equally important component of their management derives from the specialized services of vision rehabilitation, a system largely unknown to most physicians other than ophthalmologists. The remainder of this chapter gives an overview of the components of this system.

PRINCIPLES OF VISION REHABILITATION FOR THE ELDERLY

Medical rehabilitation and vision rehabilitation have many similarities. Both are comprehensive, multidisciplinary, and interdisciplinary processes that require a team approach and that move beyond the medical model to incorporate a psychosocial and (when appropriate) vocational perspective. The physical therapist and occupational therapist have their counterparts in the O & M instructor and the rehabilitation teacher of the vision rehabilitation system. Low vision aids (vision enhancement) and technologic alternatives to vision (vision substitution) can be considered the "orthotics" and "prosthetics" of vision rehabilitation.

Mobility and Self-Care

Carroll's classic 1961 text on rehabilitation of the blind (29) describes the loss of mobility as "perhaps the greatest of all the reality losses of blindness." The partial or total loss of visual feedback is a major impediment to ambulation and increases the danger of falls as well as the dangerous consequences of falling, such as hip fracture (7).

The older person with a severe visual impairment or blindness has six mobility options: (a) guide dog, (b) white cane, (c) specialized mobility aids, (d) standard ambulation aids (e.g., walker), (e) wheelchair, or (f) human guide.

Guide dogs have been used by blind Americans since they were first introduced into this country in 1929 (29). The highly trained dog can provide an excellent sight substitute to a blind individual as well as a source of companionship and security. However, the training of dog and master is a protracted and complex process, and for the relatively frail older person the requisite strength and speed of walking may make it unsuitable as a mobility aid.

The long white cane that was developed by Hoover during World War II to improve the mobility skills of newly blinded veterans (30) is really not a cane in the traditional sense of a solid support that bears weight. It is, rather, more like an antenna that extends the tactile awareness of the individual to cues beyond the reach of a standard cane (29). The thin, long cane (approximately 4 to 4½ feet for adults) is usually white except for red coloring toward its lower segment for better visibility by cars and other individuals. It is held in front of the path of ambulation and moved across the path of intended travel in either a continuous arc or by tapping at the medial and lateral edges of this arc. With appropriate training by a certified O & M instructor (31), the white cane is an excellent mobility aid for visually impaired people of all ages. It is relatively inexpensive and many models can be folded into a smaller size when desired. One inevitable disadvantage is the stigmatizing effect of this well-recognized symbol of blindness. Some older persons, especially those in urban areas with high crime rates, may be understandably reluctant to show their vulnerability by the display of this symbol (32).

In recent years a number of new mobility aids have been developed, but they are considerably more expensive than the white cane, more difficult to learn to use, and therefore may be of value only for selected older individuals. The laser cane emits three laser beams that travel ahead of the user: one detects drops-offs or irregularities at ground level; the second indicates objects directly ahead, and the third warns of obstacles at head level (the latter is a considerable advantage in certain environments). Vibrations of specific areas of the laser cane indicate an upcoming object, and if the obstacle is at head level, a high-pitched beep is produced. Three mobility devices utilizing ultrasonic output are also available: the Russel Pathsounder (worn on the chest, leaving the hands free—an advantage for patients using wheelchairs), the Sonicguide (mounted on a pair of glasses, objects to one side produce a sound in the ipsilateral ear), and the Mowat Sensor (held in the hand, vibration indicates an upcoming object) (12).

The occurrence of neuromusculoskeletal problems in older visually impaired patients has already been highlighted, and their coexistance can make the use of the white cane painful (e.g., arthritis of the wrist or fingers) or ineffective (e.g., painful hip or knee problems, neurogenic or myogenic lower extremity weakness). Under these circumstances, a more traditional ambulation aid such as a straight cane, quadruped cane, or walkerette may be more appropriate. The walkerette offers some advance tactile information, and its frame protects the user from contact with objects at a distance equal to that of the outstretched arm. In the presence of more severe physical impairments, a wheelchair may be the only resource for some patients, but safety in propulsion will then be dependent on the degree of remaining vision.

The human guide is an alternative to any of these mobility aids, whether on a temporary or regular basis. The technique of "sighted guide" should be learned by any practitioner who is likely to encounter visually impaired patients in his or her practice. In this procedure, the visually impaired person put his or her hand around the arm of the guide just above the level of the elbow and then walks a step behind so that the guide's arm position will give advance notice of rises or falls in the upcoming terrain. A backward elbow movement can warn the blind person of the need to step behind the guide due to a narrow passageway or the presence of oncoming people (15).

The effects of visual loss on self-care abilities are obvious and potentially devastating. Formerly routine tasks such as selecting clothing, cooking, doing laundry, and grooming become formidable impediments to a sense of social adequacy that is already compromised by the loss of mobility outside the familiar limits of the home environment. These ADL-homemaking deficits are addressed by the rehabilitation teacher. Ingenious techniques and simple devices allow even a totally blind person to identify specifically colored socks, shirts, or dresses.

Raised markings on kitchen dials can facilitate cooking, and practical tips make it possible to perform such potentially daunting and even dangerous tasks as boiling water, pouring a glass of wine, and eating without knocking over filled glasses or spilling food. These activities require advance planning and some reorganization of closet, kitchen, and bathroom. When the visually-impaired person is not living alone, the roommate, spouse, or significant other needs to be made aware of these changes and must cooperate in keeping the home environment as consistent as possible.

Vision Enhancement

Most older patients who are visually impaired or legally blind have at least some degree of residual visual function, and enhancing this remaining vision to maximum effect is the primary goal of so-called low vision aids (33). These can be divided into: (a) magnifiers, (b) enlarged print, (c) field expanders, (d) illumination devices, (e) antiglare devices, and (f) contrast enhancing devices.

When standard eyeglasses for near or far vision do not provide adequate acuity, the most available, affordable, and practical visual enhancement device is a magnifier. High-power spectacles, the most common type of magnifier, focus reading material at a closer than usual distance from the eye. Hand-held magnifiers (Fig. 28.1) come in many sizes and shapes; some include a built-in

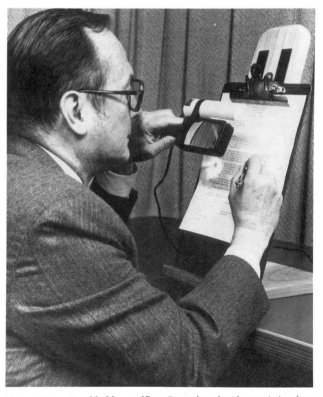

Figure 28.1. Hand-held magnifier. Reproduced with permission from Eschenbach Optik, Weston, Conn.

source of incandescent or (most recently) halogen light (Fig. 28.2). Stand magnifiers are less portable than hand-held magnifiers, and their distance from reading material is fixed; however, for elderly patients with arthritic hand deformities or tremors due to cerebellar or extrapyramidal disorders, they may be particularly useful when placed on a desk or table. Built-in illumination is also available in many models. As a rule, magnifiers can benefit patients whose central visual acuity is as low as 20/800 (15). Telescopic magnifiers are another option, although they are less frequently used than other magnifiers. Small hand-held monocular telescopes for distance vision are often useful for the visually-impaired traveller who is unable to read street signs due to reduced central acuity. Telescopes for near vision are often not accepted because they cover only a very narrow field of vision (12).

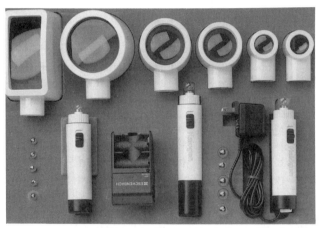

Figure 28.2. Hand-held magnifiers with halogen illumination. Reproduced with permission from Eschenbach Optik, Weston, Conn.

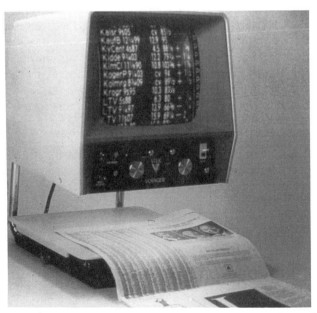

Figure 28.3. Closed-circuit television (CCTV) videomagnifier with reversal (white on black) image. Courtesy of Donald Fletcher, M.D., Tampa, Fla.

The closed-circuit television (CCTV) magnifier is one of the most valuable of all low vision devices despite its relatively high price of $1,000 to $3,000 (depending on which features are included). It consists of a television screen, a table for reading materials, and a videocamera with zoom lens that allows material to be magnified up to 60 times normal size (34), making it suitable for patients with central visual acuity as low as 20/2000. The CCTV can produce a white-on-black (reversal) image, which may facilitate reading by providing greater contrast (Fig. 28.3). It also has the advantage of allowing persons with low vision to read for relatively long periods without the fatigue experienced when using other magnification devices.

Magnification can also be accomplished without the use of the aforementioned devices. Large-print books and magazines—for example, the *New York Times* and *Readers Digest*—are readily available for older readers with impaired vision (34). Many organizations of or for the elderly or visually impaired now publish material in large-print formats. Additionally, computers can be programmed to produce large-print output on their screens or to produce large-print copies of any material.

When the patient's visual loss is related to field deficits rather than reduced central acuity, magnification devices are an inadequate solution. In these situations, prisms have been developed, which are mounted on eyeglasses and permit the user to look in one direction while simultaneously visualizing a different area; this technique has been applied to patients with AMD or those with homonymous hemianopsia. When the problem is one of peripheral field loss (glaucoma, for example), field expanders include reverse telescopes or spectacle-mounted fish-eye lenses, both of which increase the width of field by making objects appear smaller and farther away (33); this optical distortion may make their use difficult for many patients.

Devices to provide adequate illumination, to reduce glare, and to heighten contrast are simple and inexpensive, but they are extremely important methods for optimizing vision in the elderly. An appropriately strong and well-directed source of incandescent or halogen light allows the older person (whose constricted pupil admits less light) to read and do detail work with greater ease and accuracy. An even level of illumination is an often neglected aspect of the design of facilities such as nursing homes whose residents are predominantly elderly (35). Glare, a consequence of too much light or a sign of underlying eye pathology (e.g., cataracts) can be minimized with sunglasses, clip-on sun shades, a sun visor, or orange/yellow colored filters (or lenses); the latter produce their antiglare effect by blocking the blue end of the light spectrum (15). Contrast enhancement can be achieved by using bold print pens and paper with extra-dark lines. Another writing aid is the typoscope or signature guide—a rectangular black template whose

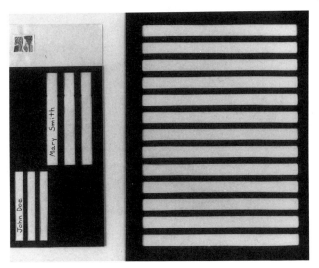

Figure 28.4. Writing guides (typoscopes) for letters and envelopes. Reproduced with permission from Stanley F. Wainapel, M.D., M.P.H.

apertures are located to facilitate filling out checks, addressing envelopes, or writing letters (Fig. 28.4).

Vision Substitution

For those older individuals whose vision is so poor that it cannot benefit from magnification or field expanding aids, various substitute skills can be exploited to preserve maximal functional independence. The distinction between vision enhancement and vision substitution is not clear-cut. One could easily include the mobility techniques already discussed above as vision substitutes, especially since guide dogs are generally used only by persons who are totally blind; but the white cane is a tool shared by those with moderate impairment and with total loss of vision. Similarly, some of the resources outlined below may well benefit many persons with lesser degrees of visual impairment.

Loss of the ability to read is a profoundly isolating aspect of blindness. The difficulty in learning the tactile language of Braille for older persons is exacerbated by diminished two-point discrimination, which renders their fingertips less able to distinguish the small six-dot "cells" that are the basis of Braille. This technique is useful in younger blind individuals, but is of relatively limited value in geriatric patients. Fortunately, many books and magazines are now available in recorded formats. The National Library Service for the Blind and Physically Handicapped, a branch of the Library of Congress, maintains an extensive selection of books on flexible disc or 4-track tape, and it provides qualified individuals with record or tape players free of charge. Other companies offer recordings of selected literature, often read by celebrated actors or authors, which can be played on any standard cassette player. A portable cassette player should be standard equipment for every blind or severely visu-

ally impaired older person with sufficient manual ability to operate its controls.

Another advance that has had a positive impact for the visually impaired older person can be described as "talking technology." Synthetic speech output has resulted in talking watches, clocks, calculators, and scales, to name but four of the most common applications of the technique. Sphygmomanometers, thermometers, and blood glucose meters have been similarly adapted, making it more feasible for a visually impaired hypertensive or diabetic person to monitor blood pressure or blood glucose. Most of these devices are financially accessible to most elderly persons. More complex technologies such as the Kurzweil reader (which reads print and converts it into synthetic speech) are too costly to be practical for the vast majority of older persons. However, the availability of software allowing voice output on personal computers may be helpful for older people with previous computer experience.

SUMMARY

Rehabilitation Medicine and modern Vision Rehabilitation were born almost simultaneously and under similar circumstances: the crisis precipitated by unprecedented numbers of young wounded soldiers from the battlefields of World War II whose limb amputations, spinal cord injuries, and visual losses demanded prompt attention in order to allow them to return to American society as productive citizens. Both systems required multidisciplinary teams and both developed special techniques and technology to meet the needs of their clientele. In the postwar period, their relationship remained very close; in fact, the first nonmilitary blindness rehabilitation center was established in 1948 at the Hines VA Hospital within that facility's Department of Physical Medicine and Rehabilitation (36). Over the next 40 years these two disciplines have gone their own way and each has added immeasurably to the quality of life of countless physically and visually handicapped people throughout the world.

The "graying of America" is a new crisis precipitated not by the horrors of global war but by medical victories in the war against acute illnesses. As a result of these victories, medical science has made possible the survival of greater numbers of older persons who, through normal or pathologic aging processes, frequently develop multisystem disabilities, including visual impairments. The rise of the new specialty of Geriatrics is testimony to the significance of this trend.

The elderly person with a vision impairment presents a special challenge to all three of these disciplines, and the key to meeting that challenge will be a marriage of methodologies that transcends any single specialty. Without this marriage, older visually impaired persons will fall between the cracks of a system that should be supporting their restoration to a maximal quality of life.

References

1. Rabin DL, Stockton P. *Long-Term; Care for the Elderly.* New York, NY: Oxford University Press; 1987.
2. Nelson KA. Visual impairment among elderly Americans: statistics in transition. *J Vis Impairment Blind.* 81:331–334, 1987.
3. Tobis JS, Block M, Steinhaus-Donham C, Reinsch S, Tamaru K, Weil D. Falling among the sensorially impaired elderly. *Arch Phys Med Rehabil.* 71:144–147, 1990.
4. Stones MV, Kozma A. Balance and age in the sighted and blind. *Arch Phys Med Rehabil.* 68:85–89, 1987.
5. Lee DN, Tishman JR. Visual proprioceptive control of stance. *J Human Mvmt Studies.* 1:87–95, 1975.
6. Cohn TE, Lasley DJ. Visual depth illusion and falls in the elderly. *Clin Geriatr Med.* 1:601–620, 1985.
7. Felson DT, Anderson JJ, Hannan MT, Milton RC, Wilson PWF, Kiel DP. Impaired vision and hip fracture: the Framingham Eye Study. *J Am Geriatr Soc.* 37:495–500, 1989.
8. Altner PE, Rusin JJ, DeBoer A. Rehabilitation of blind patients with lower extremity amputations. *Arch Phys Med Rehabil.* 61:82–85, 1980.
9. Fisher R. Rehabilitation of the blind amputee: a rewarding experience. *Arch Phys Med Rehabil.* 68:382–383, 1987.
10. Wainapel SF. Rehabilitation of the blind stroke patient. *Arch Phys Med Rehabil.* 65:487–489, 1984.
11. Wainapel SF, Kwon YS, Fazzari PJ. Severe visual impairment on a rehabilitation unit: incidence and implications. *Arch Phys Med Rehabil.* 70:439–441, 1989.
12. DiStefano AF, Aston SJ. Rehabilitation for the blind and visually impaired elderly. In: Brody SL, Ruff DL, eds. *Aging and Rehabilitation: Advances in the State of the Art.* New York, NY: Springer; 1986.
13. Morse AR, Silberman R, Trief E. Aging and visual impairment. *J Vis Impairment Blind.* 81:308–312, 1987.
14. Kahn HA, Moorehead HS. *Statistics on Blindness in Model Reporting Area, 1969–1970.* Washington, DC: US Printing Office; 1973. Dept. of Health, Education and Welfare Publication 73-427.
15. Greenblatt SL. *Providing Services for People with Vision Loss.* Lexington Mass: Resources for Rehabilitation; 1989.
16. Biegel DE, Petchers MK, Snyder A, Beisgen B. Unmet needs and barriers to service delivery for the blind and visually impaired elderly. *Gerontologist.* 29:86–91, 1981.
17. Appollonio I, Frattola L, Carabellese C, Trabucchi M. The eyes and ears of the world of function. *J Am Geriatr Soc.* 37:1099–1100, 1989.
18. Linn MW, Linn BS. Self-Evaluation of Life Function (SELF) scale: a short comprehensive report of health for elderly adults. *J Gerontol.* 39:603, 1984.
19. Branch LG, Horowitz A, Carr C. The implications for everyday life of incident self-reported visual decline among people over age 65 living in the community. *Gerontologist.* 29:359–365, 1989.
20. Gillman AE. Visual handicap in the aged: self-reported visual disability and the quality of life of residents of public housing for the elderly. *J Vis Impairment Blind.* 80:588–590, 1986.
21. Marmor MF. Management of elderly patients with impaired vision. In: Ebaugh FG, ed. *Management of Common Problems in Geriatric Medicine.* Menlo Park, Calif: Addison-Wesley; 1981.
22. Kenney RA. *Physiology of Aging.* 2nd ed. Chicago, Ill: Year Book Medical Publishers; 1989.
23. Kane RL, Ouslander JG, Abrass IB. *Essentials of Clinical Geriatrics.* 2nd ed. New York, NY: McGraw-Hill Information Services Company; 1989.
24. Applegate WB, Miller ST, Elam JT, Freeman JM, Wood TO, Gettlefinger TC. Impact of cataract surgery with lens implantation on vision and physical function in elderly patients. *JAMA.* 257:1064–1066, 1987.
25. Kahn HA, Leibowitz HM, Ganley JR, et al. The Framingham Eye Study 1: outline and major findings. *Am J Epidemiol.* 106:17–32, 1977.
26. Liu IY, White L, LaCroix AZ. The association of age-related macular degeneration and lens opacities in the aged. *Am J Public Health.* 79:765–769, 1989.
27. Ferris FL. Senile macular degeneration: review of epidemiologic features. *Am J Epidemiol.* 118:132–150, 1983.
28. Faye EE. *Clinical Low Vision.* Boston, Mass: Little, Brown; 1984.
29. Carroll TJ. *Blindness: What It is, What It Does, and How to Live with It.* Boston, Mass: Little, Brown; 1961.
30. Muldoon JE. Carroll revisited: innovations in rehabilitation, 1938–1971. *J Vis Impairment Blind.* 80:617–626, 1986.
31. Walsh R, Blasch BB. *Foundations of Orientation and Mobility.* New York, NY: American Foundation for the Blind; 1983.
32. Wainapel SF. Attitudes of visually impaired persons toward cane use. *J Vis Impairment Blind.* 83:446–448, 1989.
33. Fonda GE. *Management of Low Vision.* New York, NY: Thieme-Stratton; 1981.
34. Kornzweig AL. Rehabilitation ophthalmology for the aged. In: Williams TF, ed. *Rehabilitation in the Aging.* New York, NY: Raven Press; 1984.
35. Hiatt LG. Care and design: is poor light dimming the sight of nursing home patients? *Nursing Homes.* 29:32–41, 1980.
36. Koestler FA. *The Unseen Minority: A Social History of the Blind in America.* New York, NY: American Foundation for the Blind; 1976.

29
Geriatric Hearing Loss

Martin A. Goins

Hearing loss can have a significant effect on interpersonal relationships, individual self-esteem and self-confidence, personal safety, and general sense of well-being. These effects are usually worse in the elderly population because of coexisting deterioration in other areas such as vision, smell, proprioception, and endocrine, vascular, and cognitive function. The incidence of significant hearing loss in the elderly appears to be between 25% and 50% among individuals over the age of 65 years. The different definitions of significant hearing loss and the different populations examined makes it difficult to offer a more definitive figure. However, a review of several recent large studies suggests that at least one third of persons in this country above the age of 65 years have a hearing impairment significant enough to interfere with the appreciation of speech at normal levels (1–5).

ANATOMY OF THE CENTRAL AUDITORY SYSTEM

Information is transmitted between the cochlea and the auditory area of the temporal lobe after acoustic energy is converted to nerve impulses. The ascending auditory pathways are complex and not completely understood. A description of the neural anatomy relevant to the scope of this chapter will be presented.

Acoustic information is presented into the external auditory canal and is amplified by the tympanic membrane and ossicles. The footplate of the stapes transmits the motion of the ossicles to the perilymph of the cochlea through the oval window. Thus, the acoustic energy is converted to vibratory energy within the cochlea. This causes movement of Reissner's membrane within the cochlea, which separates the scala vestibuli, a perilymph-containing cavity, from the scala media (also called the cochlear duct), an endolymph-containing cavity. The third cavity within the cochlea is the scala tympani. It is a perilymph-containing cavity and is separated from the scala media by the basilar membrane. These three chambers are present along the length of the spiral-shaped cochlea. The scala media contains the Organ of Corti and the hair cells, which are the receptor cells of the acoustic nerve. The scala media ends in a blind sac called the cecum cupulare at the apex of the cochlea. The scala vestibuli begins at the oval window (against which the footplate of the stapes rests) and communicates at the apex of the cochlea with the scala tympani through a small opening called the helicotrema. The scala tympani begins at the round window and ends at the helicotrema. Please refer to Figures 29.1 and 29.2 for a better understanding of this anatomy.

When the perilymph within the cochlea is placed in motion by movement of the footplate of the stapes, the basilar membrane and Reissner's membrane also move, resulting in stimulation of the afferent nerve fibers innervating the hair cells. There appear to be electrical and chemical changes around the hair cells, which may also play a part in nerve stimulation. The nerve impulses are then transmitted to the spiral ganglia of the eighth cranial nerve within the cochlea. The impulses then ascend through the cochlear nuclei, superior olivary complex, lateral lemniscus nuclei, inferior colliculus, medial geniculate body, and finally to the auditory cortex in the temporal lobe. There are also efferent fibers that innervate the cochlea, but these are not very well understood at present.

The vascular supply of the cochlea is through the internal auditory artery, which exits the posterior fossa through the internal auditory canal. The internal auditory artery is a branch of the anterior inferior cerebellar artery or, sometimes, the basilar artery (5–9).

TYPES OF HEARING LOSS

Hearing loss is usually classified under three general headings: conductive, sensorineural, or mixed.

Conductive hearing losses are due to disorders of the external and/or middle ear systems. These disorders interfere with the transformer mechanism of the auricle, external auditory canal, tympanic membrane, and middle ear ossicles. Examples of causes of conductive hearing

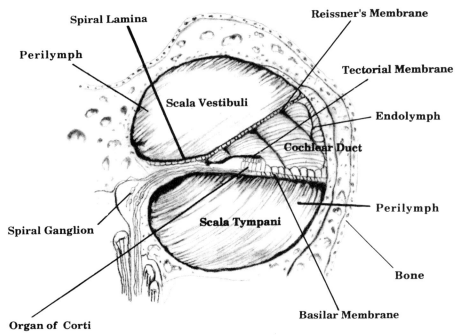

Figure 29.1. The cochlea.

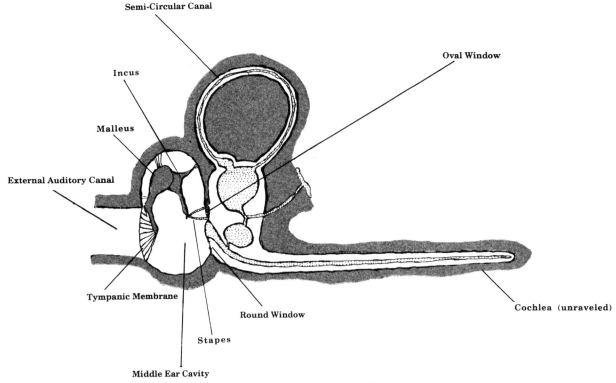

Figure 29.2. Unraveled cochlea.

loss due to external ear disorders are stenosis or occlusion of the external auditory canal (congenital or acquired), otitis externa, cerumen, a foreign body, bony overgrowth (exostosis), neoplasm, or abscess. Examples of causes of conductive hearing loss due to middle ear disorders are perforation of the tympanic membrane, hematoma, mass or foreign substance over the tympanic membrane, changes in the thickness of the tympanic membrane (such as from chronic infection), fluid or neoplasm in the middle ear space, stiffening of the joints between the three middle ear ossicles, fixation of the foot plate of the stapes within the oval window, disarticulation of the middle ear ossicles due to traumatic or chronic infectious causes, and, very rarely, congenital absence of one or more of the ossicles (10).

The cause of a conductive hearing loss can usually be found through careful history taking, physical examination, and diagnostic testing. Occasionally, an operation to examine the middle ear (an exploratory tympanotomy) becomes necessary if the cause of a significant conductive hearing loss remains unclear.

An etiologic classification of sensorineural hearing loss is demonstrated in Table 29.1. The etiologies have been divided into congenital and delayed onset. The congenital and delayed onset etiologies are each further divided into genetic and nongenetic etiologies. The genetic etiologies (congenital and delayed onset) constitute 50% of sensorineural hearing loss (11).

Conductive hearing losses can usually be treated successfully. On the other hand, sensorineural hearing losses can rarely be improved by medical or surgical intervention, even though the cause can sometimes be identified. Exceptions are: hearing loss from syphilis, which can sometimes be improved by antibiotic and steroid therapy; hearing loss from Meniere's disease, which is frequently made less severe by treatment with low-salt diet, diuretics, and other drugs and sometimes improved by surgery; and the sensorineural hearing loss

from cochlear otospongeosis (also known as otosclerosis). There are some reports that progressive sensorineural hearing loss associated with otospongeosis has been stabilized and sometimes improved after stapes surgery and after the administration of sodium fluoride (10).

DEFINITION AND TYPES OF PRESBYCUSIS

The term presbycusis generally means an otherwise unexplained sensorineural hearing loss in an elderly person. The hearing loss in presbycusis is usually approximately equal in both ears and is usually worse in the higher frequencies. There are many other causes of hearing loss in this age group, and these causes must be excluded by a complete evaluation before the diagnosis of presbycusis can properly be applied. It is not clear what effect environmental factors such as noise exposure, diet, level of physical activity, ototoxic drug exposure, and head trauma have on the development of presbycusis. The extent that metabolic factors and genetic predisposition influence the hearing impairment also is not clear. It is possible that all these factors and others contribute to the loss.

Audiograms and clinical findings identified four patterns of presbycusis. Although there is not uniform agreement that these classifications are entirely accurate,

Table 29.1. Classification of Hearing Loss[a]

I. Congenital Sensorineural Hearing Loss
  A. Genetic etiologies
    1. Hearing loss occurring alone
      a. Michel's aplasia
      b. Mondini's aplasia
      c. Scheibe's aplasia
      d. Alexander's aplasia
    2. Hearing loss occurring with other abnormalities (syndromes)
      a. Waardenburg's syndrome (deafness may be delayed)
      b. Albinism
      c. Hyperpigmentation
      d. Onychodystrophy
      e. Pendred's syndrome
      f. Jervell's syndrome
      g. Usher's syndrome
    3. Chromosomal abnormalities
      a. Trisomy 13–15
      b. Trisomy 18
  B. Nongenetic etiologies
    1. Hearing loss occurring alone
      a. Ototoxic poisoning (streptomycin, quinine, etc.)
    2. Hearing loss occurring with other abnormalities
      a. Viral infection (maternal rubella)
      b. Bacterial infection
      c. Ototoxic poisoning (thalidomide)
      d. Metabolic disorders (cretinism)
      e. Erythroblastosis fetalis
      f. Radiation (first trimester)
      g. Prematurity
      h. Birth trauma, anoxia

II. Delayed Sensorineural Hearing Loss
  A. Genetic etiologies
    1. Hearing loss occurring alone
      a. Familial progressive sensorineural deafness
      b. Otosclerosis
      c. Presbycusis
    2. Hearing loss occurring with other abnormalities (syndromes)
      a. Alport's disease
      b. Hurler's syndrome (gargoylism)
      c. Klippel-Feil syndrome
      d. Refsum's disease
      e. Alstrom's disease
      f. Paget's disease
      g. Richards-Rundel syndrome
      h. Von Recklinghausen's disease
      i. Crouzon's disease
  B. Nongenetic etiologies
    1. Inflammatory diseases
      a. Bacterial (labyrinthitis and otitis media)
      b. Viral (measles, mumps, influenza, labyrinthitis, etc.)
      c. Spirochetal (congenital and acquired syphilis)
    2. Ototoxic poisoning
    3. Neoplastic disorders (leukemia, peripheral, and central ear tumors, etc.)
    4. Traumatic injury (acoustic trauma, temporal bone fractures)
    5. Metabolic disorders (hypothyroidism, allergies, Meniere's disease, etc.)
    6. Vascular insufficiency (sudden deafness, presbycusis)
    7. Central nervous system disease (multiple sclerosis)

[a] From Paparella MM. Sensorineural hearing loss in children—nongenetic. In: Paparella MM, Shumrick DA, eds. *Otolaryngology, II.* Philadelphia, Pa: W.B. Saunders; 1980.

most practitioners find them useful. Figures 29.3 to 29.6 are examples of audiograms seen in the four patterns of presbycusis (3, 12, 13).

Sensory Presbycusis

Sensory presbycusis gives an abrupt high-frequency sensorineural hearing loss. It is thought to be secondary to atrophy of the Organ of Corti and the auditory nerve in the basal end of the cochlea. However, the atrophy may be in the supporting cells in the Organ of Corti, with secondary involvement of the nerve fibers. This type of hearing loss usually begins at middle age and is slowly progressive. The progression is only in the higher frequencies. The speech frequencies are rarely involved. Postmortem examinations have shown atrophy in the basilar turns of the cochlea only, where the higher frequency sounds are received.

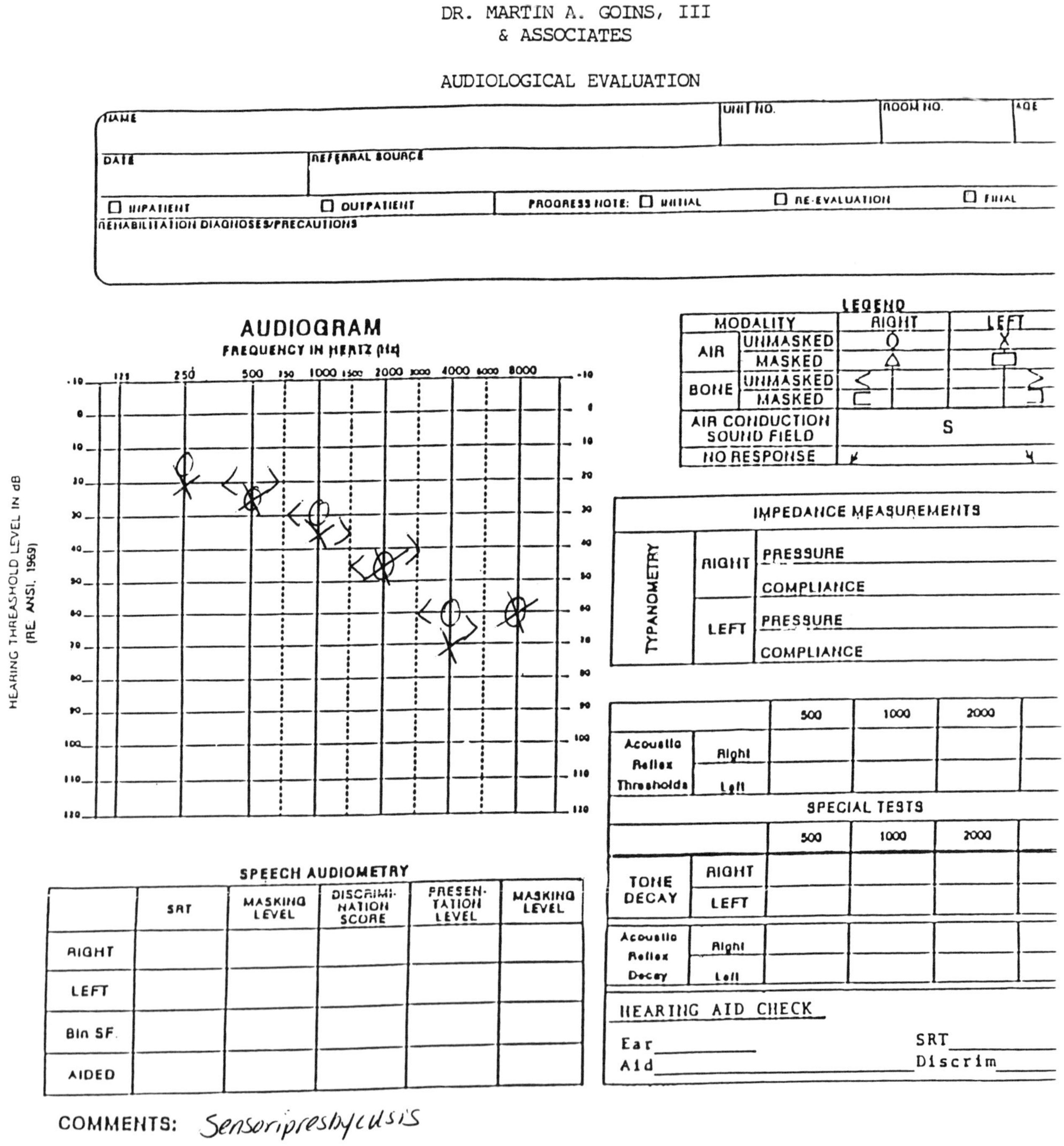
DR. MARTIN A. GOINS, III
& ASSOCIATES

AUDIOLOGICAL EVALUATION

NAME | UNIT NO. | ROOM NO. | AGE
DATE | REFERRAL SOURCE
☐ INPATIENT ☐ OUTPATIENT PROGRESS NOTE: ☐ INITIAL ☐ RE-EVALUATION ☐ FINAL
REHABILITATION DIAGNOSES/PRECAUTIONS

AUDIOGRAM
FREQUENCY IN HERTZ (Hz)
125 250 500 750 1000 1500 2000 3000 4000 6000 8000
HEARING THRESHOLD LEVEL IN dB (RE: ANSI, 1969)
-10 0 10 20 30 40 50 60 70 80 90 100 110 120

LEGEND

MODALITY		RIGHT	LEFT
AIR	UNMASKED	O	X
	MASKED	Δ	☐
BONE	UNMASKED	<	>
	MASKED	[	]
AIR CONDUCTION SOUND FIELD		S	
NO RESPONSE			

IMPEDANCE MEASUREMENTS

TYPANOMETRY	RIGHT	PRESSURE
		COMPLIANCE
	LEFT	PRESSURE
		COMPLIANCE

		500	1000	2000
Acoustic Reflex Thresholds	Right			
	Left			

SPECIAL TESTS

		500	1000	2000
TONE DECAY	RIGHT			
	LEFT			
Acoustic Reflex Decay	Right			
	Left			

SPEECH AUDIOMETRY

	SRT	MASKING LEVEL	DISCRIMINATION SCORE	PRESENTATION LEVEL	MASKING LEVEL
RIGHT					
LEFT					
Bin SF					
AIDED					

HEARING AID CHECK
Ear ______ SRT ______
Aid ______ Discrim ______

COMMENTS: Sensoripresbycusis

Figure 29.3. Audiogram of sensory presbycusis.

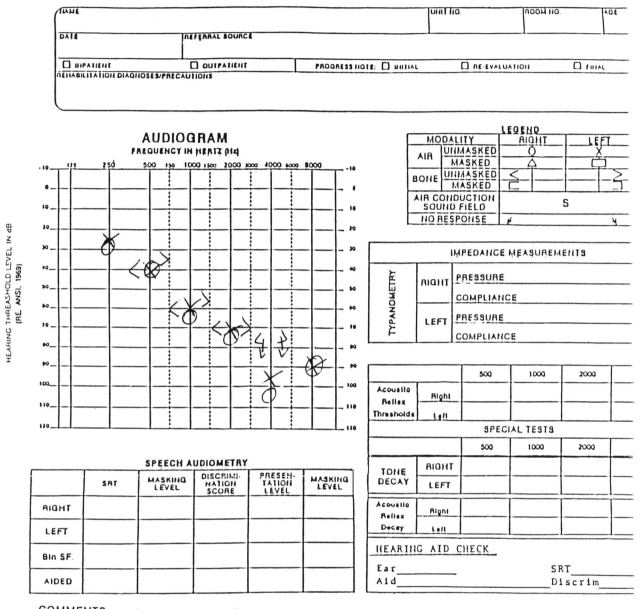

Figure 29.4. Audiogram of neural presbycusis.

Neural Presbycusis

Neural presbycusis results from the loss of ganglion cells and the regeneration of neural fibers. It usually becomes significant late in life. The impairment of speech discrimination is usually disproportionately worse than the pure tone impairments. This type of presbycusis usually results in a down sloping audiogram.

Metabolic Presbycusis

Metabolic presbycusis is sometimes called strial presbycusis. This is thought to be secondary to defects in the chemical and physical processes involved in the production of energy in the inner ear. Postmortem sections of the cochleas in these patients have demonstrated atrophy of the stria vascularis, the organ within

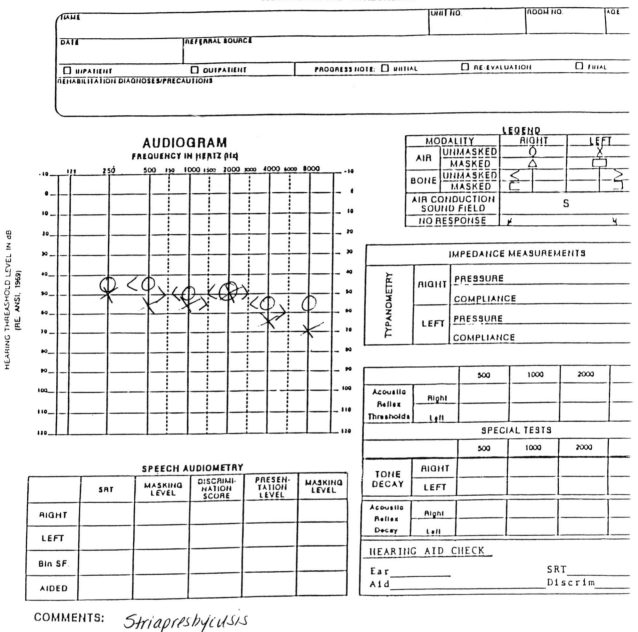

Figure 29.5. Audiogram of metabolic presbycusis.

the cochlear duct that is thought to be the sight of endolymph production and possibly the site of generation of an electrical potential necessary for proper cochlear transduction. In metabolic presbycusis, the audiogram is flat and speech discrimination is usually good. Patients with this type of presbycusis are usually excellent candidates for hearing amplification.

Mechanical Presbycusis

Mechanical presbycusis is sometimes called cochlear presbycusis. It is felt to be due to a thickening and/or stiffening of the basilar membrane without changes in the neural components of the pathway. This usually gives a straight line descending audiometric pattern.

WORKUP OF ELDERLY PATIENTS WITH HEARING LOSS

The many identifiable causes of hearing loss must be ruled out by a careful work-up before the diagnosis of presbycusis can properly be applied. The following pages outline the basic work-up of the patient with hearing loss, which can be performed by or arranged by the rehabilitative team (4, 5, 12–14).

History

1. Unilateral or bilateral.
2. Sudden or gradual.
3. Constant or intermittent.
4. Duration.
5. History of noise exposure.
6. History of ototoxic drug therapy.
7. Associated ear symptoms such as tinnitus, vertigo/

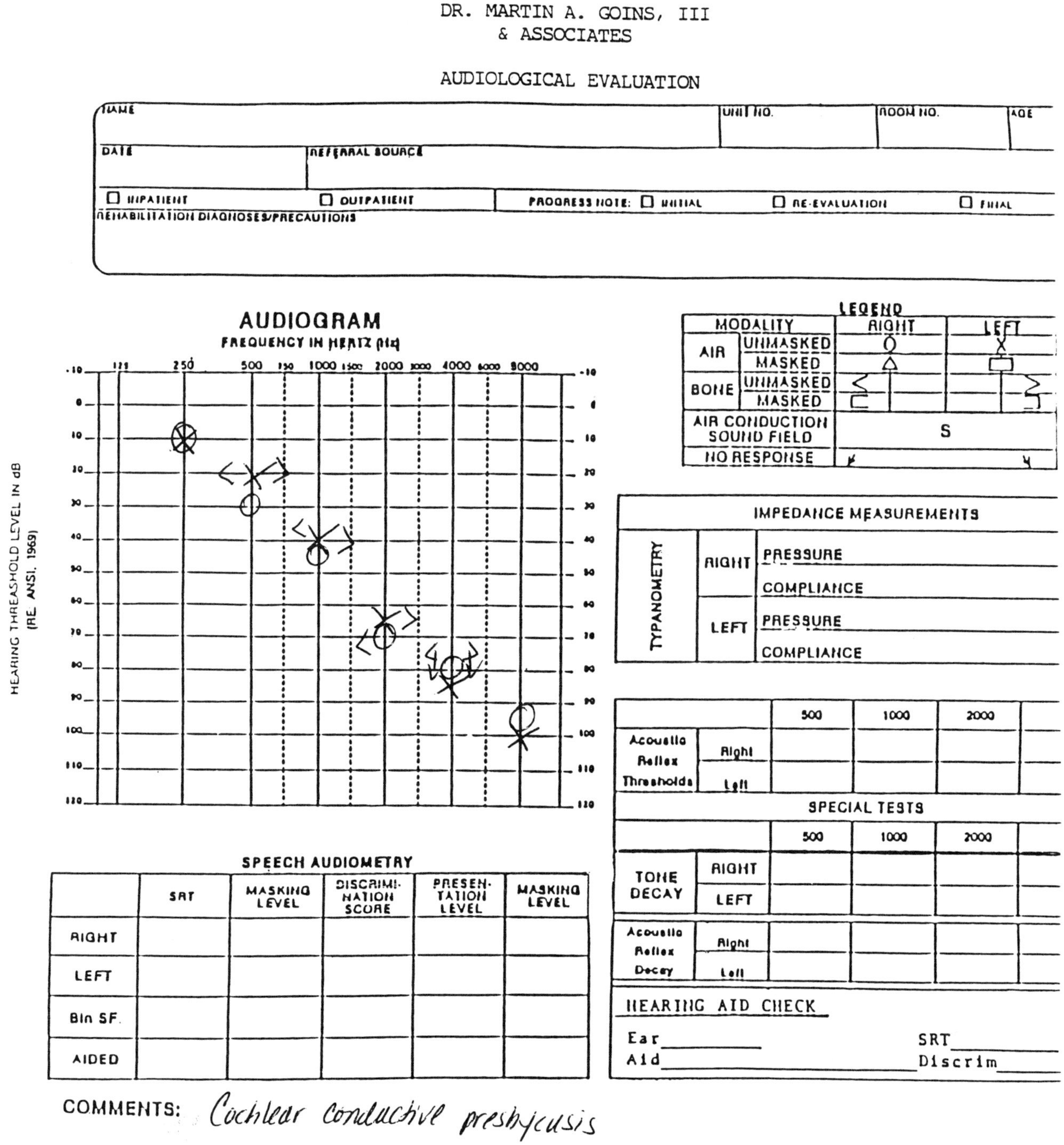

Figure 29.6.   Audiogram of mechanical presbycusis.

dizziness, ear pain, ear fullness, or ear discharge.

8. Personal history of ear disease, ear trauma, or ear surgery.
9. Family history of ear disease or hearing difficulty.
10. Any neurologic symptoms.

Physical Examination

1. Inspection of the auricle and the surrounding skin.
2. Otoscopic examination of the external auditory canal and the tympanic membrane.
3. Pneumatic otoscopy.
4. Weber tuning fork test.
   The 512 Hz fork should be placed anywhere along the anterior midline of the face from the forehead to the chin. The Weber test will lateralize to the ear with a conductive hearing loss or to the ear opposite a sensorineural hearing loss. The results are confusing if the patient has a bilateral hearing loss or mixed losses.
5. Rinne tuning fork test.
   The 512 Hz tuning fork and sometimes the 1024 Hz tuning fork are used. The sound of the vibrating tuning fork when placed over the mastoid bone is compared to the sound of the same fork 2 centimeters lateral to the meatus of the ipsilateral ear. The conduction when the tuning fork is near the meatus is through the transformer mechanism of the outer ear and middle ear to the cochlea and is therefore called air conduction. The conduction when the fork is placed over the mastoid bone is called bone conduction because the sound is transmitted directly through bone to the cochlea. Normally, air conduction is significantly better than bone conduction because of the transducer effects of the external ear and middle ear. Bone conduction will be equal to or better than air conduction in the Rinne test if the conductive hearing loss is 20 decibels or greater using a 512 Hz fork or 25 decibels or greater using a 1024 Hz fork.
6. Other tests appropriate for neurologic symptoms discovered during history taking.

Diagnostic Testing

AUDIOGRAM

Pure tone audiometry is performed by presenting the patient with pure tones of various frequencies. The commonly used frequencies are 250 Hz, 500 Hz, 1000 Hz, 2000 Hz, 4000 Hz, 8000 Hz, and sometimes 6000 Hz. The tone at each frequency is presented at various intensities, measured in decibels, until the examiner can determine the lowest decibel level at which the patient can hear the tone at that frequency 50% of the time. In a child or young adult with normal hearing, these levels should be 20 decibels or less. Various typical patterns in presbycusis will be shown later.

The tone presented to the patients in pure tone audiometry can be presented either through the external auditory canal via a headphone or earpiece or directly onto the mastoid. As explained above, the tones presented through the meatus will give air conduction results and are considered to be a measure of the conductive hearing apparatus. Tones presently directly to the mastoid bone will give bone conduction results and are a measure of the sensorineural hearing apparatus. These air conduction results and the bone conduction results are usually plotted separately on an audiogram report. Though air conduction should be better than bone conduction, audiometers are calibrated in such a way that the air conduction curve and bone conduction curve will be the same in a patient with normal hearing. If the two curves are different, the difference is called an air-bone gap and is indicative of a conductive hearing loss.

If the hearing in one ear is significantly better than the hearing in the other ear, masking may be used in the better ear while the poorer hearing ear is being tested. Masking is simply a sound that is placed into the better hearing ear so that the tones presented into the poorer ear will not be heard in the better ear and confuse the results.

Figure 29.7 is an example of a normal audiogram.

SPEECH RECEPTION THRESHOLD

The speech reception threshold (SRT) is approximately the level at which the patient can understand speech. Usually 25 double syllable words are presented to the patient by the examiner. The SRT is the lowest decibel level at which the patient is able to correctly identify 50% of the presented words. The SRT should be approximately the same as the pure tone averages between 500 Hz and 2000 Hz because this is the frequency range for most speech.

SPEECH DISCRIMINATION

The speech discrimination test uses a list of monosyllabic words, which are presented to the patient at 20 to 40 decibels above the SRT. The speech discrimination score is the percentage of words that the patient is able to correctly identify.

TYMPANOMETRY

Tympanometry is a method of measuring the mobility of the tympanic membrane. This gives indirect information on the status of the ossicles, the presence or absence of middle ear fluid, the patency of the eustachian tube, the presence or absence of a tympanic membrane perforation, and the activity of the middle ear muscles. The tympanogram is actually a graph of the compliance of the tympanic membrane as various pressures are created in the ear canal through a probe that is placed in the meatus. The graph can then be inter-

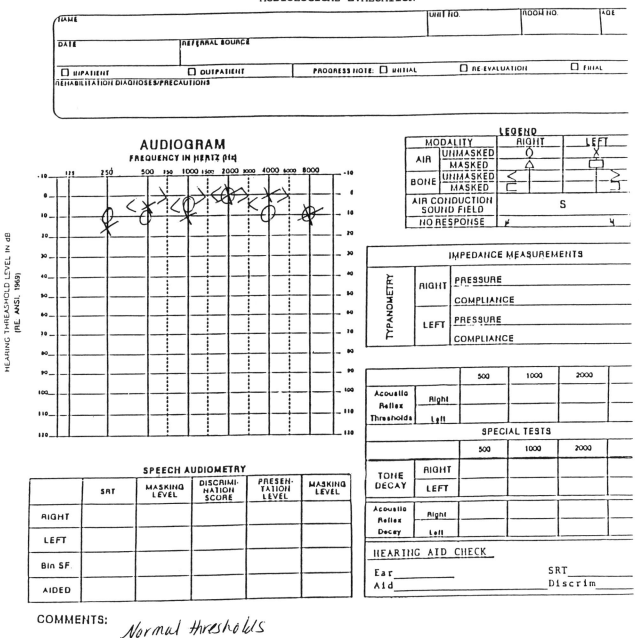

Figure 29.7. Audiogram of normal thresholds.

preted as being normal or as fitting into several categories of abnormal patterns, which can then be correlated with known causes of conductive hearing loss.

ACOUSTIC REFLEX

The acoustic reflex can be tested with the use of a tympanometer. The reflex is caused by contraction of the stapedial muscle in response to presentation of a signal approximately 60 decibels above the patient's hearing threshold. The stapedial muscle inserts into the stapes, and contraction of the muscle rotates the stapes slightly in the posterior direction and stiffens the tympanic membrane and ossicular system. This causes a change in the tympanic membrane compliance and, therefore, in the tympanogram. The acoustic reflex in normal patients occurs bilaterally, even though the sound is introduced unilaterally; therefore, the reflex can be tested ipsilaterally, i.e., in the ear where the sound is being introduced, or contralaterally. The reflex is considered normal if it occurs at 90 decibels or less above the hearing level at a specified frequency. If it does not occur until the signal intensity is 90 decibels or more above the hearing level, it is considered to be elevated. If the reflex does not occur at 115 decibels above the hearing level, it is considered to be absent. There are many situations in which the acoustic reflex is elevated or absent. These situations are somewhat confusing, and it is therefore easier to understand the conditions necessary for a normal acoustic reflex. The conditions are: the ability to hear the presented sound on the side to which it is presented, normal compliance of the tympanic membrane and ossicular system on the side being tested, and normal innervation of the stapedial muscle. Any conditions in these requirements that are not met will result in an abnormal tympanogram.

ACOUSTIC REFLEX DECAY

The acoustic reflex decay test measures the change in tympanic membrane compliance when a sound is presented to the tested ear over a 10-second period. Normally, there should be less than a 50% reduction in the compliance. Acoustic reflex decays of over 50% suggest the presence of an abnormality of the acoustic nerve or the brainstem.

BRAINSTEM EVOKED RESPONSES (BSER) OR ACOUSTIC BRAINSTEM RESPONSES (ABR)

Acoustic signals (clicks, tone pips, or tone bursts) are presented to one ear by earphones or a bone vibrator. Scalp electrodes are usually placed at the vertex and over the mastoid process. The electrical potentials resulting from the sound stimulation are received by the two electrodes, amplified, and recorded through a computer. The responses are then printed on a graph, showing five distinct positive waves. Interpretation of the BSER is based on peak latency, interpeak interval, peak amplitude, and less definitively, the appearance of the wave.

The BSER is a very reliable indicator of a retrocochlear lesion (acoustic nerve or brain). Conductive hearing losses and sensorineural hearing losses secondary to cochlear lesions can also usually be identified.

The disadvantages of the BSER are that movement artifact makes the results difficult to interpret and that the test cannot be performed if the patient has a 60 decibel or greater hearing loss in the midfrequencies.

The advantages of the BSER are that the results are independent of patient attention and sincerity. Therefore, the test can be used in infants, comatose patients, sedated patients, and malingerers. In addition, a BSER is a much less expensive test than an enhanced computed tomography (CT) scan or magnetic resonance imaging (MRI).

RADIOGRAPHIC STUDIES

Mastoid Roentgenograms

Mastoid roentgenograms can demonstrate abnormalities within the mastoid, middle ear, or internal auditory canal. Transorbital views nicely demonstrate the size and shape of the internal auditory canals. Tumors of the acoustic nerve will usually cause asymmetry of the internal auditory canals. Mastoid roentgenograms are relatively inexpensive and can usually be obtained without the patient having to make an appointment.

CT Scan

CT scans of the temporal bone show much greater detail than do plain mastoid roentgenograms. A CT scan with contrast shows bony architecture better than any other single study. Thus, bony erosion from infectious or neoplastic processes is best shown by this study. The disadvantages of the study are that it is more expensive than plain mastoid roentgenograms, an appointment is usually required to have the study, and some patients are allergic to the intravenous contrast.

MRI

The MRI study shows soft tissue details better than does the CT scan. Therefore, it is the best radiographic study to demonstrate a tumor of the brain or eighth cranial nerve. The study is even more precise with the addition of gadolinium intravenous contrast. The disadvantages of the MRI scan are that it is even more expensive than a CT scan and clinically insignificant mucosal edema may masquerade as mucosal inflammation.

REHABILITATION

Many patients with mild presbycusis only need education about the importance of noise avoidance and regular audiologic evaluations. Patients with greater degrees of hearing loss often need hearing amplification. The most common form of amplification in use today is a hearing aid.

Hearing Aids

The conventional hearing aid consists of three basic parts: a microphone that picks up the sound energy and converts it into electrical energy, an amplifier that amplifies the electrical energy, and a receiver or speaker that converts the amplified electrical energy back into sound energy that can be heard by the patient. Hearing aids can be of several different types, including the in-the-ear hearing aid, the postauricular or behind-the-ear hearing aid, the body aid, the eyeglass hearing aid, and, most recently, the implantable hearing aid. Implantable hearing aids are either completely or partially implanted. Partially implanted hearing aids require an external component. The implantable hearing aids, including cochlear implants, will be used more often as the technology improves. However, the conventional hearing aid will probably continue to be used more frequently (15–18).

Many patients who could be helped significantly by hearing aids will refuse to wear their hearing aids for various reasons. The most common reasons for this are distortion of sound by the hearing aid, difficulty in understanding the controls, inability to insert the ear canal portion of the aid because of impaired manual dexterity, inability to feel or turn the volume control knob, an uncomfortable fit, and (although it is not always admitted) vanity.

Patients who feel that they need hearing amplification are often confused about where to go to seek help. Essentially, there are three categories of providers who can dispense hearing aids: hearing aid dealers, clinical audiologists, and otolaryngologists. The hearing aid dealers usually work independently. Clinical audiologists are either independent or are affiliated with an otolaryngologist, clinic, or hospital. Most otolaryngologists today are in some way associated with an audiologist. In general, prices for hearing aids are higher if the aid is purchased from a hearing aid dealer rather than from an audiologist.

Almost all states require that a patient have medical clearance from a physician before a hearing aid is issued. It is recommended that this physician be an otolaryngologist or otologist. However, the patient may waive the medical clearance by signing a waiver form (16, 18).

Assistive Listening Devices

Assistive listening devices are devices that can help patients hear better in specific listening situations. An example of such a device is the personal amplification system that is designed for use in situations such as a live theater. These devices can be used with or without a personal hearing aid (19).

Assistive Alerting Devices and Assistive Signaling Devices

Assistive alerting devices and assistive signaling devices are similar. These are devices such as bells, buzzers, flashing lights, or vibrating devices that can alert hearing impaired people to various situations. These devices are most often used to make patients aware of doorbells, telephones, smoke detectors, turn signals within a car, cooking or laundry timers, or the cry of a baby (19).

Other Types of Assistance for the Hearing Impaired

Other examples of equipment available to help patients with hearing losses are telephone amplifiers and closed captioned television (19).

Lip Reading

In patients whose hearing is unsatisfactory after medical therapy, surgical therapy, and amplification have been considered or used, lip reading can sometimes be of benefit. It does, of course, require that the patient have adequate vision.

SUMMARY

The elderly population has a significant instance of communication difficulty, some of which is a result of hearing impairment. This communication difficulty can result in a change in the patient's general sense of well-being. The rehabilitative team can significantly improve the situation with an understanding of the relevant neural anatomy, pathophysiology, diagnostic tests, modes of therapy, and roles of associated health care providers. This knowledge will greatly aid the rehabilitative team in improving the quality of life of elderly patients with hearing loss.

References

1. Babin RW. Effects of aging on the auditory and vestibular systems. *Otolaryngol Head Neck Surg.* 4:1986, 3189–3199.
2. Boone DR, Bayles KA, Koopman CF Jr. Communicative aspects of aging. *Otolaryngol Clin North Am.* 15(2):1982, 313–327.
3. Hinojosa R, Meyerhoff WL. Presbycusis. In: Paparella MM, Shumrick DA, eds. *Otolaryngology*, II. 2nd ed. Philadelphia, Pa: W.B. Saunders; 1980.
4. Popelka GR, Gates GA. Hearing aid evaluation and fitting. *Otolaryngol Clin North Am.* 24(2):1991, 415–428.
5. Tyler RS, Tye-Murray N, Gantz BJ. Aural rehabilitation. *Otolaryngol Clin North Am.* 24(2):1991, 429–445.
6. Kennedy R, Clemis JD. The geriatric auditory and vestibular systems. *Otolaryngol Clin North Am.* 23(6):1990, 1075–1082.
7. Lee KJ. Anatomy of the ear. In: Lee KJ, ed. *Essential Otolaryngology: Head and Neck Surgery.* 5th ed. New York, NY: Medical Examination Publishing Company; 1991.
8. Neely JG, Dennis JM, Lippe WR. Anatomy of the auditory end organ and neural pathways. *Otolaryngol Head Neck Surg.* 4. 1986, 2571–2608.
9. Paff GH. *Anatomy of the Head and Neck* Philadelphia, Pa: W.B. Saunders; 1973.
10. Shambaugh GE Jr, Glasscock ME III. *Surgery of the Ear.* 3rd ed. Philadelphia, Pa: W.B. Saunders; 1980.
11. Lee KJ. Congenital deafness. In: Lee KJ, ed. *Essential Otolaryngology: Head and Neck Surgery.* 5th ed. New York, NY: Medical Examination Publishing Company; 1991.
12. Lassman FM, Hoel RL. *Audiology.* In: Adams GL, Boies LR Jr, Paparella MM, eds. *Boies's Fundamentals of Otolaryngology.* 5th ed. Philadelphia, Pa: W.B. Saunders; 1978.
13. Yanagisawa E, Lee KJ. *Audiology.* In: Lee KJ, ed. *Essential Oto-*

laryngology: Head and Neck Surgery. 5th ed. New York, NY: Medical Examination Publishing Company; 1991.

14. Silverman SR. Rehabilitative audiology. In: Paperella MM, Shumrick DA, eds. *Otolaryngology*, II. Philadelphia, Pa: W.B. Saunders; 1980.

15. Cody RC. Hearing aids. In: Paparella MM, Shumrick DA, eds. *Otolaryngology*, II. 2nd ed. Philadelphia, Pa: W.B. Saunders; 1980.

16. Kirkwood DH. In the hearing aid delivery structure, where does the ENT fit? *Hearing J.* 44(4):11–17, 1991.

17. Maniglia AJ. Implantable hearing devices: state of the art. *Otolaryngol Clin North Am.* 22(1):1989, 175–200.

18. Smriga DJ, Huber TP, Paparella MM. Developments in hearing aid fitting and delivery: a decade of revolution. *Otolaryngol Clin North Am.* 22(1):1989, 105–127.

19. Pehringer JL. Assistive devices: technology to improve communication. *Otolaryngol Clin North Am.* 22(1):1989, 143–174.

30

Issues on Medication Use and Substance Abuse in Older Adults

Hilary Siebens

Pill consumption is a mainstay in Western medicine and a part of American culture (1). Older Americans consume considerably greater amounts of medication in comparison with the rest of the population. One in eight Americans is over 65 years old, but this group received one fourth of the prescriptions written by physicians. By the year 2030, one in five Americans will be over 65 years old, and this group will be given just under one half of all prescriptions written in the United States. As well, an almost equal number of over-the-counter (OTC) preparations are consumed.

As the health care of these older persons is being scrutinized for potential improvements, several observations are especially relevant to physicians' use of medications in treating these patients. First, many older adults suffer from multiple diseases, which are being appropriately treated with multiple medications (2). However, medications are underused in certain groups of older patients (3). Second, patients may be receiving inappropriate prescriptions (4). Third, adverse drug outcomes occur frequently in older patients. The price of these reactions are high both in terms of human suffering and of actual cost (2, 5). Fourth, patients do not always adhere to medications as prescribed. This chapter reviews these points with special emphasis on polypharmacy since multiple, concurrent medication use places patients at special risk for adverse outcomes and poorer adherence.

Less is known about the problems of prescription medication abuse and other substance abuse in older persons. Alcoholism is a well-documented disease in this group. Nicotine addiction occurs, as well as tolerance and dependency on barbiturates, opiates, and benzodiazepines. Detection and treatment of these problems are important components of comprehensive geriatric rehabilitation.

A CLINICAL MODEL OF MEDICATION USE

Many factors determine actual medication use by patients (Fig. 30.1). Generally, a patient first develops symptoms. The patient may self-medicate with an OTC medication. In addition, or alternatively, the patient visits a physician. The physician may or may not correctly identify the condition causing the symptom (Decision Point A). Next, a medication may or may not be available to treat the condition. The physician may or may not give a prescription, and the prescription may or may not be the correct drug choice at the correct dosage (Decision Point B). Up to this point, two decision points—diagnosing the condition and giving a prescription—depend on physician behaviors.

The outcomes from a medication prescription depend on patient behaviors as well. Patients may take the medication(s) correctly, less than prescribed, or more than prescribed. In each case, the clinical outcome could be clinical improvement, no clinical change, or clinical deterioration.

Epidemiology of Medication Use

Research is available on only certain aspects of the above model. Studies on polypharmacy are especially important since polypharmacy is common in older patients and since the risk of adverse outcomes is increased as medication regimens become more complex (6).

Medication use varies in different residential and hospital settings. The typical person over 65 years of age living in the community, takes an average of 4.5 medications—2.3 prescription and 2.1 nonprescription (7). In the nursing home setting, an average of 7 drugs are prescribed per resident (8). One survey of an intermediate care facility clarified that 4.7 medications were received on average during the survey month even though 8.1 medications were prescribed (9). The total cost of all these medications was $9.5 billion in 1982 (10).

The medications most frequently prescribed depend on setting—outpatient, hospital, or nursing home. In the outpatient setting, 30% of prescriptions are for nonthiazide dieurtics; 14% for antiarthritics; about 12% each of beta-blockers, thiazide diuretics, and nitrates; 9%

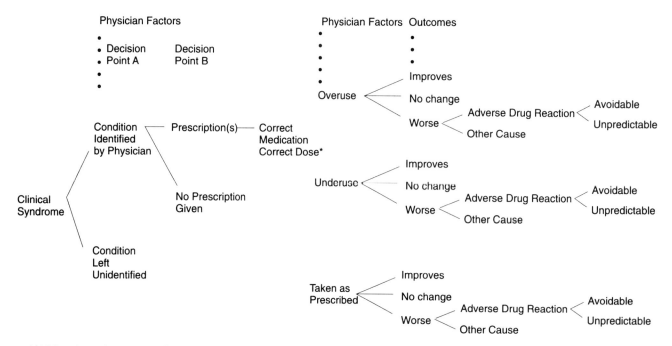

*At this point an incorrect medication and/or incorrect dosage can be given increasing the risk for poor outcome.

Figure 30.1.

for other antihypertensives; 8% for benzodiazepines, and 2% for antidepressants (11). For patients discharged from hospitals, the predominant medications include 19% cardiac agents; 9% respiratory agents; 6% diuretics and antibiotics; 5% digoxin preparations, diabetic agents, vitamins, laxatives, and narcotic analgesics, and 4% nonnarcotic analgesics (12). In nursing home surveys, psychotropic medications are the most frequently prescribed medications ranging from 61% to 86% of prescriptions (8).

Estimates suggest that OTC medications are used almost as frequently as prescribed medications in the outpatient setting (13, 14). More than half are oral analgesics. Thirteen percent are cough-and-cold preparations with the remainder including predominantly vitamins, antacids, and laxatives.

Clinical Outcomes Associated with Medication Use

Many of the medications used benefit patients or do no physical harm (though the financial cost to the patient may be high). The possibility of adverse drug reactions shown in Figure 30.1 have been studied in detail.

Several factors in older patients contribute to the high frequency of adverse drug reactions. Changes in pharmacodynamics and pharmacokinetics as persons age are starting to be more widely appreciated (see Chapter 7). The risks of drug interactions increase as the number of medications increases (6). Clinically significant drug interactions can occur with over 14 classes of medica-

tions (15). Among the most serious risks are impaired cognition and hip fracture. Medication toxicity caused altered mental status in 11% of 300 patients evaluated for mental status changes at an outpatient geriatric clinic (16). The risk of hip fracture is increased in a probable causal relationship whenever psychotropic medications are used either singly or in combination with other medications (17).

Adverse drug reactions precipitate hospital admission in 11% to 20% of admissions of persons 65 years old and above (18, 19). Studies looking at patients 75 years and older report rates as high as 33% (20). Adverse drug events (ADEs) occurring during hospitalization increase in frequency in older age groups (21). ADEs occurred in 3.7% of patients 71 years of age and older but in only 2% of patients 31 to 40 years old. The ADEs frequently involve nonsteroidal antiinflammatory and cardiovascular drugs.

Further studies will define whether or not adverse drug outcomes can be prevented more often. One estimate suggested that 70% of adverse drug reactions were predictable and generally preventable (1). Ninety-one percent of adverse drug events during 36,653 hospitalizations were directly related to a drug's pharmaceutical characteristics (21). These reactions were therefore felt to be predictable and preventable. A recent RAND study (4) of patients 65 years and older concluded that 7% to 37% of medication is overused in outpatients, and 44% to 90% is misused. Improving physician prescribing patterns would potentially decrease adverse drug reactions.

In contrast to these studies, one study identified aspirin and other nonsteriodal antiinflammatory drugs as responsible most often for adverse reactions (18). Review of the cases, however, showed that all medications were being properly used. All these data suggest closer scrutiny of outcomes of medication use, especially polypharmacy, is needed to determine which, if any, negative outcomes can be prevented.

Medication Reduction

Studies of geriatric assessment units and consult teams showed that the number of unnecessary medications and inappropriate medication choices do get reduced when comparing intervention to control groups (22, 23). However, whether these medication changes were related to the better patient outcomes is unclear.

Outcomes of reductions in medications have been studied more frequently in nursing homes. The number of nursing home medications was reduced 12% to 39% without clinical deterioration in one study (8). One 169-bed extended care unit in Canada reduced the average drug number from 8 to less than 3 per patient (24). Nursing time devoted to medication distribution decreased from 85% to 20% at another site (25). Studies such as these will be needed for outpatient and hospital settings.

Physicians' Prescribing Behaviors

Physicians are directly responsible for utilization of prescription medications and may or may not be responsible for OTC medication use. Physician prescriptions occur in response to the multiple illnesses and symptoms patients experience. However, it is also well known that physician behavior is shaped largely by drug advertising (2). This may contribute to some of the high use of medications in the management of older patients.

Physicians should also be aware that medication histories that elicit may be inaccurate. A study in Italy showed that general practitioners correctly recorded 2.9 of the 3.6 drugs their patients were taking (26). Underreporting was most often of benzodiazepines taken over a long period of time for insomnia or anxiety. In a study of hospitalized elderly, medication histories as recorded by physicians were also frequently inaccurate (27). In 60% of cases at least one medication was not recorded, and in 18% of cases three or more errors occurred.

Another challenge concerning appropriate drug use in older patients is that physicians may be undertreating some of their patients. Negative age biases do occur in treatment decisions (28). For example, age bias had lead to undertreatment of breast cancer after controlling for stage of disease, comorbidity, and functional status (29). Few studies have examined the morbidity associated with undertreatment of other clinical syndromes. A study in Italy demonstrated that in the nursing home setting some diseases are overtreated and some are neglected (3). Treatments were more frequent for illnesses that produced ongoing discomfort for the patient or staff (i.e., gastrointestinal disturbance and agitation). Undertreated were diseases in which symptoms developed only intermittently, as with exertion (i.e., chronic congestive heart failure and arthritis.) The challenge to the physician and research community in the years ahead will be to define more clearly how to avoid excessive and detrimental medication use while using medications appropriately in all instances where they can be beneficial.

Changing Physician Prescribing Behavior

Studies indicate that physicians should change their prescribing patterns for nursing home patients. The quantity of medications can be reduced, and the choice of psychoactive medication can be changed (8, 9).

There have been relatively few studies, however, evaluating methods of changing physicians' prescribing behavior. Physician prescribing patterns in the hospital setting are changed most effectively when there is close person-to-person contact with a knowledgeable pharmacist or a highly regarded faculty member in a group setting (2). The results of one study on housestaff suggested that the costs of ongoing person-to-person education would be less than imagined. One 15-minute tutorial session was sufficient to achieve impressive improvements in prescribing patterns (30).

In one of the few controlled studies of medication reduction in the outpatient setting, a small but significant reduction occurred in the mean number of drugs, the complexity, and the cost of patients' drug regimens (5). In the majority of cases, medication regimens could be simplified by stopping a drug, decreasing the dosing complexity, and substituting a safer or easier-to-administer drug. Compared to the control physicians who received no feedback, the physicians receiving recommendations changed medication use in 59% of the cases.

Physician Prescribing in the Rehabilitation Setting

Two studies have evaluated aspects of physician prescribing patterns in the rehabilitation setting. Review of 122 consecutive new outpatient referrals to a physical medicine and rehabilitation clinic identified 45 moderate drug interactions using a computer software system (31). Sixty-two percent of these interactions were not correctly identified by the physiatrists. The physiatrists falsely identified 28 other drug combinations as potential drug-drug interactions. Therefore, computer programs may become increasingly helpful in patient care. Physiatrists, along with other physicians, need to be particularly vigilant for potential drug-drug interactions in patients receiving polypharmacy treatment.

Potential simplifications of medication regimens were evaluated in another study during inpatient rehabilitation (32). Reasons to simplify were several: (a) decreased chances of adverse drug events; (b) less interference with daily activities; (c) decreased caregiver burden of dispensing medications. Discharge medications were reviewed in 91 consecutive discharges. Fifteen patients were excluded—5 were taking no medications and 10 were discharged back to an acute medical center. The mean patient age was 68+17 years. The mean daily pill-taking frequency was 4.8 excluding PRN medications. In Group A, pill frequency was less than or equal to three times a day (mean frequency 2.8, 26% of the cases). In Group B, pill frequency was over three times a day (mean frequency 6.0 times a day, 74% of cases). In Groups A, the mean number of drugs was 2.8 and in Group B, 5.5. On reviewing the dosage schedules, the authors concluded that in many cases the drug regimens could have been simplified. For example, most of the q.i.d. medications could have been decreased to t.i.d. schedules.

Patient Adherence to Medications

Patients of all age groups actually take medications as prescribed only 50% to 75% of the time (33). Adherence in older adults is also in this range (34). Complexity of a regimen is more important in nonadherence than is the number of medications (6, 33, 35, 36).

The term nonadherence rather than noncompliance describes better the circumstances under which a medication is not taken as prescribed (37). Unlike noncompliance, nonadherence does not imply that the patient is at fault. In a study of elderly outpatients, 71% of cases of nonadherence were intentional (37). Patients felt that they didn't need the medication in the dosages prescribed by the physician. Fewer patients indicated that they took less of the drug secondary to side effects or other negative consequences. The nonadherence occurred in all drug categories—in 60% of musculoskeletal drugs, in 35% of antibiotics, in 18% of gastrointestinal drugs, in 13% of psychotherapeutic drugs, in 8% of blood pressure and cardiac drugs, in 4% of potassium supplements, and in 6% of all other drugs.

Nonadherence highlights that a physician's obligation extends beyond writing an accurate prescription (35, 37). Included is establishing that the medication can be taken—that the patient understands why it is to be used, agrees to try it, knows for what side effects to watch, and has the means of purchasing and taking the pills at the correct time. One of the most important interviewing skills physicians need to achieve this is empathy: the capacity to understand what another person is experiencing from that person's perspective (38). Patients can be more honest when their feelings are understood by their physicians. In this setting, patients will be more forthright about intentions to not agree with medication use. An empathic relationship is even more important in the setting of substance abuse, which will be discussed below.

Recommendations for Medication Prescription During Rehabilitation

Several basic principles can be followed by rehabilitation personnel to safeguard against some of the medication complications discussed above (Table 30.1).

All rehabilitation team members need to have a high index of suspicion for the potential toxicities of medications taken by the patient. Medication histories are most accurate when patients and families bring ALL medication containers, including OTCs, to health care professionals to clarify the actual regimen. The indication for each medication needs confirmation either through record review or speaking with the prescribing physician. Recording accurate diagnoses is especially important when a psychotropic medication is used.

Questionable or unnecessary medications can be gradually eliminated while monitoring for clinical improvements or complications. The possibility should always be considered that a second drug has been prescribed to treat symptoms from a first medication. Medication simplification is especially appropriate during inpatient rehabilitation following acute hospital admission. Major medication changes occur during hospitalizations. Up to 40% of drugs taken at home are discontinued during acute hospitalization, and 45% of hospital medications are new (12). Reassessment of these drug regimens can easily be done during inpatient rehabilitation.

During rehabilitation, staff should monitor for evidence that medications are impairing cognitive function. Several markers for drug-induced cognitive impairment in the outpatient setting can be useful during both inpatient and outpatient rehabilitation: a suspected diagnosis of dementia; polypharmacy, often including sedative-hypnotics, and unexplained falling (16).

Table 30.1. Guidelines For Medication Use During Rehabilitation of Older Adults

Maintain a HIGH index of suspicion for medication toxicities.
Obtain accurate over-the-counter and prescription medication histories.
Review that each medication is still indicated.
Record a clear diagnosis for which each medication, especially psychotropic medication, is prescribed.
Gradually eliminate unnecessary medications.
Review that medication dosages are correct.
Simplify medication schedules as much as possible.
Clarify with patients that they are willing and able to take medications.
Educate patient and family about indications for medications and their side effects.

To improve patient adherence, physicians can adopt an approach that implies sharing responsibility for medication regimens between physicians and patients. The physician should emphasize patients' wishes and expectations and arrange for adequate education. For example, a 15-minute educational counseling session prior to discharge from a geriatric unit led to twice as much correct medication used compared with controls (39). In the outpatient setting, use of modern technologies like voice mail are in development and may improve adherence, especially in persons with memory impairment (40).

Rehabilitation personel should be aware of the Omnibus Budget Reconciliation Act of 1987 (OBRA), which affects psychotropic drug use in nursing homes (41). The regulations were designed to help avoid drug-drug interactions and the use of unnecessary medication. The OBRA regulations require that all psychotropic medications be justified by a bonfide diagnosis for which the drug is indicated and not by a symptom alone. Dosage reductions, medication holidays, and the use of nondrug behavioral treatments are required. Pharmacists have already been particularly active in decreasing polypharmacy in nursing homes (8). They can be invaluable to the rehabilitation team in other settings to help monitor medication use.

Finally, the American public is learning about the problems of overmedication in older persons. In the future, patients and their families may expect pills less readily, making physicians less likely to prescribe.

INTENTIONAL MEDICATION MISUSE AND SUBSTANCE ABUSE

Medications and many other chemical substances are misused and abused by older patients. These problems are not restricted to younger persons (42–45). One survey estimated that 10% of men and 2% of women over 60 years are chemically dependent. Another indicated an incidence between 10% and 20%. Specific figures on alcoholism suggest 5% to 15% of medical outpatient visits involve patients who suffer from alcoholism. The rehabilitation literature is increasingly documenting that alcohol and drug abuse are major causes of spinal cord injury and closed head injury in younger patients (46). While less is known about these problems in geriatric rehabilitation patients, drug misuse and abuse are likely to be related to rehabilitation problems like closed head injury, impaired cognition, and chronic pain syndromes.

Many terms are used to describe these types of clinical problems. For the sake of discussion in this chapter, the following definitions apply based on principles described elsewhere (see Table 30.2) (45, 47, 48).

1. *Medication Misuse.* Patients are using OTC or prescription medication for their intended medical uses.

Table 30.2.   Categories of Intentional Medication Misuse and Substance Abuse

I.   Over-the-Counter Medication Misuse
II. Prescription Medication Misuse or Abuse
    A. Barbiturates
    B. Opiates
    C. Benzodiazepines
III. Legal Substance Abuse
    A. Alcohol
    B. Nicotine
IV. Illegal Substance Abuse

Usage however is incorrect and not sanctioned by standards of good medical practice.

2. *Medication Abuse.* Patients are using OTC or prescription medications in characteristic nonmedical usage patterns. These patients often have a history of alcohol and other substance abuses.

3. *Substance Abuse.* The use of any chemical substance in characteristic nonmedical usage patterns. Authors use the term in different ways, oftentimes including all categories of substances: OTC medications, prescription medications, legal chemicals such as nicotine and alcohol, and illegal chemicals. The clinical problems with these four classes of chemicals are very different and therefore are each discussed separately in this chapter.

4. *Psychologic Dependence.* Patients, often with anxiety syndromes, substitute medications, such as anxiolytics, for conflict resolution. Physiologic adaptation or dependence may or may not be present as well.

5. *Physiologic Adaptation or Dependence.* Withdrawal symptoms occur when the medication or chemical substance is removed.

6. *Addiction.* The use of a chemical substance by patients is a nonmedical manner with physiologic adaptation or dependence present.

All of these problems when they occur in patients require careful management if rehabilitation is to be successful. The available information on these issues is increasing through the field of addiction medicine. The American Medical Association adopted a resolution in 1987 that all drug dependencies are diseases (48). A declaration followed in 1989 that substance abuse is our country's number one public health problem. Legal substance abuse is by far a greater health problem than is illegal substance abuse. Over 100,000 persons die of alcoholism annually and 350,000 from cigarette addiction. Only 20,000 die from illicit drug abuse (48). The problem affects all ages and all socioeconomic groups (49). For example, physicians are as vulnerable as others to chemical dependency (50, 51). The recently developed Addictive Disease Model, well-developed for alcoholism, provides a useful structure for understanding and treating addicted patients, regardless of the substance involved.

The Addictive Disease Model

The biopsychosocial disease model for addiction describes the disease as a multidimensional phenomenon (52). The model parallels the patient care model in rehabilitation medicine. Both acknowledge a close interaction of biologic, psychologic, and sociocultural components in a patient's problem. In alcoholism, biologic factors are being clarified through genetic studies and cell membrane and brain enzyme research, as well as studies of the effects of alcohol metabolites on animal behavior (52). For example, strains of mice and rats have been selectively bred to select for alcohol-related behaviors. Twin studies in humans have identified Type I alcoholics with later onset of disease and in whom environmental factors are required for the development of the disease. In contrast, in Type II alcoholics the disease starts earlier and does not require environmental factors. Also, studies have isolated condensation products that also form from the interaction of the alcohol metabolite acetaldehyde and neurotransmitters. When these condensation products are infused into brains of rats or monkeys, the animals begin to drink large quantities of alcohol. These types of research discoveries support the concept of alcoholism as an illness with critical biologic components that interact with cultural and social factors. Alcoholism no longer appears to be simply a problem of human will power, character, or morality (52).

Over-the-Counter Medication Misuse

Traditionally OTCs have been medications that would not cause serious medical problems if used incorrectly. Unfortunately, this is no longer the case for older persons (13, 14, 45). A wide array of OTCs contain significant anticholinergic properties (the antihistamines and other cold medications), which contribute to confusion, exacerbations of glaucoma, and bowel and bladder dysfunction. OTCs also contain a wide variety of aspirin-like compounds that lead to gastrointestinal bleeding, iron deficiency anemia, and renal dysfunction. Self-medication with antacids containing calcium carbonate is associated with constipation and gastric hypersecretion. Chronic laxative abuse leads to worsening constipation and obstipation. Some OTCs contain alcohol and caffeine, contributing potentially to oversedation or worsening of hypertension, dysrythmias, and anxiety syndromes.

Little is known about the actual prevalence of the above potential problems associated with OTCs. What is known is that OTCs are used frequently in older persons. In one survey, OTCs accounted for 40% of medications used in a survey of outpatients (53). Gross OTC medication misuse was not found, but the survey was not sufficiently detailed to detect cases of misuse associated with medical complications.

Prescription Medication Misuse and Abuse

Three categories of prescription medications used frequently in older adults are associated with misuse and even abuse. These include barbiturates, opiates, and benzodiazepines. All were associated with unrecognized drug dependency and withdrawal in one survey of psychiatric inpatients 65 years and older (54). Withdrawal symptoms were defined as unambiguous autonomic hyperactivity, including heart rate greater than 100 beats per minute and temperature greater than 37.5° C. At least three of the six other DSM-III criteria for the diagnosis of drug withdrawal had to be present including (a) nausea and vomiting, (b) malaise or weakness, (c) anxiety, (d) depressed mood or irritability, (e) orthostatic hypotension, and (f) coarse tremor of the hands, tongue, and eyelids. Withdrawal occurred in 19 cases, 21% of admissions. However, withdrawal was diagnosed and treated in only 9 cases. Medical intensive care transfer was required in one of the diagnosed cases and in 3 of the 10 unrecognized cases. Two of the unrecognized cases were transferred to medical units for treatment of fever and delirium. Appropriate recognition and treatment of the 10 undiagnosed cases may well have prevented these emergent medical transfers. Since these withdrawal signs and symptoms can occur 2 weeks to even 4 weeks after drug cessation, patients may already be in rehabilitation programs when these symptoms develop. Rehabilitation physicians therefore need to always keep in mind the possibility of drug withdrawal in patients who develop these signs and symptoms.

These prescription medications were also found to be abused in a survey of a high-risk community-based elderly population (55). Of note, a 60% correlation was found between prescription drug abuse and previous or active alcoholism.

Several factors may contribute to misuse or abuse of these categories of medications. Many older patients—41% percent in one community survey—have symptoms that are psychiatric, described often as mostly "nerves" (53). There can be trouble sleeping, irritability or impatience, shortness of breath, or pain in differing body parts (47). In fact, anxiety disorders are more common than diabetes mellitus in primary care offices (47). Physicians may not know how to best treat these problems and use medications such as barbiturates and benzodiazepines without, or in lieu of, other needed interventions.

Many physicians do not feel comfortable with psychiatric symptoms, and families and patients alike may not permit psychiatric evaluations. The results may be an overreliance on psychotropic medications by physicians not experienced with such drugs. The data on these issues are more intuitive than empirical, however (45).

In recent years, anxiety disorders have been classified more clearly. Several of the more common disorders may be seen in rehabilitation patients: a panic disorder with or without agoraphobia, adjustment disorder with anxious mood, generalized anxiety disorder, and posttraumatic stress disorder (47). Management of these as well as milder anxiety symptoms involves patient education and consideration of personality characteristics and active psychosocial stressors, as well as judicious use of medication (47). As physicians become more knowledgeable about anxiety syndromes and addictive diseases, misuse and abuse of prescription medications in older patients may decrease.

BARBITURATES

Approximately one third of all prescriptions for barbiturates are given to persons 65 years of age and older. Physicians must be aware of barbiturate dependency since withdrawal symptoms may appear during rehabilitation and since impaired cognition could result from patients using the medication at bedside without health staff awareness.

OPIATES

Opiate misuse and abuse can occur in older patients (56, 57). These drugs have sometimes been called narcotics, but this term is used nonspecifically by law enforcement officials to refer to any potent, abusable drug. There are appropriate clinical circumstances to use opiate analgesics in older patients. Usually this would be in the setting of acute surgeries or severe acute musculoskeletal pain syndromes not manageable through more conservative means. Physicians, however, must be aware that medication dependence does occur. Vigilance is required to prevent the development of severe addiction as well as withdrawal symptoms when the medications have stopped.

BENZODIAZEPINES

While benzodiazepine use is fairly common, extensive studies have shown that they are usually used for a short period of time to relieve clinically significant symptoms (58). When abuse does occur, it is usually by persons already abusing alcohol or other substances. Of concern in the geriatric population is that elderly women are the most common long-term users of low-dose benzodiazepines (59, 60). This use is often unreported to general practitioners (26). Long-term benzodiazepine treatment can be indicated in certain circumstances. It is unclear, however, if all older patients on long-term therapy, with its risks of confusion and possibly hip fracture, could benefit from alternative antianxiety therapies.

Any patient receiving long-term benzodiazepine therapy should be reassessed at regular intervals using a standard checklist to review if the medication is still indicated (47). The decision to stop benzodiazepines can be difficult but guidelines include: (a) the patient has an active chemical dependence including the use of alcohol; (b) the dose is above Food and Drug Administration recommendations for anxiety; (c) the patient is having a poor therapeutic response; and (d) the patient's behavior is impaired as seen by oversedation and/or treatment-related mental disorders such as depression. Family or friends as well can be aware of these types of problems and should be questioned about their presence (61). Discontinuation of the medication should be gradual since withdrawal symptoms can occur, especially with the shorter-acting agents. An excellent recent review discusses this process in detail (61).

Alcoholism in Older Adults

The quantity of alcohol ingestion that constitutes the disease alcoholism in older adults remains to be defined. In younger persons, four drinks a day, three days a week defines alcoholism based on the concept of hazardous consumption and thresholds from morbid risks (62). This definition, therefore, looks at outcomes other than merely significant alcohol-induced disease. The effects of alcoholism in older persons at present remain harder to quantitate since most older persons are not employed, drive less than younger persons, have symptoms from alcoholism that may be attributed to other conditions like depression and dementia, and are not suspected of being alcoholic by the public and by medical professionals.

Epidemiologic studies have established that alcoholism is present in 10% to 21% of medical hospital admissions, 5% to 15% of medical outpatient visits, and 15% to 20% of nursing home admissions (43, 44, 63). In 1984, a conservative estimate was that 1,500,000 persons over 65 years old suffer from alcoholism (44).

One of the reasons that these estimates are conservative is that older persons are often not suspected of alcoholism. In a hospital setting, house officers correctly identified 60% of persons under 60 years old but only 37% of those over 60 years old who had the disease (43). Not a single white nor female patient over 60 years old with alcoholism was identified by housestaff. Also, questionnaire screening tests like the CAGE and the Short Michigan Alcoholism Screening Test (SMAST) have been validated in younger persons and, although used to screen older persons, may not be appropriate for the older age group (63, 64). Cognitive impairment during the initial months of abstinence may well be confused with medically or drug-related delirium or dementia syndromes (see below).

While the exact prevalence of alcoholism in older

adults is not known, epidemiologic studies suggest a decline in the percentage of drinkers with age. Some controversy remains around the concept of alcoholism "burn out" with advancing age (44, 63, 65). One longitudinal study of otherwise healthy, educated, and affluent adults (N = 271, mean age 71 years old), identified 28 heavy drinkers who decreased the quantity of alcohol ingested over 7 years. Daily alcohol consumption in these persons decreased from 40 grams or higher to less than 28 grams per day. (For reference, 13 grams of alcohol is equivalent to a 12 oz beer, a 5 oz glass of wine, and 1¼ oz of 86-proof whiskey.)

PATHOPHYSIOLOGY

Reasons behind the chemical toxicity of alcohol include its complete miscibility in water, permitting wide distribution within the body, and its toxicity to all biologic tissues at certain concentrations and after repeated use. These factors are even more significant in older adults in whom total body water decreases along with lean body mass leading to a smaller volume of distribution of alcohol. The central nervous system (CNS) appears more susceptible to the toxic effects of alcohol (63).

Of particular concern in rehabilitation is cognitive function. One of the most serious consequences of alcohol's CNS toxicity is cognitive deficits both during acute intoxication and during abstinence (66). Domains of cognitive impairments during acute detoxification (up to 2 weeks abstinence) include distractibility, mild confusion, and irritability as well as all the deficits seen during intermediate (2 weeks to 2 months) and long-term (greater than 2 months) abstinence. These later deficits occur in the domains of attention, reaction time, verbal learning ability, verbal abstract reasoning, and verbal short-term memory during intermediate-term abstinence. During long-term abstinence, deficits can be seen in nonverbal abstract reasoning, visuospatial abilities, mental flexibility, and nonverbal short-term memory. Other etiologies can cause these same cognitive deficits (i.e., medication toxicities, dementias, strokes). Therefore, a high index of suspicion should always be kept when first evaluating older persons with cognitive deficits.

Persons with alcoholism become increasingly susceptible to cognitive impairment from alcohol as they age. Alcoholism may lead to premature aging of the brain (66). Impairments in learning and memory in alcoholics resemble those of nonalcoholic controls approximately 10 years older. Other impairments, however, are specific to alcoholism and are not seen in normal aging.

CLINICAL PRESENTATION

Older persons suffering from alcoholism have several characteristics similar to their younger counterparts (44, 45, 63). They tend to be male, divorced or single rather than married or widowed, black or Anglo rather than Latin or other ethnic group, and Protestant or no religion rather than Catholic, Jewish, or other religion. These older persons divide into two groups depending on recent versus distant onset of the alcoholism. Two thirds of cases have an early onset, prior to 40 years old, and survival extends beyond 60 years of age (63, 67, 68). In the remaining third of cases, alcoholism develops late in life, and a positive family history or a personal history of psychopathology are less likely. Late-life onset is associated with depression, bereavement, retirement, loneliness, marital stress, and physical illness (55, 63, 67, 68).

Older persons with alcoholism present to medical professionals with a variety of problems that all may have multiple other etiologies: recurrent falls, incontinence, hallucinations, bizarre behavior, malnutrition, social isolation, atypical dementia, self-neglect, myopathy, severe diarrhea, and accidental hypothermia. In order to be sure not to miss alcoholism as a primary or contributing cause in these syndromes, it is advisable to suspect the presence of alcoholism in any older person presenting these signs and symptoms.

Making the diagnosis of alcoholism can be difficult. Physicians have been taught to question patients on quantities of alcohol consumed. Self-reported consumption usually is not sensitive in detecting alcoholism. Better are questions about effects of alcohol on daily life as in the CAGE and SMAST questionnaires. How well these particular questions perform in older persons remains unclear. Friends and family may themselves not recognize alcohol dependence in their relative. Until further studies clarify the best method for diagnosing the disease, physicians should use interviewing questions as in the CAGE and SMAST questionnaires as well as interviewing friends and family carefully. The interviewing technique should reflect kind, nonjudgmental concern. Blood testing in cases of suspected recent ingestion should be used as well.

TREATMENT

Noncompliance by persons struggling with alcoholism is not as hopeless a situation as most physicians believe (44, 45, 63, 67, 69, 70). In younger persons, multidimentional treatment has shown short-term (6-month) improvement rates of up to 80%. Long-term improvement (abstinence of greater than 1 year) ranges from 25% to 50%. In older adults, several studies show that they are more likely to remain in treatment and maintain sobriety for longer periods than are their younger counterparts (55, 68–70).

Treatment begins with a kind confrontation by a knowledgeable physician with a spouse or significant other present if possible (44, 71). The initial empathic encounter includes clear explanations of the nature and hazards of the illness. The initial interview may be the single most effective element of early intervention (71). While older patients experience denial, confrontation is not required to the same degree as in younger patients.

Group socialization benefits patients with early or late-life onset. All interventions are best done through usual health care channels like homecare and outpatient clinics. Specific alcohol treatment programs and Alcoholics Anonymous—mainstays of treatment in younger patients—can be appropriate if older persons are being treated with other patients the same age.

Other components include patient and family education and judicious use of antidepressants and tranquilizers. Given the cognitive deficits that may occur during abstinence, it may be particularly important to be sure that cognitive demands can be met by patients during initial treatment (66). Treatment may need to progress in stages from early treatment focusing on enforced abstinence and provision of support with later treatment involving education and insight-oriented aspects of rehabilitation as patients' cognition improves.

The treatment concept of "controlled drinking" has been advocated as a feasible plan for many persons with alcoholism. However, studies have shown multiple treatment failures using this approach and, therefore, even limited use of alcohol by patients cannot be advocated. (44, 63).

THE NONBENEFITS OF ALCOHOL

Some studies to date have suggested that small amounts of alcohol can be beneficial by increasing social interaction, decreasing urinary incontinence, improving quality of behavior and relations, improving sleep, and reducing risk of myocardial infarction (72). In a survey of rehabilitation training programs, more than 50% of respondents believed that alcohol could be prescribed during inpatient rehabilitation for several reasons: worthwhile medical properties, such as vasodilation and appetite stimulation; assistance in relaxing patients, thereby facilitating socialization, and prohibition impinges on personal freedoms (46).

Recommending alcohol use as a treatment for some of these problems is not advisable. Doses yielding the "therapeutic" effects may be dangerously close to doses leading to deleterious effects such as impaired sleep and depressant effects on myocardial muscles. The only patients who truly need alcohol during rehabilitation treatment will be those chemically dependent on it.

One situation in which controlled drinking may be a more realistic treatment will be for nursing home residents that are alcoholic (45). In this instance, controlled alcohol use may be appropriate while working closely with nursing staff to control the resident's access to alcohol and facilitating liaison with alcoholic treatment facilities and Alcoholics Anonymous.

Nicotine Dependence

Older persons continue to smoke. An outpatient survey documented 21% of persons over 65 years old continued to smoke significantly (53). Rehabilitation units continue to treat patients with strokes and amputations that are older and still smoke. Studies indicate that smoking even for those over 75 years of age is associated with higher mortality (73). On the encouraging side is that smoking cessation after a stroke is associated with better health outcomes (74).

Several factors have been identified that can help patients stop smoking (75). Physicians can successfully help their patients stop if they counsel them consistently to do so (76). Various smoking cessation programs involving group support can be useful for some patients, along with other interventions reviewed elsewhere (75). Perhaps the increasing publicity that cigarette smoking is an independent risk factor for wrinkling of the skin will be useful (77). The ill effects of smoking will no longer be invisible.

Illegal Substance Abuse

Illegal substance abuse has not yet appeared as a significant problem in the studies that have evaluated substance abuse in older persons. Hopefully, illegal drug abuse will not become an issue for patients, their families and friends, and health care professionals in the future.

RECOMMENDATIONS FOR REHABILITATION STAFF

Medication and substance abuse can be problems in older persons requiring rehabilitation. This review has highlighted some of the key issues both in diagnosis and treatment. Staff should monitor closely for these types of problems, become educated on how to manage the abuse, and seek help when needed. Patient, families, and friends will all benefit from this approach, as will staff morale, confidence, and satisfaction.

References

1. Melmon KL. Preventable drug reactions—causes and cures. *N Engl J Med.* 284:1361–1368, 1971.
2. Soumerai SB, Avorn J. Efficacy and cost containment in hospital psychotherapy: state of the art in future directions. *Milbank Mem Fund Q.* 62:447–474, 1984.
3. Rozzini R, Bianchetti A, Zanetti O, Trabucchi M. Are too many drugs prescribed for the elderly after all? *J Am Geriatr Soc.* 37:89–90, 1989.
4. Brook RH, Kamberg CJ, Mayer-Oakes A, Beers MH, Raube K, Steiner A. *Appropriateness of Acute Medical Care for the Elderly.* Santa Monica, Calif: The RAND Corp; September, 1989.
5. Kroenke K, Pinholt EM. Reducing polypharmacy in the elderly. *J Am Geriatr Soc.* 38:31–36, 1990.
6. Nolan L, O'Malley K. Prescribing for the elderly part I: sensitivity of the elderly to adverse drug reactions. *J Am Geriatr Soc.* 36:142–149, 1988A.
7. Ostrom JR, Hammerlund ER, Christensen DB, Puin JB, Rethley AJ. Medication use in an elderly population. *Med Care.* 23:157–164, 1985.
8. Nolan L, O'Malley K. Prescribing for the elderly part II: prescribing patterns: differences due to age. *J Am Geriatr Soc.* 36:245–254, 1988B.

9. Beers MH, Avorn J, Soumerai SB, Everett DE, Sherman DS, Salem S. Psychoactive medication use in intermediate care facility residents. *JAMA.* 260:3016–3020, 1988.

10. Baum C, Kennedy DL, Forbes MB, Jones JK. Drug use and expenditures in 1982. *JAMA.* 253:382–386, 1985.

11. Carty MA, Everitt DE. Basic principles of prescribing for geriatric patients *Geriatrics.* 44(6):85–98, 1989.

12. Beers MH, Dang J, Hashegawa J, Tamai IY. Influence of hospitalization on drug therapy in the elderly. *J Am Geriatr Soc.* 37:679–683, 1989.

13. Abrams RC, Alexopoulos GS. Substance abuse in the elderly: over-the-counter and illegal drugs. *Hosp Community Psychiatry.* 39(8):822–823, 1988.

14. Lamy PP. Over-the-counter medication: the drug interactions we overlook. *J Am Geriatr Soc.* 30(11):S69–S75, 1982.

15. Salzman C. *Clinical Geriatric Psychopharmacology.* New York, NY: McGraw-Hill; 1984.

16. Larson EB, Kukull WA, Buchner D, Reifler BV. Adverse drug reactions associated with global cognitive impairment in elderly persons. *Ann Intern Med.* 107:169–173, 1987.

17. Ray WA, Griffin MR, Schaffner W, Baugh DK, Melton III LJ. Psychotropic drug use and the risk of hip fracture. *N Engl J Med.* 316:363–369, 1987.

18. Colt HG, Shapiro AP. Drug-induced illness as a cause for admission to a community hospital. *J Am Geriatr Soc.* 37:323–326, 1989.

19. Sinoff GD, Kohn D. Prevalence of adverse drug reactions. *J Am Geriatr Soc.* 38:772–729, 1990.

20. Ives TJ, Bentz EJ, Goiyther RE. Drug related admissions to a family medicine inpatient service. *Arch Intern Med.* 147:1117, 1987.

21. Classen DC, Pestotnik SL, Evans RS, Burke JP. Computerized surveillance of adverse drug events in hospital patients. *JAMA.* 266(20):2847–2850, 1991.

22. Epstein AM, Hall JA, Besdine R, et al. The emergence of geriatric assessment units: the "new technology of geriatrics". *Ann Intern Med.* 106:299, 1987.

23. Owens NJ, Sherburne NJ, Silliman RA, Fretwell MD. The senior care study—the optimal use of medications in acutely ill older patients. *J Am Geriatr Soc.* 38:1082–1087, 1990.

24. Gryfe CI, Gyrfe BM. Drug therapy of the aged: the problem of compliance in the roles of physicians and pharmacists. *J Am Geriatr Soc.* 32:301–307, 1984.

25. Daws DE, Bell A, Irving, P. *Extended Care Seminar.* Vancouver: British Columbia Hospitals Association; 1973.

26. Spagnoli A, Ostino G, Borga AD, D'Ambrosia, et al. Drug compliance and unreported drugs in the elderly. *J Am Geriatr Soc.* 37:619–624, 1989.

27. Beers MH, Munekata M, Storrie M. The accuracy of medication histories in the hospital medical records of elderly persons. *J Am Geriatr Soc.* 38:1183–1187, 1990.

28. Wetle T. Age as a risk factor for inadequate treatment. *JAMA.* 258:516, 1987.

29. Greenfield S, Blanco DM, Elashoff RM, et al. Patterns of care related to age of breast cancer patients. *JAMA.* 257:2766–2770, 1987.

30. Klein LE, Charache P, Johannes RS. *J Med Educ.* 56:504–511, 1981.

31. Braverman SE, Bryant PR. Potential drug interactions in a physical medicine and rehabilitation clinic. *Am J Phys Med Rehabil.* 71:224, 1990.

32. Siebens H, Martin W. Pill taking frequency after acute rehabilitation in older adults. *Gerontologist.* 29:90A, 1989.

33. Blackwell B. Patient compliance. *N Engl J Med.* 289:249–252, 1973.

34. Morrow D, Leirer V, Sheikh J. Adherence and medication instructions. *J Am Geriatr Soc.* 36:1147–1160, 1988.

35. Komaroff AL. The practitioner and the compliant patient. *Am J Public Health.* 66:833–835, 1976.

36. Eraker SA, Kirscht JP, Becker MH. Understanding and improving patient compliance. *Ann Intern Med.* 100:258–263, 1984.

37. Cooper JK, Love DW, Raffoul PR. Intentional prescription nonadherence (non-compliance) by the elderly. *J Am Geriatr Soc.* 30:329–332, 1982.

38. Bellet PS, Maloney MJ. The importance of empathy as an interviewing skill in medicine. *JAMA.* 266(13):1831–1832, 1991.

39. MacDonald ET, MacDonald JB, Phoenix M. Improving drug compliance after hospital discharge. *Br Med J.* 2:618–621, 1977.

40. Leirer VO, Morrow DG, Tanke ED, Pariante GM. Elders' nonadherence: its assessment and medication reminding by voice mail. *Gerontologist.* 31(4):514–520, 1991.

41. Smith DA. New rules for prescribing psychotrophics in nursing homes. *Geriatrics.* 45(2):44–56, 1990.

42. Johnson LK. Chemical dependency in the elderly. *J Gerontol Nurs.* 15(12):22–26, 1989.

43. Curtis JR, Geller G, Stokes EJ, Levine DM, Moore RD. Characteristics, diagnosis and treatment of alcoholism in elderly patients. *J Am Geriatr Soc.* 37:310–316, 1989.

44. West LJ. Alcoholism. *Ann Intern Med.* 100:405–416, 1984.

45. Atkinson JH, Schuckit MA. Alcoholism and over-the-counter and prescription drug misuse in the elderly. In: Eisdorfer C. *Ann Rev Gerontol Geriatrics.* 2:225–284, 1981.

46. Rohe DE, DePompolo RW. Substance abuse policies in rehabilitation medicine departments. *Arch Phys Med Rehabil.* 66:701–703, 1985.

47. McGlynn TJ, Metcalf HL. *Diagnosis and Treatment of Anxiety Disorders: A Physician's Handbook.* Washington, DC: American Psychiatric Press; 1989.

48. Smith DE. Addiction medicine and the primary care physician. *West J Med.* 152:500–501, 1990.

49. McDonald AJ, Abrahams ST. Social emergencies in the elderly. *Emerg Med Clin Am.* 8(2):443–457, 1990.

50. Siegel BJ, Fitzgerald FT. A survey on the prevalence of alcoholism among the faculty and housestaff of an academic teaching hospital. *West J Med.* 148:593–595, 1988.

51. Ikeda R, Pelton C. Diversion programs for impaired physicians. *West J Med.* 152(5):617–621, 1990.

52. Wallace J. The new disease model of alcoholism. *West J Med.* 152(5):502–505, 1990.

53. Chien C, Townsend EJ, Townsend AR. Substance use and abuse among the community elderly: the medical aspect. *Addict Diseases.* 3(3):357–372, 1978.

54. Whitcup SM, Miller F. Unrecognized drug dependence in psychiatrically hospitalized elderly patients. *J Am Geriatr Soc.* 35:297–301, 1987.

55. Jinks MJ, Raschko RR. A profile of alcohol and prescription drug abuse in a high-risk community-based elderly population. *DICP Ann Pharmacother.* 24:971–975, 1990.

56. Schuckit MA. Geriatric alcoholism and drug abuse. *Gerontologist.* 17(2):168–174, 1977.

57. Ling W, Wesson DR. Drugs of abuse—opiates. *West J Med.* 152(5)565–572, 1990.

58. Glass RM. Benzodiazepine prescription regulation autonomy and outcome. *JAMA.* 266(17):2431–2433, 1991.

59. Farnsworth MG. Benzodiazepine abuse and dependence: misconceptions and facts. *J Fam Pract.* 31(4):393–400, 1990.

60. Woods JH, Katz JL, Winger G. Use and misuse of benzodiazepines: issues relevant to prescribing. *JAMA.* 260:3476–3480, 1988.

61. Dupont RL. A physician's guide to discontinuing benzodiazepine therapy. *West J Med.* 152(5):600–603, 1990.

62. Rains VS, Ditzler TF, Blanchette PL. Recognition of alcohol dependence in the elderly. *J Am Geriatr Soc.* 37:1204–1205, 1989.

63. Atkinson RM. Alcoholism in the elderly population. *Mayo Clin Proc.* 63:825–829, 1988.

64. Ewing JA. Detect alcoholism—the CAGE questionnaire. *JAMA* 252(14):1905–1907, 1984.

65. Adams WL, Garry PJ, Rhyne R, Hunt WC, Goodwin JS. Alcohol intake in healthy elderly. *J Am Geriatr Soc.* 38:211–216, 1990.

66. Fein G, Bachman L, Fisher S, Davenport L. Cognitive impairments in abstinent alcoholics. West J Med. 152:531–537, 1990.

67. Dunham RG. Aging and changing patterns of alcohol use. *J Psychoactive Drugs.* 13:143–151, 1981.

68. Atkinson RM, Turner JA, Koffed LL, et al. Early vs. late onset alcoholism in older persons: preliminary findings. *Alcohol Clin Exp Res.* 9:513, 1985.

69. Glatt MM. Treatment results in an English mental hospital alcohol unit. *Acta Psychiatr Scand.* 37:143, 1961.

70. Hurt RD, Finlayson RE, Morse RM, Davis LJ. Alcoholism in elderly persons: medical aspects and prognosis of 216 inpatients. *Mayo Clin Proc.* 63:753–760, 1988.

71. Edwards G, Orford JW. A plain treatment for alcoholism. *Proc R Soc Med.* 70:344–348, 1977.

72. Turner RB, Bennett VL, Hernandez H. The beneficial side of moderate alcohol use. *John Hopkins Med J.* 148:53–63, 1981.

73. LaCroix AZ, Lang J, Scherr P, et al. Smoking and mortality among older men and women in three communities. *N Engl J Med.* 324(23):1619–1620, 1991.

74. Abbott RD, Yin Y, Reed DM, Yano K. Risk of stroke in male cigarette smokers. *N Engl J Med.* 315(12):717–720, 1986.

75. Sees KL. Cigarette smoking, nicotine dependence and treatment. *West J Med.* 152(5):578–584, 1990.

76. Anda RF, Remington PL, Sienko DG, Davis RM. Are physicians advising smokers to quit? *JAMA.* 257(14):1915–1920, 1987.

77. Kadunce DP, Burr R, Gress R, Kanner R, Lyon JL, Zone, JJ. Cigarette smoking: risk factor for premature facial wrinkling. *Ann Intern Med.* 114 (10):840–844, 1991.

31
Cancer Rehabilitation in the Elderly

Gail L. Gamble and Margaret R. Lie

Rehabilitation management of the elderly cancer patient is a common but increasingly complex problem facing rehabilitation practitioners today. Increased general survival rates portend a larger percentage of elderly patients, with an estimated 22% more than age 65 years by the year 2040 (1). Cancer is the second leading cause of death in men and women more than 65 years of age. There is an increased incidence of cancer among elderly patients, with more than half of all cancer deaths occurring in patients more than 65 years of age (2). However, survival rates for cancer are also increasing, which implies prolonged survivorship with disability of disease added to the increased disability of aging. Cancer, for many, is joining the category of chronic disease.

Problems of the elderly cancer patient must be assessed and managed within a different physical, psychologic, social, and, frequently, economic framework than that of the younger population. Many of these patients have already begun to face their own mortality, and "quality of life" issues may be more important than mere increased life span. The normal physiologic effects of aging, multiple comorbidities (probably including impaired physical function), and altered social or economic support will affect patient needs. Cancer treatment options have become increasingly complex, often involving multimodal approaches including surgery, radiation, and chemotherapy. The treatment-related morbidity adds significant physiologic stress to the already aging system.

Other problems for the elderly cancer patients also influence medical care and rehabilitation. There may be a delay in diagnosis; elderly patients often present with more advanced cases of some types of cancer (3). These patients tend to blame altered functions or new pain on "just getting old" and are less likely to see early medical attention. The challenges of being diagnosed, treated, and surviving a disabling cancer may impose a perceived threat to independence, which also can cause the patient to delay seeking medical attention when new symptoms occur.

This chapter includes an overview of the physiology of aging cells and organ systems and integrates these findings with current knowledge of the pathophysiology of the cancer cell. Current treatment options and the short-term and long-term effects of these treatments will also be addressed. The unique components of cancer rehabilitation, including team members, team function, and goals, will be defined with emphasis on rehabilitation management of specific conditions facing the clinician. The important aspects of pain management, psychosocial needs, and ethical issues will also be presented because they are too frequently minimized in the day-to-day management of both the cancer and the geriatric patient.

As with other areas of geriatric medicine, the approach and practice in geriatric oncology involves a broad knowledge of internal medicine, biology of aging, pharmacology, neurobehavior, psychiatry, and rehabilitation. Diagnostic and therapeutic goals should be directed toward improving the quality of life, sustaining function, and maintaining independent living.

BIOLOGIC RELATIONSHIP OF AGING AND CANCER

The medical aspects of aging and cancer are practical and perplexing issues for the clinician and geriatrician. Aging is generally regarded as a natural process of life for humans and other creatures. During the span of an individual's physical existence, aging is a biologic clock that records elapsed time. From conception to death, there are periods of rapid growth, maturation, and development as well as involution and decline. During certain phases of aging, the evidence of change or alteration is barely perceptible, yet the eventual progression to senescence or postmaturational physiologic deterioration inevitably occurs if human life remains undisturbed or uninterrupted.

Aging and senescence occur at the cellular as well as the organismic level. Normal, diploid, somatic cells from many organs and tissues can be propagated in culture. They age and senesce in vitro and exhibit biologic changes that parallel those of the intact organism. Several theories for aging have been proposed, which have been broadly classified as stochastic or developmental-genetic (4). The stochastic theory of aging identifies the accumulation of "insults" from the environment as the principle cause of cellular and organismic decline. Genetic or protein damage from radiation, toxins, and other adversities in the environment are not completely eliminated by the cell and slowly impair physiologic capacity.

The developmental-genetic theory is based on the principle that aging is part of development, which is genetically determined and programmed. Immunologic mechanisms, neuroendocrine systems, free radical formation, and intrinsic mutagenesis are several examples of developmental-genetic mechanisms that may mediate the process of aging and senescence. Although the bases of these theories are distinct, they are not mutually exclusive. In fact, a combination of these events appears to operate. However, it is difficult to distinguish the cause from the consequence of aging.

Cancer is a cellular process in which biologic control of normal growth and differentiation is lost within an organ or tissue. During physiologic aging, specific genetic events may be induced that immortalize a cell otherwise destined to undergo senescence and death. Cancer is a multistep event, which includes the stages of initiation, promotion, progression, and metastasis. Other genetic alterations must develop for the cell to be further transformed to the malignant state. At the molecular level, specific genes capable of inducing or repressing cancer have been identified and named oncogenes or tumor-suppressor genes. Normal or defective forms of these genes are inherited or acquired and are either activated or deactivated during the aging process.

Based on theories of aging and our current understanding of the development of cancer, it is apparent that aging and cancer share common properties in the cell and organism, although one is a physiologic occurrence and the other is a pathologic state. The age-specific and population-specific annual cancer incidence rates increase in older age groups for most of the major types of adult cancer. Malignant neoplasia is most frequent in persons more than age 65 years (5, 6). Although decreased cellular replication is observed in aging cells, biochemical and molecular alterations that regulate aging and senescence also participate in carcinogenesis. Thus, aging and cancer are linked although the relative probabilities of occurrence are different, such that only aging is a biologic inevitability. Nonetheless, we recognize that cancer in the elderly becomes a significant medical issue as the population ages and rehabilitation of the aging cancer patient is undertaken.

SPECIFIC TUMOR INVOLVEMENT

Lung Cancer

INCIDENCE

Half of all lung cancers occur in persons 65 years and older; lung cancer is the leading cause of cancer death in the United States for both men and women, and the incidence continues to increase sharply (7).

PATHOLOGY AND NATURAL HISTORY

Of the four main subtypes of lung cancer—adenocarcinoma and squamous, small, and large cell carcinomas—the relative proportion of squamous cell carcinoma increases with age, and this type is associated with the best 5-year survival rate. Additionally, it is virtually the only lung cancer to be detected by screening studies (8).

CLINICAL MANIFESTATIONS

At the time of diagnosis, lung cancer is usually symptomatic—a cough being the most common symptom. However, many symptoms are nonspecific and are often attributed to comorbid disease. Lack of resources or a fatalistic attitude contribute to delay in diagnosis. Regional metastases may cause hoarseness, superior vena cava syndrome, dysphagia, brachial plexus pain, and chest wall pain. Distant metastases cause bone pain, altered mental status, jaundice, or abdominal pain.

Paraneoplastic syndromes are diverse and occur with all lung cancer cell types. The most common are the syndrome of inappropriate secretion of antidiuretic hormone, Cushing's syndrome, hypercalcemia, hypertrophic osteoarthropathy, neuromyopathies, and Eaton-Lambert syndrome (7).

TREATMENT

Treatment of lung cancer is based on cell type, stage of disease, and general condition of the patient. Surgery is the primary modality for nonsmall cell carcinomas. The roles of laser therapy, chemotherapy, and radiation therapy are reviewed in general oncology texts (7, 9). Age alone should not be a criterion to deny a patient with lung cancer a diagnostic evaluation, and some studies suggest that lung cancers present at earlier stages in the elderly (10).

PALLIATIVE TREATMENT

Control of symptoms includes assistance with fatigue, lethargy, and pain management. Quality of life issues relate to life planning, activities of daily living, optimum living environment (home, nursing home, hospice), attention to the caregiver's stress, and minimizing complications of the disease and the elderly patient's treatment.

PROGNOSIS

Age alone should not be used as a prognostic indicator. The prominent role of performance status as a prognostic factor has been consistently identified (11). Hence, tumor measurement, cell type, and staging determine the anatomic extent of disease, and symptoms, performance status, and presence of comorbid disease help to define prognosis and guide the rehabilitation plan.

Colon Cancer

INCIDENCE

Colorectal cancer is the second most common malignancy in the United States, occurring most frequently in older individuals. Age is the leading risk factor for colorectal cancer; risk increases sharply at age 50 years and doubles each decade until age 80 years (12).

PATHOLOGY AND NATURAL HISTORY

Most colorectal tumors are of epithelial origin in both younger and older patients. Anatomic staging is based on location of the cancer within the large intestine and its spread to other sites. Geriatric patients present at stages similar to those of younger patients, and treatments should be based on overall medical status.

CLINICAL MANIFESTATIONS

Colorectal cancer can be cured if it is detected early. The 5-year survival rate is 90% for asymptomatic, localized lesions. Hence, routine use of inexpensive screening tests (e.g., occult blood) is important.

Symptoms usually relate to bleeding, constipation, abdominal pain, weight loss, or weakness due to anemia and are similar in all age groups. Regional metastases often spread to regional lymph nodes and adjacent organs. Distant metastases spread to bone.

TREATMENT

Therapeutic decisions are based on stage of disease and comorbid disease and not on age alone. Surgical resection is the primary treatment. In advanced disease, palliative treatment may include surgery, radiation therapy or chemotherapy, and those measures that enhance management of pain and quality of life, including laser therapy, nutritional support, and bypass procedures.

PROGNOSIS

Prognosis is determined primarily by the stage of colorectal cancer; obstruction, perforation, and rectal bleeding are poor prognostic factors.

Other Gastrointestinal Cancers

Esophageal, gastric, and pancreatic cancers occur most frequently in the later decades of life. Most gastrointestinal cancers present difficult treatment decisions in the elderly, and palliative care is of prime importance.

ESOPHAGUS

Esophageal cancer can be treated with preoperative radiation and chemotherapy as well as adequate nutritional support by way of a small feeding tube. However, the optimal treatment in the elderly continues to evolve (13).

STOMACH

Gastric cancer has been on the decline for 50 years, but the older patient remains at higher risk (14). Presenting symptoms are vague, and the disease is frequently advanced and incurable at the time of diagnosis. Adenocarcinoma accounts for 95% of gastric cancer. This type of malignancy is radiosensitive, but the normal gastric mucosa has a low tolerance to ionizing radiation. The major role of therapeutic radiation is in conjunction with chemotherapy if the patient can maintain adequate nutrition and is ambulatory. The assessment of overall performance status is more important than chronologic age in determining the value of chemotherapy.

PANCREAS

Pancreatic malignancy is a disease of the elderly; 50% of deaths are in patients more than 65 years of age, and the worldwide incidence is increasing (15).

Pain is the most frequent presenting complaint and is often severe. Weight loss, anorexia, and jaundice are also common. Vague, nonspecific symptoms are also reported frequently. However, the stage of pancreatic carcinoma is usually advanced and rarely resectable at the time of diagnosis. No treatment is standard, and even palliative treatment must be carefully considered in the frail, elderly patient for whom morbidity may outweigh benefit. Compassionate, supportive care with judicious use of analgesics and vigorous nutritional support are appropriate.

Overall, for upper gastrointestinal cancers, investigational trends favor a combination of radiation, chemotherapy, and surgery, and the favorable palliative options ease symptoms and prolong independence.

Breast Cancer

INCIDENCE

Breast cancer is the most common invasive malignant neoplasm in women and increases in incidence with advancing age (16). Approximately 50,000 women in the United States age 65 years or older are diagnosed annually as having breast cancer.

PATHOLOGY AND NATURAL HISTORY

Although distributions for stage, location, and histologic type are uniform in all age groups, hormonal effects vary with age, and there is a higher rate of response in the elderly. In contrast, chemotherapy is less effective in the elderly. The cure rate is strongly dependent on early detection; mammography screening has produced a striking decrease in mortality from breast cancer.

TREATMENT

Definitive treatment includes a choice of modified radical mastectomy, simple mastectomy, and lumpectomy, with or without radiation therapy. Lumpectomy may be performed under local anesthesia and, hence, can be used in patients with significant comorbid heart or lung disease.

METASTATIC DISEASE

The debilitating effects of metastatic spread are significant in breast cancer. The potential for cure is a lesser consideration than is quality of life.

The goal is to produce maximum palliation to relieve symptoms and keep the patient functioning for as long as possible. The basic modalities are hormonal manipulation, chemotherapy, and radiotherapy, but ultimately most interventions will fail because of evolution of resistant cells by mutation. Specific complications include local extension on the chest wall and lymphedema, especially in the setting of lymph node dissection and radiation. Brachial plexopathy represents a significant management challenge given the severe neuropathic pain usually associated with progressive weakness. Lung involvement has an impact on fatigue and energy levels. Bony metastatic disease creates a major challenge in regard to pain control and maintenance of function. The central nervous system can be involved with intracerebral metastatic disease, meningeal carcinomatosis, or spinal cord compression.

Prostate Cancer

Prostate cancer is the second most frequently occurring cancer in men more than 75 years of age (17, 18). Among men ages 55 to 74 years, prostate cancer is the third leading cause of cancer-related deaths. With careful patient selection, aggressive therapy may produce successful outcomes.

INCIDENCE

The incidence of prostate cancer increases with increasing age; fewer than 1% of cases occur in men less than 50 years old.

PATHOLOGY OF CLINICAL PRESENTATION

The common histologic entity is adenocarcinoma, and the neoplasm may be well, moderately, or poorly differentiated. Signs and symptoms depend on extent of disease, and, as tumor size increases, symptoms related to bladder neck obstruction become common. In the elderly, the symptoms associated with widespread bony metastatic disease may be misinterpreted as degenerative arthritis.

TREATMENT

Therapeutic options include observation in the early stage of disease because tumor progression often exhibits slow evolution over a period of years. Surgery, radiation therapy, hormonal therapy, and chemotherapy each offers essential treatment options and effective responses.

METASTATIC DISEASE

Local and distant metastatic disease can produce various complex and difficult clinical syndromes. Some of these include obstructive uropathy, intestinal obstruction, and lymphedema of the lower extremities. Hypercalcemia as well as anemia, thrombocytopenia, and severe bone pain occur in those patients with bony involvement. Intravascular coagulation, fibrinolysis, and hypercoagulable complications such as deep venous thrombosis are common. Spinal cord compression is a medical emergency, and timely intervention can preserve neurologic function.

Bladder Cancer

A significant increase in the incidence of bladder cancer is observed in both sexes after 65 years of age (19). The incidence is higher in industrialized countries and in cigarette smokers.

CLINICAL MANIFESTATIONS

Painless hematuria is the most common presentation in addition to dysuria.

TREATMENT

Local treatment includes intravesical instillations and partial cystectomy. Radical cystectomy with urinary diversion is a viable option even in the population more than 80 years old.

Gynecologic Malignancies

Gynecologic malignancies are a significant health problem for elderly women. These include vulvar, vaginal, cervical, endometrial, and ovarian carcinomas (20, 21). If discovered early, each of these cancers is curable. Increasing age usually correlates with more advanced stage of disease at presentation. Surgery, radiation therapy, and chemotherapy each offers effective therapeutic options for elderly patients.

In addition, comorbid disease makes treatment more difficult. Bowel and bladder dysfunction may be sequelae of these treatments, and lack of bladder control poses a great threat to independence in the elderly patient. Except for endometrial cancer, age alone has not been of prognostic significance when other factors are controlled.

Hematologic Malignancies

CHRONIC LYMPHOCYTIC LEUKEMIA

Chronic lymphocytic leukemia is essentially a disease of the elderly population and is the most common type of leukemia in patients age 50 years or older (22). Median age at onset is 60 years. Later stages of the disease are characterized by increasing susceptibility to bacterial and viral infections, anemia, and thrombocytopenia. The clinical course is variable, with duration of survival from diagnosis ranging from less than 1 year to more than 10 years. Therapy is generally reserved for symptomatic disease, and chemotherapy is the primary modality. Radiation therapy has a largely adjuvant role and is used palliatively to treat lymph nodes and compromised organ function due to obstruction and for relief of painful bony lesions.

HODGKIN'S DISEASE

Hodgkin's disease has a bimodal age distribution. The first peak is at 15 to 35 years, and a second peak is at 50 years of age or more. Despite improvements in response to treatment in the younger patient with Hodgkin's disease, the prognosis for the elderly patient remains poor. Age is the single most important prognostic factor for this disease, and elderly patients tend to have more symptoms and less adenopathy (23).

NON-HODGKIN'S LYMPHOMAS

There is a steady increase in the incidence of non-Hodgkin's lymphomas from childhood to beyond age 80 years (24). There is a marked difference in the natural history of low-grade versus intermediate and high-grade non-Hodgkin's lymphomas. Low-grade lymphoma tends to be diagnosed at more advanced stages. In contrast, higher grades are more likely to be recog-

nized when the disease is limited, but they are potentially curable with combination chemotherapy.

Because of the indolent natural history of the low-grade lymphomas, many oncologists recommend postponing therapy until patients are symptomatic.

MULTIPLE MYELOMA

The incidence of multiple myeloma increases with age (25). The highest rates are in men aged 80 years or more and women aged 70 years or more. Although the disease responds to chemotherapy in 50% to 60% of the patients, it is not regarded as curable. Therapy is, therefore, postponed until the patient has a progressive increase in monoclonal protein levels, osteoporosis, symptomatic skeletal lesions, renal insufficiency, anemia, or hypercalcemia. At present, therapy is generally continued for 1 to 2 years and then discontinued if protein levels in serum and urine have been stable for 6 months.

Acute Leukemia

In the majority of series, there has been a lower complete remission rate in elderly people compared with younger age groups (26). Once remission is attained, however, its duration does not appear to be influenced by age. The role of maintenance therapy is unclear—most trials failed to demonstrate any impact on remission duration.

SIDE EFFECTS OF CHEMOTHERAPY AND RADIATION THERAPY

Radiation Therapy

Radiation therapy frequently has curative potential in patients with local or regional disease and offers the advantage of no appreciable early mortality. Radiation treatment is not contraindicated by associated medical conditions occurring with advanced cancer, and the function of the organ of tumor origin may be preserved. This, of course, is especially important in the elderly in whom organ deterioration may already be present. The risk of a later secondary malignancy is also of less concern than in a younger patient. Radiation is frequently used as an adjunct to surgery, chemotherapy, or both and is an attractive option in this group of older patients. Disadvantages of radiation therapy include the length of time involved for curative regimens, often extending for 6 to 7 weeks. As discussed later in this chapter, dysphagia, anorexia, or mucositis are often more debilitating in the elderly (27).

Palliative radiation therapy is effective in providing relief from pain of bone metastases and neurologic deficit from brain metastases and control of local obstructive symptoms. Higher dose fractionation courses of 1 to 2 weeks duration can provide significant palliation and less time commitment than the longer, lower dose fractionation courses.

The frequency of complications of radiation therapy is related to the dose and body area exposed. Results of treatment and incidence of complications are dependent on available technology. Those patients who can be treated with more penetrating x-rays will be spared some of the complications, and the use of high-energy equipment has been associated with improved therapeutic results. Some studies suggest that the radiation effect on normal tissue is enhanced 10% to 15% in elderly persons, and those with marked physiologic decline would be most in jeopardy (28).

Side effects of radiation are reported as acute and chronic (29). Acute effects occur during treatment in proliferative or cell-renewing areas such as skin or enteral mucosa. Radiosensitivity of these sites may result in oral stomatitis, pharyngitis, dysphagia, nausea, diarrhea, or bladder or genital irritation. These symptoms are usually reversible with cellular regrowth after treatment. Late effects are related to permanent cell damage, including tissue necrosis, fibrosis, or ulceration, occasionally causing loss of vital organ function (lung, spinal cord, brain). These side effects are dose-related and, with present technology, may be avoided.

Chemotherapy

There are no direct studies of the effect of age on the pharmacokinetics of chemotherapeutic agents. However, altered drug absorption and distribution and altered liver, cardiac, and renal function would be expected to have an impact on drug absorption and distribution, thus affecting treatment.

As outlined earlier in this chapter, systemic effects of cancer in the elderly and the physiologic effects of aging may compromise chemotherapy; special emphasis should be placed on pain control, nutritional support, and aggressive supportive care.

The major limiting factor for most drugs is a toxic effect on bone marrow. Presently, dosage reductions made purely on the basis of age may adversely affect outcome.

Severe vomiting can be a cause of significant morbidity; chemotherapeutic agents and narcotics are the worst offenders. Cytopenias are frequently present and should be treated with transfusion of blood products used to alleviate symptoms. A compromised immune response carries a significant risk for the older cancer patient. Infection in the elderly has a poor outcome owing to many factors, including comorbid conditions, delay in diagnosis, slower response to antimicrobial therapy, and high incidence of adverse reactions. For many reasons, the use of empiric therapy is frequently necessary when a specific cause of infection is unknown.

Summary

Chronologic age alone should not be used to exclude patients from therapeutic approaches; for several reasons, radiation therapy may be the treatment of choice, in conjunction with a carefully planned approach utilizing adjunct surgery or chemotherapy. Substantial supportive care is imperative in the management of the older patient because of the devastating effects of the disease and its treatment. A key question to be addressed is the impact of diagnosis and treatment of cancer on the older patient's quality and quantity of life. It remains the physician's responsibility to weigh health, function, and financial and social status in formulating appropriate therapeutic plans.

REHABILITATION NEEDS OF THE ELDERLY CANCER PATIENT

Lehmann et al (30) surveyed the perceived needs of more than 800 cancer patients in outpatient clinics and found many rehabilitation issues that had been previously unidentified. Although no age-specific data were reported, approximately 25% received financial support from Medicare, and the majority of these patients were presumably old enough to receive Medicare. Interestingly, those patients with physical disability exhibited a significantly higher percentage of psychologic problems.

In a more recent study examining satisfaction with care, cancer patients expressed a high level of comfort with the technical competence provided to them and the communication ability of their primary caregiver. The least satisfaction was identified for issues pertaining to dismissal planning, home care, symptom control at home, and support for family members, all of which are concerns usually addressed by the rehabilitation team (31). When the early needs of breast cancer patients in the first month after primary therapy were assessed, the majority of problems related to physical disability limiting daily activities (32). Identification of patient needs can be difficult because patients and their families may focus on different rehabilitation issues as problems (33). This is particularly pertinent in elderly patients whose younger family members may be prime spokespersons in the clinical setting. Patients, regardless of age, have clearly identified questions not answered by the scope of the initial diagnosis or therapeutic intervention. These problems are only magnified in the elderly whose preexisting conditions may include physical disability, early fatigability, or fewer resources for home care.

The fact that the geriatric population needs to be questioned and assessed regarding functional capability has been well established (34, 35). The studies previously described demonstrate the same need for the cancer patient. Multiple instruments have been developed to objectively assess geriatric patients' functional status and ability for self-care. As with cancer patients, too frequently only the most immediate medical problem has been addressed, with the important questions as to how the elderly patient will manage at home remaining unasked and unanswered. Thus, the elderly cancer patient appears to be at greater risk for dependency, with a greater need for rehabilitation intervention by virtue of being old and having a potentially disabling illness as well.

UNIQUE COMPONENTS OF THE CANCER REHABILITATION TEAM

Although the needs of the cancer patient can be adequately met in various different program models, the cancer rehabilitation team should consist of an interdisciplinary group that has special training and skills in the treatment of cancer patients and is sensitive to the particular needs of the elderly. The rehabilitation team works closely with the patient's primary physician or oncologist to identify the patient's rehabilitation problems and to provide appropriate rehabilitation services.

Team Members

Rehabilitation team members include those on the interdisciplinary rehabilitation teams, and they are described below by their major functions.

1. *Physiatrist*
   a. Is a physician specializing in Physical Medicine and Rehabilitation
   b. Has special interest in the care of elderly, debilitated patients
   c. Introduces goals of cancer rehabilitation to patient and family
   d. Evaluates patient's physical and functional capacity and medical status
   e. Develops rehabilitation prescription, which may include management strategies for neurologically impaired limbs, neurogenic bowel and bladder dysfunction, amputation, exercise programs, pain management modalities, lymphedema control, appropriate bracing, or other rehabilitative interventions
   f. Develops a coordinated plan for patient's management with primary physician
   g. Maintains close communication among patient, team members, and primary service
2. *Cancer Rehabilitation Nurse*
   a. Is a nurse specializing in the rehabilitative care of cancer patients and who has experience in geriatric care
   b. Serves as nursing resource and liaison to patient, family, nursing staff, and team members
   c. Coordinates rehabilitation team services

   d. Provides assistance in development of bedside patient care plan (including skin, bowel, and bladder care)
   e. Coordinates development of dismissal planning
3. *Physical Therapist*
   a. Evaluates patient's physical capabilities and limitations
   b. Teaches exercise to increase flexibility, strength, and endurance
   c. Provides patient with special assistance in gait and transfer training
   d. Uses modalities to decrease patient pain and increase comfort and function
   e. Identifies needed equipment for management in the home setting
4. *Occupational Therapist*
   a. Evaluates patient's functional ability to care for self in daily life (dressing, grooming, bathing, feeding, homemaking)
   b. Assesses cognitive and perceptual skills
   c. Evaluates swallowing capabilities and retrains when possible
   d. Provides exercises to increase arm and hand strength and coordination
   e. Identifies needed equipment for home setting
5. *Chaplain*
   a. Specializes in counseling the spiritual needs of cancer patients
   b. Helps patients and families use their faith when applicable to adapt to illness and disability
   c. Provides support to rehabilitation team members when needed
6. *Dietician*
   a. Assesses patient's nutritional status and needs
   b. Recommends specific daily requirements and diet options
   c. Provides patients and families with appropriate individualized plans
7. *Social Worker*
   a. Specializes in the needs and care of the elderly cancer patient
   b. Addresses practical and emotional needs of patient and family
   c. Provides counseling and support
   d. Possesses special knowledge of insurance and reimbursement policies for health care of elderly patients
   e. Ensures an appropriate and manageable dismissal plan for patient
   f. Arranges referrals to local community resources for appropriate home health-care services and equipment
8. *Psychologist*
   a. Available for consultation with patient and family
   b. Assesses social and emotional adjustment to illness
   c. Provides intervention strategies to patients in need

d. Serves as resource to team members for difficult patient problems

Other rehabilitation professionals, such as the speech therapist, orthotist, and prosthetist may become an integral part of the rehabilitation team to meet the individual needs of a specific patient.

Each of the team members develops a special relationship with the patient and family, depending on the disability and needs. Cancer patients are frequently facing new diagnoses or new knowledge of advanced metastases. For the elderly patient, thorough understanding and difficult decision-making may be complicated by impaired hearing, fatigue from disease and multiple tests, information overload, slowed processing, or pain. Cancer team therapists, by daily contact with the patient, offer support, answer appropriate questions, alleviate patient fears, and, via continuity, assist patients through the episode of care.

Therapists' roles become blurred as the patient may choose to share spiritual concerns, pain management issues, or desire for advance directives with one team member who can then relay information to the appropriate specialist for further discussion and action. Frequently scheduled rehabilitation team meetings are vital to assess the patient's progress and, with condensed episodes of care, to ensure that appropriate dismissal planning is occurring.

One of the most important functions of team members is to serve as emotional support for each other. The elderly cancer patient usually presents a complex case, may have advanced disease, and may be vulnerable during the course of treatment. The rehabilitation team members provide continuous support for patients and family, and in turn they require emotional support themselves while repeatedly dealing with such difficult situations.

Frequent patient and family conferences are also necessary, specifically in the case of elderly cancer patients, because family members gather under usually extremely stressful conditions. There are issues of adjustment and adaptation to a new, sometimes devastating illness. Dismissal planning issues are often complex because the care may involve an elderly patient who previously lived alone, or worse, a patient who was previously the caregiver for a cognitively or physically disabled elderly spouse. These conferences enhance family education and also provide a forum to allow communication among family members when conflict occurs regarding the therapeutic or dismissal plan. It is the team's responsibility to serve as the patient's advocate and to protect the competent elderly patient's rights and opinions in a setting in which well-meaning adult children may inadvertently try to make decisions for the patient.

Goals

The main goals of the rehabilitation team are preservation and restoration of the patient's physical function, maintenance of functional independence, and return to the home setting if possible.

Equally important in the development of a program for the elderly cancer patient is flexibility of this program and emphasis on success in short-term goals. The cancer patient's status can fluctuate frequently during an episode of care; some decline may be permanent, and functional goals may need to be altered. Extensive long-term goals may be inappropriate, depending on the patient's age, extend of disease, and baseline physical condition.

Identification and management of cancer-related pain problems is a central goal of an effective rehabilitation program. Pain control is vital in order to enhance patient participation in therapies and increase functional activities. Patients may share pain concerns only with a trusted nurse or therapist and minimize these concerns to the primary physician.

Special emphasis needs to be placed on the goal of comprehensive dismissal planning. Many cancer patients are minimally disabled, and a dismissal plan that includes a follow-up visit can address interim needs. Some elderly cancer patients finish inpatient or outpatient therapeutic interventions in a state of fatigue and debilitation. Patients may have experienced severe nausea and dysphagia and exhibit a state of poor nutrition. Dismissal plans must provide options for different levels of supportive care. The key word again is flexibility. It is hoped that the cancer patient will gain strength and endurance posttreatment and require fewer services, but the reverse may also be true with advanced disease and preterminal states.

The overall goal of the cancer rehabilitation team is improved quality of life. The definition of success in cancer treatment has progressed from reports of survival, and the measurement of quality of life has been utilized increasingly (36). Quality of life issues involve the patient's feelings of self-worth, satisfaction with life, functional status or activity level, and level of symptom control. These areas are subjective, involve individual values, and when measured can be reported differently depending on who is reporting—the patient, caregiver, or physician (37). This is especially important to realize when working with the older patient whose adult child may be perceiving a higher level of quality of life for the patient when, from the patient's perspective, problems still exist. The cancer rehabilitation effort strives to enhance quality of existence for all variables listed above, keeping the patient's perception of that quality foremost.

The team's goals for dismissal planning must agree with those of the patient and family. Maximum equipment and home health-care support can be arranged for short periods of terminal home care if the patient and family are physically and emotionally capable and willing to use them. It is our belief that a family should not expend all its physical energy caring for a terminal patient at the expense of not being able to provide continued emotional support. Alternative-care settings are a viable option in such situations and should be encouraged.

FACTORS IN THE DEVELOPMENT OF A REHABILITATION PLAN

Ethical Issues

The rehabilitation practitioner and the team, including patient and family, face many ethical considerations as treatment is entertained, initiated, monitored, and finally terminated. The cancer rehabilitation team working with older cancer patients must be sensitive to particular questions raised. Should the older patient or the cancer patient be considered for intensive rehabilitation efforts and what are the goals of rehabilitation? What role is given to the rights of patient and family regarding initiation and termination of rehabilitation treatment? What are the differences in values of the elderly patient that may affect care decisions regarding rehabilitation, and how does our constricting economic environment affect the way we care for older people with a chronic progressive disease? These questions and others are frequently unspoken when deciding whom to treat and for how long.

It is of interest to review ethical considerations that pertain particularly to our own specialty during decision-making. Ours is one of few areas of medicine in which the team or physician usually decides if a patient would benefit from rehabilitation services, i.e., practitioners choose their patients (38). Rehabilitation, particularly in today's economic environment, is not a right. Therefore, the subjective values of those giving or not giving care are important. It is usually the practitioner who also decides when to terminate care (39), for the most part when a patient's functional gains have plateaued. These are important aspects because the implications for moral responsibility for patient well-being are enormous.

How are these decisions made for the older cancer patient? There is growing evidence that age alone should not be the sole criterion for excluding patients from medical care (39, 40). Treatment decisions for an elderly patient must involve the patient's own value system, especially in defining quality of life issues (41, 42). Interestingly, in many instances quality of life issues for the older sick patient are discussed in reference to termination of care, whereas in rehabilitation, quality of life in terms of comfort and relief of pain may be used as an incentive for rehabilitative interventions.

Should the assignment of do not resuscitate (DNR) orders mandating withdrawal of aggressive interventions include rehabilitation? The authors believe that, with the patient's consent, rehabilitation interventions are frequently appropriate in the terminal patient, assisting patient and family with comfort measures such as positioning, range of motion, pain management, skin care, and equipment needs.

Termination of care, sometimes a difficult decision and in other instances comfortable for all, is appropriate secondary to patient and family wishes and physician judgment that continued care would not be of benefit. Termination of physical therapy is sometimes difficult for patients to accept because functional restoration is viewed as a hopeful goal long after medical interventions have been abandoned. A useful model for ethical decision-making has been reported by Cassel (43). This involves gathering of data, examination of motives, application of existing principles, and examination of consequences as one develops the final decision. In summary, the ultimate goal of rehabilitation in the older cancer patient is to make decisions enhancing the relief of suffering (44), but it remains the patient's domain to define the word suffering and the associated needs.

Psychosocial Issues

The presence of psychologic stability and social and economic supports is a major concern in the care of the older cancer patient. Patients facing new diagnoses and prospects of prolonged treatment regimens may already be socially and economically limited. Hospital stays involving complex decision-making, complicated by treatment-associated morbidity, increase the feelings of loss of control. Accepting a new body image after years of stability, grieving over prospective loss, and facing one's own mortality can cause heightened anxiety. Depressive symptoms are common among hospitalized elderly patients and closely correlate with severity of medical illness (45).

Families of cancer patients experience their own psychosocial problems. Emotional strains, including symptoms of fear, anxiety, and depression, have been reported to be higher in spouses than patients (46). Age has also been reported to be an important variable in family stress; data suggest that family members more than 70 years of age cope less well and exhibit more mood disturbances than those 50 years old and younger (47). Interestingly, although depression and feelings of hopelessness occur in the geriatric population, studies have shown that older cancer patients adapt better to their diagnoses and report a better overall psychosocial state than do younger patients (48–50).

A useful conceptual model categorizing different levels of psychosocial needs adjustment and basic intervention strategies has been reported (51) (Table 31.1). Different levels of adaptation describe a progressive inability to cope, with level 1 patients exhibiting appropriate feelings of loss, anger, and sadness, often with good family support.

The patient in level 2 seems familiar to those who work in cancer rehabilitation settings, with patients exhibiting mild depression and increased anxiety during diagnosis and decision-making. Families demonstrate poor coping skills, either being too protective and solicitous or registering anger at team members regarding care issues and communicating poorly with the patient. This group requires and is helped by team interventions.

Level 3 patients have had a significant psychiatric history, exhibit visible signs of depression or agitation, and require early structured interventions to assist patient, family, and frequently, the health-care team. The suggested interventions are multifocal in nature. The cancer team becomes involved in discussing feelings with patient and family, concentrating on short-term attainable goals, providing structure for behavioral changes, and offering patient and family support.

Sexual issues are often neglected in the older can-

cer patient. There is a growing body of data that indicates that the diagnosis of cancer affects patient and sexual partner in adverse ways (52, 53). Anxiety, depression, and physical disability may affect sexual function and frequently are already present in the geriatric population. Rehabilitation team members should be aware of potential problems and include questions regarding sexual health in the initial assessment. Little has been written about intervention, but open discussion regarding changed body image, exercise to improve general feeling of well-being, and psychologic counseling for patient and spouse may be in order.

With increasing cancer survival rates, many geriatric patients have survival problems associated with the chronic diagnosis of cancer. Body image, chronic family stress, lower energy and activity level, and employment problems have been reported many years after the diagnosis and treatment, indicating that the quality of physical and psychologic health may be affected long-term (54). The possibility of disease recurrence with the threat of further associated disability adds to the stress of the aged population. The loss of independence—complicated by spouse disability or a single living situation and limited resources or insurance—is the ultimate survival issue for the geriatric cancer survivor. Many previously discussed areas, including physical, psychologic, and nutritional health, may be adversely affected

Table 31.1. Appropriate Psychosocial Intervention for Each Level of Adaptation[a]

Interventions	Level 1	Level 2	Level 3
Individual therapy	Brief, once a week, supportive	Two times a week; relationship oriented, grief resolution	Frequent and extended daily visits, ventilation, clarifying, limit setting, little or no dynamic/interpreting work
Behavioral approaches	Progressive muscle relaxation, can use audiotape, self-hypnosis	Relaxation training/hypnosis; improving coping strategies, reframing of negative experiences	Relaxation procedures and hypnosis only with therapist present
Family therapy	Optional support group; information and education	Support group plus occasional family therapy	Family therapy, with patient and without; sessions directive and aimed at limit setting
Psychopharmacologic	Rarely	Often necessary as requested; usually tricyclic antidepressants	Usually necessary; benzodiazepines, antidepressants, and occasionally phenothiazines
Staff issues	Usually not necessary	Staff often have difficulty dealing with family members of patient and in helping patient cope with anxiety and depression	Additional psychologic consultation usually necessary; provide ventilation/support for staff members and behavioral planning, and resolve staff splitting

[a]From Bond GG, Wellisch DK. Psychosocial care. In: Haskell CM, ed. *Cancer Treatment*. Philadelphia, Pa: W.B. Saunders; 1990:893–904. By permission of W.B. Saunders Company.

by the older cancer patient's determination to remain living independently.

The responsibility of the rehabilitation team is to assist the geriatric patient in identifying personal problems of survivorship, to develop a rehabilitation approach when feasible, and to ensure healthy independence for as long as possible. The rights of survivorship (55) (Table 31.2) apply especially to the geriatric population in which physical, social, economic, and sometimes family restrictions are already at work to limit the quality of remaining life.

Pain Management

The adverse impact of pain on the cancer patient cannot be overstated. The inadequacy of pain control is largely attributable to the failure to implement available therapies. The elderly patient and family may suffer because of inadequate knowledge and lack of understanding of this problem (56).

This is compounded by a lack of data evaluating the influence of the unique physiologic, social, and psychologic characteristics of these patients on the assessment and management of cancer pain. Chronic pain is often accompanied by affective disturbances, usually depression. These problems may be amplified in the elderly, and the older cancer patient may present a paradox of relatively reduced pain complaints but greater compromise of psychologic, social, and physical function when pain is present.

EPIDEMIOLOGY

Cancer-related pain and the fear of pain can be major deterrents to successful rehabilitation in the elderly. Physical and occupational therapy sessions are frequently cancelled if pain management is inadequate. The risk of physical side effects of immobility and deconditioning is increased. If the patient is in pain before therapy, increased physical activity is feared and avoided.

Table 31.2. American Cancer Society: The Cancer Survivors' Bill of Rights[a]

A new population lives among us today—a new minority of 5 million people with a history of cancer. Three million of these Americans have lived with their diagnoses for five years or more.

You see these modern survivors in offices and in factories, on bicycles and cruise ships, on tennis courts, beaches and bowling alleys. You see them in all ages, shapes, sizes and colors. Usually they are unremarkable in appearance; sometimes they are remarkable for the way they have learned to live with disabilities resulting from cancer or its treatment.

Modern medical advances have returned about half of the nation's cancer patients of all ages (and 59 percent for those under the age of 55) to a normal lifespan. But the larger society has not always kept pace in helping make this lifespan truly "normal": at least, it has felt awkward in dealing with this fledgling group; at most, it has failed fully to accept survivors as functioning members.

The American Cancer Society presents this Survivors' Bill of Rights to call public attention to survivor needs, to enhance cancer care, and to bring greater satisfaction to cancer survivors, as well as to their physicians, employers, families and friends:

1. Survivors have the right to assurance of lifelong medical care, as needed. The physicians and other professionals involved in their care should continue their constant efforts to be:
   - sensitive to the cancer survivors' lifestyle choices and their need for self-esteem and dignity;
   - careful, no matter how long they have survived, to have symptoms taken seriously, and not have aches and pains dismissed, for fear of recurrence is a normal part of survivorship;
   - informative and open, providing survivors with as much or as little candid medical information as they wish, and encouraging their informed participation in their own care;
   - knowledgeable about counseling resources, and willing to refer survivors and their families as appropriate for emotional support and therapy which will improve the quality of individual lives.
2. In their personal lives, survivors, like other Americans, have the right of the pursuit of happiness. This means they have the right:
   - to talk with their families and friends about their cancer experience if they wish, but to refuse to discuss it if that is their choice and not to be expected to be more upbeat or less blue than anyone else;
   - to be free of the stigma of cancer as a "dread disease" in all social relations;
   - to be free of blame for having gotten the disease and of guilt for having survived it.
3. In the workplace, survivors have the right to equal job opportunities. This means they have the right:
   - to aspire to jobs worthy of their skills, and for which they are trained and experienced, and thus not to have to accept jobs they would not have considered before the cancer experience;
   - to be hired, promoted and accepted on return to work, according to their individual abilities and qualifications, and not according to "cancer" or "disability" stereotypes;
   - to privacy about their medical histories.
4. Since health insurance coverage is an overriding survivorship concern, every effort should be made to assure all survivors adequate health insurance, whether public or private. This means:
   - for employers, that survivors have the right to be included in group health coverage, which is usually less expensive, provides better benefits, and covers the employee regardless of health history;
   - for physicians, counselors, and other professionals concerned, that they keep themselves and their survivor-clients informed and up-to-date on available group or individual health policy options, noting, for example, what major expenses like hospital costs and medical tests outside the hospital are covered and what amount must be paid before coverage (deductibles).

[a] From Spingarn N. American Cancer Society's Cancer survivors' bill of rights. *Cancer News.* 42:15, 1988. By permission of the American Cancer Society.

If the patient focuses on pain during therapy, new skills and educational information are not retained.

The risk of cancer increases dramatically with age; pain is present as an initial symptom in 40% of patients and in 70% of patients with advanced disease (57). Interestingly, in the elderly, pain prevalance rates show some decline. The elderly may experience less pain or pain patterns may be better controlled when treated. However, in a setting of increased stoicism, slowness to respond, or cognitive deficits, a careful evaluation is warranted.

PAIN ASSESSMENT

A comprehensive assessment recognizes the complex interplay between physiologic and psychologic factors and clarifies the specific needs of the individual patient. Unrelenting pain increases the burden of caregivers and often results in emotional and physical distancing from the patient. It is important to assess the environment in which the patient is living. A comprehensive needs assessment for cancer patients' families highlighted the importance of ambulation and pain control as the major concerns of patients and their families (58). The rehabilitation professional plays a role in pain assessment, particularly as pain relates to limitation of function.

ORIGIN OF PAIN SYNDROMES IN THE CANCER PATIENT

These can be summarized as follows (59, 60).

1. Pain due to direct tumor involvement
   a. Tumor invasion of bone
   b. Tumor involvement of nerve, plexus, or spinal cord
   c. Tumor involvement of viscera
   d. Other types of tumor involvement causing vascular compromise
2. Syndromes associated with cancer therapy
   a. Postsurgical syndromes such as post thoracotomy, mastectomy, radical neck dissection, and amputation pain syndromes
   b. Postchemotherapy pain
   c. Postradiotherapy pain
3. Pain caused by cancer-induced changes such as paraneoplastic syndromes, myofascial pain syndromes, constipation, bed sores, and debility
4. Pain unrelated to cancer especially from chronic musculoskeletal problems

PAIN PROBLEM

As Twycross outlined (61), pain control begins with an explanation followed by modification of pathologic process, elevation of pain threshold, interruption of pain pathways, and modification of life-style. Whatever its origin, continuous pain requires regular preventive therapy. The aim is to titrate the dose of the analgesic against the patient's pain, gradually increasing the dose until the patient is pain-free. Only in this way is it possible to erase the memory and fear of pain. The Cancer Pain Relief Program of the World Health Organization suggested the following scheme (62).

1. For mild pain, nonsteroidal antiinflammatory agent with or without an adjuvant analgesic
2. For moderate to severe pain, a weak opiate such as codeine with a nonsteroidal antiinflammatory agent
3. For severe pain, a potent opiate with morphine as the prototype, titrating to a stable dose pattern with a short half-life drug and then switching to a long-acting preparation.

In the elderly patient, a drug with a short half-life is warranted. One drug should be prescribed at a time, beginning with a low dose. Coanalgesics such as the use of a nonsteroidal drug to allow a lower dose of an opiate can be beneficial (decreasing side effects). Aggressive treatment of expected side effects such as nausea, constipation, sedation, and confusion is warranted. On occasion, in elderly patients with neuropathic pain, tricyclic antidepressants may be beneficial, and for lancinating neuropathic pain, neuroleptics may be of value. Treatment of depression and insomnia should begin with small doses of antidepressants and close monitoring for expected response. Corticosteroids such as methylprednisolone can play a major role in the elderly for anorexia, lassitude, dysphoria, and neoplastic infiltration of brain or lung, giving dramatic relief for severe headache and dyspnea.

ANESTHETIC APPROACHES

Age alone should not be a contraindication to nerve blocks for somatic or autonomic pain, and these may be valuable for refractory localized syndromes. These may be categorized by techniques including trigger-point injection; peripheral, autonomic, or central nerve block; or infusions (60).

Initially, simply listening to a patient's concerns and allowing patient control when possible may help alleviate patient anxiety. Proper bed positioning will assist in pain management via edema control, decreased skin pressure points, and decreased pressure on involved viscera. Therapeutic exercise, including gentle range of motion and stretching, helps control painful spasticity and subsequent contractures. Both spine and limb orthoses are beneficial, providing support and decreasing axial loading, which allows increased activity. Therapeutic modalities that are useful include superficial heat or cold application over secondary painful muscle spasm (in nonradiated skin areas). Transcutaneous electrical nerve stimulations (TENS) has also been helpful in the management of cancer pain and should be considered (63).

Use of appropriate adaptive equipment in the home setting (electric beds, mechanical transfer assists, wheelchairs) minimizes painful transfers and other unnecessary movements. Effective pain management in the elderly may require a multimodal approach, including analgesics combined with the other interventions described.

BEHAVIORAL APPROACHES

Relaxation, biofeedback, cognitive, and behavioral training, including hypnosis and music therapy, have been integrated into the management of cancer pain. These approaches decrease pain by their ability to modulate the affective response to painful stimuli and help to decrease the hopelessness and helplessness experienced by the elderly patient with severe pain.

SUPPORTIVE CARE

Inadequate control of pain is a common cause for readmission to the hospital, and patient and family education in the use of analgesics is imperative. This, in addition to psychologic support for patients and their families and integration of community support services, can allow the patient to remain at home for prolonged periods.

Nutrition

The nutritional status of the elderly cancer patient is an important component of rehabilitation assessment. If the patient's nutritional needs are not addressed, then the chance for a meaningful exercise program with the hope of building endurance is poor. The probability of malnutrition is high because this is a diagnosis commonly made in both the cancer and elderly populations. Anorexia, protein-calorie malnutrition, and dehydration occur in the aged and those with cancer for multiple complex reasons. The effects of aging on nutritional status are well-described elsewhere in this test (see Chapter 6).

Cancer patients are at risk for development of poor nutrition in various ways. Local tumor can mechanically obstruct oral intake (including dysphagia). Systemic effects of the neoplasm, including tumor growth, competition for body nutritional resources, or tumor-mediated metabolic derangements, may result in anorexia, weight loss, and cachexia. Cancer treatments, including surgery, radiation, and chemotherapy, may result in a severely altered nutritional state secondary to complications such as dysphagia, nausea, or vomiting; local edema within the digestive tract, or enteral cell death.

Cancer-related nutritional needs may vary widely, from zero to home parenteral nutritional support. Adequate screening and periodic reassessment are an integral part of patient care. Most oncology teams have a nutritionist available, particularly during intensive periods of cancer treatment, and screening for malnutri-

tion has become an integral part of cancer care. The rehabilitation team, however, may be following the patient on a daily basis in the hospital or as an outpatient and should be familiar with a basic nutritional screen because the effects of the cancer, various treatment modalities, age itself, and psychosocial issues take their toll (Table 31.3). Changes in status should be reported to the patient's dietician, primary caregiver, or both because treatments may need to be modified. Recently, a comprehensive text (64) was published; it reviews needs, screening methods, treatments (including tube feedings and parenteral nutrition), sample menus, and national resources. Although the text is not limited to care of the geriatric patient, the reader is referred to this excellent text for more detailed information.

Therapeutic Exercise

Much has been written regarding the elderly, severely debilitated patient with cancer. We might consider if there even is a role for therapeutic exercise in this population? We believe that therapeutic exercise plays a vital role in helping to meet the goals of cancer rehabilitation, including those of increased functional independence and quality of life.

The risks of the deconditioned state secondary to immobility involve many organ systems, and, unfortunately, as one reads through a summary of major changes in organ systems, one also sees that the decline in many cases may be associated with aging alone (Table 31.4). (65). Thus, the older patient with chronic disease, who is already at risk, needs to be particularly sensitive to immobility and to combat its effects with simple therapeutic exercise.

Can some of the negative effects be reversed in the elderly, or are the effects of immobility and aging too great to overcome? The literature on therapeutic exercise in older patients indicates that significant effects can be achieved in terms of increased cardiac conditioning (66), decreased hypertension (67), increased

Table 31.3. Brief Nutritional Screen in Geriatric Cancer Patient

Patient report
  Content/frequency of meals
  Approximate daily fluid intake
  Use of nutritional supplements
  Anorexia/nausea/vomiting
  Dysphagia
  Bowel change
  Weight change
Observed data
  Weight
  Height
  Skin turgor
  Oral hydration
  Serum albumin

Table 31.4. Changes in Organ System Influenced by Immobility and Aging[a]

Organ System	Change
Cardiovascular	Reduced cardiac output
	Decreased blood volume
	Orthostatic hypotension
Musculoskeletal	Muscle weakness
	Muscle atrophy
	Osteoporosis
Respiratory	Increased airway resistance
	Decreased minute ventilation
Nervous system	Impaired balance
	Decreased sensation
	Confusion
	Depression
	Decreased intellectual function
Genitourinary	Altered bladder function
	Urinary stasis
	Increased urinary tract infections

[a]Modified from Halar EM, Bell KR. Contracture and other deleterious effects of immobility. In: DeLisa JA, ed. *Rehabilitation Medicine: Principles and Practice.* Philadelphia, Pa: J.B. Lippincott; 1988:448–462.

pulmonary function (68), decreased osteoporosis and bone loss (69), and increased cerebral function (70). Other benefits include increased flexibility and increased social contact with associated decrease in depression (71). Muscle strength has been shown to improve with a strengthening program, even in sedentary nursing home patients between 90 and 100 years old (72).

Guidelines for exercise programs in the elderly are presented elsewhere in this text (see Chapters 21 and 22). In the older cancer patient, strenuous exercise programs may have to be modified secondary to fatigue and temporary disability related to recent surgery or radiotherapeutic and chemotherapeutic interventions. However, elderly patients with the diagnosis of at least one chronic disease who participated in a modified exercise program have been shown to increase function in areas previously mentioned as important: cardiovascular function, strength, and flexibility (73, 74). Thus, when developing a program of rehabilitation for the elderly patient, exercise should not be excluded. From simple range of motion exercises to cardiovascular fitness training, exercise should play an integral role.

MANAGEMENT OF SPECIFIC REHABILITATION PROBLEMS

Spinal Cord Compression

INCIDENCE

With improved treatment and longer survival for many cancers that occur in the geriatric age group, spinal cord compression, a potentially devastating complication, will be seen more frequently. Spinal cord compression is a medical emergency requiring prompt

decompressive laminectomy or radiation therapy. In a setting of unrelenting spine pain, with or without weakness, a high degree of suspicion should be sustained, and appropriate treatment should be initiated before loss of spinal cord function results. Most studies have shown the presence of pain for many weeks prior to the onset of motor or sensory complaints; these complaints usually evolve over a few days. Early diagnosis and prompt intervention prior to the inability to walk lead to better outcome (75). Bowel and bladder dysfunction are poor prognostic signs. In the geriatric age group particularly, radiation therapy is favored, reserving laminectomy for progression of disease or tissue diagnosis.

PROBLEMS

The spinal column with vertebral stability is the major area of concern (76). A clear understanding of anatomic relationships, site and extent of bone metastases, and extension of metastases into the epidural space or development within the intramedullary area is important.

Control of pain is also important, and radiation therapy is of value, but immediate selection of appropriate pharmaceutical agents is of paramount importance. The combination of bone pain, spinal cord compression, and radicular pain is indeed challenging in this group of patients, and aggressive pain control is appropriate in all ages.

GOALS AND TREATMENT

The goals of treatment are local tumor control, spinal stability, pain control, prevention of complications, and improved neurologic function (77). Both decompressive laminectomy and radiation therapy may produce complications. In the geriatric age group, radiation therapy is the treatment of choice when combined with aggressive and creative pain control and nutrition, particularly in those patients at risk for dysphagia or radiation-induced gastrointestinal complications.

In those patients with bowel and bladder symptoms, careful management decisions should take into consideration the age and life expectancy of the patient. One should be sensitive to the overall quality of life and not feel compelled to follow the same criteria as for investigation and treatment of traumatic spinal cord compression.

An intermittent catheterization program would be unrealistic in the older debilitated cancer patient with myelopathy whose goal is to return home. Indwelling catheterization would be appropriate in this setting, minimizing the necessity of transfers. Practical solutions should be the norm, as bladder management is frequently the limiting factor in a dismissal plan in which the patient returns home.

REHABILITATION TECHNIQUES

Spinal Stability

An appropriate level of spine stabilization can be achieved with consideration for appropriate orthoses, depending on the area of spinal column affected and degree of neurologic deficit. Emphasis should be placed on stability and pain control, with more rigid bracing (body jacket) being required for spinal immobilization.

The more extensive the brace, the greater the energy expenditure for mobility in transfers and walking. An expert fitting by an experienced orthotist is required in addition to careful adjustment and supportive encouragement to the patient. In ambulatory patients, lightweight ankle-foot orthoses and gait aids also will promote functional mobility.

Pain Control

As discussed in the sections on pain and metastatic bone disease, pain control is of primary importance to allow the patient to continue with treatment and actively participate in activities of daily living and mobility. When stability is not an issue, a less rigid corset will frequently give adequate support for good pain relief and yet allow greater flexibility of movement.

Preservation of Function

As noted above, emphasis on spinal stability, bracing, gait aids, and ankle-foot orthoses will improve function. Additionally, appropriate wheelchair cushions and adaptive equipment can contribute to quality of life. In those tumors sensitive to radiation therapy such as prostate and lymphoma, muscle reeducation and strengthening is appropriate as neurologic function returns.

Skin Care

Expert spinal orthotic fitting is imperative for comfort and prevention of skin breakdown. Likewise, foam or sheepskin mattresses and wheelchair cushions are necessary to prevent pressure ulcers and their many complications.

Bladder Management

Intermittent catheterization and progression to formal bladder retraining is appropriate in those patients with otherwise minimal metastatic or comorbid disease who are able to learn and have the energy to perform the technique. Frequently, in older patients, an indwelling catheter is the correct choice, at least initially, especially in a setting of pain and anxiety related to progression of disease.

Bowel Care

Careful attention to nutrition with prevention of constipation and diarrhea assists dramatically in patients' overall ability to participate in daily activities and better cope with treatment. The basic program includes a high-fiber diet or supplement, a bulking agent, adequate fluid intake, and a stool softener. Additional use of suppositories may be necessary on a scheduled basis, but frequent enemas should be avoided in this age group.

SUMMARY

Spinal cord compression is a medical emergency requiring immediate treatment with corticosteroids followed by prompt decompressive laminectomy or initiation of radiation therapy. The members of a rehabilitation team require a high degree of acuity when working with patients in the geriatric age group with known or unknown metastatic cancer. The application of broad rehabilitation principles can have a significant impact on the quality of life of these patients and their families.

Metastatic Bone Disease

INCIDENCE

Metastatic deposits to the skeleton are a common clinical problem; they develop in up to 70% of all patients with cancer, especially those with lung, breast, and prostate cancers (78). All of these cancers are common in the geriatric age group, and many of these patients have some compromise of their musculoskeletal system due to osteoporosis, rheumatoid arthritis, or osteoarthritis. Improvements in oncologic management of the primary tumor due to advances in chemotherapy, immunotherapy, and radiation therapy have resulted in increased survival of patients with cancer. Hence, there are more patients with compromised function of the musculoskeletal system secondary to dissemination of cancer cells. Treatment is palliative. However, aggressive management will preserve function and improve the quality of the patient's life, and a carefully planned interdisciplinary approach is necessary to achieve these goals.

PROBLEMS

The major challenges in this group of patients are pain control, loss of structural integrity, and neurologic compromise (79, 80). All of these areas require a careful evaluation of general medical problems and investigation into the role of chemotherapy, radiation therapy, surgery, and rehabilitation techniques. Functional staging of the patient with metastatic bone disease assists in developing a realistic plan and outlines goals for the treatment team, patient, and family (Table 31.5).

A method of viewing bone metastasis according to extent of disease is needed when discussing treatment

Table 31.5. Functional Staging for Metastatic Bone Disease

Treatment Goal	Treatment
Preventive	Decrease weight bearing
	Decrease torsional load
Restorative	Pain control
	Stability
Supportive	Persistent disability
	Adaptation
Palliative	Pain control and comfort

with patients and family, and Table 31.6, modified from Stoll (81), shows a stratification of bone metastasis into two main categories. This grouping of favorable and unfavorable factors helps the clinician and elderly patient be more realistic when planning future rehabilitation goals.

TREATMENT OPTIONS

Radiation and surgical therapy are the two interventions most frequently used. The usual indicators for radiation are need for pain control, loss of structural integrity, and neurologic compromise. The symptoms should be carefully assessed in conjunction with other problems relating to the disease process.

Early functional restoration may be enhanced by elective surgical procedures for pending pathologic fracture. Joint replacement, internal fixation, or cementing allow length of hospital stay to be minimized while optimizing the patient's chances for increased functional activity.

REHABILITATION TECHNIQUES

Vertebral Column

Orthoses can be used with the goals of spinal stability and pain control, and they may include halo vest, cervical post brace, Philadelphia collar, or corsets. Supports are usually made of heavy cotton or elastic with

Table 31.6. Prognostic Factors in Metastatic Bone Disease[a]

Factor	Favorable	Unfavorable
Nature of primary lesion	Indolent (prostate)	Aggressive (lung)
Recurrence-free interval	Long (>3 yr)	Short (<1 yr)
Bone lesions	Single	Multiple
System(s) involved	Single	Multiple
Vital organs involved	Absent	Present
General condition (performance status)	Good	Poor

[a]Modified from Stoll BA. Natural history prognosis, and staging of bone metastases. In: Stoll BA, Parbhoo S, eds. *Bone Metastasis: Monitoring and Treatment.* New York, NY: Raven Press; 1983:1–20.

modular components or, if necessary, a rigid body jacket if spinal stability is of concern. Issues to be considered in development of a prescription include reduction of axial loading and torque forces, enhancement of body mechanics, and use of gait aids. Recommendations for activities of daily living and mobility should also be considered.

Humerus

Stability and pain control are of greatest importance in humeral lesions. If surgical intervention is recommended, early involvement in rehabilitation is imperative to prevent contractures and improve function. Posterior shell, coaptation splints, or, for severe pain, a shoulder immobilizer may be warranted. Rehabilitation in conjunction with radiation therapy, which is well tolerated in the elderly, provides good pain control and may be the treatment of choice in patients with severe comorbid disease.

Pelvis and Femur Involvement

When the pelvis or femur is involved, the rehabilitation issues involve all mobility skills and activities of daily living. Careful evaluation of cortical integrity is necessary to decide on weight-bearing options for the patient. Surgical intervention allows early ambulation and provides dramatic pain control, and age alone is not a contraindication. Stabilization before a catastrophic fracture occurs decreases morbidity and mortality and is cost-effective. The major issues in mobility are the decrease in weight bearing, avoidance of pivoting on the involved side, and careful continued assessment of pain and its relation to activity.

Advanced Disease

For patients with spinal compression fractures and advanced disease in the ribs and long bones, pain control and comfort are paramount considerations. Deconditioning, weight loss, and poor nutrition contribute to discomfort. Simple measures such as attention to body mechanics with turning and sitting and close attention to skin care by providing full-length sheepskin or foam mattresses can help decrease pain and anxiety and promote rest. Bed positioning, a padded corset, and a reclining wheelchair are readily available and can be used in the patient's home to improve quality of life. As noted previously, control of pain at rest to allow adequate sleep is a primary goal, and reduction and control of pain with activity can be assisted with the interventions described.

Hemiplegia

INCIDENCE

Hemiplegia secondary to intracranial neoplasm is rare compared to hemiplegia resulting from cerebrovascular disease (stroke). The incidence of stroke increases with advancing age to more than 1,100/100,000 for those more than 75 years of age (82). The incidence of primary neoplasm also increases in the elderly to 20.4/100,000 up to age 75 years and then has been noted to decrease (83). However, metastasis is the most common form of brain tumor in adults (83), with lung and breast the most common primary sites in the elderly (84). Two studies showed that in those more than age 65 years, malignant astrocytoma, meningioma, and metastases to the brain accounted for more than 90% of all intracranial neoplasms (85, 86). With increasing survival of patients secondary to aggressive surgery and radiotherapy, there will probably be an increased prevalence of neurologic morbidity and its consequences.

PROBLEMS

Focal weakness or hemiparesis has been reported in several studies to be the most frequent presenting sign of intracranial neoplasm, specifically in elderly patients (87, 88). This usually is a slowly progressive deficit. In reviewing several studies on presenting symptoms in the elderly, Werner and Schold (89) found that change in mental status occurred most frequently. Other frequent symptoms were those usually associated with cerebrovascular accident such as headache, visual disturbance, and aphasia, although seizure was found to occur relatively infrequently in the older adult (89).

The differential diagnosis must not be neglected in the older patient because neoplasm can present with sudden onset via tumor hemorrhage, and cerebral metastasis can be the presenting symptom in up to 10% to 20% of older patients, mimicking stroke, which has the much higher incidence (88). Computed tomographic scanning and magnetic resonance imaging have helped differentiate these difficult cases. The cause of focal weakness is extremely important because stroke is a static deficit, and brain tumor, in spite of treatment, usually is progressive.

GOALS OF TREATMENT

When reviewing rehabilitation goals for cancer-related hemiplegia, one must consider what the likely gains are to be and develop an appropriate plan. Prognosis may limit goals. Age has been found to be a predictor of a poorer functional outcome along with previous cerebrovascular accident, incontinence, and visuospatial problems (90). Risk factors for stroke itself (systolic hypertension, coronary artery disease) are common comorbid conditions in elderly patients with cancer and can limit a patient's endurance and ability to participate in rehabilitation efforts.

Patient and family goals and capabilities must also be considered. Intensive prolonged rehabilitation with a goal of dismissal to the home may be unrealistic for an already frail elderly couple who were previously managing only marginally. For minor deficits, impairment may dissolve with the institution of steroid treatment, but it must not be forgotten that, unlike stroke, the lesion frequently recurs in spite of treatment, and complete resolution of severe symptoms is unlikely.

TREATMENT

Options for treatment of brain tumor include surgery, radiation therapy, chemotherapy, and steroids in patients of all ages. Surgery is tolerated surprisingly well in older patients in terms of survival, but neurologic morbidity postoperatively may be increased (compared to the greater plasticity of the brain of younger patients) (84). Radiation therapy is a mainstay for treatment of brain tumor, and its efficacy either alone or as an adjunct to surgery has been demonstrated (91).

Radiation therapy usually extends over many weeks, and this may be difficult for the single elderly patient without social support or resources. Concurrent disease also adds to the burden in the case of metastatic brain lesions. Radiation therapy is not without consequence, and the older patient may suffer short-term and long-term side effects listed elsewhere in this chapter. Late-onset necrosis or diffuse encephalopathy occurs as late as a year posttherapy and may be mistaken for other forms of slowing and dementia in older patients.

Chemotherapy is used for aggressive tumors but has not been shown to be of great value. Some chemotherapeutic agents can cause specific neurologic deficits, including peripheral neuropathy (vinca alkaloids) or leukoencephalopathy (methotrexate) (88). These agents are not frequently used to treat primary brain tumors, but they may play a role in the treatment of metastatic disease. When side effects occur, a confusing neurologic picture may develop in an already compromised older patient.

Finally, steroid therapy is frequently part of the treatment regimen to decrease neurologic symptoms in the elderly (92). Side effects, of course, present a risk, some of which already have an increased incidence in older patients (e.g., hypertension, osteoporosis, glucose intolerance), and such patients must be monitored closely.

REHABILITATION TECHNIQUES

For an intensive review of the rehabilitation issues in hemiplegia the reader is referred to Chapter 16 on stroke in this text. Several areas of importance will be discussed as they pertain to rehabilitation of the cancer patient.

Gait

The ability to walk has been described as important by cancer patients and their families (58). Being able to take a few necessary steps may make home management a reality for some patients. In a dense, flaccid hemiplegic patient, whose body is already suffering cachexia and other effects of systemic cancer, the increased energy requirement for walking may make the task nearly impossible.

The realistic possibility of bony metastases in the long bones of the lower or upper extremities must be considered, and the risk of pathologic fracture must be assessed before significant weight bearing through the nonparetic extremities is attempted. Pain from bony disease may prove to be a strong deterrent to weight bearing as well.

The mechanics of gait reeducation remain the same, including mastering good sitting and standing balance, weight shifting, and transfer techniques prior to initiating gait reeducation. Lower extremity orthotics can be helpful, as with other hemiplegic patients, and should be used to assist in ankle and knee control.

Upper Extremity

Depending on the location of the brain lesion, the upper extremity may be more or less affected. Rehabilitation techniques include range of motion exercises, muscle reeducation, stretching, and progression to functional activities if possible. Comfort always remains a major goal as does good positioning with elevation for avoidance of the complications of upper extremity edema, shoulder subluxation, and shoulder pain. When possible, intravenous line placement in an edematous, upper extremity should be avoided as well. Bony metastases can and do occur in the upper extremities, and particular care must be given to proper support of these areas with appropriate splinting.

Bowel and Bladder

Neurogenic bladder problems usually do not affect the patient with hemiplegia, or they resolve in the early stages. If incontinence is a problem, then use of an indwelling urinary catheter frequently helps with patient comfort and family home management. Constipation is usually the problem, if any, with bowel management, and a good program of stool softeners, increased dietary fiber, and use of suppositories may be needed.

Equipment

Coordinating the patient's needs for equipment in the home is one of the most important aspects of rehabilitation for the older patient with hemiplegia. We find these patients to be fiercely independent and stoic regarding pain or functional disability. The patient and family must learn that the use of appropriate equipment may minimize the need for outside supports and increase independent function. The appropriate fitting and use of the wheelchair within the home cannot be overemphasized. The use of items such as hospital bed,

commode, and walker may greatly increase patient comfort and enhance the quality of home care. An excellent discussion of this topic and other equipment including gait aids, bed and bathroom aids, and devices to assist with dressing and feeding has been published elsewhere (93). The rehabilitation team should assist in arranging for equipment and utilize the resources of the American Cancer Society, which in many instances offers equipment items locally to the patient free of charge.

Dysphagia

INCIDENCE

Disorders of eating and swallowing in the elderly are related to a complex mix of factors, and dysfunction may manifest itself dramatically with acute aspiration or more insidiously with malnutrition and progressive debilitation. The role of anorexia and constipation or other gastrointestinal problems needs to be clearly differentiated from dysphagia. The incidence of dysphagia in the geriatric population with cancer is quite high. The causes vary from alterations in dentition, taste appreciation, or oral swallowing mechanism to neurologic deficits relating to the disease itself. Complications occurring because of radiation therapy or chemotherapy with related mucositis are common.

Maintenance of optimal nutrition is a prime concern because of the frequent impairment noted above, and it may enhance the patient's chance of recovery. A positive nitrogen balance must be restored for the patient to undergo the rigors of chemotherapy or radiation.

PROBLEMS

Dysphagia is frequently seen in patients with head and neck or upper gastrointestinal cancer and in those patients with central nervous system involvement due to other primary or secondary disease. Those patients receiving radiation therapy that includes the oropharynx or esophagus are particularly prone to painful mucositis and *Candida* esophagitis. A detailed dysphagia evaluation and nutritional survey needs to be done in addition to the history and careful physical examination. A video fluoroscopy study complemented by an esophageal transit study is worthwhile to evaluate the presence of possible silent aspiration because this is of particular concern in the geriatric patient.

Surgical excision of structures important to swallowing has a greater influence on swallowing than does impaired mobility. Patients who have had partial or total glossectomy require individualized evaluation.

TREATMENT

The primary goal of dysphagia management is maintenance of adequate nutrition in addition to protection of the airway and maintenance of hydration. At times, alternative hydration routes, such as intravenous therapy for shorter periods or percutaneous endoscopic gastrostomy feeding tube placement, may help promote normal nutrition while dysphagia is being managed. In those tumors responsive to treatment, age alone is not a contraindication, and aggressive therapy to maintain nutrition and hydration should be implemented.

Careful dietary planning is necessary using food substitutions when possible with emphasis on varied textures and sensory input and utilization of those foods and flavors the patient most enjoys.

For those patients with pain and a dry oral mucosa, increased total fluid intake, use of papain (a proteolytic enzyme), or swabbing of the mouth before meals may be of value. Viscous lidocaine 5 to 10 minutes before a meal acts as a soothing topical analgesic.

REHABILITATION TECHNIQUES

The speech therapist and occupational therapist work closely with the patient and family and use various swallowing reeducation techniques to assist in the problem of dysphagia. Variations in texture, bite size, and head positioning can facilitate swallowing mechanisms (94). Fluids may be thickened to make swallowing easier. Increased fluid intake and frequent small meals may be more appealing to many patients in this age group. The geriatric patient also may exhibit significant cognitive or psychologic symptoms that affect ability to swallow, and careful evaluation of these functional areas is necessary (95).

Of concern are the ethical considerations involved in feedings, particularly when this involves a patient judged to be incompetent. Feeding is a true life-support system and, as such, can be interpreted as extraordinary means that may be withheld at the request of a patient or guardian; however, each case must be carefully considered on an individual basis and thoroughly understood and discussed by the health caregivers involved and the patient and family members.

SUMMARY

The evaluation and treatment of dysphagia in the geriatric cancer patient covers a wide ranging array of deficits and options, and the problems are best managed using an interdisciplinary team approach, as described by Gray et al (96).

Lymphedema

Lymphedema is a chronic progressive condition that develops if the lymphatic load exceeds the transport capacity of the lymphatic system and occurs in various degrees in patients after surgical ablation of the axillary or inguinal nodes or radiation therapy with subsequent fibrosis.

Various studies have reported incidence of lymphedema from 6% to 65%, and lymphedema may occur within weeks of a procedure or many years later. Most studies reported in the literature pertain to management of the upper extremity in postmastectomy lymphedema. However, the same basic principles apply to problems in the upper and lower extremity.

PROBLEMS

Secondary lymphedema after mastectomy is a serious long-term problem for the patient. Clodius et al (97) repeatedly emphasized the distressingly swollen arm and hand as being an ever-present sign of previous mastectomy and breast cancer. In addition to the esthetic deformity, which may considerably decrease social activities and quality of survival, there can be a feeling of tension within the arm, both acute and chronic pain syndromes, diffuse hyperesthesia, and decreased mobility of all joints of the limb. Minor injuries may lead to cutaneous lymphorrhea, with the ever-present threat of infection and septicemia. Lymphangiosarcoma is a rare complication of chronic lymphedema.

Secondary arm lymphedema with risk of recurrent tumor in the axilla is a major concern. Additionally, local skin metastases, venous obstruction, repetitive use, and sunburn or other skin trauma need to be excluded.

Unfortunately, many patients are not referred until the lymphedema is quite severe, at which time restoring normal size and function to the limb is improbable. As lymphedema progresses, irreversible changes occur as a result of tissue fibrosis and chronic interstitial inflammation. These problems are more complex in the geriatric age group than in younger patients. Additionally, in the male, associated lymphedema of the scrotum and penis can be a major source of severe pain and discomfort.

TREATMENT

Early intervention and minimization of complications is the goal of management in a patient with lymphedema. The standard treatment of lymphedema continues to be a conservative approach: use of compression devices, wrapping between pump treatments, elevation with isometric exercises of the limb, and decongestive massage if helpful. Circumferential or volumetric measurements are not always reliable, and the greatest care should be taken in recording this information as one follows the treatment program.

In addition, detailed patient education relating to meticulous care of the limb, avoidance of injury, and limitation of repetitive activities all contribute to improved function. The patient should understand that fluid reduction may take several weeks, and the key component to progress is the maintenance of external pressure on the limb, especially when the limb is dependent.

The newer microsurgical techniques, as discussed by Gloviczki et al (98), may be considered in this group of patients, but at the present time outcome has been disappointing.

REHABILITATION TECHNIQUES

After careful evaluation and exclusion of secondary metastatic involvement or infection, secondary lymphedema may be treated with a sequential pneumatic pumping device at a pressure of 60 mm Hg to 80 mm Hg for 1 hour with the arm elevated (99). This may be followed by massage, centripetal in nature, beginning proximally and moving distally. Isometric exercises of the limb combined with elevation are also used. Initially, an external elastic wrap should be applied, and the limb should be rewrapped every 4 to 6 hours, with close attention to avoiding a tourniquet effect. The pumping can be repeated twice a day while there is continued progress as noted by volumetric or circumferential measurements. Patient education should emphasize avoidance of factors that may precipitate or aggravate lymphedema. Modalities such as superficial and deep heat and warm hydrotherapy should not be used. Absolute contraindications to the use of a pneumatic pumping device are cellulitis, acute phlebitis, or recurrent carcinoma. Brawny edema is a relative contraindication because the outcome will be poor.

When the limb size has stabilized, the patient may be fitted with an appropriate elastic support garment. In postmastectomy lymphedema, a wrist to shoulder sleeve, including a shoulder cap, is most practical, with an additional gauntlet for the hand and digits. It is imperative that the patient understand the importance of maintenance of size of the limb to allow continued correct fitting of the custom garment.

Problems of compliance occur for multiple reasons, most frequently because of difficulty donning the garment, particularly on the lower extremity. In the older patient with decreased upper extremity strength secondary to arthritis or neuropathy, compliance may depend on spouse aid or home health assistance. Maintenance of the material is also important. A worn garment that does not provide a pressure of 30 mm Hg to 40 mm Hg will not control the lymphedema, and compliance will decrease. Comfort of the limb and hand are also of concern to many patients, and the sensation of compression and heat may be unacceptable. These problems can be addressed by lighter-weight fabric now available and also by requesting silk inserts for the cubital and popliteal fossa areas.

SUMMARY

Secondary lymphedema is the most common form of lymphedema and usually presents as a sequela to surgery involving the axilla or groin, and it may occur following radiation therapy to these areas. Outcome is dependent on the severity of lymphedema at the time of treatment, and it is reversible in the early stages. Emphasis should be placed on education of medical personnel and patients so that early preventive measures may be implemented.

A custom-fitted elastic pressure garment should be provided. The patient should wear it throughout the waking hours, and as fabric deteriorates, it must be replaced (every 3 to 4 months). Intermittent pneumatic compression before measuring for a new sleeve or stocking may be necessary. For patients who choose not to have a sleeve, a home pneumatic massage unit can be used daily. Diuretic therapy and salt restriction have not been shown to be very helpful. For those patients who have had recurrent episodes of cellulitis, therapy with penicillin or erythromycin 1 week per month should be considered. Each patient's treatment will need to be considered carefully depending on the overall disease, presence of metastases, and capability for successful use of a garment.

Amputation

INCIDENCE

Amputation of a limb secondary to cancer is rare; the incidence is highest among pediatric patients in the second decade of life (100). In the geriatric population, amputation for vascular disease is a more common occurrence and certainly may be a complication in a geriatric cancer patient.

PROBLEMS

Historically, advancing age and cancer diagnosis have both carried a stigma regarding the value of fitting a prosthesis, with the presumption that the survival of the geriatric or the cancer patient did not merit the expense. When comparing the survival of cancer patients and older vascular amputees, the survival of the cancer patient equals that of the elderly vascular amputee—approximately 50% at 5 years (101). Additionally, the vascular amputee patient is at 25% to 30% risk of having bilateral amputations; no data are available on this in cancer patients.

Reports have shown that the presence of coronary artery disease in patients with above-knee amputation correlates negatively with functional ambulation. However, in patients with below-knee amputation, coronary artery disease did not decrease ambulation potential (102). Thus, in the case of the older cancer patient, neither age alone nor the cancer diagnosis should deter aggressive treatment and fitting of a prosthesis.

The positive body image and increased activity from generalized conditioning have great importance for older patients, and the increased quality of survivorship cannot be overemphasized.

REHABILITATION ISSUES

Little is known specifically about rehabilitation of the older cancer amputee. In a general group of cancer amputees, Subbarao and McPhee (101) found comparable outcomes to those of the vascular amputee in terms of survival and functional ambulation status. Thorpe et al (103) found, as is the trend in standard practice with amputees, that immediate postsurgical fitting of a prosthesis and early ambulation in patients with above-knee amputations for sarcoma yielded comparable results, with an overall decrease in the duration of final prosthetic fitting time. The reader is referred to Chapter 33 in this text for details regarding postoperative rehabilitation management and prosthetic fitting of the older amputee.

What is the significance of amputation for the rehabilitation of the older patient with cancer? It has been clearly shown that an increasing level of disability increases the energy requirement and decreases the efficiency of gait (104). In assessing the appropriateness of fitting an older amputee with a prosthesis, variables such as severity of other medical conditions (including coronary artery disease), extent of disability from cancer, and level of amputation should be considered, because all may affect energy reserve.

Age or diagnosis alone should not be the limiting factor. As in many other areas of geriatric rehabilitation, social, psychologic, and economic issues need to be considered as well.

PROGRAM MODELS

Cancer rehabilitation for the older patient may be successful in various settings. Traditionally, cancer patients have been hospitalized for systemic chemotherapy or radiation treatments, and many patients received necessary rehabilitation therapies in this setting. Presently, duration of hospital stay has decreased and meeting the needs of the elderly patient has become a much greater challenge. The patients are medically more complex; they are, with increasing frequency, frail isolated outpatients, and reimbursements for rehabilitation services for older patients are increasingly scrutinized (105).

Little has actually been written regarding existing programs for cancer rehabilitation. In an early (1982) descriptive survey of cancer rehabilitation programs, 36 existing programs were in inpatient (64%), outpatient (30%), or home (6%) setting (106). With inpatient stays decreasing sharply for Medicare-age patients since the advent of prospective payment in 1983, the number of patients treated in outpatient settings has increased.

Inpatient Settings

Cancer patients can be housed within the traditional structure of the inpatient rehabilitation setting, although there are few centers specifically designated for this patient group. The traditionally integrated team approach is appropriate for patients with severe cancer-related physical impairment (hemiplegia, spinal injury) when acquisition of multiple skills is required in order to achieve increased functional independence.

Older patients frequently stay in rehabilitation units for weeks, and prior to transfer several important factors should be considered: (a) prognosis, (b) desired versus achievable functional outcome, (c) adaptability to the intense activity level on the unit, (d) physical endurance, and (e) realistic options for dismissal planning. Each of these factors may limit chances for success. It should be understood that the older cancer patient exhibits special qualities, including an often progressive rather than static disability and systemic fatigue, which may make the "up and going" attitude of many inpatient rehabilitation settings an inappropriate choice.

Inpatients may also be assessed and treated by the cancer rehabilitation team while in the general hospital setting for cancer diagnosis and treatment. The rehabilitation team then functions in a consulting capacity, working closely with the primary physician or oncology team. The individualized program is developed while the patient is receiving other treatments (107). Whether one is treating an inpatient or outpatient, the components of the integrated team assessment and planning remain essentially the same (Fig. 31.1).

Rehabilitative care also can occur within the nursing home setting; many facilities now offer both physical and occupational therapy. If a high level of care is needed, patients and families should be encouraged to utilize this option. Positive benefits include the option of physical and occupational therapy without travel for the patient, flexibility of scheduling if pain or fatigue occurs, and the provision of necessary skilled care for the patient without physically burdening the family. Payment may become an issue because Medicare benefits for extended care are limited, and few added insurance policies for elderly people cover nursing home care.

Outpatient Setting

The rehabilitation needs of the older cancer patient are not dispelled and perhaps are just beginning at the time of hospital dismissal (105). The needs to be addressed in long-term care have been summarized and include financial, personal, and home-care issues; various social supports; equipment, and transportation (105). These are the same issues raised by many elderly patients with other medical problems.

Older cancer patients can and do receive rehabilitation interventions in the form of physical and occupational therapy within the outpatient setting when the patient comes to the clinic or hospital. However, the elderly patient may suffer systemic fatigue from disease,

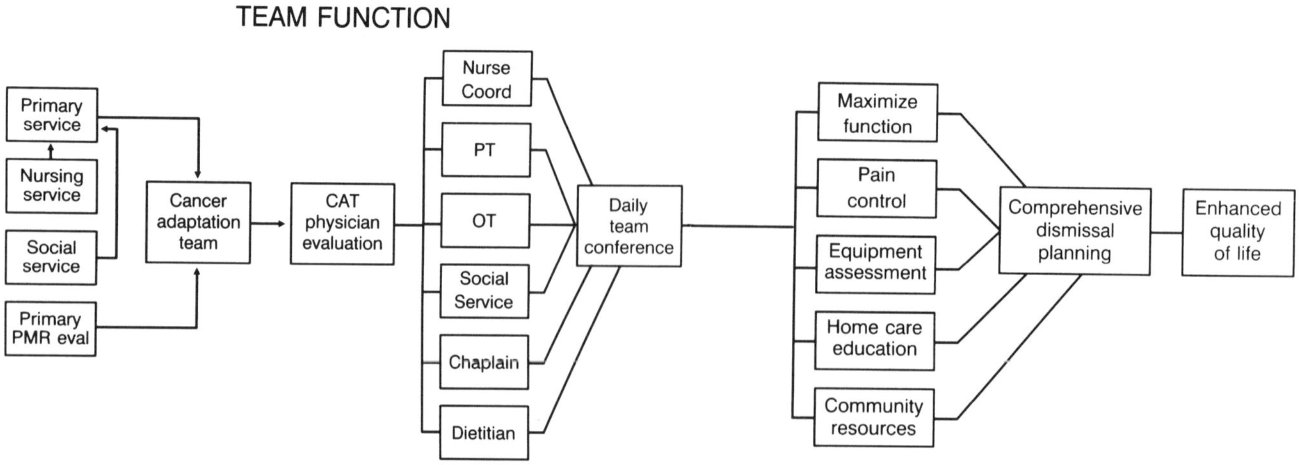

TEAM FUNCTION

Figure 31.1. Integrated team assessment. CAT, cancer adaptation team; coord, coordinator; eval, evaluation; OT, occupational therapy; PMR, physical medicine and rehabilitation; PT, physical therapy.

complicated by recovery from complex cancer treatments. Lack of social or economic supports, including transportation, may limit consistent participation. Regular monitoring of patients' conditions is warranted because older people and those with cancer do not report needs or concerns, and then perhaps they are too anxious (or unable) to hear appropriate information regarding community resources when it is given (108). New and innovative ways of patient contact and follow-up (automated telephone interview) are being investigated, and preliminary results are hopeful for an economically feasible periodic intervention to get the correct help to the needy patient promptly without burdensome clinic visits (109).

Home Care or Hospice

The authors believe that a discussion of the care of the terminally ill patient is consistent with the goals of a comprehensive cancer rehabilitation program. Quality of life issues are foremost in providing good care. Cancer rehabilitation-type services frequently maintain that quality of life.

There are many types of home-care services: nonprofit, government run, or private business concerns. Home health-care services can provide excellent assistance for an older mildly or moderately affected patient with long-term disease who lives alone or whose spouse perhaps is frail and elderly as well. Some services are reimbursable, with usually only skilled services being paid by Medicare.

Hospice care, as it has evolved in the United States, is usually a form of home care. Hospice programming has received increasing attention in recent years and detailed descriptions of the development of hospice care, first in England and now in the United States, are available (110, 111). Hospice care in the United States, for various reasons, has not mimicked the early local inpatient settings of the English system but has reflected the American patient's desires to remain at home as long as possible and still receive adequate pain management and physical and emotional support under supervision.

Hospice care has become more comprehensive and complex since Medicare certification became available in 1983. The issues surrounding this are particularly important to the elderly Medicare-age patient. With Medicare reimbursement available, rapid growth in the number of hospice programs has occurred, with a reported 516 programs in 1983 and 1,700 (600 of those Medicare-certified) in 1989 (112).

As with other government programs, the impetus for Medicare approval of hospice programs (under certain rigid conditions) appeared to be control of costly hospital stays with emphasis on home care. This is in concert with the original hospital philosophy that emphasized quality of life and palliative care, openly ignoring the aggressive investigation of concurrent medical problems.

The results of these programs as indicated by the patient and government remain equivocal. Although some studies found decreased costs, particularly in the last months of life, the only randomized study to look at two program models found no difference (113). The lack of success revolves around the rigid criteria for program and patient to be eligible for benefits (Table 31.7) (112). Those criteria have adverse consequences for the elderly cancer patient who has no certified hospice program available locally or who is unwilling to face a 6-month life expectancy. Needed home-care services, physical therapy, and occupational therapy would not be covered by Medicare, and thus the patient may not opt for needed supports. This may result in a downward clinical spiral. What is worse, the existing programs are not as highly utilized as they could be because of patient and caregiver ignorance of available services.

Table 31.7. The Medicare Hospice Benefit [a]

Patients must have a terminal illness with a life expectancy of 6 months or less and be entitled to Medicare part A insurance.

Election of the hospice benefit requires relinquishing other Medicare benefits (except for reimbursement to the patient's attending physician).

The benefit is divided into two 90-day periods and one 30-day period, for a total of 210 days.

Revocation of benefit means losing the remaining days in the benefit period.

The hospice program must continue to provide care to patients who live beyond 210 days.

The hospice is reimbursed at a daily rate that depends on the patient's level of care: routine home care, continuous home care, inpatient respite care, and general inpatient care.

More than 80% of each hospice's care days must be for home care. There is an annual payment cap for each hospice based on the number of enrolled patients.

The hospice must provide medical and nursing care, home health services, inpatient care, social work, counseling (including bereavement counseling), medications, medical supplies, durable medical equipment, and physical, occupational, and speech therapy, as needed, based on a plan for each patient.

[a] From Rhymes J. Hospice care in America. *JAMA*. 264:369–372, © 1990. By permission of the American Medical Association.

Acknowledgment. The authors gratefully acknowledge the efforts of Mrs. Eleanor Britt for typing and review of this manuscript.

References

1. Siegel JS, Davidson M. Demographic and socioeconomic aspects of aging in the U.S. *Current Population Reports, Series P-23: Special Studies.* No. 138. Washington, DC: Department of Commerce, Government Printing Office; August, 1984.
2. Silverberg E, Boring CC, Squires TS. Cancer statistics, 1990. *CA.* 40:9–26, 1990.
3. Holmes FF, Hearne E III. Cancer stage-to-age relationship: implications for cancer screening in the elderly. *J Am Geriatr Soc.* 29:55–57, 1981.
4. Cristofalo VJ. Biological mechanisms of aging: an overview. In: Hazzard WR, Andres R, Bierman EL, Blass JP, eds. *Principles of Geriatric Medicine and Gerontology.* 2nd ed. New York, NY: McGraw-Hill Information Services Company; 1990:3–14.
5. Crawford J, Cohen HJ. Relationship of cancer and aging. *Clin Geriatr Med.* 3:419–432, 1987.
6. Lipschitz DA, Goldstein S, Reis R, Weksler ME, Bressler R, Neilan BA. Cancer in the elderly: basic science and clinical aspects. *Ann Intern Med.* 102:218–228, 1985.
7. Minna JD, Pass H, Glatstein E, Ihde DC. Cancer of the lung. In: DeVita VT Jr, Hellman S, Rosenberg, SA, eds. *Cancer: Principles & Practice of Oncology.* 3rd ed. Philadelphia, Pa: J.B. Lippincott; 1989:591–705.
8. Crawford J, Cohen HJ. Relationship of cancer and aging. *Clin Geriatr Med.* 3:419–432, 1987.
9. Figlin R, Holmes E, Petrovich Z, Sarna G. Lung cancer. In: Haskell C, ed. *Cancer Treatment.* Philadelphia, Pa: W.B. Saunders; 1990:165–188.
10. O'Rourke, MA, Feussner JR, Feigl P, Laszlo J. Age trends of lung cancer stage at diagnosis: implications for lung cancer screening in the elderly. *JAMA.* 258:921–926, 1987.
11. Stanley KE. Prognostic factors for survival in patients with inoperable lung cancer. *J Natl Cancer Inst.* 65:25–32, 1980.
12. Cohen AM, Shank B, Friedman MA. Colorectal cancer. In: DeVita VT Jr, Hellman S, Rosenberg SA, eds. *Cancer: Principles & Prac-*

tice of Oncology. 3rd ed. Philadelphia, Pa: J.B. Lippincott; 1989:895–964.
13. Rosenberg JC, Lichter AS, Leichman LP. Cancer of the esophagus. In: DeVita VT Jr, Hellman S, Rosenberg SA, eds. *Cancer: Principles & Practice of Oncology.* 3rd ed. Philadelphia, Pa: J.B. Lippincott; 1989:725–764.
14. Macdonald JS, Steele G Jr, Gunderson LL. Cancer of the stomach. In: DeVita VT, Jr, Hellman S, Rosenberg SA, eds. *Cancer: Principles & Practice of Oncology.* 3rd ed. Philadelphia, Pa: J.B. Lippincott; 1989:765–799.
15. Brennan MF, Kinsella T, Friedman M. Cancer of the pancreas. In: DeVita VT Jr, Hellman S, Rosenberg SA, eds. *Cancer: Principles & Practice of Oncology.* Philadelphia, Pa: J.B. Lippincott; 1989:800–835.
16. Henderson IC, Harris JR, Kinne DW, Hellman S. Cancer of the breast. In: DeVita VT Jr, Hellman S, Rosenberg SA, eds. *Cancer: Principles & Practice of Oncology.* 3rd ed. Philadelphia, Pa: J.B. Lippincott; 1989:1197–1268.
17. Gaddipatie J, Ahmed T, Friedland M. Prostatic and bladder cancer in the elderly. *Clin Geriatr Med.* 3:649–667, 1987.
18. Perez CA, Fair WR, Ihde DC. Carcinoma of the prostate. In: DeVita VT Jr, Hellman S, Rosenberg SA, eds. *Cancer: Principles & Practice of Oncology.* Philadelphia, Pa: J.B. Lippincott; 1989:1023–1058.
19. Richie JP, Shipley WU, Yagoda A. Cancer of the bladder. In: DeVita VT Jr, Hellman S, Rosenberg SA, eds. *Cancer: Principles & Practice of Oncology.* 3rd ed. Philadelphia, Pa: J.B. Lippincott; 1989:1008–1022.
20. Hoskins WJ, Perez C, Young RC. Gynecologic tumors. In: DeVita VT Jr, Hellman S, Rosenberg SA, eds. *Cancer: Principles & Practice of Oncology.* Philadelphia, Pa: J.B. Lippincott; 1989:1099–1161.
21. Young R, Ruks Z, Hoskins W. Cancer of the ovary. In: DeVita VT Jr, Hellman S, Rosenberg SA, eds. *Cancer: Principles & Practice of Oncology.* Philadelphia, Pa: J.B. Lippincott; 1989:1162–1196.
22. Fialkow PJ, Singer JW. Chronic leukemias. In: DeVita VT Jr, Hellman S, Rosenberg SA, eds. *Cancer: Principles & Practice of Oncology.* 3rd ed. Philadelphia, Pa: J.B. Lippincott; 1989:1836–1852.
23. Hellman S, Jaffe ES, DeVita VT Jr. Hodgkin's disease. In: DeVita VT Jr, Hellman S, Rosenberg SA, eds. *Cancer: Principles & Practice of Oncology.* 3rd ed. Philadelphia, Pa: J.B. Lippincott; 1989:1696–1740.
24. DeVita, VT Jr, Jaffe ES, Mauch P, Longo DL. Lymphocytic lymphomas. In: DeVita VT Jr, Hellman S, Rosenberg SA, eds. *Cancer: Principles & Practice of Oncology.* 3rd ed. Philadelphia, Pa: J.B. Lippincott; 1989:1741–1808.
25. Salmon SE, Cassady JR. Plasma cell neoplasms. In: DeVita VT Jr, Hellman S, Rosenberg SA, eds. *Cancer: Principles & Practice of Oncology.* 3rd Ed. Philadelphia, Pa: J.B. Lippincott; 1989:1853–1895.
26. Wiernik PH. Acute leukemias. In: DeVita VT Jr, Hellman S, Rosenberg SA, eds. *Cancer: Principles & Practice of Oncology.* 3rd ed. Philadelphia, Pa: J.B. Lippincott; 1989:1809–1835.
27. Hertler AA, Crawford J, Cohen HJ. Update on cancer. *Geriatr Med Annu.* 3:1–49, 1989.
28. Crocker I, Prosnitz L. Radiation therapy of the elderly. *Clin Geriatr Med.* 3:473–481, 1987.
29. Hellman S. Principles of radiation therapy. In: DeVita VT Jr, Hellman S, Rosenberg SA, eds. *Cancer: Principles & Practice of Oncology.* 3rd ed. Philadelphia, Pa: J.B. Lippincott; 1989:247–275.
30. Lehmann JF, DeLisa JA, Warren CG, deLateur BJ, Bryant PLS, Nicholson CG. Cancer rehabilitation: assessment of need, development, and evaluation of a model of care. *Arch Phys Med Rehabil.* 59:410–419, 1978.
31. Wiggers JH, Donovan KO, Redman S, Sanson-Fisher RW. Cancer patient satisfaction with care. *Cancer.* 66:610–616, 1990.
32. Ganz PA, Schag CC, Polinsky ML, Heinrich RL, Flack VF. Re-

habilitation needs and breast cancer: the first month after primary therapy. *Breast Cancer Res Treat.* 10:243–253, 1987.

33. Grobe ME, Ahmann DL, Ilstrup DM. Needs assessment for advanced cancer patients and their families. *Oncol Nurs Forum.* 9:26–30, 1982.

34. Applegate WB, Blass JP, Williams TF. Instruments for the functional assessment of older patients. *N Engl J Med.* 322:1207–1214, 1990.

35. Lachs MS, Feinstein AR, Cooney LM Jr, et al. A simple procedure for general screening for functional disability in elderly patients. *Ann Intern Med.* 112:699–706, 1990.

36. Jones DR, Fayers PM, Simons J. Measuring and analyzing quality of life in cancer clinical-trials: a review. In: Aaronson NK, Beckmann JH, eds. *Quality of Life of Cancer Patients.* New York, NY: Raven Press; 1987:41–61.

37. Aaronson NK. Methodologic issues in assessing the quality of life of cancer patients. *Cancer.* 67(suppl):844–850, 1991.

38. Caplan AL, Callahan D, Haas J. Ethical & policy issues in rehabilitation medicine. *Hastings Cent Rep.* 17(suppl):1–20, 1987.

39. Wu AW, Rubin HR, Rosen MJ. Are elderly people less responsive to intensive care? *J AM Geriatr Soc.* 38:621–627, 1990.

40. Hosking MP, Warner MA, Lobdell CM, Offord KP, Melton LJ III. Outcomes of surgery in patients 90 years of age and older. *JAMA.* 261:1909–1915, 1989.

41. Pearlman RA. Ethical issues in geriatric care. In: Hazzard WR, Andres R, Bierman EL, Blass JP, eds. *Principles of Geriatric Medicine and Gerontology.* 2nd ed. New York, NY: McGraw-Hill Information Services Company; 1990:367–379.

42. Thomasma DC. Quality-of-life judgments, treatment decisions, and medical ethics. *Clin Geriatr Med.* 2:17–27, 1986.

43. Cassel CK. Ethical dilemmas in the clinical care of the elderly. In: Calkins E, Davis PJ, Ford AB, eds. *The Practice of Geriatrics.* Philadelphia, Pa: W.B. Saunders; 1986:93–101.

44. Cassel EJ. The nature of suffering and the goals of medicine. *N Engl J Med.* 306:639–645, 1982.

45. Koenig HG, Meador KG, Cohen HJ, Blazer DG. Depression in elderly hospitalized patients with medical illness. *Arch Intern Med.* 148:1929–1936, 1988.

46. Cooper ET. A pilot study on the effects of the diagnosis of lung cancer on family relationships. *Cancer Nurs.* 7:301–308, 1984.

47. Wellisch DK, Fawzy FI, Landsverk J, Pasnau RO, Wolcott DL. Evaluation of psychosocial problems of the home-bound cancer patient: the relationship of disease and the sociodemographic variables of patients to family problems. *J Psychosoc Oncol.* 1:1–15, 1983.

48. Cassileth, B.R., Lusk, E.J., Strouse, et al. Psychosocial status in chronic illness: a comparative analysis of six diagnostic groups. *N Engl J Med.* 311:501–511, 1984.

49. Maisiak R, Gams R, Lee E, Jones B. The psychosocial support status of elderly cancer outpatients. *Prog Clin Biol Res.* 120:395–403, 1983.

50. Ganz PA, Schag CC, Heinrich RL. The psychosocial impact of cancer on the elderly: a comparison with younger patients. *J Am Geriatr Soc.* 33:429–435, 1985.

51. Bond GG, Wellisch DK. Psychosocial care. In: Haskell CM, ed. *Cancer Treatment.* 3rd ed. Philadelphia, Pa: W.B. Saunders; 1990:893–904.

52. Wellisch DK, Jamison KR, Pasnau RO. Psychosocial aspects of mastectomy: II. The man's perspective. *Am J Psychiatry.* 135:543–546, 1978.

53. Andersen BL. Sexual functioning morbidity among cancer survivors: current status and future research directions. *Cancer.* 55:1835–1842, 1985.

54. Fobair P, Hoppe RT, Bloom J, Cox R, Varghese A, Spiegel D. Psychosocial problems among survivors of Hodgkin's disease. *J Clin Oncol.* 4:805–814, 1986.

55. Spingarn N. Cancer survivor's bill of rights. *Cancer News.* 42:15, 1988.

56. Portenoy RK. Cancer pain. *Geriatr Med Annu.* 3:50–72, 1989.

57. Baines M. Pain relief in active patients with cancer: analgesic drugs are the foundation of management. *Br Med J.* 298:36, 1989.

58. Grobe ME, Ahmann DL, Ilstrup DM. Needs assessment for advanced cancer patients and their families: a hospice program. *Oncol Nurs Forum.* 9:26–30, 1982.

59. Bonica JJ, ed. *The Management of Pain,* I. 2nd ed. Philadelphia, Pa: Lea & Febiger. 1990:400–460.

60. Foley KM, Arbit E. Management of cancer pain. In: DeVita VT, Jr, Hellman S, Rosenberg SA, eds. *Principles & Practice of Oncology.* 3rd ed. Philadelphia, Pa: J.B. Lippincott; 1989:2064–2087.

61. Twycross RG. Analgesics and relief of bone pain. In: Stoll BA, Parbhoo S, eds. *Bone Metastasis: Monitoring and Treatment.* New York, NY: Raven Press; 1983:289–310.

62. World Health Organization. *Cancer Pain Relief.* Albany, NY: WHO Publications Center USA; 1986.

63. Ventafridda V, Sganzerla EP, Fochi C, Pozzi G, Cordini G. Transcutaneous nerve stimulation in cancer pain. *Adv Pain Res Ther.* 2:509–515, 1979.

64. Bloch AS, ed. *Nutrition Management of the Cancer Patient.* Rockville, Md: Aspen Publishers; 1990.

65. Halar EM, Bell KR. Contracture and other deleterious effects of immobility. In: *Rehabilitation Medicine: Principles and Practice.* DeLisa JA, ed. Philadelphia, Pa: J.B. Lippincott; 1988:448–462.

66. Mahler DA, Cunningham LN, Curfman GD. Aging and exercise performance. *Clin Geriatr Med.* 2:433–452, 1986.

67. Seals DR, Hagberg JM. The effect of exercise training on human hypertension: a review. *Med Sci Sports Exerc.* 16:207–215, 1984.

68. deVries HA. Physiological effects of an exercise training regimen upon men aged 52 to 88. *J Gerontol.* 25:325–336, 1970.

69. Brewer F, Meyer BM, Keele MS, Upton SJ, Hagan RD. Role of exercise in prevention of involutional bone loss. *Med Sci Sports Exerc.* 15:445–449, 1983.

70. Dustman RE, Ruhling RO, Russell EM, et al. Aerobic exercise training and improved neuropsychological function of older individuals. *Neurobiol Aging.* 5:35–42, 1984.

71 Shepard RJ. The scientific basis of exercise prescribing for the very old. *J Am Geriatr Soc.* 38:62–70, 1990.

72. Fiatarone MA, Marks EC, Ryan ND, Meredith CN, Lipsitz LA, Evans WJ. High-intensity strength training in nonagenarians: effects on skeletal muscle. *JAMA.* 263:3029–3034, 1990.

73. Posner JD, Gorman KM, Klein HS, Woldow A. Exercise capacity in the elderly. *Am J Cardiol.* 57(suppl):52C–58C, 1986.

74. Thompson RF, Crist DM, Marsh M, Rosenthal M. Effects of physical exercise for elderly patients with physical impairments. *J Am Geriatr Soc.* 36:130–135, 1988.

75. Martenson JA Jr, Evans RG, Lie MR, et al. Treatment outcome and complications in patients treated for malignant epidural spinal cord compression (SCC). *J Neurooncol.* 3:77–84, 1985.

76. Bos GD, Ebersold MJ, McLeod RA, et al. Lesions of the spine. In: Sim FH, ed. *Diagnosis and Management of Metastatic Bone Disease: A Multidisciplinary Approach.* New York, NY: Raven Press; 1988:221–236.

77. Delaney TF, Oldfield EH. Spinal cord compression. In: DeVita VT, Jr, Hellman S, Rosenberg SA, eds. *Cancer: Principles & Practice of Oncology.* 3rd ed. Philadelphia, Pa: J.B. Lippincott; 1989:1978–1986.

78. Malawer MM, Delaney TF. Treatment of metastatic cancer to bone. In: DeVita VT, Jr, Hellman S, Rosenberg SA, eds. *Cancer: Principles & Practice of Oncology.* 3rd ed. Philadelphia, Pa: J.B. Lippincott; 1989:2298–2317.

79. Sim FH. *Diagnosis and Management of Metastatic Bone Disease: A Multidisciplinary Approach.* New York, NY: Raven Press; 1988.

80. Dietz JH Jr. *Rehabilitation Oncology*. New York, NY: John Wiley & Sons; 1981.

81. Stoll BA. Natural history, prognosis, and staging of bone metastases. In: *Bone Metastasis: Monitoring and Treatment*. Stoll BA, Parbhoo S, eds. New York, NY: Raven Press; 1983:1–20.

82. Broderick JP, Phillips SJ, Whisnant JP, O'Fallon WM, Bergstralh EJ. Incidence rates of stroke in the eighties: the end of the decline in stroke? *Stroke*. 20:577–587, 1989.

83. Walker AE, Robins M, Weinfeld, FD. Epidemiology of brain tumors: the national survey of intracranial neoplasms. *Neurology*. 35:219–226, 1985.

84. Cairncross JG, Posner JB. Brain tumors in the elderly. In: Albert ML, ed. *Clinical Neurology of Aging*. New York, NY: Oxford University Press; 1984:445–457.

85. Tomita T, Raimondi AJ. Brain tumors in the elderly. *JAMA*. 246:53–55, 1981.

86. Twomey C. Brain tumours in the elderly. *Age Ageing*. 7:138–145, 1978.

87. Friedman H, Odom GL. Expanding intracranial lesions in geriatric patients. *Geriatrics*. 27:105–115, 1972.

88. Posner JB, Chernik NL. Intracranial metastases from systemic cancer. *Adv Neurol*. 19:579–591, 1978.

89. Werner MH, Schold SC Jr. Primary intracranial neoplasms in the elderly. *Clin Geriatr Med*. 3:765–779, 1987.

90. Jongbloed L. Prediction of function after stroke: a critical review. *Stroke*. 17:765–776, 1986.

91. Cairncross JG, Kim JH, Posner JB. Radiation therapy for brain metastases. *Ann Neurol*. 7:529–541, 1980.

92. Graham K, Caird FI. High-dose steroid therapy of intracranial tumor in the elderly. *Age Ageing*. 7:146–150, 1978.

93. Redford JB. Assistive devices for the elderly. In: Calkins E, Davis PJ, Ford AB, eds. *The Practice of Geriatrics*. Philadelphia Pa: W.B. Saunders; 1986:166–174.

94. Logemann JA. *Evaluation and Treatment of Swallowing Disorders*. San Diego, Calif: College-Hill Press; 1983.

95. Castell DO. Dysphagia in the elderly. *J Am Geriatr Soc*. 34:248–249, 1986. Editorial.

96. Gray RP, Stefans V, Sowell TW. Rehabilitation of dysphagia in state of the art reviews. In: Maloney FP, Means KM, eds. *Rehabilitation and the Aging Population*. Philadelphia, Pa: Hanley & Belfus; 1990:105–112.

97. Clodius L, Piller NB, Casley-Smith JR. The problems of lymphatic microsurgery for lymphedema. *Lymphology*. 14:69–76, 1981.

98. Gloviczki P, Fisher J, Hollier LH, Pairolero PC, Schirger A, Wahner HW. Microsurgical lymphovenous anastomosis for treatment of lymphedema: a critical review. *J Vasc Surg*. 7:647–652, 1988.

99. Stillwell GK. Treatment of postmastectomy lymphedema. *Mod Treat*. 6:396–412, 1969.

100. Reinstein L. Rehabilitation of the lower extremity cancer amputee. *Md Med J*. 29:85–87, 1980.

101. Subbarao JV, McPhee MC. Prosthetic rehabilitation: comparison of the outcome in patients with cancer and vascular amputation of extremities. *Orthop Rev*. 11:43–51, 1982.

102. Moore TJ, Barron J, Hutchinson F III, Golden C, Ellis C, Humphries D. Prosthetic usage following major lower extremity amputation. *Clin Orthop*. 238:219–224, 1989.

103. Thorpe W, Gerber LH, Lampert M, Reed J, Sabel I. A prospective study of the rehabilitation of the above-knee amputee with rigid dressings: comparison of immediate and delayed ambulation and the role of physical therapists and prosthetists. *Clin Orthop*. 143:133–137, 1979.

104. Fisher SV, Gullickson G Jr. Energy cost of amputation in health and disability: a literature review. *Arch Phys Med Rehabil*. 59:124–133, 1978.

105. Christ G, Klein LL, Loscalzo M, Weinstein LL. Community resources for cancer patients. In: DeVita VT, Jr, Hellman S, Rosenberg SA, eds. *Cancer: Principles & Practice of Oncology*. 3rd ed. Philadelphia, Pa: J.B. Lippincott; 1989:2225–2237.

106. Harvey, RF, Jellinek HM, Habeck RV. Cancer rehabilitation: an analysis of 36 program approaches. *JAMA*. 247:2127–2131, 1982.

107. Lie MR. Principles of rehabilitation. In: Sim FH, ed. *Diagnosis and Management of Metastatic Bone Disease: A Multidisciplinary Approach*. New York, NY: Raven Press; 1988:91–97.

108. Siegel K. *Continuing Care of Cancer Patients—Concrete Needs: Progressive Report*. New York, NY: Memorial Sloan-Kettering Cancer Center; 1987.

109. Christ G, Siegel K. Monitoring quality-of-life needs of cancer patients. *Cancer*. 65:760–765, 1990.

110. Torrens PR. Hospice programs. In: Haskell CM, ed. *Cancer Treatment*. 3rd ed. Philadelphia, Pa: W.B. Saunders; 1990:904–912.

111. Billings JA. Specialized care of the terminally ill patient. In: DeVita VT, Jr, Hellman S, Rosenberg SA, eds. *Cancer: Principles & Practice of Oncology*. 3rd ed. Philadelphia, Pa: J.B. Lippincott; 1989:2237–2242.

112. Rhymes J. Hospice care in America. *JAMA*. 264:369–372, 1190.

113. Kane RL, Wales J, Bernstein L, Leibowitz A, Kaplan S. A randomised controlled trial of hospice care. *Lancet*. 1:890–894, 1984.

SECTION IV

AGING WITH A DISABILITY

32
Aging After Traumatic Spinal Cord Injury

Gary M. Yarkony

Aging was not initially considered to be a concern of those sustaining a traumatic spinal cord injury (1). Death from infections, renal failure, thromboembolism, pneumonia, pressure ulcers, and the numerous other sequelae of spinal cord injury was thought to be inevitable within days to weeks or months. The fortunate survivors were expected to die within a few years. Spinal cord injured individuals were often discharged home and given no hope for the future (2).

Fortunately, this feeling of hopelessness is no longer pervasive in the medical community. Munro, Guttman, Bors (3, 4) and other pioneers in spinal cord injury established systems of care that, along with medical advancements such as antibacterial chemotherapeutics, have led to improved medical and functional outcomes. Spinal cord injured individuals are now leading longer and more productive lives. This chapter will address the aging process and how it impacts on individuals with spinal cord injuries. It is not intended to be a review of the general principles of spinal cord injury care and rehabilitation.

SURVIVAL AFTER SPINAL CORD INJURY

Spinal cord injured individuals are surviving longer, and the causes of death have been changing with modern spinal cord care (5, 6). After the first world war, pyelonephritis was the leading cause of death (7). Spinal cord injured individuals generally died within weeks of their injury. Life expectancy after spinal cord injury has improved markedly since World War II. The life expectancy, in fact, approaches normal for many with a spinal cord injury. Although there are numerous studies with estimates of the life expectancy of spinal cord injured individuals, these studies are based on large populations. No effort is made to delve into the individuals' living situations and determine the care they receive, equipment available, and access to medical care.

Renal failure, generally associated with amyloidosis, was reported as the leading cause of death after the initial acute phase of spinal cord injury in the 1960's

(8–10). In the 1970's, renal failure was again reported as the leading cause of death although it accounted for 31% as opposed to 50% of deaths (11). It was not until 1983 that cardiovascular disease was reported the leading cause of death after spinal cord injury, followed by renal and respiratory causes (12). The authors gave estimates of life expectancy based on their statistical analysis. They estimated that a complete paraplegic at age 20 years would live for 40 years and at age 50 years would live for 15 years. For a complete quadriplegic at age 20 years, projected life expectancy was 30 years, and at age 50 years it was 9 years. They noted this to be am improvement over 1973 statistics.

These general projections cannot be applied to all spinal cord injured individuals. The person's specific situation must be assessed. The most recent study to address causes of death after a spinal cord injury studied patients during the first 7 years after injury. Pneumonia was the leading cause of death, followed by unintentional injuries and suicides, septicemia, and heart disease for the entire population studied. The leading cause of death for the entire population studied for the age groups under 25 years and between 25 and 54 years was unintentional injuries and suicides. Pneumonia was the leading cause of death for patients at all levels of injury over 55 years of age. Among quadriplegic patients, pneumonia was again the leading cause of death, while unintentional injuries, suicide, and cancer were the leading causes among paraplegic patients. During the first 6 months after injury, pneumonia was the leading cause of death, while unintentional injuries and suicides, followed by pneumonia, were the leading cause of death after 6 months. Septicemia related to severe pressure ulcers or urinary tract infections caused more deaths than expected of all age groups. This indicated to the authors of the study that many deaths after spinal cord injury are preventable with appropriate skin care, equipment, long-term follow-up, environmental modifications, and improved patient compliance (7).

The prevalance of traumatic spinal cord injury in the United States has been estimated in several studies.

Estimates vary due to disparities in the prognosis, incidence estimations (13), and sampling methods used. The most recent estimate by Harvey (14) is 721 cases per million or 177,000 spinal cord injured persons in comparison to DeVivo's (13) estimate of 906 cases per million or 222,515 persons. Other prevalence estimates range from approximately 129,000 to 276,000 persons with spinal cord injury in the United States. The institutionalized population is estimated at 2.6% (14). These studies indicate that spinal cord injury in the United States is an uncommon health care problem. This poses a problem for the aging spinal cord injured individual. Health care providers, particularly those not affiliated with regional centers where spinal cord injury is often treated, may not be familiar with the medical, psychologic, and social problems unique to a spinal cord injury.

THE OLDER NEWLY INJURED PERSON WITH SPINAL CORD INJURY

Older individuals who sustain a spinal cord injury may develop complications more frequently than those who sustain their injuries during their youth. In a recent comparison of spinal cord injured persons over 61 years of age to those younger than 30 years they were more likely to develop pneumonia, gastrointestinal hemorrhage, pulmonary emboli, and renal stones. Rehospitalization was also more common as was nursing home placement (15). Survival during the first 2 years was significantly diminished, particularly for the older neurologically complete individual (15). However, a recent study by Roth (16) comparing spinal cord injured individuals over 55 years of age with younger patients noted a significantly higher incidence of preexisting medical complications, but no difference in occurrence of medical complications.

Studies of rehabilitation outcomes support admitting the older spinal cord injured individual to a spinal cord injury rehabilitation unit (17). Of course, mental status and medical condition must be considered in the screening process. Motor function, not age, is the predominate limiting factor in the attainment of functional goals after a spinal cord injury. In complete paraplegics, however, more complex tasks such as dressing, bathing, stair climbing, and complex transfers are limited by age (17). Greater than 90% of complete paraplegics younger than 60 years can perform upper extremity dressing, while 60% of those 60 years or older can. Less than 50% of individuals over 50 years can bathe independently and do transfers or lower extremity dressing, while the majority of younger patients can perform these tasks. Individuals with the central cord syndrome do, however, have better functional outcomes at younger ages although older individuals with the central cord syndrome made significant functional improvement (18). Individuals whose age was greater than 45 years had less favorable outcomes in terms of functional independence as measured by the Barthel index, complication rate, length of stay in the hospital, and bladder continence and were less likely to be discharged home.

SPONSORSHIP OF MEDICAL CARE

Sponsorship of medical care can have a significant impact on numerous measures of rehabilitation outcome (19). Sponsorship refers to the funding source of medical payments such as private insurance, Medicare, Medicaid, or self-pay. The availability of health care services, equipment, and supplies can have a major impact during the aging process. The majority of individuals with a spinal cord injury are in constant need of medications, durable medical equipment, disposable supplies, and routine medical and radiologic follow-up. Durable medical equipment may pose a particular problem to the aging individual. Lightweight wheelchairs may not be available to them if their insurance carrier is unwilling to replace a heavier impractical but functional chair or if Medicare limits the selection of "approved" chairs to a model inappropriate for that individual. Many aging individuals may require a power wheelchair as they age but are unable to obtain financing for their equipment or have long delays in obtaining funding while their mobility becomes limited. The availability of accessible housing is often limited in the community. As the ambulatory individual relies more on the wheelchair or previously surmountable limitations in the environment now result in a limitation of accessibility, the older individual may become homebound.

Disposable medical supplies are often essential to maintain proper hygiene and perform bladder and bowel management. Both access to these supplies and the ability to finance their purchase may be limited with aging and a diminution of financial resources.

Medical follow-up for spinal cord injured persons is recommended at a minimum of an annual basis for physical examination and renal follow-up. If appropriate assistance and transportation is not available, treatable problems may be missed resulting in greater morbidity and cost.

THE AGING FAMILY

Although this chapter focuses on the aging person with a spinal cord injury, the fact that his or her family is aging as well cannot be overlooked. Spinal cord injured individuals often rely on family members for the majority of their care. Even those patients with home care provisions through their third party payor supplement the care provided. Problems arise as their children grow up and marry or leave home to attend college. One of the most unfortunate situations is the one in which a parent or spouse who has essentially assumed the entire care of the loved one ages or becomes disabled themselves and can no longer care for the child or spouse. In turn, the spinal cord injured individual cannot provide for parent or spouse. After 20 to 30 years of a relatively complication free course, pressure ulcers, contractures, and other physical and medical complications now begin to occur. Often, these situations arise in those people with limited financial resources and without private insurance. Nursing home placement may result in a newfound restriction in community accessibility, a change in health care routines, and the associated psychologic consequences. It is difficult to replace the care one has become accustomed to from a loved one with that of a hired caregiver. This situation is further compounded by turnover of personnel. Reliability has often been a problem in meeting needs on regularly scheduled shifts.

MEDICAL CONSIDERATIONS

Medical problems associated with aging may impact the life of the spinal cord injured individual in many ways. They may result in a loss of functional ability or lead to hospitalization or the need for more complex and expensive equipment. While improved longevity after spinal cord injury has resulted from improved medical care and a decrease in renal and other complications, the normal aging process is now a factor to be considered.

Degenerative joint disease is considered to be a universal occurrence by age 65 years (20) in the general population. It is unclear whether there is greater risk of developing degenerative joint disease after a spinal cord injury (21). Osteoarthritis of the shoulder or other joints of the upper extremities may cause the user of a manual wheelchair to require a power wheelchair. It may be prudent to prescribe the power wheelchair early in the course of osteoarthritis to limit the impact and progression of the disability. Osteoarthritis of the hip and other lower extremity joints may limit those individuals who remained ambulatory after their injuries. This may result in an increase in wheelchair use or total dependence on a wheelchair. Degenerative joint disease of the hips will occur in quadriplegics as well, perhaps related to limitations in movement that result in decreased synovial fluid circulation. For similar reasons, degenerative changes occur in the sacroiliac joints. Charcot's (neuropathic) joints may occur in areas distal to the lesions or in the shoulders of individuals with posttraumatic syringomyelia (22). The impact of degenerative joint disease will vary depending on the functional abilities of the patient.

Muscle mass decreases with age, resulting in decreased strength, a slowing of muscle contraction, and increased fatigue (23). Body fat content increases. This contributes to loss of strength, decreased mobility, and an increased risk of falling. Exercise may decrease but not completely prevent this muscle loss. Frail elderly individuals will benefit from strengthening exercises, but an ongoing exercise program is needed to sustain these gains (24). The effects of these changes in muscle on the spinal cord injured individual is obviously quite variable. Many spinal cord injured individuals will maintain their strength through regular exercise programs or through regular functional activities such as wheelchair propulsion. In others, this loss of muscle mass may necessitate the need for power equipment and increased assistance.

Osteoporosis below the level of the spinal cord lesion increases the risk of lower extremity fractures in spinal cord injured individuals. Surprisingly, the incidence has been reported to be less than 6% in most series (25). The trauma that causes these fractures may be minimal and may not be recognized by the individual. Fractures to the supracondylor area or shaft of the femur are most common. Management of these fractures has two aims. The fracture should heal with minimal associated complications. Splints or casts should be well padded, and mobility should be maintained to avoid further complications of immobilization such as pressure ulcers and joint contractures. Fractures should be treated in a way to maintain maximal functional independence. Open reduction and internal fixation are often difficult in the osteoporotic bone fracture but may be necessary in selected individuals (26). Bicycle ergometry training using functional electrical stimulation of the lower extremities does not increase bone mineral density (27).

Repetitive use of the upper extremities to compensate for lower extremity weakness may result in compression neuropathies. Individuals who push wheelchairs and perform other repetitive activities may develop a carpal tunnel syndrome. Activities requiring repetitive trauma to the elbow may result in ulnar nerve entrapment at the elbow. Diagnosis of these conditions may be obscured by dyesthetic pain syndrome or other musculoskeletal pain syndromes. These individuals are prone to tendonitis of the biceps and supraspinatus tendons as well. Careful physical examination, often assisted by electrodiagnostic studies, is needed to ascertain the nature of an individual's pain complaints. In addition to the standard medical management of these patients, physical and occupational therapy may determine methods to decrease this repetitive trauma. Faulty transfer techniques, improper seating in the wheelchair, and poor positioning during activities must be carefully investigated. Management is often difficult as a cessation of various functional activities that aggravate the condition is not always possible.

Intraabdominal complications are common in the aging spinal cord injured individual. Constipation and fecal impaction are by far the most common problem in the aging individual. Prevention of constipation is of course the mainstay of management of these patients (28).

This generally involves a high fiber diet, adequate fluid intake, and supplements with stool softeners as needed. Regular performance of the bowel program is encouraged. These problems often develop in individuals who decrease the frequency of bowel movements for personal convenience. Cholelithiasis has been reported to occur with increased frequency after a spinal cord injury (29). The natural history after a spinal cord injury is not known, and there are no studies to determine whether a cholecystectomy is needed in asymptomatic patients. It has been suggested that spinal cord injured individuals have an increased risk of colon cancer. This risk is hypothesized to relate to prolonged contact of fecal mutagens and the colonic mucosa due to decreased transit time (30). Further study is needed in this area as well.

Complications of the genitourinary system are common after a spinal cord injury. Traditionally, the annual follow-up visit of a spinal cord injured patient includes an annual radiologic follow-up examination. Initially, this was an intravenous pyelogram. This has largely been replaced by either a nuclear scan or a renal and bladder ultrasound, often accompanied by an abdominal roentgenogram. Recent evidence suggests that an annual exam may not be necessary and may be limited to symptomatic individuals (31). Our clinical experience indicates that many asymptomatic individuals develop renal and bladder stones. This indicates that regular renal follow-up is still needed. Several studies have suggested that spinal cord injured individuals may be at a greater risk for the development of bladder carcinoma (32, 33). Although the risk is minimal, the clinician must be aware of this possibility. Frequent urinary tract infections or an indwelling catheter may be a predisposing factor to development of bladder carcinoma. No guidelines exist for appropriate methods of screening (2).

Pressure ulcers are a complication that almost all spinal cord injured individuals develop at some time in their lives. The severity of these ulcers varies from superficial lesions that quickly resolve to severe areas requiring surgery. Their development in the lower extremities may be coincidental with the development of peripheral vascular disease. Treatment of these lesions in the extremities should be accompanied by an evaluation of the arterial system. The history of a prior ulcer and cigarette smoking may predispose the individual to development of pressure ulcers. In severe cases, pressure ulceration has lead to amputation of the extremities particularly in those individuals with chronic osteomyelitis. This generally occurs in individuals who neglect their personal care or who have underlying medical problems. There are no data to implicate aging alone as a factor in pressure ulcer development.

Ohry's hypotheses (34) that spinal cord injured persons develop cardiovascular disease and hypertension prematurely remains unproven. One study suggests a higher incidence of cardiovascular disease, hypertension, and diabetes mellitus but this has not been confirmed by multicenter studies in patients from various ethnic groups (35). Noninsulin-dependent diabetes mellitus has been reported to be increased in spinal cord injured patients. This is due to insulin resistance of unclear etiology (36). High density lipoproteins are reduced in sedentary spinal cord injured individuals as opposed to wheelchair athletes (37). This increases their risk of ischemic heart disease.

Ventilator-dependent quadriplegics are surviving longer as well (38). In a series of 199 ventilator-dependent individuals, 63% were alive at 9 years postinjury. Complications and long-term care needs remain higher for these individuals. Urinary tract infections, pneumonia, renal or bladder stones, and pressure ulcers are the most common complications and occur with greater frequency than in high quadriplegics not on ventilators. The costs of care for these individuals in the home setting particularly due to the high costs of nursing/attendant care and hospital readmissions are far higher than in high quadriplegics not on ventilators.

PSYCHOLOGIC ASPECTS

There are numerous factors that can impact upon the psychologic well-being of an aging spinal cord injured person. Although psychologic distress and cognitive dysfunction may occur with aging, their occurrence in someone with a spinal cord injury has additional consequences. Aging persons with medical or disabling conditions are at high risk for developing emotional disorders. The person's perceived health status and perceived self-sufficiency will affect adjustment with aging (39). The spinal cord injured individual's well-being is particularly affected by the loss or aging of a caregiver. Lack of financial resources will have a greater impact on their ability to care for themselves or obtain care after a spinal cord injury. Social contact with family and friends is important to maintain psychologic well-being, and this is a particular problem in a physically disabled person with access often limited by architectural and transportation barriers.

The ability to obtain employment and continue to meet the physical demands of employment is another important issue. Spinal cord injured individuals often retire early from their jobs due to the physical demands. Rossier has stated that "Paraplegics are often required to make heroic efforts to achieve results, which while spectacular and impressive within themselves cannot be repeated during a working life whose ordinary needs are already fatiguing for a normal person (40 p 87)."

Physical disabilities cause difficulties in interpersonal relationships, limit the ability to marry and have children, and increase the likelihood of divorce. Substance abuse of drugs or alcohol may impact the ability to reintegrate into society. Death from suicide clearly occurs all too commonly after a spinal cord injury.

Spinal cord injury clearly impacts three major behavioral components of health: (a) survival activities, (b) harmonious living and working environment, and (c) productivity (2). It is well known that psychologic distress can lead to further medical complications after a spinal cord injury. Depressed individuals may not follow their catheterization and turning schedules or may neglect to take their medications and thereby develop further complications. The aging process clearly will impact these individuals in a way that far exceeds aging in nondisabled individuals.

Individual counseling may be necessary at various stages during the spinal cord injured individual's life. Support groups for the families are often available at local spinal cord centers or through local spinal cord societies. Readmission to the rehabilitation hospital, outpatient therapy, or respite care for the family may aid the aging spinal cord injured person's adaptation.

SUMMARY

Aging and its impact on persons with spinal cord injury and other disabilities is an area in which extensive clinical research is underway. Hopefully this will help to answer many of the questions we have about the aging process (41). This chapter has provided an overview of many of the medical, psychologic, and social aspects of aging with a spinal cord injury. It was not meant to imply that all spinal cord injured individuals will be subject to the possible complications described. Our clinical experience and their markedly improved life span indicate that this is clearly not the case. The dedication of the developers of modern spinal cord care and the resolution of the injured persons and their caregivers has allowed spinal cord injured patients to "age" alongside other members of society.

References

1. Guttmann L. New hope for spinal cord sufferers. *Paraplegia.* 17:6–15, 1979.
2. Trieschmann RB. *Aging with a Disability.* New York NY: Demos Publications; 1987:6–32, 44–59, 106–133.
3. Freed MM. Traumatic and congenital lesions of the spinal cord. In: Koffke FJ, Lehmann JF, eds: *Krusens Handbook of Physical Medicine and Rehabilitation.* 4th ed. Philadelphia, PA: W.B. Saunders; 1990:717–764.
4. Guttmann L. *Spinal Cord Injuries Comprehensive Management and Research.* 2nd ed. Boston, Mass: Blackwell Scientific; 1976.
5. DeVivo MJ. Life expectancy and causes of death for persons with spinal cord injuries. In: Apple D, Hudsen L, eds. *Spinal Cord Injury: The Model.* Proceedings of the National Consensus Conference on Catastrophic Illness and Injury, Dec. 1989. Atlanta GA: The Georgia Regional Spinal Cord Injury Care System, Shepherd Center for Treatment of Spinal Injuries, Inc; 1990.
6. DeVivo MJ, Kortus PL, Stover SL, Rutt RD, Fine PR. Seven-year survival following spinal cord injury. *Arch Neurol.* 44:872–875, 1987.
7. DeVivo MJ, Kortus PL, Stover SL, Ruff RD, Fine PR. Cause of death for patients with spinal cord injuries. *Arch Intern Med.* 149:1761–1766, 1989.
8. Breithaupt DJ, Jousse AT, Wynn-Jones M. Late causes of death and life expectancy in paraplegia. *Can Med Assoc J.* 85:73–77, 1961.
9. Jousse AT, Wynne-Jones M, Breithaupt DJ. A follow-up study of life expectancy and mortality in traumatic transverse myelitis. *Can Med Assoc J.* 98:770–772, 1968.
10. Tribe CR. Causes of death in the early and late stages of paraplegia. *Paraplegia.* 1:19–47, 1963.
11. Geisler WO, Jousse AT, Wynne-Jones M. Survival in traumatic transverse myelitis. *Paraplegia.* 14:262–275, 1977.
12. Geisler WO, Jousse AT, Wynne-Jones M, Breithaupt D. Survival in traumatic spinal cord injury. *Paraplegia.* 21:364–373, 1983.
13. DeVivo MJ, Fine PR, Maetz M, Stover SL. Prevalency of spinal cord injury: a reestimation employing life table techniques. *Arch Neurol.* 37:707–708, 1980.
14. Harvey C, Rothschild BB, Asmann AJ, Stripling BA. New estimates of traumatic SCI prevalence: a survey-based approach. *Paraplegia.* 28:537–544, 1990.
15. DeVivo MJ, Kortus PL, Ruff RD, Stover SL, Fine PR. The influence of age at time of spinal cord injury on rehabilitation outcome. *Arch Neurol.* 47:687–691, 1990.
16. Roth EJ, Lovell L, Heinemann AW, Lee MY, Yarkony GM. The older adult with a spinal cord injury. *Paraplegia.* (In press).
17. Yarkony GM, Roth EJ, Heinemann AW, Lovell L. Spinal cord injury rehabilitation outcome: the impact of age. *J Clin Epidemiol.* 41:173–177, 1988.
18. Roth EJ, Lawler MH, Yarkony GM. Traumatic central cord syndrome: clinical features and functional outcomes. *Arch Phys Med Rehabil.* 71:18–23, 1990.
19. DeVivo MJ, Stover SL, Fine PR. The relationship between sponsorship and rehabilitation outcome following spinal cord injury. *Paraplegia.* 27:470–479, 1989.
20. Lewis RB, Applin JW. Degenerative joint disease. *Phys Med Rehabil State Art Rev.* 4:49–55, 1990.
21. Wyle EJ, Chakera TMH. Degenerative joint abnormalities in patients with paraplegia of duration greater than 20 years. *Paraplegia.* 26:101–106, 1988.
22. Rush PJ. The rheumatic manifestations of traumatic spinal cord injury. *Symp Arth Rheum.* 19:77–89, 1989.
23. Carter WJ. Effect of normal aging on skeletal muscle. *Phys Med Rehabil State Art Rev.* 4:1–7, 1990.
24. Fiatarone MA, Marks EC, Ryan ND, Meredith CN, Lipsitz LA, Evans WJ: High-intensity strength training in nonagenarians. *JAMA.* 263:3029–3034, 1990.
25. Ragnarsson KT, Sell GH. Lower extremity fractures after spinal cord injury: a retrospective study. *Arch Phys Med Rehabil.* 62:418–423, 1981.
26. McMaster WC, Stauffer ES. Management of long bone fracture in spinal cord injured patient. *Clin Orthop.* 112:44–52, 1975.
27. Leeds EM, Klose J, Ganz W, Serafini A, Green BA. Bone mineral density after bicycle ergometry training. *Arch Phys Med Rehabil.* 71:207–209, 1990.
28. Price N, Schubert ML, Vijay M. Gastrointestinal disease in the spinal cord injury patient. *Phys Med Rehabil State Art Rev.* 1:475–488, 1987.
29. Apstein MD, Dalecki-Chippenfield K. Spinal cord injury is a risk factor for gallstone disease. *Gastroenterology.* 92:966–968, 1987.
30. Frisbie JH, Chopra S, Foo D. Colorectal carcinoma and myelopathy. *J Am Paraplegia Soc.* 7:33–38, 1984.
31. Ozer MN, Shannon SR. Renal sonography in asymptomatic persons with spinal cord injury: a cost-effectiveness analysis. *Arch Phys Med Rehabil.* 72:35–37, 1991.
32. Kaufman J, Fam B, Jacobs S, et al. Bladder cancer and squamous metaplasia in spinal cord injury patients. *J Urol.* 118:967–971, 1977.
33. El Masri W, Fellows G. Bladder cancer after spinal cord injury. *Paraplegia.* 19:265–270, 1985.

34. Ohry A, Shemesh Y, Rozin R. Are chronic spinal cord injured patients (SCIP) prone to premature aging. *Med Hypoth.* 11:467–469, 1983.

35. Yekutiel M, Brooks ME, Ohry A, Yarom J, Corel R. The prevalence of hypertension, ischaemic heart disease and diabetes in traumatic spinal cord injured patients and amputees. *Paraplegia.* 27:58–62, 1989.

36. Duckworth WC, Solomon SS, Jallepalli P, Heckemeyer C, Finnern J, Powers A. Glucose intolerance due to insulin resistance in patients with spinal cord injuries. *Diabetes.* 24:906–910, 1980.

37. Brenes G, Dearwater S, Shapera R, LaPorte RE, Collins E. High density lipoprotein cholesterol concentrations in physically active and sedentary spinal cord injured patients. *Arch Phys Med Rehabil.* 67:445–450, 1986.

38. Whiteneck G. Long-term outlook for persons with high quadriplegia. In: Whiteneck G, Lammertse DP, Manley S, eds. *The Management of High Quadriplegia.* New York, NY: Demos; 1989:353–367.

39. Hazlewood MG, Fielstein EM. Psychological aspects of aging. *Phys Med Rehabil State Art Rev.* 4:19–28, 1990.

40. Rossier AB. *Rehabilitation of the Spinal Cord Injury Patient.* Summit, NJ: Ciba-Geigy; 1975:87.

41. Menter RR. Aging and spinal cord injury: implications for existing model systems and future federal state and local health care policy. In: Apple D, Hudson L, eds. *Spinal Cord Injury: The Model.* Proceedings of the National Consensus Conference on Catastrophic Illness and Injury, Dec. 1989. Atlanta, Ga: The Georgia Regional Spinal Cord Injury Care System, Shepherd Center for Treatment of Spinal Injuries, Inc; 1990:72–80.

33
The Elderly Amputee

James A. Leonard, Jr.

Who is the elderly amputee? Is this the geriatric amputee, the older person who undergoes amputation? Is this the individual who was born with a limb deficiency or had an amputation as a youngster and has now grown older? The medical literature almost exclusively discusses the former. In truth, a discussion of the elderly amputee or aging with amputation should include both of these groups.

It is best to first consider the case of the geriatric amputee for several reasons. The majority of civilian amputations are performed in the lower extremity of individuals over the age of 50 years with peripheral vascular disease. Research regarding this population of aged individuals with amputations is available to look at outcome (1–9). Many of the same complicating medical problems and prosthetic issues faced by the geriatric amputee will also be dealt with by the younger amputee who lives to retirement years.

GERIATRIC AMPUTEE

The majority of amputations performed in the United States in nonwar time are in the lower limb. Surveys have shown that the amputations most commonly occur in the sixth decade of life or later, and men usually outnumber women (6, 7, 9). About 57,000 major lower extremity amputations were performed in 1988 in nonfederal US hospitals, a number that has not changed appreciably over the last decade (10). Up to 90% or more of all amputations are due to complications of peripheral vascular occlusive disease associated with arteriosclerosis, diabetes, thromboembolism, or thromboangitis obliterans (10). Aging with an amputation for this population is a concern from day one.

Amputation Surgery

Amputation surgery is often thought of as a relatively straightforward and benign procedure. It should be viewed as a plastic or reconstructive procedure to be done by an experienced surgeon as it will impact on the patient's level of function for the remainder of his or her life (11). Amputation surgery in the elderly individual has been associated with a significant increase in mortality and morbidity. Studies of geriatric amputees have shown varying rates of postoperative mortality. Most studies conclude that there is approximately 10% mortality postoperatively (30 days) (2, 7, 8, 11, 12). An increase in mortality over that of the general population continues for up to 2 years following amputation, at which time the mortality rate of the geriatric amputee population again returns to that of the general population or is slightly better than that of the general population (4, 7, 8, 12). Geriatric amputees have also been shown to have an increased likelihood of having a second amputation in 2 (15% to 28%) (7, 8) to 5 years (28% in nondiabetics and 46% to 66% in diabetics) (8).

To reduce the increased risk in older and otherwise debilitated patients, the argument was to do one surgical procedure that accomplished primary wound healing and would not require exposure to additional surgery. This rationale, in the past, led to most lower limb vascular amputees having above-knee amputations. At the same time, it was recognized from a rehabilitation perspective that elderly below-knee amputees were more likely to walk with prostheses than were above-knee amputees. Through the efforts of a number of surgeons reviewing and writing of their amputation experience (7, 9), together with the utilization of new techniques to assess the likelihood of healing of the amputation wound (9, 13, 14), the trend has been to attempt to save the knee when appropriate and possible.

More below-knee amputations are done now in this group of patients than in the 1960's. Despite all the efforts to show the advantage of below-knee amputation, the ratio of below-knee to above-knee amputation has varied only slightly from year to year during the past decade, with about equal numbers of below-knee and above-knee amputations being done. Nationally in 1988, 32,000 above-knee amputations and 25,000 below-knee amputations were performed (10). Stern (10), reviewing the data for a tertiary teaching hospital, noted a more positive trend than the national data showed with both a reduction in the total number of lower limb amputations being performed and a significantly greater number of below-knee than above-knee amputations being done over the last several years.

Rehabilitation

It is the older individual undergoing amputation of the lower limb for vascular disease that accounts for the vast majority of patients needing prosthetic restoration and rehabilitation services in this country. Many older individuals with peripheral vascular occlusive disease who have had a lower limb amputation may also have had a history of claudication, rest pain, or gangrene. They are likely to have associated vascular disorders such as cardiovascular, cerebrovascular, or renovascular disease (15). They may have had several hospitalizations for various vascular surgical procedures attempting to save their limb. If diabetic, they may also have a significant peripheral neuropathy in addition to other medical complications associated with diabetes. The net result of these multiple medical problems is often an elderly individual who may be weak, with poor endurance, and of limited mobility.

Most amputees indicate that they want a prosthesis and wish to walk again, whether this is a realistic goal or not. Successful rehabilitation is usually thought of by the amputee as ambulating independently with a prosthesis. To what degree must amputees use a prosthesis to be successfully rehabilitated? Can all geriatric amputees use a prosthesis? How old is too old? How much should they wear a prosthesis? And once fit, how long will they continue to use them? Will coexisting medical problems or disabilities such as a stroke affect prosthetic and rehabilitation outcome? The challenge for the amputee clinic team is to answer these questions. The cost of a prosthesis has become considerable, and the amount of time necessary for the geriatric amputee to achieve maximum rehabilitation with a prosthesis can be substantial (2, 6, 9, 16). These realities mean that amputee clinic teams must establish realistic rehabilitation goals as well as develop and utilize appropriate selection criteria when prescribing prostheses.

In developing criteria, the general experience of the field with this age group is helpful. In general, a unilateral below-knee amputee who was ambulating prior to an amputation is most likely to walk with a prosthesis after an amputation. The above-knee amputee is less likely to walk. Bilateral amputees are more likely to walk if they had previously been fit with and were walking with a prosthesis before the second amputation. Bilateral below-knee amputees frequently are more successful ambulating with prostheses than are unilateral above-knee amputees. The chances of bilateral amputees with one above-knee amputation walking are small, but better if

they had successfully ambulated with an above-knee prosthesis before having the below-knee amputation. For bilateral above-knee amputees in the elderly population, wheelchair use is the most appropriate form of mobility primarily due to the significant increase in energy expenditure required to use prostheses (17, 18).

In addition to these general guidelines, contractures, history of nonwalking prior to surgery, severe cardiac disease, cognitive deficits, blindness, severe vascular disease in the other leg, and other disabilities such as stroke have all been proposed as guidelines for not fitting an older amputee with a prosthesis. It has been this author's experience that, while the above list represents significant obstacles to prosthetic restoration and rehabilitation, they must not be considered absolutes. Depending on the severity of these other problems and the objectives for prosthetic fitting it is possible to successfully fit individuals with the above problems with a prosthesis. If the goal is to achieve functional independent ambulation in the community without the use of any ambulatory aids, then success with these problems will be small. Prosthetic rehabilitation may be considered successful even if all the prosthesis is used for is transfer activities, permitting the amputee to return home to be cared for by a spouse or a family member rather than living in a nursing home. Some would consider prosthetic fitting successful if used only for cosmetic reasons if this improved the psychologic health or self-esteem of the individual. Sometimes, despite the best efforts of the clinic team, it is impossible to determine whether an amputee will use a prosthesis successfully without trying one. In this situation, the use of a provisional (temporary) prosthesis has been a helpful and less costly diagnostic tool than has a definitive prosthesis.

Prosthetic Rehabilitation Program

The rehabilitation process for the geriatric amputee is a team effort and should incorporate the same elements of a rehabilitation program as for the nongeriatric amputee. Ideally the program has four phases: preamputation, postoperative, prosthetic, and follow-up phases.

PREOPERATIVE PHASE

The preoperative phase of the program focuses on education of the patient. The goal is to provide the patient with some understanding of the process which he or she is to encounter following amputation. Instruction is provided to help the patient avoid postoperative problems such as joint contractures by using proper positioning of the extremities following surgery. Pillows under the residual limb are to be avoided to prevent promotion of flexion contracture. Information is provided regarding phantom sensation (a normal phenomenon), phantom pain, and residual limb pain, as well as prostheses and their function. The patient's physical capabilities and mobility can also be evaluated and deficits addressed preoperatively if time permits. It is frequently easier to teach patients exercises and crutch walking preoperatively when they are not bothered by postoperative pain.

POSTOPERATIVE PHASE

Postoperatively, the program addresses the same educational issues as would have been covered preoperatively if not already done. The patient should receive physical therapy postoperatively, initially at the bedside, for range of motion exercises and proper positioning to prevent contractures. As soon as the patient is able, the program is continued in the physical therapy gym to work on range of motion, strengthening, endurance training, transfer activities, ambulation, and/or wheelchair mobility.

In the postoperative period, one of the prime objectives is the management of the residual limb. For the elderly vascular amputee, the chief objective is to get the wound to heal. The use of modern diagnostic techniques will help with appropriate level selection to achieve this goal. The residual limb can be managed by the use of soft surgical dressings, compressive dressings, or rigid dressings (19). It has been our preference to use rigid removable dressings for several reasons. These dressings, if put on at the time of surgery or in recovery, can prevent the development of postoperative edema, have been said to reduce postoperative pain, aid in shaping, and provide protection for the residual limb. On many occasions, a rigid dressing has maintained the integrity of an incision during a fall at the bedside. It has been our experience that wound dehiscence in a vascular patient following trauma to the residual limb has delayed healing of the wound by up to 6 months or has required revision to a more proximal level. It is not uncommon for an elderly person to awaken in the middle of the night to get up to go to the bathroom and attempt to take a step with their residual limb only to fall on it. When questioned, patients usually comment that they thought the leg was there—the phantom sensation. It is wise to have patients use the bedrails when in the hospital and to improvise a bedrail when they go home (such as a chair at the bedside) so that, if they go to get up at night, they are slowed down until they can think about what they are doing (20). As the residual limb shrinks, socks can be added to the rigid dressing to maintain adequate fit and continue to promote shrinkage. The second choice for postoperative residual limb dressings would be compressive dressings such as elastic wraps or shrinker socks, which can be effective at shrinking and shaping the limb, but must be frequently reapplied when they become loose.

PROSTHETIC PHASE

It is possible to apply a pylon to a rigid dressing (removable or nonremovable) to provide a temporary or provisional prosthesis in the immediate postoperative period (21). If this is done, the vascular patient needs to be observed very closely to assure that not too much weight is born on the residual limb, which can lead to breakdown and delayed wound healing. It has been our experience that it is best to follow a program of early prosthetic fitting rather than immediate fitting.

The patient is usually fit with a provisional prosthesis when the incision has fully healed. The provisional prosthesis is made with materials that are easy to modify to accommodate fitting changes and has components that permit easy alignment adjustments. For the elderly amputee, the general rule regarding prosthetic prescription is that the prosthesis should be simple, lightweight, comfortable, safe, securely suspended, and easy to put on and take off.

The fit of the socket in a lower extremity prosthesis is critical, especially for the vascular patient who may also have a peripheral neuropathy and is unable to detect a poorly fitting socket before skin breakdown occurs. The fit of the socket is usually evaluated with a check socket or test socket fitting. The most commonly prescribed sockets for below-knee amputees are total contact patellar tendon bearing (PTB) or total surface bearing sockets. All sockets for this age group are usually prescribed with a liner to provide additional protection for the residual limb.

For most amputees, suspension systems for below-knee prostheses that are secure and relatively easy to manage include sleeves, supracondylar cuffs, waist belts, or supracondylar suspensions. The supracondylar suspension is simple to don, but some elderly amputees do have difficulty tolerating the pressure of the supracondylar wedge over the medial femoral condyle.

There are a number of different types of prosthetic feet available. Generally those that are lightweight are the most appropriate. Some elderly amputees do well with multiaxis feet allowing motion in several directions, but it has been our experience that feet of relatively simple design such as a SACH foot, Seattle Light foot, or equivalent prosthetic feet serve this group the best.

For the above-knee amputees it is important that they have adequate knee stability at the time of heel strike and during stance phase so that they do not fall. This can be accomplished by aligning adequate knee stability into the prosthesis when it is fabricated as well as choosing a knee with more inherent stability such as a four bar knee with extension assist, a safety knee, or, if needed, a locking knee. The amputee must also be aware that the heel height of the shoe plays an important role in knee stability of the prosthesis as well. A higher heeled shoe will make a prosthetic knee less stable by altering the alignment (relative position of the knee center and the TKA line) of the prosthesis. The socket for above-knee prosthesis should be total contact and have a quadrilateral or ischial containment design. The above-knee suspension systems that are the easiest for most geriatric amputees to manage are those that involve some form of support around the waist such as a Silesian belt, TES belt, or pelvic band and belt with hip joint. There are some drawbacks to these suspension systems, which are discussed later in this chapter.

After the amputees have received their prostheses, they need to be referred to physical therapy for appropriate gait training with the prostheses. Initially, the amputee starts out wearing the prosthesis for very short periods of time, 10 to 30 minutes, gradually increasing wearing time. Initial work is done in the parallel bars, working on weight shifting, then stride length, etc. Only after the patient has attained a somewhat normal appearing gait in the bars does the training move outside the bars, usually at first with a walker, progressing to crutches, cane, or no aid as able. The gait training should not be considered complete until the amputee has been trained on all surfaces and taught how to fall.

FOLLOW-UP PHASE

Once the amputee has been successfully fit and trained with the prosthesis, he or she should be seen in follow-up once to twice per year to assure that there are no problems and to provide routine maintenance for the prosthesis. Additional specifics of geriatric amputee programs have been well covered by other authors (20, 22–24).

THE AMPUTEE WHO GROWS OLDER

Little or nothing is written about the amputee who grows older, so one cannot turn to the medical literature for assistance when reviewing the rehabilitation management of these individuals. As is frequently the case in clinical medicine, it is our patients who are often the best teachers. Individuals such as the gentleman in Figure 33.1, a farmer who sustained an upper limb amputation at a young age and later had amputations of both lower extremities due to peripheral vascular occlusive disease, have helped frame the management of the aging amputee. As we have had to address specific prosthetic and rehabilitation needs of several of these older amputees, we have come to identify a number of recurring issues and answers that apply to many amputees. The impact of aging on the amputee appears to be changes in physiology, life-style, functional needs, and expectation. The discussion to follow is in no way intended to be a compendium of issues and answers, but should provide some suggestions and guidelines for those who will deal with this group of individuals.

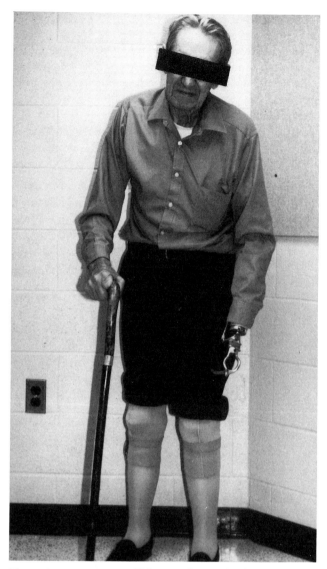

Figure 33.1. An 84-year-old farmer who sustained a traumatic left below-elbow amputation as a young man and later had a right below-knee amputation at age 77 and a left below-knee amputation at age 79 for complication of peripheral vascular disease. He was living independently at home with assistance of a housekeeper.

Aging

Williams (25) has pointed out that there are several myths about aging that are not necessarily true. In careful studies, healthy elderly individuals do not necessarily demonstrate a decline in mental or functional capabilities (25). There are, however, some physiologic changes that all elderly individuals will experience that closely parallel the biologic changes associated with inactivity (26). Lean body mass will decrease by 20% to 30% between the ages of 30 and 80 years as muscle atrophy occurs and there is increased adipose deposition. There is a loss of bone density as well, greater in women (25%) than in men (12%) (27). There are also changes in cardiac, renal, hormonal regulation, and, to a lesser degree and not as well documented, cerebral function that occur with aging. Changes in gait have also been noted with aging, including generalized decrease in trunk and associative movements; reductions in step length, cadence, vertical displacement, excursion of the leg during swing and swing to stance ratio, and a wider base of support (28). The result is a slower, more stable gait at the cost of increased energy expenditure.

Chronic Disease

Acquired chronic disease occurs more frequently as people age, with 80% of the population over 65 years having at least one condition (25). The most common of these disorders are arthritis (40%), impaired hearing or vision or both (20% to 30%), diabetes (10% to 15%), chronic heart conditions (15% to 20%), and cognitive disorders (5% or more) (25).

Individuals with amputations can expect to experience the same physiologic changes associated with aging as nonamputees and to develop the same chronic diseases. Whether amputees are at a greater risk for developing additional medical problems has not been clearly identified. Kegle (29) surveyed 134 amputees of varying ages and etiologies 6 months to 12 years following amputation to determine their functional capabilities. Seventy-four percent of the respondents identified no medical problem other than their amputation (29). The remainder reported additional medical problems such as blindness, cardiac disease, strokes, asthma, seizures, back problems, arthritis, ulcers, and renal failure (29). Some disorders such as vascular, neurologic, or rheumatologic disease may have a specific impact on the amputee, while others such as cancer, chronic pulmonary, or cardiac disease may have a more indirect effect resulting in weakness, weight loss, and general debility.

For amputees, development of an additional chronic disease may have greater implications regarding their independence than for the population at large. This is particularly true for some vascular, neurologic, or rheumatologic disorders. These disorders may initially present in such a way as to be confused as amputation-related or prosthetic management problems rather than new disorders. A few examples of how these other disorders can impact on the management and function of the aging amputee may help clarify this point.

Vascular occlusive disease may manifest itself by involving the peripheral, cardiac, or cerebral vessels. Peripheral vascular disease, presenting with claudication, may involve the amputated or nonamputated lower extremity. If the amputated lower extremity is involved, it may be mistaken as pain from a poorly fitting prosthesis or local residual limb pain interfering with ambulation. In the nonamputated leg, claudication may be the limiting factor determining whether the amputee will be able to walk with or without a prosthesis. Peripheral oc-

clusive disease may also progress on to rest pain, ischemia, and tissue necrosis. A nonhealing ulcer on the residual limb may require revision to a more proximal level or, if on the nonamputated lower limb, may necessitate a second amputation. Such revision or new amputation is likely to impact on the amputee's function.

Cardiovascular disease can be associated with a significant decrease in cardiac function making it impossible for the amputee to tolerate the increased energy expenditure required to ambulate with a prosthesis (17, 18). There may also be chronic heart failure, with fluid retention leading to fluctuation in residual limb volume making it difficult to maintain an adequate prosthetic socket fit.

Cerebral vascular accident is another manifestation of vascular disease that can have a significant functional impact on the amputee. Several authors have looked at the dual disability of stroke and lower extremity amputation in an attempt to determine prognostic factors that might predict rehabilitation outcome. Many of the studies have suggested that amputees with a below-knee amputation and fit with a prosthesis before having a stroke are more likely to continue ambulating than those who sustain an amputation following a stroke (30, 31). Others have not found this to be so (32).

In addition to stroke, other neurologic disorders such as motor neuron disease, multiple sclerosis, peripheral neuropathy, or dementia can result in an alteration in strength, balance, coordination, perception, and cognition making it more difficult or impossible for the amputee to continue to function independently. Motor neuron disease in an above-knee amputee may first present as prosthetic gait abnormalities. Vaulting on the sound (nonamputated) side, circumduction of the prosthesis during swing phase, or instability of the prosthetic knee at heel strike may be the first signs of weakness associated with the disease. Initially the problem may be considered to be a prosthetic problem with the solution being to change the prosthetic alignment or to change the prosthetic knee to increase stability; the correct prosthetic decision for the wrong reason. Only with the passage of time and the development of additional neurologic symptoms and signs will the correct diagnosis manifest itself. Changes in cognitive function as seen with dementia may require that a previously independent amputee get assistance for the once simple tasks of donning and doffing the prosthesis.

Connective tissue disorders involving the weight-bearing joints of the lower extremities may have a direct impact on the use of a lower limb prosthesis. Pain with weight bearing or painful range of motion may make ambulation with the prosthesis difficult or impossible. These disorders may affect hand function as well, which can result in difficulty with donning the prosthesis. Amputation itself may result in increased wear and tear on joints leading to the development of degenerative arthritis, as in the case of a lower limb amputee who chooses not to use a prosthesis and ambulates with crutches and develops severe degenerative changes in the shoulders necessitating wheelchair use for mobility. Osteoarthritis of the lumbosacral spine or hip joint with resulting decrease in range of motion can be disastrous for the bilateral upper limb amelic who has relied on foot use for independent activities of daily living function.

In the elderly amputee, nutrition can be an issue that has impact on prosthetic use. If, as the amputee ages, the level of activity is reduced and caloric intake is not reduced, significant weight gain may occur to the point that the prosthetic socket may be too small. More often the problem for the elderly amputee is poor nutrition with accompanying weight loss, reduction in adipose tissue, and a socket that is too large, resulting in end bearing, skin irritation, and breakdown. The experienced amputee will often attempt to compensate for loss of limb volume by adding additional limb socks, sometimes resulting in a choke syndrome. Often with weight loss it is only the distal portion of the limb that becomes significantly smaller in circumference not the proximal bony portion. If too many full length socks are added, this results in a tight fit proximally in the socket and lack of contact distally resulting in a choke. Often shortening the length of the limb socks to cover only the distal residual limb will solve the problem temporarily until the prosthetist can either refit or make a new socket as needed.

The skin of the elderly amputee is frequently thinner and more fragile than that of the younger amputee and may require additional measures to avoid irritation and breakdown, especially from shear forces. The use of a polyamide sheath, liner, or different liner materials such as silicone to reduce the shear may be necessary.

The elderly are known to fall more frequently than the young and are likely to sustain more serious injuries (8% to 40% resulting in fractures in the elderly) (33). Ideally, a lower limb amputee would never fall, but reality dictates that the amputee should expect to fall on occasion, and so all amputees should be taught how to fall safely as part of their gait training program. We have seen a number of older below-knee amputees who have come to clinic complaining of knee pain and prosthetic fit problems who have sustained what they considered to be a relatively minor fall days to weeks prior to being seen. The typical complaint was that of knee pain and the feeling that they were going too deeply into the socket and the prosthesis seemed to be short. The problems persisted despite the addition of more limb socks. In the clinic, the foot of the prosthesis was also noted to be externally rotated and the fit of the socket appropriate. Examination in all cases demonstrated hip joint irritability and a short limb with x-ray films showing a hip fracture. Most patients were treated with total hip re-

placement and were able to resume ambulation with their prosthesis.

Prosthetic Modifications for Lower Limb Amputees

PROSTHETIC MODIFICATIONS

There are no standard modifications that should or must be made to lower limb prostheses to accommodate for changes that can be seen with aging. Indeed, many amputees will go their entire lives and never require anything special done to their prostheses. They will continue to use the same type of prostheses they used as young people. For some this will not be the case. Because of disease, additional disability, or frailty, modification will need to be made to allow continued prosthetic use. The modifications to be made are usually

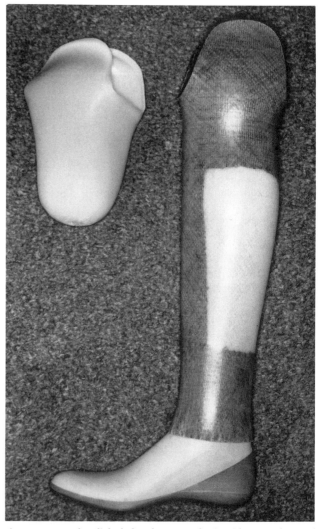

Figure 33.2. Ultra light below-knee prosthesis with SACH foot, gel liner, and hollow laminated shank reinforced with carbon graphite fibers (black).

very specific and suited to meet the needs of an individual amputee. Often the problems presented require ingenuity and patience on the part of the amputee team and especially on the part of the prosthetist.

BELOW-KNEE AMPUTEE

In the majority of situations, no modifications may be necessary for the prosthesis of typical below-knee amputees. Far and away the greatest concern expressed by the elderly amputee, new or old, is regarding the weight of their prosthesis. Many amputees who have done well for many years with a conventionally constructed prosthesis that may weigh as much as 5 or even 6 pounds find this weight intolerable as their strength and endurance fade. Lightweight components, construction techniques (Ultra light design, hollow shanks, Figs. 33.2 and 33.3), use of lightweight materials (carbon fibers, thermoplastics, titanium), and lightweight prosthetic feet can reduce the

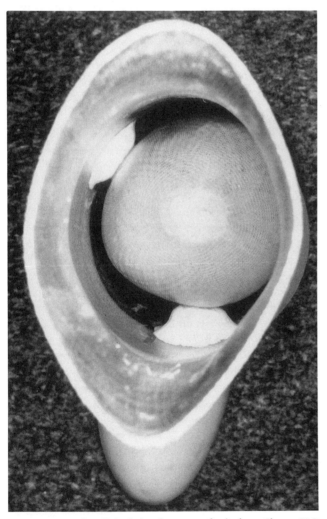

Figure 33.3. Ultra light below-knee prosthesis from Figure 33.2 looking up into the socket from the ankle through the hollow shank at the bottom of the laminated socket.

weight of the prosthesis to a few pounds or less. Improved suspension, however, may be as or more important than reducing the overall weight of the prosthesis. With many forms of suspension there is an up and down movement of the prosthesis on the residual limb, pistoning, that occurs during the gait cycle. The more pistoning that occurs, the greater the sensation of heaviness of the prosthesis the amputee experiences. Improving suspension alone will often help reduce the sensation of the weight of the prosthesis by reducing pistoning. There are several simple ways to improve below-knee prosthetic suspension including adding an elastic waist belt to a prosthesis with a supracondylar cuff, adding an elastic or rubber sleeve to a prosthesis with a supracondylar cuff or supracondylar suspension, or replacing a supracondylar cuff or waist belt with a sleeve. Most elderly amputees are readily able to manipulate the sleeve and find it provides a secure form of suspension for their prostheses.

For below-knee amputees, limited hand function whether due to weakness, arthritis, hemiparesis from a stroke, or the presence of prosthesis (Fig. 33.1) can result in problems with donning or doffing a below-knee prosthesis with some forms of suspension. We have observed this to be true especially with some of the sleeve suspensions. The addition of tabs or loops to the sleeves aids in pulling up the sleeves for such individuals, allowing the amputee to continue to be independent and not require the assistance of another (Fig. 33.4). Straps attached to the proximal medial and lateral brims of the socket aid in pulling the socket on the limb, but more importantly permit the individual with limited hand function to independently roll down the suspension sleeve and remove the prosthesis. (Fig. 33.5). The manner in which the sleeve can be rolled down with these straps has given rise to their name "Banana" straps—the sleeve is rolled down in a fashion very similar to peeling a banana.

Some below-knee amputees will have worn their prostheses as young adults with a hard socket (without a liner). As they get older, they may develop fragile skin, a more bony residual limb from weight loss, or a peripheral neuropathy. To provide greater protection for the residual limb and a more comfortably fitting socket, use of a liner may become appropriate. Also, it may become appropriate to switch from a heavier multiaxis dynamic foot used for ambulation on uneven terrain to a lighter more stable foot to provide a more secure stance and gait with improved proprioception.

Development of severe arthritis and/or ligamentous instability of the knee joint on the amputated side may require the addition of a thigh corset to the prosthesis to accomplish either some reduction in weight bearing through the involved knee or external support for the lax joint

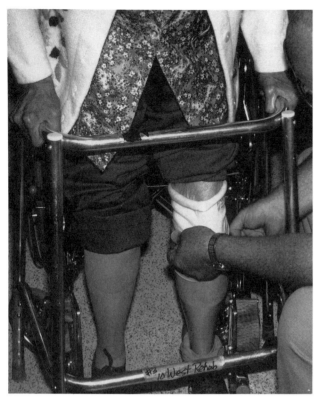

Figure 33.4. Elderly bilateral below-knee vascular amputee requiring assistance to pull up the latex rubber sleeve suspension on her left prosthesis. This woman was later able to don her prostheses independently after the addition of tabs to her rubber sleeve suspensions.

ABOVE-KNEE AMPUTEE

Many above-knee amputees will have worn prostheses with suction sockets when younger. Reduced hand function may result in difficulty with donning and doffing the prosthesis for an above-knee amputee who previously did well with a suction socket. There may be difficulty pulling into the prosthesis completely. This may result in residual limb pain proximally or distally with or without skin irritation or breakdown due to improper positioning of the limb in the socket.

Difficulty donning the suction socket may also occur with disorders that result in reduced hip or low back range of motion preventing the patient from bending over to pull into the socket. Often a simple device that compensates for poor hand function or extends the patient's reach (Figs. 33.6 and 33.7) will solve the problem.

More often than not, the elderly patient who can no longer pull into a suction socket because of poor hand function, limited range of motion, or poor balance is switched to a prosthesis with a different type of suspension such as a Silesian belt, pelvic band and belt with hip joint, or a TES belt to permit easier donning. This change, although solving the donning problems, frequently results in a new prosthetic problem. The am-

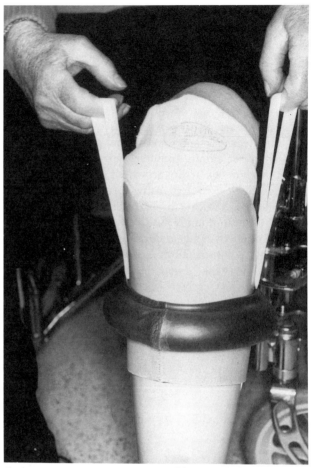

Figure 33.5. "Banana" straps added to below-knee prosthesis. These straps make it easier for the amputee to pull on the socket and also help in rolling down the neoprene rubber sleeve (rolled black tube at base of straps).

putee may don the prosthesis with the correct orientation of the foot relative to the residual limb, but after a few steps it may be noted that the foot of the prosthesis has become internally rotated and the orientation of the knee has also changed such that it is no longer in the line of gait progression. This may result in gait deviations that include circumduction of the prosthesis during swing phase and/or vaulting on the nonamputated limb during stance to aid in clearing the floor with the prosthesis during gait. These gait deviations result in an increased energy expenditure during walking, which may have the effect of reducing limited walking efficiency in some amputees to a point where ambulation is no longer practical or safe.

A solution for the potential drawbacks of switching to a belt-suspended above-knee socket has been the use of a hypobaric sock in place of the conventional limb sock. This sock permits the advantages of using a socket worn and donned with a sock while at the same time giving some of the advantages of a suction socket. The silicone band on the sock provides a seal to limit air movement in the socket, thus giving suction, while the friction of the band tends to limit internal rotation of the prosthesis on the residual limb, maintaining proper orientation.

In a postpolio patient, another solution to the problem of donning the above-knee suction socket was accomplished by modifying the suction socket by using a very flexible inner socket surrounded by a rigid frame with a blood pressure cuff bladder sandwiched inbetween. This patient noted decreasing strength in the upper extremities felt to be related to postpolio. A more conventional socket design with belt suspension was not successful due to the presence of a severe scoliosis. The use of a flexible liner and the air bladder permitted easy donning following which the bladder was inflated resulting in a beltless suspension similar to the patient's previous suction socket.

Many above-knee amputees will have also used hydraulic or pneumatic knees with their prostheses. These types of knee units allow the prosthesis to adapt to varying cadence or speeds of walking. These knee units are excellent and durable but also significantly heavier and may be less stable than those units typically chosen for older amputees. If an above-knee amputee's strength, endurance, balance, proprioception, or stability de-

crease, it may be necessary to change the knee unit for a more stable one to assure safety and reduce weight. The same considerations may need to be given to changing from more sophisticated prosthetic feet to those of simpler and lighter design.

SUMMARY

Some have been pessimistic about fitting the geriatric amputee with prostheses as they believe that prosthetic use is limited at best and at worst may contribute to the loss of the other lower extremity (34). Most, however, are positive to the idea of considering prosthetic restoration for the elderly (1, 16, 23, 35). Several long-term studies have shown reasonably successful use of prostheses after several years, although there is often a decrease in the amount of walking done by these patients when compared to the time when they were first fit (1, 36). The best answer is that prosthetic restoration

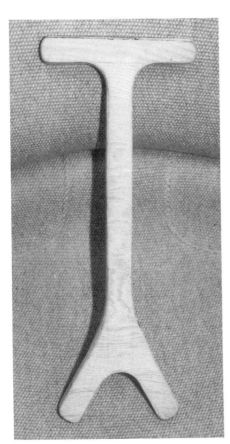

Figure 33.6. Assistive device to extend the reach and compensate for weak grasp of an above-knee amputee to aid in donning a suction socket.

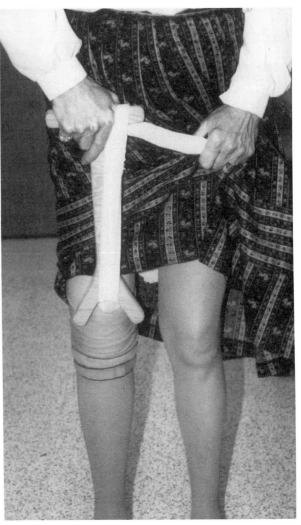

Figure 33.7. Above-knee amputee using assistive device in Figure 33.6 to assist pulling her residual limb into a right above-knee suction socket with a pull sock.

and rehabilitation for the geriatric amputee is a very individualized process that must take into account the patient's health, physical condition, motivation, and support systems. Although these elderly amputees may have limited and different functional goals compared to the younger amputees, it is still appropriate to consider prosthetic restoration and rehabilitation.

The young amputee who ages is not limited in ability to walk or function in life so much by his or her amputation level, but more by the acquiring of other diseases or disabilities. The impact of chronic disease on the amputee population may be greater than for the general population. Additional disease will often alter the amputee's functional abilities and require new compensations that may be difficult for the amputee to achieve. With a bit of ingenuity and perseverance, the amputee clinic team can assist the elderly amputee with prosthetic modifications and adaptations that will allow continued independent function and improved quality of life.

References

1. Brodzka WK, Thornhill HL, Zarapkar SE, Malloy JA, Weiss M A. Long-term function of persons with atherosclerotic bilateral below-knee amputation living in the inner city. *Arch Phys Med Rehabil*. 71:895–900, 1990.

2. Couch NP, David JK, Tilney NL, Crane C. Natural history of the leg amputee. *Am J Surg*. 133:469–473, 1977.

3. Dove HG, Schneider KC, Richardson F. Rehabilitation of patients following lower extremity amputation: an analysis of baseline, process and outcome. *Am Corr Ther J*. 36:94–102, 1982.

4. Harris PL, Read F, Eardley A, Charlesworth D, Wakefield J, Sellwood RA. The fate of elderly amputees. *Br J Surg*. 61:665–668, 1974.

5. Helm P, Engel T, Holm A, Kristiansen VB, Rosendahl S. Function after lower limb amputation. *Acta Orthop Scand*. 57:154–157, 1986.

6. Kerstein MD, Zimmer H, Dugdale FE, Lerner E. What influence does age have on rehabilitation of amputees? *Geriatrics*. 30:67–71, 1975.

7. Kihn RB, Warren R, Beebe GW. The "geriatric" amputee. *Ann Surg*. 176:305–314, 1972.

8. Mazet R. The geriatric amputee. *Artif Limbs*. 11:33–41, 1967.

9. Malone JM, Moore WS, Goldstone J, Malone SJ. Therapeutic and economic impact of a modern amputation program. *Ann Surg*. 189:798–802, 1979.

10. Stern PH. The epidemiology of amputations. *PMR Clin NA*. 2:253–261, 1991.

11. Malone JM. Complications of lower extremity amputation. In: Moore WS, Malone JM, eds. *Lower Extremity Amputation*. Philadelphia, Pa: W.B. Saunders; 1989.

12. Mandrup-Poulsen T, Jensen JS. Mortality after major amputation following gangrene of the lower limb. *Acta Orthop Scand*. 53:879–884, 1982.

13. Moore WS, Malone JM, eds. *Lower Extremity Amputation*. Philadelphia, Pa: W.B. Saunders; 1989.

14. Piotrowski JJ, Bernhard VM. Noninvasive methods of determining amputation levels. In: Ernst CB, Stanley JC, eds. *Current Therapy in Vascular Surgery*. 2nd ed. Philadelphia, Pa: B.C. Decker; 1991.

15. Kerstein MD, Zimmer H, Dugdale FE, Lerner E. Associated diagnoses complicating rehabilitation after major lower extremity amputation. *Angiology*. 25:536–547, 1974.

16. Katrak PH, Baggot JB. Rehabilitation of elderly lower-extremity amputees. *Med J Aust*. 1:651–653, 1980.

17. Fisher SV, Gullickson G. Energy cost of ambulation in health and disability: a literature review. *Arch Phys Med Rehabil*. 59:124–133, 1978.

18. Waters RL, Perry J, Chambers R. Energy expenditure of amputee gait. In: Moore WS, Malone JM, eds. *Lower Extremity Amputation*. Philadelphia, Pa: W.B. Saunders; 1989.

19. Leonard JA, Andrews KL. Rigid removable dressings, immediate postoperative prostheses, and rehabilitation of the amputee. In: Ernst CB, Stanley JC, eds. *Current Therapy in Vascular Surgery*. 2nd ed. Philadelphia, Pa: B.C. Decker; 1991.

20. Mort M. *Retraining for the Elderly Disabled*. Dover, NH: Croom Helm; 1985.

21. Moore WS, Hall AD, Lim RC. Below the knee amputation for ischemic gangrene. Comparative results of conventional operation and immediate postoperative fitting technique. *Am J Surg*. 124:127–134, 1972.

22. Brown PS. The geriatric amputee. *Phys Med Rehabil State Art Rev*. 4:67–76, 1990.

23. Clark GS, Blue B, Bearer JB. Rehabilitation of the elderly amputee. *J Am Geriatr Soc*. 31:439–448, 1983.

24. Warren M. The problem of the aged amputee. *Postgrad Med J*. 33:436–443, 451, 1957.

25. Williams TF. The aging process: biological and psychosocial considerations. In: Brody SJ, Ruff GE, eds. *Aging and Rehabilitation Advances in the State of the Art*. New York, NY: Springer; 1986.

26. Granger CV. Goals of rehabilitation of the disabled elderly: a conceptual approach. In: Brody SJ, Ruff GE, eds. *Aging and Rehabilitation Advances in the State of the Art*. New York, NY: Springer; 1986.

27. Cape RT. Overview. In: Cape RT, Coe RM, Rossman I, eds. *Fundamentals of Geriatric Medicine*. New York, NY: Raven Press; 1983.

28. Lewis CB. *Aging: The Health Care Challenge*. 2nd ed. Philadelphia, Pa: F.A. Davis; 1990.

29. Kegel B, Carpenter ML, Burgess EM. Functional capabilities of lower extremity amputees. *Arch Phys Med Rehabil*. 59:109–120, 1978.

30. OConnell PG, Gnatz S. Hemiplegia and amputation: rehabilitation in the dual disability. *Arch Phys Med Rehabil*. 70:451–454, 1989.

31. Varghese G, Hinterbuchner C, Mondall P, Sakuma J. Rehabilitation outcome of patient with dual disability of hemiplegia and amputation. *Arch Phys Med Rehabil*. 59:121–123, 1978.

32. Altner PC, Rockley P, Kirby K. Hemiplegia and lower extremity amputation: double disability. *Arch Phys Med Rehabil*. 68:378–379, 1987.

33. Tideiksaar R. *Falling in Old Age: Its Prevention and Treatment*. New York, NY: Springer; 1989.

34. Davis WC, Blanchard RS, Jackson FC. Rehabilitation of the geriatric amputee: a plea for moderation. *Arch Phys Med Rehabil*. 48:31–36, 1967.

35. Childress DS. Technology for functional ability and independent living. In: Brody SJ, Ruff GE, eds. *Aging and Rehabilitation Advances in the State of the Art*. New York, NY: Springer; 1986.

36. Holden JM, Fernie GR. Extent of artificial limb use following rehabilitation. *J Orthop Res*. 5:562–568, 1987.

34

Pediatric-Onset Disabilities

Maureen R. Nelson and Michael A. Alexander

"Let each become all that he was created capable of being: expand, if possible, to his full growth, and show himself at length in his own shape and stature, be these what they may."
—Thomas Carlyle.

Until recently, adults with pediatric-onset disabilities often have been neglected by the medical profession. There are few data on long-term outcome or on the proper care of their long-term medical needs. These individuals continue to have difficulty in obtaining medical care that meets their needs and desires. Only recently has there been an emerging interest in their long-term rehabilitation and medical care. In past years, many of these individuals spent their lifetime in institutions or isolated at home and died relatively young because of missed medical problems, delayed care, and/or limited health care resources.

CEREBRAL PALSY

Of the many childhood-onset disabilities, cerebral palsy (CP) has been followed the longest. In this chapter we will use it as the main teaching example, and most of what can be said about problems in those with CP can be said about those with many other pediatric-onset disorders.

A study looking at access to health care in adults with CP interviewed 100 patients older than age 30 years. Over 90% of those interviewed reported increasing physical disability with aging, particularly with mobility, urination, and digestion problems. Forty-two percent reported dental problems, and 35% believed that their condition interfered with their opportunity to form a sexual relationship and perform sexually. Fifty-eight percent reported some feeling of depression, and 50% had obtained professional help. Forty-three percent of these patients reported problems with accessibility to health care (1).

Musculoskeletal Problems

The physical working capacity of people with physical disabilities decreases over time because of poor mechanical efficiency and repeated trauma. In adults with CP, seizures adding to frequent falls contribute to aging arthropathy. There is a higher frequency of contractures and osteoporosis (2). Early onset of arthritic changes further complicates preexisting mechanical inefficiency.

A survey of 90 adult patients who were between 30 and 71 years old with CP in the community at large revealed several common skeletal complaints (3). Chronic back pain was a frequent complaint of wheelchair users and was believed to be due to poor sitting posture. Ninety-six percent of the wheelchair users were found to have contractures, and 80% had scoliosis. Approximately 60% of current wheelchair users had walked in the past, most having stopped as teenagers because of inefficiency in gait or from problems of increasing age. Some did not cease walking until they were 45 years old. Thirty-five percent of those surveyed had been community ambulators since they were children (3).

Scoliosis is one of the common musculoskeletal problems seen in adults with cerebral palsy. The scoliotic curve may progress after skeletal maturity, may continue to deform into adulthood, and may progress both above and below previous spinal fusion levels. Curves in nonambulatory patients with poor sitting balance are more likely to progress after skeletal maturity (4). A retrospective study of institutional patients with CP followed for 4 to 40 years after skeletal maturity showed that curves progressed the most in patients who had the largest degree of curvature at skeletal maturity. These investigators found a rate of progression of 1.4 degrees per year if the curve was greater than 50 degrees at skeletal maturity and 0.8 degrees per year if the curve was less than 50 degrees at skeletal maturity. They also found that the largest curves at skeletal maturity were found in spastic quadriplegic patients with thoracolumbar and lumbar curves, and again, particularly in those who were bedridden (5).

The cervical spine has been reported to be a problem in patients with CP in adulthood. In a survey of 90 adult patients, 67% complained of neck pain, and many were found to have early degenerative joint disease of the cervical spine region (3). There have been several studies that present the problem of cervical spondylosis and myelopathy in adult patients with CP. Myelopathy often presents with decreasing strength and loss of bladder control. This problem is seen in people who have used their neck muscles as a body lever for heavy work such as to move themselves. Adults with CP appear to be particularly susceptible because of frequent and severe stress on their neck, particularly in athetoid patients (6–8) who use their head to move themselves in bed and on the floor. This problem has also been reported in three patients with spastic CP and profound mental retardation who developed symptomatic cerebral spine impairment between the ages of 29 and 33 years (9). A common theme in each of these descriptions is that of a history of repetitive forceful flexion and extension of the cervical spine. A delay in diagnosis in these patients can be avoided if there is a high index of suspicion for vague symptoms with slow intermittent deterioration. It is our experience that a laminectomy has a low success rate in advanced cases. Avoidance of hyperextension of the neck by use of a firm but well-padded collar may be helpful.

Several studies have also looked at the natural history of hip dislocation in the patient with CP. Cooperman studied 38 noninstitutionalized patients with spastic quadriplegic CP and found 51 dislocated hips, 9 of which had been reduced. After a mean follow-up of 18 years in this patient population with an average age of 26 years, he found that only four patients were ambulating, and they were using assistive devices. These four patients had normal intelligence and a level pelvis. Of 18 hips that were unilaterally dislocated and not reduced, 12 had pelvic obliquity and scoliosis. Of 7 patients with unilateral hip dislocation that was reduced, only 2 had pelvic obliquity and scoliosis. Fifty percent of the dislocated hips in this series were reported as painful (8).

A study by Skoff (10) looked at total hip replacement surgery in patients with neuromuscular impairment including CP. He reviewed 9 patients with 12 hips replaced with an average patient age of 42 years. After an average follow-up of 3.5 years, all patients reported decreased pain with increased range of motion and increased function. The patients who were institutionalized were more easily cared for, and there were no major complications.

Howard et al (11) reviewed 85 patients, 6 to 28 years old, to study the natural history of spontaneously dislocated hips in patients with CP. They found that of 44 bilateral hemiplegic patients, at least one hip was dislocated in 59%. None of the patients with dislocated hips were able to walk without assistive devices, and 18 were unable to walk at all. Additionally, 9 of the 18 in the group with normal hips were unable to walk. Of 29 diplegic patients, they found that one patient had a dysplastic hip, and another patient had bilaterally dislocated hips. Both of these patients were able to walk with assistive devices. Lastly, they looked at 12 patients with unilateral hemiplegia, none of whom had any type of hip dysplasia or instability and all of whom could walk independently (11). One should follow hips in the adult patients with CP on an annual basis when there is a known dislocation or subluxation. Nonambulatory patients with a dislocated hip will often develop pain over time. The use of nonsteroidal medications and avoidance of overaggressive range of motion programs is mandatory as late hip reduction has a low salvage rate. Therapy should only be provided to maintain enough range of motion to facilitate hygiene.

Spastic deformities of feet and toes have been described, which can become problems in adulthood. These include hallux valgus, metatarsus adductus, and flexion contractures. Additionally, some cases of cavus foot caused by surgical overcorrection of a tight heel cord with resultant muscle imbalance have been reported (12, 13).

Dental Problems

In adults with CP, there is a high incidence of dental problems. People with CP have a higher than usual incidence of enamel hypoplasia of their teeth, tooth decay, gingivitis, malocclusion, bruxism, and temporomandibular joint dysfunction. In adulthood, bruxism, particularly in athetoid and spastic cerebral palsy patients, can lead to temporomandibular joint dysfunction. Additionally, use of candy as a reward in childhood and syrup-based medications lead to increased incidence of tooth decay in childhood. Decreased fine motor ability for activities of daily living (ADLs) leads to decreased dental hygiene to prevent decay and plaque.

Chronic drooling can be a problem in cerebral palsy. There are several procedures to minimize this, including diverting salivary flow from the parotid glands by surgically creating tunnels to the tonsillar fossa and resecting the submandibular glands. An alternative method is resecting the submandibular gland with bilateral parotid duct ligation, which has been found to have excellent results (14). Both of these procedures are associated with the complication of increased plaque accumulation with increased risk of gingival disease.

Bowel and Bladder Problems

Bowel and bladder problems frequently occur in nonambulatory adults with CP. In a study by Murphy et al (3), it was found that the more severely disabled patients had decreased their fluid intake so that they could decrease their toileting. This led to constipation and occasional stress incontinence in some patients. Constipation, diverticulosis, and hemorrhoids have a higher than usual incidence in these patients. In a survey by Thomas, Bax, and Smyth (15) 56% of young adults with CP had bowel problems, and 53% reported incontinence. Yokoyama et al (16) in a study of 132 patients with CP between the ages of 5 and 59 years (mean, 23.2 years) found 31.8% had urinary incontinence, 14.4% had decreased urinary stream, and 16.7% had a urinary tract infection. They found that patients with poor ambulation had the highest incidence of urinary incontinence and decreased urinary stream. Yokoyama et al could not prove that these patients had bladder dyssynergia on the basis of urodynamic studies (16). In our experience, women with CP restrict fluids and try to hold off voiding until they get home at day's end. Increased risk of urinary tract infection has been reported in patients with poor hygiene and chronic constipation. It is recommended that renal function be carefully watched over time and that annual urinary checkups, particularly in the nonambulatory adult with CP, be considered.

Skin Problems

With aging, the skin loses elasticity and is more easily injured. Circulation changes contribute to poor skin healing. It should not be surprising that with aging, decubitus ulcers have also been reported in this population. These ulcers are associated mostly with restricted movement and poorly fitting wheelchairs, shoes, or braces. These can not only be painful and socially undesirable but decubiti can also be very expensive as well as life-threatening.

Dystonia

Progressive dystonia has been reported in seven adult patients with CP. A study in Israel found that dystonia and/or spastic paraparesis appeared or worsened in patients between the ages of 14 and 40 years after a long static period of disease. Five of these seven cases were Ashkenazi Jews in whom idiopathic dystonia is reportedly more frequent. Those authors, therefore, hypothesize that CP may perhaps trigger clinical expression in a gene that has incomplete penetrance (17).

Use of Anesthesia

Use of general anesthesia poses an increased risk in patients with CP. Posture, as well as contractures and movement disorders, may lead to positioning problems on the table. Cervical osteoarthritic changes present a risk to the spinal cord with neck extension during intubation. Because of an increased incidence of gastroesophageal reflux, as well as poor laryngeal and pharyngeal reflexes, patients need to be intubated. Patients with a seizure disorder who are on anticonvulsants may have increased hepatic enzyme activity with a concomitant change of their responsiveness to anesthetic drugs. There is an increased risk of pulmonary problems in people with CP, as well as an increased risk of intraoperative hypothermia, so temperature monitoring and heating must be carefully done (2). Weak cough and poor swallow postoperatively predispose these patients to aspiration pneumonia.

Sexuality and Pregnancy

Physicians were surveyed regarding sexuality in their developmentally disabled patient population. Forty-eight percent of the physicians rarely or never discussed sexuality with either the patients or their caretakers. Forty-five percent of the physicians did not recommend contraception to disabled men, and 29% did not recommend it to disabled women, although 59% did provide this information for their general patient population. Thirty percent to 40% of the physicians did not know if their disabled patients were sexually active (18).

A retrospective study of pregnancies in women with CP was done looking at eight obstetrical charts as well as 34 women admitted at a university hospital. Twenty-one of these 42 women were pregnant at least once, and 20 of them had mild to moderate CP (19). There were a total of 35 pregnancies in this group, with 24 term live births. Obstetric outcome was found to be similar to the general population with all patients going into spontaneous labor, with a mean postpartum stay of 3.5 days in patients with vaginal delivery and 5 days in patients with cesarean section (19). In reviewing the charts of 14 infants of mothers with cerebral palsy, seven were born by cesarean section and seven vaginally. Six of 13 term babies needed supplemental oxygen, and one had meconium aspiration (as did the one 32 week preterm baby). Mean apgar scores were 7.5 and 8.7, and all babies were of appropriate size for their gestational age. The only abnormalities found in these 14 babies were two abnormal hip exams, three cases of mild hypotonia, and two cases with respiratory problems (20).

Cognitive Effects

Because the brain insult of CP is usually rather diffuse, impaired cognitive function is the most common associated deficit of cerebral palsy if one includes mental retardation, learning disorders, and thought process difficulties (21). Mental retardation is associated with 30% to 70% of patients with CP, and there tends to be an increased risk of mental retardation with a higher number of motor-impaired extremities. Of adults with CP with similar motor handicaps and other problems, people with an IQ greater than 70 are more likely to be successfully employed (21). No specific pattern of change in intellectual abilities has been reported with aging; however, deterioration is possible because of superimposed disease.

Cognitive impairment continues to be a problem. Some patients who are very alert and socially responsive may appear to have higher cognitive function than they actually possess, and therefore they may become frustrated with the efforts of programs or people who assume that they have a higher cognitive function than is true. An adult with CP may master a job after special training, but when promoted to a new job may find her- or himself overwhelmed. On the other extreme, patients with severe motor involvement frequently are assumed to have a lower cognitive ability than they actually possess. This is equally frustrating for them. There have been reports of patients in institutions who were classified as retarded finally receiving recognition for higher cognition when they were found to laugh at bawdy jokes (22). It is difficult to perform intellectual tests in a severely motor impaired person; however, using motor-free or revised tests, it is possible. Any severely physically handicapped adult with CP needs to have such testing (23).

Communication Problems

Communication also can be a problem for the adult with CP. The communication problems in CP tend to be in three groups: motor production of speech, actual language and central processing, and, lastly, hearing loss. One person with CP may have any combination of these problems. Deafness has been found in 6% to 16% of patients with CP (21), and in one series, 22% of adults with CP were found to have mild to moderate hearing problems. Because of the combination of the aforementioned problems as well as cognitive deficits, it is frequently difficult to properly assess these problems. Many patients would benefit from augmentative communication systems; however, these often are not available, particularly for use at home even if they are available for school use. It has been found that once a person is out of the school system there is even less access to this type of assistance (15).

Activities of Daily Living

Thomas, Bax, and Smyth (15) studied restrictions in activities of daily living. They found that 71% of young adults with CP had restrictions in mobility, 60% in toileting, 65% in hand function, 67% in dressing, and 55% in feeding. Additionally, they found that these young adults were also limited in their ability to cook, prepare food, and manage their own finances. The authors felt that the patients could have done better but had low expectations of themselves, as did their families and healthcare professionals. In a study by Murphy et al (3) of 90 adult patients with CP, they found that ability to perform activities of daily living did not decrease with age.

Medical Care Problems

It has been widely documented that there is a decreased access to medical care in patients with CP after their school years are completed. A study by Thomas, Bax, and Smyth (15) in the United Kingdom found that regular hospital treatment for people with CP decreased from 49% before age 18 years to 22% after age 18 years. They found that young adults with CP had regular contact with a general physician in only 20% of cases and no contact in 18% of the cases. These people had reported themselves that their physical condition had deteriorated since they left school, with reported decreased mobility and worsening of contractures. Additionally, they had a decrease in dental care, as well as a decrease in physical therapy, occupational therapy, and speech therapy. In an unpublished study by Steven Buchrach (1990) from Delaware, both physicians and patients were surveyed to evaluate medical care for adults with disabilities. Forty-six percent of those adults contacted were currently receiving no medical care. Twenty-eight percent that were receiving care were not satisfied with it. Of the physicians interviewed, 85% said they had an accessible office; however, only 67% had a ramp, only 50% had grab bars in the restrooms, and only 25% had an elevator. Physicians concerns with regard to their seeing disabled patients were listed as time taken per visit by 28%, medication compliance by 17%, keeping appointments by 20%, and follow-up by 22%. Additionally, a lack of insurance was mentioned by 23% of those surveyed. Only 6% of the adults with disabilities contacted reported that they had no method of payment. Difficulty was reported by these adults in entering their physician's offices, that ramps were often too steep or unavailable, bathrooms were not accessible, and transportation was unreliable. Additionally, at times they could only enter through a back door and had no space to move in an exam room and did not have help to transfer onto an exam table.

McCluer (6) described several potential problems for the physician in interacting with an adult with CP (6). Decreased communication an verbal skills make an accurate history difficult to assess, as physicians may not be accustomed to understanding variations in speech in a patient with CP. Additionally, an accurate neurologic exam in some patients is difficult, and so minor changes may be missed. It has been described that a patient's own description of his or her previous level of function tends not to be believed unless a reliable witness confirms the patient's report. Additionally, new neurologic symptoms may not be appreciated by a physician who is unaccustomed to examining adults with childhood-onset disability and who may attribute symptoms to the disease itself rather than a new finding. Many physicians have insufficient training and experience with behavior problems. There may be negative stereotyped attitudes toward patients who appear different from the typical office patient. In communicating with the patient, a physician may improperly assume that the patient is unable to understand him or her. The physician may then not bother to speak to the patient or may become patronizing. Additionally, as noted previously, if the patient is very verbal, the physician may assume that the patient has more cognitive function than is actually present. The problems between patient and physician are not all one-sided. There is a lack of information on the part of the patients as to whom and when they can go for various services. They may not understand how payment is handled. Lack of mobility and knowledge of how long it takes to get to an office leads to arriving late for appointments. Maximizing available information can be extremely valuable to one's patient and community. This dispersal of information can be both through the adults with CP and through the medical community.

Social Problems

Social problems can also be found in adults with CP. In a 1982 survey of young adults, 49% of an able-bodied control group believed that they had a satisfactory social life with a good number of social contacts, whereas only 21% of young adults with disabilities agreed with this statement. Twenty-nine percent of those with disabilities believed they had a limited social life. The same study showed that 46% of the disabled young adults stated they had no special friend, which was true of only 21% of the controls (24).

Infrequent contacts with friends, which may remain at a superficial level, as well as visible disabilities evoking negative attitudes in others, contribute to the decrease in socialization. Lack of mobility and a lack of social skills can lead to social isolation (24). Additionally, along with a disability is the prejudice in our culture against anyone who is different. An encouraging sign, however, is a study in 1989 of a national cohort followed for 36 years, which showed that the psychosocial status of these former patients at age 36 followed those of the national norms even though when they were younger they had shown problems (25). Along with this may be a need for an emphasis on socialization, leisure activities, and social confidence, along with sex education in school programs. Sex education, especially regarding the specifics of a person's own specific physical abilities and limitations, is appropriate except for those who are severely and profoundly mentally retarded (21).

Employment

Employment in adulthood is obviously a major concern. Studies have shown that two thirds of those

with CP who hold a job went to regular school and most obtained a high school or higher degree. Most individuals with CP who went to special schools worked in sheltered workshops and only rarely in competitive jobs (26). In a study looking at the factors that differentiated between those who are employed and those who are not employed, it was found that an IQ over 70, attendance at a regular school, and physical ability, along with increase in independence in daily activities, and lower age were significant factors. It was found that the most important factor in working to attain competitive employment was the medical diagnosis. Other important factors were personal determination, as well as family support (27).

Work opportunities also have evolved from the traditional sheltered workshop to competitive jobs and now on-the-job-training and work-in-industry programs. Work-in-industry programs are regular working environments with an acknowledgment that the person with a disability will likely have a slower rate of work. This gives a more normal environment as well as more diverse work requiring various skills (21).

A recent German study (28) evaluating vocational status of 102 patients with CP showed that 23% were fully employed during the study, 19 of whom were moderately to severely physically disabled. The researchers concluded that achievement of full occupation was determined less by the severity of disability than by intellectual potential. They advocated mainstreaming into regular education as the best assistance to vocational status in the future.

A survey by O'Grady et al (27) in 1985 of adults in California with CP showed that 65% had been employed at some time, with 57% having been competitively employed. Only 28% were currently employed, and 35% had never been employed. This 72% unemployment rate in adults with CP compares with a 5.8% overall unemployment for the general population in that same region. The investigators found that the type of employment (competitive versus sheltered) was best predicted by medical diagnosis; best being in spastic hemiplegics with mild to moderate involvement who had a higher IQ and education in a regular school by the high school level (27).

OTHER DIAGNOSES

Down Syndrome

Patients with Down syndrome are more likely to develop epilepsy in adulthood than is the general population. This is believed to be related to degenerative neuronal changes (29). Coyle et al (30) report that the brains of virtually all patients with Down syndrome over the age of 40 years have pathologic findings diagnostic of Alzheimer's disease, including neurofibrillary tangles and neuritis plaques. These researchers point out that there is a controversy over whether this is associated with cognitive deterioration in patients with Down syndrome. It is known that cognitive deterioration is not invariably present in older individuals with Down syndrome.

There are several common orthopedic complaints found in adults with Down syndrome, particularly involving the neck, lower extremities, spine, and pelvis. The fact that many of these patients have ligamentous laxity is thought to be a significant contributing factor to these problems. Along with the ligamentous laxity, joint dislocation is commonly found; however, this is not usually a severe problem. Atlantoaxial instability has been reported in 9% to 20% of individuals with Down syndrome, and pain is a common symptom. Neurologic change may be associated with this. All patients with Down syndrome should have radiographs evaluating the C1-C2 region. Surgical stabilization can be performed in patients with significant C1-C2 instability. Additionally, degenerative changes of the cervical spine have been noted in this population. In one study, this was present in 50% of adults over age 25 years (31). Another orthopedic abnormality seen in individuals with Down syndrome is scoliosis with approximately 50% of the curves in the thoracolumbar region. These curves seldom require operation, as they do not progress after adulthood. Hip subluxation and dislocation have been reported. In the study of 162 patients, eight adult patients were found to have degenerative joint changes in the hip and were treated with nonsteroidal antiinflammatory medications. Six of these patients developed side affects including severe gastrointestinal bleeding in two patients; therefore, it is recommended that extreme caution be used in prescribing nonsteroidal medication in this population (31). The same study showed 36% of the patients with significant patellofemoral disorders that were symptomatic in approximately two thirds of the patients. The main problems contributing to patellofemoral instability appear to be ligamentous laxity and genu valgum. That study also reported common deformities of the ankle and feet, with 80% of the patients in their series having pronated flat feet and approximately 25% of the patients showing rigid pes planus and marked hallux valgus (31).

Spina Bifida

Patients with spina bifida have a dramatically increased life expectancy over that of 20 years ago. Medical problems that may arise in these patients as adults include hydromyelia, tethered cord, symptomatic Arnold Chiari syndrome, and inclusion dermoids, all of which can be treated operatively. One must be aware of the possibility of shunt failure and watch for the symptoms: decreased level of consciousness, headaches, eme-

sis, change in motor level, upper extremity weakness, facial diplegia, and even coma. Urinary and renal status need to be carefully monitored and treated as they can continue to change with age. Additionally, with increasing age of patients with long-term use of assistive devices, arthritis, rotator cuff injury, and entrapment neuropathies can be seen as complicating factors (32).

Duchenne Muscular Dystrophy

In Duchenne muscular dystrophy, it has been demonstrated that there is an increased incidence of upper gastrointestinal dysfunction. Signs and symptoms of this dysfunction include nasal quality of voice, dysphasia, choking while eating, needing to clear the throat during and/or after eating, heartburn, and vomiting during or after meals. Nonambulatory patients with Duchenne muscular dystrophy were found to have heartburn more frequently than ambulatory patients. Severity of skeletal muscle weakness and smooth muscle disease are related to the upper gastrointestinal symptoms (33). With changes in technology there also have been an increased number of patients with Duchenne muscular dystrophy living to an older age, including those who are on ventilator support at least part of the time (34).

SUMMARY

As medical professionals, how can we promote the best status of cerebral palsy patients, and others with pediatric-onset disabilities, for their future as adults? Probably by gradually increasing their decision-making involvement and responsibility. Beginning with very small decisions, increasing their responsibility for themselves, and encouraging the rehabilitation team, family, and schools to do the same. Interpersonal skills and education need to be stressed to them throughout their growth to adulthood. Career guidance should be available and should be informed and based on our knowledge of the long-term outcome for their disability. Practical daily living skills should be instructed. As mentioned earlier, education in regular schools maximizes a person's possibilities for competitive employment. Additionally, we need to remember that social skills can compensate for many physical and intellectual deficits, and therefore, we should encourage the development of these along with the more traditional education and therapy goals. We need to make sure that information is available to these individuals and their families throughout their lifetime of care. Our responsibility as physicians is in preventing medical complications and giving the best possible medical treatment throughout their lifetimes. The pediatric physiatrist must help in the transition of pediatric care to adult medical care. One of our main responsibilities is remembering that the cute child with cerebral palsy will become an adult with cerebral palsy, and therefore, we need to be sure that all involved in their care keep this long-term view in mind as well.

References

1. O'Grady RS, Fleischmann S, Lankasky K. A project to determine the medical and psychosocial problems of adults with cerebral palsy, and their access to and use of health services. *Dev Med Child Neurol.* 31:36, 1989.
2. Rubin IL, Crocker AC. *Developmental Disabilities: Delivery of Medical Care for Children and Adults.* Philadelphia, Pa: Lea & Febiger; 1989.
3. Murphy KP, Molnar G, Lankasky K, Fleischmann S. Medical and functional status of adults with cerebral palsy. *Dev Med Child Neurol.* 31(suppl):59, 1989.
4. Ferguson RL, Allen BL Jr. Considerations in the treatment of cerebral palsy patients with spinal deformities. *Orthop Clin North Am.* 19:419–425, 1988.
5. Thometz JG, Simon SR. Progression of scoliosis after skeletal maturity in institutionalized adults who have cerebral palsy. *J Bone Joint Surg.* 70:1290–1296, 1988.
6. McCluer S. Cervical spondylosis with myelopathy as a complication of cerebral palsy. *Paraplegia.* 20:308–312, 1982.
7. Fuji T, Yonenobu K, Fujiwara K. Cervical radiculopathy or myelopathy secondary to athetoid cerebral palsy. *J Bone Joint Surg Am.* 69A:815–821, 1987.
8. El-Mallakh RS, Rao K, Barwick M. Cervical myelopathy secondary to movement disorders: case report. *Neurosurgery.* 24:902–905, 1989.
9. Reese ME, Msall ME, Owen S, Pictor SP, Paroski M. Acquired cervical spine impairment in young adults with cerebral palsy. *Dev Med and Child Neurol.* 31(suppl):59, 1989.
10. Skoff HD, Keggi K. Total hip replacement in the neuromuscularly impaired. *Orthop Rev.* 15:154–159, 1986.
11. Howard CB, McKibbin B, Williams LA, Mackie I. Factors affecting the incidence of hip dislocation in cerebral palsy. *J Bone Joint Surg.* 67B:530–532, 1985.
12. Bleck EE. Forefoot problems in cerebral palsy—diagnosis and management. *Foot Ankle.* 4:188–194, 1984.
13. Bleck EE. Where have all the cerebral palsy children gone? The needs of adults. *Dev Med Child Neurol.* 26:674–676, 1984.
14. Brundage SR, Moore WD. Submandibular gland resection in bilateral parotid duct ligation as a management for chronic drooling in cerebral palsy. *Plastic Reconstr Surg.* 83:443–446, 1989.
15. Thomas AP, Bax MCD, Smyth DPL. *The Health and Social Needs of Young Adults with Physical Disabilities.* Oxford, England: MacKeith Press; 1989. Clinics in Dev Med No 106.
16. Yokoyama O, Nagano K, Hirata A, Hisazumi H, Izumida S. Clinical evaluation for voiding dysfunction in patients with cerebral palsy. *Jpn J Urol.* 80:591–595, 1989.
17. Treves T, Korczyn AD. Progressive dystonia and paraparesis in cerebral palsy. *Eur Neurol.* 25:148–153, 1986.
18. Salvato J, O'Neill ML, Sulkes S. Physician's management of sexuality in persons with developmental disability. *Dev Med Child Neurol.* 31(suppl):59, 1989.
19. Bengston L, Winch R, Fitzsimmons J, McLaughlin J, Budden S. Obstetric outcome of women with cerebral palsy. *Dev Med Child Neurol.* 31:37, 1989.
20. Winch R, Bengston L, McLaughlin J, Fitzsimmons J, Budden S, Hickock D. Neonatal status of infants born to women with cerebral palsy. *Dev Med Child Neurol.* 31:37–38, 1989.
21. Thompson GH, Rubin IL, Bilenkin RM. *Comprehensive Management of Cerebral Palsy.* New York, NY: Grune and Stratton; 1983.
22. Sienkiewicz-Mercer R, Kaplan SB. *I Raise My Eyes to Say Yes. A Memoir.* Boston, Mass: Houghton Mifflin Company; 1989.
23. McCarty SM, St James P, Berninger VW, Gans BM. Assessment of intellectual functioning across the life-span in severe cerebral palsy. *Dev Med Child Neurol.* 28:369–372, 1986.
24. Anderson EM, Clarke L. *Disability in Adolescence.* London: Methuen; 1982.
25. Pless IB, Cripps HA, Davies JMC, Wadsworth MEJ. Chronic physical illness in children: psychological and social effects in adolescents and adult life. *Dev Med Child Neurol.* 31:746–755, 1989.
26. O'Reilly DE. Care of the cerebral palsied: outcome of the past and needs for the future. *Dev Med Child Neurol.* 10:447–452, 1968.
27. O'Grady RS, Nishimura DM, Kohn JG, Bruvold WH. Vocational predictors compared with present vocational status of 60 young adults with cerebral palsy. *Dev Med Child Neurol.* 27:775–843, 1985.
28. Stadler D. What has become of them? The careers of the physically handicapped—a model study. *Rehabilitation (Stuttg).* 23:120–123, 1984.
29. Thomas P. Special adults: new challenge to primary care MD's. *Medical World News.* 68–81, Feb 24, 1986.
30. Coyle JT, Oster-Granite ML, Gearhart JD. The neurobiologic consequences of Down syndrome. *Brain Res Bull.* 16:773–787, 1986.
31. Lawhon SM, Ballard WT, Hays KR. Orthopaedic aspects of Down syndrome. *Contemp Orthop.* 20:395–403, 1990.
32. Alexander MA, Steg NL. Comprehensive management of myelomeningocele. *Arch Phys Med Rehabil.* 70:637–641, 1988.
33. Jaffe KM, McDonald CM, Ingman E, Haas J. Symptoms of upper gastrointestinal dysfunction in Duchenne muscular dystrophy: case control study. *Arch Phys Med Rehabil.* 71:742–744, 1990.
34. Alexander MA, Johnson EW, Petty J, Stauch D. Mechanical ventilation of patients with late-stage Duchenne muscular dystrophy management in the home. *Arch Phys Med Rehabil.* (6):289–292, 1979.

35

Poliomyelitis

Lauro S. Halstead

Although our understanding of the late effects of polio is still far from complete, what we do know about long-term polio survivors provides us with some intriguing insights and challenges to our concepts of aging.

This chapter will explore some of these insights and challenges, which provide an important philosophic perspective in the rehabilitation of postpolio patients who are having new health problems regardless of their chronologic age.

A survey by the National Center of Health Statistics in 1987 found there were more than 640,000 people in the United states who had experienced paralytic polio (1). Thus, despite the virtual elimination of new cases since early 1960s, paralytic polio remains one of the most prevalent neuromuscular diseases in this country. Of this population of 640,000, it is now believed that more than 50% are having new health problems related to their old polio 30 to 40 years after the acute episode (2). These include excessive fatigue, progressive weakness, pain, loss of function, and less commonly, muscle atrophy. These problems previously escaped widespread attention of the medical community because it was not until recently that enough cases from the big epidemics of the 1940s and 1950s had survived to begin experiencing new, residual effects after having achieved a plateau of neurologic and functional recovery. This large concentration of polio patients who survived the big epidemics is now mostly middle-aged, but ranged from 24 years to 86 years in one survey (3). As this population ages, an unknown number of survivors who have not yet had new problems can be expected to experience polio-related late effects. Furthermore, the residual effects of polio in the others may get worse as they age, compounded by common medical conditions that affect the elderly such as hypertension, heart disease, stroke, and arthritis. To prepare for this growing problem in the next few decades, we will present a brief overview of the etiology, diagnosis, and management of the late effects of polio.

POSSIBLE CAUSES OF POSTPOLIO COMPLICATIONS

Acute Polio and Premature or Accelerated Aging

The pathophysiology of acute polio provides important clues to some possible causes for the new neurologic changes characteristic of late effects of poliomyelitis. It may also suggest which management strategies are most likely to help an aging population.

Acute poliomyelitis, caused by one of three RNA viruses of the enterovirus group, invades the spinal cord of only 1% to 5% of the persons infected. Here, the virus's predilection for motor neurons in the lateral anterior horns produces a variable amount of paralysis. Regardless of the extent of paralysis, the virus typically infects over 95% of motor neurons due to its widespread dissemination throughout the central nervous system. After this invasion, cells either die or shed the virus and regain a normal or near normal appearance. A possible explanation for motor neuron dysfunction recurring decades later is that these recovered motor neurons may remain more susceptible to insults later in life.

Once the virus has invaded the central nervous system, the extent of neurologic and functional recovery is determined by the number of motor neurons that: (a) survive unimpaired, (b) recover and resume their normal function, and (c) develop terminal axon sprouts to reinnervate muscle fibers left orphaned by the death of their original motor neurons. This terminal axon sprouting enables either an uninvolved or a recovered motor neuron to adopt up to seven additional muscle fibers for every muscle cell innervated originally. Through this process, a single motor neuron that originally innervated 100 muscle fibers could conceivably innervate 700 fibers. As a result, the survivors of acute polio may be left with a few, significantly enlarged motor units doing the work previously performed by many units. Because this mechanism of neurophysiologic compensation is so effective, a muscle can retain normal strength even after 50% of the original motor neurons have been lost. However, the overworked anterior horn cells' control over a greater than normal percentage of muscle function may cause them to succumb prematurely to the aging process, resulting in pronounced weakness beginning as early as the fourth decade and steadily worsening with advancing age. Thirty to 40 years after recovery, the giant motor units appear to have lost their ability to sustain all of the terminal sprouts supplying so many muscle fibers. Consequently, the number of muscle fibers driven by each motor neuron declines, and the polio survivor experiences new weakness and other symptoms of neurologic dysfunction. If this pathophysiologic process is correct, then the overworked motor unit may be a paradigm for accelerated or premature aging of other organs or body parts, as we shall see below.

Residual polio

Musculoskeletal disuse, musculoskeletal overuse, or motor unit dysfunction may act singly or together to produce progressive weakness, the cardinal symptom of postpolio complications. Their potential interactions and complications are illustrated in Figure 35.1. Musculoskeletal disuse leads to atrophy, weakness, contractures, and diminished endurance, complications thoroughly studied in other groups with sedentary life-styles or neuromuscular lesions. Overuse, however, is less well understood although studies suggest relationships between the number of motor units, muscle damage, and exercise intensity and duration (4), but the extent to which a primary muscle defect is weakening some polio survivors remains unknown. Overuse has a cumulative effect over time; chronic mechanical strains on joints, liga-

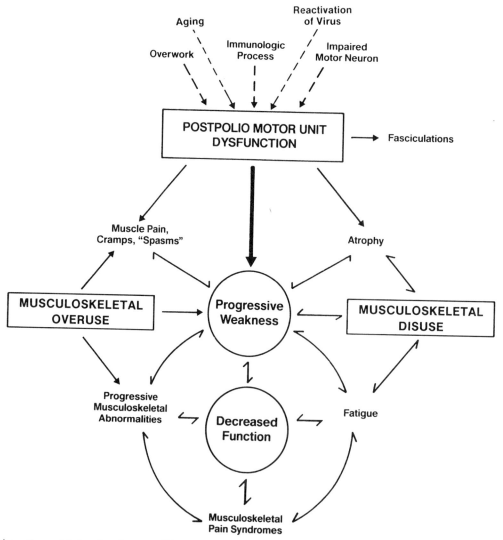

Figure 35.1. Schematic model showing three possible causes for the late neuromuscular and musculoskeletal complications of polio and their interactions.

ments, and soft tissues that have not been supported well for 30 or more years produce a self-perpetuating cycle of further complications. Recognizing overuse complications early and implementing effective interventions by middle age may avert severe postpolio disablement in old age.

It is motor unit overwork, eventually causing neuronal dysfunction, that provides the most plausible theory for why new motor unit dysfunction can occur so many years after recovery from acute illness. The giant motor units characteristic of muscles reinnervated after acute polio increase the metabolic demand on the remaining motor neurons. According to this theory, neurologic dysfunction results from this increased metabolic load after a critical number of years. Several clinical studies and electromyographic (EMG) data indirectly support the overuse theory.

Both Windebank and co-workers (2) at the Mayo Clinic and Maynard (5) found that, in persons with similar neurologic involvement, new weakness occurred more often in the weight-bearing muscles of the legs than in the nonweight-bearing muscles of the arms, and those limbs affected the most by the original disease were the most susceptible to new weakness. In subjects with about the same residual loss, Perry et al (6) observed that compared with asymptomatic polio survivors, symptomatic patients had a less efficient gait; both the intensity and contraction duration of extensor muscles were increased. More recently, Agre and co-workers (7) found that symptomatic postpolio subjects had evidence of more severe original polio involvement by history, were weaker and capable of performing less work than were asymptomatic subjects, and recovered strength less readily than did controls.

In electrophysiologic studies, Wiechers (8) and Dalakas et al (9) have found neuromuscular transmission abnormalities suggesting that the giant motor neurons may not be able to sustain indefinitely the metabolic demands of all their sprouts. As a result, individual terminals slowly deteriorate and reinnervated muscle fibers drop off. The more muscle fibers lost, the more apparent is the slowly progressive weakness.

Related to the overwork theory, the original viral attack of the anterior horn cells may have left some motor neurons functional but impaired, making them more vulnerable to dysfunction as time passes. Tomlinson (10) observed many neurons smaller than normal in the spinal cords of persons who survived long after the acute polio episode. Consistent with Bodian's findings (11), his observation led him to conclude that the protein synthetic mechanisms of any cell invaded by polio are likely to be permanently damaged. Possibly, then, prolonged overwork with increased metabolic demand of the greatly enlarged motor units compounds injury to the motor unit sustained during acute infection.

Although there is less evidence to support other

hypotheses, they warrant mention as possible contributors to postpolio complications. Does premature aging of the polio survivor cause new neuromuscular changes? Normally, motor neurons do not die out in significant numbers until the seventh decade (12). Polio survivors with fewer anterior horn cells to begin with, however, might suffer a disproportionate loss of clinical function if the relatively few giant motor units shrink or more anterior horn cells die. This hypothesis conceivably explains new weakness in some polio patients, but remains unsubstantiated by muscle biopsy changes such as group atrophy that would reflect the new loss of whole motor units. Also, several studies have failed to show a positive relationship between the onset of new weakness and chronologic age (2, 13). Instead, the determining variable is the length of the interval between onset of polio and the appearance of new symptoms. New difficulties should steadily increase as the polio population ages if major motor neuron loss is occurring.

Another hypothesis proposes immunologic involvement. Ginsberg et al (14) recently described significant alternation in CD4+; subsets in both symptomatic and asymptomatic postpolio subjects when compared with normal controls, supporting the possibility that immunologic factors may contribute to late disease progression. Dalakas et al (15, 16) have reported preliminary evidence of a lymphocytic response in muscle biopsies and IgG oligoclonal bands in the cerebrospinal fluid (CSF) of some symptomatic patients, whereas asymptomatic patients had no oligoclonal bands in their CSF. Because these patients have not responded to immunosuppressant therapy, however, whether such evidence of immunologic involvement can explain postpolio weakness remains uncertain.

Is it possible that polio virus or viral fragments lie dormant until they are reactivated by some unknown trigger? Polio virus can cause persistent asymptomatic infection in animals, but persistent infection has not yet been demonstrated in human studies (17).

Perhaps polio-related changes in the spinal cord are compromising motor neuron function. Pezeshkpour and Dalakas (18) observed active inflammatory gliosis, neuronal chromatolysis, and axonal spheroids in the spinal cords of polio patients who died many years after acute infection, but of other causes. Do these changes represent a primary lesion in the cord or a response to a lesion in the distal axon?

Finally, there is an intriguing suggestion by Rudman (oral communication, 1990) that the "growth hormone (GH) menopause" may be a risk or precipitating factor in the development of postpolio syndrome (PPS). It has been shown that GH secretion drops off dramatically in approximately one third of normal adults over the age of 40 (19). This results in a fall in Somatomedin C (SmC), which plays an important role in muscle cell protein synthesis, the proliferation of muscle satellite cells, and the regeneration of peripheral nerve sprouting. In a preliminary, unpublished survey, SmC was normal in a group of 12 asymptomatic older polio survivors and low in 9 of 10 symptomatic postpolios. A study is being planned to evaluate the effect of giving replacement GH on muscle size, strength, and endurance in symptomatic postpolio subjects.

PATIENT CHARACTERISTICS

Typical characteristics of postpolio patients with new health problems, originally identified in surveys (2, 13, 20, 21), have been confirmed by observation in the many postpolio clinics that have opened recently. The experience of one of these clinics, the Postpolio Clinic at the Institute for Rehabilitation and Research in Houston, Texas, is summarized in Tables 35.1 through 35.5. Most postpolio patients were women (66%), caucasian (92%), married, well-educated, and working outside the home. The majority of patients were middle-aged, the median age 45 years and the range from 24 to 86 years, and had contracted polio at a median age of 7 years (range 3 months to 44 years). The median interval between onset of polio and onset of new health problems was 31 years. Although this interval is similar in other studies, it has ranged from 2 to 8 decades (9, 13).

The factors most closely associated with risk for developing new problems are age and severity at onset of acute polio. The older the patient and the more severe the symptoms, the greater the risk for developing new neurologic symptoms 25 to 30 years later. Occasionally, however, a patient with apparently very mild polio initially and excellent clinical recovery still presents with typical postpolio symptoms.

Table 35.1. Most Common New Health and Functional Problems for 132 Consecutive Patients with Confirmed Polio[a]

	N	%
Health problems		
Fatigue	117	89
Muscle pain	93	71
Joint pain	93	71
Weakness:		
Previously affected muscles	91	69
Previously unaffected muscles	66	50
Cold intolerance	38	29
Atrophy	37	28
Cramps	24	18
Fasciculations	16	12
ADL problems[b]		
Walking	84	64
Climbing stairs	80	61
Dressing	23	17

[a]Reprinted with permission from Halstead LS. Late complications of poliomyelitis. In: Goodgold J, ed. *Rehabilitation Medicine*. St. Louis, Mo: Mosby; 1988:322.
[b]ADL = activities of daily living.

Although postpolio symptoms usually begin insidiously, specific events that are more frequent among elderly populations often precipitate recognition of polio-related health problems. Such a precipitating event—a period of bedrest, weight gain, a fall, or minor accident—would not cause as great a decline in health and function in persons who never had polio. Another triggering mechanism is the development or exacerbation of unrelated medical problems, such as diabetes. The frequency of such problems increases with aging.

What are the new, polio-related, health and functional problems most often reported by polio survivors? Table 35.1 lists the most common new health and functional problems found in 132 consecutive patients seen over a 1-year period at the TIRR Postpolio Clinic. All patients were carefully evaluated to confirm the diagnosis of polio and rule out nonpolio causes for their new symptoms. Although specific complaints differ somewhat from one clinic to another, the Houston patients most often experienced a cluster of complaints (Table 35.2): weakness, functional loss, pain, and fatigue. New atrophy, while relatively uncommon (28%), tended to occur only in conjunction with four or more other problems.

Weakness and Functional Loss

Weakness is most prominent in muscles most severely involved in the original illness, but may also occur in muscles believed to have been spared previously. Functional capacity tends to diminish in direct proportion to muscle weakness. If functional reserve was already marginal, additional muscle weakness can result in marked functional incapacity. A patient's ability to compensate for random, scattered motor deficits by unconventional muscle and joint movements may have adequately masked abnormal function until late-onset weakness of a critical muscle disrupted this delicate balance. The result? A disproportionate amount of functional loss. Walking, climbing stairs, and other activities requiring endurance may become more difficult if the legs are involved. Although polio survivors with presumably normal upper extremities may have been essentially "walking" with their arms for years, they may find ambulating, driving a car, transfers, or even dressing progressively exhausting. Patients typically also find that recovering from strenuous activity takes longer than it formerly did. And, exertion may seriously compromise breathing in persons with initial pulmonary weakness, especially at night.

Respiratory Impairment

In addition to weakness of respiratory muscles, impairment may be triggered by decreased compliance of respiratory tissue, progressive scoliosis, recurrent pul-

Table 35.2. Number of Problems and Frequency of Persons Experiencing Each New Problem for the Six Most Common Problem Areas for 132 Postpolio Patients[a]

# of Problems	# of Persons (%)	New Health Problems[b]					
		F	P	W	FL	CI	A
2	11 (8%)	4	7	4	3	2	0
3	22 (17%)	17	15	14	11	1	2
4	51 (39%)	48	46	45	45	4	7
5	36 (27%)	33	32	33	32	18	16
6	12 (9%)	12	12	12	12	12	12
Totals	132 (100%)	114	112	108	103	37	37

[a]Reprinted with permission from Halstead LS. Late complications of poliomyelitis. In: Goodgold J, ed. *Rehabilitation Medicine.* St. Louis, Mo: Mosby; 1988:333.
[b]F = fatigue; P = pain in muscles and/or joints; W = weakness in previously affected and/or unaffected muscles; FL = functional loss in walking, climbing stairs, dressing, etc.; CI = cold intolerance; A = new atrophy.

monary infection, and smoking. In the geriatric population, respiratory impairment from polio may be exacerbated by emphysema or chronic bronchitis resulting from a lifetime of smoking or exposure to occupational hazards. As in the acute phase of polio, respiratory failure is still the most feared complication because, unlike other complications, it is not benign and can ultimately lead to death if left untreated.

At greatest risk for serious late-onset pulmonary complications are those who had severe respiratory involvement during the acute illness, requiring ventilatory assistance. Also at high risk are those who developed thoracic spine deformities. Several preliminary studies suggest that as many as 18% to 38% of polio survivors who were successfully weaned off a respirator after acute illness now require ventilatory assistance full or part-time (22). The long-term prognosis for those who were not ever weaned completely from a ventilator appears favorable (23). More than half of patients interviewed 21 to 30 years after acute polio reported that the respiratory treatment needed had not changed since 1 year after polio onset; 27% believed impairment had worsened, and 17% felt it had improved; only four needed more daily respiratory support than formerly (23).

Fatigue

In addition to exhaustion related to physical exertion, postpolio patients also report generalized fatigue, described as a marked change in energy level, endurance, and sometimes mental alertness. Previously, everyday activities had been performed without any special effort. Postpolio fatigue usually occurs in the afternoon and early evening. When patients "hit the wall," they must stop what they are doing, rest, and take a short nap whenever possible.

Pain

When pain occurs, it is felt in the muscles, joints, or both. Occasionally, pain takes the form of hypersensitivity and a sensation of crawling or cramping, espe-

cially at night. Otherwise, it is experienced as a deep, aching pain similar to the muscle pain experienced during acute polio. Physical activity and cold temperature tend to aggravate the pain. Although weight bearing often produces the joint pain, it is rarely accompanied by swelling or inflammation.

The location of pain depends primarily on the patient's method of locomotion (Table 35.3 and Table 35.4) (24, 25). In many patients, muscle and joint pain appears to result directly from abnormal body mechanics that are compensating for muscle weakness and skeletal abnormalities. Consequently, the remaining innervated muscles carry increased work loads. Abnormal, excessive forces on unstable joints and supporting tissues increase the energy expenditure required to perform a given task. These costs accumulate silently over many years until they cross a critical threshold and produce painful muscles, joints, and ligaments.

DIAGNOSIS BY EXCLUSION

No serologic, enzymatic, or electrodiagnostic test is able to distinguish symptomatic from asymptomatic postpolio patients. Despite growing evidence suggesting that the major pathologic process in postpolio syndrome is motor unit dysfunction, no existing objective method can predict who might become symptomatic in the future or monitor the progress of the underlying pathology in the person who is already symptomatic. As polio survivors age, there is no way of knowing for sure how many, if not all, of them will develop postpolio symptoms. Nor is there any way to predict how much their everyday functioning will be impaired by the imposition of postpolio symptoms on coexisting medical disorders and side effects from medication. Differential diagnosis is still very much by exclusion, but is exclusion a realistic goal in a geriatric population?

Because postpolio complications are diagnosed by exclusion, and elderly patients are particularly susceptible to having other medical, orthopedic, or neurologic conditions that could be causing or aggravating the pre-

Table 35.3. Prevalence of Chronic Pain by Method of Locomotion in 114 Postpolio Patients[a]

Method of Locomotion	Number	Number with Pain	% with Pain
Ambulatory no brace (Independent)	67	56	84
Ambulatory with brace (Independent)	12	11	92
Ambulatory with crutches (Independent)	21	21	100
Wheelchair locomotion (Independent)	7	7	100
Wheelchair locomotion (Need personal assistance)	7	7	100
Total	114	102	90

[a]Reprinted with permission from Smith LK, McDermott K. Addressing causes versus treating effects. In: Halstead LS, Wiechers DO, eds. *Research and Clinical Aspects of the Late Effects of Poliomyelitis.* White Plains, NY: March of Dimes Birth Defects Foundation; 1987:122.

Table 35.4. Location of Chronic Pain by Method of Locomotion in 114 Postpolio Patients[a]

	Number	Percent
Independent ambulators with or without lower extremity orthoses	79	69
Back	37	47
Hip	19	24
Diffuse lower extremity	18	22
Other (neck, shoulder, knee, ankle)	31	39
Locomotion performance using crutches or wheelchairs	35	31
Neck and shoulders	18	51
Back	13	37
Glenohumeral joint	11	31
Elbow	6	17
Wrist and hand	9	26
Other (lower extremity and head)	15	43

[a]Reprinted with permission from Smith LK, McDermott K. Addressing causes versus treating effects. In: Halstead LS, Wiechers DO, eds. *Research and Clinical Aspects of the Late Effects of Poliomyelitis.* White Plains, NY; March of Dimes Birth Defects Foundation; 1987:334.

senting symptoms, an interdisciplinary evaluation is essential. The initial evaluation team should include a physician, physical therapist, and social worker and referrals to other medical specialists should be made as needed to rule out nonpolio-related causes. In addition to a careful history and physical examination, appropriate laboratory studies, x-ray films, electromyography (EMG/NCV studies), psychosocial evaluation, and a functional assessment of gait, orthotic needs, and strength and endurance of key muscle groups are crucial. Standard screening tests such as an SMA 24 or thyroid panel, however, have not proven to be helpful or cost-effective.

Patients who had respiratory impairment during acute polio or have a history of pulmonary disease should also undergo pulmonary function studies and measurement of arterial blood gases. Complaints suggesting respiratory impairment include shortness of breath, exertional dyspnea, daytime somnolence, early morning headache, sleep disturbance, and sleep apnea. Asympto-

matic patients with normal test results should be reevaluated at least once a year. Patients with nighttime sleep disturbances, especially dyspnea or apnea, and with elevated PCO_2 should undergo sleep studies or at least evaluation of nighttime oxygen saturation, with ear oximetry (22). Central and obstructive sleep apnea should also be differentiated by sleep studies.

The results from all diagnostic tests should be collated to determine whether the patient meets three major criteria necessary for making a diagnosis of postpolio syndrome. These are: (*a*) objective evidence of a prior episode of paralytic polio; (*b*) a characteristic pattern of recovery and neurologic stability before the new problems began; (*c*) exclusion of other medical, orthopedic, and neurologic conditions that could cause the presenting symptoms.

The diagnosis of paralytic polio usually can be confirmed by examining, whenever possible, the original medical records; eliciting a credible history of an acute, febrile illness producing motor but no sensory loss; noting whether other members of the patient's family or neighbors had had a similar illness; and by observing certain features during physical examination and electromyography. One very characteristic feature is the presence of focal, asymmetric weakness or atrophy. Electromyography should reveal changes consistent with chronic denervation and reinnervation characteristic of previous anterior horn cell disease. Other changes on routine EMG compatible with prior polio include increased amplitude and duration of motor unit action potentials, an increased percentage of polyphasic motor units, often of long duration, and a decrease in the number of motor units on maximum recruitment in weak muscles.

The second criterion for establishing a diagnosis of postpolio syndrome, a specific pattern of recovery and neurologic stability preceding the onset of new problems, is so characteristic that its absence makes aging-related and other medical disorders much more likely explanations for the patient's symptoms. This pattern, depicted in Figure 35.2, includes a period of functional and neurologic stability lasting at least 20 years (26). At least one of the new problems should include nondisuse weakness. One clue to nondisuse weakness is diminished function despite maintenance of the usual level and intensity of activity. Weakness in a geriatric patient who has become much less active after retirement, coupled with muscular atrophy normally occurring during the seventh decade, may not be related to prior polio.

The third criterion is the most difficult to satisfy in an elderly patient. A history of paralytic poliomyelitis does not exempt anyone from getting the chronic illnesses, diseases, or psychiatric disturbances that afflict the general population, and particularly, an aging population. When medical, orthopedic, or neurologic conditions coexist with postpolio problems, a similar set of overlapping signs and symptoms may occur. Compression neuropathies, radiculopathies, degenerative arthritis, disc disease, obesity, anemia, diabetes, thyroid disease, and depression are some common examples. But ruling out all possible causes of the symptoms is impractical and prohibitively expensive. Furthermore, as shown in Figure 35.1, the original problem may be impossible to identify when, for example, weakness triggers a chain reaction of other complications, regardless of the underlying etiology. Nevertheless, because nondisuse weakness is such an important indicator of postpolio syndrome, and different etiologies dictate very different management strategies, every attempt should be made to differentiate postpolio weakness from other possible causes including amyotrophic lateral sclerosis (ALS).

Despite some similarities between postpolio weakness and ALS, major differences found during clinical and laboratory evaluation (Table 35.5) facilitate differential diagnosis (27). Because some patients who had polio have been diagnosed as having ALS, clinicians have speculated that antecedent infection with polio might predispose one to developing ALS later in life (28–30). It is now believed that ALS was misdiagnosed in some

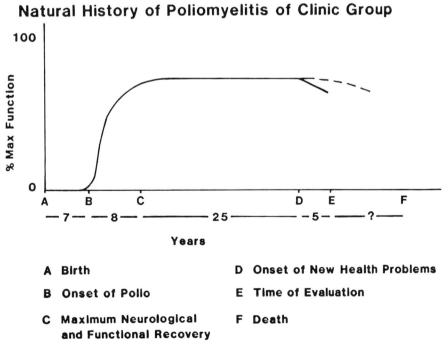

Figure 35.2. The natural history of polio based on data from patients evaluated in the Post Polio Clinic, Houston, Texas.

Table 35.5. Comparison of Clinical and Laboratory Findings in Patients with Late Polio and Amyotrophic Lateral Sclerosis (ALS)[a]

Patients	Clinical Findings					
	Weakness	Bulbar Sxs	Fasciculations	Long Tract Signs	Sensory Changes	Prognosis
ALS	Often symmetrical, generalized	Common	Common	Very common	Absent	Rapid, downhill course; death 3–5 years
Postpolio	Asymmetrical focal	Rare	Occasional	Very rare	Absent	Loss of strength at 1% per year

Patients	Laboratory Findings[b]			
	DNA Repair	CPK	EMG	Muscle Biopsy
ALS	Abnormal	Frequently elevated	Fibs and PSW ↑↑+, fasciculations +++ MUP—rarely >10mV, fiber density ↑ jitter/blocking ↑, neurogenic jitter often present	Group atrophy common; scattered angulated fibers; inflammation rare
Postpolio	Normal	Occasionally elevated	Fibs and PSW + fasciculations + MUP— often >10mV, fiber density ↑↑↑ jitter/ blocking ↑, neurogenic jitter rare	Group atrophy uncommon; inflammation in 40%

[a]Adapted from Dalakas MC. Amyotrophic lateral sclerosis and postpolio: differences and similarities. In: Halstead LS, Wiechers DO, eds.: *Research and Clinical Aspects of the Late Effects of Poliomyelitis.* White Plains, NY: March of Dimes Birth Defects Foundation; 1987:74.
[b]PSW = positive sharp wates; MUP = motor unit potential; Fibs = fibrillations; + = one plus, +++ = three plus; ↑ = increased; ↑↑↑ = markedly increased; Sxs = symptoms.

patients with a protracted course. Had these patients been evaluated today, most would probably be diagnosed as having postpolio syndrome (31).

NOSOLOGY

Because diagnostic criteria remain nonspecific and pathognomonic tests unavailable, a consistent diagnostic name has not yet been established for new health problems associated with former polio. Indeed, several pathologic processes may interact at any given time to produce similar, overlapping symptoms (Fig. 35.1), especially in the geriatric patient. Use of a general rather than a precise diagnostic term takes into account the impossibility of determining a distinct origin for each new symptom. One heterogeneous term often used is postpolio syndrome, a diagnosis reserved for those patients whose symptomatology indicates motor unit dysfunction accompanied by variable musculoskeletal overuse. Not every polio survivor complaining of weakness, however, can be classified as having postpolio syndrome. This diagnosis should be made only after a trial of closely supervised exercise to rule out disuse weakness.

A more specific diagnostic term for postpolio complications is postpolio progressive muscular atrophy (PPMA). Only patients who have documented, objective evidence of neuromuscular deterioration and evidence on muscle biopsy of active denervation in the form of scattered angulated fibers qualify for this diagnostic category (9). A less restrictive but similar term to PPMA is postpolio motor neuron disease (PPMND).

MANAGEMENT

As soon as other medical, orthopedic, and neurologic diagnoses have been excluded, new health problems related to former polio must be identified and managed to enable the elderly person to continue functioning at home as independently as possible. The problems that warrant the earliest attention include muscle weakness, pain, respiratory failure, and psychologic issues. In many cases, alleviating these problems will require gradual changes in life-style which the physician must persuade the patient to accept.

Weakness

Depending on whether weakness is exacerbated by inactivity or overuse, a trial of progressive exercise or rest and support, respectively, should be instituted. Several studies (32, 33) have shown improved strength in response to carefully supervised exercise programs for polio survivors with new weakness. Since the effects of exercise on such muscles are unknown, however, longterm maintenance or strengthening exercises are recommended only in those muscles in which clinical or EMG evidence of prior polio involvement is absent. Exercising muscles initially damaged by polio may increase the risk of accelerating motor unit dysfunction and produce overuse weakness.

The aim with overuse complications is to reduce mechanical stress, support weakened muscles, and stabilize abnormal joint movements. When patients have been pushing themselves and their muscles to maximum performance daily, a change in life-style with less stress and better support of weakened muscles has often slowed the decrease in strength, prevented further deterioration, and in some cases, actually reversed symptoms. However, even those patients who have overuse weakness can benefit from some kind of formal exercise program within the limits of comfort and safety. This program can range from gentle stretching and yoga to aerobic training. Alba and co-workers (34) found that 66% of 35 postpolio survivors were able to attain normal cardiopulmonary levels during exercise using a Monarch arm ergometer, Quinton treadmill, or Collins chair ergometer. The remainder of the subjects were unable to obtain a normal range of work capacity due to focal or generalized fatigue in their extremities or improper biomechanical techniques during exercising. Therefore, when prescribing more vigorous exercise, select any repetitious activity that appeals to the patient but doesn't cause undue pain or muscle fatigue. Weakness or discomfort that takes several hours to subside is a good indicator of excessive activity. An ideal form of exercise for the elderly postpolio patient is swimming; it not only avoids the stresses and microtrauma of other types of exercise but also readily accommodates concurrent musculoskeletal conditions such as degenerative joint disease that become so prevalent with aging.

Pain

Pain management is designed to compensate for years of abnormal and excessive forces on unstable joints and supporting tissues. Conservative measures such as decreased activity, better support of unstable joints and weakened muscles, improved biomechanics of the body during common daily activities, supplemented by low doses of antiinflammatory medications, moist heat, and transcutaneous electrical nerve stimulation (TENS) usually help alleviate pain. Life-style modifications and improved biomechanics should be emphasized and the use of pain medication discouraged.

Cervical pillows, lumbar rolls, gluteal pads, dorsallumbar corsets, and heel lifts can help modify abnormal biomechanics. In addition, the musculoskeletal mechanics of sitting, standing, walking, sleeping, and other daily, repetitive activities at work must be corrected. The basic orthotic principle applied in the management of other neuromuscular disorders also apply to relieving pain related to polio. Patients needing an orthosis that combines strength with lightness may benefit from the new plastics and lightweight metals if they can be convinced to trade in their old heavy braces. Frequently, patients prefer to repair and use these old braces than to start over again with new ones. Others may resist using any kind of brace support for cosmetic reasons.

Reductions in stress, activity, and weight are lifestyle changes that have the most impact on reducing pain. These strategies may be the most difficult to accomplish, however, because they often require developing behaviors very unlike the old, familiar ways of coping. Essential is altering the pace and intensity of discretionary activities and learning new ways to gain more control over when and how activities are performed. The elderly postpolio patient may have already begun this process after retirement and may have the additional advantage of fewer demands to juggle than the patient who is employed full-time. Nevertheless, retired persons may still need to clarify and accept their own limitations and negotiate with family and friends when and how activities will be performed to accommodate these limitations.

Respiratory Impairment

Referral to a pulmonologist, preferably with experience in neuromuscular diseases, is indicated for managing respiratory problems. Supplemental oxygen alone is sufficient to alleviate many patients' symptoms when nighttime desaturation has been documented. Others may experience marked improvement in both day and nighttime symptoms on a trial ventilatory assistance at night. The pneumo-wrap or raincoat and chest cuirass are the most practical means of providing nighttime ventilatory assistance. Alternatives that are not so readily available or practical include intermittent pressure with a Bennett mouth seal, nasal continuous positive airway pressure (C-PAP), and the iron lung. Few patients will benefit from tracheostomy, which should be avoided if possible (35). Every patient with impaired pulmonary function and a history of recurrent respiratory infections should receive flu vaccines yearly and Pneumovax at least once.

Psychologic Issues

Emotional responses to experiencing new medical problems related to polio can be as traumatic and disabling as the physical problems. Although they may experience any combination of denial, anger, frustration, and hopelessness, postpolio patients generally exhibit one of three distinct categories of psychologic responses: (a) those who do not regard themselves as handicapped, regardless of the extent of involvement and presence of obvious deformities; (b) those who feel disabled now, but who never did in the past, even during the acute illness; and (c) those who feel that, because they are experiencing polio for the second time, the are "twice cursed."

Polio survivors may resist making life-style changes to accommodate weakness, fatigue, and other postpolio symptoms because they have worked so hard to overcome the initial paralysis and achieved a high level of functional performance and personal fulfillment. They no longer perceive themselves as handicapped and believe, even if some disability remains, that they have won; the long struggle with polio was over. Instead, new limitations unexpectedly and abruptly developed 25 to 40 years later. But patients still expect to regain lost function and feel better by persevering and working harder when better advice may be to slow down.

To overcome this combination of denial and personal history of successful coping and reluctance to try something new, the physician can help the patient modify old familiar coping mechanisms. For example, have the old brace repaired after the patient's first visit rather than prescribing a new one. Beginning with a minor, acceptable intervention may prepare the patient to make necessary major changes later. A patient who has been ambulatory for 35 years may reject buying a wheelchair but agree to use a cane or restrict wheelchair use to the airport. The wheelchair may become more acceptable, however, as the patient learns that the cane is helpful but insufficient to relieve symptoms. Polio survivors may also reject anything that publicly advertises handicapped status. Changes that enable them to retain some sense of control, such as displaying a handicap placard on the dashboard when desired instead of getting handicapped license plates, may enhance compliance.

PROGNOSIS

Since all evidence suggests that the pathologic processes involved are benign, postpolio syndrome is not life-threatening unless there is severe pulmonary involvement or a swallowing disorder. Dalakas et al (9) found an average loss of strength of 1% per year in 27 persons followed for a mean of 8.2 years. This represents a rate of natural progression, since no one in the group studied was being treated to combat or modify the weakness. If weakness is in part due to overwork of the motor unit combined with musculoskeletal overuse, then interventions designed to reduce the metabolic demand on the overextended motor unit could conceivably alter this rate of decline. Although the long-term effects of such interventions remain to be studied, many clinicians have reported that patients who conscientiously adjust their life-styles do improve, often increasing strength and stabilizing function.

Nevertheless, while many patients experience only minor weakness and mild annoyance from associated symptoms, others experience profound weakness, diminished functional capacity, and as a result, social isolation as well as greater risk of developing osteoporosis, fractures, contractures, depression, and other disabling conditions.

SUMMARY

We can only speculate about how these late complications will affect geriatric survivors; relatively few who survived the large epidemics of the 1940's and 1950's have attained their sixties and seventies, and postpolio problems have been widely recognized for study only in the past 7 years. Similarly, no group has been followed long enough to estimate the mean survival time. Future study of postpolio patients promises not only to shed light on the many unanswered questions about pathologic mechanisms, best forms of treatment, the role of exercise, and long-term prognosis, but also to reveal much about the aging process in other disabled groups. Furthermore, health care workers and policy makers should keep in mind that thousands of people who survived paralytic polio will continue to survive well into the 21th century, joining an ever-growing pool of elderly citizens.

References

1. National Health Survey. *Prevalence of Selected Impairments (Series 10)*. Washington, DC: US Dept of Health and Human Services. In press.
2. Windebank AJ, Daube JR, Litchy WJ, et al. Late sequelae of paralytic poliomyelitis in Olmsted County, Minnesota. In: Halstead LS, Wiechers DO, eds. *Research and Clinical Aspects of the Late Effects of Poliomyelitis*. White Plains, NY: March of Dimes Birth Defects Foundation; 1987.
3. Halstead LS, Rossi CD. New problems in old polio patients: results of a survey of 539 polio survivors. *Orthopedics*. 8:845–850, 1985.
4. Herbison GJ, Jaweed MM, Ditunno JF. Exercise therapies in peripheral neuropathies. *Arch Phys Med Rehabil*. 64:201–205, 1983.
5. Maynard FM. Differential diagnosis of pain and weakness in Postpolio patients. In: Halstead LS, Wiechers DO, eds. *Late Effects of Poliomyelitis*. Miami, Fla: Symposia Foundation; 1985:33–44.
6. Perry J, Barnes G, Granley JK. Post polio muscle function. In: Halstead LS, Wiechers DO, eds. *Research and Clinical Aspects of the Late Effects of Poliomyelitis*. White Plains, NY: March of Dimes Birth Defects Foundation; 1987:315–328.
7. Agre JC, Rodriguez AA. Neuromuscular function: comparison of symptomatic and asymptomatic polio subjects to control subjects. *Arch Phys Med Rehabil*. 71:545–551, 1990.
8. Wiehcers DO, Hubbell SL. Late changes in the motor unit after acute poliomyelitis. *Muscle Nerve*. 4:524–528, 1981.
9. Dalakas MC, Elder G, Hallett M, et al. A long-term follow-up of patients with postpoliomyelitis neuromuscular symptoms. *N Engl J Med*. 314:959–963, 1986.
10. Tomlinson BE, Irving D. Changes in spinal cord motor neurons of possible relevance to the late effects of poliomyelitis. In: Halstead LS, Wiechers DO, eds. *Late Effects of Poliomyelitis*. Miami, Fla: Symposia Foundation; 1985:57–72.
11. Bodian D. Motoneuron disease and recovery in experimental poliomyelitis. In: Halstead LS, Wiechers DO, eds. *Late Effects of Poliomyelitis*. Miami Fla: Symposia Foundation; 1985:45–56.
12. Tomlinson BE, Irving D. The numbers of limb motor neurons in the human lumbosacral cord throughout life. *J Neural Sci*. 34:213–219, 1977.
13. Halstead LS, Wiechers DO, Rossi CD. Late effects of poliomyelitis: A national survery. In: Halstead LS, Wiechers DO, eds. *Late Effects of Poliomyelitis*. Miami, Fla: Symposia Foundation; 1985:11–32.
14. Ginsberg GH, Gale MJ, Rose LM, Clark EA. T-Cell alternations in late postpoliomyelitis. *Arch Neurol*. 46:487–501, 1989.
15. Dalakas MC, Sever JL, Fletcher M, et al. Neuromuscular symptoms in patients with old poliomyelitis: clinical, virological and immunological studies. In: Halstead LS, Wiechers DO, eds. *Late Effects of Poliomyelitis*. Mianmi, Fla: Symposia Foundation; 1985:73–90.
16. Dalakas M. Post polio syndrome: clues from muscle and spinal cord studies. In: Munsat TL, ed. *Post Polio Syndrome*. Boston, Mass: Butterworth-Heinemann; 1990:39–65.
17. Miller JR. Prolonged intracerebral infection with poliomyelitis in asymptomatic mice. *Ann Neurol* 9:590–596, 1981.
18. Pezeshkpour GH, Dalakas MC. Pathology of spinal cord in postpoliomyelitis muscular atrophy. In: Halstead LS, Wiechers

DO, eds. *Research and Clinical Aspects of the Late Effects of Poliomyelitis.* White Plains, NY: March of Dimes Birth Defects Foundation; 1987:229–236.

19. Rudman D, Feher AG, Nagras HS, et al. Effects of human growth hormone in men over sixty years old. *N Engl J. Med.* 323:1–6, 1990.

20. Frick NM. Demographic and psychological characteristics of the post-polio community. Presented at the First Annual Conference on the Late Effects of Poliomyelitis; October 1985; Lansing, Michigan.

21. Halstead LS, Rossi CD. New problems in old polio patients: results of a survey of 539 polio survivors. *Orthopedics.* 8:845–850, 1985.

22. Fischer DA. Poliomyelitis: late respiratory complications and management. *Orthopedics.* 88:891–894, 1985.

23. Alock AJW. Respiratory poliomyelitis: a follow-up study. *Can Med Assoc J.* 130:1305–1310, 1984.

24. Smith LK, McDermott K. Addressing causes versus treating effects. In: Halstead LS, Wiechers DO, ed. *Research and Clinical Aspects of the Late Effects of Poliomyelitis.* White Plains, NY: March of Dimes Birth Defects Foundation; 1987:121–134.

25. Smith LK. Current issues in neurological rehabilitation. In: Umphred DA, ed; *Neurological Rehabilitation.* 2nd ed. St. Louis Mo: CV Mosby; 1990:509–528.

26. Halstead LS, Rossi DC. Post polio syndrome: clinical experience with 132 consecutive outpatients. In: Halstead LS, Wiechers DO, eds. *Research and Clinical Aspects of the Late Effects of Poliomyelitis.* White Plains, NY: March of Dimes Birth Defects Foundation; 1987:13–26.

27. Dalakas MC. Amyotrophic lateral sclerosis and post-polio: differences and similarities. In: Halstead LS, Wiechers DO, eds. *Research and Clinical Aspects of Late Effects of Poliomyelitis.* White Plains, NY: March of Dimes Birth Defects Foundation; 1987:63–80.

28. Pierce-Rhuland R, Patten BM. Repeat study of anticedent events in motor neuron disease. *Ann Clin Res.* 13:102–107, 1981.

29. Poskanzer DC, Cantor HM, Kaplan GS. The frequency of preceding poliomyelitis in amyotrophic lateral sclerosis. In: Norris FH Jr, Kurland LT, eds. *Motor Neuron Diseases: Research on Amyotrophic Lateral Sclerosis and Related Disorders.* NY: Grune & Stratton; 1969:286–290.

30. Zilkha KJ, *Proc R Soc Med.* 55:1028–1029, 1962. Discussion.

31. Brown S, Patten BM. Post-polio syndrome and anyotrophic lateral sclerosis: a relationship more apparent than real. In: Halstead LS, Wiechers DO, eds. *Research and Clinical Aspects of the Late Effects of Poliomyelitis.* White Plains, NY: March of Dimes Birth Defects Foundation; 1987:83–98.

32. Feldman RM. The use of strengthening exercises in post-polio syndrome: Methods and results. *Orthopedics.* 1985:889–890.

33. Grimby G, Einarsson G. Muscle morphology with special reference to muscle strength in postpolio subjects. In: Halstead LS, Wiechers DO, eds. *Research and Clinical Aspects of the Late Effects of Poliomyelitis.* White Plains, NY: March of Dimes Birth Defects Foundation; 1987:265–274.

34. Alba A, Block E, Adler JC, et al. Exercise testing as a useful tool in the physiatric management of the post-polio survivor. In: Halstead LS, Wiechers DO, eds. *Research and Clinical Aspects of the Late Effects of Poliomyelitis.* White Plains, NY: March of Dimes Birth Defects Foundation; 1987:301–314.

35. Bach JR, Alba AS, Bodofsky E, et al. Glossopharyngeal breathing and non-invasive aids in the management of post polio respiratory insufficiency. In: Halstead LS, Wicchers DO, eds. *Research and Clinical Aspects of the Late Effects of Poliomyelitis.* White Plains, NY: March of Dimes Birth Defects Foundation; 1987:99–114.

36
Aging with Multiple Sclerosis

Nancy D. Cobble, Jan R. Miller, Jim Grigsby, and Judy C. Lane

Multiple sclerosis (MS), a demyelinating disease of the central nervous system (CNS), is the most common disabling neurologic disease diagnosed in young adults. Given that life span for these patients is nearly normal, the issues of aging with MS will eventually confront most patients, their families, and health care providers.

ETIOLOGY, PATHOLOGY, NATURAL HISTORY

The etiology of MS remains obscure. Exposure to a common environmental factor (probably viral) appears to trigger a dysregulated immune response in a genetically susceptible individual (1–5).

In MS, white matter lesions continuously appear, resolve, and recur, leaving residual areas of damage scattered throughout the CNS (Fig. 36.1). Initially, the blood-brain barrier is disrupted permitting hematogenous lymphocytes to enter the brain and spinal cord. Then, during an immune-mediated inflammatory process, my-

elin is stripped from axons, but the axons remain intact. Astrocytes produce glial fibers, eventually giving the older plaque a firm, sclerotic texture. The name multiple sclerosis refers to the end-stage appearance of "many scars" (1, 2, 4, 6, 7).

Neurologic dysfunction results from partial, complete, or intermittent nerve conduction block through demyelinated areas. Relapsing/remitting or progressive signs and symptoms reflect the accumulation of multiple CNS lesions causing impaired neuronal output, distorted sensory input, and slowed or uneven central processing. Spinal cord disease causes the greatest physical disability. Common lesion locations and symptoms are:

- Optic nerves—optic neuritis
- Cerebrum, especially periventricular and frontal lobe—cognitive, behavioral, and motor planning problems
- Spinal Cord, especially cervical—weakness; spasticity; incoordination; sensory disturbances; and bowel, bladder, and sexual dysfunctions
- Brain Stem—vertigo, nystagmus, extraocular muscle impairments, dysarthria, and dysphagia
- Cerebellum, basal ganglia—ataxia and tremor.

Other common MS symptoms include fatigue, heat sensitivity, autonomic dysfunctions, and pain. Less frequent are seizures, paroxysmal phenomena, and movement disorders (1, 7–9).

The course of MS is initially relapsing/remitting in 85% of cases, but with increasing age and duration of disease a progressive course becomes more common. Remission may occur because of resolution of inflammation, partial remyelination, alternative routing of nerve transmission, or resumption of altered conduction through the demyelinated axon. Also, progression may clinically appear to stabilize for a time in spite of the fact that silent lesions continue to form. Silent lesions may be primarily edematous and thus may not interfere with nerve transmission. Also, lesions located in CNS areas with reserve capacity may remain asymptomatic. Over time, however, as residual demyelination accumulates and

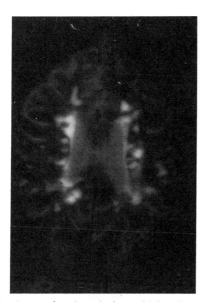

Figure 36.1. Scattered periventricular multiple sclerosis lesions seen on cerebral magnetic resonance imaging.

reserve CNS function diminishes, the disease often becomes clinically progressive (1, 6, 10, 11).

Prognosis is variable and unpredictable, ranging from patients who are asymptomatic for a lifetime to others who progress within months (1, 3, 12, 13). Although onset later in life is associated with a less favorable outcome, prognosis in general for MS patients is not always bad. For instance in one survey, at least 60% remained ambulatory with single support after 25 years (14). Life expectancy is only slightly reduced, and mortality is usually due to unrelated causes or complications of debilitation.

MANAGEMENT—DIAGNOSIS AND MEDICAL TREATMENT

Multiple sclerosis is diagnosed twice as often in women as in men, with onset most often between the ages of 20 and 40 years. The highest incidence occurs in the early fourth decade, but the highest prevalence occurs in the fifth decade as cases accumulate with the aging of the MS population (1, 3, 5). The diagnosis of MS remains a clinical one, based on history and neurologic exam demonstrating multiple, multiphasic white matter lesions. Laboratory tests provide supportive evidence of (a) multiple lesions, [evoked potentials, magnetic resonance imaging (MRI)], (b) blood brain barrier disruption (gadolinium MRI), (c) abnormal CNS immune activity or myelin breakdown (cerebrospinal fluid analysis), and (d) the absence of a better explanation. Differential diagnoses include normal aging (15), CNS neoplasms, infections, postinfectious encephalopathy, stroke, connective tissue vasculitides, cervical spondylopathy, Arnold Chiari malformation, peripheral neuropathies, and metabolic abnormalities (such as vitamin B_{12} or thyroid deficiency (1, 6, 7, 13).

There is no cure for MS. Medical treatment attempts to alter disease activity by shortening exacerbations and slowing or preventing progression. Most standard and experimental treatments use various immunomodulating interventions, consistent with the theory that MS results from immune dysregulation (1, 16, 17). However, new treatable disease activity can be difficult to identify. Not all new MS lesions are symptomatic, and not all new systems represent new lesions. Previously silent lesions may become symptomatic when nerve conduction is adversely affected by extraneural conditions such as heat or fatigue (1, 10).

High-dose pulse steroids are used for their antiinflammatory and immunosuppressive effects to shorten the duration and lessen the morbidity of MS exacerbations (1, 16–19). The protocol followed at the Rocky Mountain Multiple Sclerosis Center (250 mg intravenous methylprednisolone q.i.d. over 4 days) permits a drug steady state level to be attained within 36 hours. Side effects of high-dose steroids include insomnia, mood change, psychosis, gastritis, hypertension, electrolyte and glucose abnormalities, acne, infection, aseptic necrosis, steroid dependence, or fluid retention followed by diuresis that can overdistend a marginal bladder (20, 21). Chronic long-term steroids are not indicated since disease activity eventually resumes despite continued use and risks (osteoporosis, cataracts, and steroid myopathy) increase. Repetition of pulse steroids may be more beneficial over time with less cumulative risk.

When MS is refractory to corticosteroids, other forms of immunosuppression such as azathioprine and cyclophosphamide are sometimes used. Disease progression resumes within months and side effects are more serious including hemorrhagic cystitis, pneumonitis, alopecia, infection, liver dysfunction, gonadal suppression, and induction of neoplasia (17, 21). The efficacy of these treatments is still being evaluated (1, 16, 17). Indications for use of immunosuppressive drugs do not change with the age of the patient, but underlying medical conditions in older patients may complicate the use of these agents (22). Our clinical impression is that benefits decrease as age increases. Other immune regulators such as beta-interferon are being intensively studied and show early promising beneficial effects.

Medications for common MS symptoms are listed in Table 36.1. All use of medications requires a thorough understanding of the differences for the aging patient in drug metabolism, distribution, and elimination, as well as a sensitivity to the issues of polypharmacy (23–29).

MANAGEMENT—REHABILITATION

Neuromuscular and Sensory Impairments

With MS, faulty nerve conduction through demyelinated CNS axons results in a variety of motor, coordination, and sensory impairments (1, 8, 10). Aging brings additional degenerative changes in the nervous system: a general slowing of central processing, slowing of peripheral nerve conduction velocity, loss of motor units and peripheral nerve fibers, and degeneration of neurons controlling movement, and muscle tone (23).

WEAKNESS

Weakness in MS is due to upper motor neuron (UMN) lesions; initial strength often fatigues rapidly, further impairing performance in functional activities. This fatigability may be related to difficulty sustaining repetitive action potentials through the demyelinated axon (1, 8, 10). Aging adds to weakness with partial lower motor neuron denervation and muscle atrophy (23). Aging muscles can improve in strength and endurance with exercise, but UMN weakness appears to be irreversible (1, 23). Exercise is important to promote general fitness and prevent or reverse disuse atrophy for the aging MS

Table 36.1. Medications for Symptom Management in Multiple Sclerosis

Drug/Dose	Symptom	Common Side Effects	Age-Related Side Effects
Baclofen: 5–20 mg bid–tid	Spasticity	Weakness, sedation, confusion	Increased side effects
Diazepam: 2–10 mg bid–qid	Spasticity	Weakness, sedation, confusion, dysphoria	Increased half-life and side effects, especially sedation. Dysphoria Disequilibrium. Paradoxical reactions; agitation, insomnia
Clonazepam: 0.25–1 mg qd–tid	Ataxia/tremor Spasticity	Weakness, sedation, confusion, dysphoria, ataxia	Increased half-life and side effects
Carbamazepine: 100–300 mg qd–qid	Dysesthesia Paroxysmal symptoms	Weakness, sedation, confusion, bone marrow suppression	Potential adverse anticholinergic, antidiuretic effects; can aggravate cardiovascular disease
Tricyclic antidepressants: Low–moderate	Dysesthesia Sleep disturbance Depression Emotional incontinence	Sedation, confusion, anticholinergic effects: dry mouth, urinary retention, blurred vision, constipation	Increased sensitivity to anticholinergic effects including agitation. Adverse cardiovascular effects; orthostatic hypotension
Amantadine: 100 mg bid	Fatigue	Dopaminergic effects: confusion, hallucinations, nightmares, spasticity, ankle edema, livedo reticularis	Increased side effects including delirium, dementia
Oxybutynin: 5 mg bid–qid	Bladder hypersensitivity	Anticholinergic effects	Increased side effects

patient. Range of motion and functional activities should also be encouraged for all patients (1, 23, 30).

SPASTICITY

Spasticity (increased muscle resistance to passive stretch, hyperactive deep tendon reflexes, and clonus) results from UMN lesions. The severity of spasticity ranges from a mild "catch" to painful mass spasms. Treatment includes the elimination of noxious sensory input and the use of physical interventions (stretch, cold, positioning), nerve/motor point, and medications. Spasticity may provide useful support to patients during transfers or walking so that functional activities actually decline when spasticity is reduced. Treatment must thus be based on the patient's functional abilities (1, 30).

INCOORDINATION, TREMOR, DYSMETRIA, ATAXIA

In MS, lesions in the cerebellum, cerebellar connections, brainstem, and spinal cord can result in ataxia, intention tremor, head or trunk titubation, ataxic breathing patterns, or dysarthria. Medications are not reliably helpful. Physical interventions emphasize compensatory strategies, stabilization of affected body parts, and balance and coordination retraining (1, 8, 30). Aging adds a general slowing of coordination and decreased agility (23).

FATIGUE AND HEAT INTOLERANCE

MS-related fatigue is distinctly different from that experienced by healthy adults. Patients may experience "time of day" fatigue (usually afternoon and evening), minimal activity fatigue, or a sense of continuous exhaustion. The mechanism of fatigue in MS is unknown. Disabling fatigue limits physical or cognitive performance, even in patients with otherwise mild symptoms. Interventions include moderate exercise, adequate sleep, planned rest breaks, energy conservation/work simplification, adaptive equipment, handicapped parking, and medications (1, 8, 30). Fatigue is also seen as part of aging, primarily due to diminished cardiopulmonary reserves that decrease activity tolerance. Exercise can improve activity tolerance in older people (31).

About 50% of MS patients experience intensified symptoms when exposed to internal or environmental heat. Thus, fevers must be treated quickly, and vigorous physical activity should be performed in cooler environments with frequent breaks to avoid internal overheating (1, 8). Air conditioning becomes a legitimate medical expense. The elderly are more vulnerable to both hypothermia and hyperthermia because of loss of homeostatic temperature-regulating controls, including decline in effectiveness of the autonomic nervous system, decrease in sweat gland function, and regional loss of insulating subcutaneous fat (23).

SENSORY IMPAIRMENTS AND PAIN

A variety of sensory deficits with both aging and MS impair the ability of patients to perceive and adapt to environmental changes. Sensory problems in MS may be experienced as vague numbness or decreased perception of vibration, temperature, and proprioception. Distortions of sensations such as tightness, swelling, tingling, burning, trigeminal neuralgia, and Lhermitte's phenomena (electric sensations upon neck flexion) can become distressingly painful (1). Aging adds a gradually decreasing ability to perceive most sensations and an increasing pain threshold (23).

Impairments in the special senses can also occur. In MS, optic neuritis and extraocular muscle dysfunction result in loss of visual acuity, double vision, or nystagmus. The degree of impairment in visual acuity and visual tracking may fluctuate with the patient's level of fatigue or exposure to heat (1). Aging brings loss of visual acuity, higher threshold for light perception, decrease in lens adaptation for near vision, and diminished color perception (23). Hearing loss due to demyelinating lesions of the eighth cranial nerve is rare. However, presbycusis, the multifactorial deterioration of hearing with aging, is common. Early recognition and treatment of hearing impairments can help prevent social estrangement, especially in the presence of cognitive deficits. Taste and smell gradually diminish in the elderly, but are only occasionally affected in MS (1, 23).

Other Organ Systems

GENITOURINARY SYSTEM

In MS, bladder dysfunction can result from lesions anywhere along the central neuroaxis, including the autonomic nervous system. Symptoms of frequency, urgency, and incontinence occur with either an overactive bladder or with spillover of residual urine from a retentive bladder. Hesitancy, retention, and recurrent infections are frequent with bladder-sphincter dyssynergia (voiding obstruction by simultaneous bladder and sphincter contractions) (1). The geriatric patient can also experience a variety of changes that individually are not likely to cause incontinence or retention, yet which may become symptomatic when present in combination or with additional disease (23). With both aging and with MS, medications, limited mobility, and constipation can add to these problems. Bladder symptoms should not be accepted in order to promote effective voiding and prevent incontinence, urosepsis, and renal damage (1, 23).

Sexual dysfunction in MS can result from CNS lesions directly affecting sexual function with impaired genital sensation, altered desire or experience of orgasm, problems in achieving or sustaining an erection or ejaculation, or insufficient vaginal lubrication. Sexual dysfunction can also occur due to fatigue, impaired mobility, bowel and bladder problems, medication side effects, and psychologic issues (1, 30). Most healthy elderly retain some degree of sexual interest and capability (23).

GASTROINTESTINAL SYSTEM

Swallowing disorders in MS may be due to cranial nerve and frontal lobe involvement resulting in difficulty with the coordination, fatigability, timing, and sequencing of oral manipulation and swallow (1). With aging, weakness of pharyngeal peristalsis results in residual material remaining in the pharynx after the swallow. Also, there is reduced tone and motility of the esophagus. Esophageal dysmobility can be associated with achalasia, dysphagia, hiatal hernia, and gastroesophageal reflux (23). Dysphagia therapy involves dietary modification, positioning, presentation compensations, and oral-motor exercises.

Both spinal cord MS lesions and normal aging may result in slowed motility of the stomach and intestine causing constipation. MS lesions can also impair rectal sensation. Contributing factors to constipation in the aging MS patient include poor dietary habits, physical inactivity, medication side effects, depression, weakness of abdominal muscles, postponement of defecation due to immobility, and fluid restriction to control bladder symptoms. Bowel incontinence usually results from dietary indiscretion, impaction, viral gastrointestinal illness, severe bilateral brain lesions, or loss of rectal sensation. Patients can usually regain regular bowel function by means of a good bowel program (1, 23).

CARDIOVASCULAR AND PULMONARY SYSTEMS

In aging there are physiologic declines in pulmonary and cardiovascular capacity and a corresponding decrease in maximal oxygen consumption and work tolerance. With exercise it is possible to improve cardiopulmonary fitness, increase maximal oxygen consumption, decrease the oxygen cost of activity, and decrease fatigability (23, 31). MS does not directly affect the cardiopulmonary system except for a variety of changes in autonomic regulation (9). However, the aging MS patient may be at increased risk for deconditioning when physical dysfunction limits the capacity for aerobic exercise.

The respiratory system may be compromised in severe MS by diaphragmatic and accessory respiratory muscle weakness, fatigue, spasticity, and ataxia, resulting in restrictive or irregular breathing and ineffective cough (1).

MUSCULOSKELETAL SYSTEM

Musculoskeletal mechanical discomfort in the aging MS patient can occur when there is abnormal use, positioning, and overuse of joints and weak or spastic muscles. These problems can aggravate the degenerative arthritic conditions common to the elderly. Interventions attempt to improve posture and activity patterns and lessen spasticity (1). In the more disabled aging MS patient, the risk of osteoporosis increases due to disuse, lack of weight bearing on long bones, and repeated treatment with steroids. Not only falls, but sometimes transfers, stretching, or other physical interventions can cause fractures.

Cognitive Dysfunction and Affective Disorders

COGNITIVE DYSFUNCTION

Cognitive impairment is relatively common among persons with multiple sclerosis. It is estimated that 50% to 70% of MS patients develop some degree of cognitive dysfunction (32), ranging from minimal impairment of discrete intellectual functions to widespread and severe deficits. Cognitive changes may progress independently of physical disability. The diversity observed among MS patients presumably reflects the interaction of a number of factors including location, size and number of lesions, premorbid state, and the aggressiveness of the disease.

Because MS is characterized primarily by the widespread and scattered deep white matter demyelination of axons, patients do not ordinarily demonstrate the circumscribed disorders of language and cognition that are characteristic of focal cortical lesions. Instead, much of the cognitive impairment presumably reflects the disruption of long fiber tracts connecting the cortex with various structures of the limbic system, basal ganglia, and reticular formation. General intelligence seems to change only gradually over time; automatic, overlearned verbal skills are resistant to impairment, while complex nonverbal abilities are more likely to be affected.

Deficits in memory are perhaps the most serious problems for many persons with MS (33). The variability in memory deficits found among patients may be more a function of the anatomic distribution of lesions rather than of the overall severity of the disease. Short-term (working) memory appears to be affected in large part as a consequence of decreased speed and capacity of information processing (33–36). With delayed recall, some evidence suggests that retrieval processes may be more involved than acquisition and storage.

Some MS patients demonstrate cognitive dysfunction characteristic of frontal or prefrontal area disorder (34, 35, 37, 38). Lesions that isolate the frontal or prefrontal cortex result in a decreased capacity to independently initiate and carry out purposeful, goal-directed activity and to inhibit irrelevant or inappropriate behavior. These problems reflect deficits in what is often described as the "executive" or organizing function of the brain. Such patients demonstrate a relatively passive intellectual and behavioral style with difficulties in independent organization, planning, carry through, active problem-solving, abstract conceptualizations, and flexibility of thinking. Distractibility and perseveration probably reflect an inability to direct and control attention and information processing. Slowed information processing may lead to deficient performance on a wide range of tasks, especially those that are timed, novel, or complex. MS patients with significant frontal lobe disorders also demonstrate markedly defective insight. They are unable to reflect on their limited capacities and fail to anticipate the possible consequences of their actions, leading to unsafe, impulsive behavior. These patients do not deliberately engage in disorganized behavior, nor are they deliberately insensitive to the needs or viewpoints of others. What appears to be depression or lack of motivation may actually be a compromised capacity to initiate and regulate one's own behavior. Difficulties of this kind are subtle in the early stages, but substantial problems may develop over time and are often confusing for care providers.

Just as cognitive dysfunction is common but not ubiquitous among MS patients, many, but not all older persons demonstrate varying degrees and kinds of cognitive impairment. Many healthy elderly perform quite well in various aspects of learning and memory. Cognitive tests thought to reflect "crystallized" intelligence (tasks that rely on overlearned abilities and require little novel problem-solving) are generally well done. These include tests of general information, vocabulary, and practical verbal reasoning.

However, several cognitive problems have been associated with normal aging. In particular, the elderly have been found to have increased difficulty with timed, novel, and complex tasks, thought to be measures of so-called "fluid" intelligence. Neuropsychologic studies of the elderly have demonstrated problems in working memory, in speed and capacity of central information processing (36), and in frontal lobe functioning (39, 40). The underlying basis for these findings in normal aging appears to involve a structural-functional decline throughout much of the brain and, importantly, of the frontal lobes and pathways and connections to the frontal lobes (7, 41–44). Older adults are capable of new learning but at a slower rate, with more rehearsal or cuing. In general, the more complex the task, the greater the age effect. Thus, the aging MS patient, who may already have some degree of frontal lobe dysfunction, is at greater risk for the development of significant cognitive disturbances.

AFFECTIVE DISORDERS

Affective disorders in MS may be related to severity or location of lesions or to other neurobiologic factors (45, 46). Psychiatric morbidity has been reported to be higher than among comparably disabled patients (patients with rheumatic or other neurologic conditions not involving the brain) (45). Depression, irritability, euphoria, and emotional lability are observed in a substantial number of MS patients, and there is also evidence of an increased incidence of bipolar affective disorders.

Depression, affecting between 27% and 54% of MS patients (47), is often moderately severe. Multiple factors contribute, including CNS neurobiologic changes and the emotional impact of functional loss, social isolation, frequent illness, and threat of future losses. Depression is also relatively common among apparently normal aged individuals. Depression in the elderly may present with classic mood and vegetative signs and symptoms, but may also be accompanied by nonspecific somatic complaints, anxiety, agitation, or the appearance of dementia (23, 48). Antidepressants are useful, but should be monitored closely for side effects in the aging MS patient. Psychotherapy may be helpful for patients with sufficient insight.

Euphoria in MS patients presents as an inappropriate cheerfulness incongruent with the individual's circumstances. It may coexist with depression, the latter being disguised by the patients euphoric demeanor. Euphoria often heralds a significant change in personality, consistent with the significant cerebral atrophy found in these patients (45), presumably affecting the orbital frontal cortex and limbic areas. There is no known treatment for euphoria, nor is it clear that it requires treatment.

Emotional lability may take two forms among MS patients. For some, the affect expressed is the same as that experienced, but the emotion is expressed too easily and too intensely. Other MS patients may suddenly express emotions that bear little relationship to their actual feeling. Patients may be puzzled, embarrassed, and frustrated by this emotional dyscontrol. Low-dose amitriptyline has been found effective with such pathologic laughing or weeping (26).

Disabilities—Mobility, Activities of Daily Living, Communication

As patients age and as MS duration lengthens, mobility becomes more difficult. In MS, gait difficulties arise from weakness, spasticity, ataxia, fatigability, incoordination, slowed reaction times, and (when there are frontal lobe pathway lesions) impaired motor planning (1). In normal aging, degenerative changes in the motor, vestibular, proprioceptive, and visual systems lead to a decreased sensitivity to movement and compromised ability to maintain an upright posture (23, 49). These changes lead to a general fear of moving and a susceptibility to falls. Gait training and lightweight walking aides help decrease energy cost and increase speed, balance, efficiency, endurance, and safety. Plastic ankle orthotics can enhance toe clearance and knee control. A lightweight wheelchair or motorized three-wheeled scooter may be useful (initially on a part-time basis) for long distance mobility. Proper wheelchair prescription for size, support, positioning, and adaptive features is essential for optimal wheelchair mobility (1, 30).

Activities of daily living, including self-care skills (such as eating, dressing, hygiene) and homemaking may consume inordinate amounts of time and energy and may become unsafe. Training with appropriate techniques, equipment, and energy conservation/work simplification strategies helps patients improve function, efficiency, and safety (1).

Communication disabilities in MS include problems in both reception and expression. Impaired vision and slowness in central auditory processing for both visual and verbal input can interfere with reception. Upper extremity sensorimotor problems can impair written expression, and dysarthria can hinder verbal expression. Slowness of central processing also presents as word finding difficulties. The pragmatics of language (keeping track of topic, taking turns, verbosity, responsiveness to social conversational cues) may be affected by cognitive deficits (1).

PSYCHOSOCIAL ISSUES

The psychosocial issues faced by people who are aging with MS are related to age and developmental life stage at onset, duration of disease, and the variable course and uncertain outcome of the disease (1, 50, 51).

Life Stage At Onset

Younger adults who develop MS are in the midst of establishing careers and families. Because of the unpredictability of MS, life is disrupted, even when initial symptoms are quite mild.

People who have grown older with active MS may have been prevented from developing the resources needed to meet the additional demands of aging. Financial, interpersonal, and personal resources are depleted over time from long-term demands of living with a chronic illness. Aging brings additional and multiple losses in health, function, relationships, and financial security (23). Often the older person who was diagnosed with MS 30 or more years ago has not had much medical, psychologic, or rehabilitative care, because they have heard or assumed that "nothing can be done for MS." These patients frequently function below their potential, without the benefit of modern adaptive equipment and techniques. On the other hand, individuals who have successfully adapted to living with MS have already developed well-tested coping skills to better meet the challenges of aging. Also, if MS stabilizes over time, as it often can, then a person may experience relative stability in his or her later years. The less dramatic and more predictable declines of aging may actually seem less problematic (52).

The newly diagnosed older adult is dealing with later life issues, possibly expecting a time of relative freedom or planning how to conserve resources through retirement years. The older person has already built up his or her resources and developed an established coping style. For those who assume that physical decline is an expected part of aging, the occurrence of MS may be easier to accept, especially when compared to the younger person who considers disability to be unexpected (53). However, accommodation to the new demands and variable impairment of MS is generally more difficult because the older person tends to have fewer physical, functional, and environmental reserves (23, 50, 52).

Adjustment Process

Adjustment to MS is a dynamic, lifelong process as variable as the disease itself. The process can involve several phases through which people move, not always in a predictable order. Emotional reactions to new losses include shock, anger, fear, loss of self-esteem, and guilt. Frequently people will not or cannot acknowledge symptoms, but instead continue attempts at "living as usual" despite impaired function. In a healthy adjustment process, people become able to grieve over losses, express appropriate anger, and deal with anticipatory anxiety over potential disability, dependency, rejection, or abandonment. They acknowledge the reality of having MS, both to themselves and to others, and also become able to redefine a sense of self with MS as a part of life (1). However, patients often report that new losses recall the same emotions and distress as the initial diagnosis or first physical changes, even after decades. Thus, when new exacerbations occur later in life, patients may feel inadequate, guilty, or ashamed that they have not adjusted "once and for all" at an earlier time. Patients and families can be helped by being allowed to reexperience feelings and issues, to reaffirm gains in adjustment and integration, and to not be "perfectly" adjusted.

Overall, people are more likely to experience a better adjustment to disability if they have more stable disease; greater financial and community resources; appropriately supportive family, friends, and religious faith; more diverse sense of self, and the ability to value remaining function.

Families and other support systems play a critical role in the well-being of the patient, by providing emotional support, social connections, and physical assistance. Family members face emotional and social experiences similar to those of the patient—anxiety, denial, depleted financial resources, change in family roles, and social isolation. In the face of the chronic stress of illness and despite good intentions, unhealthy family responses can range from overprotection to neglect or even abuse. Underlying dysfunctional family dynamics make adjustment more difficult (1, 23, 54).

Aging family members who are caregivers may be experiencing a decline in their own energies and abilities just as the need for care may be increasing (23, 53). Appropriate intervention for the older family dealing with MS involves mobilizing inhome services, financial help, and respite care; teaching compensatory skills for declining physical function, and helping patients and family members understand and support patients' actual abilities. Families may need guidance in developing new roles and support systems. Although older families have had a longer time to develop stability and cohesiveness, acknowledgement of marital problems is probably less common, given the social stigma from past generations. Yet the need to recognize and communicate openly about anger, guilt, depression, and fears of abandonment and dependency is important. The disabled spouse may need counseling in how to reciprocate for assistance received from loved ones and attendants in order to maintain self-esteem and to learn how to help the caregiver feel valued. MS family members and caregivers should be encouraged to seek sufficient respite from caregiving to maintain outside interests and to continue social activities. Effective interaction between the patient and spouse can be fostered by understanding their usual means of coping, lifelong roles, and support networks and by enhancing positive coping behaviors (55).

Social connectedness in general is linked to life satisfaction, promptness in seeking medical attention, fewer medical problems, greater function, and less depression (23), yet a sense of alienation from self and others is often experienced in the aged and also in MS patients. Opportunities for aging MS patients to develop social relationships are threatened by decrease in personal mobility, lack of adequate transportation, adjustment problems, a change in home (often to a more physically supported environment), death of spouse or friends, and loss of mutually interesting activities. Also, it can be difficult for others to understand how MS affects a person. A person with MS often lives on the borderline between feeling well and ill, sometimes changing from hour to hour, and some of the most disabling symptoms (such as fatigue) are invisible.

In addition to physical environmental barriers, society often provides attitudinal barriers that create handicaps out of disabilities (56). Many people with MS attempt to conceal impairments in order to avoid the minority status and social devaluation associated with being disabled. In addition, persons with MS often face another form of discrimination—the attitude that, since MS is progressive and incurable, "why provide treatment or care?" Additional biases and societal attitudes exist toward the aging, with and without disabilities (57). Being old in today's society often carries negative stereotypes that most elderly persons are senile, rigid, resistant to change, unproductive, infirm, dependent, emotionally disengaged, and nonsexual. However, it is well-established in gerontologic research that old age is a time of great variability both within and among individuals (23, 58, 59). Handicapping sequelae of ageism include the devaluation of disabled elderly persons, by themselves as well as others, lack of interest in their problems, and limited opportunity for access to appropriate rehabilitative care (23).

Vocation

Employment usually becomes modified to less time or intensity and too often is lost entirely due to the disabilities caused by MS and fears in both patients and employers. Primary factors impacting vocation are mobility, fatigue, cognition, upper extremity impairments, bladder dysfunction, visual losses, communication disorders, transportation difficulty, and depression (60). However, the demographics of MS suggest better employability than might be expected since most MS patients have strong educational backgrounds, normal life span, minimal cognitive involvement, and generally good prognosis for only mild to moderate disability over time.

Vocational issues need to be addressed early in the course of the disease since it is easier to maintain rather than to resume employment. Once on disability benefits, the person with MS is unlikely to return to work when faced with the real threats of variable disease course and the likelihood of recurrent periods of time when they will be unable to work. Most people with MS who remain in their original vocation are older, better educated, male, less disabled, and are in managerial or professional positions (61). Vocational adaptations and work-enhancing conditions have been found to include physical accessibility and conveniently arranged equipment; cool environments; the use of self-pacing, intermittent rest periods and adjusted work schedules; emotional support from family and friends; stress management skills, and a positive attitude (30, 60, 62). Vocational rehabilitation programs help people obtain adaptive equipment and training to remain employed or to explore new career objectives and job structures such as job sharing, supportive employment, or homebound employment. Age alone does not affect productivity or effectiveness. In fact, the older person has the advantage of a longer work history and greater experience in a particular position to draw from when making accommodations (63).

Avocation and Recreational Activities

People with MS may pursue many types of recreational activities by planning for the effects of time of day and environmental temperature to avoid fatigability and heat sensitivity (1, 30). Individuals with more restrictive disabilities may participate in special recreational programs sponsored by local communities, senior or MS organizations, or such organizations as PAW (Physical Access to the Wilderness). Recreational pursuits may need to be further emphasized as a means of productive involvement in living when vocational or volunteer pursuits are no longer feasible.

Finances

MS is costly to patient and to society; costs increase with severity of disability. Expenses deal with medical and rehabilitative care, personal care attendants, special adaptive and durable medical equipment, architectural housing modifications or change in home, and lost wages (64). Many patients lose health care insurance coverage when they are no longer able to work, through divorce, or when they are dropped by their current insurance company. Many are not able to become insured again. The younger person with active MS almost always remains a drain on family resources or needs public assistance programs in order to survive financially. The person who acquires MS at a later age may be more financially prepared to handle some of the costs, but also may be devastated by the need to spend savings on medical and supportive costs.

IMPLICATIONS FOR HEALTH CARE PROVIDERS

Given the irreversibility of both multiple sclerosis and aging, the ultimate goal of medical care is not to effect cure, but rather to maintain optimal health, prevent complications, minimize societal and environmental handicaps, and maximize function.

Good health care for the aging MS patient involves the management of the multiple symptoms and medical problems, the enhancement of decreased physiologic reserves, the avoidance of iatrogenic illness (23, 28, 65), the adaptation of the medical and rehabilitation environment to the aging MS patient (1, 66–68), and the prevention of medical complications. Any new symptoms require special attention and must not be attributed to "just MS," or "just aging" (1, 23).

For best physical function, it is important to encourage maximal physical activity, while acknowledging the reality of fatigue. Exercise should be prescribed and professionally monitored. Since the energy required to perform simple activities (walking, for instance) represents a larger percent of total aerobic capacity with age and increasing neurologic disability, even routine activities can produce a physical conditioning effect (1, 23, 69). Often the most motivating and most effective exercise and skills training takes place in the context of functional activities. Because debilitation secondary to periods of inactivity and illness may occur earlier, be more severe, and be harder to reverse in the aging MS patient, early mobilization and active rehabilitation should be provided after illness, injury, surgery, or any enforced bedrest (1, 23, 69).

In order to provide the most effective long-term care for the aging MS patient, the patient's support system must be identified and cared for, with special attention to the health and fitness of the primary caregiver. Family and friends should be encouraged to understand the effect on the aging MS patient of fatigue and other variable symptoms and capabilities. Function can change rapidly—day to day, even minute to minute. Participating in rehabilitation may foster more realistic expectations by the patient him or herself and by important others. Being able to maintain the greatest range of valued options for the patient and family is often dependent on the opportunities to make appropriate housing modifications, acquire appropriate adaptive equipment, receive adequate physical support with personal care and household maintenance, and obtain transportation at a reasonable cost (1, 23, 70).

Psychologic intervention with the older MS patient can be useful in managing affective disorders or in dealing with later life themes of cumulative losses, the struggle to remain independent, concern over family relations, the maintenance of self-esteem and sexuality, and a review of past life and preparation for the end of life (56, 66). Counseling can also include issues of sexuality, stress management, and living wills. Such psychotherapeutic work is enhanced by the tendency for people to become more introspective and concerned about the meaning of one's life with age (71). On the other hand, insight may decrease if frontal cognitive problems increase.

Cognitive issues should be addressed directly. Commonly, patients fear the benign forgetfulness of aging or MS as a sign that they are becoming demented or are going crazy. Gaining an understanding of the true nature and severity of their problems and of compensatory management strategies can be helpful to patients and families. When severe frontal lobe problems are present, it is necessary to help families and caregivers change their expectations and interpretations of these patients' behavior. At some point the legal and ethical issues of competence will need to be addressed. In order to help patients function to their best, families and caregivers need to simplify the physical environment, develop routines, and provide consistent, direct, ongoing, and concrete cues and structure (72, 73).

Aging with MS often results in multiple, progressive losses. Comprehensive, accessible medical and rehabilitative care (1, 68) can have a life-long effect in helping people who are aging with MS optimize health and learn the skills and develop the resources to minimize losses and maximize functional capacities.

References

1. Cobble ND, Wangaard C, Kraft GH, Burks JS. Rehabilitation of the patients with multiple sclerosis. In: DeLisa, JA ed. *Rehabilitation Medicine, Principles and Practice*. Philadelphia, Pa: J.B. Lippincott; 1988.
2. Ellison GW. Multiple sclerosis: why? *Biomed Pharmacother*. 43:327–333, 1989.
3. Gorelick P. Clues to the mystery of multiple sclerosis. *Postgrad Med*. 85:125–134, 1989.
4. Rodriguez M. Multiple sclerosis: basic concepts and hypotheses. *Mayo Clin Proc*. 64:570–576, 1989.
5. Wynn DR, Rodriguez M, O'Fallon WM, Kurland LT. Update on the epidemiology of multiple sclerosis. *Mayo Clin Proc*. 64:808–817, 1989.
6. McDonald WI, Barnes D. Lessons from magnetic resonance imaging in multiple sclerosis. *Trends Neurosci*. 12:376–379, 1989.
7. Adams RD, Victor M. *Principles of Neurology*. 4th ed. New York, NY: McGraw-Hill; 1989.
8. Kelly R. Clinical aspects of multiple sclerosis. In: Vinken PJ, Bruyn GW, Klawans HL, Koetsier JC, eds. *Handbook of Clinical Neurology, XLVII, Demyelinating Diseases*. Amsterdam: Elsevier Science Publishers; 1985.
9. Nordenbo A, Boeson F, Anderson EB. Cardiovascular autonomic function in multiple sclerosis. *J Auton Nerv Syst*. 26:77–84, 1989.
10. Kocsis JD, Waxman SG. Demyelination: causes and mechanisms of clinical abnormality and functional recovery. In: Vinken PJ, Bruyn GW, Klawans HL, Koetsier JC, eds. *Handbook of Clinical Neurology, XLVII, Demyelinating Diseases*. Amsterdam: Elsevier Science Publishers; 1985.
11. Willoughby EW, Grochowski E, Li DKB, Oger J, Kastrukoff LF, Paty DW. Serial magnetic resonance scanning in multiple sclerosis: a second prospective study in relapsing patients. *Ann Neurol*. 25:43–49, 1989.
12. Goodkin DE, Hertsgaard D, Rudick RA. Exacerbation rates and adherence to disease type in a prospectively followed-up population with multiple sclerosis. Implications for clinical trials. *Arch Neurol*. 46:1107–1112, 1989.
13. Swanson JW. Multiple sclerosis: update in diagnosis and review of prognostic factors. *Mayo Clin Proc*. 64:577–586, 1989.
14. Percy AK, Nobrega FT, Okazaki H, Glattre E, Kurland LT. MS in Rochester, Minn: a 60-year reappraisal. *Arch Neurol*. 25:105–111, 1971.
15. Fazekas F, Offenbacher H, Fuchs S, et al. Criteria for an increased specificity of MRI interpretation in elderly subjects with suspected multiple sclerosis. *Neurology*. 38:1822–1825, 1988.
16. Carter JL, Rodriguez M. Immunosuppressive treatment of multiple sclerosis. *Mayo Clin Proc*. 64:664–669, 1989.
17. Sibley WA, ed. *Therapeutic Claims in Multiple Sclerosis*. 2nd ed. New York, NY: Demos; 1988.
18. Durelli L, Cocito D, Riccio A, et al. High-dose intravenous methylprednisolone in the treatment of multiple sclerosis: clinical-immunologic correlations. *Neurology*. 36:238–243, 1986.
19. Kesselring J, Miller DH, MacManus DG, et al. Quantitative magnetic resonance imaging in multiple sclerosis: the effect of high dose intravenous methylprednisolone. *J Neurol Neurosurg, Psychiatry*. 52:14–17, 1989.
20. Seale JP, Compton MR. Side effects of corticosteroid agents. *Med J Aust*. 144:139–142, 1986.
21. *AMA Drug Evaluation*. Chicago, Il: American Medical Association; 1983.
22. O'Callaghan JW, Brooks P. Disease-modifying agents and immunosuppressive drugs in the elderly. *Clin Rheum Dis*. 12:275–289, 1986.
23. Clark GS, Murray PK. Rehabilitation of the geriatric patient. In: DeLisa JA, ed. *Rehabilitation Medicine, Principles and Practice*. Philadelphia, Pa: J.B. Lippincott; 1988.
24. Delafuente JC, Stewart RB, eds. *Therapeutics in the Elderly*. Baltimore, Md: Williams & Wilkins; 1990.
25. Hulme A, MacLennan W, Ritchie RT, John VA, Shotton PA. Baclofen in the elderly stroke patient, its side-effects and pharmacokinetics. *Eur J Clin Pharmacol*. 29:467–469, 1985.
26. Schiffer RB, Herndon RM, Rudick RA. Treatment of pathologic laughing and weeping with amitriptyline. *N Engl J Med*. 312:1480–1482, 1985.
27. Salzman C, ed. *Clinical Geriatric Psychopharmacology*. New York, NY: McGraw-Hill; 1984.
28. Siebens H. Medications in older adults: adverse and therapeutic effects on cognition in the rehabilitation setting. *Top Geriatr Rehabil*. 5(3):20–25, 1990.
29. Williams P, Rush DR. Geriatric polypharmacy. *Hosp Prac*. Feb:109–120, 1986.
30. Erickson R, Lie MR, Wineinger MA. Rehabilitation in multiple sclerosis. *Mayo Clin Proc*. 64:818, 1989.
31. Siebens H. Deconditioning. In: Kemp B, Brummel-Smith

K, Ramsdell JW, eds. *Geriatric Rehabilitation.* Boston, Mass: Little, Brown; 1990.

32. Heaton RK, Nelson LM, Thompson DS, Burks JS, Franklin GM. Neuropsychological findings in relapsing-remitting and chronic-progressive multiple sclerosis. *J Consult Clin Psychol.* 53:103–110, 1985.

33. Rao SM, Leo GJ, St. Aubin-Faubert P. On the nature of memory disturbance in multiple sclerosis. *J Clin Exp Neuropsychol.* 11:699–712, 1989.

34. Beatty WW, Goodkin DE, Monson N, Beatty PA, Hertsgaard D. Anterograde and retrograde amnesia in patients with chronic progressive multiple sclerosis. *Arch Neurol.* 45:611–619, 1988.

35. Beatty WW, Goodkin DE, Beatty PA. Frontal lobe dysfunction and memory impairment in patients with chronic progressive multiple sclerosis. *Brain Cognition.* 11:73–86, 1989.

36. Baddeley A. *Working Memory.* Oxford, England: Oxford Science Publications; 1986.

37. Rao SM. Neuropsychology of multiple sclerosis: a critical review. *J Clin Exp Neuropsychol.* 8:503–542, 1986.

38. Rao SM, Hammeke TA, Speech TJ. Wisconsin Card Sorting Test performance in relapsing-remitting and chronic-progressive multiple sclerosis. *J Consult Clin Psychol.* 55:263–265, 1987.

39. Kaye K, Grigsby J, Robbins LJ, Korzun B. Prediction of independent functioning and behavior problems in geriatric patients. *J Am Geriat Soc.* Vol 38:1304–1310, 1990.

40. Mittenberg W, Seidenberg M, O'Leary DS, DiGiulio DV. Changes in cerebral functioning associated with normal aging. *J Clin Exp Neuropsychol.* 11:918–932, 1989.

41. Fuster JM. *The Prefrontal Cortex: Anatomy, Physiology, and Neuropsychology of the Frontal Lobe.* New York, NY: Raven Press; 1989.

42. Haug H, Barmwater U, Eggers R, et al. Anatomical changes in aging brain: morphometric analysis of the human prosencephalon. In: Cervos-Navarro J, Sarkander HI, eds. *Neuropharmacology.* New York, NY: Raven Press; 1983.

43. Jacobs L, Grossman L. Three primitive reflexes in normal adults. *Neurology.* 30:184–192, 1980.

44. Gur RC, Gur RE, Obrist WD, Skolnick BE, Reivich M. Age and regional cerebral blood flow at rest and during cognitive activity. *Arch Gen Psychiatry.* 44:617–621, 1987.

45. Ron MA, Logsdail SJ. Psychiatric morbidity in multiple sclerosis: a clinical and MRI study. *Psychol. Med.* 19:887–895, 1989.

46. Horner WG, Hurwitz T, Li DKB, Palmer M, Paty DW. Temporal lobe involvement in multiple sclerosis patients with psychiatric disorders. *Arch Neurol.* 44:187–190, 1987.

47. Minden SL, Schiffer RB. Affective disorders in multiple sclerosis: review and recommendations for clinical research. *Arch Neurol.* 47:98–104, 1990.

48. Blazer D. Depression in the elderly. *N Engl J Med.* 320:164–166, 1989.

49. Brummel-Smith K. Falls and instability in the older person. In: Kemp B, Brummel-Smith K, Ramsdell JW, eds. *Geriatric Rehabilitation.* Boston, Mass: Little, Brown; 1990.

50. Kivnick HQ. Disability and psychosocial development in old age. *Rehabil Counseling Bull.* 29:123–134, 1985.

51. Robinson I. Managing symptoms in chronic disease: some dimensions of patients' experience. *Int Disabil Stud.* 10:112–118, 1988.

52. Treischman RB. *Aging With A Disability.* New York, NY: Demos; 1987.

53. Rankin SH, Weekes DP. Life-span development: a review of theory and practice for families with chronically ill members. *Scholarly Inquiry Nurs Prac.* 3:(1)3–22, 1989.

54. Huston PG. Family care of the elderly and caregiver stress. *Am Fam Phys.* 42:671–676, 1990.

55. Dewis ME, Chekryn J. The older dyadic family unit and chronic illness. *Home Health Care Nurse.* 8:42–48, 1990.

56. Vash CL. *The Psychology of Disability.* New York, NY: Springer; 1981.

57. Zola IK. Aging and disability: toward a unifying agenda. *Gerontology.* 14:365–387, 1988.

58. Rowe JW, Minaker KL. Geriatric medicine. In: French CE, Schneider EL, eds. *Handbook of The Biology of Aging.* New York: NY: Van Nostrand Reinhold; 1985.

59. Willis SL. Towards an educational psychology of the older adult learner: intellectual and cognitive bases. In: Buren JE, Schaie KW, eds. *Handbook of the Psychology of Aging.* New York, NY: Van Nostrand Reinhold; 1985.

60. Gulick EE, Yam M, Touw MM. Work performance by persons with multiple sclerosis: conditions that impede or enable the performance of work. *Int J Nurs Stud.* 26:301–311, 1989.

61. LaRocca N, Kalb R, Scheinberg L, Kendall P. Factors associated with unemployment of patients with multiple sclerosis. *J Chron Dis.* 38:203–210, 1985.

62. Marsh GG, Ellison GW, Strite C. Psychosocial and vocational rehabilitation approaches to multiple sclerosis. *Ann Rev Rehabil.* 4:242–267, 1983.

63. Dunn DV. Vocational rehabilitation of the older disabled worker. *J Rehabil.* 47:76–81, 1981.

64. Inman RP. Disability indices, the economic costs of illness, and social insurance: the case of multiple sclerosis. *Acta Neurol Scand.* 101:46–55, 1984.

65. Mold JW, Stein HF. The cascade effect in the clinical care of patients. *N Engl J Med.* 314:512, 1986.

66. Kemp B, Brummel-Smith R, Ramsdell JK. *Geriatric Rehabilitation.* Boston, Mass: Little, Brown; 1990.

67. Hartke RJ. The older adult's adjustment to the rehabilitation setting. In: Hartke RJ, ed. *Psychological Issues in the Physical Rehabilitation of the Disabled Older Adult.* Rockville, Md: Aspen Publishers; 1991.

68. Cobble ND, Burks JS. The team approach to the management of multiple sclerosis. In: Maloney FP, Burks JS, Ringel SP, eds. *Interdisciplinary Rehabilitation of Multiple Sclerosis and Neuromuscular Disorders.* Philadelphia, Pa: J.B. Lippincott; 1985.

69. Rowe JW, Wang S. The biology and physiology of aging. In: Rowe JW, Besdine RW, eds. *Geriatric Medicine.* Boston, Mass: Little, Brown; 1988.

70. Reschovsky JD, Newman SJ. Adaptations for independent living by older frail households. *Gerontologist.* 30:543–552, 1990.

71. Butler RN, Lewis MI. *Aging and Mental Health.* St. Louis, Mo: CV Mosby; 1982.

72. Rentz DM. The assessment of rehabilitation potential: cognitive factors. In: Hartke RJ, ed. *Psychological Issues in the Physical Rehabilitation of the Disabled Older Adult.* Rockville, Md: Aspen Publishers, 1991.

73. Luria AR. *Higher Cortical Functions in Man.* 2nd ed. New York, NY: Basic Books; 1980.

SECTION V

REHABILITATION AND CARE

37
Rehabilitation Team: Process and Roles

Gary S. Clark

"Teamwork: Coming together is a beginning;
Keeping together is progress;
Working together is success."
—Henry Ford

Teamwork is prerequisite for both rehabilitation and geriatrics. The basic philosophy and process of rehabilitation involves a "continuing and comprehensive team effort, (1)" while geriatrics similarly mandates a multidisciplinary health care team (2) with interdisciplinary teamwork (3). In fact, T. Franklin Williams, M.D. (4) maintains that "the rehabilitation philosophy and approach should be at the heart of geriatric medicine." It logically follows that geriatric rehabilitation also embraces the concept of teamwork; the American Geriatrics Society Public Policy Committee, in its Position Statement on Geriatric Rehabilitation (5), states explicitly that "an interdisciplinary approach should be used in the delivery of comprehensive geriatric rehabilitation services." Rothberg (6) traces the evolution of health care teams in response to an increasingly complicated health care delivery process and postulates that the team concept evolved as a compromise between the benefits of specialization and the need for continuity and comprehensiveness of care.

DEFINITIONS AND CONCEPTS

Foley et al (7) characterize a geriatric health care team as a group of professionals with diverse training and skills who meld their joint expertise for the benefit of the individual patient or client and who provide support for the individual members who constitute the team. Halstead (8) similarly defines a team as a group of two or more health professionals from different disciplines who share common values and work toward common objectives. He further defines team care as coordinated, comprehensive care provided by persons who integrate their observations, expertise, and decisions. Teamwork may be viewed as a special form of interactional inter-

dependence between health care providers who merge different but complementary skills or viewpoints in the service of patients and in the solution of their health problems (3).

The simplest form of a health care team uses the *multidisciplinary approach*, where each team member contributes his or her discipline-specific skills, resulting in a summation of individual member's contributions. There is no intrinsic need for a team member to learn skills or knowledge of other disciplines or of group process (9). Multidisciplinary teams have been utilized for health care in multiple settings and contexts, including rehabilitation and geriatrics (2, 9). However, the *interdisciplinary approach* is considered the more appropriate (and presumed more effective) model for both geriatrics and rehabilitation (3, 10). An interdisciplinary team utilizes overlapping skills and knowledge of team members of different disciplines to obtain a synergistic effect whereby the outcome is enhanced and more comprehensive than the simple aggregation of individual efforts. (9, 10). Keys to effective interdisciplinary team functioning include frequent and consistent communication among team members, patient, and family, as well as joint planning and action with shared responsibility for outcomes (3, 10).

Given the integral nature of the team to both geriatrics and rehabilitation, it might be assumed that the utility and efficacy of this instrument (7) has been extensively studied. Halstead (8) surveyed the literature up to 1976 regarding team care in chronic illness and determined that, although there had been numerous anecdotal and descriptive articles extolling the virtues of team care, there were relatively few controlled and comparative studies using team care as a treatment variable. Analysis of the latter suggested that coordinated team care was more effective than was fragmented care, with improved or maintained functional status. However, Halstead concluded that generalizability was severely limited due to differing process and outcome variables, types of patients and settings, and even terminology. He also noted that team care is not a single, homogenous treatment variable, but rather a broadly defined, heterogeneous concept encompassing many elements (8). Others have also expressed concern over the lack of description of standards for calibration, reliability or reproducibility regarding team composition, education and development, functioning, or effectiveness (7). Although the interdisciplinary team approach demonstrates face validity and perceived efficacy for geriatric rehabilitation, further investigation of standardized formats (with specific protocols for membership, training, functioning, etc.) in various treatment settings is needed to objectively substantiate benefit and cost-effectiveness.

TEAM DYNAMICS

Effectiveness of a group or team can be assessed in terms of its success in completing assigned tasks or work, as well as its ability to function cohesively as a group of independent individuals (7). A number of characteristics of effective work teams have been described (11):

- informal, relaxed atmosphere with considerable participatory discussion,
- team goals and objectives understood and accepted by all members,
- mutual nonjudgmental listening with open expression of feelings,
- constructive criticism and nonacrimonious disagreement among team members,
- consensus decision-making with clear task assignments,
- flexible, nondominating leadership, and
- self-analysis and self-consciousness regarding team function/effectiveness.

A team practicing these characteristics has developed a built-in feedback mechanism to regularly reassess (and maintain or improve) its process and outcomes (10). The development or restoration of effective team functioning is referred to as team building (12).

Team Building

Tsukuda (3) references the "technology of team development" as having derived from a variety of theoretical bases, including general systems, communication sciences, group dynamics, and organizational development. She maintains that teams must acquire a number of key skills and concepts to facilitate collaborative development of rules governing their function, which in turn may improve team performance. Critical concepts include knowledge and skills in management, group process, interpersonal communication, and interdisciplinary interaction (3). Necessary team tasks include role negotiation; building effective working relationships between members; developing procedures for goal-setting, problem-solving, decision-making, and task assignment, and establishing a supportive environment that facilitates open communication among team members (3, 10).

All too frequently, teams devote little or no time or attention to the style and manner of their functioning or to training members to work as coordinated teams (6). Another frequent error is focusing primarily on interpersonal problems rather than on the development of a structure of appropriate operating policies and procedures (3). Newly formed teams should designate specific meetings devoted to becoming familiar with each other's expertise and perspectives and to developing an organizational and operational structure (10).

While the need for team building is obvious in the developmental phases of a nascent health care team, it is also critical when there is turnover or addition of new members to the team (3, 10). To avoid future conflicts, new team members must not only understand and commit to the team process, but also have the opportunity to contribute to (and thereby develop ownership of) team goals (3).

Communication

Establishing and maintaining intrateam communication has been identified as the key to an effective team (10). To effectively and appropriately solve problems and make decisions, the team requires accurate and timely information, which is freely communicated among team members (7). A number of barriers to effective team communication have been identified including autonomy; personality conflicts; role ambiguity; conflicting perceptions of authority, power and status; differing educational backgrounds and knowledge base, as well as hidden agendas (13). Yet another potential impediment to accurate information interchange is variable understanding and definition of basic rehabilitation terminology (14).

Since communication is a dynamic and ongoing process, teams must constantly work to maintain, if not improve, their skills (7). This most appropriately occurs as part of team building, requiring conscious effort and commitment to minimize and overcome barriers to effective communication (10).

Leadership

Although the physician typically is accorded formal titular leadership of most health care teams by virtue of ultimate responsibility for care provided and/or regulatory requirement, this does not necessarily translate to consistent operational leadership (3). In fact, interdisciplinary team dynamics are usually characterized by flexible or shifting leadership (3, 7). Rather than a single leader, there may be multiple leaders (acting in varied roles as initiators, facilitators, or encouragers) or sequential leaders (such as during a team conference) (7, 10). This is not to say that a health care team can function effectively without leadership, as responsibility must be assumed for developing a care plan, assigning tasks, and monitoring to ensure attainment of goals (3). Lundborg (15), who maintains that leadership skills can be learned, developed, and enhanced, has described a number of qualities of a leader:

- knows where he or she is going,
- knows how to get there,
- has courage and persistence,
- can be believed,
- can be trusted not to "sell out" a cause for personal gain,
- makes the mission seem important, exciting, and possible to accomplish
- makes each team member's role in the mission seem important, and
- makes each team member feel capable of performing his or her role.

Lundborg (15) also stresses the importance of such additional leadership skills as articulateness, the ability to inspire faith in followers, and an aptitude for engendering and preserving morale.

The leadership role(s) and process need to be clarified as part of the team building process, particularly with regard to the process of decision-making. Although decision-making has traditionally been imbued in the titular leader, there is an impetus "to have decisions made as close to the source of the problem as possible, and by those who have the relevant information, regardless of their role or location in the organizational hierarchy (16). Clinically this translates to team members with the most knowledge concerning a patient and the particular situation having primary responsibility (or at least major input) in the decision process. The decision-making process includes determining what needs to be decided, who should participate in making the decision, who will implement the decision, and who should be informed about the decision (3). This obviously requires an effective communication process, with both structured meetings (e.g., team conferences) and informal information exchanges and discussions.

Role Expectations

Each team member is a member of several reference groups (7), each of which promulgates formal and informal expectations and rules of conduct that influence individual behavior. For example, therapists may belong to one or more professional discipline organizations (at the local, state, and national levels) and to special interest groups corresponding to certain disability categories, as well as their peer groups in the rehabilitation program or at their facility. These various groups may impose ambiguous, conflicting, or overloading expectations, resulting in multiple loyalties for individual team members, which may in turn impact on team functioning (7).

In addition to such externally imposed behavioral standards and expectations are internally generated role expectations, incorporating one's personal and professional self-image, interpretations (often inaccurate) of collegial perceptions, and perceived expectations of peer responses in similar situations. A further contributing factor is the degree of understanding of professional skills, knowledge, and responsibilities of colleagues from different disciplines, which is frequently limited, flawed, and biased (7).

Also contributing to potentially conflicting team member role expectations is the considerable overlap of clinical ability and expertise between disciplines. While such overlap is desirable in an interdisciplinary team setting, there is nonetheless increased potential for conflict, duplication of efforts, and difficulty reaching agreement on professional boundaries and responsibilities (3). To avoid such problems, the team building process should include adequate time and focus on defining and communicating expectations of various team members, anticipating and resolving possible areas of conflict. Role negotiation and task differentiation should result in clear delineation of behavioral and performance expectations for each team member, correlated with necessary skills and experience (3). An important concept for team members to embrace is the interdependency of team members and the value of each member's contributions. An effective team consists of a cohesive group of professionals with different but complementary skills, who trust and respect the expertise of other team members and adopt the team mission (3).

Team Barriers

Barriers to effective teamwork can occur at the level of individual members, the team itself, or the organizational setting in which the team functions (3). A number of potential barriers have already been referenced, such as communication difficulties or conflicts in role expectations.

At the level of the individual, the most common (and difficult) barriers are attitudinal. Our educational system for health care professionals tend to be rigid and standardized, with separate curricula for each discipline, emphasizing unique bodies of expertise (3, 6). As a result, health care professionals may receive little formal exposure to skills and expertise of other disciplines (particularly areas of shared ability), let alone formal training in the conceptual and operational aspects of health care teams. This may be a contributing factor to Rothberg's (6) lament regarding health care professionals' lack of trust in the professional judgment of colleagues from other disciplines (an underlying tenet of interdisciplinary team functioning) and their assignment to teams in spite of lack of commitment to or understanding of concepts of team functioning. Another potential problem relates to ego rewards and job satisfaction, especially when dealing with a clientele where cure is not feasible and gains may be limited (6). Other potential arenas for conflict that interfere with team function include sexism, racism, generation gaps, and income or status differentials between disciplines.

Team problems often occur as a result of lack of attention to or analysis of the style and manner of team functioning, both at the outset (team building) and in periodic evaluation of performance (team maintenance) (6). Other frequent issues include lack of clarity of roles, personality conflicts, lack of clearly defined (and accepted) goals, communication difficulties, and disagreements over leadership and the distribution of authority (2, 3).

The setting in which a team functions can also influence its cohesiveness and effectiveness (3). The facility or organization imposes its own structure and expectations, with standards of conformity that may be at odds with team-derived procedures. Limited resource allocation (staff, equipment) to accomplish identified goals may also prove a barrier to team functioning. Along the same lines, a poor working environment or frequent turnover of staff may result in poor team morale and interfere with team effectiveness.

TEAM SETTINGS

The concept of the team approach for health care in general and rehabilitation in particular can be applied at the various levels and settings of health care delivery. However, the ease, consistency, and efficacy of team functioning will vary significantly across levels of care.

The hospital represents the most traditional health care setting for rehabilitation services, both on the acute medical/surgical services and the inpatient rehabilitation unit. Rehabilitation involvement usually begins while the patient is on the acute floor, via consultation to initiate therapy treatment. In this setting, the therapist must interact with the other members of the medical/surgical team. This typically includes the medical/surgical nurse, attending physician, and various other acute care staff. The limited, intermittent nature of the rehabilitation therapists' involvement makes it difficult to achieve an interdisciplinary format. Interaction with other treating

health care professionals is often limited to medical record entries and conversations with nursing staff. On units with a consistently high volume of referrals for therapy (e.g., orthopedics), there is greater opportunity for more consistent interaction (and accordingly, teamwork), particularly if a satellite therapy program is established with full-time therapists present. There are examples of more highly developed team approaches to identifying and addressing problems in older hospitalized patients, such as Geriatric Consultation Teams (17–19) and Geriatric Evaluation Units (20, 21). Such programs provide much of the structure and process needed for effective team functioning (e.g., focus of efforts, role delineation, communication).

The hospital-based rehabilitation unit (or free-standing hospital-level rehabilitation facility) provides the ideal setting for interdisciplinary team functioning. Treatment protocols are well established for comprehensive evaluation of the patient (and family) by each discipline, with sharing of findings and treatment strategies among all team members and subsequent joint goal setting and treatment plan formulation (1). Team members work in proximity to each other and interact regularly, both informally (e.g., in hallways, treatment areas) and in a more structured format in team meetings. Lengths of stay of patients are long enough (weeks) to develop good rapport and stable relationships with patients and their families. There is a tendency to develop an identity and esprit de corps among team members, with shared pride in team accomplishments (e.g., patient improvement, with ability to return home).

Rehabilitation programs established within skilled nursing facilities (nursing homes) also afford opportunities for interdisciplinary teamwork, as the structure and process is similar to that of acute care (hospital) based units or facilities, albeit at a lower intensity (22). In more generic long-term care facilities, there is evidence of the potential for benefit with use of a structured team approach (23). However, this benefit was observed more in patients with potential for significant improvement (medical or functional), which does not apply to the majority of long-term residents (24).

Outpatient (ambulatory care) rehabilitation treatment settings offering multiple therapies may be hospital or rehabilitation facility-based or free-standing, such as Comprehensive Outpatient Rehabilitation Facilities (CORF's). In these settings, the rehabilitation team is again working in close proximity to each other and in coordinated treatment programs. The team process and functioning is comparable to the inpatient acute rehabilitation unit or facility, with similar opportunities for interdisciplinary collaboration. Specialized outpatient rehabilitation programs for elderly individuals with disabilities, termed Day Hospitals, provide individual and group therapy in conjunction with social and recreational activities (25, 26).

Finally, rehabilitation services may be provided in patients' homes by various public and private community agencies (e.g., County Public Health Department, Visiting Nurse Association). These home-based services are usually in conjunction with and coordinated by a community nurse, per physician prescription. The team process tends to be multidisciplinary, with less structure or intensity than other levels of care (27). Individual health care professionals are more autonomous regarding individual patient treatment plans, with communication routinely via written reports and by phone for problem discussion and resolution. However, in the continuing evolution of varying levels of care and settings for rehabilitation, home-based comprehensive rehabilitation programs with acute hospital-level intensity have been developed (28). A well-structured rehabilitation team visits the home regularly (up to daily), including therapists, rehabilitation nurses, social worker, and physiatrist. Since treatment incorporates the patient and family directly, this setting offers an excellent opportunity for significant and continuing patient/family input into treatment planning and goal-setting.

TEAM COMPOSITION

While the composition of the team is somewhat standardized for most inpatient (hospital-based) rehabilitation programs (1), there is lack of consensus regarding geriatric teams, particularly in less traditional settings, such as long-term care facilities, outpatient, and home-based programs (7). Health care team membership is most appropriately determined based on skills necessary to address the identified problems; unfortunately, all too often teams consist of only those disciplines readily available within the organization (3). As a result, existing team members may be forced to try to expand their skills to cover the gap, perhaps with less than ideal results. Other options may include recruitment of additional team members (usually a lengthy and uncertain process) or acquiring needed experts via consultative or temporary agency contracts. The latter strategies have obvious ramifications for team building, communication, cohesiveness, consistency, and function.

A concept utilized most frequently with geriatric health care teams is that of core and extended teams (3, 7). In this context, the core team usually consists of the primary care physician (e.g., geriatrician), nurse, and social worker. Extended team members variably could include rehabilitation therapists, activities therapist, dietician, pharmacist, family, consulting physicians, clergy, psychologist, administrators, and volunteers. Various extended team members may be included in the core team for individual patients or programs (3).

Applying this construct to rehabilitation (and geriatric rehabilitation) health care teams, the core team would typically include the physician (e.g., physiatrist), rehabilitation nurse, physical therapist, occupational therapist, speech and language pathologist, and social worker, as well as the patient and his or her family (1). Depending on the setting and needs, a rehabilitation extended team could consist of a clinical or neuropsychologist, recreational therapist, dietician, consulting physicians, vocational counselor, prosthetist or orthotist, respiratory therapist, and cognitive therapist, among others.

Individual rehabilitation and geriatric rehabilitation programs and facilities will typically evolve their own composition for core and extended teams, based on their scope of services and patients' needs. The process of integrating core and extended teams may well necessitate more involved and ongoing team building, particularly with respect to roles, communication, and decision-making (7). Moreover, disability or population-specific rehabilitation teams (e.g., spinal cord injury, orthopedic, traumatic brain injury, pediatric) may develop even more specialized core teams and expanded extended teams. Unique versions of core and extended teams may also be observed in alternative (subacute) rehabilitation settings, such as ambulatory (outpatient), Skilled Nursing Facility (SNF) or nursing home, and home-based community programs.

Following is a brief summary of the areas of expertise and focus of the various health care professionals in the context of participating on the interdisciplinary geriatric rehabilitation team (1, 10).

Physical Therapy

The physical therapist is primarily concerned with improving mobility, with a major emphasis on safe independence (i.e., minimizing the risk of falling). Areas of focus accordingly include strength, endurance, balance, coordination, and joint range of motion. Therapeutic modalities may be employed to help decrease muscle spasm or pain, enhance stretching, or facilitate muscle strengthening. Examples of such modalities include superficial heat or cold, deep heat (diathermy), electrical stimulation, massage, and hydrotherapy. Assistive devices may serve to improve stability and safety with ambulation, such as various types of canes, crutches and walkers, or orthoses (braces). Training is progressive across various levels of mobility as appropriate, such as turning and moving in bed, transferring (in and out of bed, on and off toilet, etc.), locomotion via wheelchair, as well as ambulation on uneven surfaces (sidewalks, gravel, curbs, ramps) and stairs. Patient and family needs and concerns are factored into realistic goal-setting; a visit to the patient's home is often invaluable for focusing training on needs within that specific environment and provides an opportunity for recommendations to achieve barrier-free accessibility.

Occupational Therapy

Achieving functional independence with various self-care skills is the major emphasis of the occupational therapist. Training may encompass such activities of daily living (ADLs) as eating, swallowing, grooming, bathing, dressing, and toileting/personal hygiene, as well as various community skills (often referred to as Instrumental Activities of Daily Living or IADL). Examples of the latter include shopping, phone use, cooking, washing dishes, doing laundry, paying bills, and balancing a checkbook. The occupational therapist concentrates on requisite abilities in upper extremity range of motion, strength, coordination, and dexterity, as well as visual-perceptual and cognitive skills. Training to circumvent underlying impairments may include adoptive techniques and a variety of assistive devices (e.g., long-handled reacher, button hook, built-up handles of utensils for easier grip). Instruction in joint protection or energy conservation techniques is provided as appropriate. Upper extremity orthotics (splints) may stabilize and protect painful or weak wrists or facilitate holding and using utensils. Home environment modifications often significantly improve safety and functional ability.

Speech and Language Pathology

While the obvious focus of the speech/language pathologist is on neurologic communication deficits, other areas of attention include swallowing evaluation and training for dysphagia, audiologic evaluation, speech training postlaryngectomy (esophageal speech or prosthetic larynx), and language-based remediation for cognitive deficits. Therapy is provided for patients with various syndromes of dysphasia, dyspraxia, or dysarthria, with involvement and training of family or significant other in conjunction with the patient. A variety of adaptive techniques and assistive devices (including augmentative communication) can be utilized.

Rehabilitation Nursing

The key to an effective inpatient rehabilitation program is the expertise and performance of rehabilitation nurses in reinforcing and practicing various functional tasks learned in the therapies. This helps to extend the several hours of therapy per day into a 24-hour "therapeutic milieu." This requires significantly more time than traditional medical/surgical nursing, as it takes longer to supervise, assist, and encourage patients through their ADLs than to just do for them. Other major areas of input from rehabilitation nursing include attention to and instruction in proper skin care, education in appropriate medication use, and evaluation and management of bowel/bladder dysfunction. Rehabilitation nurses represent the most frequent, if not the primary, team contact with a patient's family and serve a key role in

family education and training in preparation for discharge.

Social Work

The social worker is usually the principal liaison with the patient and family and helps to establish open channels of communication with the rest of the team. Effectiveness in disposition planning requires ready access to a variety of vendors for various prescribed assistive devices and adaptive equipment, as well as a working knowledge of community services (such as visiting nurse or aide services, home-based therapy, Meals-On-Wheels, etc.). In this way the social worker ensures that the rehabilitation process is continuing and coordinated beyond the hospital inpatient phase. Other key functions of the social worker include family education and counseling regarding the impact of a disabling condition on family dynamics and functioning and adaptation to persisting impairments.

Clinical and Neuropsychology

Depending on the nature of the underlying disabling condition, the psychologist may conduct screening or more detailed testing of intelligence and cognitive functioning, perceptual skills, manual dexterity, personality and mood characteristics (including depression), and problem-solving abilities. This critical information is provided to the rehabilitation team to factor into realistic goal-setting and treatment strategy formulation. Other roles for the psychologist include more focused and in-depth patient and family counseling (as well as group counseling), particularly with regard to adaptation to disability, sexual dysfunction, or depression. The psychologist can also serve as a resource for the rehabilitation team with regard to team dynamics, conflict management, and role negotiation.

Recreational Therapy

The recreational therapist can serve an important role in a rehabilitation program with respect to developing or enhancing leisure activity skills. Not only does this make the often arduous rehabilitation process more pleasant and tolerable, but it also encourages more structured leisure time planning for older individuals who may have lost family, friends, or significant others. Group activities often include games, movies, arts and crafts, and trips into the community. This affords additional opportunities for socialization and developing new friendships, with positive benefits in morale and motivation.

Nutrition

The dietician, while not routinely a member of the core rehabilitation team, provides a valuable service with regard to adequate nutrition. Many older individuals with disabling conditions are transferred to a rehabilitation unit with marginally adequate nutrition, which is inadequate in the face of the significantly enhanced exercise and activity levels in an active rehabilitation program. This may be further compounded by dysphagia, requiring special consistencies of food and liquid or augmentative feeding via gastrostomy or parenteral hyperalimentation. In such situations, the dietician works closely with the rehabilitation nurse, occupational therapist, and physician to ensure appropriate nutrition and with the patient and family regarding education and instruction in special dietary needs and administration.

Case Management

A relatively new team member/role, usually part of the core team, is the case manager. This individual typically has a health care background (e.g., nurse, therapist, social worker), but is not directly involved in providing health care services to the individual he or she represents. It is the case manager's responsibility to represent the patient's/family's interests and to advocate on their behalf regarding appropriate, timely, and effective treatment. The case manager will also interact (and intercede) with the patient's insurance carrier regarding authorization of needed treatment and equipment and timely feedback regarding treatment outcomes.

Medicine

The physiatrist, specializing in Physical Medicine and Rehabilitation, is the physician who by regulation, training, and tradition provides medical leadership and guidance to the rehabilitation team. This is most consistently true for acute inpatient rehabilitation programs and facilities, but less uniformly in subacute settings (SNF, outpatient programs, home-based care) (22). While the physiatrist serves as the primary physician for many geriatric rehabilitation programs, geriatricians have also become increasingly involved in this component of the spectrum of geriatric practice (most often at the subacute level).

The physiatrist typically performs a consultative evaluation of patients with disabling conditions while they are on the acute medical/surgical service. The major focus of this assessment is to determine the reversibility of the disability and the intensity of rehabilitation intervention (1). An older patient very deconditioned from severe, prolonged, and often multiple illnesses may not be able to tolerate the intensity of an acute (hospital level) rehabilitation program, but may be more appropriate for an SNF (nursing home) based unit (22). Patients with less severe disabilities may be most effectively managed in an outpatient or home-based program, with periodic physiatric follow-up evaluation to monitor progress and adjust the therapy intervention as needed.

When a patient is transferred to a Diagnostic Related Groups (DRG) exempt rehabilitation unit or facility, the physiatrist is usually the attending physician, admitting the patient to his or her service. Responsibilities include a comprehensive assessment of the patient with regard to medical status and needs, determination of the severity and reversibility of disability, prescription of a comprehensive rehabilitation treatment program, and ongoing coordination of care rendered (1).

In the context of providing primary inpatient care, the physiatrist must manage the often complicated medical care of older patients. Not only do these individuals typically manifest multiple comorbid conditions, but they also tend to be discharged expeditiously from the medical/surgical (DRG-based) service: the "quicker and sicker" phenomenon (29). Frequent and close monitoring of medical status is critical to anticipate and prevent (ideally) or promptly recognize and treat such complications as orthostatic hypotension (e.g., from dehydration, medication side effect), skin breakdown (decubitus ulcer due to impaired mobility), thromboembolic phenomena (related to immobilization prior to transfer), or cardiovascular decompensation with anginal syndrome or congestive heart failure (as a result of increased activity and exercise in therapies) (22). While the physiatrist may determine the need for consultation from any of a variety of medical/surgical specialists to assist in the evaluation and management of complex clinical situations, he or she retains the ultimate authority and responsibility for decisions regarding treatment.

As the de facto team leader, the physiatrist is responsible for coordinating the rehabilitation program in conjunction with the medical management (10). As such, he or she will contribute to the discussion of a patient's physical, functional, and psychosocial status; participate in realistic goal-setting; assist with patient and family education; monitor and maintain medical stability to enable the patient to fully participate in therapies; formulate a timely and appropriate discharge plan, and prescribe necessary postdischarge continuing care (1). He or she will typically follow the patient after discharge on a periodic basis to continue to monitor progress in ongoing therapy programs, with modification of the treatment plan as necessary.

Physician leadership and coordination functions are comparable in subacute rehabilitation settings such as outpatient, SNF and home-based programs.

Patient and Family

While the patient and his or her family are appropriately considered members of the core team, their role and degree of actual participation is often not well defined or documented (7). Their level and frequency of interaction with the team and focused discussion of the treatment program is typically less than that of the health professional team members. Levels of input and interaction range from one-to-one contact with individual team members (often unstructured, during therapy sessions), to scheduled family conferences with the entire team (structured, relatively infrequent). Patient and family contributions to the team process of goal-setting accordingly tend to be limited, primarily occurring early during the evaluation process when they are asked about their goals and concerns. Subsequently, their input may be primarily feedback and reaction to team-determined goals and treatment strategies, either directly to individual health professionals or to the team as a whole in a family conference. Purtilo (30) explores somewhat divergent philosophies regarding patient autonomy and self-determination, conflicts arising from structural and environmental barriers, and differing expectations between the patient and the health care team. She identifies several structural factors related to team dynamics that tend to form barriers to a patient's ability to remain actively involved in goal and treatment plan formulation. For example, a patient may be:

- *too involved* with multiple team members and activities to identify or pursue alternative treatment options (fatigued, overwhelmed),
- *too anxious* to risk conflicts with the team, since he or she is dependent on their interest and willingness to treat,
- *too grateful* for this treatment opportunity to reject or question it,
- *too outnumbered* (and intimidated) by the health care professionals to effectively effect change in the treatment process, or
- *too convinced* that the team, as experts, knows best what is appropriate.

While the health care professional team does have the advantage of expertise and experience in observing outcomes of treatment with other patients, it is still appropriate and important to acknowledge and, to the extent reasonable and feasible, incorporate patient/family-identified goals into the treatment plan. This will help to ensure that in addition to the reactive factors listed previously, the patient and his or her family will be actively invested and committed to the rehabilitation process.

TEAM ATTITUDES AND BIASES

Because of their nature and dynamics and their degree of control over the patients they treat, rehabilitation teams (and health care teams in general) must constantly be on guard against counterproductive or harmful attitudes and biases affecting their work. As discussed, patients and their families typically place their trust in the rehabilitation professionals as the experts who know what's best for them. The tendency is to accept and adopt team decisions and attitudes with little challenge. This entails a prime responsibility on the part of the rehabilitation team to ensure unbiased, objective, and nonjudgmental decision-making and interactions (30).

Beneficence versus Paternalism

Purtilo (30) describes beneficence as "acts which contribute positively to the welfare of others, as well as acts intended to prevent or remove harm," sometimes interpreted as honoring patient preferences. Since patients and their families may be unrealistic or inappropriate (in the opinion and experience of the team) in their goals and desires, the rehabilitation team may feel justified in overruling the patient's wishes to accomplish greater benefit or prevent harm. This process has now become paternalistic, in the presumption that the team's judgment should take precedence over the patient's (30). While limited paternalism (31) or paternalism with permission (32) may be defensible in situations of high uncertainty, with diligent consideration of and respect for the patient's wishes, teams must ensure that "the least restrictive, least humiliating, and least insulting alternative has been selected (31)." A team that imposes its own structure and goals out of convenience or by routine, without consideration or respect for patient concerns, has become inappropriately autocratic.

Certain types of "hateful" (33) patients have been described, who may provoke intense feelings of repugnance, anger, and revenge in health professionals. Rehabilitation teams must maintain a conscious check and balance system to preclude coercion or punishment of a patient who does not conform to the team's wishes or expectations or challenges a team decision. A case manager may fulfill this role, acting as an advocate on behalf of the patient. Team dynamics may interfere with recognizing or disciplining a member acting in a revengeful manner (perhaps to protect a colleague or avoid team censure), resulting in inappropriate neglect and tacit complicity (30).

Arrogance and Self-Fulfilling Prophecies

As acknowledged (by patients) and self-perceived experts, health care professionals may develop an unwarranted elitism, with the danger of patronizing and arrogant attitudes. An indication of this tendency is the presumptive familiarity many health professionals practice by calling patients by their first names without specific permission from them. Alternatively, staff may dehumanize a patient by referring to him or her as "Bed 14A" or "the left hemi in 502." This represents the antithesis of the holistic, empathetic, and compassionate philosophy of rehabilitation. In fact, there is an increasing tendency to avoid using the term patient with its obvious and latent connotations and substitute client or just individual. This approach helps to reinforce the patient's (client's) role as a fellow team member, actively involved in decisions affecting his or her care.

Often unrecognized by the rehabilitation team is the possibility of intimidation of a patient and his or her family in the setting of a family conference. They are surrounded (literally) and outnumbered by the multiple health professionals, who usually have a set agenda and limited time frame to conduct the meeting. One strategy to try to minimize trepidation is to conduct the initial family conference as a series of one-to-one discussions with various staff members; once the patient and family know and are more familiar with the team, there is less risk of intimidation. Another unprofessional indication of arrogance or lack of respect on the part of staff is when team members eat or write notes during the family conference, conduct side conversations, or convey disinterest by facial expression, tone of voice, or body language.

Teams must also be cognizant of the potential for projecting personal value systems on patients, judging them based on staff-generated standards. A latent idiosyncrasy of the team process is the danger of generating self-fulfilling prophecies, whereby a patient judged not to have potential will not receive the extra attention or effort accorded another patient (felt to have a good prognosis). In a similar manner, the patient perceived as uncooperative or undeserving ("hateful") (33) will tend to be treated summarily by the team and discharged quickly, while the cooperative, likeable ("cute") patient is kept longer because staff enjoy working with him or her. Contributing to this negative team dynamic is the bandwagon mentality, with an outspoken team member influencing the attitudes and decisions of the rest of the team.

Jargon and Hidden Biases

While jargon, or inappropriate use of professional terminology (not understood by the lay patient and family), may be simply an unconscious habit of health professionals, it may also reflect arrogance or lack of respect. To avoid a further impediment to effective communication and education of the patient and family, team members must monitor each other's language to minimize use of perplexing words and phrases.

Another unrecognized but disparaging tendency of health care workers is the inadvertent use of what Rubenfeld (34) has termed disabilityisms, or biased phrases that connote negative images concerning individuals with disability. Johnson (35) cites a classic example of the phrase "confined to a wheelchair" or "wheelchair bound," which produces an image of ropes and chains binding someone to a wheelchair. In reality, a wheelchair is mobility-facilitating and liberating; without it an individual with a disability would indeed be bound and immobile.

Other examples include the term "victim of an illness," which likens a disease to a crime or "afflicted with/suffers from," which connotes significant pain and distress. Butler (36) coined the term ageism to describe biased perceptions of older people by their younger counterparts, as well as perceptions of old age by older persons themselves. Williams (4) maintains that use of such terms as the elderly and the aged depersonalize and stereotype perceptions of older individuals. The same objection holds for such terms as the disabled, arthritics, or the brain injured.

Conflict versus Complacency

With health care teams there is a delicate balance between complacency and conflict. The former suggests a blind acceptance without questioning, analyzing, or striving to improve. Teams can get into ruts or routines, actively resisting new ideas or alternative approaches because "it's always been done that way." There is a risk of intolerance of dissent on the part of other team members, let alone a patient and family. The other end of the spectrum is a team rife with conflict and discontent, without coordination and collaboration, which can prove even more dangerous for the patients they attempt to treat. The ideal team, as referenced earlier, is one which is dynamic and self-critical and willing to challenge itself to improve its function. A perennial concern with health care teams in general is that of staff burnout, with declining effectiveness, deteriorating morale, and cynicism. Part of the periodic and ongoing team building process attempts to forestall such cycles.

Empowerment

The ultimate goal and challenge for a rehabilitation team is to foster independent functioning, physically, socially, and emotionally. This empowerment process requires tailored but diminishing assistance and support, encouraging appropriate risk-taking (referred to as the dignity of risk). While the rehabilitation team cognitively may be concerned about the risks involved with letting an older individual return home alone, they must factor in his or her wishes and not arbitrarily impose their personal value systems and assumptions. The team's responsibility is to maintain a morally responsible approach (30) by demonstrating respect for individuals' welfare as reflected in their choices and, in rare instances, for their welfare instead of their choices (37).

It is appropriate that the rehabilitation team, functioning as a referral-based service, should adopt the philosophy of Continuous Quality Improvement (CQI) (38), and strive to exceed the expectations of their customers (persons with disabilities and their families). Team members must bear in mind that the team's ultimate success and effectiveness will be judged in the context of outcomes of care of the individuals they treat.

References

1. Clark GS, Bray GP. Development of a rehabilitation plan. In: Williams TF, ed. *Rehabilitation in the Aging.* New York, NY: Raven Press; 1984:125–143.
2. Schmitt MH. The team approach in the elderly. In: Calkins E, Davis PJ, Ford AB, eds. *The Practice of Geriatrics.* Philadelphia, Pa: W.B. Saunders; 1986:14–19.
3. Tsukuda RA. Interdisciplinary collaboration: teamwork in geriatrics. In: Cassel CK, Reisenberg DE, Sorensen LB, Walsh JR, eds. *Geriatric Medicine.* 2nd ed. New York, NY: Springer-Verlag; 1990:668–675.
4. Williams TF. Rehabilitation: goals and approaches in older people. In: Rowe JW, Besdine RW, eds. *Geriatric Medicine.* 2nd ed. Boston, Mass: Little, Brown; 1988:156–143.
5. AGS Public Policy Committee. Geriatric rehabilitation. *J Am Geriatr Soc.* 38:1049–1050, 1990.
6. Rothberg JS. The rehabilitation team: future directions. *Arch Phys Med Rehabil.* 62:407–410, 1981.
7. Foley CJ, Libow LS, Charaton FB. The team approach to geriatric care. In: Hazzard WR, Andres R, Bierman EL, Blass JP, eds. *Principles of Geriatric Medicine and Gerontology.* 2nd ed. New York, NY: McGraw-Hill; 1990:184–191.
8. Halstead LS. Team care in chronic illness: critical review of the literature of past 25 years. *Arch Phys Med Rehabil.* 61:507–511, 1976.
9. Melvin JL. Interdisciplinary and multidisciplinary activities in the ACRM. *Arch Phys Med Rehabil.* 61:379–380, 1980.
10. DeLisa JA, Martin GM, Currie DM. Rehabilitation medicine: past, present, and future. In: DeLisa JA, Currie DM, Gans B, Gatens P, Leonard JA Jr, McPhee M, eds. *Rehabilitation Medicine: Principles and Practice.* Philadelphia, Pa: J.B. Lippincott; 1988:3–24.
11. McGregor D. *The Human Side of Enterprise.* New York, NY: McGraw-Hill; 1960:232–235.
12. Dyer WG. *Team Building: Issues and Alternatives.* Reading, Mass: Addison-Wesley, 1977.
13. Given B, Simmons S. Interdisciplinary health care team: fact or fiction? *Nurs Forum.* 15:116–184, 1977.
14. Wanlass RL, Reutter SL, Kline AE. Communication among rehabilitation staff: "mild," "moderate," or "severe" deficits? *Arch Phys Med Rehabil.* 73:477–481, 1992.
15. Lundborg LB. What is leadership? *J Nurs Admin.* 12:32–33, 1982.
16. Beckhard R. Organizational issues in the team delivery of comprehensive health care. *Milbank Q.* 50:287–316, 1972.
17. Saltz CC, McVey LJ, Becker PM, Feussner JR, Cohen HJ. Impact of a geriatric consultation team on discharge placement and repeat hospitalization. *Gerontologist.* 28:344–350, 1988.
18. Campion EW, Jette A, Berkman B. An interdisciplinary geriatric consultation service: a controlled trial. *J Am Geriatr Soc.* 31:792–796, 1983.
19. Blumenfield S, Morris J, Sherman FT. The geriatric team in the acute care hospital: an educational and consultation modality. *J Am Geriatr Soc.* 30:660–664, 1982.
20. Rubenstein LZ, Abrass IB, Kane RL. Improved care for patients on a new geriatric evaluation unit. *J Am Geriatr Soc.* 29:531–536, 1981.
21. Kerski D, Drinka T, Carnes M, Golob K, Craig WA. Post-geriatric evaluation unit follow-up: team versus nonteam. *J Gerontol.* 42:191–195, 1987.
22. Clark GS, Siebens HC. Rehabilitation of the geriatric patient. In: DeLisa JA, Currie DM, Gans B, Gatens P, Leonard JA Jr, McPhee M, eds. *Rehabilitation Medicine: Principles and Practice.* 2nd ed. Philadelphia, Pa: J.B. Lippincott; 1993.
23. Feiger SM, Schmitt MH. Collegiality in interdisciplinary health teams: its measurement and its effects. *Soc Sci Med.* 13A:217, 1979.
24. Evers HK. Multidisciplinary teams in geriatric wards: myth or reality? *J Adv Nurs.* 6:205, 1981.
25. Cummings V, Kerner JF, Arones S, Steinbock C. Day hospital service in rehabilitation medicine: an evaluation. *Arch Phys Med Rehabil.* 66:86–91, 1985.
26. Fisk AA. Comprehensive health care for the elderly. *JAMA.* 249:230–236, 1983.
27. Pesznecker BL, Paquin R. Implementing interdisciplinary team practice in home care of geriatric clients. *J Gerontol Nurs.* 8:504, 1982.
28. Portnow J. Innovations in community and home-based rehabilitation. Presented at Annual Assembly of the American Academy of Physical Medicine and Rehabilitation; October 30, 1991; Washington, DC.
29. Felsenthal G, Cohen BS, Hilton EB. Panagos AV, Aiken BM. The physiatrist as primary physician for patients on an inpatient rehabilitation unit. *Arch Phys Med Rehabil.* 65:375–378, 1984.
30. Purtilo RB. Ethical issues in teamwork: the context of rehabilitation. *Arch Phys Med Rehabil.* 69:318–322, 1988.
31. Childress JF. Ensuring care, respect, and fairness for elderly. *Hastings Center Rep.* 14:27–31, 1984.
32. Cross AW, Churchill LR. Ethical and cultural dimensions of informed consent: case study and analyses. *Ann Intern Med.* 96:110–113, 1982.
33. Groves JE. Taking care of the hateful patient. *N Engl J Med.* 298:883–887, 1978.
34. Rubenfeld P. Ageism and disabilityism: double jeopardy. In: Brody SJ, Ruff GE, eds. *Aging and Rehabilitation: Advances in the State of the Art.* New York, NY: Springer; 1986:323–328.
35. Johnson EW. Editorial. *Am J Phys Med Rehabil.* 70:1, 1991.
36. Butler RN. Age-ism: another form of bigotry. *Gerontologist.* 9:243–246, 1969.
37. Caplan AL. Informed consent and provider-patient relationships in rehabilitation medicine. *Arch Phys Med Rehabil.* 69:312–317, 1988.
38. *1993 Joint Commission Accreditation Manual for Hospitals.* Oakbrook Terrace, Il: The Joint Commission on Accreditation of Healthcare Organizations; 1992.

38

Assistive Devices and Environmental Modifications

Karen J. Kalupa, Sunanda Apte-Kakade, and Steven V. Fisher

The potential for disability increases with aging. Simple assistive devices and environmental modifications can increase independence and improve quality of life. Applied engineering and technology can be key factors in extending older patients' quality of life.

This chapter provides a brief overview of this topic. It includes environmental adaptations, clothing modifications, mobility aids, driving aids, communication devices, adaptive equipment, and community resources.

ENVIRONMENTAL ADAPTATIONS

Kitchen

The kitchen area should be conveniently planned and tailored to the person's needs (Fig. 38.1). Creative rearranging can frequently substitute for expensive remodeling. Organization of work areas saves energy as well as time. Examples include a cutting board placed over a pulled-out drawer to lower a work surface, a pegboard installed to hang items vertically, and a cookie sheet used as a carrying aid. Items in the kitchen should be stored so that they can be retrieved without causing safety problems. Place knives in holders rather than in the bottom of a drawer and store heavy things low. Utensils should be stored in the area in which they are first used. For example, place the coffee pot or teapot near the sink since the first step in using such items involves obtaining water. To eliminate opening and searching cabinet shelves, use the back of a door for storage of canned goods. If hand function is limited, set cabinet and drawer handles at a 45-degree angle for easy grasp (1).

The most convenient refrigerator-freezer combination is the side-by-side double door model. Slide-out and revolving shelves increase accessibility. Use turntables on lower shelves to retrofit a standard refrigerator. A built-in wall oven and a separate cooktop provide better accessibility. If there are three or four burners in a cooktop stove, they should be in a staggered pattern to reduce the danger of reaching over front burners. In order to slide hot items directly to the countertop, it is best to have the most used oven shelf at the level of the countertop. An electric hotplate, electric skillet, toaster oven, or microwave oven are alternatives to a standard oven (2). Cooking can be made safer by the use of barbecue tools and long matches. A cookie sheet placed under an oven baking dish improves safe portability. Rather than carry a pot to the sink to drain, use a slotted spoon to remove food from hot liquids (1).

Three quarters of the time spent in a kitchen is at the sink. Washing dishes can be accomplished from a sitting position. Nonslip strips on the floor near the sink can reduce the risk of slipping on water. A hand-held reacher eliminates the need for use of a stool to reach objects on high shelves. There are hundreds of gadgets and work-saving ideas for kitchen activities. Occupational therapists should be consulted for their extensive expertise in this regard.

Bathroom

The bathroom may be the most essential room in the house, but it is often the most inaccessible. Compromise is usually necessary for the older or impaired person to maintain independence in the bathroom. A device is available to permit a wheelchair to be temporarily narrowed by a few inches for access through a bathroom door.

Elevating the toilet seat 3 to 6 inches improves leverage for regaining the standing position, especially when there is lower extremity weakness or limited motion of the hips and knees (Fig. 38.2). Structures such as a towel bar, the edge of a sink, and the toilet tank should not be used as an assist to come to standing. The sink edge can be slippery, especially when wet, and the towel bar can separate from the wall. The use of a nonslip grab bar, ideally in a color that contrasts with the wall,

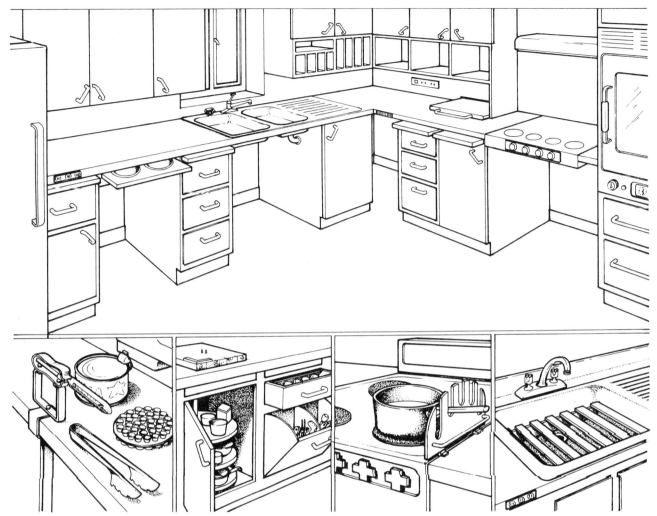

Figure 38.1.   Kitchen with multiple adaptations.

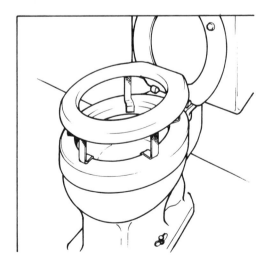

Figure 38.2.   Elevated commode seat.

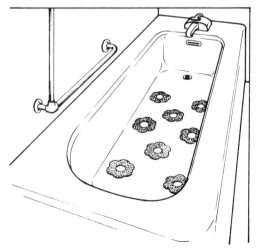

Figure 38.3.   Tub with nonslip surface and grab bars.

is best. Nonslip adhesive strips can be placed alongside the sink and toilet (Fig. 38.3). Commode chairs with wheels may be placed over a toilet to prevent slippage on water. For use of the bathroom at night, a light and an unobstructed path from the bedroom to the bathroom are necessary. A commode chair that conceals its actual purpose can be placed in the bedroom.

A single lever faucet, which requires only very light pressure rather than twist knobs, is easier to use at the sink and bathtub. An extended handheld shower hose can convert a bathtub to a shower to improve safety and independence. Tub seats make transfers to the bathtub safer and eliminate the need to stand during a shower. A cabinet below a sink can be removed to permit wheelchair accessibility. The exposed pipes under a sink should be insulated to prevent burns (Fig. 38.4).

Living Room

The primary function of a living room chair is to provide firm yet comfortable body support. Since many older people tend to fall backward when attempting to sit, the chair should be stable. It should have arms to provide for upper extremity comfort and assistance for sitting and standing. It should be high enough to provide ease in standing. A 3- or 4-inch elevation of seat height may help an older person to sit safely and rise independently. The height of the chair seat can be increased with blocks under the legs, with chair lifters, or with an extra cushion. If a cushion is added to the chair, it can be stabilized by inserting a piece of nonslip carpet tape between the cushion and the seat. For comfort, a footstool can be used if a person's feet do not reach the floor. The table next to the chair should be at a convenient height. Having easy access to a lamp, a remote control for a television, and a portable phone provide increased safety and independence in the living room.

Bedroom

A person should be able to control lighting, heating, and ventilation independently. A telephone should be beside the bed. An intercom or bell can be used to summon a caregiver. A nightlight in the bedroom, as well as in the bathroom, is very helpful (1) (Fig. 38.5).

The bed must be comfortable and should be situated to allow a person to look out a window or into a hallway. The best way to determine the optimum height for the bed is by trial and error. Screw-in legs, blocks, or an extra mattress may be used to increase the height of the bed. If the bed is higher than needed, the legs can be sawed shorter. A firm mattress is a prerequisite for good body support, as well as for safe and smooth transfers. An adjustable bed that raises the upper part of the body can improve independence by easing the change of positions in order to read, write, and watch television (Fig. 38.6). The typical rental hospital bed is usually too high for independent transfers, however.

A sliding board may be used to achieve a seated lateral transfer when a standing transfer is not possible. An overhead trapeze and side rails may improve the ability to roll and sit up to prepare for transfers in specific cases (Figs 38.7 and 38.8). Persons with severe impairment who require maximum assistance for transfers may need a Hoyer lift to transfer. The Hoyer lift is a hydraulic lifting device that can be operated by one person.

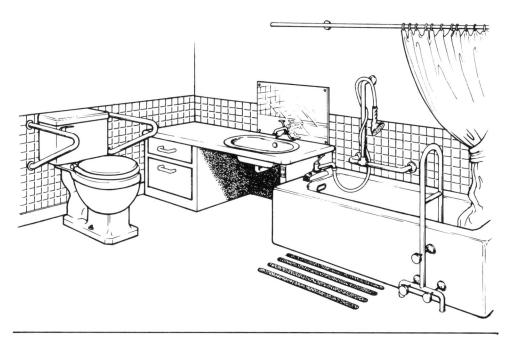

Figure 38.4.   Bathroom with modifications.

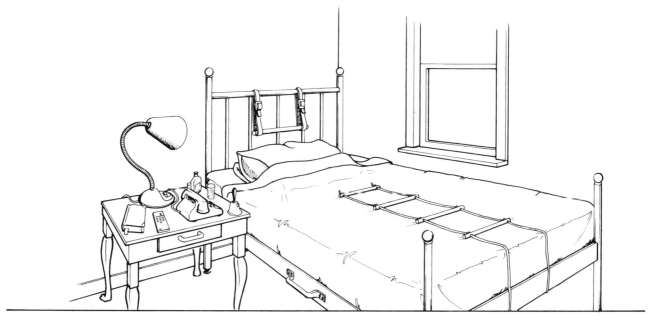

Figure 38.5.   Bedroom with modifications.

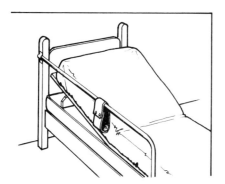

Figure 38.6.   Adapted bed with side rail, strap and elevating headboard.

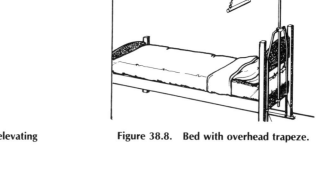

Figure 38.8.   Bed with overhead trapeze.

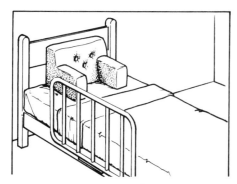

Figure 38.7.   Bed with side rail and support cushion.

An electric blanket does not add much weight, can be easily controlled, and may add significant comfort. Thermal weave blankets are lightweight and provide warmth and ventilation. A blanket support can be put under the bedclothes to take the weight of the bedding off the feet.

Laundry Room

Easy care permanent-press clothing and sheets simplify laundry chores. Many new laundry products including stain removers and fabric softeners eliminate handscrubbing or ironing. A washing machine is convenient, but it is not necessary if there are only small amounts of laundry. Wringing out clothes and drying

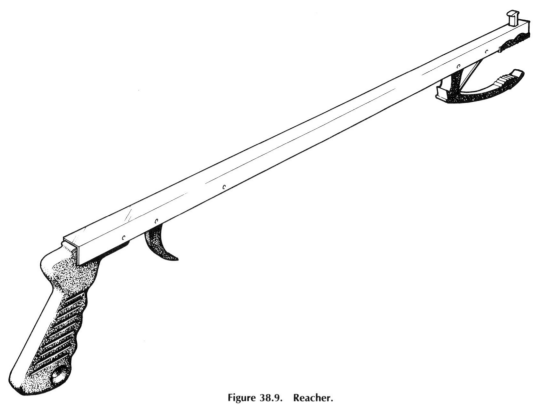

Figure 38.9. Reacher.

are greater problems than washing; a dryer may be the more useful appliance (1). The washer and dryer controls should be easy to read and manipulate. If reach is limited, long-handled tongs or a reacher can be used to retreive items (Fig. 38.9). A top-loading washing machine is usually most appropriate for someone who works from a standing position. The dryer should be adjacent to the washer. If installed on a platform, bending and stooping are minimized. A front-loading washing machine allows someone in a wheelchair to use the washer and transfer clothes to the dryer easily.

Removing items from the dryer while they are still warm reduces the need for ironing. An ironing board that pulls down from the wall is easier to set up and fold back if installed at a proper working height, which is 2 inches below the elbow. It is not necessary to use a heavy iron. Heat and stem do most of the work. A cord holder can help keep the cord out of the way. Use of a lower temperature allows a slower ironing speed without the risk of scorching the fabric (1).

CLOTHING MODIFICATIONS

Clothing adaptations can accommodate the physical changes of aging. Ease in donning and doffing clothing minimizes energy cost and fatigue. Clothing should fit easily over the head and allow for freedom of movement. It should not create pressure or constriction. It should be constructed of materials that are easy to care for and wrinkle-resistant. If putting on clothing is difficult, very simple changes can help. Hook and loop tape is an excellent adaptation with multiple uses. This item can be inexpensively obtained from most sewing and notion stores. Hook and loop tabs can be sewn under the front of a shirt to eliminate buttoning; it can also be used to make waistbands adjustable. It can be applied to bras at the front opening, and it can be used on the fly-front of men's trousers. Garments that have a front opening are the easiest to use. The larger the opening, the greater the freedom of movement (Fig. 38.10). Buttonhooks, available with different types of handles depending on the person's grasp, can be useful for dealing with small buttons (2) (Fig. 38.11). Patterns for sewing easy-to-wear clothing are widely available.

Donning shoes or stockings requires agility and mobility. There are many aids and techniques that can help. Longer, looser fitting socks are often easier to manage. Tubular socks, which do not have a shaped heel, are best when it is difficult for a person to put a heel in position. When limited flexion makes reaching the feet impossible, a long-handled shoehorn can be helpful. Some long-handled shoehorns have a spring at the point where the handle and shoehorn join, which is helpful if the ankle is limited in motion. Some people find it easier to put on stockings while lying on the bed. A stocking aid may be useful (Fig. 38.12). Elastic shoelaces can convert a tie shoe into a slipon shoe.

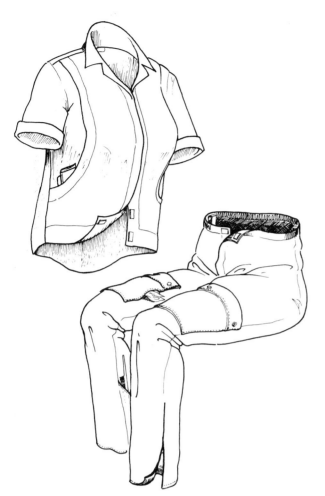

Figure 38.10.   Clothing adaptations.

With increasing age, the foot becomes wider and less flexible. Elderly people generally require a wider shoe with a soft, flexible sole, a soft upper, and a low heel. High heels or crepe-soled shoes may increase the risk of falling.

MOBILITY AIDS

Mobility is a significant quality of life issue. Impairments that cause limited mobility affect the entire spectrum of functional activities including self-care, homemaking, shopping, recreation, and socialization. The risks of falls and subsequent injury are increased in the elderly. Appropriately prescribed and fitted mobility aids are critical for the overall rehabilitation process.

Cane

A cane is the most often used simple mobility device. It should be of the proper length and have a comfortable, appropriate handle. There are three methods used to determine the proper length of a cane, as follows: (a) it should equal the distance from the distal wrist crease to the ground when the patient is standing erect, wearing shoes and with the arms relaxed (3); (b) it should equal the distance from the greater trochanter to the ground; and (c) it should be a length such that when its tip is placed on the ground, 15 cm in front of and to the side of the tip of the shoe, the elbow is flexed at 30 degrees (4). There is controversy regarding the best method of measurement; however, the first method mentioned may be superior because wrist crease to ground measurement is more consistent (3). The correct cane height should provide maximum support and comfortable use.

The cane tip is fitted with a minimum 1.5-inch diameter rubber tip with concentric ring to prevent slipping. The tips should be periodically checked for wear and cleanliness. Special tips for ice are also available. If additional stability is required, a three-prong or four-

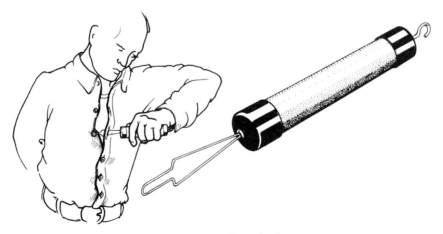

Figure 38.11.   Buttonhook.

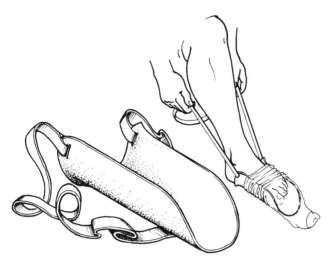

Figure 38.12. Sock aid.

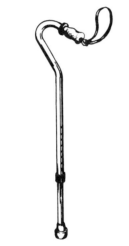

Figure 38.13. Single point cane.

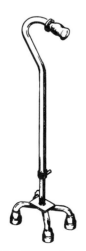

Figure 38.14. Narrow base quad cane.

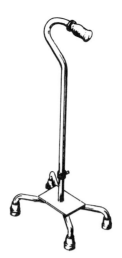

Figure 38.15. Wide base quad cane.

prong cane can be used with narrow or wide base of support (Figs. 38.13, 38.14, and 38.15).

If the elderly person has a hand impairment, a functional handle rather than a straight cane is preferred. A built-up or molded handle accommodates finger flexion limitations and allows weight bearing evenly over the entire palm.

A cane may function as an aid for balance by increasing the base of support and giving sensory feedback. It may function to reduce weight bearing on the contralateral lower extremity by providing weight bearing through the upper extremity. Some people, however, have difficulty in using the cane in the contralateral hand, especially if it is the nondominant hand. They derive some benefit from unilateral usage. Use of the cane in the opposite hand is most commonly used for ambulation following lower extremity fractures, amputation, stroke, or arthritic involvement of the lower extremity. Use of a cane may improve balance and compensate for visual and proprioceptive losses.

Crutches

If additional support is required, crutches may be used instead of canes. The length is adjusted according to the third method described with canes. Underarm crutches should not contact the axillae during weight bearing to avoid brachial plexus pressure neuropathy. Contoured crutch hand grips, molded of neoprene sponge, provide a soft, comfortable grip (Fig. 38.16). Underarm crutches should also have a rubber axillary pads for comfort (Fig. 38.17). If the wrist or hand is painful, a platform piece can be added to shift the weight bearing from the wrist and hand to the elbow and forearm (Fig 38.18). The Loftstrand or forearm crutch is loosely attached to the forearm by a metal cuff so that the user's hand can be free for activities when not specifically using the crutch for weight bearing (Fig. 38.19).

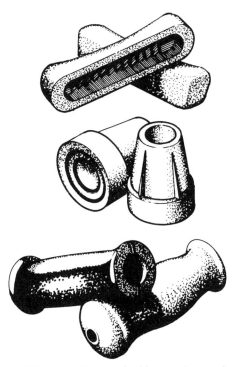

Figure 38.16.   Hand grip and rubber tips for crutches.

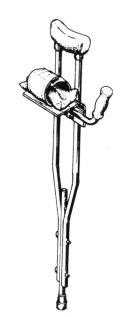

Figure 38.18.   Platform crutch.

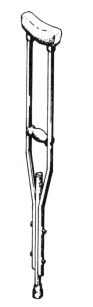

Figure 38.17.   Axillary crutch.

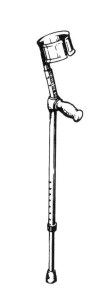

Figure 38.19.   Forearm crutch.

Canes and crutches can be used either in one hand or bilaterally, depending on the need. Gait instruction may be required for stairs and ramps.

Walkers

When a cane or a crutch does not offer enough stability, a walker may be prescribed. A walker is a four-point mobility aid that offers significant support. The pick-up walker (Fig. 38.20) is lifted and moved forward, followed by the user's advancement. This provides very slow, nonreciprocal gait. The reciprocal walkers allow a reciprocal walking pattern and provide more support. A wheeled walker (Fig. 38.21) may be used for patients who have difficulty lifting and manipulating conventional walkers. It provides a faster gait. This walker may

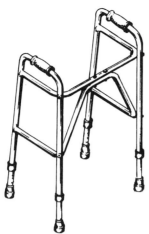

Figure 38.20. Pickup walker.

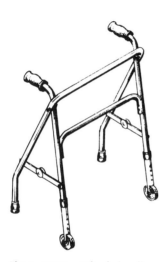

Figure 38.21. Wheeled walker.

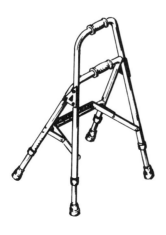

Figure 38.22. Hemiwalker.

be more difficult to control, is less stable, and does not operate easily on thick carpet. Generally, wheeled walkers have wheels in the front and crutch tips on the back legs. A glide walker has wheels on all four legs and does not provide adequate stability. Walkers can be used for both functional outdoor ambulation as well as limited indoor use. Older persons may prefer the walker to crutches or canes due to the fear of falling. A hemiwalker (Fig. 38.22) is a compromise between a cane and a walker, offering a wide base of support for stability similar to a walker, yet allowing one-handed ease of handling similar to a cane.

Wheelchairs

For patients who are unable to ambulate or have limited endurance, the wheelchair provides mobility. Wheelchairs allow elderly persons to be more functional, leaving both hands available for various activities of daily living (5). However, a wheelchair should not be considered simply a "geriatric chair." A wheelchair must be physician-prescribed after a thorough evaluation of the potential user, including age, body build, weight, disability, prognosis, functional skills, and preferences. Seat position, height, width, depth, back angle, and contour should be considered to achieve optimum fitting. Incorrect fit may result in poor posture, joint deformities, restriction of general mobility, pressure sores, circulatory impairment, and discomfort. A standard wheelchair has 24-inch or 26-inch rear wheels and 8-inch front casters. The wheelchair frame is available in various weights. The arm rest may be either full length or desk-type to allow the user to sit closer to a standard table or desk. Arm rests may be fixed, removable, or adjustable in height (Fig. 38.23). The wheelchair may be equipped with or without leg rests, which can be detachable, swing away, with or without an elevating mechanism. The foot rest has a foot plate, which is adjustable with optional heel and toe loops (Fig. 38.24). The tires are commonly made of solid rubber for ease of propulsion on smooth hard surfaces. Pneumatic tires are recommended for outdoor use. Brakes are either of the toggle or lever type. Brake extensions are available for easier reaching (Fig 38.25). The rear wheels have hand rims for propulsion. Friction rims, as well as knobs, are available to improve ease of propulsion for elderly persons with hand weakness or deformities (Fig 38.26). Antitipping devices are available to prevent backward or forward tipovers. A seat belt is an important safety option. Higher back wheelchairs are available for persons with diminished balance or needing increased support.

For people who have use of only one arm, such as a hemiplegic or an unilateral arm amputee, one-arm-drive chairs are available, but usually not practical. A wheelchair that is lower allows the user to propel the chair using the uninvolved foot against the floor. Am-

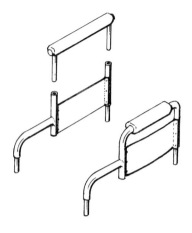

Figure 38.23. Arm rests.

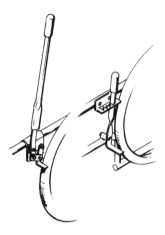

Figure 38.25. Brake extension.

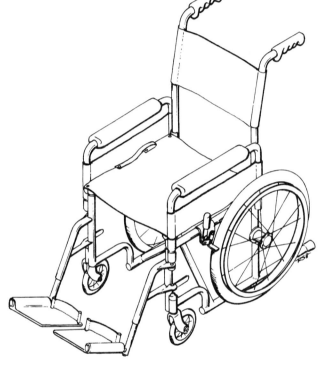

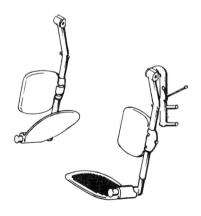

Figure 38.24. Leg rests.

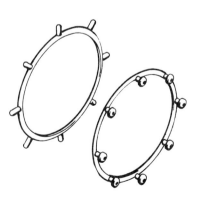

Figure 38.26. Rims.

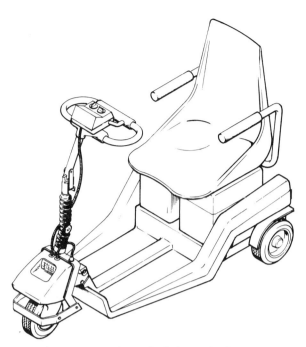

Figure 38.27. Three-wheeled motorized scooter.

putee chairs have the wheel axle set posteriorly to accommodate the shift of the center of gravity of bilateral lower limb amputees. Motorized wheelchairs are prescribed for persons who are unable to propel a wheelchair due to upper limb involvement or severely reduced endurance. It is important to ascertain that the elderly person is mentally alert and has adequate vision, sitting balance, and motor control for the safe operation of a motorized wheelchair. The motorized wheelchair is heavy, does not fold, and is difficult to transport in a motor vehicle. Hand control adaptations are available for individuals with poor hand function. A three-wheel motorized wheelchair scooter is useful for persons with adequate sitting balance who are able to stand to transfer (Fig. 38.27).

Architectural changes may be necessary for wheelchair use. These include widened doorways and installation of ramps. The recommended slope is no greater than one inch rise in one foot of ramp length (6). Guard rails are recommended on the ramps. A chairlift may be installed on a stairwell, though the cost is significant. Elderly persons frequently need help not only transferring into a car, but also loading the wheelchair. Community-assisted wheelchair transport is available as an alternative in many cities. Lightweight wheelchairs are becoming a frequently prescribed option. The lighter chair is somewhat easier to maneuver and is much easier to lift into a motor vehicle, which is important for the caregiver.

A wheelchair cushion must be individually prescribed and should be part of the overall wheelchair prescription. Elderly patients who are primarily wheelchair dependent are at risk for the development of decubitus ulcers. Wheelchair cushions should be considered a medical necessity for the elderly person who depends on a wheelchair for mobility. The three main functions of a wheelchair cushion are the following: (*a*) to relieve pressure in anatomic areas vulnerable to breakdown by distributing the body weight away from bony prominences; (*b*) to stabilize the body for upper extremity function; and (*c*) to maintain posture. The cushion must be waterproofed and easily cleaned. The proper cushion is dictated by the features desirable for the specific elderly person (7).

DRIVING AIDS

In the United States, by the year 2000, one out of every three drivers will be 55 years of age and older. The aging process decreases visual acuity, increases sensitivity to glare, decreases color discrimination, and decreases peripheral vision. These impairments may be compounded by various diseases, deconditioning, medication effects, dementia, and psychosocial issues. Errors commonly experienced by the elderly include problems with merging, yielding right of way, negotiating intersections, quick maneuvering, and reading traffic signs. Modifications to the automobile can only partially address some of these driving skill concerns. A driving evaluation on a regular basis, now required in only eight of the 50 states, can be coupled with modifications and assistive devices for the automobile, as well as driving education and use of compensatory techniques (8, 9).

There are multiple devices to aid in automobile entry and exit. Built-up key handles ease turning with diminished finger function. A handle on the rain gutter of the car aids in transferring in and out of the car. Small ramps allow a wheelchair to be rolled into the back seat rather than lifted into the car. Manual or electric wheelchair loaders are available to load the wheelchair into the car behind the front seat. A fully automatic cartop wheelchair carrier is also available. Assistive devices for the steering wheel, such as a spinner knob for one-handed care operation and hand controls for controlling the accelerator, brake, and dimmer switches, are just a few examples of possible driver control adaptations (4).

Seat cushions, including backrests and contoured seat supports, provide comfort and seating stability. Larger mirrors located outside of the automobile as well as a wide angle mirror attached to the usual rearview mirror allow greater visibility if neck mobility is reduced. It should be stressed that, as in the prescription of any adaptive equipment, an assessment by a qualified driving evaluator is mandatory for successful prescription and safe use of these adaptive devices.

COMMUNICATION DEVICES

The need to communicate is a basic human desire. For reading, proper lighting and/or magnification stands

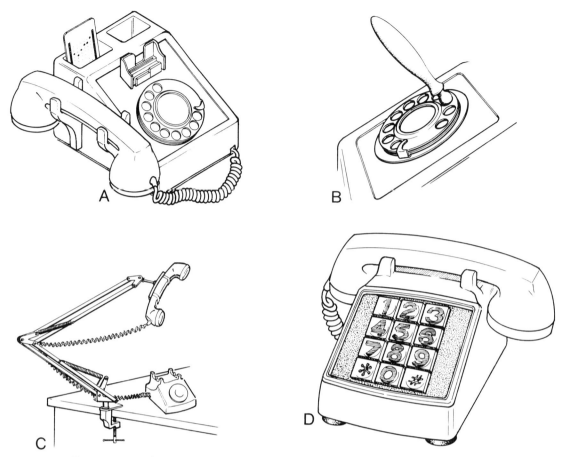

Figure 38.28.   Adapted telephones. A. Card dialer. **B.** Dialing adapter. **C.** Receiver extension.
D. Giant button adapter.

are available for persons with reduced vision. Large print additions of many books and magazines are available in bookstores and most public libraries. Machines that project pages or books on walls for further magnification are also available. There are many forms of book-stands as well as elaborate electric-powered page turners for persons having problems positioning reading materials or turning pages.

For writing, such simple aids as a felt tip pen, which needs less pressure, can be utilized. For ease in holding a pen, an enlarged handle can be made or purchased. Electric typewriters and word processors can be used with very limited upper extremity function. Either the left or right hand can be utilized singly, and books are available to teach one-handed typing. A tape recorder can be a valuable aid when writing is impossible (1).

Adapted telephones have become common (Fig. 38.28). The telephone company offers a special needs division for people with disabilities. Free publications are available. For the hearing impaired, there is an amplifying handset with adjustable volume control. There are multiple adaptations for holding the handset. If this is not possible, a lightweight headset is available. There are telephones with large, more visible pushbutton

numbers. There are various types of dialing systems available to reduce the need for locating and dialing individual numbers. There are phones that store hundreds of numbers. A card dialer telephone is available. When the user cannot recognize a name, a photo may be used on the card, which is introduced into the telephone for automatic dialing.

A TTY, teletypewriter, is available for the hearing impaired (10). It permits typed messages to be transferred through regular telephone services. Auditoriums, theaters, and churches can be equipped with laser-directed sound transmission to headset amplifiers for the hearing impaired.

There are telephone systems that allow the disabled person to press a transmitter device worn as a necklace, which activates the central telephone dialer to call a previously programmed number and transmit a previously recorded distress message. This serves a safety function and allows a sense of security.

Speaking aids include spelling boards, picture charts, sign language, fingerspelling, portable miniature typewriters, and the electrolarynx, to name a few. Information and training should be sought through speech language pathologists.

ADAPTIVE EQUIPMENT

Orthoses can be used in the older person for many reasons. The basic purposes of orthoses are to prevent or correct deformity, to enhance or substitute for function, to support the weight of a body part, and to protect a fragile or injured structure (11). The orthosis must have a well planned design in order to accomplish a specific purpose. There are two types of orthoses: static, with no movable parts, and dynamic, with movable parts. A static orthosis may be protective, supportive, or corrective in design. It may be prescribed to protect a weak muscle from being overly stretched (11). It can support an inflamed joint. It may substitute for weak muscles by supporting the joints. Static orthoses should hold the body part in the most functional position for the person's needs. Dynamic splints may be required for skeletal substitution, to support bones and joints; for muscle balance; to counteract the deforming forces of paralyzed muscles, for joint motion, to preserve existing joint motion when a deforming potential contracture is present, or to increase joint motion where it may already be restricted (11). Any dynamic orthosis must be designed and constructed to provide specific forces to achieve the goals intended (12).

Geriatric patients may not tolerate orthotic devices well secondary to fragile skin, prominent bones, prominences, etc. A change to larger size clothing or change in footwear may be needed to incorporate the orthosis.

An orthotic device may be somewhat uncomfortable when first worn, so that the goal of comfort may not be attained immediately. Orthoses must be individually prescribed and custom-fabricated to suit the person's individual needs and goals. A "universal" or "off the shelf" orthosis is less than ideal under most circumstances.

All orthotic devices and aids should be frequently inspected and reevaluated by a knowledgeable health care provider, as needs and equipment change over time.

Upper Extremity Supports/Orthoses

The following devices provide proximal support to the upper extremity. The suspension sling is a device that supports the upper extremity with cuffs that fit around the elbow and wrist. These cuffs are suspended from a spring, which is attached overhead, some from a rod that attaches to the wheelchair and some attached to a floorstand (Fig. 38.29). These are infrequently used, but are valuable for some patients to assist with eating when the arm is paretic, requiring gravity assist proximally. It may also be useful in reducing shoulder subluxation in difficult situations where other measures fail.

Arm slings can decrease shoulder subluxation in patients with brachial plexus injury, hemiplegia, and other similar disabilities (Fig. 38.30). Some support and im-

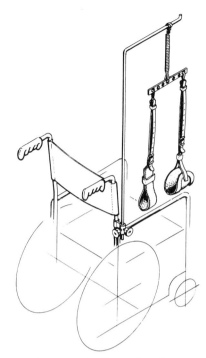

Figure 38.29. Suspension sling.

mobilize the entire arm; others support only the shoulder, leaving the lower arm and hand free for function. Some slings are commercially available. A therapist should check the sling for size and comfort frequently. A properly prescribed sling does not diminish function or create additional problems such as edema in a dependent hand. Wheelchair arm troughs provide an alternative to the use of a suspension sling for a wheelchair-bound older person. They are an arm rest attached over the regular wheelchair arm. Some have special contouring to hold the hand in a particular position and can be elevated (Fig. 38.31). Use of a clear plexiglass lapboard allows the older person to see his whole lower body, supports a weak arm, and provides a work surface for a wheelchair-bound person (Fig. 38.32).

Shoe Modifications

Specific shoe modifications are best determined when the physician and the orthotist evaluate the person simultaneously. In most instances, the goal is to accommodate the abnormal foot and improve the biomechanics rather than to correct the abnormality itself. Heel and sole lifts are prescribed to compensate for a leg length discrepancy (13). A lift of three-eighths-inch or less can be used under the heel inside a suitable shoe. If the lift is more than 1 inch, both heel and sole elevations are recommended. Foot deformities such as bunions are quite common in the elderly. A shoe with an extra wide toe box provides room for most toe deformities. However, customizing the toe box may be necessary for severe toe

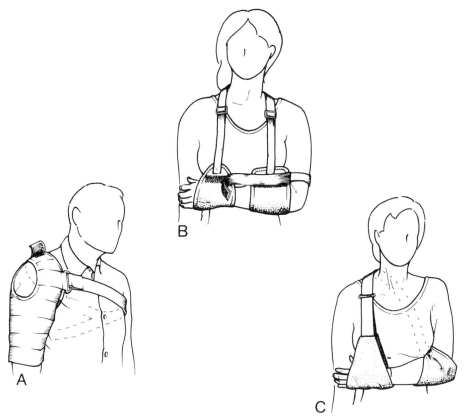

Figure 38.30.   Arm slings.   A. Shoulder support sling. **B.** Full arm sling. **C.** Cuff-type arm sling.

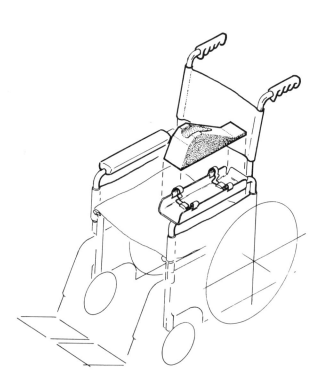

Figure 38.31.   Arm trough with elevating foam insert.

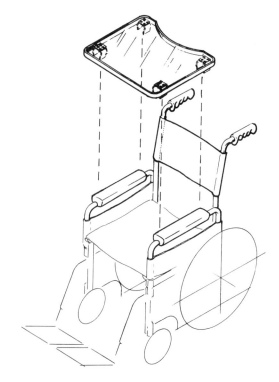

Figure 38.32.   Removable acrylic lapboard.

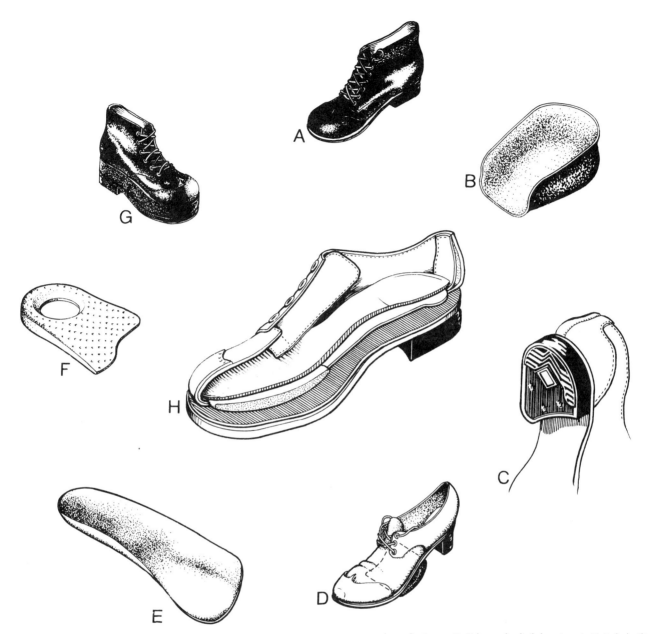

Figure 38.33. Shoe modifications. A. Thomas orthopedic boot. **B.** Corrective heel cup. **C.** Thomas heel. **D.** Rocker bottom shoe. **E.** Plas- tazote orthopedic insert. **F.** Calcaneal relief shoe insert. **G.** Sole built- up shoe. **H.** Orthopedic shoe.

deformities. For painful heel spurs and plantar fascitis, a heel cushion or plastazote insert may be useful.

Impairment of sensation in the foot occurs commonly in peripheral neuropathies. Such conditions may require, in addition to regular foot care, a fitted total contact insole for proper pressure distribution (14). The metatarsal heads receive high pressure during weight bearing. A metatarsal bar on the outside of the shoe with the high point located proximal to the metatarsal head will help relieve pressure on the metatarsal heads.

Arthritic problems causing foot deformities are common in the elderly. The goal of a properly fitting shoe is to improve comfort and reduce skeletal stress and repeated joint trauma. A severely deformed or pain-

ful foot may require a custom-made shoe (Fig. 38.33). Follow-up evaluation after shoe prescription is important to ensure that the desired effect has been achieved.

Spinal Orthoses

Spinal compression is a major site of fracture associated with bone loss in the elderly. Spinal orthotics can be used as a temporary measure for pain control. Since immobilization is thought to further exacerbate osteoporosis, the orthotic device should be discontinued as soon as possible. The purpose of spinal bracing is to decrease pain, to protect against further injury, to assist weak muscles, and to prevent or help correct a deformity (15). These objectives are gained through the biomechanical effects of trunk support, motion control, and spinal realignment (16). The corset is the most common lumbosacral support and, of all orthotics, it is prescribed approximately 44% of the time in the United States (17). A corset offers only minimal support; however, it reminds the wearer to maintain adequate posture. For more rigid bracing, a lumbosacral orthosis of the "chair back brace" type offers more support in multiple planes. The Williams back brace controls primarily extension or lordosis, as well as minimal lateral control. An extension brace such as the Jewett should be carefully considered in the older person since it may place excessive hyperextension forces on the lower lumbar vertebrae, inducing posterior element fractures or exacerbating degenerative arthritis. When a brace is prescribed, a program of reconditioning and mobilization for the elderly must be recommended simultaneously. Effective use of these orthoses depends upon proper application. For the older person, hook and loop closures will ease donning and doffing; however, assistance may be required.

COMMUNITY RESOURCES

There are millions of people who have mobility problems. Modern medicine, engineering, and technology have made it possible for those who have a disability to participate more fully in community activities. However, modern building design and construction have been influenced more by aesthetics than by practical considerations of accessibility. Few able-bodied people can appreciate the feelings of frustration and even humiliation created by lack of access. Free movement in and out of buildings such as houses, offices, schools, theaters, and post offices is a right taken for granted by the able-bodied, but access can be exasperating for those using assistive devices (18).

In the United States, the first significant official recognition of need for recommendations in the Building Code occurred in 1961 with the recommendation by the President's Committee on Employment of the Handicapped. Studies were conducted that provided the groundwork for such subsequent legislation as the Housing Act of 1964 and later acts in 1968, 1973, and 1974, which incorporated in-depth specifications.

Architectural Barriers Act

The Architectural Barriers Act, passed by Congress in 1968, specified that all federally funded buildings must be designed and constructed to provide access to physically handicapped persons. Compliance with the Act was less than effectively achieved during the 6 years that followed, and in 1974, the Architectural and Transportation Barriers Compliance Board, Section 502 of the previous year's Rehabilitation Act, was amended. It recommended federal funds be withheld or suspended if construction of any building or facility had not been carried out in accordance with the Act. Despite these acts, there is considerable variance throughout the country in the enforcement and the functioning of the responsible agencies (18).

Ramps should be constructed in conjunction with the main staircase of a public building so that the disabled person need not use a segregated entrance. The accessibility of a building cannot be separated from that of the surrounding terrain and general environment. Adaptations such as curb-cuts, ramps, and widened doorways can actually benefit many persons, including the elderly, those using mobility devices, and people pushing baby strollers (18).

Americans with Disabilities Act

The Americans with Disabilities Act (ADA) became law on May 22, 1990. Under this act, millions of citizens with disabilities will be protected from discrimination and will be guaranteed greater access to employment, transportation, and communication systems. This legislation extends the 1964 Civil Rights Act, which bars discrimination on the basis of race, sex, and national origin, as well as expanding a 1973 law that bars discrimination against those with disabilities by the federal government, its contractors, or entities that receive federal funds. The Americans with Disabilities Act provides new opportunities as businesses begin seeking ways to enhance accessibility. Key components of this legislation include the following.

EMPLOYMENT

Businesses with 25 or more employees must accommodate the disabled within 2 years, with the provisions extending to businesses of 15 or more employees within 4 years. In addition to physical accessibility, provisions include adjusting work schedules and, in some cases, supplying assistance as well as prohibiting discrimination in hiring on the basis of facial disfigurement (18).

PRIVATE SERVICES

The ADA prohibits service establishments, such as doctors' offices, restaurants, hotels, stores, and theaters, from discriminating in provision of services; for example car rental agencies would be required to fit cars with hand controls. The ADA requires that any newly constructed or renovated service buildings be accessible, such as hotels, stores and restaurants, and places of employment (18).

PUBLIC TRANSPORTATION

The ADA mandates that public transportation systems provide accessibility to wheelchairs. New buses must be accessible with lifts or other devices; old buses are exempt from retrofitting. Special services must be phased in to provide for those unable to use the regular system (18).

TELECOMMUNICATIONS

The ADA requires telephone companies to provide oral relay services to persons with hearing or speech impairments, who input and receive written messages, within 3 years.

Penalties for violating the ADA include injunctions for employers to halt their bias and backpay for victims of discrimination who have been fired or have been passed over for promotion. There are provisions for exemptions to be granted to businesses that can demonstrate that the required changes would be too costly, too disruptive, or substantially alter the way they do business. For example, taxicabs are not required to be accessible. Cab drivers are, however, required to accept a wheelchair as a piece of luggage.

The older or disabled person as a consumer must consistently bring obstacles and hazards to the attention of responsible individuals such as business owners, storekeepers, restaurant owners, theater managers, museum directors, and government officials. The most effective action can be implemented by the determined public as they are the persons who are most affected by inadequate access (18).

References

1. Hale G. *The Source Book for the Disabled.* New York, NY: Paddington Press Ltd; 1979.
2. Slonaker DM. *Guide to Independent Living for People with Arthritis.* 2nd ed. Atlanta, Ga: The Arthritis Foundation; 1988.
3. Sainsbury R, Mulley GP. Walking sticks used by the elderly. *Brit Med J.* 284:1751, June 12, 1982.
4. Friedmann LW, Capulong ES. Specific assistive aids. In: Williams TF, ed. *Rehabilitation in the Aging.* New York, NY: Raven Press; 1984:315–329.
5. Todd SP Jr, ed. *J Rehab Res & Devel, Clini Suppl* No. 2, March 1990:1–116.
6. Britell CW. Wheel chair prescription. In: Kottke FJ, and Lehmann JF, eds. *Medicine and Rehabilitation.* 4th ed. Philadelphia, Pa: W.B. Saunders; 1990:548–563.
7. Zacharkow D. *Wheelchair Posture and Pressure Sores.* New York, NY: Charles C Thomas; 1984.
8. Okada SH. Should Miss Daisy drive. *Geriatr Rehabil Preview.* 2:1, 7, 1990.
9. Retchin SM, Cox J, Fox M, Irwin L. Performance-based measurement among elderly drivers and non-drivers. *J Am Geriatr Soc.* 36:813–819, 1988.
10. Pehringer JL. Assistive devices: technology to improve communication. *Otolaryngol Clin North Am.* 22:143–174, 1989.
11. Trombley CA. *Occupational Therapy for Physical Dysfunction.* 2nd ed. Baltimore, Md: Williams & Wilkins; 1983:265–266, 288.
12. Ziegler EM. *Current Concepts in Orthotics.* Chicago, Il: Bell, Stromberg & Harris; 1984:32–38.
13. Bistevins R. Footwear and footwear modifications. In: Kottke FJ, Lehmann JF, eds. *Handbook of Physical Medicine and Rehabilitation.* 4th ed. Philadelphia, Pa: W.B. Saunders; 1990:967–975.
14. Hicks JE, Leonard JA, Nelson VS, Fisher SV, Esquenazi A. Prosthetics, orthotics and assistive devices. 4. Orthotic management of selected disorders. *Arch Phys Med Rehabil.* 70:S10–S217, 1989.
15. Lucas BD. Spinal orthotics for pain and instability. In: Redford JB, ed. *Orthotics, Etcetera.* Baltimore, Md: Williams & Wilkins; 1980:123–152.
16. Luskin R, Berger N. Prescription principles. In: *Atlas of Orthotics: Biomechanical Principles and Application.* American Academy of Orthopedic Surgeons; St. Louis, Mo: CV Mosby; 1975.
17. Perry J. The use of external support in the treatment of low back pain. JBJS. 52A:1440–1442, 1970.
18. Ruben B. ADA approval guarantees rights for persons with disabilities. *OT Week.* 4:2–10, June 7, 1990, 2 & 10.

39

INPATIENT EPISODIC CARE SETTINGS

I/Geriatric Rehabilitation Unit
Paul T. Diamond, Donna H. Butler, and Gerald Felsenthal

In the past decade, the number of individuals over the age of 65 years rose by 18.9% and currently represents 12.4% of the total United States population (1). Approximately 25% of these individuals have major activity limitation resulting from chronic illness (2). This population accounts for a large percentage of the patients in a general inpatient rehabilitation unit. From 1980 to 1990 the number of individuals over 75 years of age increased by over 30%, while the number of those over 85 years of age increased by more than 40% (2). These individuals, known as the old-old, present unique needs that are the focus of the specialized geriatric rehabilitation unit.

Normal aging is accompanied by physiologic changes, which affect endurance, performance, and ability to learn. During aging there are declines in short-term memory and performance time (3). There is a 5% to 10% reduction in maximal oxygen consumption each decade after the age of 25 (4). Decreases in muscle mass and responsiveness to beta-adrenergic modulators limit physical work capacity (5). From the age of 25 years to 75 years there is an expected 40% to 60% decline in upper extremity vibration sense and leg flexion and a 20% to 40% decline in a variety of functional activities including rising from a chair with support, foot dorsiflexion, donning a shirt, managing a large button, zipping a garment, speed of handwriting, and cutting with a knife (3). A high prevalence of chronic illness further limits abilities. Fifty-three percent of people over the age of 85 years have a history of arthritis, 16% have coronary heart disease, and 44% have hypertension (2). Approximately 50% are hearing impaired, and almost 30% are visually impaired (2). All of these changes, whether considered normal or pathologic, affect these individuals' abilities to tolerate therapies, the rate at which they make gains, and ultimately the functional goals obtained.

The specialized geriatric rehabilitation unit attempts to address the multiple needs of the very elderly in order that they may achieve the greatest functional outcomes possible. Successful rehabilitation must include a comprehensive evaluation and treatment of the patient's multiple impairments, ongoing modifications in therapy prescriptions, physical evaluation, and possible alteration of environment, and an emphasis on follow-up health care and community services. Physicians, therapists, nursing staff, social workers, and all student health professionals require training and experience in the care of the elderly.

CANDIDATE SELECTION

Appropriate candidate selection is necessary for successful rehabilitation. Medicare guidelines stipulate that appropriate candidates for an inpatient rehabilitation unit must require 24-hour medical and nursing supervision (6). It should be expected that their rehabilitation will yield beneficial goals in a reasonably predictable period of time. Finally, successful candidates must be able to tolerate at least 3 hours of therapy each day although Medicare guidelines allow acceptance of a patient to build enough endurance to meet this time requirement. These criteria, on the surface, appear nonnegotiable. However, identifying those individuals who will, in fact, make substantial gains in therapy and defining legitimate goals of rehabilitation can be complex in the more debilitated geriatric population.

When patients are referred for admission, they are evaluated by an attending physiatrist along with a Physical Medicine and Rehabilitation (PM&R) houseofficer or nurse. In cases where an older patient on initial consultation shows evidence of impaired mental status and/or poor participation in acute hospital therapies, we routinely make follow-up visits. During the early phase of acute hospitalization, the elderly are prone to delirium (7) secondary to medications, medical illness, recent surgery or simply due to a lack of familiar surroundings. High rates of depression are found in patient groups commonly receiving inpatient rehabilitation (8). Depression should be treated since those patients receiving treatment have been found to perform significantly better on measures of physical and cognitive rehabilitation (9). Prolonged hospital stays can foster learned helplessness. These problems can be successfully addressed using the comprehensive rehabilitation approach. Therefore, to deny acceptance to a rehabilitation unit based on one assessment or secondary to poor progress early on may exclude many appropriate candidates.

The effectiveness of inpatient rehabilitation of patients with dementia is controversial. Some studies suggest that dementia portends a poor rehabilitation outcome (10, 11). Yet, it would be a mistake to deny rehabilitation to all patients with dementia without considering the overall clinical and social situation (12). For example, a patient with severe dementia who has sustained a hip fracture and is without weight bearing or other restrictions has the potential to return to premorbid functioning without the need to learn new skills. Rehabilitation efforts are not limited to the patient, but include appropriate environmental modification, the ed-

ucation of caregivers, and the establishment of comprehensive home support services. In this scenario, goals can be attained even in the more cognitively impaired patients.

Some rehabilitation units deny admission to elderly individuals who may be discharged to a nursing home. However, increased independence in self-care and mobility can enhance self-esteem and quality of life, regardless of one's disposition, and decrease the care burden of the nursing staff.

ADDRESSING THE SPECIAL NEEDS OF THE ELDERLY

A study of the demographics of our geriatric rehabilitation unit revealed that the most common primary diagnosis was cerebrovascular accident followed by fracture (Table 39.1A). Deconditioning was the fourth most common diagnosis, comprising 11% of admissions (13). The mean age was 74.1 years. What characteristics and needs distinguish this group of patients and how do we begin to address them?

Special Assessment Programs on the Geriatric Rehabilitation Unit

Comprehensive medical and rehabilitation assessment
Medication assessment and training
Visual and auditory evaluations
Cognitive assessment
Bladder and bowel training
Fall prevention
Nutrition assessment
Skin care
Equipment assessment and prescription

The elderly often present with a history of multiple medical problems. A retrospective study of our geriatric rehabilitation unit revealed that approximately 50% of the patients admitted over a 6-month period developed at least one medical complication during the course of their stay (14). Optimal medical management of these conditions can enhance gains made in rehabilitation. Therefore, efforts are made to ensure that comprehensive medical care is provided. Though daily rounds serve well to investigate the patients' current complaints and medical status, it is frequently necessary for a physician to evaluate the patient at various times of the day, especially at the time of admission to the rehabilitation unit. Frequent communication between the physiatrist and therapists is essential. The patient's primary physician is involved in his or her care. As a result, it is possible to reduce the impact of the patient's illnesses on participation in therapy (13).

The elderly are commonly subjected to polypharmacy, including prescription as well as over-the-counter

Table 39.1A. Primary Diagnoses, Levindale Geriatric Rehabilitation Unit[a]

	Patients	
Diagnosis	n	%
Cerebrovascular accident	28	34.1
Other cerebral lesions	7	8.5
Fractures	10	12.2
Deconditioned	9	11.0
Arteriosclerotic cardiovascular disease	5	6.1
Parkinson syndrome	5	6.1
Cancer	3	3.7
Spinal cord lesion	3	3.7
Amputation	2	2.4
Arthritis	2	2.4
Multiple sclerosis	2	2.4
Peripheral vascular disease	2	2.4
Chronic obstructive pulmonary disease	1	1.2
Multiple lacerations	1	1.2
Pain syndrome	1	1.2
S/P total knee surgery	1	1.2

[a]Reprinted with permission from Felsenthal G, Cohen BS, Hilton EB, Panagos AV, Aiken BM. The physiatrist as primary physician for patients on an inpatient rehabilitation unit. *Arch Phys Med Rehabil*. 65:375–378, 1984.

medications. Unfortunately, these same individuals are especially susceptible to adverse effects from these medications as a result of the alterations in pharmacokinetics associated with aging. In addition, underlying cognitive impairment greatly increases the risk of delirium associated with the use of sedatives and other medications with anticholinergic properties. Medications should be carefully reviewed at the time of admission. Efforts are made to simplify the medical regimen by eliminating unnecessary medications and choosing equivalent medications that may be taken less frequently in order to enhance compliance. An integral part of the rehabilitation process includes training patients and their caregivers in proper administration of medications. The purpose of each medication as well as potential side effects are reviewed. Memory aids are used if necessary. This process of simplification and education can be instrumental in return to independent living (15).

Given the high prevalence of sensory impairment in this population, the initial history and physical exam should include screening for visual and hearing impairments. Frequent referrals are made to audiology for the prescription of hearing aids. Ophthalmology consultation is also available.

It is estimated that dementia occurs in less than 1% of individuals between the ages of 65 years and 70 years, but increases to more than 15% in those over the age of 85 years (5). Therefore, formal cognitive screening and assessment plays a major role in the geriatric rehabilitation unit. A clinical psychologist, speech pathologist, and occupational therapist participate in the patient's cognitive evaluation. The geriatric physiatrist contributes to this process by ensuring that consideration is given to all reversible causes of dementia and that appropriate medical evaluation is pursued if indicated. Major depression, a recognized cause of pseudodementia, is seen in 10% to 20% of the elderly in acute and long-term care facilities (16). Appropriate diagnosis and treatment can enhance participation and progress in therapies.

Formal monitoring, evaluation, and treatment of bladder and bowel problems are an integral part of the rehabilitation process. Urinary incontinence in the elderly is multifactorial (17) and can be studied best in the inpatient setting. Medical/surgical evaluations are obtained when indicated. Various management options include the use of timed voiding schedules, condom catheters, adult diapers, and in certain cases, intermittent catheterization or indwelling catheters. Fecal incontinence may also respond to various interventions (18). Fourteen percent of individuals over 85 years of age living in the community have functional limitations that make the use of a toilet difficult (2). Prescription of appropriate adaptive equipment can be of great benefit. The preservation of bladder and bowel continence enhances self-esteem and may facilitate return home.

The elderly are at an increased risk of falling. The annual incidence of falls in individuals 70 years of age living at home increases from 25% to 35% over the next 5 years of life (19). A majority of these falls occur at home during ambulation and simple transfers. Recurrent falls have severe implications; they are thought to be a contributing factor in the need for nursing home placement in 40% of cases and result in approximately 9,500 deaths each year in individuals over the age of 65 years (18). Therefore, a comprehensive evaluation of an individual's risk of falling and appropriate preventative interventions is an important component of any geriatric rehabilitation program. Gait abnormalities are common in the elderly and increase the risk of falls (20). The etiology of these abnormalities can be multifactorial, and therefore a careful clinical assessment on the part of the physiatrist is also indicated. Attempts are made to correct visual and hearing impairments and to ensure that clothing fits properly and that foot wear is safe. Therapists conduct home visits to assess potential hazards in the home environment and to make recommendations regarding home adaptive equipment such as stair rails and transfer bars.

Malnutrition is seen commonly in the elderly. It is estimated that 17% to 65% of the elderly admitted to acute care hospitals are malnourished (21). Since most patients admitted to the geriatric rehabilitation unit are referred from an acute care setting, the nutritional status of each patient should be assessed by a nutrition specialist. Efforts are made to ensure adequate caloric intake to meet the increased needs during rehabilitation, with dietary modifications as indicated by swallowing abilities.

Pressure ulcers are seen in 3% to 11% of hospitalized elderly; the associated mortality is high (22). A thorough skin survey is performed on each admission to our rehabilitation unit by a team of specialized nurses. Treatment plans are implemented in consultation with the physician, and progress is monitored closely.

ESTABLISHING A REHABILITATION ORIENTED ENVIRONMENT

How do we address the problem of motivating our patients to put forth the great effort needed to achieve functional goals? We begin by emphasizing the functional significance of all the therapeutic activities we ask our patients to perform. We discourage ageism and elderly entitlement, the perception that age equals the right to be dependent on others. Inactivity and apparent apathy are confronted, rather than ignored, in a supportive manner. We attempt to maintain good morale on the unit, which helps motivate not only our patients but the entire rehabilitation staff. Frequently we see close bonds form between staff and patients that further help foster participation and progress in therapies. The patient's family is made aware of possible functional outcomes so that they may encourage rehabilitation efforts without feeling compelled to assist out of fear or guilt. Finally, an emphasis is placed on open communication. Patients should feel comfortable telling their therapists what they wish to gain from therapies. Just as importantly, the rehabilitation staff should effectively communicate their expectations to each patient.

The interior layout of our unit has been nicely designed for inpatient rehabilitation. Semiprivate patient rooms are large, allowing wheelchair accessibility. Each room contains a separate bathroom with commode and sink. The sinks lack vanities so that a wheelchair can roll under them, enabling the patient to perform grooming and hygiene activities at the sink rather than bedside. The unit has separate tub and shower rooms in order to ensure safe, supervised retraining of bathing. Specially designed telephones with large red numbers and hearing aid compatibility are kept at each bedside table for training. Large instruction sheets are placed over each patient's bed to inform nurses and family members of their current level of function and special precautions such as dietary restrictions.

Patients' rooms are located in a circle around the day area. The nurses' station is located centrally between the day area and a second large area where therapies are provided. This design allows the patients easy access to all areas of the unit, encourages interaction between patients and staff, and allows the nursing staff better visibility of the entire unit from their station. Several features are designed to provide reality orientation on the unit. Ideally, rooms should vary in appearance in order to ease visual identification. On our unit, patient rooms and entry doors are painted various colors. Patient names are posted outside each room. Personal bulletin boards are provided, and families are encouraged to bring in photos and other personal items. Large clocks and calendars are also located in each room. The central day area has an orientation board with the date, current weather, and next holiday. Our institution also has its own "radio station" that broadcasts recent local and world news and makes announcements such as scheduled events and birthdays.

Unit policies have been designed to encourage the relearning of self-care skills, both in and out of therapies, and to facilitate social interaction. At the time of admission, each patient is assigned an appropriate wheelchair to afford mobility. Patients are encouraged to remain outside their rooms during the day and wear the clothing they typically wear at home. The centrally located day area provides them with a pleasant area to interact with the other patients and staff. Communal dining provides a significant amount of time for socialization for patients as well as family members who usually visit at the supper hour. Many new friendships, which often last long after discharge, are formed. Since endur-

ance is often limited in the elderly, multiple short therapy sessions are scheduled in place of the more common twice a day scheduling. Rest times are incorporated into the patients' schedules to further enhance the benefits of therapy. Simultaneous physical and occupational therapy are offered in the gymnasium to maximize outcomes. In addition to the more routine physical and occupational therapy department equipment, specific seating devices and gait surfaces should be available. Other facilities include an activities of daily living (ADL) kitchen, washer and dryer, and ideally an ADL apartment where patient and family can practice independent living under unit supervision.

SUMMARY

As can be seen, the geriatric rehabilitation unit differs from the standard unit in many respects. Early on, fundamental changes in the principles used during the selection process yield an older, more impaired patient population. Special programs are in place to assess and meet the increased needs of this elderly population. The design of the unit and structuring of therapies are meant to optimize the older patients' ability to benefit from rehabilitation. Finally, all members of the rehabilitation team are experienced in the care of the geriatric patient.

Several studies have reviewed and supported the efficacy of specialized geriatric assessment and rehabilitation units (23–30). The economic benefits of keeping our elderly out of nursing homes can be measured in billions of dollars. No dollar value can be placed on the restoration of dignity and independence to our elderly.

References

1. Kineannon CL. Changing population patterns. In: Hoffman MS, ed. *The World Almanac and Book of Facts 1990*. New York, NY: Pharos Books; 1990:550.
2. Statistical abstract of the United States 1990. *The National Data Book*. 110th ed. Washington, DC: US Department of Commerce, Bureau of the Census; 1990.
3. Katzman R, Terry RD. Normal aging of the nervous system. In: Katzman R, Rowe, JW, eds. *Principles of Geriatric Neurology*. Philadelphia, Pa: F.A. Davis; 1992:18–58.
4. Morley JE, Reese SS. Clinical implications of the aging heart. *Am J Med*. 86:77–110, 1989.
5. Davis Conference. Moderator: Geokas MC. Discussants: Lakatta EG, Makinodan T, Timiras PS. The aging process. *Ann Intern Med*. 113:455–466, 1990.
6. Health Care Financing Administration. Inpatient rehabilitation hospital care: Section 3101.11(D). *Medicare Intermediary Manual: Part 3. Claims process*. Transmittal No. 1293, 3-38.8–3-38.9, 1986.
7. Lipowsi ZJ. Delirium (acute confusional states). *JAMA*. 258:1789–1792, 1987.
8. Lingam VR, Lazarus LW, Groves L, Oh SH. Methylphenidate in treating poststroke depression. *J Clin Psychiatry*. 49:151–153, 1988.
9. Fedoroff JP, Robinson RG. Tricyclic antidepressants in the treatment of poststroke depression. *J Clin Psychiatry*. 50:18–23, 1989.

10. Schuman JE, Beattie EJ, Steed DA, Merry GM, Kraus AS. Geriatric patients with and without intellectual dysfunction: effectiveness of a standard rehabilitation program. *Arch Phys Med Rehabil.* 62:612–618, 1981.

11. Caradoc-Davies TH. Medical profiles of patients admitted to a geriatric assessment and rehabilitation unit. *NZ Med J.* 100:557–559, 1987.

12. Uhlmann R, Larson E, Rees T, Koepsell T, Duckert L. Relationship of hearing impairment to dementia and cognitive dysfunction in older adults. *JAMA.* 261:1916–1919, 1989.

13. Felsenthal G, Cohen BS, Hilton EB, Panagos AV, Aiken BM. The physiatrist as primary physician for patients on an inpatient rehabilitation unit. *Arch Phys Med Rehabil.* 65:375–378, 1984.

14. Felsenthal G, Aiken BM, Cohen BS. Incidence of medical problems in a geriatric inpatient rehabilitation unit. *Md State Med J.* 33:110–13, 1984.

15. Felsenthal G, Glomski MA, Jones D. Medication education program in an inpatient geriatric rehabilitation unit. *Arch Phys Med Rehabil.* 67:27–29, 1986.

16. Blazer D. Depression in the elderly. *N Engl J Med.* 320:164–166, 1989.

17. Resnick NM, Yalla SV. Management of urinary incontinence in the elderly. *N Engl J Med.* 313:800–805, 1985.

18. Tobin GW, Brocklehurst JC. Faecal incontinence in residential homes for the elderly: prevalence, etiology and management. *Age Ageing.* 15:41–46, 1986.

19. Tinetti ME, Speechley M. Prevention of falls among the elderly. *N Engl J Med.* 320:1055–1059, 1989.

20. Sudarsky L. Geriatrics: gait disorders in the elderly. *N Engl J Med.* 322:1441–1446, 1990.

21. UCLA Conference. Moderator: Morley JE. Discussants: Mooradian AD, Silver AJ, Heber D, Alfin-Slater RB. Nutrition in the elderly. *Ann Intern Med.* 109:890–904, 1988.

22. Allman RM. Pressure ulcers among the elderly. *N Engl J Med.* 320:850–853, 1989.

23. Applegate WB, Akins D, Vander Zwaag R, Thoni K, Baker MG. A geriatric rehabilitation and assessment unit in a community hospital. *J Am Geriatr Soc.* 31:206–210, 1983.

24. Lefton E, Bonstelle S, Frengley JD. Success with an inpatient geriatric unit, a controlled study of outcome and follow-up. *J Am Geriatr Soc.* 31:149–155, 1983.

25. Liem PH, Chernoff R, Carter WJ. Geriatric rehabilitation unit: a 3 year outcome evaluation. *J Gerontol.* 41:44–50, 1986.

26. Rubenstein LZ, Josephson KR, Wieland GD, English PA, Sayre JA, Kane RL. Effectiveness of a geriatric evaluation unit: a randomized clinical trial. *N Engl J Med.* 311:1664–1670, 1984.

27. Rubenstein LZ, Wieland D, English P, Josephson K, Sayre JA, Abrass IB. The Sepulveda VA geriatric evaluation unit: data on four-year outcomes and predictors of improved patient outcomes. *J Am Geriatr Soc.* 32:503–512, 1984.

28. Murphy PJ, Rai GS, Lowy M, Bielawska C. The beneficial effects of joint orthopaedic-geriatric rehabilitation. *Age Ageing.* 16:273–278, 1987.

29. Sainsbury R, Gillespie WJ, Armour PC, Newman EF. An orthopaedic geriatric rehabilitation unit: the first two years experience. *NZ Med J.* 99:583–585, 1986.

30. Boyd RV, Compton E, Hawthorne J, Kemm JR. Orthogeriatric rehabilitation ward in Nottingham: a preliminary report. *Br Med J.* 285:937–938, 1982.

II/Geriatric Assessment Unit
Joseph J. Gallo

Rehabilitation teams have pioneered geriatric assessment principles through emphasis on restoration and maintenance of function. The rehabilitation process, after all, begins with assessment of the patient's strengths and weaknesses. Although the elder is rather vulnerable to disability from many processes, social as well as physiologic, correction or compensation of seemingly trivial deficits can have a direct effect on the quality of life of older persons. This section describes the domains of geriatric assessment, composition of interdisciplinary teams, and literature on geriatric assessment and rehabilitation units.

Multidimensional assessment expands the traditional medical evaluation to include assessment of cognitive status, affective state, function [activities of daily living (ADLs)], and social support, in addition to the physical examination. Economic factors, elicitation of patient values, and formulation of appropriate preventive strategies may also be included as domains of multidimensional assessment (1–4). The effect of a medical diagnosis on the elder's function in these domains must be considered; for example, multidimensional assessment is useful in evaluation and rehabilitation of

the patient in various stages of recovery following a stroke (5).

GERIATRIC ASSESSMENT AND REHABILITATION TEAMS

Geriatric assessment units have been called the new technology of geriatrics (6). The settings in which geriatric assessment takes place are varied and include inpatient units, outpatient clinics, consultation services, rehabilitation units, and, in the United Kingdom, day hospitals. In a survey of geriatric assessment units affiliated with a medical school or Veterans Administration hospital, providing rehabilitation services was cited as a major activity (6). Many geriatric assessment teams consist of a core team of a physician, nurse, and social worker. Other professionals, including dietitians, occupational therapists, physical therapists, and dentists, as well as medical and surgical subspecialists, may be part of the core team.

After evaluation, findings, consultations, and any special studies are reviewed by the team. The team leader focuses activities of the team and ensures that opinions of team members are expressed. Well-functioning teams require periodic definition of their goals and roles to maintain appropriate performance (7). To be useful, recommendations are as specific as possible; an example is the format utilized by the University of Washington, which includes recommendations regarding medical condition, mental health, daily routine, medications, nutrition, household tasks, transportation, housing, finances, and the patient's effect on the family (8, 9). The recommendations are presented to the patient, family, and primary care physician.

ADMISSION

Criteria to guide selection of patients for geriatric assessment units have yet to be precisely defined. It seems that geriatric assessment is most effective for a targeted group of elders. Patients who are not too sick and not too well, sometimes referred to as the frail elderly, appear to benefit to the greatest extent, especially when assessment is combined with treatment and rehabilitation (10). The frail elderly may have health conditions that require frequent hospitalizations, medication, and visits to physicians' offices. In addition, the frail elderly are often functionally dependent and at risk for institutionalization.

Specific conditions have been used as criteria of exclusion for geriatric assessment. These include those indicating imminent death, long-standing psychotic disorders, well-evaluated irreversible dementia progressed to a degree that the patient can perform no more than three ADLs and long-term nursing home patients. Patients who may be appropriate for admission to a geriatric assessment unit are those with at least one family member or surrogate willing to participate in assessment, those in whom nursing home placement is contemplated, and those with functional impairment who are clinically stable.

LITERATURE REVIEWED

In 1973, Williams and associates at the Monroe Community Hospital Evaluation-Placement Unit in Rochester, New York, reported that, following team assessment, more than half of the patients needed further diagnostic, therapeutic, or rehabilitative efforts before final disposition. Three fourths of the patients referred for rehabilitation were able to be discharged home. In all, two thirds of the patients were able to be discharged home or to care other than a nursing home. The conclusion was that, in some cases, patients could stay at home after rehabilitation when nursing home placement had previously been considered the only option (11).

Applegate and colleagues reported the results of a randomized, controlled clinical trial of a geriatric assessment unit in a rehabilitation hospital (12, 13). Patients in the trial received care from community physicians;

there was no specialized follow-up care. Eligible patients were felt to be at risk for nursing home placement with potentially reversible functional impairment. Patients also had to be able to give informed consent to a randomized study. Patients with unstable medical problems, with survival estimated to be less than 6 months, and in whom nursing home placement was felt to be inevitable were excluded. Average length of stay in the unit was 24 days. Subjects were predominantly female and white.

Patients were stratified into high and low risk groups by asking the question, "If you were discharged today, where would you go?" Patients who anticipated nursing home placement were considered high risk. They had longer hospital stays, greater severity of illness, and were more dependent in ADLs. Patients receiving intensive assessment and rehabilitation in the unit, especially those in the high risk group, were less likely to be institutionalized at follow-up when compared to control group patients who received care from community physicians. Patients in the intervention group also had improved in performance of ADLs compared to the controls. Patients in the low risk stratum had improved survival as well (12).

Rubenstein and coworkers (14, 15) at the Sepulveda Veterans Administration Medical Center reported on the results of a randomized study of a geriatric evaluation unit. Patients in the unit received care from an interdisciplinary team and after discharge were followed in an outpatient geriatric clinic. Patients in the control group had access to the same services but continued to be cared for by acute care physicians. Inclusion criteria included age over 65 years and a persistent medical, functional, or social problem that put the patient at risk for institutionalization. Patients with severe dementia, poor ADL function, terminal illness, or who had no social support were excluded. Subjects were predominantly male and white.

Patients who were cared for in the unit showed lower mortality than did a control group at 1 year of follow-up (48% versus 24%). More unit patients were able to be discharged home compared with control patients. Unit patients had fewer days spent in institutions after discharge when figured per years survived. In addition, unit patients had greater improvement in functional status. The number of drugs prescribed decreased, and unit patients had five times as many new diagnoses made. The investigators believed that improved functional status and morale contributed to improved survival; in addition, positive staff expectations may have affected discharge location (14).

Liem and associates (16) at the Little Rock and North Little Rock Veterans Administration Hospitals created a geriatric evaluation unit in conjunction with a geriatric rehabilitation unit. Roughly 10% of patients admitted to the hospital were seen in consultation, and

75% of these were recommended for assessment in a 10-bed geriatric evaluation unit. These patients underwent comprehensive assessment, and at discharge 40% were able to live at home. Half of these patients were transferred to the geriatric rehabilitation unit from which they were discharged when maximum rehabilitative potential was achieved. Leading diagnoses treated included stroke, congestive heart failure, and dementia.

Following a period of rehabilitation, averaging 70 days, 77% went home and 23% went to a nursing home. Mental status and the availability of caretakers were important predictors of patient placement. Mortality was inversely correlated with the ADL level. This study did not use a control group, so it is unclear whether patients would have done well even without treatment in a specialized unit.

SUMMARY

Studies of the efficacy of a multidomain approach to geriatric assessment are, for the most part, favorable although relatively few studies incorporate a control or comparison group (17). It does appear, however, that an approach that considers the special needs of the elderly can be effective in reducing unnecessary institutionalization and disability.

References

1. Gallo JJ, Reichel W, Anderson L. *Handbook of Geriatric Assessment.* Rockville, Md: Aspen Publishers; 1988.
2. Kane RA, Kane RL. *Assessing the Elderly: A Practical Guide to Measurement.* Lexington, Mass: Lexington Books; 1981.
3. Granger CV, Gresham GE, eds.: *Functional Assessment in Rehabilitation Medicine.* Baltimore, Md: Williams & Wilkins; 1984.
4. Applegate WB, Blass JP, Williams TF. Instruments for the functional assessment of older patients. *N Engl J. Med.* 322:1207–1214, 1990.
5. Kelly JF, Winograd CH. A functional approach to stroke management in elderly patients. *J Am Geriatr Soc.* 33:48–60, 1985.
6. Epstein AM, Hall JA, Besdine R, et al. The emergence of geriatric assessment units: the "new technology of geriatrics". *Ann Intern Med.* 106:299–303, 1987.
7. Campbell LJ, Cole KD. Geriatric assessment teams. *Clin Geriatr Med.* 3:99–109, 1987.
8. Reifler BV, Larson E, Cox G, et al. Treatment results at a multispecialty clinic for the impaired elderly and their families. *J Am Geriatr Soc.* 29:579–582, 1981.
9. Reifler BV, Eisdorfer C. A clinic for the impaired elderly and their families. *Am J Psychiatry.* 137:1399–1403, 1980.
10. National Institutes of Health Consensus Development Conference Statement. *Geriatric Assessment Methods for Clinical Decision-making.* Washington, DC: October 19–21, 1987.
11. Williams TF, Hill JG, Fairbank ME, et al. Appropriate placement of the chronically ill and aged: a successful approach by evaluation. *JAMA.* 226:1332–1335, 1973.
12. Applegate WB, Miller ST, Graney MJ, et al. A randomized, controlled trial of a geriatric assessment unit in a community rehabilitation hospital. *N Engl J Med.* 322:1572–1578, 1990.
13. Applegate WB, Akins DE, Elam JT. A geriatric assessment and rehabilitation unit in a rehabilitation hospital. *Clin Geriatr Med.* 3:145–155, 1987.
14. Rubenstein LZ, Josephson KR, Wieland GD, et al. Effectiveness of a geriatric evaluation unit: a randomized trial. *N Engl J Med.* 311:1664–1670, 1984.
15. Rubenstein LZ, Abrass IB, Kane RL. Improved care for patients on a new geriatric evaluation unit. *J Am Geriatr Soc.* 29:531–536, 1981.
16. Liem PH, Chernoff R, Carter WJ. Geriatric rehabilitation unit: a 3-year outcome evaluation. *J Gerontol.* 41:44–50, 1986.
17. Rubenstein LZ. Geriatric assessment: an overview of its impacts. *Clin Geriatr Med.* 3:1–15, 1987.

III/Geriatric Psychiatric Unit
Jeffrey Lafferman

The practice of inpatient psychiatry among elderly patients is generally thought of in the environment of an acute general hospital. The high rate of concurrent medical problems in the elderly psychiatric inpatient and the special attention needed to assist in activities of daily living (ADLs) in these patients have resulted in geropsychiatry units. The appropriateness and usefulness of the geropsychiatry inpatient unit in the chronic hospital setting is discussed in this section.

LEVEL OF CHRONIC CARE

The hospital level of care for chronic illness is a poorly understood resource in our health care system. Chronic level is a misnomer because it is not chronic; in fact, most inpatient stays in the hospital for care of chronic illness are approximately 60 days. It is a lower level of care than acute care as reflected by lower staffing patterns, generally 5 hours of staff care per patient per 24 hours in the chronic hospital compared to 6.5 hours of staff time per patient per 24 hours in the acute hospital. The staff is also composed of fewer registered nurses (RNs) with a greater proportion of licensed practical nurses (LPNs) and nursing assistants. However, level of chronic care is substantially more intense than skilled level of care that provides 2.5 hours of staff time per patient per 24 hours with an even greater reliance on LPNs and nursing assistance (Department of Nursing, Levindale Hebrew Geriatric Center and Chronic Hospital, unpublished data). The chronic level of care is used for patients who require extended care following acute hospital stays such as daily medication management, specialized beds for decubitus care, ventilators for maintenance and weaning, intravenous antibiotics over an extended period of time, physical rehabilitation, and intravenous analgesia. With the stricter utilization review of acute hospital stays in the face of tightening diagnosis related groups (DRGs) and the aging of the population requiring more complicated care, use of chronic hospitals will undoubtedly be increasing.

PATIENT POPULATION

The elderly patients who require inpatient psychiatric care are a diverse group with psychiatric disorders often complicated by concurrent cognitive and medical disorders. The patient best served in a psychiatric service in the chronic hospital is the fragile elderly patient with coexisting medical and cognitive disorders that subsequently result in deterioration of ADL skills needed for independent living. The presence of psychiatric disorders in a medically fragile population has been speculated to result in greater disability and possibly result in custodial care that would not otherwise be necessary (1). Treatment of psychiatric disorders in a fragile group of elderly inpatients who deteriorate from independent functioning would ideally be managed by nursing staff that is supportive in providing assistance with ADLs while simultaneously being rehabilitative in promoting return of lost ADL skills as medical debility and psychiatric symptoms improve in treatment. Nursing staff in chronic hospitals are already trained in this technique and are willing to provide ADL support for total care patients that psychiatric nursing in the acute general hospital psychiatric units often are unwilling to do.

The reliance upon interdisciplinary care as a cardinal feature in geropsychiatry is also well represented in the skills of staff members already present in the chronic hospital and affiliated long-term care institutions. Medical consultants are already available as needed for the elderly population. Expressive arts therapists trained as therapists are ideal in working with patients who are not very verbal or overly somatic. Psychiatric occupational therapists are useful in continually assessing functional abilities as patients progress and can be extremely helpful in distinguishing functional versus organic disabilities. The role of social workers to educate families and perform discharge planning is already present. Physical therapy is in place in rehabilitative and custodial care. In fact, the role of treating psychiatric disorders by the staff of the chronic hospital is already present, but not well coordinated to treat the elderly psychiatric patient.

As a community resource, the psychiatric rehabilitation service in the chronic hospital is ideal for servicing the nursing home resident who has become so behaviorally problematic that custodial care is not possible. The presence of mental health problems in residents of nursing homes is largely ignored, and as a rule the psychiatric illness does not receive attention until the symptoms erupt and become disruptive to the normal ebb and flow of custodial care. The resident who deteriorates in the nursing home from psychiatric illness despite psychiatric treatment that is provided on site could benefit by admission to the chronic hospital. Often, it is the resident with medical and cognitive complications who needs much ADL support who is in need of a psychiatric admission and could benefit from an inpatient service in a chronic hospital. Special attention is deserving of the nursing home resident with Alzheimer's disease who has excess disability, meaning overlapping depression with progressive dementia. When agitation results as a consequence of depression in a patient with Alzheimer's disease, it is commonly attributed to the dementia, and neuroleptic trials might be used causing a great disservice to the patient. In the wake of the Omnibus Budget Reconciliation Act (OBRA) (2) 1987 regulations, this will hopefully be avoided. Thorough psychiatric evaluation is necessary to make the diagnosis, and an inpatient admission can be used if the agitation is severe or the patient is very frail.

PSYCHIATRIC SERVICE AS RESOURCE FOR GENERAL HOSPITAL

The psychiatric service of a chronic hospital could also be an important resource for the general hospital where elderly hospital patients are often suffering psychiatric complications causing excess physical disability (3), for example, the case of a depressed cardiac patient with anorexia and anergia. Patients of this type might not ordinarily be accepted into general hospital psychiatric units because of advanced physical disability. Additionally, shortening length of stays may be a factor in both medical patients who fail to progress because of psychiatric complications as well as psychiatric inpatients in the general hospital who might need an extended stay to recover. In both these cases, transfer to a chronic hospital psychiatric service would be helpful.

The psychiatric service of a chronic hospital might also be an important resource for psychiatric outpatients in the community. However, residents in the community who are otherwise physically healthy and independent would best be served in general hospital psychiatric units. Those elderly who are disabled and cognitively impaired and living in the community in sheltered housing, living with companion care, or attending day care would be best suited for the chronic hospital when they deteriorate behaviorally. Those who might need nursing home placement after being psychiatrically stabilized would also benefit from admission to the chronic hospital psychiatric unit.

In contrast to the acute general hospital, chronic hospital has the potential for providing less intense services and longer hospital stays. The decline of general hospital stays through DRG mechanisms and prepayment for usual anticipated stays is often inconsistent with good psychiatric care, even when psychiatric treatment is applied efficiently. The fragile elderly patient may not need the intensity or service offered in the acute general hospital as seclusion rooms, close one-to-one observation, and intense nursing psychosocial support are not required. Instead, the cognitively impaired psychiatric patient may require safety restraints to prevent falls or combative behavior and supportive nursing intervention to provide ADL care. Administratively, the average bed day charge per hospital day is less expensive in the chronic hospital, generally about two thirds the cost of the acute hospital day.

The Psychiatric Rehabilitation Unit at Levindale Hebrew Geriatric Center and Hospital has been developed to meet the needs of the elderly who need inpatient psychiatric treatment along with complicating cognitive and medical problems. The PsychRehab Unit was started July, 1989, and at present we have expanded to 20 beds. Geriatric psychiatrists are the medical attendings. Patients are admitted using acute hospital criteria on the premise that patients ill enough for acute care always will warrant a less intense level of care. Examples of admission criteria are failure of outpatient treatment, severe progression of the psychiatric disorder associated with psychosis or dangerousness to self, usually by severe anorexia and weight loss or self-neglect in ADLs. The physical plant includes 10 semiprivate rooms surrounding a common area with an adjoining nursing station that connects to a large day area, half of which is for dining and the other half set up like a large living room. The milieu of the unit is structured activity with regularly scheduled group therapies and activities. Expressive arts therapy and psychiatric occupational therapy are heavily represented to encourage nonverbal expression followed by verbal interpretation. Occupational therapy and physiatry consult on most patients for assessment and treatment of physical and self-care deficits. Neuropsychologic assessment is available for patients who need cognitive assessments. Patients are assessed in multidisciplinary care plan meetings once every 2 weeks to document continued need for stay. Continued need is based upon having unmet goals. Those who are making progress toward their goals are continued in the program. Those who do not progress toward their goals are reassessed in a week and, if judged by the team to have no likelihood of progression, are discharged.

Discharge planning occurs in each team meeting. Group homes and sheltered housing are used regularly instead of nursing homes for patients who can live semiindependently.

In the first 6 months of clinical activity, the average patient age was 78 years. There was an average number of six diagnoses, psychiatric and medical, per patient. The average length of stay was 28.3 days per patient. Comparing this to the nearby metropolitan University Hospital geropsychiatry unit, the average patient age was 68.1 years, and the average length of stay in this acute hospital geropsychiatry unit was 26.7 days. Generally one half of the referrals come from the community and acute hospitals and one half come from nursing homes. Further information about patient outcome is pending; however, it is this author's impression that robust improvement is seen in approximately one third of the cases with another one third showing moderate improvement.

The long-term care center has been undergoing a transformation from retirement home to a hospital providing care using a medical model. Acute care hospitals now limit length of stay to control hospital costs. The elderly patient will be unable to recover from acute illness in the time allowed, and as a result chronic hospitals will emerge as a valuable resource to provide continuing care. The effect of the emerging need for the chronic hospital will drive the regionalization of health care resources. Local residents in the community who need less intense medical services may be triaged to chronic hospitals in an attempt to reduce costs. More likely, however, diagnosis and treatment may be initiated in the acute general hospital prior to the transfer of patients to community chronic hospital for less intensive ongoing care. The organization of a psychiatry service in the chronic hospital is likely to be widespread to meet the needs of the growing elderly population with a high prevalence of neuropsychiatric disorders.

References

1. Rovner BW, German PS, Broadhead J, et al. The prevalence and management of dementia and other psychiatric disorders in nursing homes. *Int Psychogeriatr.* 2:13–24, 1990.
2. House of Representatives: Report 100-495 (1987) Omnibus Budget Reconciliation Act of 1987, Conference report to accompany HR 3545. Washington, DC: US Government Printing Office; 1987.
3. Warshaw GA, Moore JT, Freidman SW, et al. Functional disability in the hospitalized elderly. *JAMA.* 248:847–850, 1982.

40
Community-Based Rehabilitation for the Elderly

Janet C. Frank and Lawrence S. Miller

There is a range of outpatient rehabilitation services, which vary by site, organizational setting, purpose, and perhaps, effectiveness. The focus of this chapter is to outline the basic ways in which outpatient rehabilitation services are delivered to older adults, with discussion centering on factors that fall into the broad categories of access, acceptability, and appropriateness.

Access includes not only the actual existence of services, but also the ability to use these available services. Rural and urban differences are noted, as well as limitations due to income differences, public and private medical coverage, and provider behavior. Given such limitations, appropriate referrals to community-based rehabilitation programs are discussed.

Acceptability relates to the provision of user-friendly services that are perceived as beneficial by the client. Acceptability moves beyond traditional patient satisfaction types of measures such as waiting time and staff courtesy. Today, concerns of cultural sensitivity of program goals, staff behavior, and ethical issues such as self-determination come within the realm of acceptability.

Appropriateness of community-based rehabilitation programs incorporates the identification of a target population, the match of service needs of the person with the service availability and organizational structure most suitable to meet the needs, the necessary types of staff with the required expertise, and the required linkages to other aspects of the social and medical care network, in addition to family and informal care providers. Evaluation of patient care outcomes are often based on the assumption that proper services have been rendered.

At the outset it is important to note the values or biases of the authors. We believe that outpatient rehabilitation programs hold an important position in the continuum of rehabilitative care, as well as in the long-term care system in general. Geriatric medicine encompasses the functional approach principle, the guiding principle of rehabilitative medicine. There are natural bridges and alliances between the two. However,

these two areas also share a lack of adequately trained health professionals, reimbursement for care, and awareness of potential contributions to improved quality of life of the older adult.

The organization of the chapter includes an introduction that discusses the philosophy of geriatric rehabilitation. The second section provides a review of access, acceptability, and appropriateness factors of home care, day care, and several types of outpatient rehabilitation programs. These factors are contrasted by type of program. We also examine the potential of providing rehabilitative services through regular medical care by the primary physicians of older adults. Finally, we establish some guiding principles to address the optimal setting, staffing, and programmatic components for geriatric outpatient rehabilitation.

PHILOSOPHY OF GERIATRIC REHABILITATION

The standard approach to rehabilitation is well-known among physiatrists and other rehabilitation professionals. Attention to the patient's functional abilities, utilization of allied health professionals, and use of the team approach in patient management are fundamental. Physicians with expertise in geriatric medicine also embrace these primary principles of patient care management. However, most physicians, including physical medicine and rehabilitation specialists, have not received specialized geriatrics training. (Refer to Chapter 43) All health care professionals who wish to be involved in the care of geriatric patients with functional impairments must bear in mind several important considerations.

The first consideration is the use of a holistic approach with the patient. Although this is routinely accepted in general rehabilitation, the need to pursue the assessment comprehensively is of much greater importance with the elderly person. The primary physician must look not only at the functional problem, but also at medical, pharmacologic, cognitive, and psychosocial issues. Specifically, if a patient presents with symptoms of fatigue or impaired balance, it is important for the physician to carefully evaluate the medical status, as well as the patient's current medications. Patients with cognitive impairment require an evaluation so that a determination of cognitive deficits, reversible or progressive, can be made. Psychologic issues are important since patients' functional complaints mask the primary problem, for example a significant depression. The social setting and environment of the patient are important in determining whether or not the patient can live in the current situation, taking into account the social supports required and the predicted rehabilitation outcome. Elderly patients themselves may be unrealistic concerning their own strengths and adaptive capacities or reluctant to admit to a tenuous living situation because they may fear limited or untenable alternatives. Therefore, it is important to augment information about the patients' living situations by involving significant others, such as family, friends, and/or neighbors, in setting realistic goals and treatment plans.

Many older adults have chronic illnesses that cause progressive deterioration in function. Unfortunately, both the person and the provider may attribute these gradual losses to aging, being reluctant to either refer or take advantage of helpful rehabilitation services. The rehabilitation goal in these cases is to decrease the rate of decline and maintain current functioning levels. Other older people may score at high functional levels during assessment on measures of independence, self-care, and mobility; however, in performing these day-to-day types of activities they may experience difficulty. The goals of rehabilitation in such cases are to reduce the effort expended. When basic activities of daily living (ADLs) are accomplished with more ease and less fatigue, this may allow the senior to lead a more active life-style, thereby improving quality of life.

Rehabilitation specialists experienced in working with younger patients will immediately note the differences in disease patterns between the young and old. Older adults often have multiple chronic diseases and suffer from deconditioning due to required bedrest related to their illnesses or more sedentary life-styles in general. The multiplicity of disease, altered presentation of acute events, and the close interaction of medical, social, and psychologic factors in the older person's life lead to difficulties in identification of problems and formulation of the care plan. The rehabilitation team must recognize that, although the causes of the older person's disability may be attributed to the primary diagnosis combined with significant comorbidities, improvements in a few of these causes may be sufficient to improve function (1).

Iatrogenic events are common in the elderly. The frail elderly person is at particular risk for adverse effects during medical care since protective reserve capacities in organ functioning may be greatly diminished. These factors may have far-reaching impact on an older person's ability to participate fully in the rehabilitation process. While the frail elderly will often be able to maximize rehabilitation potential, it may be at a slower rate over a longer period of time while experiencing more plateaus in the improvement process than will a younger adult. This time factor, in addition to health care reimbursement policies, can disadvantage the elderly adult who may not have rehabilitation coverage for a time period necessary to reach optimal recovery.

The incorporation of the team approach to care is another important consideration in community-based rehabilitation. Utilization of well-trained allied health professionals, nursing staff, and aides is critical to delivery of high quality community rehabilitation services. The physician may have a more remote role in some community-based programs, such as home health, compared to inpatient programs. Typically, the greater the distance the care delivery site is from the medical center setting, the less the physician provides hands-on care. The physician develops and manages the care plan and evaluates the patient at appropriate intervals. The team, usually via the nurse, keeps the physician informed. (Refer to Chapter 37)

In general, there is an acute shortage of all types of rehabilitation team professionals for both inpatient and community-based programs (2). The practical results of these personnel shortages are larger caseloads, vacant positions, and lengthy recruitment efforts. The staff shortages are even more critical in rural areas (3).

Most nursing and allied health professionals have had limited academic exposure to concepts and clinical issues of geriatric medicine. There are gerontologic nurse practitioner programs and a new added qualifications exam for physical therapists, but currently there are relatively few members of the rehabilitation team who have received special training in geriatric medicine.

The focus and expertise of the geriatric rehabilitation team is different, by necessity, from other types of specialized therapists and nursing professionals. One would not expect the same results in working with sports medicine physical therapists or occupational therapists with a special interest in hand therapy. The health care team must have a strong interest and concern for helping the elderly patient improve or maintain function. The team must recognize the frailty of the older person; common conditions such as hearing impairment often hinder the older person's ability to work with the rehabilitation team members. Informal care providers are a tremendous resource for the rehabilitation team working with the elderly. They often become ad hoc team members, providing key assistance in implementing the care plan. (Refer to Chapter 37)

A PUBLIC HEALTH ANALYSIS OF COMMUNITY-BASED REHABILITATION PROGRAMS

Home-Based Geriatric Rehabilitation Programs

Home-based rehabilitation is defined as a service or set of services dispensed in the home, determined by comprehensive assessment, with the goal of improving the function or well-being of the patient and caregiver (4).

ACCESS TO SERVICES

Over the past decade, home-delivered medical and social services have been expanding in recognition of perceived cost savings as well as need. Increased demand for home health services has been driven by earlier hospital discharges due to the prospective payment system. Improvements in transportable technology have also increased the type and range of home health services. However, highly technical, labor-intensive services delivered in the home are not cost-effective compared to delivery of these same types of services in an institution, such as an inpatient unit (5).

All communities, large and small, have access to some combination of home health rehabilitation services. In rural communities, the services available may be limited in scope and number, with possibly one agency administered by the local county health department delivering services countywide.

An advantage to these potential limitations appears to be in the coordination of services. The "one-stop shop" approach of the umbrella agency reduces the potential for communication problems and interagency gaps in services. Often in rural areas, the same staff perform multiple functions within their agency. Staff turnover often does not occur at the same rate as in urban settings. This provides staff continuity, both with patients as well as in team relationships within the agency and related institutions in the geographic area.

While it is probable that the quality of personal contact and coordination of services is as good, if not better, than those generally delivered in urban areas, the rural service setting has some definite drawbacks. One limitation is the actual types of services available. Since the technology and additional training for therapists may have high costs, a minimum number of patients are needed to warrant the expense (4). The number of patients available in a rural catchment area may not provide the economic incentive for initiation of important

therapy programs or the income to sustain the services once initiated.

Another limitation in rural areas is a result of staffing patterns and personnel issues. Staff may be required to cover wide geographic areas. The quality of training of rural-based home health service professionals meets minimum licensure requirements, but may not be comparable to urban areas where job selection and pay are more attractive (6). Due to limited numbers of therapists, there may be no opportunity for patients to switch if a patient receives inferior services from a particular therapist, even if the patient or family complains to the agency. We are not aware of studies of the quality of care or patient outcomes of urban versus rural service delivery.

Payment for home health rehabilitation services is accomplished by a combination of public and private sources. Public funding for home care services is provided primarily by Medicare, with substantial limitations. Medicare provides skilled home care, primarily targeted for limited services postacute illness. These Medicare-funded services include skilled nursing services, rehabilitation therapists' services, and home health aides. Agencies contend with burdensome paperwork necessary to document the services provided and the Medicare accepted rationales for service; however, they often receive claim denials for services long-since delivered to their clients.

The Medicare policy approach is too limited, both in scope and length of services. Rehabilitation service programs are designed to address functional limitations that are the residual of acute illness. The individualized care plan is formulated with the impairments, resources, and reasonable achievement goals established with patient and family input. The service package is functionally specific. Services are discontinued when the patient no longer shows improvement.

The curative focus of Medicare funding falls short of providing adequate care to the chronically ill. This statement is universally accepted by geriatric health policy specialists. Such disservice is strikingly clear in addressing the issues of a maintenance level service provision to protect and sustain the functional gains achieved during the rehabilitation phase of chronic illness. The perversity of the present reimbursement system is that, once improvement plateaus, a new exacerbation of the condition, a new "acute" event, is required for services to be covered. The new event may have been avoided, thousands of dollars saved, and human trauma alleviated if maintenance services had been in place.

The role of the private community physician as a monitor of functional status is important in this setting. However, the private physician's potential to protect is also held in check by the same acute-care focus of the major funding source. Lack of clinical training in both rehabilitation and geriatric medicine, ageism, and lack of awareness of reimbursable services hinder the primary care physician in this important role.

In addition to Medicare service provision, home rehabilitative services are also publicly funded by Medicaid for the "categorically needy," recipients of Supplemental Security Income (SSI) for the aged, blind, and disabled. According to Rowland and Lyons (7), the disabled elderly are more likely than the nondisabled elderly population to receive Medicaid benefits, with about 30% of them receiving such assistance. Forty states have opted to extend Medicaid coverage to the "medically needy," providing additional services such as physical therapy (PT), occupational therapy (OT), speech pathology, and audiology (8). The Medicaid waiver program was introduced in 1981 in an effort to reduce institutional long-term care costs by shifting the site of care to the home. Title XX of the Social Security Act and Title III of the Older Americans Act both provide adjunctive support services, such as home-delivered meals, personal care, and homemaker assistance (9). The Department of Veterans Affairs furnishes eligible veterans the Home Based Health Care (HBHC) program, which has similar service coverage as Medicare but can be provided for longer periods of time (8).

Given the range of public support, it is surprising to note that all public funding accounts for only one third of the payments for all home health services and community-based services (8). The public sources for home rehabilitation services are augmented by private funds, both in the form of private insurance coverage and out-of-pocket expenses. With few exceptions, private insurance coverage mirrors Medicare coverage, with the emphasis on skilled care in response to acute medical problems. Personal care and attendant and homemaker services are usually provided as informal care by spouses and other family members. Personal assistance, provided informally, supplements required skilled rehabilitative services.

The limiting factors in provision of informal services are availability and task burden. Personal care services are more often purchased by those disabled elderly who live alone or are more severely disabled and do not have adequate family resources. Only 20% of elderly with two to three ADL limitations purchase such services, compared to almost 40% of those elderly with limitations in four to five ADLs (10). These services usually are not reimbursable through either public or private insurance and therefore are paid directly by the elderly or their families. Accordingly, access to this type of rehabilitation support is limited by income availability. There are striking racial differences in utilization of formal home services, with whites more often purchasing services than other races. While minority aging health services research is in its infancy, the various utilization patterns most likely represent a combination of cultural preferences, differences in family availability due to living situations, and lower incomes resulting in reduced purchasing power.

ACCEPTABILITY

Home health rehabilitation services are convenient and provide assistance to the disabled older adult with residual impairments. A major advantage of the home setting is the ability for the professional team to recommend environmental supports to compensate for ADL limitations. In the initial home assessment, the team considers environmental adaptations, such as grab bars, ramps, or bathroom fixtures, that can provide day-to-day assistance. These home adaptation devices are utilized in addition to the biomechanical assistive equipment and strengthening exercises provided by the therapists.

Services provided in the home setting are generally acceptable to the disabled elderly and their families. Most importantly, there are no transportation problems. Some elderly may not be comfortable having people in their home; they may find the treatment protocols too strenuous, or they may not like a particular therapist or aide. However, the major problem is that the therapy benefits may be too short or too limited.

APPROPRIATENESS

Targeting patients for home-based rehabilitation programs has been identified as a key factor in providing suitable and effective services. Appropriate targeting includes not only the opportunity for medical management, but also adequate cooperative support resources provided by family or paid caregivers. A primary patient group for home rehabilitation is one that will benefit from continued care in the home setting as a transition upon discharge from acute rehabilitation programs or the hospital. Since the "three-hour rule" for reimbursable therapy sessions does not hold true for home rehabilitation, it may be most appropriate for elderly who do not have the stamina for the rigor of inpatient services (11).

A second group is the frail elderly whose functional level will deteriorate if such services are not utilized. In this category, rehabilitation is actually being used as a preventive health service. Unique to geriatrics, this application embraces the restorative functions of traditional rehabilitative services to protect from serious illness or delay inevitable functional decline. For example, the physician can identify the condition and recommend physical therapy or review of medications, thereby avoiding a fall and possible hip fracture.

ROLE OF THE COMMUNITY PHYSICIAN

The primary care physician is usually the only person with ongoing long-term contact in the position of monitoring patient status and ordering the needed services. It is virtually unknown how many primary care physicians make such referrals or whether the referrals are driven by patient and family problem identification or by the physicians' own evaluation methods. It is probably rare in either case; the problem is usually identified after the acute event.

Bannerman (12) has identified three critical roles for the physician in private practice. The first relates to referral for rehabilitation for a precipitous decline in function resulting from an acute event such as a stroke or hip fracture. The second type of referral is required posthospitalization for any condition due to reduced stamina and functional decline as a result of the illness and the iatrogenic consequences of bedrest. The third situation that requires referral is the gradual decline of the community-dwelling older person. This effort must be focused at the older adult in a maintenance phase postformal rehabilitation services, as well as at the older community resident who has not previously received rehabilitation services.

The primary care physician is hampered in fulfilling the prevention role by both medical training and the reimbursement system. Since rehabilitative and geriatric medicine content, philosophy, and clinical training are the exception rather than the rule in medical school curricula, many physicians who provide care to the elderly do not possess this specialized knowledge. The core of this knowledge is the functional approach to care rather than the curative focus of modern medicine. Currently, about 4,200 internal medicine and family practice physicians hold the certificate for added qualifications in geriatric medicine. Physicians who specialize in rehabilitative medicine, physiatrists, number about 3,500. Of these, less than 150 physiatrists specialize in geriatric care.

Since there are not adequate numbers of practicing geriatricians to provide total care to the current or future older populations, efforts have focused on these physicians serving in a consultative role to practicing physicians. Current research aimed at influencing primary care provider behavior has focused on the preventative or monitoring role in the care of the older person. In one study, older adults attended a health fair at which they received a comprehensive medical and social screening by a multidisciplinary geriatric specialist team. Care recommendations identified were communicated to both the senior and the primary care physician for follow-up. These physicians were later contacted on the disposition of the recommendations. It was found that many simply had not been acted upon. A special review of the factors contributing to the inaction on physical therapy recommendations revealed that the physicians receiving the referrals did not understand the following: what physical therapy referrals were being ordered, the reimbursement potential to them for ordering the services, and the potential benefit to their patients for this service (A. Mayer-Oakes,. personal communication, 1992).

A second study, in progress, is identifying factors that influence physician's implementation of geriatric assessment recommendations on four target conditions: falls, urinary incontinence, depression, and functional decline. The recommendations as they relate to falls and functional impairment have particular relevance to community-based rehabilitation. After a comprehensive screening and assessment, recommendations are given both to the patient and the primary physician. The goals of the study are to identify factors that impede the physician's implementation as well as the patient's follow-through. This type of research provides a more thorough understanding of physician-patient behaviors (13).

EVALUATION RESEARCH

Rehabilitation services delivered in the home have been evaluated in a number of studies, with inconclusive results. Improved patient care outcomes have not been consistently identified as a goal. Approximately 30 clinical trials of home care have not actually investigated rehabilitative service programs. Various results have been shown in survival, improvement of ADLs, mental functioning, nursing home and hospital utilization, and service costs. Consistently positive results have been attained in improved life satisfaction and social interaction (8, 9, 14).

Day Care Programs

Day care programs have a range of models, varying from social to medical-rehabilitation. Common characteristics across models include ambulatory or wheelchair ambulator clients, group treatment settings, and drop-off clients, hence the borrowing of the term day care from the childcare arena. In recognition of the problems employees experience in both eldercare and childcare, some innovative businesses have developed combined programs offering services to both older family members and young children of employees.

ACCESS TO SERVICES

In general, day care programs tend to be located in large urban cities, nestled in health or social service agencies that offer a number of types of service delivery programs. In 1987, it was estimated that there were about 1,400 day care sites in the United States, representing a considerable increase from the 250 or so identified in 1978 (15). There can be much variation from one day care program to another. Day care programs do not offer a set service package, but represent different orientations and models, ranging from a psychosocial model to a medical-rehabilitation model (16). Transportation services are included in most program models, demonstrating a recognition of the mobility problems associated with the frail elderly.

The target population differs across program models; independent groups use the psychosocial model programs while the more frail elderly are involved in medical-rehabilitation models. The caregivers of dementia patients use day care programs as respite care or, literally, day care during work hours.

Private funding sources include client fees and private endowments to the centers. Public funding for day care programs is a state option. When selected for inclusion, funding is through the Social Security Act's Title XX for the social model programs and Title XIX (Medicaid) via the waiver option for the medical service model or the Older American's Act (15). Each model has conflicting legislative mandates directing the focus, service package, and personnel requirements. These regulatory restrictions create an artificial separation between the social service and medical-rehabilitative needs of the elderly patient—a major drawback in creating the holistic atmosphere required for geriatric rehabilitation (17).

ACCEPTABILITY

For those seniors who require medical-rehabilitative services but have limited informal family support, day care programs offer a viable community-based option. However, older adults attending day care programs due to cognitive impairments may not provide a good patient mix with others receiving rehabilitation for specific physical impairments. From a consumer viewpoint, there is not adequate information on patients' and families' satisfaction levels with geriatric rehabilitation services delivered via day care programs.

APPROPRIATENESS

The match between rehabilitation needs and program services is critical in the selection of a particular day care program. For those seniors who depend on employed caregivers, day care-based rehabilitation programs may be the only community-based alternative.

For a rehabilitative service to be identified as appropriate, it needs to meet the goals of maximizing the patient's functioning levels and improving the independent living skills, given any residual impairment. To date, there are no comparative studies of patient outcomes from day care programs compared to other types of community-based rehabilitation programs.

Outpatient Rehabilitation Clinics

Outpatient programs share similarity with day care-based programs in that patients come into the facility for treatment. Comprehensive outpatient rehabilitation addresses a range of patient needs with more extensive therapies and services available. Outpatient rehabilitation programs are often linked to a larger inpatient rehabilitation center or hospital, but can also be free-standing facilities in the community. The range of services available is vast, from highly specialized physical therapy to multiple services, often delivered in the team approach.

ACCESS TO SERVICES

Outpatient rehabilitation programs have increased in number over the past decade. According to annual surveys completed by the American Hospital Association, 46% of all hospitals in 1989 had organized outpatient programs, compared to 27% of hospitals in 1980 (2). In 1981, Medicare Part B payments, previously limited to hospital outpatient rehabilitation units, were extended to separate or free-standing outpatient rehabilitation facilities. The Omnibus Reconciliation Act of 1980 provided for a type of certification, the Comprehensive Outpatient Rehabilitation Facility (CORF), which extended these Medicare benefits to services received remote from the hospital. In 1991, there were 193 CORFs in the United States according to the Health Care Financing Administration (2). In 1987, Medicare initiated the coverage of similar skilled services received in non-CORF rehabilitation facilities although an annual reimbursement limit is placed on allied health services (18).

Free-standing rehabilitation outpatient programs are more available in urban settings. In rural areas, outpatient rehabilitation programs are located at regional medical centers or attached to separate rehabilitation inpatient hospitals. Rural outpatient programs, which cover a wide geographic catchment area, offer a range of basic therapeutic services. Specialized physical therapy private practice offices, available in urban areas, are virtually nonexistent in rural communities.

Transportation is the major access barrier for the elderly utilizing community-based services; the use of outpatient rehabilitation services is no exception. Rural communities serving wide regional areas often utilize shuttle vans for the rehabilitation patients. While these transportation services are valuable and essential in accessing service, additional costs are incurred in a variety of ways. Some are obvious; for example, additional time is required for pick-up and delivery routes. The extra physical exertion required for the travel to and from the service site may be overwhelming to the patient.

Outpatient rehabilitation services are funded primarily by Medicare. The skilled nature of services delivered to the constantly improving patient is the canon for reimbursement by Medicare. Covered services include medical/physician services; nursing services; allied health services, including PT, OT, speech therapy (ST), and recreational therapy (RT); psychosocial services; some medications and assistive devices; and only one home evaluation visit (18). Because of the strict review and frequent denial of reimbursement for services rendered, evaluation of rehabilitation potential is critical to program continuity. Often, referrals are made and patients accepted only when Medicare coverage is considered certain. We have discussed above the differences with which older adults present and the various types of needs that could be fulfilled if given the opportunity. The low-income medically indigent are limited in their ability to access outpatient rehabilitation services since Medicaid is not a primary funding source for such services in most states (2). Private insurance also covers outpatient rehabilitation services, subject to copayment and deductible policies of the plan. Health Maintenance Organizations (HMOs) may contract with outpatient rehabilitation programs if these services are not provided inhouse since HMOs generally attempt to contain costs by limiting expensive inpatient care whenever feasible.

ACCEPTABILITY

Like other forms of community-based rehabilitation, outpatient programs vary in goals, structure, and resources. If older adults are referred and accepted, they usually will be able to take advantage of a wide array of services as long as they have transportation. The menu of services is selected and coordinated specifically to meet the improvement goals identified for the individual patient. Patients who receive rehabilitation services in outpatient clinics may have been recently discharged from an inpatient rehabilitation setting. Outpatient services bridge the gap of services necessary to improve function once the patient is medically stabilized and no longer requires the 24-hour monitoring of the inpatient unit.

APPROPRIATENESS

Comprehensive rehabilitation outpatient clinics offer the widest array of services staffed by a team of allied health rehabilitation specialists and auxiliary health personnel available outside the inpatient unit. Since these team members deliver care under one roof, there are additional opportunities for team communication and service coordination that may not occur in home-delivered program offices. It is unknown whether differences in service delivery and relative costs result in patient outcomes such as improved functioning (19).

Evaluation of outcomes in all types of community-based rehabilitation presents difficult challenges to health services researchers. Kane and Kane (14) reviewed evidence of the effectiveness of community-based long-term care services, specifically home care and day care. Although differences between programs could obliterate any meaningful grouping for comparison purposes, meta-analysis evaluation questions improved patient outcomes and cost-effectiveness of all community-based rehabilitation-oriented long-term care programs. Whether this is due to true outcome deficits or exemplifies the difficulty in evaluation design of community-based programs is unknown. The common-sense notion

that these team-delivered services improve patient functioning has not yet been proven by research studies.

IS THERE AN 'OPTIMAL' SETTING FOR COMMUNITY-BASED GERIATRIC REHABILITATION?

It appears that the deeper the inquiry into programmatic differences of outpatient rehabilitation, the more elusive is the answer to the optimal setting or service package for delivery of geriatric rehabilitation. There are a number of principles that define the standards of outpatient geriatric rehabilitation programs.

The Team Principle

This hallmark in general rehabilitation is critical in the delivery of high quality geriatric rehabilitation services. The team members have important professional perspectives in addressing problems presented by the whole person. The concepts of interdisciplinary communication and coordination of services and resources are inherent in the team principle. Team members can be housed within the service agency or available on a contractual/consultative basis.

The Self-Determination Principle

Involvement of the elderly patient and family is an important factor in geriatric rehabilitation. The patient's perspective is crucial in selecting the type of outpatient rehabilitation service, determining appropriate rehabilitation goals, creating needed motivation, and protecting informal medical care and social support networks already in place. While this principle holds true for all age groups, the elderly person often has a very clear view of what factors are most important in recovery.

The Patient-Service Match Principle

Appropriate targeting of the patient for a particular service is a paramount consideration. This principle goes beyond assigning required types of therapies to meet patient goals; it includes matching the service delivery mode to the patient's needs and resources. For example, if the patient enjoys the stimulation of being with other people, an outpatient facility should be chosen over home therapy services if there is a choice. This principle has important limitations, which include rural differences in service availability and denial of service access due to reimbursement policies or income inadequacy, as well as minority and culturally-sensitive service availability.

The Cost-Effectiveness Principle

The cost-effectiveness studies undertaken to date have focused on comparing service costs across inpatient and outpatient settings. For example, the publicly-funded Medicaid waiver programs are designed to provide community-based services instead of those based in an institution, such as a nursing home. The problems with this approach are multiple, the greatest concern being the poorly funded nursing home care benefit to which home care programs are being compared. An additional fundamental concern is conceptual in nature; these types of services are not equal substitutes, but are sequential in nature, given the expected deterioration of functioning over time with multiple chronic illnesses.

Cost-effectiveness needs to be extended to include training of health professionals in principles of geriatric medicine, as well as in preventive approaches in geriatric care. We cannot afford to continue funding the aftermath of preventable problems. This focus also supports and maintains functional gains achieved in rehabilitation programs. The functional outcome approach of geriatric rehabilitation seeks to improve mobility, self-care behaviors in the basic ADLs, and instrumental activities of daily living (IADLs). Improved functioning in these levels is seen as beneficial in reducing illness and hospitalization episodes, in addition to mobilizing the patient's support systems.

The Principle of Proven Benefit

Evaluation research has failed to provide unequivocable data on the benefits of outpatient rehabilitation programs. Program effectiveness must be proven. Benjamin (20) calls for a four-part approach for future evaluation research, as briefly outlined below. While Benjamin's proposal addresses issues in home care evaluation, we have adapted his approach to outpatient geriatric rehabilitation programs.

• Reconceptualizing Effectiveness

By more clearly defining the objectives of the specific geriatric rehabilitation intervention and broadening our ideas about outcomes to include a range of patient and caregiver variables, we will identify realistic and comprehensive goals by which the program can be judged.

• Respecifying Populations

This approach calls for an examination of within group differences, which may have created spurious or suppressed program research results. It recognizes that service populations with varying needs and differences in potential benefits will likely alter the aggregated impact data gathered in intervention studies.

• Specifying Interventions

Fundamental to outcome evaluation, the specific components of service delivery must be clearly identified in operational terms. Combinations of services delivered must also be examined from an interactional viewpoint, recognizing that provision of one type of service may influence another.

• Understanding Care Settings

Different types of delivery sites, including the home, have a great deal of variation, which may be influencing evaluation research. It is important to take into account how care setting characteristics hinder or facilitate geriatric rehabilitation programs.

SUMMARY

By incorporating the above approaches into future evaluation research on geriatric rehabilitation programs and health services research in general, we will be able to more clearly examine whether programs are achieving reasonable outcomes and meeting stated goals. We are constantly under scrutiny to provide care of high quality with fewer and fewer resources at hand. The functional and restorative approach to care may be built into primary patient care practices, utilizing geriatric rehabilitation principles. This integration would address staff shortages, lack of appropriate referrals, care plan support, and improve the geriatric prevention concepts of care. With increasing numbers of older adults in our future, we must provide adequate geriatric rehabilitation services.

References

1. Coogler C. Geriatric rehabilitation. In: Fletcher G, Banja J, Jann B, Wolf S, eds., *Rehabilitation Medicine.* Philadelphia, Pa: Lea & Febiger: 1992:299–312.
2. Sliwa J, ed. *Outpatient Rehabilitation Services.* Chicago, Ill: American Hospital Publishing; 1991.
3. Moser E. The special needs of the rural client. *Caring.* February: 18–20, 1992.
4. Keenan JM. In-home geriatric rehabilitation. In: Kemp B, Brummel-Smith K, Ramsdell J, eds. *Geriatric Rehabilitation.* Boston, Mass: Little, Brown; 1990:357–370.
5. Weissert WG. Seven reasons why it is so difficult to make community-based long-term care cost effective. *Health Serv Res.* 20:423–433, 1985.
6. Berke D. Delivering home care in rural areas: results of a nationwide survey. *Caring:* February: 4–7, 1992.
7. Rowland D, Lyons B. The elderly population in need of home care. In: Rowland D, Lyons B, eds. *Financing Home Care.* Baltimore, Md: The Johns Hopkins University Press; 1991:3–26.
8. Wieland D, Ferrell B, Rubenstein LZ. Geriatric home health care. In: *Clinics in Geriatric Medicine,* VII. Philadelphia, Pa: W.B. Saunders; 1991:645–663.
9. Rubenstein LZ, Kaiser F. Functional limitations and home care requirements. In: Rowland D, Lyons B, eds. Baltimore, Md: Johns Hopkins University Press; 1991:87–103.
10. Lewin/ICF, Inc. and Brookings Institution. *The Estimated Cost of a Proposed Home Care Program,* Background paper 16. Baltimore, Md: Commonwealth Fund Commission on Elderly People Living Alone; 1989.
11. Johnston M, Miller L. Cost-effectiveness of the medicare three-hour regulation. *Arch Phys Med Rehabil.* 67:581, 1986.
12. Bannerman C. Rehabilitation in private practice. In: Kemp B,

Brummel-Smith K, Ramsdell J, eds. *Geriatric Rehabilitation*. Boston, Mass: Little, Brown; 1990:339–346.

13. Reuben DS, Hirsch J, Chernoff Y, et al. An outreach program to address the health needs of a low-income frail, elderly population: project safety net. *Gerontologist*. In press.

14. Kane RL, Kane RA. *Long-Term Care: Principles, Programs and Policies*. New York, NY: Springer; 1987.

15. Haber D. *Health Care for an Aging Society: Cost-Conscious Community Care and Self-Care Approaches*. New York, NY: Hemisphere Publishing Corporation; 1989.

16. O'Brien C. *Adult Day Care: A Practical Guide*. Monterey, Calif: Wadsworth Health Sciences Division; 1982.

17. Brody S. Impact of the formal support system on rehabilitation of the elderly. In: Brody S, Ruff G, eds. *Aging and Rehabilitation*. New York, NY: Springer; 1986.

18. Ratner D, Strum J. Reimbursement and Financial Management. In: *Outpatient Rehabilitation Services*. Chicago, Ill: *American Hospital Publishing*; 1991.

19. Keith R. The comprehensive treatment team in rehabilitation. *Arch Phys Med Rehabil*. 72:269–274, 1991.

20. Benjamin AE. An overview of in-home health and supportive services for older persons. In: Ory M, Duncker A, eds. *In-Home Care for Older People*. Newbury Park, Calif: Sage Publications; 1992.

41

Protecting the Employability of the Working Elderly

Donald E. Shrey and Norman C. Hursh

The escalating number of older workers in the work force signals a clear need for industry to examine the relationship between the aging process, disability incidence, productivity, and health care costs. While demographic trends of the aging population are well documented, the impact of an aging work force on business and industry is highly complex and far less understood. Older workers represent the fastest growing segment of the nation's work force. With fewer individuals entering the work force over the next decade, older workers represent a potentially valuable resource in an expanding economy. However, the aging process is often accompanied by functional losses and increasing incidence of impairment and disability that result in work disruption, loss of productivity, and escalating health care costs.

This chapter will discuss the following questions related to the older worker who experiences an impairment or disability:

- How is the work potential of older workers impacted by aging, impairment, and disability?
- How can industry reduce the personal and economic costs of work-related injury and disability?
- What are the disability management interventions available to industry to reduce work disruption, sustain productivity, and enhance quality of work life for older workers with injury or disability?

THE AGING WORKER: DEMOGRAPHICS AND STATISTICS

Older individuals represent the fastest growing segment of the general population and the work force. In 1984, there were 28 million elderly in the United States, representing 12% of the population. Older individuals are expected to comprise 13% of the US population by the year 2000 and 21% of the population by 2030, including over 51 million people (1). This dramatic increase is a result of several factors, including increased life expectancy, an aging baby boom population, improved medical care available to increasing numbers of people, and an increased adherence to fitness and healthy life-styles.

While the number of individuals entering the work force is decreasing due to a lower birth rate, the number of older workers in the work force, proportionately, is increasing. Between the years 1982 and 2000, the number of workers between 18 and 34 years of age will decrease 12%. However, the number of individuals between 35 and 54 years of age will increase 53% (2). The significance for industry is that a projected economic expansion will result in 16 million new jobs by the year 2000, with older workers representing a valuable labor pool resource.

The correlation between aging and disability prevalence is significantly high (3). Older individuals have a disability rate eight times that of individuals under 45 years of age (4). In addition, the older person is more likely to experience multiple and chronic impairments, as well as a higher degree of disability (5). The annual number of days of restricted activity due to illness increases from 16 for individuals between 25 and 44 years of age, to 26 for individuals between 45 and 64 years of age. In addition, 35% of older workers have a disability serious enough to limit working, housework, or involvement in a major life activity (5).

An aging work force is one that has increased impairment and disability incidence. Two-thirds of individuals with work disability are over 40 years of age (6). The frequency and rate of secondary work limitations, occupational disability, and total disability are greater after 55 years of age than for any other work group (7). This has significant implications for employers concerned with work disruption and productivity loss, health care utilization and cost containment, and escalating worker compensation costs (8).

Illnesses and disabilities with the greatest impact on work and day-to-day functioning are chronic disabilities, which include hypertension, hearing and visual impairment, heart disease, diabetes, and arteriosclerosis (9). Aging is also accompanied by increases in progressive and cumulative disability, such as degenerative disc disease, carpal tunnel disorders, and arthritis. Cumulative trauma disorders impact work through fluctuating and cyclical periods of work disruption and progressively greater use of sick time and other health care benefit utilization.

The aging process of older workers is also associated with physical, emotional, and sensory developmental losses in areas such as memory, judgment, reaction time, and intellectual or cognitive ability. The functional losses experienced by older persons are typically viewed as an accepted and expected part of aging. The reality is that developmental losses are highly selective, variable, and gradual across individuals and the aging process itself. Jobs requiring physical strength, endurance, and rapid work pace realize the greatest decline in performance with aging (9). However, physical effort, ability, and performance, even across age groups, are highly individualized factors. Additionally, the impact of functional losses for the older worker is dependent on the work activity of the individual. Management, service, or information technology positions are less affected by developmental loss or physical decline than are jobs that are physically labor intensive.

Older workers are often viewed as more accident prone and susceptible to injury. While accidents, injury, and acute impairments are often associated with the aging process, they actually decrease with age (9, 10). Hester (11) found that injuries account for 35% of disabilities between 45 and 54 years of age but only 20% of disabilities between 55 and 64 years. More important to employers and industry is that older workers are less resilient, take longer to recuperate, and, therefore, experience longer periods of work disruption when injured or disabled. For the employer, older worker injury and impairment results in loss of productivity, uncertainty about worker availability, potential for extended leave, and costs associated with recruiting, selecting, hiring, and supervising new workers.

Older workers and individuals with a disability are often conceptualized as the "aged" or the "disabled" and viewed as a homogeneous group with similar and stereotypical characteristics (12). The older worker is portrayed as having reduced reaction time, slower in learning new tasks or keeping up with technologic advances, unable to adjust, reacting poorly to stress, and losing memory, intelligence, and so forth. In reality, older workers, as well as the elderly in general, are a very heterogeneous group (1). The functional losses associated with aging are highly variable in terms of individual performance differences, and, for many, functional abilities may be as well maintained as in younger workers (13).

Losses and impairment do occur with increasing incidence, but develop over a span of time. The variability between individuals actually increases with age (12). The heterogeneity of the aging work force dictates that assessment and development of vocational potential be individualized to best determine how available work return options and health care resources may be tailored to the individual.

CURRENT ISSUES

Disability Costs

Management of escalating health care costs is becoming an increasing concern for all employers. Older workers represent a segment of the work force with escalating health care cost liability due to the higher incidence of illness and chronic disability. It is estimated that between $98 billion and $362 billion are spent annually on overall health care services, with 50% spent on older individuals (14, 15).

Work-related injuries related to the aging process, including cumulative trauma disorders, represent a large percentage of medical claims. For example, degenerative disc disease, common in individuals between 40 and 60 years of age, costs industry between $10 billion and $14 billion annually in lost production, employee turnover, and medical reimbursement (16). The average cost of a worker's compensation claim rose from $8,811 in 1988 to $9,225 in 1989 (*The Wall Street Journal*. July 16, 1990:B1, B3.)

Once out of work due to injury or illness, older workers stay out longer than younger workers (17) and develop increased dependence on public and private health care systems. If they receive income maintenance benefits such as Social Security Disability Insurance (SSDI) or Long Term Disability (LTD), there is little financial incentive to return to work. Studies consistently document that less than 1% of individuals receiving SSDI benefits return to work and leave the benefit roles. Reliance on income transfer benefit systems such as SSDI or LTD is very costly, with approximately $22.7 billion in 1989 and $24 billion in 1990 paid in SSDI benefits alone (18).

With increasing numbers of older workers with disability or impairment, demand on both income and medical benefit programs such as SSDI, LTD, Medicare, and Medicaid will increase sharply. As the work force ages, it becomes imperative to manage rapidly escalating costs (14).

Economic and Employment Market Characteristics

Between 1988 and 2000, the US economy is expected to grow by 30%. While this statistic represents continued economic growth, trends are not as dynamic as in previous decades. During this time, the labor force is experiencing lower retirement ages among workers, fewer people entering the work force, and a greater proportion of older individuals in the work force.

Over the next decade, the labor market will experience greater changes from a strong manufacturing and industrial market to a service and information technology market (19). It is projected that by the year 2000, the service field will provide 90% of all new jobs, with business service and health service industries accounting for the greatest increase in countable jobs (20).

A shift to service industries will reduce the need for workers to be involved in work that has a high physical demand and a corresponding high risk for injury and cumulative trauma. The emphasis and expansion in the service and information technology area will require a work force armed with a range of new skills and specialized abilities. Workers must take advantage of training and retraining opportunities to remain marketable to employers. This presents a challenge to older workers who are often reluctant to participate in retraining or who view themselves as unable to profit from training. The challenge, however, is placed equally on the employer to orient workers to the economic changes and to identify training and retraining methods responsive to the workers' learning styles, while providing incentives for workers to take advantage of the training opportunities.

Technologic Impact

The economy is also shaped by rapid technologic developments. For the older worker, technology represents both challenge and opportunity. Technologic applications rapidly displace old jobs with new ones, with skill obsolescence occurring as jobs become outdated. Older workers must be receptive to exploring how their skills transfer to new jobs and how to utilize existing training resources to keep pace with technologic advances.

Technology also creates opportunities for individuals who experience impairment or decline in functional capacities. Jobs and work sites can be "engineered" to reduce ergonomic barriers to performance or modified to accommodate functional deficits. Technology has developed assistive devices that accommodate disability and augment functional abilities. Examples include adapted computer keyboards to accommodate physical disabilities and enhanced keyboards for data entry personnel to prevent carpal tunnel syndrome.

Older workers with impairments and disabilities will need to be flexible in adapting to new jobs and retraining and receptive to technologic accommodations that enhance performance and promote work retention. As the need for workers increases, it will become more feasible for employers to retrain older workers who are physically unable to perform former jobs. Employers must

integrate reasonable accommodations, work retention planning, and training and retraining as the normal course of doing business.

Vocational Rehabilitation Practice

The philosophy of rehabilitation is congruent with the needs of older workers with disabilities. Unfortunately, the practice of rehabilitation has not been responsive to the need (12). Persons over 45 years of age represent only 23% of state vocational rehabilitation caseloads, compared to 50% to 60% of the population with impairments (2, 10). Vocational rehabilitation services for elderly disabled persons are presently limited or nonexistent (21), and older workers (over 45 years of age) with a disability have not been served when otherwise eligible. Sax and Bauman (3) site the lack of adequate information about aging and disability available to vocational rehabilitation counselors and incorrect conclusions about work capacity and potential for employment as critical deterrents for vocational rehabilitation's involvement with older workers. Rehabilitation and health care professionals categorically accept functional loss, physical decline, injury, and dependence as part of the aging process.

Older workers with disabilities represent a group for whom disability is a common experience and for whom services are least provided (6). It is obvious that clarification is needed with respect to the roles, responsibilities, and policies of vocational rehabilitation, health care systems, and labor and industry. Rehabilitation services for disabled and impaired workers appear to be cost-effective over time, and employers should view rehabilitation as a viable cost containment effort with older workers (22).

ATTITUDINAL BARRIERS TO WORK RETENTION

Although chronic disability, cumulative trauma, and developmental losses result in work disruption and jeopardize ongoing employability for older workers, there are several barriers that play a far more significant role in successful and sustained work performance for older workers with impairments or disability. These barriers include stereotypical attitudes about the older person, public policy decisions that reflect disincentives for the individual to attempt work, and barriers in the work environment itself.

Employer Attitudes

The attitude of employers, health care professionals, and the older worker toward aging and disability is the most significant and pervasive barrier. Older workers face systematic stereotyping and discrimination based solely on chronologic age, a bias identified as ageism (23). Ageism is not a benign or static concept, but an active and instrumental belief system that impacts social interaction, employment practice, health care management, and public policy (24).

Employer attitudes toward the older worker affect hiring and promotion decisions as well as efforts to develop realistic work return options when faced with progressive disabilities. Employers view the older worker with a disability as less capable, inflexible, unwilling to be retrained, lacking physical skills, and as a factor contributing to increased health care costs (14). Decisions about hiring older workers are based on judgments about productivity, injury risk, adaptability, potential health care and insurance costs, memory and judgment, and age-related employment costs (5, 22). Additionally, when an individual is considered for employment, employers often view the older worker as having fewer years of future employment and, subsequently, of less worth to the company (14).

Bauman (2) reported findings of an employment age discrimination study, which indicated that eight of 10 Americans believe most employers discriminate against the older worker. Six of 10 employers believe older workers are discriminated against in the work force. Age discrimination was found to be the most frequently cited case brought to the Equal Employment Opportunity Commission (EEOC) Board (2).

Attitudes of Health Care Professionals

Ageism is particularly limiting when it affects the level and type of services offered by rehabilitation professionals, health care providers, and health benefit systems. Although rehabilitation philosophy is well suited to working with the older person with a disability, vocational rehabilitation counselors demonstrate a high degree of age bias and tend to view older persons more negatively than younger individuals (10, 23). Younger persons are viewed as more likely to have significant years of work life ahead of them; older individuals are faced with increasing functional loss, illness, and withdrawal from vocationally productive activity (23). The potential for return to normalcy, independence, and self-sufficiency for an older worker with an impairment is considered unlikely. Moreover, it is viewed as acceptable and expected that the older person will have an inability to perform up to previous standards or levels of functioning after rehabilitation (5).

When the functional disability or impairment that is present in older workers requires a work site modification or negotiations with union and management representatives, counselors often resist contacting employers to develop labor/employer relationships (25). The full range of vocational rehabilitation services is not made available to the older worker who may desire to continue work.

Attitudes of Older Workers with a Disability

The relevance of negative attitudes, stereotypes, and ageism among medical and rehabilitation professionals and society as a whole is that these attitudes and values are then transmitted to the older worker (23). Older workers, in turn, internalize the negative social judgments and conclusions about their own worth, productivity, and potential (5) and develop a lower self-concept. They may perceive their role as a worker as being incapable, unproductive, and less desirable.

Older persons with impairments or disabilities are often placed in "double jeopardy" according to Rubenfeld (26) since they are faced with multiple stereotypes. There is a similarity of attitude toward individuals who age and those who have a disability. Each group is seen as dependent, having problems with coping, and unable to adjust. The impaired aged are seen as sick, ill, or disabled. The stereotypes associated with aging are compounded by the experience of a disability. The perception of illness further restricts employment practice and health care efforts (22).

In effect, attitudinal barriers become more overwhelming and restricting than developmental losses and chronic and progressive impairments experienced by the older worker. Ageism masks the reality that a wide range of individual differences exist and that the older worker with an impairment experiences adaptive skills as well as losses. It further conceals the fact that the worker requires individual planning skills if capacities and potentials are to be maximized (27).

Despite the social implications of disability, many older workers who experience functional loss, cumulative trauma, or injury want to work. Work serves an important economic, social, and psychologic function at a time in life when the individual experiences other losses.

Lower expectations about adaptive capabilities, level of functioning, and future potential are instrumental in shaping health benefit structure and health care system response: the response to the older worker with an injury or impairment is viewed in medical and economic terms rather than through rehabilitation or disability management efforts. Societal response to the elderly has been a result of ageism: provide social security, medical insurance, income maintenance, and support, rather than rehabilitation needed to promote independence, productivity, and self-sufficiency.

DISABILITY MANAGEMENT PROGRAMS IN INDUSTRY

As individuals live and work longer, the health care problems associated with aging are expected to increase (13). Because business and industry will rely on older workers to fill new jobs, they must recognize and take responsibility for the disability, impairment, and performance characteristics that accompany aging. Several employers have developed responsive programs that utilize the potential that the older worker brings to the work force and that must be considered as the individual works and ages.

Recent literature has described several creative work retention programs for older workers. Coberly (28) described industrial policy and programs that emphasize work retention up to and beyond normal retirement age as alternatives to lay-offs and costly early retirement incentives. Atlantic Richfield and Northern Natural Gas Company utilize job-sharing and part-time work variations, where two workers may share the same job or have specified responsibilities for half a job. This allows a person to make the transition to fewer hours while retaining benefits and continuing contributions to the pension fund and, therefore, the tax base.

Several companies have formal or informal programs directly responsive to injury or disability through job modification, job transfer, or retraining programs as alternatives to disability retirement (3, 28). The US Postal Service was able to return workers to modified jobs despite the fact that they had retired on disability. Stouffers, General Dynamics, and Xerox, recognizing the high physical demand impact of certain work activities, have formal programs of evaluation and job transfer of older workers to less physically demanding jobs. Such programs reduce the impact of injury, prolong the working life of the employee, and continue worker productivity in a position commensurate with functional abilities (3). Similarly, General Electric found it cost-effective to retrain older workers whose skills had become obsolete through technologic advances rather than hire and retrain younger workers (3).

While the programs and policies cited above respond to the aging worker in general, there are also more comprehensive disability management programs in industry that respond to injury, disability, and illness on the job.

Disability management programs in industry represent a proactive, comprehensive, and multidisciplinary approach to resolving work disability and subsequent costs. They often include prevention, rehabilitation, and treatment interventions to control personal and economic costs of injury and disability. Employer control and responsibility in the planning and coordination of interventions and services seems to be the key to successful disability management programs. Model disability management programs have been implemented in such industries as 3M (29), Kimberly-Clark Corporation, Control Data Corporation, and Volvo Corporation (30). Shrey (31–34) described the coordinated and structured methods for controlling worker injury and reducing work disruption through use of prevention, education, labor and management collaboration, early return-to-work planning, and related processes. Significant cost savings

have been reported in studies by Sears Roebuck and Company, Aluminum Company of America (ALCOA), and E.I. duPont (35).

Industry-based disability management programs have the capacity to assess individual vocational potential and design work return programs to maximize functional abilities (31). The increasing numbers of older workers experiencing chronic and progressive disability are often denied the benefits of such programs. As a result, many will never attain their employment potential.

Disability Management: Strategies and Interventions

A variety of strategies, programs, and interventions exist for reducing the impact of disability on the older worker's capacity to perform work. The primary components of a disability management system discussed in this section include the following: Disability Case Management, Medical Management, Disability Resolution Process, Rehabilitation Plan Development, and Work Return Transition/Worker Retention Programs. These primary program components are highly relevant to a multidisciplinary service systems concept, targeting employer obligations under the Americans with Disabilities Act (ADA).

DISABILITY CASE MANAGEMENT

Assessment, as a generic process, has traditionally been used with older individuals as a diagnostic tool to identify the presence and extent of a disability. There has been little recognition and less application of assessment methods in prevention, planning, and rehabilitation of older workers who experience functional loss, cumulative or progressive disability, or acute traumatic injury. Medical and health care planners are often unaware of the multiple evaluation functions that can assist older workers, and subsequently, assessment has been more a medical intervention than an ongoing rehabilitation option.

To be effective in evaluating older workers, assessment must recognize that work disruption or declining productivity is a function of the kinds of work performed, the characteristics of the work setting, and the changing functional abilities of the worker. There are several assessment strategies that can be used instrumentally with older workers to enhance vocational potential. These methods include transferability of skills analysis, work site risk analysis, and vocational evaluation.

Transferable Skill Analysis

The analysis of transferable skills is a formal process that considers the individual's education and work experience to identify a range of jobs in which same or lesser skills are required; similar tools, equipment, or machinery are used; and the same materials, procedures, subject matter, or services are involved. The objective of a transferable skills analysis is to identify jobs that are compatible with the individual's present or expected functional capacity.

For many older workers there is gradual loss of specific functional abilities due to functional loss or cumulative trauma that is experienced over an extended period of time. Analysis of transferable skills during this time can identify performance abilities not affected by impairment. The skill transfer analysis process will specify skills, knowledge, and abilities that may transfer to jobs and job tasks, equipment, machines, or work fields that are within the individual's residual functional capacity.

Assessment of transferable skills is also important when technologic change or a changing labor market results in job skills or entire jobs becoming obsolete. The prospect of change or participating in retraining can be traumatic for the older worker who may have little confidence in his or her ability to learn or profit from retraining. Analysis of transferable skills facilitates the older worker's smooth transition to related jobs, demonstrates that older individuals may presently be able to perform the essential job tasks within the new job, and utilizes the retraining approach that complements the individual's preferred learning style.

Work Site Risk Analysis

In addition to evaluating worker skills, information about the job and work site must be analyzed. Using job and task analysis and ergonomic evaluation techniques, work site risk analysis assesses the degree of compatibility between the job activities and work environment demands and the individual's functional capacities.

Ergonomic evaluation examines the motion, movement, body mechanics, and effort requirements involved in the use of tools, equipment, and machinery within the specific work setting. Job analysis is a more comprehensive description of the job activities, including functions, methods, techniques, and procedures used in performing the job; the worker characteristics such as skills, knowledge, and abilities needed; and a description of the results of the work effort in terms of goods, service, or products.

The goal of work site risk analysis is to identify and reduce or remove elements that constitute work hazards for the worker. The analysis includes recommendations regarding job accommodations and job or work site modifications or adaptations to machines or tools. Work site risk analysis also delineates the use of assistive or augmentative devices to enhance productivity and includes recommendations for technologic mod-

ifications required to substitute mechanical or electronic adaptations for physical effort requirements of the job.

Little consideration is given to the reasonable accommodations that can be made to respond to the older worker's impairment. Employers often view accommodations or modifications as too expensive (14) although studies have demonstrated that over 50% of accommodations cost under $100. Technology is available to provide assistive and augmentative devices, modify job and work site equipment, and adapt work site barriers to accommodate declining abilities. However, existing technology to respond to work disruption related to disability and impairment has not been systematically applied in industry.

Vocational Evaluation

Vocational evaluation is a comprehensive, systematic process designed to identify and explore vocational alternatives and maximize the vocational potential of the individual. For the older worker with a disability, vocational evaluation provides multiple functions as outlined in Figure 41.1.

Vocational evaluation is particularly useful for the older worker who may experience a period of work disruption due to injury and discovers that their previous job becomes unavailable or unrealistic. Other workers may benefit from vocational evaluation when productivity is decreasing and accommodations, job transfer, or other adjustments are needed. The function of evaluation is to delineate the multiple options available, identify the services needed to promote work retention, and develop an industrial rehabilitation plan resulting in sustained employment.

The evaluation process results in an Individualized Modified Reemployment Plan (IMRP) to reduce work disruption, return the worker to suitable work activity, and promote sustained employment in a satisfying job.

Disability Case Manager

Disability Case Management may be considered an alternative management support system for controlling injury and disability problems. Within the context of disability management services, the defined duties of the case manager are based on the specific interventions, programs, and services required to facilitate the employer's management of workers with disabilities. Tasks performed by the case manager typically focus on resolving barriers to safe and productive work performance. For example, the case manager may be responsible for obtaining multidisciplinary evaluations such as job analysis, independent medical examination, functional capacity evaluation, vocational evaluation, psychologic assessment, and so forth of older workers with impairments to identify specific work disability and job handicap problems in order to identify relationships between

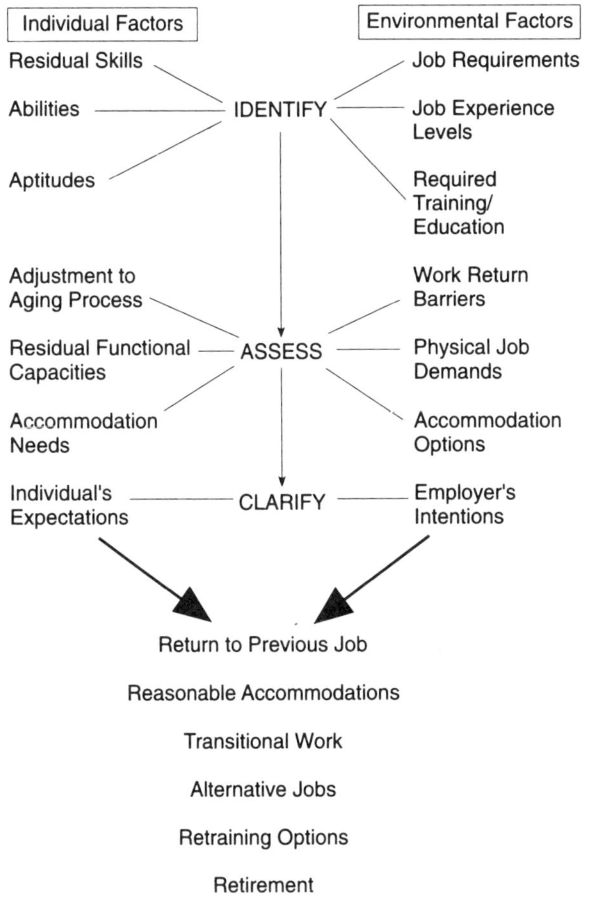

Figure 41.1. Vocational evaluation of individual and environmental factors.

job demands and older workers' mental and physical capacities.

Work disability involves medical, legal, ergonomic, vocational, psychosocial, and labor relations issues. Resolving issues of work disability requires a high level of coordination, decision-making, and planning. Therefore, interdisciplinary collaboration among labor-management resources and community-based services is an essential component of effective case management. The case manager functions as a liaison among managers, physicians, safety personnel, labor organizations, insurance carriers, and others, while carefully orchestrating work return and worker retention planning activities for older persons with disabilities.

MEDICAL MANAGEMENT

Many case managers provide medical management services for impaired employees to ensure quality rehabilitation and treatment outcomes. Typically, Medical Management involves the close monitoring of employees with prolonged work disruptions, such as those having greater than 3 months projected time loss or injured workers experiencing excessive hospitalizations. The case

manager is often responsible for making visits to physicians and treatment programs, functioning as a liaison between the employer, other community treatment providers, and the impaired worker. The case manager may accompany injured workers to physician office visits for examinations or for independent medical evaluations. Likewise, the case manager may be required to make visits to homebound impaired workers to monitor the recovery process and to facilitate planning activities for return to work.

DISABILITY RESOLUTION PROCESS

The Disability Resolution Process is a key component of industrial rehabilitation and disability management. This multidisciplinary process involves the coordination of objective medical, functional capacity, psychologic, and vocational evaluations for older workers with disabilities. Ideally, the case manager arranges and coordinates multiple evaluations, as dictated by the older worker's specific needs. Once the worker's capabilities, motivations, and work qualifications have been comprehensively assessed, work environment information must be obtained through a formal job analysis.

As previously discussed, there are a variety of job analysis approaches, some of which are rather basic and informal and others which are relatively complex and intricate. Generally, the Disability Resolution Process requires a formal analysis of tasks associated with a specific job or group of jobs in order to identify what the older worker does; the purpose of performing each job task; the tools, equipment, and processes used in the performance of the job; physical demands required of the older worker performing the job; knowledge, skill, and experience level required to safely and accurately perform the job; and other measurable and descriptive information.

The written job analysis report serves as an accurate, objective, functional job description. Accommodations cannot be made in the absence of this information. Job analysis information may be made available to treating physicians when projecting safe work return dates for older workers with injuries. The job analysis report may also be used when developing on-site work return transition and modified duty options for older workers with disabilities.

The purpose of the Disability Resolution Process is to resolve any questions or issues involving the relationship between the older employee's physical/mental job demands and the worker's capacities to successfully perform competitive employment. Both overestimation and underestimation of the worker's capabilities can result in unnecessary prolongation of disability and subsequent costs. If the physician overestimates the worker's physical capabilities, premature return to work may result in reinjury. More commonly, the physician conservatively sets return to work restrictions that greatly underestimate a patient's physical capabilities, thus delaying the restoration of function. Consolidation of information from the functional capacity evaluation, medical/psychologic impairment evaluation, and vocational assessment helps substantiate the older worker's medical impairment, disability, and job handicap.

The outcome of the Disability Resolution Process is the identification of realistic, attainable options for resolving questionable or unknown disability and work performance problems. Such options may include job-site redesign, reasonable accommodations, rehabilitation engineering, ergonomic job restructuring, assignment of temporary modified duty, or referral to treatment or rehabilitation programs.

REHABILITATION PLAN DEVELOPMENT

Rehabilitation plans enhance communication and service coordination through clearly defined goals, objectives, and responsibilities. The Rehabilitation Plan also serves as a tool to evaluate the progress of the worker as well as the quality of services provided by insurance, medical, and rehabilitation providers.

In formulating rehabilitation plans for older workers with disabilities, three important tasks are accomplished. The first is to determine what obstacles prevent employment or worker retention and what must be done to remove these barriers. In order to make this determination, knowledge of the older worker's capabilities, physical job demands, and the relationship between these two factors is identified (e.g., the Disability Resolution Process). Second, the older worker with a disability and the employer must be made aware of any incongruence between job demands and worker functional capacities and available options for remediating these differences. The third step involves development of a schedule that provides for evaluation of success at definite points. This helps the older worker to pace his or her own progress, making adjustments as needed. The Rehabilitation Plan serves as the key instrument in the coordination of disability management activities for older persons with disabilities.

WORK RETURN TRANSITION/WORKER RETENTION PROGRAMS

Some of the most effective disability management systems in industry promote the development of on-site work return transition/worker retention (WRT) programs. It is highly desirable for employers to develop and implement such programs in order to prevent work disruptions among older employees with medical impairments that affect work performance; promote a safe and timely return to work among impaired workers on medical leave, workers' compensation, or long-term disability; and accommodate older workers in alternative jobs.

The success of WRT programs is not only dependent upon their actual design, but also on corporate policy, labor relations issues, and a host of other conditions. Once these critical factors are considered, the degree of success in a WRT program is only limited by available resources and the employer's creativity, flexibility, and imagination. Clearly, the most effective WRT model in industry is characterized by its adaptation of work hardening and physical conditioning concepts. These concepts reflect a highly structured, productivity-oriented evaluation, treatment, and work practices education program that uses real work tasks to increase strength, functional capacity, and stamina in order to perform work safely and productively.

The development of a successful worker-job fit is a function of both the capabilities of the older worker and the requirements of the job. In a significant number of cases, job modifications such as tool redesign, utilization of aids or adaptive devices, or job-site restructuring are effective methods for enabling an older individual with a disability to perform essential job tasks. These same interventions can be utilized in a preventive manner to identify and redesign jobs that are likely to result in work-related injuries and disabilities. The participation of ergonomists, allied health professionals, and vocational rehabilitation specialists in the development of disability management programs and individual accommodation interventions is imperative. Such a multidisciplinary effort is required in order to avoid an overreliance on medical model interventions, which seek to remove the older individual's symptoms without regard to the possibilities for accommodation that may exist in the work environment.

On-site work return transition and worker retention programs, when properly designed, are far superior to clinic-based work hardening services. The goal of these programs is to promote worker retention among employees with work performance problems resulting from a physical impairment or an earlier return to work among employees with physical restrictions. WRT programs are designed to provide a therapeutic work environment that promotes a gradual increase in the worker's strength and endurance. The case manager may coordinate and manage the work return transition and worker retention program in collaboration with vocational rehabilitation specialists, physical therapists, ergonomists, managers, and supervisors.

ADA: IMPLICATIONS FOR OLDER PERSONS WITH DISABILITIES, EMPLOYERS AND REHABILITATION SERVICE PROVIDERS

The Americans with Disabilities Act (ADA), signed into law by President Bush in July, 1990, affects over 40 million persons with disabilities. This law is considered by many to be the most important US civil rights legislation in recent history. When considered in the context of injury and disability trends among older workers, this act has important implications for rehabilitation professionals, employers, and others as new legal incentives for employers to develop disability management programs emerge. The law is intended to extend civil rights protection similar to that found in other civil rights legislation related to race, sex, age, and ethnicity to individuals with disabilities. Regulations have been developed by the federal Equal Employment Opportunity Commission, which is also responsible for disseminating information to employers regarding their responsibilities under the ADA, which became effective July, 1992.

The ADA has important implications for older workers with disabilities. The employment-related provisions of the act, under Title I, covers all employers with 25 or more employees and will cover all employers with 15 or more employees by 1994. The act utilizes the definition of "individual with a disability" originally put forth in the Rehabilitation Act of 1973.

Specifically, Title I of ADA prohibits discrimination against a "qualified" individual with a disability in making an employment decision. A "qualified" individual under the act is one who meets the definition of disabled and can perform the "essential functions" of the job with or without reasonable accommodation. ADA does not define the term "essential functions," but this same language was utilized in the Rehabilitation Act of 1973 to avoid individuals being disqualified as a result of their inability to perform functions that were considered of marginal importance to overall job function.

Given these provisions of the law, employers will be required to be very specific in regard to the essential tasks and functions required of a "qualified" applicant for any position for which they hire. Moreover, employers will need to enumerate those qualifications in writing prior to advertising, interviewing, or hiring. There will be a legal incentive for employers to consider job restructuring and job modifications that could both eliminate marginal tasks from the job description and enable otherwise "qualified" individuals with specific limitations to perform the "essential" functions of a job.

The United States has recently witnessed an unprecedented increase in the cost of health care in general and work-related disability and illness in particular. In the American health care system this has translated into direct costs to business, industry, and government, which have significant implications for the stability of the US economy. Additionally, the passage of ADA, prohibiting discrimination in employment practices toward individuals with disabilities, requires that employers prepare to demonstrate compliance in less than 2 years. In this environment, it is becoming increasingly obvious that employers need to establish policies and procedures for the management of disability and illness among workers when employability is threatened. Employer-based programs utilizing interdisciplinary collaboration to intervene with both workers with disabilities and their work environments will characterize companies that successfully respond to the challenges of this changing business environment.

SUMMARY

Health care and demographic trends indicate a compelling need to protect the employability of the working elderly. Despite the myths and misperceptions of older workers' capacities to perform competitive employment, the aging process does not necessarily pose an economic burden to employers. Proven disability management strategies and interventions have important implications for controlling the personal and economic costs of injury and disability in the work place. This chapter describes many essential features of proactive disability management systems that have profound implications for employers, health care providers, and the millions of working elderly. The future implementation of disability management concepts in industry will facilitate the retention of older workers and the years of skills and experience they bring to the US labor force.

References

1. Lewis K. Persons with disabilities and the aging factor. *J Rehabil.* 55(4):12–13, 1989.
2. Bauman NJ, Anderson JC, Morrison MH. Employment of the older disabled person: current environment, outlook, and research needs. In: Brody S, Ruff G, eds. *Aging and Rehabilitation: Advances in the State of the Art.* New York, NY: Springer; 1986.
3. Sax EB, Baumann NJ. Options for equality of services for the older worker with a disability. In: Perlman LG, Austin GF, eds. *The Aging Workforce: Implications for Rehabilitation.* Alexandria, Va: National Rehabilitation Association; 1987.
4. Kemp B, Brummel-Smith K, Ramsdell J. *Geriatric Rehabilitation.* Boston, Mass: College-Hill Press; 1990.
5. Myers JE. Challenges for the older worker in the rehabilitation process. In: Perlman LG, Austin GF, *The Aging Workforce: Implications for Rehabilitation.* Alexandria, Va: National Rehabilitation Association; 1987.
6. Blake R. Disabled older persons: a demographic analysis. *J Rehabil.* 47(4):19–27, 1981.
7. Holland BE, Falvo DR. Forgotten: elderly persons with disability—A consequence of policy. *J Rehabil.* 56(2):32–35, 1990.
8. Shrey DE, Bruyere SM. Disability management in industry: a joint labor-management process. *Rehabil Counsel Bull.* 35(3):227–242, 1991.
9. Robinson PK. Age, health, and job performance. In: Birren JE, Robinson PK, Livingston JE, eds. *Age, Health, and Employment.* Englewood Cliffs, NJ: Prentice-Hall; 1986.
10. Myers JE. Rehabilitation of older workers. In: *Rehab Brief.* Washington, DC: Department of Education, National Institute of Handicapped Research; 1983.
11. Hester EJ. The need for rehabilitation services among older workers. In: Perlman LG, Austin GF, eds. *The Aging Workforce: Implications for Rehabilitation.* Alexandria, Va: National Rehabilitation Association; 1987.
12. Bozarth JD. The rehabilitation process and older people. *J Rehabil.* 47(4):28–32, 1981.
13. Williams TF. The aging process: biological and psychosocial

considerations. In: Brody S, Ruff G, eds. *Aging and Rehabilitation: Advances in the State of the Art.* New York, NY: Springer; 1986.

14. Nash BE. The state of the art: an overview of the world of work. In: Perlman LG, Austin GF, eds. *The Aging Workforce: Implications for Rehabilitation.* Alexandria, Va: National Rehabilitation Association; 1987.

15. Williams TF, Jones PW. Rehabilitation in our aging society. *Aging.* 350:2–3, 1985.

16. McAbee RR, Wilkinson WE. Back injuries and registered nurses. *AAOHN J.* 36(3):106–112, 1988.

17. US Department of Labor. *Labor Market Problems of Older Workers.* Washington, DC: US Department of Labor, 1989.

18. Social Security Administration. *SSA/90—Annual Report to the Congress.* Washington, DC: United States Department of Health and Human Services; 1990.

19. US Department of Labor. Outlook 2000: the major trends. *Occup Outlook Q.* Spring:3–7, 1990.

20. Williams W, Rice BD. *The Future Workplace: Implications for Rehabilitation.* Hot Springs, Ar: Arkansas Research & Training Center in Vocational Rehabilitation; 1987.

21. Salmon HE. Theories of aging, disability and loss. *J Rehabil.* 47(4):44–50, 1981.

22. Becker G, Kaufman S. Old age, rehabilitation, and research: a review of the issues. *Gerontologist.* 28(4):459–468, 1988.

23. Benedict RC, Ganikos ML. Coming to terms with ageism in rehabilitation. *J Rehabil.* 47(4): 10–18, 1981.

24. Barry JR. Challenges of the future. *J Rehabil.* 47(4):94–95, 1981.

25. Dunn DJ. Vocational rehabilitation of the older disabled worker. *J Rehabil.* 47(4):76–81, 1981.

26. Rubenfeld P. Ageism and disability: double jeopardy. In: Brody SJ, Ruff GF, eds. *Aging and Rehabilitation: Advances in the State of the Art.* New York, NY: Springer; 1986.

27. Brody S, Ruff G. *Aging and Rehabilitation: Advances in the State of the Art.* New York, NY: Springer; 1986.

28. Coberly S. Keeping older workers on the job. *Aging.* 349:23–36, 1985.

29. Davidson G. *Private sector efforts to control disability-related health costs.* Presented at Meeting on Economics of Disability, US Department of Education, National Institute of Handicapped Research; April, 1985; Washington, DC.

30. Galvin D. Health promotion, disability management, and rehabilitation at the workplace. *Interconnector.* 6(2):1–6; 1983.

31. Shrey DE. Disability management: an employer-based rehabilitation concept. In: Scheer S, ed. *Assessing the Vocational Capacity of the Impaired Worker.* Rockville, Md: Aspen Publications; 1990.

32. Shrey DE. The employer: a key force in man Ageing disability. *Disabil Manag.* 1(2):3–5; 1988.

33. Shrey DE. Managing disability hinges on strong labor relations. *The Greater Cincinnati Business Record.* July:2–8, 1990.

34. Shrey DE. Managing disability in the work place. *Disabil Manag.* 2(2):2–3; 1989.

35. Hinds KF. *Workers Compensation Cost Control: A Maverick Approach.* Pensacola, Fla: Ability Management Associates Publications; 1988.

SECTION VI

EDUCATIONAL AND LEGAL ASPECTS

42

Geriatric Rehabilitation Research: State of the Art and Future Projections

Kevin M. Means and Felicia D. Sankey

The geriatric population is undergoing rapid growth and significant changes. Increased life expectancy due to public health improvements, life-style changes, and new developments in medical care and technology, among other factors, have resulted in a marked decline in mortality rates from previously fatal diseases and an increase in the proportion of the population over the age of sixty-five years (1). The most rapidly growing segment of this group are those age 85-years and older. Many of the significant improvements in health and health care have occurred due to the advancement of biomedical research. Increasing our understanding of human biologic mechanisms and application of this knowledge to extend longevity and enhance the quality of life have long been major goals of biomedical research. Relatively recently, biomedical researchers have focused their efforts on the problems of the geriatric population (2).

Prior to the 1960s, the growth of the geriatric population had not yet gained extensive attention from researchers, policy makers, or significant sources of funding for biomedical research. Legislation establishing the National Institute on Aging (NIA) within the National Institutes of Health (NIH) was enacted by the US Congress in 1974. Since that time, there has been a dramatic expansion of interest in and support for research in gerontology, the study of normal aging, and for geriatrics, the study and treatment of diseases and disorders associated with elderly persons. Technologic advances are facilitating new discoveries at the molecular and cellular level. Increases in the quantity and quality of knowledge in gerontology have challenged existing concepts of aging. This in turn has led scientists to the development of new and expanding theories on the biologic, psychologic, and sociologic aspects of how and why we age. Important aspects of our aging population, including information and projections about growth, characteristics, and needs, are more accurate due to improved epidemiologic methods and data collection (3). Many clinical research studies are testing the application

of this expanded knowledge in aging and the control of age-associated conditions. Advances in gerontology and geriatric research directly affect the clinical care of older persons.

A related but underutilized research area of potential importance to the geriatric population is the discipline of medical rehabilitation research. A large percentage of the geriatric population either demonstrate or are at risk for multiple, chronic disabling conditions. Our understanding of the etiology, pathophysiology, treatment, and prevention of these conditions and the effects of their interaction has lagged behind our understanding in other areas of biomedicine. However, continued growth of the geriatric population with a high incidence and prevalence of disability, coupled with the fact that this population already accounts for a disproportionately high expenditure of both personal and entitlement health care costs, suggests that improved control of these conditions by preventive and rehabilitative strategies will be imperative. Basic, clinical, and applied medical rehabilitation research provide the impetus for the development of these strategies.

STATE OF GERIATRIC REHABILITATION RESEARCH

Recent evidence suggests that medical rehabilitation research in general and medical rehabilitation research as applied to problems of aging and the elderly in particular are areas of relative deficiency in medicine (4–7). Many factors account for this deficiency. Perhaps most important is the growing shortage of research scientists actively involved in geriatrics and rehabilitation-related disciplines. Other factors include the following: limited exposure of rehabilitation professionals to the area of geriatrics during their training; a lack of formal skills, such as statistical analysis, necessary to conduct research; and characteristics of the academic and clinical environment that represent barriers to research. These barriers include a general limitation of adequate resources to support research studies, a lack of senior researchers and opportunities for collaboration, and a traditional tendency of many academic departments to assign a relatively low priority to research activities (8–10). This shortage has been recognized by the leadership of many rehabilitation and geriatric professionals, which has led to increased attention and formulation of strategies for improvement (11–14).

Survey of Current Research Literature

INTEREST AREAS

In an attempt to determine the extent of the relative deficiency of geriatric rehabilitation research, we conducted a survey of geriatric research articles in the medical literature. For survey purposes, three general areas of interest were identified: (a) rehabilitation research articles with emphasis on aging or the elderly; (b) geriatric medicine research articles with rehabilitation emphasis; and (c) research articles in nongeriatric journals that cover geriatric rehabilitation topics. Due to the diversity of professional disciplines involved in rehabilitation and/or aging and the wide variety of journals potentially comprising the geriatric rehabilitation literature, such a survey was challenging. An equally difficult task was defining what actually constituted a geriatric rehabilitation article. In order to obtain a representative sample of recent research literature and to identify recent trends, broad definitions of geriatric rehabilitation articles were used. When possible, we selected peer-reviewed journals that we felt were representative of research published by research scientists and practitioners in specific disciplines. This survey was not intended to be an exhaustive review of the entire body of geriatric or rehabilitation literature. Some general medical and nursing journals were also surveyed.

SURVEY METHODOLOGY

The methodology used for all three areas of interest was similar in that the survey was conducted by one or both of the authors of this chapter and that an identical survey period was used. For all journals included in the survey, issues published from July 1989 through June 1992 were reviewed. Only original research and review articles meeting the specific criteria below were included. All editorials, letters to the editor, case reports, and brief reports were excluded. The specific review criteria for articles included varied according to the particular survey area of interest.

To evaluate the content, quantity, and topic distribution of rehabilitation research articles pertaining to the geriatric population, the following criteria were used: (a) geriatric-specific articles were defined as articles that

specifically included the words geriatrics, aged, aging, elderly, old, or older in the title or abstract; and (b) geriatric-related articles were defined as articles that did not mention the above words in the title or abstract, but did mention the words nursing home, long-term care, or dementia in the title or abstract or included the words geriatrics, aged, aging, elderly, old, or older as key words.

In order to determine rehabilitation emphasis among journals in the geriatric medicine literature, somewhat different review criteria were used: (a) rehabilitation-specific articles were defined as articles that specifically included the word rehabilitation in the title or abstract; and (b) rehabilitation-related articles were liberally defined as articles that did not mention the word rehabilitation in the title or abstract, but did mention any of the following words in the title or abstract: disability, handicap, disabled, impairment, functional, mobility, activities of daily living, exercise, strength, activity, balance, range of motion, nerve or muscle stimulation or conduction, prosthesis, orthosis, or assistive device. Articles that mentioned in the title or abstract any of several disorders (listed in Table 42.1) commonly seen in elderly patients and in the rehabilitation team setting were also considered to be rehabilitation-related.

To determine the quantity and content of geriatrics, rehabilitation, or geriatric rehabilitation research articles in the nongeriatric medical and nursing literature, a combination of the above criteria were used as follows: (a) geriatric rehabilitation-specific articles were defined as articles that specifically included the word rehabilitation *and* either of the following words in the title or abstract: geriatric(s), aging, aged, elderly, old, or older; (b) geriatric rehabilitation-related articles were defined as articles that were either geriatric-related *or* rehabilitation-related but did not meet the criteria in (a) above; (c) geriatric-related articles were defined as above for the rehabilitation literature; and (d) articles considered to be

Table 42.1. Common Disorders Seen in the Geriatric Rehabilitation Team Setting[a]

Amputation	Joint replacement
Arthritis	Lymphedema
Burns	Neuropathy
Cancer	Osteoporosis
Cardiovascular disorders	Pain syndromes (acute)
Chronic pain	Parkinson's disease
Chronic pulmonary disease	Peripheral vascular disease
Contractures	Postural disorders/falls
Deconditioning	Pressure sores
Disk disorders	Spinal cord injury
Fracture	Spinal stenosis
Head injury	Stroke
Immobility	Trauma

[a] Adapted from Reichel W. *Clinical Aspects of Aging.* 3rd ed. Baltimore, Md: Williams & Wilkins; 1989:184.

rehabilitation-related were defined as above for the geriatric literature.

Rehabilitation Research with Emphasis on Aging or the Elderly

The journals reviewed for this area were: the *Archives of Physical Medicine and Rehabilitation* (Arch PM&R), the *American Journal of Physical Medicine and Rehabilitation* (Am J PM&R), *Physical Therapy* (Phys Ther), the *American Journal of Occupational Therapy* (Am J OT), and *Rehabilitation Nursing* (Reh Nurs). The *Archives of Physical Medicine and Rehabilitation* is the official journal of the American Congress of Rehabilitation Medicine, an interdisciplinary organization of rehabilitation professionals, and the American Academy of Physical Medicine and Rehabilitation, the professional society of physicians in this specialty. The *Archives of Physical Medicine and Rehabilitation* is published monthly. The *American Journal of Physical Medicine and Rehabilitation* is the official journal of the Association of Academic Physiatrists and is published bimonthly. *Physical Therapy*, the official journal of the American Physical Therapy Association, a professional organization of physical therapists, is published monthly. The *American Journal of Occupational Therapy* is the official professional journal of the American Occupational Therapy Association and is published monthly. *Rehabilitation Nursing*, published bimonthly, is the official journal of the Association of Rehabilitation Nurses.

RESULTS

The *Archives of Physical Medicine and Rehabilitation*

We reviewed a total of 389 articles in 36 issues. Of this total, 25 (6.4%) articles specifically mentioned geriatric, aged, aging, elderly, old, or older in the title or abstract. Eight (2.1%) articles mentioned the words nursing home, long-term care, or dementia in the title or abstract or included geriatrics, aged, aging, elderly, old, or older as key words. Among geriatric rehabilitation topics identified were standing balance [1], falls [5], therapeutic exercise [5], amputation [2], stroke rehabilitation [1], spinal cord disorders [3], rehabilitation of renal dialysis patients [1], pressure sores [1], geriatric rehabilitation abroad [1], geriatric emotional dysfunction [1], physical disability [1], physical medicine and rehabilitation residency training [1], gait [3], prospective payment for rehabilitation [1], and comparison of rehabilitation outcome [1]. The institutional affiliations of the various authors of these geriatric-specific and geriatric-related articles ranged from academic departments of physical therapy, epidemiology, physiology, social work, anatomy, family practice, medicine, physical medicine and rehabilitation to special research centers within various academic and clinical institutions.

The *American Journal of Physical Medicine and Rehabilitation*

A total of 149 research articles were reviewed. Four (2.7%) articles specifically mentioned geriatrics, aged, aging, elderly, old, or older in the title or abstract. None of the articles mentioned the words nursing home, long-term care, or dementia in the title or abstract or included geriatrics, aged, aging, elderly, old, or older as key words. Among geriatric rehabilitation topics identified were mobility [1], posthip fracture [1], peripheral vascular disease [1], and aging and rehabilitation in renal disorders [1]. The contributing authors' departmental affiliations included anatomy, orthopedic surgery, and rehabilitation medicine.

Physical Therapy

A total of 241 research articles were reviewed. Twelve (5%) articles specifically mentioned geriatrics, aged, aging, elderly, old, or older in the title or abstract. Only 2 (0.8%) articles mentioned the words nursing home, long-term care, or dementia in the title or abstract or included geriatrics, aged, aging, elderly, old, or older as key words. Topics addressed included balance performance [4], postural changes in the elderly [2], range of motion and age [1], walking patterns in the elderly [2], motor performance [1], physical therapy in nursing homes [1], attitudes toward the elderly [1], and hand function [1]. The authors of these geriatric topics represented affiliations with departments of physical therapy, kinesiology, rehabilitation medicine, physical education and human movement studies, orthopedics, and general medicine, in addition to a special clinical center. One author had no specified affiliation.

The *American Journal of Occupational Therapy*

A survey of 258 research articles revealed 18 (7%) articles that specifically mentioned geriatrics, aged, aging, elderly, old, or older in the title or abstract. In addition, 7 (2.7%) articles mentioned geriatric-related topics. Among the geriatric topics covered were therapeutic exercise [4], technology and computers and the elderly [2], activity and the elderly [1], fear of falling [1], family care of the elderly [2], mobility skills [1], needs of cognitively impaired elderly [1], long-term care and federal policy [1], empowerment [1], cultural diversity and older adult needs [1], gerontology education and occupational therapy [1], ethics, long-term care, and occupational therapy [1], occupational therapy in the Veterans' Administration (VA) [1], geriatric mental health [1], role assessment and physical disability [1], independent living alternatives [1], private practice occupational therapy in nursing homes [1], day care [1], and spatial disorientation and Alzheimer's disease [1]. The authors included occupational therapists in clinical or academic departments of occupational therapy. One of the authors was an officer of the American Occupational Therapist Association, and one author was a physical therapist. An academic department of geography was represented as well.

Rehabilitation Nursing

Eight (7.5%) articles of 107 mentioned geriatrics, aged, aging, elderly, old, or older specifically, while 4 (3.7%) were about geriatric-related topics. The topics of the geriatric-specific and geriatric-related articles included teaching the elderly [1], joint self-care [1], sexuality [1], family caregiving [1], rehabilitation nursing [1], self-medication [1], functional assessment [1], activity intolerance in stroke patients [1], use of restraints [2], fall prevention [1], and correlation between mini-mental state examination scores and activities of daily living status in dementia patients [1]. All of the authors of these articles were nurses with various affiliations at academic and clinical institutions.

DISCUSSION

Rehabilitation Nursing, although it contained a relatively small number (8) of geriatric-specific research articles during the survey period, had the highest percentage of these articles of all of the rehabilitation journals reviewed. Table 42.2 shows that, compared to *Rehabilitation Nursing, Archives of Physical Medicine and Rehabilitation* with the largest number of geriatric-specific articles [25] and *American Journal of Occupational Therapy* with the next largest number of geriatric-related articles [19] had similar but lower percentages of geriatric-specific research articles (6.4% and 7.4% respectively). *Physical Therapy* and the *American Journal of Physical Medicine and Rehabilitation* had lower percentages of geriatric-specific articles (5.0% and 2.7%, respectively). Figure 42.1 shows that there was only a slight increase in the total number of rehabilitation research articles published in these journals from 1989 through 1992. On a percentage basis, the number of geriatric-specific and geriatric-related articles in the rehabilitation literature during the same period was essentially unchanged. The

most commonly represented departments of the primary authors were academic departments of nursing, occupational therapy, physical therapy, and rehabilitation medicine. Few primary authors were from a department of physical medicine and rehabilitation.

SUMMARY

There is a paucity of articles with an emphasis on aging or the elderly in the rehabilitation literature, and this pattern does not appear to be changing. Although some of the more traditional rehabilitation disciplines are publishing in the literature, they are still grossly underrepresented.

Geriatric Medicine Research with Rehabilitation Emphasis

JOURNALS

The journals reviewed for this area were: the *Journal of the American Geriatrics Society* (J Am Geriatr Soc), the *Journal of Gerontology* (J Gerontology), *The Gerontologist,* and *Geriatric Nursing.* The *Journal of the American Geriatrics Society,* published monthly, is the official journal of the American Geriatrics Society, an organization comprised primarily of physicians with an interest in geriatric medicine. The *Journal of Gerontology* and *The Gerontologist,* each published bimonthly, are both official peer-reviewed journals of the Gerontological Society of America, a large and diverse organization of biologic, behavioral, and social scientists as well as scientists and practitioners from other clinical disciplines. The *Journal of Gerontology* allocates space for research articles equally among the four major scientific divisions of the parent organization's membership: biologic sciences, medical sciences, psychologic sciences, and social sciences. Clinical research articles, rehabilitation or otherwise, from this journal would therefore not ever be expected to exceed 25% of the total number of articles, the allocation for medical sciences. *Geriatric Nursing* is a peer-reviewed nursing journal that bimonthly publishes scientific research articles and articles of general clinical interest.

RESULTS

Journal of the American Geriatrics Society

We reviewed a total of 363 articles in 36 issues. Using the above liberal criteria, 6 (1.7%) rehabilitation-specific articles and 73 (20%) rehabilitation-related articles were identified. This included 46 (12.7%) of the total articles that mentioned rehabilitation-related words in the title or abstract and 27 additional articles that mentioned specific rehabilitation disorders in the title or abstract. Among the specific rehabilitation topics identified were: neuropathy [1], arthritis [1], fracture [5], head

Table 42.2. Survey of Rehabilitation Literature

Journal[a]	No. of Articles	Geriatric-Specific	Geriatric-Related
Arch PM&R	389	25(6.4%)	8(2.1%)
Am J PM&R	149	4(2.7%)	0(0.0%)
Phys Ther	241	12(5.0%)	2(0.8%)
Am J OT	258	18(7.0%)	7(2.7%)
Reh Nurs	107	8(7.5%)	4(3.7%)
Totals:	1144	67(5.9%)	21(1.8%)

[a]Arch PM&R = *Archives of Physical Medicine and Rehabilitation;* Am J PM&R = *American Journal of Physical Medicine and Rehabilitation;* Phys Ther = *Physical Therapy;* Am J OT = *American Journal of Occupational Therapy;* Reh Nurs = *Rehabilitation Nursing.*

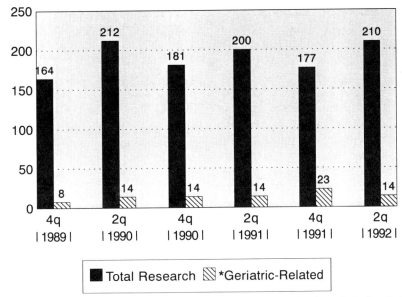

N = 1144 Articles   *includes geriatric-specific and geriatric-related articles

Figure 42.1.   Rehabilitation literature. (Arch PM&R; Am J PM&R; Am J OT; Phys Therap; Rehab Nurs). N = 1144 articles (nongeria- tric-related articles not shown); 2q = 1st through 2nd quarters; 4q = 3rd through 4th quarters.

injury [2], immobility [1], osteoporosis [1], Parkinson's disease [2], postural disorders and falls [2], pressure sores [3], pain [1], stroke [1], and amputation [1]. The affiliations of the various authors of these geriatric rehabilitation and related articles ranged from academic departments of geriatric medicine, family practice, psychiatry, surgery, epidemiology, rehabilitation medicine, nursing, physiology and physical therapy to special clinical and research centers within various academic or clinical institutions and governmental agencies.

The Journal of Gerontology

A total of 444 articles in 18 issues were reviewed. No articles specifically mentioned rehabilitation in the title or abstract. Sixty-two (14%) rehabilitation-related articles were identified. This included 42 (9.5%) articles that mentioned rehabilitation-related words in the title or abstract and an additional 20 (4.5%) articles that mentioned specific rehabilitation disorders in the title or abstract. Among the specific rehabilitation topics identified were the following: arthritis [1], fracture [4], osteoporosis [1], postural disorders and falls [10], and pain [4]. Affiliations represented by the authors of these articles were academic departments of geriatric medicine, physical therapy, internal medicine, preventive medicine, neurology, community medicine, kinesiology, psychiatry, epidemiology, nursing, sociology, physiology, and physical therapy. Special institutes for research and governmental agencies were also represented.

The Gerontologist

A total of 315 research articles were reviewed. None of the articles specifically mentioned rehabilitation in the

title or abstract. There were 48 (15.2%) rehabilitation-related articles identified. This included 43 articles (13.7%) that mentioned rehabilitation-related words in the title or abstract and 5 articles (1.6%) that mentioned specific rehabilitation disorders, such as Parkinson's disease, stroke, and postural disorders and falls. Institutional affiliations of the authors of these articles included social work, psychology, psychiatry, health education, internal medicine, health services, health policy, gerontology, nursing, physical education, geriatric medicine, education, and family practice. Aging and geriatric clinical and research centers as well as clinical institutes and projects for the elderly were also represented.

Geriatric Nursing

One hundred forty-three research articles in 18 issues were reviewed. Only 1 article (0.7%) specifically mentioned rehabilitation in the abstract. Twenty-six articles (18.2%) were rehabilitation-related. Three articles (2.1%) mentioned rehabilitation-related words in the title or abstract, and 15 articles (10.5%) mentioned specific rehabilitation disorders. Among the specific rehabilitation topics identified were postural disorders and falls [4], pain syndromes [4], head injury [2], pressure sores [2], stroke [1], osteoporosis [1], exercise/activity [1], functional mobility [1] and Parkinson's disease [1]. Only two of these articles were written by primary authors without a nursing degree. The degree status of one author could not be determined. Eighteen of the primary authors were from academic departments, 11 from nursing schools or departments of nursing, and 7 from nonnursing departments. The remainder of the primary authors represented nursing in clinical institutions, geriatric centers, nursing homes, and special research centers and projects.

DISCUSSION

There has been a steady increase in the quantity of geriatric research as evidenced by the increase in numbers of articles in virtually all of the journals included in the survey. The number of rehabilitation-specific articles in the geriatric literature was negligible, considering the large number of articles surveyed and the duration of the survey period. Using our liberal criteria for inclusion as a rehabilitation-related article, there appears to be an increase in their absolute number, ranging from a late 1989 low of 26 to a high of 41 in 1991. However, Table 42.3 and Figure 42.2 reveal that, when viewed on a percentage basis, there is only a very slight increasing trend among rehabilitation-related articles—14% in 1989, 20% in 1990, and 16.3% in 1992. Because of the liberal criteria used, it was not always easy to clearly identify a specific rehabilitation topic among the rehabilitation-specific and rehabilitation-related topics. This is because some articles may have made references to terminology or techniques common within the rehabilitation setting although the primary emphasis of the article was not about a common rehabilitation topic. The distribution of specific rehabilitation topics was somewhat predictable, with inclusion of many rehabilitation disorders common in the geriatric population. The relative lack of attention to geriatric

Table 42.3. Survey of Geriatric Literature

Journal[a]	No. of Articles	Rehabilitation-Specific	Rehabilitation-Related
J Gerontology	444	0(0%)	62(14%)
J Am Geriatr Soc	363	6(1.7%)	73(20.1%)
The Gerontologist	315	0(0%)	48(15.2%)
Geriatric Nursing	143	1(0.07%)	26(18.2%)
Totals:	1265	7(0.6%)	209(16.5%)

[a]J Gerontology = *Journal of Gerontology*; J Am Geriatr Soc = *Journal of the American Geriatrics Society.*

rehabilitation, reflected by the small number of articles addressing rehabilitation topics such as exercise, arthritis, and mobility impairment, was surprising.

The relatively low percentage of rehabilitation-specific and rehabilitation-related articles may have several explanations. The primarily general medical and nursing or basic science background of the editorial boards, parent organizations, and readership of the geriatric journals surveyed would indicate that there are many more nonrehabilitation research papers competing for acceptance and publication. Most of the articles were written by authors in primary care medical specialties, basic scientists, and other researchers from nonrehabilitation academic departments or clinical settings. These nonrehabilitation professionals and settings may have been lax in adopting a rehabilitation orientation, in formulating rehabilitation-related research questions, or in collaborating with rehabilitation colleagues. This orientation has been somewhat slow to develop, but is apparently

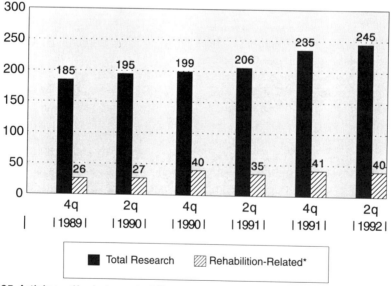

N = 1265 Articles *includes rehabilitation-specific and rehabilitation-related articles
2q = 1st through 2nd quarters; 4q = 3rd through 4th quarters

Figure 42.2. Geriatric literature. J Gerontol; J Am Geriatr Soc; The Gerontologist; Geriatr Nurs. N = 1265 articles (includes rehabilitation-specific and rehabilitation-related articles); 2q = 1st through 2nd quarters; 4q = 3rd through 4th quarters.

gaining in emphasis in the medical and nursing scientific community. Very few of these articles were written by researchers in specific rehabilitation departments. This could be due to the relatively small numbers of researchers in these disciplines or perhaps due to an inability to or preference for not publishing in the geriatric literature.

SUMMARY

The number of rehabilitation-related articles in the geriatric literature is increasing slowly in absolute numbers, but not significantly as a percentage of the total number of research articles. The small number of rehabilitation-specific articles, rehabilitation topics, and primary authors from specific rehabilitation departments or disciplines in our survey results suggests a modest emphasis on rehabilitation in this literature or a tendency of researchers active in geriatric rehabilitation research not to publish extensively in this literature.

Coverage of Geriatric Rehabilitation Topics by Nongeriatric Medical and Nursing Research Journals

A sampling of nongeriatric journals were reviewed for this area, including the *New England Journal of Medicine* (NEJM), the *Journal of Family Practice* (J Fam-Pract), the *Journal of the American Medical Association* (JAMA), and the *Journal of Nursing Research* (Nurs Res). Both the *New England Journal of Medicine* and JAMA are well-established, extensively read general medical journals published weekly. JAMA is the official journal of the American Medical Association, a professional organization of physicians. The *Journal of Family Practice* is the official journal of the Association of Departments of Family Medicine, the North American Primary Care Research Group, and the Society of Teachers of Family Medicine. The *Journal of Family Practice* is published monthly. Family practice and its affiliated organizations value a comprehensive clinical approach that is broad in scope. The family practice literature would be expected to include a variety of clinical research topics, including geriatrics and rehabilitation. *Nursing Research*, published semimonthly, contains original research primarily from nurse investigators.

RESULTS

The *New England Journal of Medicine*

A total of 827 NEJM articles in 63 issues were reviewed. None of these articles specifically mentioned both aging or related terms and rehabilitation in the title or abstract. Fifteen (1.8%) geriatric-related or rehabilitation-related articles were identified. This included 1 article that mentioned geriatric-related words and 14 articles that mentioned rehabilitation-related

words in the title or abstract or discussed rehabilitative aspects of specific disorders. Among the disorders and topics included were osteoporosis [3], disability in Parkinson's disease [1], exercise [3], low back pain [2], geriatric functional assessment [1], rheumatoid arthritis [1], geriatric gait disorders [1], spinal cord injury [1], falls and hip fracture [1], and dysphagia [1]. Most of the primary authors (53%) were affiliated with academic departments of geriatric medicine or internal medicine [8]. Other academic departments represented were epidemiology, biostatistics, or public health [2]; neurology [2]; endocrinology [1], and cardiology [1]. One primary author was from the department of rehabilitation medicine of a federal health facility, the National Institutes of Health.

The *Journal of the American Medical Association*

A total of 573 articles in 37 issues were reviewed over a 3-year period from July 1989 through June 1992. Two of the 573 articles (0.35%) specifically mentioned both aging or related terms and rehabilitation in the title or abstract. Twenty-seven (4.7%) geriatric-related or rehabilitation-related articles were identified. This included 19 articles (3.3%) that were considered to be geriatric-related and eight articles that mentioned rehabilitation-related words in the title or abstract or mentioned and discussed rehabilitative aspects of specific rehabilitation disorders. Among the rehabilitation topics covered by these articles were exercise and fitness [7], drug therapy [3], delirium [2], phlebothrombosis after hip arthroplasty [2], depression and function [2], dementia [1], health and medical care in nursing homes [2], coronary heart disease [1], incontinence [1], pain [1], patient satisfaction [1], restraints in the nursing home [1], visual impairment [1], pressure sores, geriatric assessment and hip fracture [1], and hyperthermia [1]. Eight of the primary authors (27.5%) were affiliated with academic departments of geriatric medicine or internal medicine. Eight articles were by primary authors from special public and private institutes or centers for research. Other institutional departments represented by the primary authors included epidemiology or public health [3], psychiatry [3], special centers or homes for the aged [3], family medicine [2], and obstetrics and gynecology [1].

The *Journal of Family Practice*

A total of 265 articles in 36 issues were reviewed. None of the 265 articles specifically mentioned both aging (or related terms) and rehabilitation in the title or abstract. Fifty-two (19.6%) geriatric-related or rehabilitation-related articles were identified, including 26 (9.8%) geriatric-related articles and 16 (6%) rehabilitation-related articles. A variety of rehabilitation-related topics were covered. These included drug therapy and adverse effects [5], dizziness [1], health services delivery [4], hypercholesterolemia [3], quality of life [2], ethics [2], pain [2], infectious diseases [2], depression [2], and nursing home health [2]. Most of the primary authors of the geriatric and rehabilitation-related articles reviewed were affiliated with academic departments of family medicine.

The Journal of Nursing Research

One hundred forty-four research articles in 36 issues were reviewed. None of the articles specifically mentioned both aging or related terms and rehabilitation in the title or abstract. Nineteen (13.1%) of the articles were either geriatric-related [7] or rehabilitation-related [12]. Among the specific topics identified were dementia [3], health care delivery [2], head injury [2], pressure sores [2], stroke [1], osteoporosis [1], exercise/activity [1], functional mobility [1], and Parkinson's disease [1]. All of the geriatric rehabilitation-related articles were written by nurses as primary authors associated with academic schools or colleges of nursing [8], mental health nursing [1], and medicine [1].

DISCUSSION

The total number of research articles published in the general medical and nursing journals surveyed has increased over the past 3 years. This trend was also seen in the rehabilitation and geriatric literature. Table 42.4 and Figure 42.3 reveal that the number and percentage of geriatric-related and rehabilitation-related research articles published over the same time period was very low, with no evidence of an increasing trend. The virtual absence of rehabilitation articles (2.1%) from these general medical and nursing journals was predictable. Interestingly, the number of geriatric-related research articles was also very small (2.9%), even using our liberal criteria for geriatric research articles. Of the four journals surveyed, the *Journal of Family Practice* had the highest percentage (9.8%) of geriatric-related articles, and *NEJM* had the lowest (0.1%). *Nursing Research* had the highest percentage (8.3%) of rehabilitation-related articles, while *JAMA* had the lowest (1.4%). *JAMA* was the only journal among the 4 surveyed that had any geriatric rehabilitation articles (2 articles; 0.4%).

As discussed above, we experienced similar difficulty in identifying geriatric, rehabilitation, and geriatric rehabilitation articles. The criteria used were admittedly subjective, but an attempt was made to be as inclusive as possible. The distribution of specific rehabilitation topics was somewhat predictable, with inclusion of many rehabilitation disorders common in the geriatric population. Among the rehabilitation-related topics covered in the articles, the most common single topic was exercise and fitness (11 articles), followed by articles on various types of drug therapy (8). *JAMA* had the widest variety of topics covered, including 7 articles on exercise and fitness. The *NEJM* and *Nursing Research* tended to include articles on more traditional rehabilitation topics, such as spinal cord injury, head injury, low back pain, hip fracture, arthritis, and pressure sores. These traditional topics were not among the most frequently covered. Articles on common and important geriatric rehabilitation topics, such as arthritis, stroke, hip fracture, and falls, were conspicuously underrepresented. Most of the articles were written by authors in geriatric or internal medicine, family medicine, and academic departments of nursing and by researchers from special research centers or clinical institutions for the aged. Virtually none of the authors were from rehabilitation disciplines. As was noted in the geriatrics and rehabilitation literature, very little cross-publication exists in the four journals among researchers in geriatric medicine or geriatric nursing, primary care medicine or general nursing, and researchers from the various rehabilitation disciplines. This suggests either limited opportunities for cross-publication, limited scientific collaboration among specialties and disciplines, or a lack of researchers in all disciplines with interests that overlap the areas of geriatrics and rehabilitation.

SUMMARY

Although the number of research articles published in the four general medical and nursing journals reviewed is increasing, the number of geriatric and

Table 42.4. Survey of General Medical and Nursing Literature

Journal[a]	No. of Articles	Geriatric Rehabilitation	Geriatric-Related	Rehabilitation-Related
JAMA	573	2(0.4%)	19(3.3%)	8(1.4%)
J Fam Pract	265	0(0.0%)	26(9.8%)	4(1.5%)
NEJM	827	0(0.0%)	1(0.1%)	14(1.7%)
Nurs Res	144	0(0.0%)	7(4.9%)	12(8.3%)
Totals	1809	2(0.11%)	53(2.9%)	38(2.1%)

[a]JAMA = Journal of the American Medical Association; J Fam Pract = Journal of Family Practice; NEJM = New England Journal of Medicine; Nurs Res = Journal of Nursing Research.

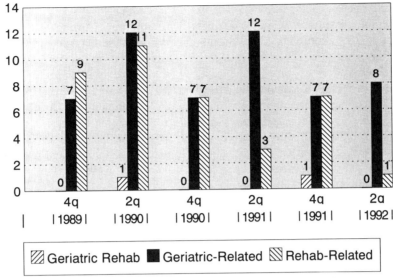

Figure 42.3. General medical and nursing literature. (JAMA; J Fam Pract; New Engl J Med; Nurs Res). N = 1809 articles; (non-geriatric or rehabilitation articles not shown); 2q = 1st through 2nd quarters; 4q = 3rd through 4th quarters.

rehabilitation-related articles has remained at a relatively low percentage. This trend is most likely due to the general, primary care medical and nursing focus of the authors, the journals, their editors, parent organizations, and readership. This lack of emphasis was expected for rehabilitation-related articles, but the small percentage of geriatric-related articles was surprising. This suggests that there is little interface among geriatric and rehabilitation researchers or little interest in geriatric rehabilitation research among the editorial boards or readership of these journals.

FUNDING SOURCES FOR GERIATRIC REHABILITATION RESEARCH

Traditional Public Funding Sources

The NIA has been a mainstay of funding for aging-oriented research since its creation by Congress in 1974 as one of the National Institutes of Health. The NIA supports biomedical, clinical, behavioral, and social research and training initiatives related to aging and diseases, disorders, and special problems of older persons. The NIA funds several intramural research and training programs, including the Gerontology Research Center and the Epidemiology, Demography, and Biometry Programs. The extramural programs funded by the NIA include Biomedical Research and Clinical Medicine, Behavioral and Social Research Program, and Neuroscience and Neuropsychology of Aging. Grant awards provided by the NIA support research and research training.

These contract awards are given for animal, cellular, and data research resource development and support. Awards are also given for research resource development and support of community populations of older people. Grants and awards provided by the NIA include research project grants (R01); program project grants; center core grants; Research Career Development Awards; National Research Service Awards; First Independent Research Support and Transition (FIRST) Awards; Small Business Innovation research grants; Teaching Nursing Home Awards; Alzheimer Disease Research Center Grants; Special Emphasis Research Career (SERCA) Awards; Academic, Clinical Investigator, Physician Scientist, and Geriatric Leadership Academic Awards; cooperative agreements; research and development contracts; and Academic Research Enhancement (AREA) Awards.

The National Institute on Disability and Rehabilitation Research (NIDRR), formerly the Vocational Rehabilitation Administration, was established by Congress in 1978. It developed as an outgrowth of the Rehabilitation Research and Demonstration Program. It is part of the Office of Special Education and Rehabilitative Services in the Department of Education. The NIDDR provides grants to the public and private sector for research of rehabilitation theory and practice. It seeks to promote independence in individuals with disabilities through the rehabilitation process. Among its programs are the Rehabilitation Research and Training Centers, Rehabilitation Engineering Centers, Field Initiated Research, Research and Demonstration Projects, Research Fellowships, Research Training and Career Development grants, Dissemination and Utilization grants, Innovation grants, Technology Assistance, Small Business Innovative Research grants, International Program, Interagency Activity, and Regional Disability and Business Technical Assistance Centers.

The Department of Veterans Affairs Rehabilitation Research and Development (Rehabilitation R&D) Service is one of the three R&D Services in the Veterans Health Services and Research Administration. Although the Rehabilitation R&D does not provide grants, it does support research and development of rehabilitation projects for veterans who are physically handicapped. The priority areas of the Rehabilitation R&D include prosthetics, amputations, and orthotics; spinal cord injury; and communication, sensory, and cognitive aids. Additionally, specific programs are sponsored by special Rehabilitation R&D centers throughout the United States. Areas of interest include the use of medical engineering technology for disabled veterans, functional problems of aging, functional electrical stimulation in spinal cord injured patients, development and distribution of new devices clinically and commercially, and promotion of research results in the scientific community in the United States and abroad.

Private Funding Sources

The private sector is an important source of support for biomedical research. Although a comprehensive list of individual sources is beyond the scope of this chapter, the interested reader is referred to reference books such as the *Foundation Reporter*, 1993, 24th Edition (B.R. Romaniuk, editor) or *The Foundation Directory*, 1993 15th Edition (S. Olson, editor) for additional information. Philanthropic institutions such as the Charles A. Dana, John A. Hartford, Brookdale, and Greenwall foundations provide funding for areas including neglected problems of the elderly, recruitment and training of geriatric academicians, and geriatric biomedical research. Special interest organizations and foundations such as the American Federation for Aging Research and the American Association of Retired Persons' Andrus Foundation, as well as numerous corporate foundations such as Allied-Signal, Inc., Sandoz Foundation, Merck Company Foundation, Pfizer, Inc., and the Travelers Company Foundation, are sources of private support for research in aging. Private funding from these sources has been utilized very little in the past for rehabilitation research.

The National Center for Medical Rehabilitation Research

Despite the existence of public and private research funding opportunities including those listed above, past experience has shown that funded rehabilitation research has continued to represent a small proportion of all biomedical research, a fraction of the amount needed to meet the growing demand for reduction and prevention of disability and chronic disease in an aging society. Rehabilitation research scientists as a group have been small in number and relatively limited in experience. Due to the diverse, interdisciplinary nature of rehabilitation and its related disorders, it has been difficult to develop and sustain a research strategy and agenda as focused as some other areas of biomedicine. The absence of a major centralized funding agency, such as one of the National Institutes of Health, has also been a limiting factor.

At the national level, increasing awareness of this problem led to legislation signed into law in November, 1990, establishing the National Center for Medical Rehabilitation Research (NCMRR). The NCMRR exists as a separate research center within the National Institute of Child Health and Human Development (NICHD) of the NIH. In 1991, a National Advisory Board on Medical Rehabilitation Research was chartered, and a research plan for the NCMRR has been developed. Prior to the NCMRR, support for medical rehabilitation research had been dispersed among many areas of the NIH, such as the NIA. Researchers wishing to compete for these funds were competing for a very limited part of an overall budget with higher priorities in nonrehabilitation areas. The NCMRR will help to provide a focus for basic and clinical research and training for scientists, engineers, and others seeking to restore or enhance the function of persons with physical disabilities.

The NCMRR funded over $600,000 in Fiscal Year 1991, and announced broad funding objectives in February 1992. These objectives included requests for research projects and research and fellowship training applications in the areas of mobility enhancement, assessment and measurement, assistive devices, behavioral systems, treatment effectiveness, and body systems research in medical rehabilitation. Although no specific age group has been targeted, these objectives include research on many problems applicable to the elderly population. For example, in April 1993, the NCMRR announced an ongoing program interest in applications for research funding in the area of restitution of ambulation following disability from neurologic disorders.

Among the tasks that remain for the developing NCMRR is the establishment of a permanent scientific review panel with rehabilitation expertise for the purpose of judging and approving submitted rehabilitation proposals. The scientific peer review panel is essential to the NIH application and funding process; a panel with such expertise is needed to ensure that meritorious rehabilitation proposals will be successful. Prospective or established researchers with an interest in geriatric rehabilitation research will find the NCMRR a welcome addition to funding source options, previously very limited.

FUTURE RESEARCH NEEDS FOR GERIATRIC REHABILITATION RESEARCH

Demographic trends indicate a continued rapid increase in the elderly population due to increasing life expectancy. A corresponding increase in the incidence and prevalence of age-associated chronic diseases is also anticipated. These factors suggest that the number and proportion of individuals at risk for disability in the population will likely increase. The elderly are disproportionately represented among the disabled population. It is estimated that at least 80% of the elderly population will develop one or more impairments, with resultant decreased function (1). According to the National Health Interview Survey, some of the leading causes of disability among noninstitutionalized persons include the following: orthopedic impairments, arthritis, heart disease, hypertension, visual impairments, diabetes, interverterbral disk disorders, nervous disorders, hearing impairments, and cerebrovascular disease (3). These disabling conditions and impairments commonly occur in the elderly. Therefore, the advancement of geriatric rehabilitation with a focus on disability prevention and treatment is imperative. Expanded efforts and interest in the area of geriatric rehabilitation research will facilitate this advancement.

One reason for the paucity of rehabilitation research activity is a relative lack of medical rehabilitation research in general. In an effort to identify and address factors that contribute to this challenge, an interdisciplinary Task Force on Medical Rehabilitation Research was formed under the auspices of the NIH in 1990. Its purpose was to investigate major activities and areas of scientific concentration of rehabilitation professionals and to review issues affecting the field of rehabilitation medicine. According to Task Force findings, inadequate attention has been given to the impact of the disabilities or impairments on the performance or functional capacity of the affected person. The limited amount of research that has been done has concentrated mainly on disability that has resulted from certain types of impairment. One area of major interest to the Task Force was geriatrics. Included in the Task Force findings and further substantiated by our work for this chapter was the absolute paucity of geriatric research.

Among the recommendations made by the Task Force were that studies be conducted to identify the following: the relationship between aging and disability onset, possible markers of functional limitations in the elderly, risk factors of limited mobility including falls, factors affecting functional capacity and actual performance level in the elderly, and effective rehabilitation interventions. Our findings that rehabilitation research has received inadequate support and attention agree with those of the Task Force. As mentioned above, even the most researched topics in our survey of the geriatric and rehabilitation literature, falls and therapeutic exercise, represented only a fraction of the total number of research articles. The amount of research must increase in order to meet the growing scientific and societal demand for expansion and application of this knowledge.

SUMMARY

There is an obvious disparity in the expanding demand for and supply of rehabilitation services to the geriatric population. An increase in both the quality and quantity of research to establish valid and reliable interventions, instruments to measure functional capacity, and innovative clinical trials are desperately needed. This challenge can most effectively be met by collaboration among interdisciplinary teams of clinical and basic scientists, more efficient technology, and consistent financial support of research and education.

References

1. AMA Council on Scientific Affairs: societal effects and other factors affecting health care for the elderly. *Arch Intern Med.* 150:1184–1189, 1990.
2. Sachs GA, Cassel CK. Biomedical research involving human subjects. *Law, Medicine & Health Care.* 18:234–243, 1990.
3. Butler RN. An agenda to extend and enhance life. *Geriatrics.* 46:13–14, 1991. Editorial.
4. Kyes K. NIH releases rehabilitation report. *Rehab Management.* April/May:85–87, 1990.
5. Becker G, Kaufman S. Old age, rehabilitation, and research: a review of the issues. *Gerontologist.* 28:459–468, 1988.
6. Kirby RL. Excellence in rehabilitation through research. *Am J Phys Med Rehabil.* 70(suppl):S7–S8, 1991.
7. Abdellah FG. Public health aspects of rehabilitation of the aged. In: Brody SJ, Ruff GE, eds.: *Aging and Rehabilitation: Advances in the State of the Art.* New York, NY: Springer Publishing Co; 1986:47–61.
8. Moloney TW, Paul B. Building the future of geriatrics. *J Am Geriatr Soc.* 39:425–428, 1991.
9. Grabois M, Fuhrer MJ. Physiatrists views on research. *Am J Phys Med Rehabil.* 67:171–174, 1988.
10. Herbison GJ. Research: ends, setting, environment, activities, resources, creativity, health. *Arch Phys Med Rehabil.* 65:112–114, 1984.
11. Braddom RL. Why is physiatric research important? *Am J Phys Med Rehabil.* 70(suppl):S2–S3, 1991.
12. AGS Public Policy Committee. Geriatric rehabilitation. *J Am Geriatr Soc.* 38:1049–1050, 1990.
13. Stolov WC. Rehabilitation research training. *Arch Phys Med Rehabil.* 65:54, 1984.
14. American Physical Therapy Association environmental statement. *Phys Ther.* 72:378–394, 1992.

43

Outcome Studies and Analysis: Principles of Rehabilitation That Influence Outcome Analysis

M.G. Stineman and C.V. Granger

Outcome analysis asks questions such as: What kind of life is there for the patient following diagnosis and definitive treatment of a condition that has long-term effects on health and functioning? What is left when cure is not possible?

A thoughtful plan of care for any disabled or frail older person must include rehabilitation designed to maximize the independence and life satisfaction of the individual. This is achieved through a team effort to restore, optimize, and conserve an individual's social status, psychologic well-being, and physical functioning. Clinicians may overlook this sequence of priorities, considering it outside the realm of their care responsibilities. One reason for this attitude may lie in the traditional emphasis, at all levels of medical training, on the pathophysiologic and morphologic causation of disease (impairment). This is exemplified by the impairment-based coding schemes used to classify patient diagnoses that are listed in the *International Classification of Diseases (ICD-9-CM)* (1). Yet a classification system that includes causative factors of disease, disability, and handicap needs to distinguish among them because the causative factors of disease are not the same as those of disability or of handicap.

In the case of chronic disease, a classification system must include the concepts of impairment, disability, and handicap, as defined by the World Health Organization (2). Impairment is a composite of anatomic, physiologic, mental, and psychologic deficits at the organ level, as coded in the ICD-9-CM. Disabilities arise as a result of impairment operating at the "person level," representing restrictions in the manner or range of activities considered normal by our functional standards. Disability is measured by activities of daily living (ADL) and instrumental activities of daily living (IADL) scales. Handicaps (resulting from impairment and disability or impairment alone) exist at the societal level. Handicaps manifest as social role disadvantages. Social and cultural factors such as age and sex modify role performance. Since handicaps are influenced by social role norms and social policy, problems related to social disadvantage should be distinguished from problems arising either from activity restrictions (disability) or from organic dysfunction (impairment).

Classification systems for coding and analyzing chronic disease and disability are underdeveloped compared with systems for coding acute pathologic entities. There is a significant variation in the way similar disabilities are identified and in the way the results of rehabilitative interventions are measured. The aging process influences the manifestations of organ impairment, personal disability, and social handicap in a manner that the results of rehabilitation interventions are altered.

PRINCIPALS OF AGING THAT INFLUENCE OUTCOME ANALYSIS

Physiologic Changes with Age

Bortz (3) reviewed the biologic changes attributed to aging and demonstrated the close similarity between most of these changes and those associated with inactivity. For example, the bodily changes of astronauts during periods of weightlessness parallel changes resulting from inactivity, such as enforced bedrest (Table 43.1). Further, Bortz suggests that insofar as changes may be due to disuse, they are then subject to correction. In particular, he states: "Certainly one of the most fundamental measurements that we can apply to ourselves is the maximum oxygen consumption (VO_2max), which ultimately describes the ability of the organism to transport oxygen from the atmosphere through the intermediate conduits, finally to the enzymatic reactions for which it is the spark." (3, p. 1203)

Numerous researchers have shown that the VO_2max

Table 43.1. Changes in Biologic Functions in Response to Aging, Inactivity, Weightlessness, and Exercise[a]

Function	Aging	Inactivity	Weightlessness	Exercise
Vo$_2$ max	Decreased	Decreased		Increased
Cardiac output	Decreased	Decreased		Increased not for older
Systolic BP[b]	Increased		Increased	Decreased
Orthostatic tolerance	Decreased	Decreased	Decreased	Increased
Body water	Decreased	Decreased	Decreased	
RBC[b] mass	Decreased	Decreased	Decreased	
Thrombosis	Increased	Increased		Decreased
Serum lipids	Increased	Increased		Decreased
HD[b] lipoprotein	Increased over age 80			Increased
Lean body mass	Decreased	Decreased	Decreased	
Muscle strength	Decreased	Decreased	Decreased	Increased
Calcium	Decreased	Decreased	Decreased	
Glucose tolerance	Decreased	Decreased		Increased
EEG[b] dominant frequency	Decreased	Decreased		Increased

[a]This table is developed from data presented in Bortz WM. Disuse and aging. *JAMA.* 248:1203–1208, 1982.
[b]BP = blood pressure; RBC = red blood cell; HD = high density; EEG = electroencephalogram.

declines with age (4) at about 1% per year. DeVries (5), Dehn and Bruce (6), and others, however, have shown that a program of physical activity markedly alters this decline. From the data of Hodgeson (7), one can calculate that a conditioning program for the inactive can recapture 40 years' worth of Vo$_2$max (8). It seems unlikely that any future drug treatments or physician-directed techniques will be of such benefit.

Progressive weakness commonly occurs with increasing age. This weakness contributes to a higher incidence of falls and functional deficits. Although some rehabilitation practitioners hesitate to prescribe high resistance exercises to elderly people because of increased cardiac stress, in those who can tolerate it such training has been shown to lead to significant increases in muscle strength, muscle size, and functional mobility up to the age of 96 years (9). Such exercise programs might be used to partly reverse age-related weakness. Many studies attest that the loss of bone mass that occurs with age can be decelerated through increased physical and weight-bearing activities (10). Thus, a major principle in rehabilitation of the older person is that carefully designed activities can alter the rate of decline expected with age and restore function lost through disability.

It is unrealistic to expect the same level of outcome for the oldest as for the youngest, even given apparently similar degrees of impairment. Such expectations may disadvantage older people unless therapeutic means compensate for the aging process itself. Rehabilitation outcome expectation must be scaled to the physiologic and psychologic reserves of the individual.

Impairments in Older People

Arthritic disorders, stroke, hip fracture, and lower limb amputation represent some of the most common disabling conditions in older persons entering rehabilitation programs. Arthritis is one of the most common chronic conditions in the oldest-old (10). Fractures, often associated with osteoporosis, are also extremely common. By the age of 90 years, one in three women will have suffered a fractured hip (10). The majority of stroke patients seen in medical rehabilitation are older. For instance, 76% of 7,905 stroke patients, drawn from the Uniform Data System for Medical Rehabilitation, were 65 years of age or older (11). Seventy-five percent of all amputations occur in those over the age of 65 years (12). Although disabilities resulting from physical trauma, such as spinal cord or head injury are more commonly seen in the young, they also occur in the old. Spinal cord injury at an older age, compared to younger, is more likely to result in more severe functional deficit (13). Approximately 15% of elderly people have some form of dementia (14). Neurologic diseases such as parkinsonism, nutritional problems, pulmonary problems, and cardiac disease are all common in the elderly and influence a patient's ability to tolerate rehabilitation.

Because of the high degree of comorbidity, functional deficits in older people usually arise as a result of complex interactions between multiple disorders. This complexity distinguishes the rehabilitation of older people from that of younger people who more commonly have a single impairment leading to a particular pattern of disability. In the older person, earlier impairments may have had little consequence until the stress of a new disorder upsets his or her ability to compensate. Disability assessment and rehabilitation in older people, therefore, can be more complex.

Age-Related Changes in Social Experience

In older people, habits are long-standing and may be hard to change (15). An individual who has lived a long life as an able-bodied person may view aids, such as walkers needed for safety, as demeaning or unattractive. These attitudes are reinforced by a society in which negative myths and ageist stereotypes are perpetuated by cruel jokes, the mass media, and even developmental and rehabilitation instructional texts that overlook the needs of older people (16). According to Jung, a person's search for meaning in life shifts from quests for independence and belonging in early years to more macroscopic reflections in old age (17). Thus, the older person may tend to look for meaning in past memories rather than investigate new challenges and social experiences. Rehabilitation must reverse the withdrawal that may become pronounced in some people as they age.

The astute clinician must be prepared to diagnose agoraphobia (the fear of leaving familiar surroundings) in appropriate cases. Older people may not want to leave their homes and families. The rehabilitation setting with its many strangers may become frightening and unfamiliar. For rehabilitation to be effective, the patient must accept challenges and look toward the future rather than the past, continued life rather than impending death, gain rather than loss, and activity rather than inactivity. Rehabilitation practitioners must understand and overcome attitudinal stumbling blocks commonly held by patients, families, and rehabilitation staff that can interfere with effective rehabilitation of the elderly person (18).

Changing Institutions and the Status of Older Persons

Economic constraints and major changes in methods of medical reimbursement influence patient entitlement to medical services, including hospital length of stay (LOS). The severity of illness at discharge from hospitals has increased since implementation of the Medicare prospective payment system (PPS), resulting in patients being less functional at hospital discharge (19). In the case of hip fracture, there is evidence that functionally-dependent patients are at greater risk for premature hospital discharge and prolonged institutionalization post-PPS compared to pre-PPS (20). Functional status deficits are associated with increased mortality and greater chance of long-term institutionalization (21–23).

Nearly one quarter (22.9%) of people over the age of 65 years require some assistance in ADLs or IADLs (24, 25). The percentage of ADL-dependent persons jumps sharply in those who are over 85 years of age, and IADL deficits are even more prevalent (26). These oldest-old represent the single fastest-growing segment of the population. Adult children, often the primary caregivers of older parents, also age and often become less able to provide custodial support. Family size is shrinking; and women, the traditional caregivers, are now more frequently in the work force (27). Many elders live alone and do not have support after hospital discharge.

In part because of the implementation of Medicare's PPS based on Diagnosis Related Groups (DRGs) (28), acute hospitalization LOS has fallen, and medical instability at hospital discharge has increased (29). There is some evidence that risk for nursing home placement, particularly in certain high-risk elderly populations, has increased post-PPS (29, 30). A more systematic assessment of the readiness of a patient to leave the hospital, combined with appropriate referral to medical rehabilitation, can forestall some of these problems. Reductions in the LOS of acute hospitalizations are not necessarily detrimental if postacute care services, such as comprehensive inpatient rehabilitation (CIR), are mobilized to enhance recovery of function. CIR, in select cases, can compensate for the falling LOSs occurring on acute hospital services by providing time and treatments specifically designed to assist those with or without caregivers to regain the capacity to function independently.

Medical rehabilitation is becoming an increasingly vital component of health care due to the ever growing numbers of disabled elderly people. Based on 1987 dollars (31), Medicare costs for the oldest-old are projected to increase six-fold by the year 2040. Successful containment of these costs will relate to the medical establishment's ability to minimize the effects of those age-related disorders that lead to disability and the need for long-term care. Postacute care rehabilitation services represent a means to lessen the prevalence of disability in our aging population. The process of rehabilitation involves patient assessment and work toward the achievement of specific goals. Rehabilitation outcome assesses the extent to which those goals are achieved.

SETTINGS FOR REHABILITATING THE OLDER PATIENT

Rehabilitation service delivery should be stratified to allow entry of patients at the level of intensity most appropriate to specific needs. Patients should then undergo rehabilitation in a coordinated, continuous manner. Figure 43.1 shows a simplified level-flow diagram for the case of an elderly individual who experiences functional deficits as a result of hospitalization for acute illness. As shown, the routing of individuals through various rehabilitation settings depends on the answers to

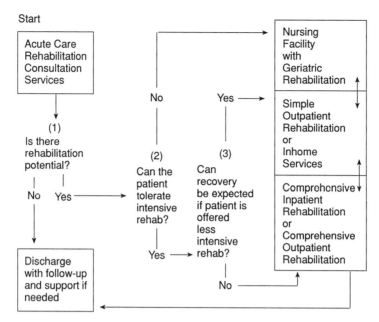

Figure 43.1. Flow chart for entry and movement through geriatric rehabilitation services. Clinical questions (nonboxed elements) are asked in sequence as numbered. Each care phase/intervention mode is boxed. Although outcome should be measured in a comparable way across settings, each setting generates a unique set of expectations relative to this measurement.

a series of questions. Entry criteria, outcome expectation, and costs differ for each intensity level. Mildly disabled patients might be served sufficiently by outpatient rehabilitation services or by inhome services if transportation is a problem. Moderately to severely disabled patients with disability of abrupt onset, such as stroke, amputation, or multiple trauma, usually need the highly coordinated and structured approach of interdisciplinary CIR. Extremely frail or profoundly disabled patients may be more effectively treated in a slower paced but more prolonged rehabilitation program available in a specialized geriatric rehabilitation nursing home unit (32). Regardless of initial intensity, follow-up is as important to rehabilitation as to general medical care. The level of care concept is critical, but few studies compare the relative benefits of each setting. Further research in this area is imperative.

Compared to younger patients, elderly disabled patients tend to receive fewer consultative services while in the inpatient rehabilitation setting. Once discharged to the community, they receive more home support and rehabilitative services (33). This implies that older patients need a more prolonged, but possibly less intensive, rehabilitation approach. In addition to restorative rehabilitation, it is important to consider the need for continuing supportive community services. There is evidence that the use of personal care attendants by elderly disabled people living in the community reduces the need for rehospitalizations (34). Whether in the community or institutional setting, the environment should encourage the achievement and maintenance of the highest possible level of autonomy, independence, and life in-

volvement. The degree to which the environment is socially stimulating will enhance functional performance, independent of capability (35, 36). The functional capacity of an older person who performs consistently below ability will likely deteriorate to the level of performance. An active life-style improves performance, thus maintaining functional capacity longer.

Each rehabilitation setting has its own set of outcome expectations, treatment objectives, and methods of reimbursement. While standards exist for practice in specialized hospitals such as CIRs and geriatric evaluation units (GEUs) within hospitals, care standards are less formalized in other settings. Most research concentrates on CIRs or GEUs. Few studies support rehabilitation and/or geriatric assessment in noninpatient settings. Those that do exist reveal conflicting results (37). It is possible that the treatment effects of outpatient or consultation rehabilitation services in isolation are small, only becoming evident when combined with other phases of rehabilitation. Rehabilitation must operate as a fully coordinated, multiple-intensity effort across all phases of illness and disability.

The important components of care in geriatric rehabilitation programs are similar, regardless of the setting. They include the following:

1. Minimization of the disabling effects of deconditioning by beginning rehabilitation programs as early as possible;
2. Recognition of the needs of elderly persons and development of a true appreciation of their personal worth and dignity;

3. Assurance of contact time between patients and staff in terms of physical and verbal interchange;
4. Development of rapport between the patient/family and rehabilitation team;
5. Balancing treatment modalities, such as range of motion, ambulation, ADL/IADL training, cognitive orientation, and exercises;
6. Prescription of and training in the use of adaptive equipment and environmental adaptations;
7. Patient and caregiver educational programs;
8. Communication between the physician, therapists, and nurses within the rehabilitation setting and those in other care phases, both prerehabilitation and postrehabilitation;
9. Program completion driven by realistic goals coordinated and reinforced within each rehabilitation phase; and
10. Establishment of strong follow-up and coordination between all rehabilitation services and the acute and chronic care phases.

Specific approaches are necessary to encourage the application of rehabilitation principles to all phases of care. They include the following:

1. Identifying patients at risk of functional deterioration;
2. Designing prophylactic programs within hospitals, nursing homes, and the community to conserve function;
3. Managing patients in ambulatory medical care settings who are experiencing early functional limitations, including those related to intellectual decline;
4. If possible, correcting functional limitations due to acute illness in order to prevent them from progressing further;
5. Referring patients with functional limitations that are not readily reversible to a medical rehabilitation facility, the consultation acute hospital rehabilitation service, or outpatient teams;
6. Training lay persons or family caregivers in optimal modes of care designed to reinforce coping behavior and encourage the disabled elderly person to continually maintain self-care skills; and
7. Developing respite and day-care programs for disabled elderly to assist family caregivers and serve as a potential social and therapeutic focus for the older person.

OUTCOME ANALYSIS APPLIED TO GERIATRIC REHABILITATION

Assessment

The core of geriatric rehabilitation is case management. The case manager must use the most perti-

nent information that, in the case of nonacutely ill geriatric patients, relates to assessment of the patient's functional, cognitive, and psychosocial status. While a very large number of variables may be collected, decisions have to be made concerning what to measure or not to measure. Problems of orientation, cognition, communication, and psychosocial adaptation modify physical functioning. Screening tests of varying applicability exist to address these areas (38).

The most objective targets for rehabilitation intervention involve deficits in the ADL functions of selfcare. Particularly in noncurable, therefore chronic conditions, treatment endpoints can be evaluated in terms of outcomes in personal functioning. Depending on patient need and circumstance, rehabilitation goals may be limited to the ADLs or extend into the more complex IADLs. Small gains in the ability to handle tasks of daily living can lead to enormous benefits for the patient and may mean the relief of a considerable burden of care for family members and the community. Standardized assessment instruments are required to quantify functional change in order to justify the program of care by demonstrating its benefit. To fully understand and treat functional deficits, it is important to undertake a thorough neuromuscular examination. Findings on physical examination, however, may not be sufficiently sensitive to identify functional status deficits, such as walking ability (39). Specific ADL and IADL deficits are best identified by directly observing the performance of each functional task.

There are many functional assessment instruments and scales. The presence of IADL deficits only implies a less severe disability. ADL deficits imply more severe disability. The Functional Assessment Screening Questionnaire (FASQ) was developed to identify and follow patients with early or minimal to moderate disability in an ambulatory care setting (40–43). Functions evaluated include selected items of personal care, instrumental household activities, leisure-time/socialization activities, occupationally-related activities, and travelling.

For more disabled persons who experience not only IADL difficulties but also dependencies in the ADLs, the Functional Independence Measure (FIM) was developed through a task force dedicated to finding a national consensus instrument (44, 45). This instrument represents a minimum data set, is easy to apply, and does not require specialized clinical skills. Derived from the Barthel Index (46), the FIM is constructed with seven levels of function—two in which no human helper is required and five in which progressive degrees of help from another person are described. Eighteen items are defined within six areas of functioning: self-care, sphincter management, mobility, locomotion, communication, and social cognition. An individual's functional status in the home setting is a strong indicator of the degree to which services are needed either in the home (47) or in other more formal rehabilitation programs.

Outcome Perspectives

In the World Health Organization's conceptual model, pathology at the organ level generates disability at the person level, which ultimately produces handicap, expressed at the societal level (2). Each of these spheres has different descriptors requiring specific analysis and interventions (Fig. 43.2). Within the domain of handicap, which represents the social manifestations of impairment and disability, there are three primary perspectives: those of the patient, of the family, and of society (Fig. 43.3). Each perspective encompasses many potential goals and domains of measurement. The measurement of rehabilitation outcome in the elderly must encompass not only the magnitude of change in some measurable state, such as functional status, but also the relevance of the particular change across these three perspectives. Any attempt to measure the value of rehabilitation should include all three perspectives. In health services research, outcome utility is theoretically measured as a compromise between increased quality of survival achieved through rehabilitation and the cost of services. Developing a universally meaningful measure of survival quality is made more difficult, but more comprehensive, with the inclusion of all three perspectives.

Rehabilitation from the perspective of the patient enhances personal dignity, autonomy, and independence. The priority is social role fulfillment and independent living achieved through improved functional performance. Role objectives must be consistent with the personal value system inherent in the individual's mood, judgment, and reactions. Role objectives can not be stereotyped, since success of rehabilitation depends on the extent to which the staff sets therapeutic goals congruent with the personal goals of the patient. Factors we designate as important outcome markers are merely proxies for the ultimate objective, which is the enhancement of a patient's life in a way that is meaningful to him or her. In visualizing this perspective, the clinician asks, "How did the patient perceive that his or her life satisfaction changed as a result of the rehabilitation?"

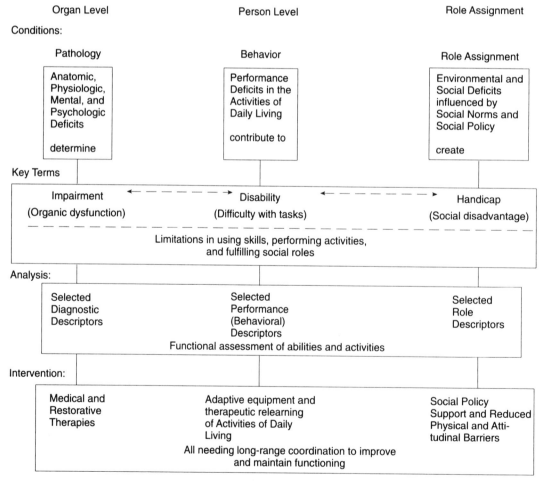

Figure 43.2. Outcome measurement in rehabilitation. Modified from Gresham GE, Granger CV. *Functional Assessment in Rehabilitation Medicine.* P. 20. Copyright 1984 Williams & Wilkins Co., Baltimore, Md.

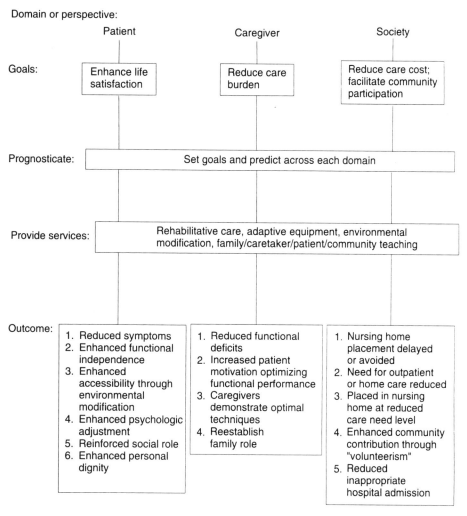

Figure 43.3.   Outcome domains for handicap in the elderly.

Rehabilitation from the perspective of the family or caregiver reduces care burden, generates potential economic savings, and helps redefine a role for the patient within the family. Improvements in function translate into reduced need for care. The central role of functional status in quantifying care burden is reflected by its use in the Resource Utilization Groups (RUGs) classification system for long-term care, used for nursing home reimbursement (48). The research leading to this case-mix system demonstrated that the number of hours of custodial care needed directly relates to severity of the functional status deficit. Reduction of care burden, expressed as hours of care per unit time saved, translates into dollars saved if such care had been purchased. Reduced care burden is achieved in three ways. The first is patient-specific; the patient realizes increased functional status. The second is caregiver-specific; the caregiver learns optimally effective care techniques designed to minimize physical and emotional strain. The third is environment-specific; the physical environment is modified so that the patient functions with greater independence.

While reduced care burden can be expressed monetarily, it is difficult to express the family's value of increased physical and social functioning in dollars (49). There may be an enhanced capability of the patient to assume former or new roles within the family. In the case of elderly persons, such roles may include home management in addition to the physical or psychologic support of other members of the family. Patterns of care and support optimally should be reciprocal and symbiotic. Many older people can contribute to their families and communities.

From the perspective of society, rehabilitation generates potential economic savings and helps reestablish individuals within the social mainstream. Reduction of care burden also translates into economic savings by reducing the dollars needed to care for the person. The greatest savings occur when a patient achieves sufficient functional recovery to avoid permanent institutionalization. Thus, the cost of rehabilitation can be considered an investment yielding future savings.

Approximately 70% of Medicare patients admitted to CIR are discharged to their own homes following rehabilitation (50). Lehmann and colleagues (51) estimated that if the rehabilitation of stroke patients avoids the need for permanent institutionalization, assuming institutionalization would have been permanent, then cost of rehabilitation would be recouped in 21.5 months by reduced expenditure for nursing homes. The degree of functional impairment and the availability of adequate social, environmental, and economic supports interact to determine the likelihood of home placement. The more disabled a person is, the greater the external support needed for community living. At some level of functional severity, the economic and/or personal costs of maintaining an individual in the community equals the costs of institutionalization. The relative costs of alternative care strategies, while remaining sensitive to the individual's personal desires, must be considered in placement issues. The degree of independence needed for community discharge depends directly on the household and community social supports available.

Outcome Expectations for Older Persons

Outcome and its prediction can only be viewed implicitly as representing the cumulative impact of many events, not just that of the rehabilitation intervention (52). Without employing an experimental design, changes that occur during rehabilitation cannot be absolutely attributed solely to that intervention. There are few well-designed, randomized control trials of CIR. Designing such experiments when services already exist raises ethical issues, since in such studies individuals who would otherwise be entitled to services would be denied. In contrast, it has been possible to experimentally test the effectiveness of GEUs, since, until recently, they did not represent the usual care standard. Because GEUs incorporate certain rehabilitation principles into a somewhat different setting, these analyses give insight into the effectiveness of rehabilitation in general. Rubenstein and colleagues (53) demonstrated that patients randomized to a Veterans Administration GEU had significantly lower mortality, less chance of being discharged to a nursing home, fewer rehospitalizations, and were more likely to realize functional improvement, compared to controls receiving usual acute hospital treatment. Applegate et al (37) had similar findings studying a GEU in a community rehabilitation hospital. However, the effect of the community GEU on patient mortality and function was less marked. This was in part attributed to lack of follow-up care in a specialized geriatric clinic. The effect of rehabilitative home services on functional status has not been conclusively demonstrated since results of trials have been inconsistent (37, 54).

There are numerous descriptive studies of CIR outcome. Studies across all diagnoses almost universally demonstrate that patients, regardless of age, can improve functionally during CIR. Kauffman, Albright, and Wagner (55), studying a cohort of elderly hip fracture patients over the age of 90 years, found that even some of the most elderly can achieve gains with appropriate rehabilitation. Although older amputees more frequently have complicating conditions—such as cardiac or peripheral vascular disease—than do younger amputees, many do extremely well in prosthetic training (12). Below-knee amputees, even if bilateral, improve more than above-knee amputees. Tabuena and colleagues (56) found that, even in the case of elderly patients with limited stamina, a large proportion of above-knee amputees fitted with ultra light polypropylene prostheses could learn to ambulate independently. Watson (13) reported functional gains in some elderly quadraplegics up to the age of 87 years.

Most studies suggest that elderly people are functionally less resilient (57–61). Some describe little, if any, difference in the aged (62, 63). There is evidence that elderly people experience a longer recovery than do younger persons, but that they can eventually make comparable recoveries (60). There is a strong association between undiagnosed depression and failure to recover premorbid function in the elderly (64). Although severe mental status deficits represent a relative contraindication to rehabilitation, some patients demonstrate improvements in mental status once in the stimulating environment of geriatric rehabilitation (65). Transient metabolic or pharmacologic disturbances can generate reversible mental status deficits. Pseudodementia, depression, or transient metabolic disturbances can easily masquerade as dementia. The rehabilitation potential of elderly patients with misdiagnosed cognitive limitation is easily missed.

Prospective Outcome Indicators

The capacity to predict outcome based on a patient's initial presentation underlies medical practice. Knowledge of those patient characteristics that are associated with various outcomes can enhance clinical decision-making. Stroke has been the most frequently studied impairment. Through outcome analysis we ask: what are the outcomes and benefits of caring for disability consequent to hemiparesis that justify large expenditures? What influences do age and physiologic parameters (including impairment) have on functional outcome?

From a review of the literature, Dombovy and colleagues (66) created a set of factors that appear related to functional outcome after stroke. Poor outcome is associated with coma at onset, incontinence 2 weeks poststroke, poor cognitive function, severe hemiparesis, no motor return within 1 month, previous stroke, perceptual-spatial disorders, significant cardiovascular disease, large deep lesions on computed tomography (CT) scan, and nonfocal neurologic signs. Other possibly negative factors are hemisensory deficit, left hemiparesis, advanced age, language disorders, lack of a close family member, poor financial resources, and more than 30 days from onset of stroke. Jongbloed (67) reviewed 33 studies and identified that the following factors had adverse prognostic effects: older age, history of prior stroke, urinary and bowel incontinence, and visual-spatial deficits. Functional outcome was not shown to be related to either sex or hemisphere of stroke. The functional status admission score was a strong predictor of discharge functional status, but its relationship to improvement in function was unclear. Findings regarding the prognostic value of severity of paralysis and onset-admission delay were ambiguous.

When making a prognosis, the clinician considers not just the isolated list of prognostic indicators, but rather judges how the many diagnostic elements interact to influence outcome. To simulate the process of clinical decision-making statistically, it is necessary to use multivariable techniques such as regression modeling. Based on patient characteristics, these statistical techniques can generate either an estimate of outcome, such as a discharge functional status score, or the probability of an event occurring, such as home discharge. Although regression analyses are extremely powerful, there are many methodologic issues that need to be considered in the development and application of outcome models (68). Statistical models of outcome have not yet shown high enough correlations between estimated and actual occurrences to predict individual outcomes. Variables found predictive of functional outcome vary somewhat depending on the definitions used, the influence of the other factors being considered, and the statistical methods employed to drive the model. Statistical relevance, a criterion used in model building, sometimes differs from clinical relevance. A good model must be both clinically relevant and statistically sound. Such models will eventually become valuable adjuncts to rehabilitation management and research.

Models will make it possible to identify combinations of patient characteristics that are relevant to particular rehabilitation outcomes. For instance in stroke, four items appear repeatedly in various combinations as prognostic indicators of function at discharge from rehabilitation and/or follow-up. These elements, easily obtained on history and physical examination, include upper extremity motor function, truncal stability, continence, and proprioception (69–75). In addition to these physical examination items, cognitive factors play an important role in stroke outcome. A model based on the performance on a series of psychologic tests designed specifically to examine perceptuomotor function explains a moderate portion of variance in the stroke patient's Barthel Index at discharge from rehabilitation (76).

Applying regression analysis to study hip fracture patients, Jette and colleagues (60) found that increased age, intertrochanteric fracture, discharge to nursing home, and poor premorbid emotional status were associated with poor functional outcome at 6 months postdischarge. A second analysis indicated that increased contact with one's social network, avoidance of rehospitalization, and good cognitive status were associated with improved recovery of walking ability at 1 year posthospital discharge (61).

Like functional outcome, the likelihood of home placement is in part predictable. Granger and colleagues (77, 78) reported the results of a study of outcomes in stroke rehabilitation for 539 patients from 17 inpatient rehabilitation facilities. A logistic regression analysis was carried out through a maximum likelihood procedure. After adjusting for age, sex, and hemiparesis on admission to hospital rehabilitation, the odds ratio showed that a person with independent bowel control had a 3.2 times greater odds of living in the community compared to a person dependent in that function. An individual independent in either bowel control and eating or bowel control and grooming was approximately six times more likely to be living in the community than a person dependent in those functions. An individual independent in bowel control, eating, and grooming had a better than 10-fold increased odds of living in the community at 6-month follow-up. The odds ratios are illustrated in Table 43.2. There is also strong evidence that married patients are more likely to achieve home discharge (79–81). The protective capacity of marriage appears particularly strong for males.

Economic Issues

Because of limited resources, today's health care policy is increasingly driven by the dual agendas of cost-containment and service justification through outcome analysis. Methods of reimbursement increasingly dictate entitlement, and thus, economics can override clinical criteria in deciding who gets admitted to rehabilitation. The restructuring of heath care in the United States mandates the development of methodologies to monitor the influences of changing health care policies on management decisions and patient outcomes (82). Ellwood (83) defines outcome management as "a technology of patient experience designed to help patients, payors, and providers make rational medical care-related choices based on better insight into the effect of these choices on the patient's life." Particularly in the case of elderly people

Table 43.2. Odds Ratio for Living in the Community at Follow-up for Individuals Functioning Independently in Bowel Control, Eating, Bladder Control, and Grooming vs Individuals Dependent in These Activities at Admission[a]

Independent Activities	Odds Ratio	Confidence Intervals[b]
Bowel control	3.2	3.1, 3.3
Bowel control and eating	6.0	5.7, 6.2
Bowel control and grooming	6.2	5.9, 6.4
Bowel control, eating and grooming	11.5	11.0, 12.1
Bowel control, eating, grooming and bladder control	14.1	13.3, 14.9

[a] From Granger CV, Hamilton BB, Gresham GE, Kramer AA. The stroke rehabilitation outcome study, Part I: general description. *Arch Phys Med Rehabil.* 69:102, 1988.
[b] Confidence intervals are at the 0.95 level.

approaching the end of their lives, it is important to seek a balance between medical approaches designed to prolong life and those intended to enhance life quality.

The specific methods of reimbursement differ from region to region. In general, to receive Medicare reimbursement, inpatient or outpatient goals must be considered functionally significant. Correcting an asymptomatic gait disturbance, such as recurvatum of the knee, might be difficult to justify in the very-old person since it would take approximately 20 years of walking for degenerative changes to occur. Meal preparation skill might be more easy to justify since this capacity directly impacts on independence (84). It is likely that modes of reimbursement will change in the near future.

Existing case-mix measures are inadequate for rehabilitation because they were developed on different patient populations. The clinician and policy analyst need to be aware of the potential incentives created by any proposed changes in reimbursement. Certain case-mix measures could generate incentives with the potential to erode care equity. For example, the concept of quality-adjusted life years (QUALYs) represents a recently proposed method of cost-effectiveness analysis for general medicine. QUALYs compare the relative worth of medical procedures or services by assigning a single numeric value weighed by expected survival time and quality of life. QUALYs imply that the lives of older people and disabled people have less value. The former have fewer years to live, and the latter presumably have a lower quality of life. However, if used to allocate rehabilitation resources, QUALYs may be detrimental to the oldest and most disabled. This method might appear well-suited for rehabilitation, since it incorporates a concept of life quality. The concept that the old have less time to benefit (lower priority for care) is central. The value of living or quality of life for the individual, given a particular state of health, is measurable and can be inferred from community opinion developed through consensus (85).

Quality of outcome must not be overlooked in favor of placement speed. In one setting, where prospective payment was applied to CIR services, LOS decreased, but 64% more patients were discharged to

nursing homes compared to before initiation of prospective payment (86). There is evidence that the PPS, as designed by Medicare for acute hospitalizations, is an inadequate method of reimbursing for rehabilitation. The use of rehabilitation resources is better justified by functional status at presentation (87, 88). Johnston and Miller (89) analyzed the impact of the "three hour rule" on rehabilitation outcome. This policy mandates that patients in rehabilitation units receive 3 hours of therapy daily. They found that there was increased cost but no measurable benefit. This underscores the importance of grading service intensity to the needs of patients rather than to a legislated standard.

Medical accountability requires outcome analysis. A useful approach to the development of cost-effective care is to examine variations in both the process and results of rehabilitation through analyses of large databases. Through relating variations in rehabilitation outcome to different care approaches, professionals can design maximally cost-effective services, while avoiding economic incentives that are detrimental to patient benefit. Rehabilitation practices based on scientific principles that explain the individual's potential for benefit will be cost-responsible. Through research and outcome analyses, rehabilitation professionals must develop methods to justify services. Otherwise, external agencies will legislate cost reduction strategies insensitive to the subtleties of clinical knowledge. The development of appropriate modes of quality assurance and reimbursement strategies must be deliberate, careful, and metered (90).

SUMMARY

In conclusion, approaching a person from a functional perspective means analyzing problems using organic, psychologic, and social circumstances in combination to account for limitations in function. The therapeutic plan for reducing these limitations must attempt to preserve the person's appropriate roles and activities by means of medical and physical restoration, psychologic training, and the bolstering of social supports. This type of approach is appropriate in the care of elderly patients because their illnesses are commonly the result of intertwined organic, psychologic, and social factors. To achieve fulfillment, one's life experience must extend beyond oneself and include active participation in family activities and community life (16, 91). Recapturing this sense of active participation enhances self-concept. The result should be a widening and enrichment of the individual's life. Each older person has woven a unique life tapestry of physical growth, physical decline, illness, intimacies, experiences, dreams, losses, defeat, and achievement. His or her style of coping has been developed and seasoned through the decades and will influence the way in which he or she responds to functional disability and rehabilitation. The geriatric rehabilitation team needs to adjust its approaches to optimize the motivation of patients who use many different coping strategies. As yet, there is no outcome analysis system that can account for the myriad of outcome possibilities.

References

1. Practice Management Information Corporation. *International Classification of Diseases, 9th Revision, Clinical Modification (ICD-9-CM.* Los Angeles, Calif: PMIC; 1991.
2. World Health Organization. *International Classification of Impairments, Disabilities, and Handicaps (ICIDH).* Geneva: World Health Organization; 1980.
3. Bortz WM. Disuse and aging. *JAMA.* 248:1203, 1982.
4. Lakatta E. Alterations in the cardiovascular system that occur in advanced age. *Fed Proc.* 38:163, 1979.
5. DeVries H. Physiologic effects of an exercise training regimen upon men aged 52–88. *J Gerontol.* 25:325, 1970.
6. Dehn MM, Bruce RA. Longitudinal variations in maximal oxygen uptake with age and acivity. *J Appl Physiol.* 33:805, 1972.
7. Hodgeson J. *Age and Aerobic Capacity of Urban Midwestern Males.* Minneapolis, Minn: University of Minnesota; 1971. Thesis.
8. Bortz WM. Effect of exercise on aging—effect of aging on exercise. *J Am Geriatr Soc.* 28(2):49–51, 1980.
9. Fiatarone MA, Marks EC, Ryan ND, et al. High-intensity strength training in nonagenarians. Effects on skeletal muscle. *JAMA.* 263(22):3029–3034, 1990.
10. Fiatarone MA, Evans WJ. Exercise in the oldest old. *Top Geriatr Rehabil.* 5(2):63–77, 1990.
11. Granger CV, Hamilton BB, Fiedler RC. Discharge outcomes after stroke rehabilitation. *Stroke.* 23(7):978–982, 1992.
12. Clark GS, Blue B, Bearer JB. Rehabilitation of the elderly amputee. *Clin Conf.* 31(7):439, 1983.
13. Watson N. Pattern of spinal cord injury in the elderly. *Paraplegia.* 14:36, 1976.
14. Terry RD, Katzman R. Senile dementia of the Alzheimer type. *Ann Neurol.* 14:497, 1983.
15. Liang MH, Partridge AJ, Eaton H, et al. Rehabilitation management of homebound elderly with locomotor disability. *Clin Geriatr Med.* 4(2):431–439, 1988.
16. Benedict RC, Ganikos ML. Coming to terms with ageism in rehabilitation. *J Rehabil.* 47(4):10–18, 1981.
17. Bozarth JD. The rehabilitation process and older people. *J Rehabil.* 47(4):28–30, 1981.
18. Hesse KA, Campion EW, Karamouz N. Attitudinal stumbling blocks to geriatric rehabilitation. *J Am Geriatr Soc.* 32:747, 1984.
19. Rogers WH, Draper D, Kahn KL, et al. Quality of care before

20. Fitzgerald JF, Fagan LF, Tierney WM, et al. Changing patterns of hip fracture care before and after implementation of the prospective payment system. *JAMA.* 258(2):218–221, 1987.
21. Narain P, Rubenstein LZ, Wieland GD, et al. Predictors of immediate and 6-month outcomes in hospitalized elderly patients. The importance of functional status. *J Am Geriatr Soc.* 36:775–783, 1988.
22. Morris JN, Sherwood S, Gutkin CE. Inst-Risk II: an approach to forecasting relative risk of future institutional placement. *Health Serv Res.* 23(4):511–536, 1988.
23. Pompei P, Charlson ME, Douglas RG. Clinical assessments as predictors of one year survival after hospitalization: implications for prognostic stratification. *J Clin Epidemiol.* 41(3):275–284, 1988.
24. National Center for Health Statistics. *The 1979 Health Interview Survey.* Hyattsville, MD: NCHS; 1979.
25. Department of Health and Human Services. *The 1982 Long-Term Care Survey.* Washington, DC: DHHS; 1982.
26. LaPlante MP. *Data on Disability from the National Health Interview Survey, 1983–1985.* An InfoUse Report. Washington, DC: National Institute on Disability and Rehabilitation Research; 1988.
27. Brody EM. Parent care as a normative family stress. *Gerontologist.* 25(1):19–29, 1985.
28. Fetter RB, Shin Y, Freeman JL, Averill RF, Thompson JD. Case mix definition by diagnosis-related groups. *Med Care.* 18:1–53, 1980.
29. Kahn KL, Draper D, Keeler EB, et al. *The Effects of the DRG-Based Prospective Payment System on Quality of Care for Hospitalized Medicare Patients.* Santa Monica, Calif; RAND, 1992. R-3931-HCFA.
30. Fitzgerald JF, Moore PS, Dittus RS. The care of elder patients with hip fracture. Changes since implementation of the prospective payment system. *N Engl J Med.* 319:1392–1397, 1988.
31. Schneider EL, Guralnick JM. The aging of America: impact on health care costs. *JAMA.* 263(17):2335–2340, 1990.
32. Adelman RD, Marron K, Libow LS, et al. A community-oriented geriatric rehabilitation unit in a nursing home. *Gerontologist.* 27(2):143–146, 1987.
33. Stineman M, Maschiocchi C, Brody SJ. An age-based comparison of service utilization patterns by rehabilitation patients. *Gerontologist.* 26(Special Issue):22A, 1986. Abstract.
34. Townsend J, Piper M, Dyer S, et al. Reduction in hospital readmission stay of elderly patients by a community based hospital discharge scheme: a randomised controlled trial. *Br Med J.* 297(6647):544–547, 1988.
35. Avorn J, Langer E. Induced disability in nursing home patients: a controlled trial. *J Am Geriatr Soc.* 30(6):397–400, 1982.
36. Kellman HR, Lilienfeld AM, Gifford AJ. An experiment in the rehabilitation of nursing home patients. In *Chronic Disease and Public Health.* Baltimore, Md: Johns Hopkins Press; 1966.
37. Applegate WB, Miller ST, Graney MJ, et al. A randomized, controlled trial of a geriatric assessment unit in a community rehabilitation hospital. *N Engl J Med.* 322(22):1572–1578, 1990.
38. Applegate WB, Blass JP, Williams TF. Instruments for the functional assessment of older patients. *N Engl J Med.* 322(17):1207–1214, 1990.
39. Tinetti ME, Ginter SF. Identifying mobility dysfunctions in elderly patients. Standard neuromuscular examination or direct assessment? *JAMA.* 259(8):1190–1193, 1988.
40. Granger CV, Gresham GE, eds.. *Functional Assessment in Rehabilitation Medicine.* Baltimore, Md: Williams & Wilkins; 1984.
41. Granger CV, Seltzer GB, Fishbein CF. *Primary care of the Functionally Disabled.* Philadelphia, PA: J.B. Lippincott; 1987.
42. Seltzer GB, Granger CV, Wineberg D. Functional assiessment: bridge between family and rehabilitation medicine within an ambulatory practive. *Arch Phys Med Rehabil.* 63:453, 1982.

43. Millard RW. Functional assessment screening tool questionnaire: application for evaluating pain-related disability. *Arch Phys Med Rehabil.* 70:308–307, 1989.

44. Granger CV, Hamilton BB, Keith RA, et al. Advances in functional assessment for medical rehabilitation. *Top Geriatr Rehabil.* 1(3):59, 1986.

45. Hamilton BB, Granger CV, Sherwin FS, et al. A uniform natioanl data system for medical rehabilitation. In: Fuhrer MJ, ed. *Rehabilitation Outcomes: Analysis and Measurement.* Baltimore, Md: Brookes; 1987.

46. Mahoney FL, Barthel DW. Functional evaluation: Barthel Index. *Md State Med J.* 14:61–65, 1965.

47. Fortinsky RH, Granger CV, Seltzer GB. The use of functional assessment in understanding home care needs. *Med Care.* 19(5):489–497, 1981.

48. Fries BE, Cooney LM. Resource utilization groups. A patient classification system for long-term care. *Med Care.* 23(2):110–122, 1985.

49. Bennett AE. Cost-effectiveness of rehabilitation for the elderly: preliminary results from the community hospital research program. *Gerontologist.* 20(3):284, 1980.

50. Gornick M, Hall MJ. Trends in Medicare use of post-hospital care. *Health Care Financing Rev.* Ann Suppl:27, 1988.

51. Lehmann JF, Delateur BJ, Fowler RS, et al. Stroke: does rehabilitation affect outcome? *Arch Phys Med Rehabil.* 56:375, 1975.

52. Fuhrer MJ. *Rehabilitation Outcomes: Analysis and Measurement.* Baltimore, Md: Brookes; 1987.

53. Rubenstein LZ, Josephson KR, Wieland GD, et al. Effectiveness of a geriatric evaluation: a randomized clinical trial. *N Engl J Med.* 311(26):1664–1670, 1984.

54. Liang MH, Partridge AJ, Gall V, et al. Evaluation of rehabilitation component of home care for homebound elderly. *Am J Prev Med.* 2(1):30–34, 1986.

55. Kauffman TL, Albright L, Wagner C. Rehabilitation outcomes after hip fracture in persons 90 years old and older. *Arch Phys Med Rehabil.* 68:369–371, 1987.

56. Tabuena A, Vachranukunkiet T, Idiculla AA, et al. Clinical experience with ultra lightweight polypropylene prosthesis for geriatric above-knee amputee. *Arch Phys Med Rehabil.* 65:624, 1984. Abstract.

57. Carey RG, Seibert JH, Posavac EJ. Who makes the most progress in inpatient rehabilitation? An analysis of functional gain. *Arch Phys Med Rehabil.* 69:337–341, 1988.

58. DeLisa JA, Miller RM, Melnick RR, et al. Stroke rehabilitation: Part I. Cognitive deficits and prediction of outcome. *Am Fam Phys.* 26(5):207–214, 1982.

59. Groswasser Z, Cohen M, Costeff H. Rehabilitation outcome after anoxic brain damage. *Arch Phys Med Rehabil.* 70(3):186–188, 1989.

60. Jette AM, Harris BA, Cleary PD, et al. Functional recovery after hip fracture. *Arch Phys Med Rehabil.* 68:735–740, 1987.

61. Magaziner J, Simonsic EM, Kashner TM, et al. Predictors of functional recovery one year following hospital discharge for hip fracture: a prospective study. *J Gerontology* 45(3):M101–M107, 1990.

62. Feigenson JS. Outcome studies and guidelines for alternative levels of care. Current concepts of CBVD. *Stroke.* 12(3):372–375, 1980.

63. Heinemann AW, Roth EJ, Cichowski K, et al. Multivariate analysis of improvement and outcome following stroke rehabilitation. *Arch Neurol.* 44:1167–1172, 1987.

64. Harris RE, Mion LC, Patterson MB, et al. Severe illness in older patients: the association between depressive disorders and functional dependency during the recovery phase. *J Am Geriatr Soc.* 36(10):890–896, 1988.

65. Liem PH, Chernoff R, Carter WJ. Geriatric rehabilitation unit: a 3-year outcome evaluation. *J Gerontology.* 41(1):44–50, 1986.

66. Dombovy ML, Basford JR, Whisnant JP, et al. Disability and use of rehabilitation service following stroke in Rochester, Minnesota, 1975-1979. *Stroke.* 18(5):830–836, 1987.

67. Jongbloed L. Prediction of function after stroke: a critical review. *Stroke.* 17(4):765–776, 1986.

68. Merbitz C, Morris J, Grip JC. Ordinal scales and foundations of misinference. *Arch Phys Med Rehabil.* 70:308–312, 1989.

69. Jimenez J, Morgan PP. Predicting improvement in stroke patients referred for inpatient rehabilitation. *Can Med Assoc. J.* 121:1481–1484, 1979.

70. Loewen SC, Anderson BA. Predictors of stroke outcome using objective measurement scales. *Stroke.* 21(1):78–81, 1990.

71. Prescott RJ, Garraway MB, Akhtar AJ. Predicting functional outcome following acute stroke using a standard clinical examination. *Stroke.* 13(5):641–647, 1982.

72. Sandin KJ, Smith BS. The measure of balance in sitting in stroke rehabilitation prognosis. *Stroke.* 21(1):82–86, 1990.

73. Shah S, Vanclay RF, Cooper B. Efficiency, effectiveness, and duration of stroke rehabilitation. *Stroke.* 21(2):241–246, 1990.

74. Smith ME, Garraway WM, Smith DL, et al. Therapy impact on functional outcome in a controlled *trial* of stroke rehabilitation. *Arch Phys Med Rehabil.* 63:21–24, 1982.

75. Wade DT, Skilbeck CE, Hewer RL. Predicting Barthel ADL score at 6 months after an acute stroke. *Arch Phys Med Rehabil.* 64:24, 1983.

76. Novack TA, Haban G, Graham K, et al. Prediction of stroke rehabilitation outcome from psychologic screening. *Arch Phys Med Rehabil.* 68:729, 1987.

77. Granger CV, Hamilton BB, Gresham GE, Kramer AA. The stroke rehabilitation outcome study, Part I: general description. *Arch Phys Med Rehabil.* 69:506–509, 1988.

78. Granger CV, Hamilton BB, Gresham GE, Kramer AA. The stroke rehabilitation outcome study, Part II: relative merits of the Barthel Index score and a four-item subscore in predicting patient outcomes. *Arch Phys Med Rehabil.* 70:100–103, 1989.

79. DeJong G, Branch LG. Predicting the stroke patient's ability to live independently. *Stroke.* 13(5):648–655, 1982.

80. Kelly-Hayes M, Wolf PA, Kannel WB, et al. Factors influencing survival and need for institutionalization following stroke: the Framingham Study. *Arch Phys Med Rehabil.* 69:415–418, 1988.

81. Lehmann JF, DeLateur BJ, Fowler RS, et al. Stroke rehabilitation: outcome and prediction. *Arch Phys Med Rehabil.* 56:383, 1975.

82. Tarlov AR, Ware JE, Greenfield S, et al. The Medical Outcomes Study: an application of methods for monitoring the results of medical care. *JAMA.* 262(7):925–930, 1989.

83. Ellwood PM. Special report. Shattuck Lecture—outcomes management: a technology of patient experience. *N Engl J Med.* 318(23):1549–1556, 1988.

84. Felsenthal G. Rehabilitating older patients: primary care evaluation, treatment, and resources. *Geriatrics.* 44(1):81–90, 1989.

85. LaPuma J, Lawlor EF. Quality-adjusted life-years. Ethical implications for physicians and policy makers. *JAMA.* 263(21):2917–2920, 1990.

86. Evans RL, Hendricks RD, Bishop DS, et al. Prospective payment for rehabilitation: effects on hospital readmission, home care, and placement. *Arch Phys Med Rehabil.* 71(5):291–294, 1990.

87. Hosek S, Kane R, Garney M, et al. *Charges and Outcomes for Rehabilitative Care: Implications for the Prospective Payment System.* Santa Monica, Calif: RAND Corporation; 1986. R-3424-HCFA.

88. Stineman MG, Williams SV. Predicting inpatient rehabilitation length of stay. *Arch Phys Med Rehabil.* 71:881–887, 1990.

89. Johnston MV, Miller LS. Cost-effectiveness of the Medicare three-hour regulation. *Arch Phys Med Rehabil.* 67:581–585, 1986.

90. Epstein AM. The outcomes movement—Will it get us where we want to go? *N Engl J Med.* 323(4):266–270, 1990.

91. Abdellah FG. Public health aspects of rehabilitation of the aged. In: Brody SJ, Ruff GE, eds. *Aging and Rehabilitation: Advances in the State of the Art.* New York, NY: Springer; 1986.

44

Medical Education in Geriatric Rehabilitation

Arthur M. Gershkoff

Contemplate the future of the health needs for the disabled elderly. In the next 50 years, the number of persons over 85 years old will triple to about 15,000,000. More than one third of these oldest-old currently need assistance in basic activities of daily living (ADLs) or mobility. The incidence of stroke and other disabling diseases may decline, but to what degree? The total numbers of persons surviving stroke, multisystem disease, hip fracture from falls, and other complex conditions will inevitably soar. Who will evaluate patients for rehabilitative services and ensure that they are provided fairly and appropriately? How can these services be provided most cost-effectively and efficiently, reaching the widest possible population that might benefit from them?

As the number of elderly continues to grow, it is imperative that our society increase the numbers of physicians interested and effective in dealing with the problems of this population. Critical areas of education, where knowledge and skills in rehabilitation as applied to older persons are essential, include the following: assessment of the functional status of individuals; assessment of the potential of acutely or chronically ill persons to improve function; recognition of the effect of medical, cognitive, and pharmacologic problems on the rehabilitation process; and evaluation of services that promote maximum functional recovery.

The above-mentioned critical areas apply to three major populations of disabled elderly including persons with acute, self-limited illnesses; those who survive acute illnesses, though with residual permanent impairments; and those with congenital disorders or impairments acquired in younger years. Additionally, geriatric rehabilitation includes prevention or slowing of functional decline in elderly persons with mild, minor musculoskeletal disorders, as well as the prescription and supervision of physical fitness programs for the well elderly (1).

This chapter discusses resources available to aid medical students and physicians in developing such knowledge and skills and in gaining exposure to the elderly in various rehabilitation settings. Methods for developing critical values and attitudes about the care of geriatric patients are also examined. The disciplines of geriatric internal medicine and family practice (geriatric medicine) and physical medicine and rehabilitation (PM&R) both offer significant resources to the medical community for these purposes.

RESIDENCY AND FELLOWSHIP TRAINING REQUIREMENTS

The Directory of Graduate Medical Education Programs (2) specifies topics related to geriatric rehabilitation in the training program requirements for several specialties and subspecialties. PM&R residencies are required to include general training in diseases, impairments, and functional limitations seen in older populations. Additional specific topics encompass the common disease processes that result in functional impairment in the elderly. In a recent survey of PM&R residency training programs, Anderson and Felsenthal (3) found that residents averaged 8.8 weeks of exposure to inpatient geriatric rehabilitation services and 5.9 weeks of outpatient geriatric experience. Robinson and associates (4) found that, while only 22% of PM&R programs have required rotations on geriatric rehabilitation units, 49% of patients seen by residents inpatient rehabilitation units are 65 years or older.

The "Special Requirements for Programs in Geriatric Medicine," developed jointly by the American Board of Family Practice and the American Board of Internal Medicine for postresidency geriatric medicine fellowships, stipulate that fellows acquire specific knowledge and skill in geriatric rehabilitation, including those aspects applicable to patients with orthopedic, rheumatologic, cardiac, and neurologic impairments (2). Further requirements specify familiarity with the use of physical medicine modalities, exercise, functional activities, assistive devices, environmental modification, patient and family education, and psychosocial and recreational counseling. Like PM&R, geriatric medicine training includes the development of team leadership skills. Interaction with PM&R is not required as part of training, but PM&R is a specialty that is listed as desirable as a part of the patient care team. A survey of geriatric medicine fellowships in 1982 revealed that 44% of the programs included rehabilitation inpatient units as training sites (5).

Educational objectives in geriatric rehabilitation for geriatric medicine fellows have been further specified within guidelines developed jointly by the American Academy of Physical Medicine and Rehabilitation and the Education Committee of the American Geriatrics Society (6) (Table 44.1). Similarly, a survey of PM&R residency program directors for the American Board of Physical Medicine and Rehabilitation has produced a list of "Topics in Geriatrics for Residents in PM&R." (7) (Table 44.2). While not a formal part of PM&R residency requirements, this list has served as a guide to some PM&R departments in structuring the clinical and didactic training in geriatric issues for their residents.

Neurologists, orthopedists, general internists, and rheumatologists also have training requirements involving rehabilitation. Neurology residents are required to have opportunities to learn the basic principles of physical medicine and rehabilitation and disorders of aging as they affect the nervous system. Orthopedic surgery residents are required to study rehabilitation of neurologic injury, orthotics, and prosthetics. Internal medicine residents are expected to develop familiarity with utilization of rehabilitation services, usually through consultations with rehabilitation professionals on non-internal medicine rotations. Knowledge of physical and occupational therapy is a requirement for rheumatology subspecialty training (2).

Therefore, medical students and residents of other specialties may learn about geriatric rehabilitation through PM&R departments with residencies or internal medicine or family practice departments with geriatric medicine fellowship programs. Other experiences may be available through neurology, rheumatology, or orthopedic surgery departments in specific settings.

EDUCATIONAL MATERIALS

Knowledge in PM&R and geriatric medicine is interrelated; each provides expertise helpful to the other. Geriatric medicine textbooks abound and offer thorough discussions of medical problems frequently encountered on the rehabilitation unit. Usually, at least one chapter covers general rehabilitation issues. The major PM&R textbooks include general chapters on geriatric rehabilitation. Other chapters involve rehabilitation techniques and technologies appropriate for the elderly, as well as the rehabilitation of disease processes.

Table 44.1. Training Objectives: Training of Geriatrics Fellows in Rehabilitation[a]

1. The trainee will be familiar with methods used to assess patients with physical impairments and disability, including screening musculoskeletal and neuromuscular examinations and the appropriate use of instruments that measure ADL's and IADL's; and to assess the extent of the disability and the patient's remaining functional capacity. The extent of deterioration by comparison with previous capacity will be determined, using historical information from the patient and family.

2. The trainee will be able to evaluate the patient's psychosocial setting, cognitive function, affect, and communication ability, and to determine the effect these may have on rehabilitation and discharge potential.

3. The trainee will be familiar with the professional ability, expertise, and specific role of each member of the rehabilitation team: physiatist, physical therapist, occupational therapist, speech pathologist, social worker, psychologist, and nurse. As in other geriatrics settings, the trainee will work with other team members in regularly scheduled conferences.

4. The trainee will learn how to develop, review, and revise each patient's rehabilitation goals, including discharge planning, in consultation with other team members, the patient and family. Objectives for each goal will be the responsibility of individual team members, according to his or her expertise.

5. The trainee will become familiar with the principles and physiology of therapeutic exercise, including indications and contraindications.

6. The trainee will become familiar with the techniques of bracing and with the use of equipment such as canes, walkers, wheelchairs, and adaptive devices.

7. The trainee will become familiar with the assessment and rehabilitation of those conditions most frequently seen in geriatric patients:
   A. Disabilities caused or aggravated by immobilization, including inactivity, deconditioning, restricted activities, malnutrition, and adverse drug reactions;
   B. Stroke, including characteristics of right- and left-sided lesions;
   C. Parkinson's syndrome;
   D. Arthritis, with impaired mobility of the back, knees, hips, shoulders, or other joints;
   E. Spinal stenosis;
   F. Paget's disease;
   G. Osteoporosis;
   H. Cervical spondylosis;
   I. Fractures of the hip, arm, or vertebrae;
   J. Joint replacement of the knee or hip;
   K. Lower extremity amputation, stump care, and indications and contraindications for prosthetic devices; and
   L. Cardiopulmonary rehabilitation in the management of ischemic heart disease, chronic lung disease, and postoperative recovery.

[a]Reproduced with permission of the American Geriatrics Society.

Textbook chapters that offer an overview of the field include "Rehabilitation and the Aged," by Redford in Reichel's *Clinical Aspects of Aging* (8); "Rehabilitation of the Geriatric Patient," by Clark and Siebens in DeLisa's *Rehabilitation Medicine: Principles and Practice* (9); "Ger-

Table 44.2. Topics in Geriatrics for Residents in PM&R[a]

1. Anatomic and physiologic changes associated with old age.

 A. Anatomical and physiological changes, particularly in neuromuscular, musculoskeletal, and cardiovascular pulmonary systems.

 B. Response to medications (pharmacologic and clinical), particularly the effects of drugs commonly used in the practice of physiatry.

2. Diagnosis and management of specific disorders.

 A. *Common disabilities of the aged:* stroke, Parkinson's disease, ischemic cardiovascular disease, peripheral vascular disease/amputations, cervical and lumbar spondylosis, rheumatoid arthritis, postsurgical total joint replacements, foot problems in the elderly, chronic lung disease, decubitus ulcer (causes, care, and various treatment protocols).

 B. *Disabilities sometimes occurring in the elderly:* (may present special problems, or occur in younger persons who reach old age): multiple sclerosis, spinal cord injury, cancer/blood dyscrasias (including ostomy care), renal disease, burns, neuromuscular diseases, cerebral palsy, poliomyelitis.

 C. *Disorders of Communication and Special Senses:* aphasia, dysarthria and related disorders, deafness, ophthalmologic disorders seen in the elderly.

 D. *Psychological disorders:* Alzheimer's disease and various acute and chronic dementias, depression—all aspects, psychological aspects of chronic pain and behavior disorders in the elderly, psychological problems of terminal illness.

3. Interaction of multiple disease processes and disabilities and their effects on functional assessment in management.

4. Psychosocial problems of old age.

 A. Issues of guardianship and autonomy.

 B. General issues, especially with respect to funding sources.

 C. Implications of placement in custodial facilities.

 D. Environmental barriers both in public and private homes.

5. Methods of accident prevention: epidemiology of accidents in the elderly, particularly falls.

6. Physical fitness training in the elderly: physiology and training methods.

7. Capabilities of various community environments to provide attainment of rehabilitation goals and maintenance of function in the elderly.

 A. Home care agencies.

 B. Rehabilitation oriented nursing homes.

 C. Skilled care nursing facilities.

 D. Custodial care nursing facilities.

 E. Boarding homes.

 F. Life care communities.

 G. Acute care hospitals.

 H. Rehabilitation hospitals.

 I. Private Homes.

 K. Hospice Care.

8. Capabilities of various personnel to provide elder care, including physical therapy, occupational therapy, and speech therapy. Knowledge of training of aides and families to take care of dependent elderly at home.

[a] Reproduced with permission of J. Redford as developed from a survey of residency training directors for the American Board of Physical Medicine and Rehabilitation, Rochester, Minn: 1988.

iatric Rehabilitation Management," by Lee and Itoh in Goodgold's *Rehabilitation Medicine* (10); and "Physiatric Rehabilitation of the Geriatric Patient," by Hong and Tobis in *Krusen's Handbook of Physical Medicine and Rehabilitation* (11). Besides this textbook, other recent texts encompassing geriatric rehabilitation care include the following: *Rehabilitation in the Aging*, edited by Williams (12); *Rehabilitation of the Older Adult*, by Andrews (13); *Aging with a Disability*, by Trieschman (14); *Geriatric Rehabilitation*, edited by Kemp, Brummel-Smith and Ramsdell (15); *Aging and Rehabilitation: Advances in the State of the Art*, edited by Brody and Ruff (16); and *Aging and Rehabilitation II: The State of the Practice*, edited by Brody and Pawlson (17).

Geriatric rehabilitation is also covered in self-directed educational materials developed by the American Geriatrics Society (AGS) and the American Academy of Physical Medicine and Rehabilitation (AAPM&R). The *Self-directed Medical Knowledge Program* of the AAPM&R includes extensive sections that describe the rehabilitation of specific disorders affecting elderly populations, including nerve and muscle disorders, joint and connective tissue diseases, musculoskeletal and soft tissue disorders, amputations, cardiovascular diseases, pulmonary diseases, cancer, and brain disorders including stroke (18). The Study Guide for Geriatric Rehabilitation (19) comprises four sections: social, attitudinal, and economic factors (20); diagnosis and management of acquired disabling disorders (21); mid-life and late-life effects of early life disabilities (22) and assessment, preservation, and enhancement of fitness and function (23).

Until 1989, the AGS published a comprehensive, medically-oriented geriatric bibliography, revised every two years. The 1989 update (24) includes 10 articles under "Care Option: Rehabilitation," seven under "Stroke Rehabilitation," and a few others related to rehabilitation scattered under the headings of specific disorders.

A concise, useful review of rehabilitation issues is contained in the *Geriatric Review Syllabus*, a self-directed learning program published by the AGS (25). Topics include mobility and self-care deficits, modalities, assistive devices, rehabilitation environments, reimbursement, and medical complications seen during rehabilitation assessment (26). Other sections of the syllabus review functional assessment, falls and immobility, geriatric physiology, geriatric medical disorders, and ethical and psychosocial issues. The syllabus includes a comprehensive annotated bibliography.

An important conference sponsored by the United States Department of Health and Human Services and Department of Education entitled "Rehabilitation and Geriatric Education: Perspectives and Potential" was held in December, 1988 (27). During this conference an attempt was made to identify resources and approaches to geriatric rehabilitation within many disciplines. A considerable effort was made to explore common ground and conflict between PM&R and geriatric medicine. Many disciplines were represented, including medical specialties, allied health professionals, and nonprovider experts in geriatric and gerontologic issues. The conference report identifies strengths and weaknesses of geriatric medicine and PM&R; in the Executive Summary, key points that each discipline emphasizes to the other are identified. Ten key references from each discipline, of value to the other, are listed. Specific recommendations are made regarding implementation of educational programs in geriatric rehabilitation at all levels, as well as to foster clinical research. Topics from this conference are further elaborated in the text *Aging and Rehabilitation II: The State of the Practice* (17).

ACADEMIC GERIATRIC MEDICINE, PM&R, AND GERIATRIC REHABILITATION

Vivell and associates (28) state that the key to affecting practice patterns, attitudes, and skills of medical undergraduates and young physicians in caring for the elderly is the presence of a highly visible, core faculty of geriatricians with skill and interest in teaching. The same can be said for geriatric rehabilitation. Both geriatric medicine and PM&R offer advantages and disadvantages for training clinicians to become teachers in this field. Geriatric medicine has a stronger research foundation than does PM&R, but often limited clinical and didactic exposure to PM&R during fellowship training. Virtually all PM&R residents experience care of the elderly in rehabilitation settings, learning to apply principles of PM&R in that context (4). Both geriatric medicine and PM&R offer extensive training in functional assessment and team-oriented care. Thus, both disciplines offer a substantial basis upon which academic clinicians interested in geriatric rehabilitation can build knowledge and expertise.

Identification of faculty with skill and interest in geriatric rehabilitation is a critical issue. In a recent survey of PM&R training programs (4), only about one third of PM&R geriatrics faculty had experienced formal fellowship level training in geriatric medicine or rehabilitation or had passed the geriatric medicine examination. The other two thirds can be assumed to have gained their expertise, like this author, from extensive clinical exposure during and after residency, continuing medical education, or research. One fourth of PM&R residency programs in the study also had nonphysician faculty with geriatric or gerontologic expertise.

Current estimates and projections of geriatric faculty identify a critical shortage in all major specialties (29). According to a recent survey (30), academic internists, family practitioners, neurologists, psychiatrists, and physiatrists spend about half of their faculty time in clinical work and only 14.3% of their time in research. Only 7.6% of geriatric physiatrists' faculty time is spent

in research. The survey demonstrated limited involvement of physiatrists in four areas: teaching medical school geriatrics courses, faculty development, health services delivery research, and behavioral and social research. The time-consuming clinical and teaching responsibilities of geriatrics faculty of all specialties may restrict expansion of the research base for geriatric medicine as a whole (31). Geriatric rehabilitation as an academic field may suffer unless research-oriented faculty can be identified and supported (4).

Less than 5% of medical students complete a clinical rotation in geriatric medicine (27). The limited number of teaching faculty interested in older patients is a major factor that restricts medical students from contact with the field and restrains the growth of geriatric medicine in general (27, 31, 32). Despite their popularity in some allied disciplines, courses focusing on older patients seem to have low visibility in many medical schools. PM&R and geriatric medicine courses are usually not required, and they compete poorly against other medical school electives. Few students have the specific interest to request an elective in geriatric medicine or geriatric rehabilitation.

Recently, increasing numbers of geriatric fellowship positions, geriatric medicine departments in hospitals and medical schools, and review courses indicate growing interest in geriatric medicine. More internists and family physicians have completed fellowships and are capable of teaching about geriatric issues. However, the impact of this activity on geriatric rehabilitation is not clear, as rehabilitation, particularly for specific physical impairments, often constitutes only a small part of the training.

Steinberg (33) identifies the critical need for clinical and didactic exposure of PM&R residents to disease processes and disabilities in the elderly. The teaching methods he suggests include lectures and seminars, taught by faculty outside of the PM&R department if necessary, and case-by-case clinical contact. He recommends that all staff physicians of PM&R departments participate in teaching in this area, but that a designated physician should develop and organize training materials and programs. Teaching hospital inpatient services, outpatient clinics, and consultation services are all excellent sources of contact with older patients for exposure to geriatric rehabilitation. Private doctors' offices, home health care units, and nursing homes are potential learning environments if sufficient professional supervision and direction is provided (33).

The AAPM&R has a special interest group (SIG) in geriatric rehabilitation numbering 122 physiatrists. The Geriatric SIG organizes advanced educational programs presented at the AAPM&R annual meeting for physicians and allied health practitioners. Many of these practitioners also teach residents and medical students. As in geriatric medicine, usually a maximum of one or two faculty per medical school are involved in geriatric rehabilitation.

Added qualifications for geriatric medicine by examination now exist in internal medicine and family practice. Some have suggested that the American Board of Physical Medicine and Rehabilitation (ABPM&R) offer this conjointly with the other two specialty boards (34). To date, physiatrists are not eligible to take the examination for added qualifications without being board certified in one of the other specialties. A multitude of geriatric medicine review courses have been offered in preparation for this examination. Most of these provide only limited didactic exposure to issues in geriatric rehabilitation for internists and family physicians. However, virtually all such courses offer in-depth discussions of critical basic science and clinical topics of value to physiatrists involved in the clinical practice and teaching of geriatric rehabilitation.

Fellowship training in geriatric rehabilitation through PM&R departments is virtually nonexistent. Recent surveys identify only one or two fellowship training sites in the United States (3, 29).

EDUCATIONAL SETTINGS

Several settings offer training opportunities in geriatric rehabilitation. General rehabilitation units in major teaching hospitals and their community hospital or freestanding rehabilitation hospital affiliates offer exposure to elderly patient populations. Typical problems include stroke, orthopedic, and neuromuscular disorders. Geriatric assessment units in major teaching hospitals offer exposure to older populations with functional deficits from a variety of causes, often precipitated by acute medical illness or deterioration of preexisting health. Patient care in the former setting is usually provided by physiatrists, while care in the latter setting is usually provided by geriatricians. Both provide consultative care, including functional assessment and direction of rehabilitative services, to older adults in acute medical settings, outpatient settings, and nursing homes. Medical students and residents receive training in all of these settings, but most intensively in geriatric assessment units, rehabilitation units, and PM&R and geriatric medicine inpatient consultation services.

Limitations in the populations served by these specialties should be considered. In some hospitals, geriatric assessment units emphasize acutely ill patients or patients with acute intercurrent illnesses. Patients with congenital or early developmental disorders may be seen rarely and may be cared for by other specialists. In contrast, some rehabilitation hospitals and units admit highly selected populations and reject patients who will need nursing home placement, regardless of potential for improvement. The presence of both units in the same hospital may bias the setting in which elderly patients need-

ing rehabilitation receive care. This will affect the experiences of students and residents who rotate on one unit but not the other. Referral patterns may be of critical importance to ensure a balanced mix of elderly patients with a representative cross-section of illnesses and rehabilitation potentials on either unit. Consultative services often expose students and residents to a broader mix of patients; they are more likely to encounter patients rejected, as well as patients accepted, for subsequent treatment in the geriatric medicine or rehabilitation unit.

Other specialties are involved in rehabilitation-oriented training. Neurology is concerned with stroke and other neurologic problems. Orthopedics provides postoperative and recuperative care in some settings to predominantly elderly populations with fractures and joint replacements. Rheumatology is involved with treating and rehabilitating patients with arthritides. Training in each of these specialties generally limits exposure to rehabilitation issues to disease processes falling within its area of expertise. In contrast, residency training in PM&R involves extensive exposure to elderly patients in all of these areas.

A key factor for the enhancement of education of students and residents rotating in any of these settings is the availability and utilization of appropriate consultants. Most physiatrists receive significant training in internal organ system disease, but not to the depth of a board certified internist. Indeed, Robinson's survey (4) documents that in most PM&R training programs physiatrists consult non-PM&R geriatrics specialists in a high proportion of their cases involving elderly patients. Geriatricians may develop fundamental skills in coordinating the rehabilitation of patients with common problems, but are likely to require consultative assistance from physiatrists or other specialists for patients with more complex problems, developmental disabilities, or complex, multiple disabilities. Even physicians double-boarded in PM&R and internal medicine may occasionally need a consultant! Units run by other specialists have similar needs. For example, orthopedists may have trouble managing hip fracture patients who also have strokes, while neurologists on stroke units may need assistance in managing stroke patients with fractures. Without consultants, students may develop a jaded view of the rehabilitation potential of patients with diseases not commonly seen on the unit on which they rotate.

Exposure to the rehabilitation team is an essential component of the educational process on all levels of medical education in geriatric rehabilitation. This is structured differently in various settings. In geriatric medicine, the team is often limited to a geriatrician, nurse, and social worker, and usually does not include allied health disciplines such as physical and occupational therapy (35). Team-oriented care in orthopedics and neurology usually includes physical therapy. Rheumatology-oriented teams often include occupational therapy. Multidisciplinary teams in general rehabilitation hospitals include all of these and may also involve speech, vocational, and recreational therapists. Thus, students, residents, and fellows rotating on different specialties may be exposed to teams with different skill levels, treatment methods, and organizations for making decisions. As long as there is adequate supervision and inclusion of the student in team meetings, all of these can provide legitimate exposure to team process.

The nursing home has considerable potential as a geriatric teaching setting (36, 37). Many patients will make varying degrees of recuperation or functional improvement if adequate resources are available to them. Therefore, experience in this environment may benefit the physician developing skills in geriatric rehabilitation. However, exposure to nursing home patients without adequate supervision is likely to lead to frustration and negative attitudes (33, 38). Physicians who have a broad perspective on the role of the nursing home in geriatric care can point out often subtle progress that individual patients make. Unless this is clearly taught, the student or resident risks acquiring the mistaken belief that the elderly in general have poor rehabilitation potential.

Students and residents can learn to evaluate and treat higher-functioning noninstitutionalized older patients with rehabilitation problems in outpatient geriatrics settings. Lavizzo-Mourey and associates (39) have described the organization and personnel requirements necessary to run a longitudinal outpatient geriatrics program for internal medicine residents. They document an increase in the likelihood that residents so trained will question patients about functional status, mental status, and social issues. This benefit would obviously be of great value to any physician in training concerned with geriatric rehabilitation. One interesting aspect of their program is the requirement that all residents be videotaped interviewing patients, with the videotape subsequently critiqued by geriatrics and psychiatry attendings.

ALTERING STUDENT ATTITUDES TOWARDS GERIATRIC REHABILITATION

A major problem in medical education and health care is the relative lack of interest in geriatric issues among medical students, residents, and practitioners (40). The prejudice against the elderly and low expectations of the elderly, termed ageism, (41) is commonplace. This is true in both acute medical settings (42, 43) and rehabilitation units (44, 45). Student contact with teaching staff and other personnel harboring such views is likely to perpetuate these attitudes. How can medical schools counteract this?

Exposure to issues of disability, chronic illness, and rehabilitation in the preclinical years may help medical students develop broader sensitivity and more appropriate health-promoting attitudes to rehabilitative concerns. In general, the earlier the initial exposure, the better (46). Actual empathetic contact with the elderly—particularly the well elderly—is more effective at altering attitudes than cognitively oriented learning emphasizing acquisition of technical knowledge (47). Experience with healthy elderly persons who are functioning in the community helps to counteract negative attitudes toward aging. However, this does not address the issue of rehabilitation potential following illness or decline. Probably the best way to instill positive attitudes regarding rehabilitation potential following illness is to provide direct contact with elderly persons who have been seriously or catastrophically ill and recovered and who responded positively to rehabilitative services. Videotapes or audioslide shows that condense months of patient progress towards recovery into minutes are a helpful substitute, worthy of inclusion into clinical as well as preclinical coursework (42).

The opportunity for medical students of all levels to interview ill patients under supervision can be a powerful learning tool that emphasizes not only pathophysiology and differential diagnosis, but also the broader experience of the psychosocial context of the patient's illness. By supervising the interview process, the instructor can observe student-patient interactions and assist the student's progress in the process of gathering, processing, and interpreting medical information (48). The use of this teaching method with elderly persons in rehabilitation settings constitutes a direct, nondidactic way to expose students to issues in geriatric rehabilitation. The instructor may also identify ageist attitudes. If this takes place in a setting where only limited rehabilitation resources are available or the instructor lacks knowledge of rehabilitation resources, the experience may be negative, suggesting that little can be done to overcome or adjust to disability. However, if the patient receives treatment in an environment where resources are readily available and the instructor is knowledgable about rehabilitation potential, such a supervised interview experience will tend to build more positive attitudes toward geriatric rehabilitation.

This author has worked extensively with third and fourth year medical students, most of whom have been assigned to a largely geriatric service in a free-standing rehabilitation hospital as part of a required 2-week clerkship in PM&R. Students are required to evaluate patients on admission and to follow them during the remainder of the clerkship. The student is responsible for writing the history, physical examination, and medical problem list. This is reviewed with the resident and attending physician, who develop the nursing orders, therapy orders, and rehabilitation problem list. Students also follow a limited number of patients already admitted. This author attempts to assign, wherever possible, a mix of patients with different disabilities or illness processes and various potentials for improvement. Students are assigned at least one patient with a reasonable likelihood of being discharged during the 2-week clerkship. Didactic sessions on patient evaluation, rehabilitation management, gait, and electrodiagnosis complement the clinical exposure. Students are encouraged to observe patients in therapies, follow medical problems, and participate in the multidisciplinary team conference. In this author's opinion, the most powerful learning experiences of the clerkship are the evaluation of newly admitted patients and ongoing assessment of medical status, adjustment to disability, and progress in rehabilitation.

Other environments may be appropriate to enable students to develop a more positive outlook toward rehabilitation potential, a key attitudinal issue in geriatrics. Holzman and associates (49) found that general attitudes toward older patients and attitudes toward rehabilitation potential improved in both a required month-long family practice clerkship in which 5 half-days were spent in a nursing home, and a 6 half-day concentrated elective in geriatric issues emphasizing contact with a largely healthy population. The first group emphasized clinical experience, while the second group emphasized didactic lectures, simulation experiences, and material specifically designed to develop empathy toward the elderly. There was no significant difference in the end result between the two groups.

Several simulation games have been developed to sensitize students to geriatric issues. The "Aging Game" (50) portrays issues of disability and dependency in a very negative way. The purpose is to facilitate students experiencing for themselves the neglectful and demeaning way society often deals with the sick, dependent, and disabled elderly. Although the program is documented to provide some positive sensitization, its long-term impact on medical student attitudes has not been established. Two board games developed include "Geriatrix," a role playing simulation game for medical students (51) and "The Road of Life," which has been tested on nonmedical, as well as medical, audiences (52). Other simulation experiences include using earphones designed to mimic severe hearing deficits, eyeglasses altered to mimic cataracts or homonymous hemianopsia, and restriction of mobility to a wheel chair. All of these have limited value in medical education unless combined with actual clinical and didactic exposure to geriatric medicine or geriatric rehabilitation.

SUMMARY

A variety of educational opportunities now exist for students to learn about geriatric rehabilitation. For maximal impact on attitudes, exposure should occur early, ideally in the preclinical years. This should include both didactic sessions about geriatric issues and gerontology and at least limited contact with healthy elderly persons or ill persons with potential to improve. Development of clinical skills and further refinement of attitudes requires exposure to disabled elderly with potential to improve their functional status in settings where they have access to necessary rehabilitation services. Such settings include primarily inpatient units (rehabilitation units and selected geriatric assessment units) and consultative services run by PM&R and geriatric medicine. Nursing homes, outpatient clinics, and home care may also offer appropriate training sites, provided there is an appropriate mix of patients and proper supervision by experienced clinicians interested in rehabilitation and committed to teaching.

For PM&R residents, geriatric rehabilitation educational objectives can be achieved through a combination of organized didactic lectures on medical and rehabilitation issues related to the elderly and clinical rotations on both inpatient units and consultation services under the supervision of faculty interested in this area. A broad mix of patients with geriatric disabilities is necessary and is easily achievable within most residency programs.

For geriatric medicine fellows, education in rehabilitation requires clinical exposure to settings where patients receive assessment of functional potential, followed by the actual provision of necessary therapy services. Didactic lectures on selected rehabilitation topics and clinical rotations on inpatient PM&R services help to achieve these objectives. Close contact with a physiatrist in the role of consultant or member of the geriatric assessment and treatment team is of value.

All physicians who work with the elderly need to be sensitized to rehabilitation issues. Primary care physicians of all specialties need to develop the capability to identify functional deficits in their patients. If they cannot determine the appropriateness of rehabilitation services to correct such deficits, then they need to know how to obtain consultation and how to refer patients for evaluation or therapy. In the future, all physicians, regardless of specialty or training, will need to work together to ensure that the elderly have access to rehabilitation services that benefit them.

ACKNOWLEDGMENT. The author wishes to thank Dr. John B. Redford for his insightful, resourceful constructive criticism of an early draft of this chapter.

References

1. Steinberg FU. Principles of geriatric rehabilitation. *Arch Phys Med Rehabil.* 70:67–68, 1989.
2. American Medical Association. *1991–1992 Directory of Graduate Medical Education Programs.* Chicago, Ill: American Medical Association; 1991.
3. Anderson JM, Felsenthal G. Residency training in physical medicine and rehabilitation I: clinical and didactic experience. *Arch Phys Med Rehabil.* 71:372–375, 1990.

4. Robinson KM, Friedman RH, Kazis LE, Moskowitz MA, Steel RK: Geriatrics training in physical medicine and rehabilitation. *Am J Phys Med Rehabil.* 72:67–74, 1993.

5. Robbins AS, Vivell S, Beck JC. A study of geriatric training programs in the United States. *J Med Educ.* 57:79–86, 1982.

6. American Geriatrics Society. *The Training of Geriatrics Fellows in Rehabilitation.* (Approved by the Board of Directors) New York, NY: American Geriatrics Society; November, 1988.

7. Redford J. *Topics in geriatrics for residents in PM&R.* Rochester, Minn: Developed from a survey of residency training directors for the American Board of Physical Medicine and Rehabilitation, 1988.

8. Redford J. Rehabilitation and the aged. In: Reichel W, ed. *Clinical Aspects of Aging.* 3rd ed. Baltimore, Md: Williams & Wilkins; 1989:177–187.

9. Clark GS, Siebens HC. Rehabilitation of the geriatric patient. In: Delisa JA, Gans BM, Currie DM, et al, eds. *Rehabilitation Medicine: Principles and Practice.* Philadelphia, Pa: J.B. Lippincott; 1988:642–665.

10. Lee M, Itoh M. Geriatric rehabilitation management. In: Goodgold J, ed. *Rehabilitation Medicine.* 5th ed. St. Louis, Mo: C.V. Mosby; 1988:393–406.

11. Hong C, Tobis JS. Physiatric rehabilitation of the geriatric patient. In: Kottke FJ, Lehmann JF, eds.: *Krusen's Handbook of Physical Medicine and Rehabilitation.* 4th ed. Philadelphia,Pa: W.B. Saunders; 1990:1209–1216.

12. Williams TF, ed. *Rehabilitation in the Aging.* 2nd ed. New York, NY: Raven Press; 1984.

13. Andrews K. *Rehabilitation of the Older Adult.* Baltimore, Md: Edward Arnold; 1987.

14. Trieschman RB. *Aging with a Disability.* New York, NY: Demos Publications, 1987.

15. Kemp KB, Brummel-Smith K, Ramsdell JW, eds. *Geriatric Rehabilitation.* Boston, Mass: Little, Brown; 1990.

16. Brody SJ, Ruff GE, eds. *Aging and Rehabilitation: Advances in the State of the Art.* New York, NY: Springer; 1986.

17. Brody SJ, Pawlson LG, eds. *Aging and Rehabilitation II: The State of Practice.* New York, NY: Springer; 1990.

18. Maly BJ. The third edition: self-directed medical knowledge program (SDMKP) 1993. *Arch Phys Med Rehabil.* 74:S-397–S-398, 1993.

19. Geriatric Rehabilitation. *Arch Phys Med Rehabil.* 74:S-399–S-425, 1993.

20. Gershkoff AM, Cifu DX, Means K. Geriatric rehabilitation: 1. social, attitudinal, and economic factors. *Arch Phys Med Rehabil.* 74:S-402–S-405, 1993.

21. Cifu DX, Means K, Curry D, Gershkoff AM. Geriatric rehabilitation: 2. diagnosis and management of acquired disabling disorders. *Arch Phys Med Rehabil.* 74:S-406–S-412, 1993.

22. Curry D, Gershkoff AM, Cifu DX. Geriatric rehabilitation: 3. mid- and late-life effects of early-life disabilities. *Arch Phys Med Rehabil.* 74:S-413–S-416, 1993.

23. Means K, Curry D, Gershkoff AM. Geriatric rehabilitation: 4. assessment, preservation, and enhancement of fitness and function. *Arch Phys Med Rehabil.* 74:S-417–S-420, 1993.

24. Rosenthal MJ. Geriatrics: an updated bibliography. *J Am Geriatr Soc.* 37:894–910, 1989.

25. Beck JC, ed. *Geriatrics Review Syllabus: A Core Curriculum in Geriatric Medicine, 1991–1992 Edition.* New York, NY: American Geriatrics Society; 1991.

26. Erickson RV. Principles of rehabilitation. In: Beck JC. ed. *Geriatrics Review Syllabus: A Core Curriculum in Geriatric Medicine, 1991-1992 Edition.* New York, NY: American Geriatrics Society; 1991:73–88.

27. Pawlson LG, Brody SJ, cochairmen. *Rehabilitation and Geriatric Education: Perspectives and Potential: Conference Report, December 4–7, 1988.* McLean, Va: The Circle, Inc.; 1989.

28. Vivell S, Robbins AS, Solomon DH, Beck JC. Education in the clinical years: delusion or reality. *Bull NY Acad Med.* 61:520–533, 1985.

29. Reuben DB, Bradley TB, Zwanziger J, et al. The critical shortage of geriatrics faculty. *J Am Geriatr Soc.* 41:560–569, 1993.

30. Reuben DB, Bradley TB, Zwanziger J, et al. Geriatrics faculty in the United States: who are they and what are they doing? *J Am Geriatr Soc.* 39:799–805, 1991.

31. Maloney TW, Paul B. Building the future of geriatrics. *J Am Geriatr. Soc.* 39:425–428, 1991.

32. Vivell S, Solomon D, Beck JC. Medical education responds to the 20th century's success story. *J Am Geriatr Soc.* 35:1107–1115, 1987.

33. Steinberg FU. Education in geriatrics in physical medicine residency training programs. *Arch Phys Med Rehabil.* 65:8–10, 1984.

34. DeLisa JA. Certificates for added/special qualifications: status report and implications for the field. *Am J Med Rehabil.* 68:172–178, 1989.

35. Brody SJ. Geriatrics and rehabilitation: common ground and conflicts. In: Brody SJ, Paelson LG, eds. *Aging and Rehabilitation II: The State of the Practice.* New York, NY: Springer; 1990:9–29.

36. Butler RN. A disease called ageism. *J Am Geriatr Soc.* 38:178–180, 1990.

37. Pawlson LG. Clinical education in the nursing home: opportunities and limits. *J Med Ed.* 57:787–791, 1982.

38. Cooney LM. An "editorial" look at geriatrics. In: *Proceedings of the Regional Institute on Geriatrics and Medical Education.* Washington, DC: American Association of Medical Colleges 1983:97–101.

39. Lavizzo-Mourey R, Beck LH, Diserens D, Day S, Johnson J, Forciea MA, Sims RV. Integrating residency training in geriatrics into existing outpatient curricula. *J Gen Intern Med.* 5:126–131, 1990.

40. American Medical Association. Council on Scientific Affairs: Societal effects and other factors affecting health care for the elderly. *Arch Intern Med.* 150:1184–1189, 1990.

41. Butler RN. The teaching nursing home. *JAMA.* 245:1435–1437, 1981.

42. Sherman FT. A medical school curriculum in gerontology and geriatric medicine. *Mt Sinai J Med.* 47(2):99–103, 1980.

43. Goodwyn JS. Geriatric ideology: the myth of the myth of senility. J Am Geriatr Soc. 39:627–631, 1991.

44. Hesse KA, Campion EW, Karamouz N. Attitudinal stumbling blocks to geriatric rehabilitation *J Am Geriatr Soc.* 32:747–750, 1984.

45. Benedict RC, Ganikos ML. Coming to terms with ageism in rehabilitation. *J Rehabil.* 47(4):10–18, 1981.

46. Birenbaum A, Aronson M, Seiffer S. Training medical students to appreciate the special problems of the elderly. *Gerontologist.* 19:575–579, 1979.

47. Coccaro EF, Miles AM. The attitudinal impact of training in gerontology/geriatrics in medical school: a review of the literature and perspective. *J Am Geriatr Soc.* 32:762–768, 1984.

48. Engel GL. The deficiencies of the case presentation as a method of clinical teaching: another approach. *N Engl J Med.* 284:20–24, 1971.

49. Holtzman JM, Beck JD, Coggan PG. Geriatrics program for medical students: II. impact of two educational experiences on student attitudes. *J Am Geriatr Soc.* 27:355–359, 1978.

50. McVey LJ, Davis DE, Cohen HJ. The 'Aging Game': an approach to education in geriatrics. *J Am Geriatric Soc.* 262:1507–1509, 1989.

51. Hoffman SB, Brand FR, Beatty PG, Hamill LA. Geriatrix: role-playing game. *Gerontologist.* 25:568–572, 1985.

52. Menks F. The use of a board game to simulate the experiences of old age. *Gerontologist.* 23:565–568, 1983.

45

Legislation and Regulations Affecting Rehabilitation of the Aging Patient

Richard E. Verville and Erwin G. Gonzalez

Rehabilitation practice with an aged patient is impacted by a number of very specific areas of law that are national in scope. These include statutes adopted by legislative bodies and regulations promulgated by governmental and private agencies. The enactment of Medicare law in 1965 began a process that has resulted, more than 25 years later, in literally thousands of provisions of law. The changes relate directly or indirectly to providing care for patients over 65 years of age as well as for the disabled who are under 65 years old. These legal principles impose direct regulations, such as conditions of care, which must be met in order to participate in the Medicare program. Due to the economic impact of reimbursement and payment provisions, Medicare indirectly affects how services are rendered. As a result of the growth and the size of the Medicare program, a number of policies affecting practice in general were created by the US Congress. Among these are the Professional Review Organization (PRO) quality and review program, the fraud and abuse provisions related to referrals and joint ventures, and physician practice data banks intended to gather information on licensing and malpractice grievances against physicians. In addition, national regulatory activity has been fueled by the Medicare and Medicaid programs, which resulted in the evolution of private accreditation agencies such as the Joint Commission on Accreditation of Health Care Organizations (JCAHO) and the Commission on Accreditation of Rehabilitation Facilities (CARF). Medicare relies heavily on accreditation by such private agencies as a basis for participation. As such regulatory activities have grown in number and scope, they have created specialty-specific requirements, as in the case of rehabilitation. Often, the purpose of these systems is benevolent or benign; however, their implementation has created restrictions that cause difficulty in compliance for professionals and administrators in the medical rehabilitation field.

Some of the regulatory programs are applicable only to facilities and services that involve Medicare patients, while others, such as accreditation, are generic in nature. Many Medicare regulations often become generic because they ultimately affect an entire program, not just the services rendered to Medicare beneficiaries.

THE AGED AND THE HEALTH CARE INDUSTRY

It is estimated that by the year 2020, the average life span of Americans will be 82 years for females and 74.2 years for males. In the same year, there will be an estimated 52 to 57 million people over 65 years of age and 6.7 to 8.6 million people over 85 years (Fig. 45.1). This aging population is subject to increasing incidence of disability and is more likely to require long-term health care. It is estimated that 3% to 6% of those over 65 years will reside in nursing homes, while 12% to 16% will remain at home with assistance. The estimated numbers are higher for those 85 years and over, with 15% to 25% residing in nursing homes, 31% to 37% at home with help (1). The burden of medical expenditure for the elderly is widely known. By the year 2020, the health care expenditure rate will double the 1987 rate, to the extent that in 1989 expenditure reached almost $599 billion, or 11.5% of the gross national product (GNP). This represents an increase of 10% to 14% each year for the next 5 years, so that by 1995, expenditure will reach one trillion dollars, and by the year 2000, health care allocation will approximate 15% of the GNP (2) (Fig. 45.2).

Several governmental programs are at risk due to the increasing cost of providing those programs and overruns in expenditure. The Medicare trust fund is no exception. Actuaries are predicting that Medicare's hospital trust fund will be depleted by 2005 unless drastic actions are taken. It is reported that despite a healthy income of 69.2 billion dollars in 1988 and expenses of only 53.3 billion dollars, by the turn of the century, expenses will increase to 205 billion dollars, while income

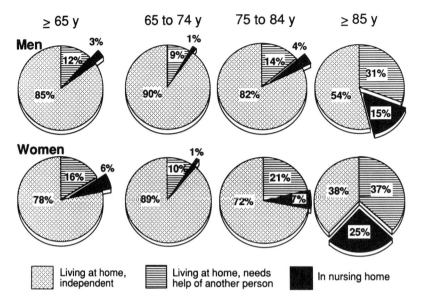

Figure 45.1. Percentage of population by age group and sex that live at home independently, live at home but require help of another person, or reside in a nursing home. Redrawn with permission from Schneider EL, Guralnik JM. *JAMA.* 263:2335–2340. Copyright 1990, American Medical Association.

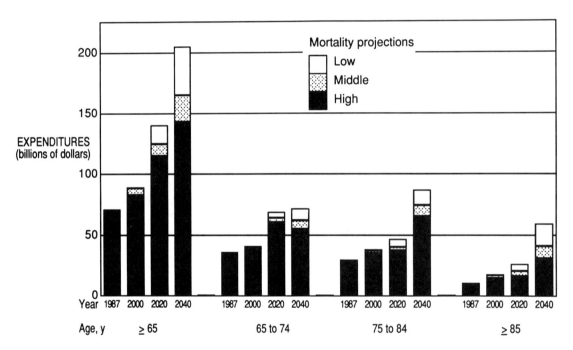

Figure 45.2. Actual (1987) and projected Medicare expenses in 1987 dollars by age group. Average Medicare expenses per person were obtained from data from the Health Care Financing Administration. Cost projections are based on low, middle, and high mortality as-sumptions from the US Bureau of Census. Redrawn with permission from Schneider EL, Guralnik JM. *JAMA.* 263:2335–2340. Copyright 1990, American Medical Association.

will be about 171 billion dollars (3). In anticipation of such a calamity, a priority item for recent administrations and the current administration is to decrease expenses, including health care. The consequences of such cutbacks are now being felt across the health care industry, as well as by consumers.

LEGISLATION AND REGULATIONS AFFECTING CARE SETTINGS

Much medical rehabilitation care is furnished in an inpatient hospital system, though institutional outpatient services, home care, skilled nursing facility rehabilitation services, and office-based practice have grown substantially in the last decade. Inpatient hospital care for the aged patient is more prevalent than for the non-aged. Therefore, the Medicare law has a very significant impact on the practice of rehabilitation in an inpatient hospital setting.

In 1983, at the prompting of the Executive Branch, Congress passed legislation that totally reshaped the method by which Medicare pays for inpatient hospital services. That law, referred to as the Prospective Payment System (PPS), establishes a fixed payment amount for each inpatient case. The payments vary in amount as determined by the diagnosis applicable to the patient (3). The amount paid is representative of the average cost per case for each diagnostic category or the Diagnostic Related Group (DRG) system. The law created a separate Medicare payment system for rehabilitation hospitals and distinct rehabilitation units of general hospitals. They are not paid a specific amount for each case from the PPS system.

To qualify for payment outside of PPS (DRG exemption), a hospital or unit must apply to the federal government for certification as a rehabilitation institution. Success in this endeavor is critical to economic success and growth since the payment amounts allowed are substantially greater for care furnished in certified institutions than in those not certified. Nonexempt facilities are paid under the DRG system. DRG number 462 is a rehabilitation DRG category with a 13.9-day average length of stay in 1993, with a cost calculation rate that is less than the cost calculated for distinct part rehabilitation units.

The major regulatory criteria that must be met in order to become certified include patient mix, distinct cost accounting and administrative structure, contiguousness of beds, comprehensiveness of services, and medical direction (4). Specifically, to be certified as an exempt DRG unit, at least 75% of patients cared for in the first full fiscal year prior to application for exemption must be from one or more of 10 diagnostic categories as follows: stroke, spinal cord, amputation, multiple trauma, fracture of femur (hip fracture), brain injury, arthritis, burns, congenital deformities, and neurologic disorders. A unit must establish that its beds, services, and cost-accounting system are separate from the remainder of the hospital. Patients must be under close medical supervision and receive rehabilitation nursing, physical therapy, and occupational therapy. Other services must also be furnished as needed (5). The medical director must be a qualified physician who has had 1 year of internship and at least 2 years of training or experience in rehabilitation management of inpatients requiring rehabilitation.

Hospitals wishing to participate in the Medicare program must also comply with the general Medicare conditions of participation. Some of those conditions include specific requirements for rehabilitation (6). Medicare deems a hospital to be in compliance with their conditions of participation if a hospital is accredited by JCAHO. Consequently, the JCAHO standards for inpatient rehabilitation have become almost obligatory as hospitals desire to participate in the Medicare program. The JCAHO standards for inpatient rehabilitation are voluminous; very specific provisions are required for each service offered including occupation therapy, physical therapy, rehabilitation medicine, and nursing (7). These JCAHO provisions also deal specifically with the role of referring physicians in the care of patients admitted to rehabilitation units where another physician directs patient care on the unit (8). This provision has a substantial impact on physician practice in rehabilitation.

CARF has also developed accreditation standards for inpatient rehabilitation care. These standards are also recognized by the Medicare program for purposes of meeting some of the separate requirements related to obtaining exemption from the DRG law. However, CARF standards do not serve as a general substitute for Medicare hospital conditions of participation as do JCAHO standards. Both CARF and JCAHO accreditation are usually sought by most rehabilitation hospitals and units. The CARF standards are voluminous, highly specific, and influence rehabilitation practice in many ways. For instance, CARF standards indicate criteria for the frequency of physician visits for rehabilitative and general medical services. The current standards require at least daily visits by physicians who are responsible for rehabilitation on days when therapy is rendered and require the attending rehabilitation physicians to be responsible for primary medical services (9). Where a physician furnishes both medical and rehabilitation services, a daily visit is expected. Such standards undergo frequent review due to their impact on practice.

In 1978, the Comprehensive Outpatient Rehabilitation Facility (CORF) benefit was established by amendment to the existing Medicare statute. This created a new Medicare benefit and a new category of medical provider in rehabilitation. CORF is defined as a free-standing facility that furnishes a comprehensive range of services to disabled persons in need of outpatient care at a fixed location and under the direction of a physician (10). Like inpatient facilities, there are specific regulations that have been developed by the Department of Health and Human Services (DHHS) in order for a facility to be able to participate under the Medicare program. Such requirements include that at least physical therapy, psychologic or social services, and physician services are furnished to the patient (11). The CORF must have the presence of a physician to provide medical policies and develop a treatment plan, although a referring physician can also establish the plan (12). The Medicare law also includes conditions of participation for free-standing facilities that are not part of a hospital or a nursing facility and that furnish only a specific service such as physical therapy or speech therapy.

It is common knowledge that the setting and arrangements in which medical care is provided have changed dramatically in recent years. This has occurred because of increased costs despite limited budgets of payors. In an effort to reduce costs, payors have stimulated, and in some cases required, changes in settings in which care is delivered. Outpatient care in particular has been emphasized. To achieve efficiency in case management, particularly in outpatient care, joint ventures have increased. The federal government, as well as many state governments, has explicitly adopted policies that are based on competition in the health care field. These procompetition policies have encouraged evolution of various entrepreneurial joint ventures. Such arrangements have raised concern about improprieties and the potential for windfall profits as a result of explicit or implicit referrals or similar arrangements by physicians who may have a financial interest in these ventures. The public concern has focused on the potential for overutilization of services and abuse in payment systems because they might be related to a referral rather than a service.

As a result of those concerns, Congress has passed legislation and the DHHS has developed policies and regulations under the Medicare and Medicaid laws to regulate ventures in which there is remuneration of any type, direct or indirect, for the referral or receipt of referral of patients (13). These regulatory provisions apply to compensation arrangements between professionals and providers, ownership of providers by professionals, and ventures between clinics or group practices. While regulatory provisions are concerned primarily with the economic arrangements between individuals and entities in health care, they also have a substantial impact on the care settings being utilized. Physicians are well advised to check with their legal counsel before entering into ventures in which Medicare patients are served. On July 29, 1991, the DHHS issued final regulations in the Federal Register, which narrowly define certain arrangements not subject to legal challenge, such as where compensation for services is at market value. Among these are ownership in health entities where not more than 40% of the ownership or revenue of the venture come from those with referral power or those doing business with the provider (14).

THIRD PARTY PAYMENT: GENERAL REGULATION

Most medical care is financed by third parties such as private insurance carriers and government-sponsored insurance or programs. Medical rehabilitation is no different than other forms of medicine in this respect. It is paid for by third parties, generally in the form of reimbursement for services rendered. Payment may also be in the form of prospectively fixed rates paid in advance or fixed payments based on the number of patients seen. The determination of payment amounts and conditions of payment involve both regulations and regulatory processes that are written in both public and private laws. Since most care for the aged is financed by Medicare, the payment law involved relative to the aged is most often public. However, private insurance supplements Medicare, and therefore, payment is also regulated by private contract and insurance law. The regulatory issues involved in third party payment are similar, regardless of whether the payment system is public or private. The issues include the following: the method by which payment amounts are created, the process used for payment, the services and products covered by the payment system, the conditions under which payment is made, and the legal system used for appeals by aggrieved providers of service to contest failure to pay. These payment issues do differ somewhat, depending upon whether the service is institutional or professional.

Institutional payments are cost-based with limits, subject to fiscal limits, while professional payments could be based upon actual or prevailing charges in the market area or derived from specified schedules of fees. Payment may also involve discounted amounts negotiated with payors and involve a reduction of regular charges or fees.

The law that establishes third party payment also involves definitions of covered services. Medicare has elaborate regulations, guidelines, and policies defining the specifics of covered services. The DHHS has a process in place for the consideration of coverage matters. The policy applies to the question of coverage of new services or technologies, as well as existing services or technologies that are deemed costly and questionable as to their effectiveness. For example, coverage guidelines for cardiac rehabilitation programs in inpatient and outpatient settings were recently developed. The Health Care Financing Administration (HCFA), which administers the Medicare program, has also developed coverage policies to guide the operations of its claims processing contractors in each state.

The existing Medicare law involves an appeal process regarding denials for payments to either institutions or professionals. The process includes federal court litigation for aggrieved claimants. Medicare uses different systems of appeal depending on whether the payment is under Part A of Medicare, which finances inpatient hospital, skilled nursing facility care, and home care, or Part B, which finances outpatient care of all types, such as physician services, medical equipment, and all other professional and laboratory services.

MEDICARE HOSPITAL PAYMENT LEGISLATION AND REGULATION

Rehabilitation hospital and units are paid on a cost reimbursement basis subject to a target rate, which often serves as a ceiling (15). The rate of payment is increased by an inflation factor that Congress often determines annually by statutory provision. The annual rate of increase ranges between 4% and 5%. This target rate is derived from the average cost per case of the hospital in a base year predetermined by regulation, divided by the number of patients discharged in that given year. The current base years used for all hospitals and units in existence prior to 1984 are 1982, 1983, or 1984. For those coming into existence after 1984, the base year is their first year of operation. The rate was intended to be updated by a percentage equaling the annual rate of increase in a collection of hospital cost items referred to as the hospital market basket; however, due to budgetary considerations, Congress has annually fixed a lesser rate. The legislation and regulations permit hospitals to seek, on a case-by-case basis, exceptions in their rates based on changes in the case mix of patients cared for or in the types and cost of programs. This process has been successfully pursued by some hospitals; however, it is a lengthy and costly effort. Hospitals may also seek a revised base year determination by the HCFA. Legislation was introduced in 1992 to allow a hospital to elect 1988 as a base year, but it was not enacted (16).

The HCFA had funded a number of studies to determine if a prospectively determined fixed price comparable to the DRG system of payment would be feasible for all hospitals and units that are exempted from the DRG law. Congressional testimony by Gail Welinsky, the HCFA Administrator, to the House Ways & Means Committee on May 10, 1990 suggests that such a reform is not likely in rehabilitation in the near future. The HCFA and Office of Management and Budget have also been considering the proposal of legislation to authorize a consolidation of payment for all postacute care into a single payment made to the acute hospital from which the patient is discharged. This payment would cover up to 90 days of postacute care of any type. Such a proposal is opposed by many in the rehabilitation community because acute hospitals, having received a fixed amount in payment, would have an incentive to lessen the cost of care furnished and reduce inpatient rehabilitative care.

As a condition of payment, Medicare regulations for inpatient hospital care also require that a patient must receive at least 3 hours per day of physical therapy, occupational therapy, or in special circumstances, other rehabilitation services such as speech therapy. All of these must be under the close supervision of a physician (17). HCFA has recently clarified that this rule is only a screen,

which triggers further review to determine if inpatient rehabilitative care was necessary and therefore covered. The 3 hour rule could not be used as a basis for payment denial under this HCFA policy.

MEDICARE PHYSICIAN PAYMENT LEGISLATION AND REGULATION

Physician services are covered under Medicare legislation if they are medically necessary and appropriate (18). There are three bases of payments as follows: the lesser of the actual charge, the customary charge of a providing physician, and the prevailing charge for the service in a given geographic area. Prevailing charges have been subject to growth limitations since 1972. However, physicians were allowed to bill patients directly for services rendered and were entitled to be paid by the patient at the level of the actual charge up until 1985. At that time, physician charges were frozen, with only slight increases allowed in subsequent years. This limitation is referred to as the Maximum Allowable Charge (MAC).

Legislation was enacted in 1989 that created a radically new payment system referred to as the Resource Based-Relative Value System (RBRVS) (19). The system involves a schedule of fees established on a national basis with some limited geographic variation. Relative values are given for most of the Medicare physician services and multiplied by a dollar conversion factor and varied by a geographic index.

Under the new legislation, relative values are established by types of services, which are defined by using codes developed by the American Medical Association (AMA). Some examples of services defined in codes are hospital visits, office visits, electromyography (EMG) and other electrodiagnostic services, and physical medicine modalities.

The relative value for each service is given a weight relative to the norm of 1. The weights were developed through an elaborate cross-specialty consultative process conducted by Harvard under a grant from HCFA (20). Physical medicine and rehabilitation services were evaluated as part of this process. The relative value is multiplied by a conversion factor to determine the fee schedule amount.

Generalists and specialists performing identical procedures will be paid the same amounts for the same procedure under the new system. This approach is very different from prior law, which permitted a specialist to receive more than a generalist for a similar service.

Geographic differentials for similar service will not vary as much as those allowed under the current law. While the RBRVS fee schedule has a geographic adjustment factor to reflect variations in cost of practice and general cost of living, the practice cost variations will not be commensurate with the current variations in payment. In general, the variation in payment will be only about 10% to 15% above and below the average payment, with urban areas receiving positive adjustments and rural areas negative ones. The factors included in determining the variation in practice cost are office rent, salaries of nonphysician employees, malpractice premiums, and the cost-of-living differential. The boundaries of geographic areas have not as yet been established. In the meantime, the current payment localities will be used in the initial phase of implementation.

In order to control increasing program costs, the dollar conversion factor is updated each year. This is based upon how expenditures in a prior year compare to a previously determined expenditure target for physician services for that given year. If the target was exceeded, the conversion factor will be reduced by an amount proportionate to the excess. This system is referred to as the Volume Performance Standard Program.

On November 25, 1991, the HCFA issued a final regulation implementing the fee schedule legislation. The effective date of the fee schedule was January 1, 1992. The conversion factor for the fee schedule for 1992 is $31.00. To determine the fee to be paid, conversion factor is multiplied by the relative values for each service after they are geographically adjusted. The proposal has new definitions of hospital and office visit codes and services. The different levels of service for visits are similar in number to the existing Current Procedural Terminology (CPT) coding system, but the content definitions are more precise and focus upon the complexity of the medical decision-making. While the Physician Payment Review Commission recommended to HCFA the inclusion of a modifier for services to people with mental or physical impairments, the HCFA proposal did not include this approach.

The midlevel hospital visit code for an initial visit has total Relative Value Units (RVUs) of 3.04, and for the follow-up visit the midlevel code has a 1.42 RVU. On average, payments would be about $94 for the midlevel initial visit and $44 for the midlevel follow-up visit. EMG services for one limb are valued at 2.33 RVUs or about $72 on average and 4.08 RVUs or about $126 for two limbs. These estimates are not geographically adjusted.

There are also RVUs for all physical modality codes, and they are very low, none equaling the norm of 1. Electrical stimulation therapy has an RVU of .44 and prosthetic training one of .70, resulting in fees on average of about $14 and $22 per service, respectively.

As previously discussed, the existing law permits direct billing to patients up to a certain limit. The limit is based upon the amount billed for a particular service during the base year 1985. The new law limits patient billing to a percentage of the new fee schedule as follows:

1. 1991: limited to 125% of the fee schedule,
2. 1992: 120% of the fee schedule, and
3. 1993 and thereafter: 115% of the fee schedule.

The new system is not going to be easier for physicians; however, it should be more equitable, since unreasonably wide differentials in payment based upon geography and on type of service will be eliminated. Payment for services in rural and less populated parts of the country will be increased. Likewise, payment for medical care, particularly medical evaluation and management services or cognitive services, will be enhanced. For example, visits with patients will be paid at greater rates. However, the new system will pay the same amount to a nonspecialist and a specialist for the same service, such as managing rehabilitative care for an amputee or stroke patient or care for a fracture rendered by an orthopedic surgeon versus a general practitioner.

The new system will pay physicians in their first 4 years of furnishing service to Medicare patients between 80% and 95% of the fee schedule and will reduce payments for outpatient visits and other services in hospitals or CORFs by about 20%. Legislation pending in 1993 would repeal this unfair provision and it is likely to be enacted.

The Medicare program regulates payment for services rendered by professionals through creating screening criteria, which Medicare contractors or carriers use to process claims. The screening criteria are applied to claims both before and after payment. If the screening criteria are not met by a claimant, then payment is suspended; additional documentation may be required of the claimant, and further review could be taken by the carrier. In rehabilitation, such a screen was initiated by most carriers that suspends payment for physicians' services to all claims when more than 12 physician visits are billed for each 30 days of inpatient rehabilitation care. All suspended payments are then subject for further claim review. At present, HCFA is developing a uniform set of criteria to review claims exceeding this visit parameter, as it is required to do by a 1990 amendment to the Medicare statute.

If after review, a claimant is denied payment on claims exceeding $500, an appeal may be filed with an administrative law judge. Thereafter, if the judge denies payment and claims exceed a $1000, a claimant may seek a federal court to review the claim.

Screens are also applied to most outpatient physical therapy services utilizing a variety of threshold limits for number of visits, keyed in with specific International Diagnostic (ICD-9) Codes. Screens are also applied to specific forms of medical equipment.

PROFESSIONAL SERVICES OF OTHER PRACTITIONERS

Medicare and private insurance all recognize physician services and pay them directly for such services. Other practitioners of rehabilitation are also paid directly for their services and have similar regulatory mechanisms to cope with regarding payment. Psychologists are now paid directly as a result of amendments to Medicare in 1989, including services furnished in rehabilitation settings. However, the initial HCFA ruling was such that direct payment does not apply in any inpatient setting. This was remedied by Congress in 1990, and payment now includes inpatient services. Physical therapists and occupational therapists are paid directly for their services in their offices or in a patient's home, but not for services furnished in institutional settings such as hospitals or skilled nursing facilities. Such institutional services are covered, but payments are made to the institution. Mental health services by clinical social workers are also paid directly under the Medicare program. These services will be governed by the relative value fee schedule though payments are not generally similar.

FUTURE LEGISLATIVE DIRECTION: LONG-TERM CARE

The Medicare Catastrophic Coverage Act of 1988 expanded coverage to protect aged beneficiaries from excessive out-of-pocket expenditures for lengthy, expensive care. The Act eliminated beneficiary coinsurance payments for hospitalization and eliminated the 90-day limit on hospitalization. The program also reduced coinsurance payments for skilled nursing care, eliminated the prior hospitalization requirement for skilled nursing care, and expanded coverage in a skilled nursing facility to 150 days a year and spell of illness. Respite care for individuals who were providing home care to others, such as spouses, was provided on a limited basis. Unfortunately in 1989, the law was repealed because elements of the beneficiary population objected strongly to the financing system used. Yet, long-term care, chronic illness, and the need for long-term care insurance is still a priority among the lobbying organizations for the elderly and the Congress. The 1988 bill made modest efforts in the direction of long-term care benefits by liberalizing existing Medicare skilled nursing and home care programs, but the bill did not address chronic care needs of the geriatric patient.

The Pepper Commission, a bipartisan body created by the 1988 legislation that survived repeal, issued a report in September 1990 on comprehensive health care needs entitled, "A Call for Action." In its report, the Commission estimated that about 10 million Americans are chronically disabled, and four million are so severely disabled that they cannot live independently. The Commission recommends federal insurance for long-term care regardless of the income of the person needing care. An extension of federal insurance would cover 3 months of nursing home and community-based care without limitation. Long-term nursing home stays would be covered for the severely disabled under a public program financed by the federal and state governments in a manner comparable to the Medicaid financing.

The Commission's recommendations include a major emphasis on the role of case managers in the delivery of long-term care services. Under the Commission proposal, case managers would allocate services and monitor service delivery within a budget allocated to each case manager for each patient. The effect of a case manager system would be to limit the freedom that providers and professionals have in furnishing services and shaping care plans.

Long-term care obviously affects patients needing rehabilitation; most long-term care beneficiaries are over 65 years of age. Most rehabilitation professional and lay interest groups have endorsed federal legislation to finance long-term care. In the next decade, this is the area of federal legislative concern that is most likely to affect rehabilitation of the geriatric patient. It may also result in tighter control and management of the allocation of resources to all postacute care, since Congress and the Executive Branch remain focused on reducing the costs of care.

References

1. Schneider EL. The aging of America. *JAMA*. 263:2335–2340, 1990.
2. Stimmel B. The study and practice of medicine in the 21st century. *Mt Sinai J Med*. 57:11–24, 1990.
3. Verville R. Medicare rate setting. *J Legal Med*. 6(1):85, 1985.
4. 42 CFR §412-23(b), §412.25, §412.29.
5. 42 CFR §412-23(b)(4), §412.19(c).
6. 42 CFR §482.56.
7. Joint Commission on Health Care Organizations. *1990 Accreditation Manual for Hospitals*. Oakbrook Terrace, Ill: Joint Commission on Health Care Organizations; 1990:177–192.
8. Joint Commission on Health Care Organizations. *1990 Accreditation Manual for Hospitals*. Oakbrook Terrace, Ill: Joint Commission on Health Care Organizations; 1990:0.190, Standard 3.3.2.
9. *1991 Standards Manual for Organizations Serving People with Disabilities*. Commission on Rehabilitation Facilities. Standard A.9.
10. 42 CFR §485.51.
11. 42 CFR §485.58.
12. 42 CFR §485.58(a).
13. Social Security Act. Section 1128 B.
14. Proposed safe harbor regulations. *Federal Register*. July 29, 1991;56(146):35952 et.seq.
15. Social Security Act. Title 18, Section 1886(a)(b).
16. House bill H.R. 4262, introduced by Mr. Moody and Mrs. Johnson.
17. *Medicare Hospital Manual*. Section 211, Transmittal 582; February, 1990.
18. Social Security Act. Title 18, Section 1832.
19. Social Security Act. Title 18, Section 1848.
20. Hsiao WC, Braun PB, Becker ER, Thomas SR. The resource-based relative value scale. *JAMA*. 258:799–802, 1987.

46

Legal Aspects of Geriatric Rehabilitative Care

Bill Allen and S. Van McCrary

Health care practitioners frequently have concerns about what they perceive to be potential legal issues in the treatment and rehabilitation of their patients. One common set of issues includes the legal requirements of informed consent for medical and rehabilitative procedures, including patients' capacity to consent to such interventions. When rehabilitation is no longer a reasonably attainable option, legal issues regarding the abatement of life-sustaining treatment and advance directives related to such abatement sometimes cause concern among caregivers. In this chapter, we will discuss some of the basic legal issues with which all health care providers in hospitals, nursing homes, and other rehabilitative facilities should be familiar. We have attempted to make this discussion meaningful for persons unacquainted with legal terminology, and we hope that it will reduce some of the anxiety about the law that is often found among health care providers.

Before discussing substantive legal issues, we will briefly explain two general features of law. The reader should bear in mind that the discussion that follows is conditioned by these important points. First, most of the legislation on advance directives and guardianship varies from state to state, and the holdings of courts are binding only within the boundaries of their particular jurisdictions. Therefore, local guidance must be sought for a reliable and detailed legal opinion on specific aspects of the law in the reader's jurisdiction. The discussion in this chapter will clarify general trends in the law and provide the reader with an analytical framework adequate to address the specific details of the law in his or her jurisdiction. The reader should use caution when generalizing our discussion into his or her jurisdiction. Second, although many states have passed legislation regarding abatement of treatment, including natural death acts, living will statutes, and durable powers of attorney for health care decision-making, such statutes are not the only sources of law that apply to these issues. Case law—the holdings of court cases—may give persons rights

to refuse treatment that are not provided by statute. Although some court holdings interpret statutes, other cases develop legal rights independent of legislative statutes (i.e., common law and constitutional rights). Even case law from other jurisdictions, although not binding, may have important persuasive impact on particular court decisions.

If the uncertainty regarding legal issues in this discussion causes the reader discomfort, we urge health care professionals to consider the similar uncertainty inherent in medical practice. In law as in medicine, some degree of uncertainty is an inevitable consequence of the subject matter. Although we qualify many of the statements in this chapter in deference to variation within individual states, the trends that we identify are important guides because they reflect ways that the law is adapting to changing societal views of these issues. Many times these changes are simply a formalization into law of emerging ethical consensus. Thus, we will at times also discuss ethical issues with particular relevance to the legal issues we encounter.

INFORMED CONSENT, PATIENTS' COMPETENCE, AND THE RIGHT TO REFUSE TREATMENT

Informed consent is generally defined as "the willing and uncoerced acceptance of a medical intervention by a patient after adequate disclosure by the physician of the nature of the intervention, its risk and benefits, as well as of alternatives with their risks and benefits" (1 p. 41). Three basic elements must be satisfied before consent can be said to be appropriate: adequate disclosure, voluntariness, and competence. Disclosure is judged adequate by two standards that vary according to state: first, the professional practice standard, which requires disclosure of information commonly provided by competent practitioners in the community or speciality; and second, the reasonable person standard, which requires disclosure of sufficient information to allow reasonable persons to make prudent choices on their own behalf (1). The reasonable person standard was first articulated by the courts in 1972 in *Canterbury v. Spence* (2). Although not accepted in all states, the reasonable person standard is supported by the ethical principle of autonomy and allows greater deference to patient self-determination. In accord with ethical and legal scholars, we suggest that responsible practitioners should use the reasonable person standard (1, 3). In order to be ethically and legally acceptable, consent must also be voluntary, i.e., obtained without coercion or undue influence. Health care providers should be aware of the possibility of coercive influence by patients' family members as well as by other health care providers. Valid consent also requires that the consenting patient be competent to make such decisions. We will discuss issues of competence later in this section of the chapter.

The legal concept of informed consent is derived from the common law right of self-determination, as first articulated in 1914 in *Schloendorff v. Society of New York Hospitals* (4). The *Schloendorff* court characterized this right by the statement: "Every human being of adult years of sound mind has a right to determine what shall be done with his body." A necessary legal principle of informed consent that has emerged from *Schloendorff* and subsequent cases is the right to refuse medical treatment. This right of competent patients to refuse medical treatment applies even when such refusal is certain to result in the patient's death. In general, courts have concluded that a patient's right to refuse treatment prevails over various other state interests that might mitigate against such a refusal. These interests include the preservation of life, the protection of the patient's survivors, the prevention of suicide, or supporting particular views of the ethical integrity of the medical profession and health care institutional policies (5).

This right of autonomous patients to refuse treatment has been upheld even in cases in which the refusing patient was not terminally ill. In *Bouvia v. Superior Court* (6), for example, a competent 28-year-old quadriplegic, bedridden patient with severe cerebral palsy and painful, crippling arthritis sued to remove the nasogastric feeding tube inserted by the hospital medical staff against her expressed written instructions. In overruling the lower court's decision to refuse her petition to remove the feeding tube on the basis that the feeding tube could allow her to live an additional 15 to 20 years, the California Second District Court of Appeals held that the lower court ". . . mistakenly attached undue importance to the *amount of time* possibly available to petitioner, and failed to give equal weight and consideration for the *quality* of that life; an equal, if not more significant, consideration." The rationale for legal recognition of a patient's right to refuse medical treatment finds

compelling expression in the holding of the *Bouvia* court (6 p. 305):

"Here Elizabeth Bouvia's decision to forgo medical treatment or life-support through a mechanical means belongs to her. It is not a medical decision for her physicians to make. Neither is it a legal question whose soundness is to be resolved by lawyers or judges. It is not a conditional right subject to approval by ethics committees or courts of law. It is a moral and philosophical decision that, being a competent adult, is hers alone."

Thus, Bouvia was allowed to refuse treatment if she still desired to do so. After the case was heard by the court, it was discovered that Bouvia had never received a thorough medical evaluation for pain relief. She later underwent such an evaluation, received appropriate analgesia, and then reconsidered her refusal of feeding. Thus, in addition to emphasizing the extent of the right to refuse treatment, the *Bouvia* case also highlights the importance of adequate pain control for critically ill patients who seek abatement of treatment.

The right to refuse treatment has also been extended to patients lacking current capacity to make medical decisions. Courts in almost all states have reached this conclusion (7). Some courts have recognized the right to refuse medical treatment not only for patients who have lost medical decision-making capacity but also for patients who never possessed that capacity. The rationale for recognizing an incapacitated patient's right to refuse treatment was expressed in the case of *Superintendent of Belchertown State School v. Saikewicz* (8 p. 428):

"To protect the incompetent person within its power, the state must recognize the dignity and worth of such a person and afford to that person the same panoply of rights and choices it recognizes in competent persons."

Before we describe various means for implementing an incapacitated patient's right to refuse treatment, we will discuss criteria for determining patients' competence or capacity to make medical decisions. In many cases a patient's incapacity will be obvious, due to unconsciousness, acute dementia, delusional behavior, etc. In other cases, incapacity may be less obvious, or patients may slip in and out of states that render them incapacitated (so-called waxing and waning competence). It is also important to remember that competence is a task-specific concept. This means that persons may be incompetent to perform certain functions and yet to be fully competent to do other tasks. Thus, an individual declared by a court to be incompetent to manage his or her legal or financial affairs may yet retain the capacity to make medical decisions, including refusal of treatment.

No precise formula exists for assessing capacity, but we find the following guidelines helpful. General criteria for judging a patient's medical decision-making capacity require that the patient be able to comprehend and communicate the relevant medical information, to reason and deliberate about health care choices, and to make such choices on the basis of some goals and values (1). The judgment as to whether a patient meets these criteria must not be based on whether the patient's decision agrees with the physician's recommendation or with the decision that a reasonable person would make. If the patient's comprehension and choice satisfies the guidelines we have described, the fact that the ensuing decision does not agree with the physician's values or the values of the patient's family does not mean that the patient lacks capacity to make medical treatment decisions. A patient's understanding does not have to be near-perfect in order for him or her to possess sufficient capacity to make health care decisions.

Courts have not articulated a consistent test for judging a patient's capacity to consent to or to refuse medical treatment. In the past, physicians commonly have determined patients to be incapacitated when the patient's decision was contrary to physicians' advice. Courts often acceded to this practice or appointed a proxy who was likely to agree to the treatment recommended by the physician. More recently, however, courts have recognized that a patient's refusal of physician-recommended treatment is not an adequate legal basis for a determination that the patient is without capacity to make medical decisions (9, 10). For example, in the case of 77-year-old Rosaria Candura, a Massachusetts appeals court upheld her right to refuse amputation of a gangrenous leg, even though the court recognized that she was confused on some subjects. In its affirmation of her capacity to refuse treatment, the court noted that no one had questioned her capacity when she originally granted her assent to the amputation, but only later, when she withdrew it (7).

THE RIGHT TO DIE AND ADVANCE DIRECTIVES

Widespread media coverage of court cases, such as those involving Karen Ann Quinlan and Nancy Cruzan, has popularized the phrase right to die. The phrase first came to general public attention during the *Quinlan* case in 1976 (11). In *Quinlan*, a New Jersey court became the first to allow the disconnection of mechanical ventilation from a patient in a persistent vegetative state. Casual use of the phrase right to die, however, may engender more confusion than enlightenment. The right to die in fact encompasses numerous legal rights and ethical guidelines—expressed in court cases, statutes, and ethical treatises—that compose a complex constellation of legal issues, possible medical scenarios, and corresponding obligations by health care providers. The growing recognition of the right of incompetent pa-

tients to refuse medical treatment has led to the development of specific legal means to exercise that right. Collectively, these means have been summarized under the general term advance directive.

An advance directive is a means of preserving a person's right to medical decisions under circumstances in which the individual has lost the immediate capacity to make such decisions personally. Advance directives allow persons to anticipate the treatments he or she would accept or refuse in given circumstances. Such directives also frequently allow patients to designate another person as their legal surrogate decision-maker. Advance directives may take various forms, including living wills, durable power of attorney, treatment plans formulated with a physician upon diagnosis of an illness anticipated to have a critical or terminal phase, and hospice plans of care. All state statutes authorizing living wills and durable powers of attorney for health care expressly provide physicians, surrogate decision-makers, and health care institutions legal immunity from criminal or civil liability for implementing patient or surrogate directives to abate life-sustaining treatments.

The fact that a patient has not executed an advance directive does not preclude abatement of treatment for incapacitated patients. Physicians legally may implement a patient's previously expressed wishes even if those wishes were not formally executed in a legal document. Even if the patient has never expressed his or her wishes, treatment may be abated if it is either deemed in the best interests of the patient or it is determined that continued treatment is futile. If no binding precedent or statutory authorization exists in the jurisdiction, a court may find support for abatement of treatment implied in the common law right of competent patients to refuse treatment, especially if the patient either expressed his or her wishes concerning life-sustaining treatment prior to losing capacity or designated an appropriate surrogate decision-maker. Some states have no cases addressing issues of abatement of treatment. In such states, case law from other jurisdictions can be highly persuasive. Courts in many jurisdictions have allowed withdrawal of life-sustaining treatment in incompetent patients based on previous statements the individual made to family or friends indicating that they would not want to receive such treatment (12).

In many states, even close family members have no formal *legal* right to make health care decisions for an incompetent patient in the absence of a durable power of attorney. However, it is common practice in most health care institutions to allow an incapacitated patient's family members to consent to medical procedures or abatement of treatment, so long as there is no reasonable suspicion of ulterior motives on the part of family members. This practice has been approved by the President's Commission for the Study of Ethical Problems in Medicine and Biomedical and Behavioral Research. Until recently, the only legally sufficient way to obtain authority for family consent to withhold or withdraw treatment was either to petition a court to appoint a family member as the patient's legal guardian or to obtain court approval of the family's consent. Such guardianship procedures can be burdensome, expensive, and time-consuming for patients and their families (13). In some cases, patients have died while awaiting judicial resolution of their petitions, thus effectively depriving them of their right to self-determination and in some cases causing additional suffering by the patient and family. A small but growing number of courts have sanctioned the medical custom of permitting family consent to abatement of treatment. Some states have passed family consent laws that formally authorize family members to act as surrogate decision-makers under certain conditions. Some of these statutes prescribe a hierarchy of legal authority among a patient's relatives in the event there is conflict among family members.

LIVING WILLS

A living will is a document recording an individual's preferences and values concerning medical treatment—including the withholding or withdrawal of life-sustaining procedures—in the event that person loses capacity to make health care decisions. These documents vary widely in specificity. On one extreme, the living will may merely express the patient's general desire to be kept alive by extraordinary or heroic measures in the event of a terminal or irreversible condition or unacceptable quality of life. The usefulness of such documents is often limited due to the difficulty of defining what treatments are to be considered extraordinary or heroic. More specifically, living wills may designate particular treatments that the patient wants withheld or withdrawn—for example, mechanical ventilation and artificial nutrition and hydration—as well as the circumstances under which these instructions apply. Such specific documents are considerably more helpful to clinicians than those using vague, general language. In addition to specific directives for treatment alternatives, living wills may contain statements of the patient's general values that give guidance useful to physicians and surrogate decision-makers under circumstances that cannot be anticipated in the document. For example, a patient who places great importance on avoiding long-term continued existence in a vegetative state can declare that preference to be the primary criterion of his or her quality of life.

Living will forms are commonly distributed by such groups as Choice in Dying and the Hemlock Society. These forms contain standard categories of language attesting to the signer's competence at the time of execution and his or her preference that treatment be abated

when it would only prolong death or when no reasonable possibility of recovery exists. Such forms typically allow space for specific personal directions about desired or undesired modes of treatment, as well as space to designate a surrogate decision-maker (e.g., a durable power of attorney). A nationwide survey by the American Medical Association (AMA) in 1988 found that 15% of persons responding had completed some form of advance directive and that 56% of those surveyed had notified family members of their preferences regarding the use of life-sustaining treatment (14). The public education requirements contained in the Patient Self-Determination Act may stimulate an increase in the number, variety, and sophistication of living wills. Whether or not the patient has an advance directive, the health care team should converse with the patient at appropriate points in the course of treatment in order to clarify the patient's wishes and assure that the patient is aware of the possible medical options and ramifications of his or her medical directives.

All living wills are not executed by means of standardized forms. A number of persons have carefully drafted personalized living wills to reflect their particular values for medical decision-making and to expand the specificity of their instructions to the extent they can anticipate specific medical outcomes. Living wills and other advance directives sometimes provide instructions for treatment or abatement of treatment in a wider range of circumstances than imminent death, including comas, persistent vegetative states, and other forms of critical illness.

More than 40 states have now enacted living will, natural death, or medical treatment decision legislation specifying the legal right of incapacitated patients to refuse or to request life-sustaining treatment and otherwise exercise their right of self-determination regarding health care decisions. Many of these statutes limit abatement of treatment to patients with terminal conditions in which death is imminent. However, a rapidly-growing minority of state statutes also allow abatement of treatment for patients who are irreversibly comatose or in a persistent vegetative state. Since many persons would strongly prefer that their lives not be prolonged in the event of irreversible vegetative states, this trend is welcome and appropriate. Most states' natural death acts also allow designation of a surrogate decision-maker of the patient's choice. Some of these statutes, however, only allow the surrogates named in the living will to make medical decisions that do not entail abatement of life-sustaining treatment.

Living wills enable patients to give legal expression to treatment choices and values as a guide for physicians and surrogates in cases of the patient's later incapacity. It is impossible, however, for living wills to anticipate all of the complex circumstances that may affect medical decision-making in particular cases. Therefore, durable powers of attorney offer the best means of implementing patients' preferences in most cases.

DURABLE POWERS OF ATTORNEY

For centuries, the common law has allowed an individual to designate a representative with the legal authority to execute binding financial transactions on his or her behalf. Formally granting such legal authority on one's personal representative is said to confer power of attorney. The scope of authority granted can be as broad or as narrow as the grantor chooses to specify in the document. The agent to whom one grants power of attorney is not required to be a lawyer; any competent adult can be granted power of attorney. Conventional power of attorney, however, is not useful for handling the affairs of incompetent persons because the agent's authority, by definition, expires upon the incapacity of the grantor. Thus, following the grantor's loss of capacity under a conventional power, decisions and transactions concerning the incapacitated person's affairs require court appointment of a guardian.

As noted previously, however, court appointment of a guardian can be time-consuming, expensive, and a significant emotional burden. In addition, there is no guarantee that a court will appoint as guardian the same person that the incapacitated person would have chosen. Parties commonly disagree about the best interests of the incapacitated person, resulting in a challenge to the appointment of a guardian. Thus, in view of these problems with guardianship, the law recognized the need for a power of attorney that continues in the event of the grantor's incapacity—the durable power of attorney. A durable power of attorney allows the grantor to convey legal decision-making authority that does not expire upon the grantor's loss of capacity.

Every state has adopted legislation allowing designation of a durable power of attorney. A number of these state statutes do not explicitly address whether the scope of a durable power of attorney includes the authority to make health care decisions on behalf of another, although it is likely that they are broad enough to include health care decisions (13). Most states, however, specifically authorize execution of a durable power of attorney for health care decisions. The trend toward authorizing surrogate health care decisions for incapacitated persons by means of a durable power of attorney is reflected in a nonbinding portion of Justice O'Connor's opinion in the *Cruzan* case (15). She endorsed the wisdom of state statutes that specifically authorize medical treatment decisions by surrogates under a durable power of attorney, noted some state courts' suggestions that a general durable power of attorney includes authority for health care decisions, and expressed her view that states' recognition of surrogate decision-makers may be constitutionally required to protect patients' liberty interests in refusal of medical treatment.

Two standards have been articulated to guide substantive decisions by surrogates under durable powers of attorney—substituted judgment and best interests. The substituted judgment standard requires that the surrogate make the same decision that the incapacitated person would have made if he or she were able to choose. The best interests standard recognizes that some persons will not have considered their health care preferences or at least will not have told anyone about such preferences. In such cases the decision-maker must attempt to make a decision that is in the patient's best interests from a more objective social viewpoint. The President's Commission has strongly recommended that substituted judgment be the guiding standard whenever possible because it better implements the value of promoting individual self-determination (16). We will discuss these standards in greater detail later in the chapter.

In many cases a family member will be the representative granted a durable power of attorney. Family members often will be the best persons to implement the substituted judgment standard because they are usually in the most advantageous position to know the patient's expressed treatment preferences, how to interpret those preferences in a manner consistent with the patient's values, and what the patient would decide in circumstances about which the patient did not express preferences. As the US Supreme Court noted in the *Cruzan* case (15 p. 2856), however, ". . . there is no automatic assurance that the view of close family members will necessarily be the same as the patient's would have been . . . while competent." In addition, some patients may not have family members who are available, willing, or sufficiently knowledgeable to execute a durable power of attorney. Unfortunately, it is not uncommon for family members to have ulterior motives—such as financial gain—that may affect their treatment decisions. Health care providers should be aware of this possibility, but should use caution when drawing such conclusions in order to respect the autonomous choices of the patient. It is not sufficient that financial gain, such as inheritance, result from the medical decision. For ulterior motives to be a compelling factor in a decision, a sustained pattern of disregard for expressed patient preferences should be established. An individual may appoint a friend, neighbor, or any competent adult as a surrogate medical decision-maker under a durable power of attorney.

Most states' statutes authorizing a durable power of attorney for medical decisions have not provided adequate guidance for how to proceed in cases in which the authorized surrogate is either unwilling, unavailable, incapacitated, or unconscionably ignoring the patient's previously expressed preferences. Several states allow an individual to designate successive substitutes to replace surrogates who will not or cannot acceptably perform the function. Only New York, Indiana, and Florida, however, in their durable power of attorney statutes adequately specify procedures for invalidating the durable power of attorney of a surrogate who has lost capacity to carry out his or her duties (e.g., mental instability) or who insists on decisions incongruent with the patient's prior directives. All states have statutory provisions for obtaining a court-appointed guardian, which should be sought in the event the patient's designated surrogate abuses the authority of a durable power of attorney for health care decisions.

ISSUES CONCERNING DO NOT RESUSCITATE ORDERS

Do not resuscitate orders (DNR) are physician orders mandating that some or all methods of cardiopulmonary resuscitation (CPR) not be applied to a patient. DNR orders are thus not advance directives themselves, but are often the result of written advance directives or oral discussions with patients or families. Sometimes, however, patients or families are not consulted about their desire for CPR. Liability concerns among physicians and health care institutions may contribute to attempted resuscitation even in cases of medical futility or against patients' wishes. The so-called slow codes or light blue codes—methods of providing CPR in ways that assure it will not be successful—may reflect this fear of liability. Not only are such tactics unethical, they are unnecessary for protection from legal liability. CPR is not appropriate treatment for patients who are likely to die from the primary disease in a relatively short time or for irreversibly comatose patients unless mitigating circumstances are present. A common example of such circumstances is the case of the out-of-town relative who is flying in to bid the patient farewell. Such cases clearly demand that implementation of decisions to abate treatment be delayed and that CPR be provided as necessary, on a short-term basis only.

Documentation in the medical record of the incapacitated patient's previous request to have CPR withheld or documentation of the authorized surrogate's decision to withhold CPR is adequate protection against liability. Communication of the DNR status selected by a patient or legitimate surrogate must be made clear to the entire health care team. Thus far New York is the only state that has enacted a very detailed statute to clarify legal implementation of DNR orders. By specifying that all patients admitted to a hospital are presumed to consent to CPR in response to cardiac or respiratory arrest, however, the New York statute may seem to require CPR or treatment even in cases in which it would be futile, unless the patient or authorized surrogate has consented to a DNR order. Although the law clearly allows patients and legitimate surrogates the right to refuse CPR by means of DNR orders and encourages physicians to address the issue with patients, it may reinforce rather than mitigate the application of CPR in cases of futility when patients or surrogates have had no opportunity to consent to DNR orders.

It is critically important to keep in mind that simply having an advance directive does *not* necessarily mean that a DNR order should be entered for a patient. Advance directives can request a maximal or intermediate level of treatment, as well as refusing it. Similarly, it is important to remember that advance directives are *never* operative so long as the patient is competent and able to express his or her preferences. Full informed consent for all proposed medical procedures must be obtained from any patient possessing capacity to make health care decisions.

INTERPRETING PATIENTS' PREFERENCES

Health care professionals attempting to follow the preferences expressed in an advance directive may find it difficult to interpret the meaning of the directive when applying it to specific circumstances. As Areen (13 p. 230) points out, advance directives, ". . . no matter now detailed cannot possibly anticipate the full range of difficult treatment decisions that may have to be made." By anticipating specific possibilities in the course of treatment and discussing them with the patient in light of the patient's advance directive prior to treatment, physicians may minimize or avoid vexing problems of interpretation if the patient should later lose capacity. A physician should ask the patient to clarify preferences expressed in an advance directive in view of possible developments and either document such clarifications in the record or ask the patient to alter the directive accordingly. Simply talking with the patient about preferences before an untoward event occurs may be the best way to avoid problems.

The language found in many of the forms circulated by interested groups is general and in some cases utilizes popular distinctions increasingly considered inappropriate in ethical analysis of treatment abatement. It is notoriously difficult to define terms like heroic and extraordinary. Distinctions between withholding and withdrawing life-sustaining treatment or between heroic and nonheroic or ordinary and extraordinary means may seem conceptually clear in the abstract, but they vary by context and begin to blur in the requirements of clinical practice. The consensus emerging among medical ethicists and legal authorities was reflected by the New Jersey Supreme Court in its 1985 opinion in the case *In Re Conroy* (17 p. 1233–1235):

We emphasize that in making decisions whether to administer life-sustaining treatment. . . . the primary focus should be the patient's desires and experience of pain and enjoyment—not the type of treatment involved. Thus, we reject the distinction that some have made between actively has-

tening death by terminating treatment and passively allowing a person to die of a disease as one of limited use in a
legal analysis of such a decision-making situation. *** The
ambiguity inherent in this distinction is further heightened
when one performs an act within an overall plan of non-
intervention, such as when a doctor writes an order not to
resuscitate a patient. *** For a similar reason, we also reject
any distinction between withholding and withdrawing life-
sustaining treatment. *** Moreover, from a policy standpoint it might well be unwise to forbid persons from discontinuing treatment under circumstances in which the
treatment could permissibly be withheld. Such a rule could
discourage other families from even attempting certain types
of care and could thereby force them into hasty and premature decisions to allow a patient to die. *** The terms
"ordinary" and "extraordinary" have assumed too many
conflicting meanings to remain useful. *** Further, since
. . . the continuum is constantly shifting due to progress
in medical care, disagreement will often exist about whether
a particular treatment is ordinary or extraordinary. In addition, the competent patient generally could refuse even
ordinary treatment; therefore, an incompetent patient theoretically should also be able to make such a choice when
the surrogate decision-making is effectuating the patient's
subjective intent.

Thus, a substantial consensus exists that there is no moral
or legal distinction between withdrawing and withholding life-sustaining treatments and that terms like extraordinary treatment and heroic measures are not useful ways of analyzing medical treatment decisions.

One previously controversial issue has been that of
whether artificial hydration and nutrition are somehow
different from other life-sustaining treatments. Some
natural death statutes prohibit withholding or withdrawal of hydration and nutrition, even if the patient's
advance directive expressly requests it. Most states' statutes, however, allow abatement of nutrition and hydration just as they would allow removal of mechanical
ventilation or any other treatment. Similarly, most courts
deciding the issue have held that abatement of nutrition
and hydration should be allowed along with other types
of medical interventions, reasoning that a nasogastric or
gastrostomy tube is no less artificial, mechanical, or intrusive than other forms of life-sustaining treatment. This
position is strengthened by the usual circumstances in
which such decisions arise—patients in a persistent vegetative state. A few ethicists have argued that provision
of food and water has sufficient symbolic value as an act
of human caring that it should never be discontinued
(18). For most ethicists, however, this argument fails to
recognize the intrusive nature of the technology providing artificial nutrition and hydration, as well as the argument that vegetative patients are incapable of receiving benefit, even from food and water, since they are
incapable of ever experiencing their environment. Thus,
the consensus of the ethical community is that the discontinuation of artificial hydration and nutrition is *not*

immoral. This position allows those who feel strongly
about the moral importance of feeding to continue to
provide treatment, without imposing their views on the
majority who see such actions as providing no benefit.
Further, some terminally ill, sentient patients can be extremely burdened by continued provision of hydration
and nutrition. Many end-stage cancer patients refuse food
and water during their final days of life, and research
has demonstrated that they are often much more comfortable than if nutrition and hydration were continued
(19). Thus, there are compelling arguments for not
forcing any patient to accept hydration and nutrition.

The case of a stroke patient who cannot swallow
and will eventually recover, yet who refuses tube feeding
and hydration, may be distinguishable from cases in which
terminally ill patients refuse nutrition and hydration. In
such cases, a physician may understandably be more reluctant to honor the patient's refusal in view of the possibility that this refusal is based on temporary depression and the fact that the patient is not terminally ill. In
addition, the effects of the stroke on the patient's ability
to communicate may make it much more difficult to determine whether the patient can exhibit the elements of
capacity necessary to recognize the validity of the patient's refusal. In such a case, the physician should exhaust all measures for treatment of depression and ensure that the patient's refusal is clear and based on a
clear understanding of the consequences. Ultimately,
however, it is possible that even a stroke patient whose
inability to swallow is temporary may competently refuse artificial nutrition and hydration—just as any competent patient may refuse any form of treatment (10).

A strong legal trend is underway to treat nutrition
and hydration as any other medical intervention. However, courts in three states may continue to run counter
to this trend—New York, Washington, and Missouri. In
the *Cruzan* case (15), the Missouri Supreme Court articulated a rule that would virtually prohibit the removal
of nutrition and hydration, although the current Attorney General of Missouri has modified his position on
this issue since the case was decided. The laws of New
York and Washington State remain similarly unclear.
Although the US Supreme Court's opinion in the *Cruzan* case did not provide legally binding precedent on
the question of food and hydration, a majority of the
Justices in *Cruzan* expressed the view that nutrition and
hydration are equivalent to other forms of medical care.
This view is thus highly persuasive regarding cases of
this type.

When an advance directive offers inadequate or no
specific or explicit guidance as to what a patient would
want done under the circumstances, the physician or the
surrogate decision-maker must attempt to preserve the
incapacitated patient's autonomy by applying the principle of substituted judgment. The doctrine of substituted judgment entails an attempt to determine what the

patient would choose if he or she were not incapacitated. As the Illinois Supreme Court explained (20 p. 299):

> Under substituted judgment a surrogate decision maker attempts to establish, with as much accuracy as possible, what decision the patient would want if he were competent to do so. Employing this theory, the surrogate first tries to determine if the patient had expressed explicit intent regarding this type of medical treatment prior to becoming incompetent. *** Where no clear intent exists, the patient's personal value system must guide the surrogate.

Missouri, New York, and Florida limit the doctrine of substituted judgment by applying a higher-than-usual standard of evidence to cases where substituted judgment is an issue. When hearing cases of treatment abatement, other states use the standard named preponderance of the evidence—the typical standard in civil cases. This standard is satisfied if the weight of evidence is 51% or better; that is, if more evidence than not favors a particular determination. In contrast, Missouri, New York, and Florida currently apply the standard known as clear and convincing evidence. Under this standard, evidence must be greater than a preponderance but need not meet the highest standard of beyond a reasonable doubt—the standard applied in criminal cases. Therefore, in Missouri, New York, and Florida it may be more difficult to discontinue life-sustaining treatment unless the patient's wishes have been clearly expressed in a manner that is verifiable—either by written advance directive or sworn testimony of persons with whom the patient conversed about his or her choices.

Critics of substituted judgment argue that determining the preference of an incapacitated patient is too speculative, suggesting instead decision-making based on what the majority of persons or an average person would choose in similar circumstances. The majority of courts have chosen to apply the substituted judgment standard, the rationale for which is found in the opinion of the *Saikewicz* case (8 p. 428):

> Individual choice is determined not by the vote of the majority but by the complexities of the singular situation viewed from the unique perspective of the person called on to make the decision. To presume that the incompetent person must always be subjected to what many rational and intelligent persons may decline is to downgrade the status of the incompetent person by placing a lesser value on his intrinsic human worth and vitality.

The legal duty to base health care decisions for an incapacitated patient on the principle of substituted judgment prevails as long as one has an adequate basis for determining what the patient's wishes would be under the circumstances. The ethical principle underlying the legal duty of substituted judgment is autonomy. As the basis decreases for determining what the patient's choice would be if competent, however, the ethical analysis must begin to shift from the principle of autonomy toward the principle of beneficence. The legal standard for implementing the principle of beneficence is the doctrine of the patient's best interest. The Supreme Court of New Jersey formulated a three-part legal test combining substituted judgment and best interest approaches in the *Conroy* case. This analysis has become widely influential in other court decisions since its articulation in 1985 (17), as follows:

1. If it is clear that the patient would have refused treatment under the circumstances, the decision should not be based on what a reasonable or average person would have done, but what the particular patient would have done if not incapacitated.
2. If it is not clear, but there is some trustworthy evidence that the patient would have refused treatment, and the decision-maker is satisfied that the burdens on the patient (pain and suffering) clearly outweigh the benefits of continued life with the treatment, treatment may be terminated.
3. In the complete absence of reliable evidence that the patient would have rejected the treatment, and the burdens of treatment outweigh the benefits of continued life, with such pain that continuing the treatment would be inhumane, treatment may be terminated.

In later cases, the New Jersey Supreme Court (21) concluded that the latter two tests were not applicable to patients in persistent vegetative states on the basis that it is impossible to ascertain and assess either the pain or pleasure such patients experience. In such cases, the court held that treatment may be refused by a family or close friend without resorting to a court-appointed guardian.

LEGAL STATUS OF ADVANCE DIRECTIVES

A common myth in health care settings is that advance directives are not legally binding on health care providers but are merely advisory guidelines relying on moral obligations. Patients' advance directives have the full force of the law behind their enforcement. Courts and most state legislatures recognize patients' preferences expressed in advance directives and allow abatement of treatment based on those choices or on the decision of an appropriate surrogate. In some cases, physicians and hospitals have been forced by courts to implement advance directives or faced liability for failure to heed them. Some state statutes limit their legal status to situations involving terminal illness or imminent death, thus excluding patients in vegetative states. Other statutes, however, do not limit abatement of treatment to persons whose conditions are terminal, but also include severe, *irreversible* conditions such as quadriplegia and persistent vegetative state. Many of these statutes require certification by independent physician(s) that death is imminent or that a patient's condition is terminal or irreversible. Even in states where statutes effectively prohibit abatement of treatment from patients with irreversible but not terminal conditions, this does not mean that patients' decisions to abate treatment are not accorded legal status. Many states have court decisions that convey rights broader than those allowed by statute. Even if no such court decision exists in the patient's jurisdiction, the increasing number of cases in other jurisdictions across the nation that allow abatement of treatment for nonterminal patients are likely to be highly persuasive precedent.

The provisions of the Patient Self-Determination Act buttress the legal status of advance directives in a substantial, if indirect, way. This federal statute, which took effect in December of 1991, requires hospitals, skilled nursing facilities, home health agencies, hospice programs, and health maintenance organizations that receive Medicaid or Medicare funding to provide each patient written explanations of the individual's medical decision-making rights according to the state's statutes and court rulings. The explanation must include the individual's right to make medical decisions, to accept or to refuse medical treatments, to specify preferences in advance directives, and to be informed about the institution's policies on implementation of specific patient preferences. Moreover, covered institutions are required to document in each patient's medical record whether that patient has an advance directive and to educate institutional staff and the public about advance directives. Noncompliance with these provisions entails mandatory loss of all Medicare and Medicaid funding. Although the Act does not confer legal validity on advance directives beyond what state legislatures or courts have already provided, it clearly signals Congress' intent that patients be informed of the medical decision rights recognized in their states, including transfer to other institutions if the hospital's policy does not accommodate particular aspects of the patient's prospective treatment directives.

CONFLICT BETWEEN PATIENT DIRECTIVES AND PROFESSIONAL OR INSTITUTIONAL POLICY

Generally, particular physicians and institutions are not legally obligated to carry out directives against their will, at least if transfer of care to another physician or institution is feasible. For example, although holding that the surrogate of a patient in a persistent vegetative state can refuse nutrition by nasogastric tube, the Massachusetts Supreme Court did not require the hospital to remove the tube against its policy (22). The patient's family was required to move him to a hospital willing to remove the tube. In some states, the physician's moral obligation to facilitate a transfer to an institution that will honor the patient's rights has been reinforced by

making it a legal duty as well. We believe this is appropriate policy that should be adopted in all states, given the extreme difficulty of obtaining transfer of patients in such cases.

Thus, in the event transfer is impractical or impossible or if institutional policy has not been adequately disclosed, the rights of patients to refuse treatment may override the positions of specific practitioners or institutions. The New Jersey Supreme Court required a nursing home to discontinue artificial feeding, reversing a lower court's decision that would have allowed the facility to maintain artificial feeding until the patient could be transferred to another facility (23). The court based its conclusion on the fact that the nursing home had not adequately informed the patient or her family about its policy on artificial feeding until the family requested that it be discontinued. Because the facility had not informed the family of its policy in advance and because it would be an extreme burden, if not an impossibility, to find another facility that would accept her, the court resolved that ". . . to allow the nursing home to discharge Mrs. Jobes if her family does not consent to continued artificial feeding would essentially frustrate Mrs. Jobes' right of self-determination." The court implied that such a hospital policy might be enforceable if it gave the patient notice of its policy at admission. The requirements of the Patient Self-Determination Act may help to avoid such situations by requiring advance disclosure.

Private health care institutions have more freedom than public ones to transfer patients whose advance directives are against their policies. In the *Bouvia* case discussed earlier (6), a California state court granted removal of a nasogastric feeding tube from a competent 28-year-old acute cerebral palsy, quadriplegic patient in continuous pain from degenerative arthritis against the hospital's conception of ethical standards of the medical profession. Because the hospital's status as a public facility required it to accept her as a patient, the court concluded that the hospital could not refuse to implement her decision to remove the nasogastric tube by transferring her to another hospital that would do so. The California Supreme Court refused to consider an appeal of this decision.

VALIDITY OF ADVANCE DIRECTIVES

Advance directives may be revoked or revised by the patient at any time, as long as the patient has the decisional capacity to do so. In some states, the statute mandates that the advance directive expires after a certain number of years, thus requiring patients to update them. In most states, advance directives are legally effective indefinitely. However, it remains advisable to update directives as preferences change or become more clear, and physicians should actively encourage patients to do so. Many states' advance directive statutes assert that an advance directive executed in another state in compliance with the law of the other state is valid in the state where the patient finds himself or herself. If there is a conflict among the two states, however, it is not clear that a directive authorized by the state in which it was executed will be allowed when the state authorizes measures not allowed in the state where the patient is being treated. The potential for this problem, especially for retirees who move out of the state where their advance directive was executed or for travelers, is illustrated by the decision of a Missouri state appellate court (24). The Missouri court prevented the father and guardian of a patient in a persistent vegetative state from moving his daughter from Missouri to Minnesota for consultation with a nationally recognized neurologist on the grounds that the father was searching for a jurisdiction that would allow abatement of life-sustaining treatment. The reader should keep in mind, however, that Missouri is in the minority regarding these issues. Nevertheless, the traveler should maintain awareness of such problems and take appropriate steps to ensure that his or her preferences are documented as carefully and explicitly as possible when traveling in states with varying laws regarding these issues.

Most states specify some formalities required for statutory advance directives. For example, most states require written advance directives to be witnessed by a specified number of persons. States frequently prohibit employees or parties with financial interests in the admitting facility from serving as witnesses or surrogate decision-makers. In most cases, the advance directive is not required to utilize specifically authorized language. Some states, however, do require exact and exclusive conformity to a standard document given in the statute, and specify that any other form will not be valid. It is plausible, but not guaranteed, that a court would base a decision in such cases on a common law right to refuse treatment and utilize a noncomplying advance directive as evidence of the incapacitated patient's prior wishes. An answer to that question would ultimately be decided by a court's reading of legislative intent behind the statute, as well as the prevailing political views of the state.

SUMMARY

In spite of significant variation among jurisdictions, several emergent trends can be recognized in summary of the current state of the law on these issues. The common-law right of self-determination, augmented by constitutional rights of privacy and liberty, entails the right of adult autonomous patients to refuse treatment, including life-sustaining treatment. Such a patient's right to refuse treatment does not end upon the patient's loss of immediate capacity to make decisions personally. Through various types of advance directives, including legally authorized surrogate decision-makers, incapacitated patients' treatment decisions can be legally implemented, including the right to refuse or withdraw life-sustaining treatment. The distinction between withholding and withdrawing treatment has no legal significance. Less formal prior expressions of an incapacitated patient's treatment wishes may be recognized as valid evidence by courts, even without a living will or durable power of attorney. Appropriately authorized termination or withholding of life-sustaining treatment on behalf of an incapacitated adult is extremely unlikely to result in criminal or civil liability for the attending physician. Physicians, therefore, may utilize these legal developments to facilitate dialogue concerning patients' treatment preferences and thereby help to preserve the autonomy and dignity of their patients under difficult circumstances without undue concern about liability.

References

1. Jonsen AR, Siegler M, Winslade WJ. *Clinical Ethics*, 2nd ed. Macmillan; New York, NY:1986.
2. *Canterbury v Spence*, 464 F2d 772 (DC Cir) (1972).
3. Faden PR, Beauchamp, TL. *A History and Theory of Informed Consent.* Oxford University Press; New York, NY: 1986.
4. *Schloendorff v. Society of New York Hospital*, 211 NY 125, 129–30, 105 NE 92, 93.
5. *Bartling v Superior Court*, 163 Cal App 3d 186, 209 Cal Rptr 220 (1984).
6. *Bouvia v Superior Court*, 179 Cal App 3d 1127, 225 Cal Rptr 297 (1986), *review denied* (Cal June 5, 1986).
7. Weir RW, Gostin L. Decisions to abate life-sustaining treatment for nonautonomous patients. *JAMA.* 264:1846–1853, 1990.
8. *Superintendent of Belchertown State School v Saikewicz*, 373 Mass 728, 370 NE 2d 417 (1977).
9. *In the Matter of Quackenbush*, 156 NJ Super 282, 383 A2d 785 (1978).
10. *Lane v Candura*, 6 Mass App Ct 377, 376 NE 2d 1232 (1978).
11. *In re Quinlan*, 137 NJ Sup 227, 348 NJ 801, modified and remanded, 70 NJ 10, 355 A2d 647, cert denied., 429 US 922 (1976).
12. *In re Eichner*, 102 Misc2d 184, 423 NYS 2d 580 (Sup Ct 1979), modified sub nom, *Eichner v Dillon*, 73 AD2d 431, 426 NYS2d 517 (App Div 1980), modified, 52 NY2d 363, 438 NYS2d 266, 420 NE2d 64 (1981).
13. Areen J. The legal status of consent obtained from families of adult patients to withhold or withdraw treatment. *JAMA*, 258:229–235, 1987.
14. McCrary SV, Botkin. Hospital policy on advance directives. *JAMA.* 262:2411–2414, 1989.
15. *Cruzan v Director, Missouri Dept of Health*, 110 S Ct 2841 (1989).
16. President's Commission for the Study of Ethical Problems in Medicine and Biomedical and Behavioral Research. *Deciding to Forego Life-Sustaining Treatment.* US Government Printing Office; Washington, DC: 1983.
17. *In Re Conroy*, 98 NJ 321, 486 A2d 1209 (1985).
18. Callahan D. Public policy and the cessation of nutrition. In: Lynn J, ed., *By No Extraordinary Means.* Expanded ed. Bloomington, Ind: Indiana University Press; 1989.

19. Schmitz P, O'Brien, M. Observations on nutrition and hydration in dying cancer patients. In: Lynn J, ed., *By No Extraordinary Means.* Expanded ed. Bloomington, Ind: Indiana University Press, 1989.

20. *In re Estate of Longeway,* 133 Ill2d 33, 549 NE2d 292 (1989).

21. *In re Peter,* 108 NJ 365, 529 A2d 419 (1987).

22. *Brophy v New England Sinai Hospital, Inc.,* 398 Mass 417, 497 NE 2d 626 (1986).

23. *In re Jobes,* 180 NJ 394, 529 A2d 434, 450 (1987).

24. *In re The Matter of Christine Busalacchi, Incapacitated and Disabled,* 1991 No App Lexis 315.

47

Ethical Issues in Caring for the Elderly

John D. Banja

The principal bioethical preoccupations of our era concerning elderly health care consumers involve the extent to which they can make compelling demands for medical services in a society that is increasingly disposed toward containing health care costs and the form of respect and extent of moral responsibility due elderly persons. As rehabilitation focuses a significant dimension of its energies and resources on the needs of disabled elderly persons, its present and future are inextricably linked with various philosophic questions with which this chapter will be concerned, such as: why is determining the allocation of care to elderly persons so contentious in our society? What obstacles prevent a public philosophy or social consensus on society's obligations toward the elderly? How should society respond to the needs and requests of the elderly, both in terms of national health policy as well as in terms of more mundane considerations involving living arrangements, supervision, and so forth? How can the freedoms and dignity of elderly persons be preserved when the intellectual and physical decline associated with aging frequently compromises the authentic expression of those freedoms? All of these questions involve moral beliefs or values about the relationship between elderly persons and the society in which they live.

This chapter will begin by philosophically examining how certain social and political norms and beliefs perpetuate a variety of ethical problems over establishing fair and just practices in allocating care for elderly disabled persons. First to be explored will be identifying those factors that disenable a broadbased, transgenerational commitment to the health care needs of elderly disabled persons.

ETHICAL DILEMMAS IN ALLOCATING CARE TO THE ELDERLY

Few health care providers are unaware of the intense pressures that currently seek to diminish and contain health care expenditures. In recent years, professional concern has been focused on a number of disturbing factors that cumulatively suggest an acute economic instability within our health care system. These indications include a failure to curb excessive inflation in health care; the availability, utilization, and continuing development of sophisticated but expensive medical technologies; the availability and successful utilization of life-saving interventions, which may prolong, without meaningfully improving, the lives of irreversibly ill persons; the demand for better qualified but higher salaried health care professionals; and the continuing suspicion about frequently practiced, though theoretically questionable, interventions (1–3).

A remarkably different climate existed in health care only 25 years ago. When Lyndon Johnson signed the Medicare Act into law in 1965, he said, "No longer will older Americans be denied the healing miracle of modern medicine. No longer will illness crush and destroy the savings that have so carefully been put away over a lifetime so that they might enjoy dignity in their later years." (*Atlanta Journal and Constitution*, July 29, 1990:A-16.) The moral underpinnings of Johnson's sentiments were as genuine as they were compelling; that is, elderly persons living on fixed but frequently modest incomes should not have to suffer the indignity and perversity of losing access to health care. The moral connection of the Medicare Act to the Johnsonian vision of the "Great Society" was that health care is a social right, that its distribution should depend on human need rather than the ability to pay, and that it should be available to all.

Only 10 years would pass, however, before health policy analysts began forecasting the bankruptcy of Medicare by the year 2000 unless serious measures were implemented either to increase Medicare's operating budget—which accrued from social security taxes—or to significantly curtail its expenditures. By the advent of the Reagan administration, which adamantly opposed raising taxes, dealing with the spiraling costs of Medicare took the form of curtailing Medicare payments to hospitals by implementing the diagnosis related group (DRG) method of reimbursement. This strategy, which appeared in 1983, limited Medicare's payments to participating hospitals to a predetermined amount of money, reflecting reasonable or average costs a hospital would incur for a Medicare beneficiary's treatment given the diagnosis (4, 5).

Although rehabilitation remains DRG-exempt at the time of this writing, numerous reports suggest that some form of prospective payment system will be instituted (6). Consequently, it is important to evaluate the degree of success that cost constraint measures have experienced in meeting the objectives of reducing health care costs.

Although there is little question that cost constraint mechanisms such as DRGs have accounted for significant reductions in inpatient expenditures, the principal moral concern they invite is that no method other than rationing health services will ultimately ensure the financial stability of the health care system in the United States (2). While no one would object to cost containment measures that identify and halt wasteful and inefficient practices, strident voices in health care policy predict that the cessation of wasteful and inefficient practices will not be nearly enough to maintain the solvency of our health care system (7). This position maintains that our society is rapidly approaching the point where the seemingly limitless consumptional capacity of the American health care consumer, coupled with a seemingly irreversible inflationary spiral in medicine, will utterly exhaust the capacity of any financing mechanism to keep apace (*Atlanta Journal and Constitution*. July 29, 1990:A-16). There is no alternative, these analysts claim; the health care system must learn to say no to its consumers. Subsequent fears have become very prominent that the elderly comprise a group to whom no will be said most often.

One of the boldest suggestions for setting limits in health care has been made by Daniel Callahan (7), who proposes using age as a criterion in allocating expensive, life-sustaining technologies. Callahan opposes such allocations beyond a certain age—which he places around 80 years—as disruptive to the economic welfare of a health care system that he believes is thoroughly out of control. He remarks that "It is time for the pretense that old age can be an infinite and open frontier to end and for the unflagging, but self-deceptive optimism that we can do anything we want with our economic system to be put aside." (7 p. 222) While Callahan purports to direct his arguments for restraining the allocation of care only with regard to the provision of life-sustaining technologies, he reveals an attitude towards rehabilitation that is hardly ingratiating:

> Even low-technology approaches to noncurable chronic problems can be enormously expensive if used by enough people . . . The most troubling problems in that respect may well be posed by advances in rehabilitation. Even now, rehabilitation for stroke is labor-intensive, difficult, and often of uncertain outcome . . . The ongoing development of

sophisticated prosthetic devices and computer-assisted methods of helping the partially paralyzed, paraplegic and quadriplegic do not promise to lower costs, and neither does their likely extension to use among the elderly. If such developments as these are even to be possible, it is hard to envision how they can financially coexist with continuing investment in life-extending treatments (7 pp. 149–150).

Callahan's book, *Setting Limits*, contains a carefully articulated and sustained series of arguments on age-related, health care rationing as the most fair and just allocation strategy, given the alternatives and constraints of the American political system. Other commentators, however, bristle at the notion that the American health care consumer will have to accept the inevitability of rationing. They ask why, in a country known for its wealth and frivolous spending, can't Americans summon a firmness of moral purpose and change those economic and spending practices so that health care, which is obviously one of our nation's most cherished resources, is supplied to everyone.

The inspiration for this latter position derives from the Judeo-Christian respect for life and the universally shared opinion on the desirability of health and physical function. Health is not only desired for its own sake, but also is a necessary prerequisite for the realization of employment, recreation, and securing the necessities of life. To deny a person health care due to an inability to pay exhibits a perverse disrespect for that person's humanness (8). Consequently, if health care allocation in the United States is presently threatened by severe economic scarcity—as evidenced by some 40 million Americans who are unable to purchase health insurance—then a rethinking of the moral values that underpin our social commitment to human dignity and identifying the resources to finance that commitment is imperative. As we so value health in our country, financing its care must become a major priority in accordance with time-honored values that insist on human dignity, the right to life, and the right to health care (9).

The social status of elderly persons, especially those with disabilities, presents a paradigm test case of this "respect for persons" position. Many, if not most, elderly persons are unable to justify their worth or define their social value through familiar utilitarian measures that understand human worth through employment, paying taxes, raising a family, occupying civic leadership positions, and so on. While many elderly persons live vital and energetic lives, their frequent disassociation from those activities most closely identified with economic productivity leaves questions about their worth and value intrinsically related to issues over their personhood. That is, elderly persons possess an inherent right and dignity because they are persons. Thus, if their rights and dignity are to be respected, then our society cannot deprive the elderly of their needs, especially when those needs so frequently and predictably involve health care.

This argument is at once inspiring, yet the plight of the elderly—as well as other special interest groups in our society such as the homeless, the mentally ill, and the economically disadvantaged—vividly suggests that this argument has failed to persuade the body politic to undertake appropriate measures to allocate adequate resources for persons in serious need. A recent body of literature explains the failure to establish a formula for allocating health care and other social goods as largely resulting from a culturally entrenched resistance to a public or communitarian philosophy that articulates a theory of the value of human life, its inherent dignity, and its ultimate meaning and proper ends (10, 11). Such a theory would presumably discuss what it is about human life that makes it distinctive, valuable, and worthwhile. It would establish whether the mere possession of human DNA bestows unconditional worth on human life or whether additional factors such as one's social contributions qualify certain lives as more valuable than others. The theory would also identify or recommend the proper ends of human life by explaining in what excellence of character consists and what would count as virtuous conduct towards satisfying the conditions for living ethically or with a view to goodness. Therefore, the theory would define or at least clarify our social roles and the nature and extent of our moral obligations toward one another by identifying those ideals and social aspirations that are demonstrably conducive to the good life.

Yet, Americans have historically resisted articulating a philosophical theory of what it means to be human that, in turn, prescribes our ethical obligations toward one another. Indeed, the very notion of deriving such a system of obligations from a moral theory based on a vision of human nature is repugnant to our political identity and heritage. In its commitment to liberal values, American society rejects the notion of a culturally mandated or historically enshrined notion of oughtness that prescribes a system of moral imperatives. As Richard Rorty provocatively observes, "a liberal society is one which has no ideal except freedom, no good except a willingness to see how (free and open) encounters go and to abide by the outcome. . . . and no purpose except to make life easier for poets and revolutionaries." (12 p. 13) Our liberal spirit is inherently opposed to any person or institution's defining what will permanently count as one person's moral obligations to someone else since the liberal mindset is forever worried about the emergence of a politically coercive force that wishes, for once and for all, to structure society and allocate that society's goods according to a particular value system (13, 14). Thus, instead of establishing a moral theory that defines the value, nature, and goals of human life and then defining one's duties within that theory, liberal governments establish a rights-oriented society wherein citizens are empowered to define their own vision of

goodness and what will count as their moral duties (10). As such, it is hardly accidental that our society is an ethically pluralistic one since tolerance of opposing values—so long as the exercise of such values does not significantly endanger others—is an inevitable corollary of liberal ideals.

The influence of liberal values and the various conflicts that have occurred among liberals over the proper role of government have had enormous repercussions within the context of disability. The sum and substance of those repercussions is a confusion over determining whether a person's misfortune in experiencing a disability should or should not invest that individual with certain privileges over and beyond what nondisabled persons enjoy. Egalitarian liberals believe that a proper function of government is to determine a scheme of redistributing social goods according to a vision of economic rights. To the egalitarian liberal, a disabled person has a right to enjoy the goods of his society and, to the extent that his or her disability interferes with the enjoyment of that right, government has a duty to redistribute goods—a process that inevitably assumes the form of taking from those who have to provide for those who do not. The libertarian liberal, on the other hand, is revolted by this notion of economic rights. Libertarians believe that life's being unfair to one person does not provide that person with special entitlements that must be accommodated or responded to by others (15). To the libertarian, governmental power becomes misdirected and misappropriated when it seeks to create special entitlements that necessitate a departure from the principles of a free market economy and the right of ownership of private property. What sustains the argument between libertarians and egalitarians, however, is that neither wants to discourse in terms of a vision of the common good or those purposes and ends that are common to all human beings, but rather within a dialogue based on rights and entitlements that first and foremost respect the separateness, uniqueness, and individuality of human beings (11).

The point of this discussion is to show that the reluctance of our society to develop a coherent moral or ethical comprehension of the meaning and value of human life and how health, disease, aging, and disability affect that value inevitably invites a series of intractable problems over what entitlements disabled persons might claim (7). While our egalitarian values dispose us to provide emergency, lifesaving care for everyone—as evidenced by the heroic efforts to save persons who have sustained catastrophic injury or who are born with severe congenital abnormalities—our libertarian values confuse us over what levels of resource allocation are subsequently owed to disabled persons as a function of their inherent worth and dignity. We remain confused because neither egalitarian nor libertarian schemes rest on a philosophical account of what that worth and dignity mean. Therefore, although it is paradoxical, it is not peculiar that Medicare will spend tens of thousands of dollars for livesaving intensive care for a stroke patient, but not pay for home care, architectural changes, technologic aids, or even prescription drugs the individual may require after rehabilitation. Indeed, the fact that elderly patients must first spend their life's savings and become impoverished to qualify for Medicaid nursing home coverage is a notorious example of the liability of a sociopolitical ideology that emphasizes individualism over a theory of collective responsibility towards preserving human dignity (16).

Furthermore, it is worth noting that whereas the moral relationship between governmental insurers and insureds is confused by liberal values, the private payor sector of the health care industry sees its relationship to health consumers as a purely contractual one. The private payor understands its moral obligation to insureds as a requirement to perform to the letter of the coverage explicitated in the insurance policy. The insured is not morally entitled to anything beyond that promised in the policy since exceeding those policy limits imperils the financial welfare of the insurer, its profit-generating capacity, and its financial commitment to investors. Consequently, whether one speaks of governmental or private reimbursement for health care, the economic welfare of the industry has superseded in importance what in other societies would be a social ethic or politics of the common good that determines the nature and limits of society's obligations to allocate goods. To the extent, then, that governmental sources of insurance are perplexed over locating and ethically justifying revenues necessary to meet the admittedly expensive spectrum of health care consumers' needs and to the extent that the private payor is unwilling to insure an individual who presents a potential risk for an expensive claim, the future of the American health care consumer, and especially the elderly, is clearly precarious.

DECISION-MAKING AMONG THE ELDERLY

What has been discussed thus far is a reluctance of the political will to rank and allocate social goods according to a theory of the meaning and worth of human life. Rather than articulate a public philosophy or consensual vision of the meaningful life by which our social goods would be prioritized, our society has instead opted for personal liberties or freedoms by which individuals would define their own values and what would count as goods in those lives. In effect, rights become invented as the political mechanisms of self-determination and through which one's relations to others are structured and the significant benefits of life secured.

Philosophers discuss two types of rights, negative and positive (17). Negative rights are those that assure the rights holder of noninterference. These rights guarantee freedom of access, noncoercion, and nondiscrimination. Thus, persons may have the right of freedom of expression, commerce, privacy, religious preference, and so on, which enable them to exercise their personal values without fearing unreasonable intrusions from others. While negative rights are at the heart of libertarian ideals in ensuring noninterference or freedom from unreasonable governmental intrusion, positive rights are entitlements to certain social goods that bind others to respond. Thus, if I have a positive right to X, someone in society has a correlative duty to assist me in securing X. For example, women presently have a negative right to abortion in the United States since they are protected from someone's interfering with their having an abortion (although they cannot compel a physician to give them an abortion). On the other hand, the hospitalized patient who unexpectedly goes into cardiac arrest has a positive right in the form of anticipating cardiopulmonary resuscitation from persons who have undertaken a duty to care for him.

Within the context of allocating care to elderly persons with disability, a rights question that has been contemplated over the last few pages is whether and to what extent such persons have a positive right to health care. As the foregoing has shown, persons in our society have only the barest claim or positive right to health care in the form of emergency care to save their lives (and, even then, not always) or to certain types of care in public health clinics (assuming they are poor enough to qualify). Otherwise, the extent to which individuals can access health care is largely determined by their ability to maintain insurance coverage or to pay for that care out of pocket (18).

Nevertheless, another and very important way of examining the rights of citizens is asking about their exerting whatever rights they unequivocally enjoy regardless of whether those rights are negative or positive. Examining this issue means digressing from the question of what society owes individuals in economic terms and examining those duties society *already assumes* in respecting and preserving whatever constitutionally acknowledged rights are available to anyone who can reasonably lay claim to them.

To the extent that old age and/or disability can compromise an individual's capacity or function, then that person's capacity as a rights holder is jeopardized. Persons do not give up their legal rights because they become old or enfeebled; however, the onset of physical or intellectual impairment may interfere with their ability to exert those rights or may expose them to others who, for a variety of reasons ranging from the well-intentioned to the perverse, might violate those rights. What, then, are the crucial considerations that need to occur among health professionals in respecting and protecting the rights of the elderly disabled?

This question is most often answered by referring

to the legal notion of competency. In law, competency denotes an individual's capacity to make a legally compelling claim or to anticipate that his or her rights expressions will be respected by others. An incompetent person cannot exert legal authority, but must depend on a guardian or proxy to make decisions or must have made rights claims prior to the onset of his or her incompetency, such as through executing a durable power of attorney or a living will (19). It is important to note that while many individuals may be globally incompetent, such as individuals with advanced Alzheimer's disease, many people may be competent in one domain but not in another (20). Thus, an individual may be competent to execute a will but not to operate a business; competent to consent to medical treatment but not to drive an automobile; competent to stand trial but not to raise a family. Hence, an individual's competence may be affected cognitively, physically, or both. The stroke patient with global aphasia would not be deemed competent to consent to or refuse medical treatment, while the intellectually intact but motorically impaired elderly person might no longer be competent to drive an automobile.

When health providers encounter situations wherein the competence of a patient is in doubt, they should secure consent for treatment from, or have the patient's decision corroborated by, the patient's guardian or proxy (21). Usually this individual will be the patient's nearest next of kin, although identifying this person may be difficult in certain cases. For example, many elderly patients may have been living alone for many years with what best appears to be a few distant relatives spread out over the country. Or, the person closest to the patient may not be a blood relative but a companion or friend who has lived with or intimately known the patient for years. In difficult situations like these, two considerations are important. First, the legal and moral comprehension of the proxy's role is that he or she make the decision *the patient would make* if the patient were capable of rational decision-making (22). The proxy should function as the patient's mirror-image or deputy and, in making the decision believed to be the one the patient would make, thus preserve the patient's right of self-determination. Second, every health provider should be familiar with the common law or statute in his or her jurisdiction that lists who may serve as a proxy. By avoiding reliance on an inappropriate person as the patient's proxy, the provider is not exposed to liability for nonconsensual treatment (21). Unfortunately, it is an open question in many states as to who can serve as proxy since some states have not addressed proxy identification issues at all, whereas other states have used vague terminology such as "nearest next of kin" (21). Thus, in a case where a never married, elderly person who lived alone is accompanied to the hospital by his two sisters and three brothers, the identity of his nearest next of kin is ambiguous. If these persons were to disagree among themselves about which treatment should or should not be provided, to whom should the health provider acquiesce?

In instances where the law is unclear as to who can function as proxy for health care decisions, an appropriate court will make the identification, often after hearing and evaluating arguments from various persons as to who is best qualified to serve (23). A court may appoint an individual as a temporary proxy if the ward is expected to regain competence at some future date. However, while temporary proxy appointment may be appropriate for certain incompetent rehabilitation consumers such as those with traumatic brain injury, the court's appointment of a proxy or guardian for elderly rehabilitation consumers is likely to be life-long, owing to the probability that the elderly person's decision-making impairment is permanent and irreversible (23).

While the law's intention of respecting the rights of persons through the mechanism of proxy appointment is admirable, the nature of that legal process is repulsive to many people. The formal judicial declaration of a person as incompetent may seem callous and heartrending; the decision as to who is best qualified to serve as proxy may be marked by conflicts among family members; and the legal proceedings themselves may be adversarial, time-consuming, expensive, and intimidating.

There is a growing literature that questions the moral spirit of a society whose method of protecting the rights of elderly health consumers assumes such a rigidly formal approach (23, 24). While the legal adjudication of competency may sometimes be the most appropriate and expedient remedy to a difficult situation, a judicial solution may not always be the most advisable. For instance, research indicates that elderly persons frequently are uncomfortable with and resist legal measures such as executing living wills and instead prefer to trust their family members to decide what is best for them (24).

The first objective of both morality and law in proxy appointments is to preserve the integrity of the incompetent's decisions. A paradoxical research finding, however, is that many elderly persons would prefer that a family member or friend make a substituted judgment when the crucial time comes for decisions (25). Analogously, just as many elderly persons may prefer to entrust their future decisions to their loved ones rather than make those decisions prior to the onset of incompetency, so, too, health professionals might argue that adverting to the courts and their legalistic paradigms of competency determinations and formal proxy/guardian appointment misses an important dimension of trust in provider-patient relationships. Obviously, health consumers need to be able to trust their physicians, nurses, and allied care providers to anticipate their best interests, which may occasionally mean that many elderly persons would rather their health care providers decide what will count as benefits and burdens in their lives.

Another argument opposing a legalistic framework for managing the patient's decision-making impairment is that competency is but one element in the conceptual architecture of autonomy. Competency determinations are important in instances when the consequences of an individual's decision-making have serious impact on his or her welfare or the welfare of others. Thus, a competency determination may be indicated when impaired cognition compromises the validity of an individual's decisions over medical care, finances, and so forth. Many elderly persons, however, may not need to make these kinds of decisions at all; or if they do, they might be capably assisted by friends or family. One must recognize that the overriding concern in the legal appointment of a proxy or guardian is the integrity of that individual's intentions towards preserving the welfare of the incompetent person; that is, that the proxy will make the decisions the incompetent would make if he or she were capable of doing so. Obviously, proxies ought not have a personal interest or agenda at stake that might constitute a conflict of interest (22). If the court's competency hearings primarily seek to assure that these considerations are in place, then these activities are superfluous when elderly persons already enjoy and benefit from the assistance of trustworthy, though not court-appointed, decision-making helpers.

A more practical concern for an elderly person is respecting dignity and the right to choose with regard to more mundane aspects of day-to-day living, such as dressing, shopping, entertainment, hobbies, and other interests. Because physical infirmities that accompany aging are frequently misinterpreted as including mental infirmities, the elderly person's intellectual functioning may be profoundly underestimated. This may not only result in the formation of attitudes toward elderly persons that ignore whatever intellectual capacities are present, but may also result in omitting measures that seek to maintain or improve those capacities (26, 27). The paternalistic attitude of the clinician or family member who simply assumes the elderly person needs assistance in making any and every decision is a notorious example of this tendency.

Collopy (28) has offered a thoughtful list of polarities embedded within the autonomy construct to which health professionals should be sensitive. These polarities embody different aspects of autonomy and encourage the health professional to be more appreciative of the nuances of autonomous function. A superficial approach to thinking about autonomy may not only imperil whatever autonomous functioning is present among elderly persons, but may dangerously assume its presence when it is actually absent.

A brief listing of these autonomy polarities is as follows:

1. *decisional versus executional*: recognizing that a person may not be able to execute certain physical tasks such as are involved in activities of daily living, but may certainly be able to make decisions about them;
2. *direct versus delegated*: recognizing that while direct decision making is an obvious suggestion or attempt at independent, autonomous function, a person may also be acting autonomously by delegating decision making to someone else.
3. *competent versus incapacitated*: recognizing that a seemingly unreasonable desire or preference may not necessarily imply incapacity or incompetence.
4. *authentic versus inauthentic*: recognizing that a seemingly logical or reasonable decision may nevertheless not be an authentic expression of a person's desires; coercion, emotional upheavals, and impulsivity may cause a person to function inauthentically by engaging in "choices and activities that are seriously out of character, discontinuous with personal history and present values, lacking self-possession and self-understanding."
5. *immediate versus long-range*: recognizing that careful thought and consideration need to be given to how short-range preferences may or may not imperil long-range goals; this consideration can be especially problematic in rehabilitation since short-range expressions of autonomy may jeopardize long-range objectives;
6. *negative versus positive*: recognizing that negative rights or rights of noninterference are substantially different from positive rights or rights whose expression compels a response from someone else.

Autonomy is not a neatly definable concept whose connotations are easily operationalized. However, if we recognize that respecting the autonomy of the elderly—which encompasses their right to choose what will count as benefits and burdens in their lives—is a significant expression of our respect for them as persons, then appreciating the textures and complexities of autonomy becomes a moral imperative.

THE ELDERLY, THE FUTURE, AND THE VIABILITY OF REHABILITATION

Rehabilitation is classically defined as the restoration of function. Within the context of care for elderly persons, this definition carries two important considerations: the realization of functional restoration is generally thought to make a meaningful difference in the elderly person's life, and rehabilitation consumers and the society in which they live appreciate and desire that difference. These assumptions are obviously independent from one another. An individual can experience what to his or her clinicians constitutes a successful rehabilitation, only to allow those functional gains to be lost to subsequent depression, lassitude, or indifference. It is important to recognize that independence must not be regarded as a given, but rather as an option whose possibility and desirability must impress not only the consumer but also the society that opts to allocate and regulate rehabilitation services (29).

As one contemplates the interface of rehabilitation services with the needs of elderly persons, the conditional worth of rehabilitation services becomes apparent. Obviously, rehabilitation would not proceed with a functionally vegetative Alzheimer's patient since this individual would have no rehabilitation potential. Yet, the word potential reminds one of the need to define the practical realization or objective of that potential as well as its inherent desirability. What criteria should be used to determine when the restoration of function should be pursued in a given case? In what context is the restoration of function meaningful rather than pointless? Under what circumstances other than financial ability might one elderly person receive considerable rehabilitation whereas another receive less, and could those differing allocations be justified according to an objective, consensually validated professional standard of care rather than the subjective impressions of disparate rehabilitation providers (30)?

Clearly, if rehabilitation is to be valued, it must be congruent with society's estimate of the needs of elderly persons and society's willingness to allocate resources to accommodate those needs. Without these social endorsements, rehabilitative care would seem extravagant, exotic, or simply incomprehensible. What is worrisome as one contemplates the future of rehabilitation services are those observations that, seemingly correctly, assert that our society has been unable to find a meaningful place in public discourse for suffering and decline in life (7). This inability casts a shroud of ambiguity over our moral obligations to elderly disabled persons since the absence of a social comprehension of suffering and decline in life undermines our confidence in defining an appropriate attitude or compass of moral responsibilities toward elderly disabled persons. If disability and aging are not valued within the moral fabric of our society, we can only expect to remain befuddled about the intrinsic value or utility of rehabilitation, either for the disabled or for the elderly at large.

These problems were anticipated within a broader discussion of aging in the form of two alternative views on the meaning of becoming elderly. The perspective of the 1950s and 1960s seemed principally one that accepted a disengagement theory of aging, wherein an individual distanced himself or herself from the affairs of

employment, family rearing, civic responsibilities, and social life proportional to his or her increasing years (31). The social role of elderly persons represented by this view was seen as an anticipation of, and resignation to, the inevitability of age-related infirmities or impairments, a belief that younger persons were more deserving of social benefits than older persons, and a peaceful capitulation to the inevitability of death. According to this perspective, the value of functional restoration to an elderly person already beset by some musculoskeletal or neurologic impairment might be suspect since such benefit would be diminished by the already present devaluation of that individual's life as a function of advanced age.

The modernist perspective emerged as a backlash to the disengagement theory and proclaimed that the inevitability of physical and intellectual decline with age is a fallacy and that "although death is inevitable, the course of the aging process is not." (32 p. 17) Modernists abhorred the disengagement theory as defeatist and biologically inaccurate. They perceived old age as but another stage on life's way—one that has the potential to be as fulfilling, productive, and enjoyable as any of the preceding ones. For the modernist, rehabilitation would be understood as similar to any kind of acute or subacute medical intervention that seeks to reverse the disabling consequences of a condition that hinders a person's capacity to be productive and lead a fulfilling life. Indeed, the political trappings of the modernist view would brand any attempt to deprive the elderly of rehabilitation as perverse and discriminatory.

Because both the ageist and modernist approaches are social ideologies as well as presumptive theories about the biologic reality of aging, both are rendered problematic by numerous counterexamples and cultural dispositions that question the rhetoric, factual accuracy, and sociopolitical visions assumed by these ideologies. Thus, the ageist perspective is certainly repulsive in its almost morbid resignation to the inevitability of age-related decline and death; yet, the acceptance of death as a natural event of life smacks of realism and psychologic health. On the other hand, a defiant rejection of a biologic decline with increasing age as touted by the modernists represents a remarkable example of denial. If, as John and Matilda Riley claim (32), it is fallacious to believe that an aging decline is inevitable, then one might expect persons to live forever or, perhaps, expect that elderly persons would someday die but from nothing at all. Still, it is obviously true that the modernist perspective presents an optimism about one's elderly years that can be enormously conducive to affirming life's bountiful potential and realizing its joys.

The moral situation regarding the value and allocation of rehabilitation services to elderly persons might very well situate itself within the ageist-modernist dispute, insofar as the elderly disabled must surely be struck by the limits of life but can just as well be impressed by possibilities and benefits that life extends throughout its duration. If, however, life as well as the benefits of rehabilitative therapies and technologies has limits, how does one establish the point at which those limits are reached and when extending beyond those limits becomes unreasonable and counterproductive?

Perhaps three solutions to these questions, along with their accompanying liabilities, are worth noting. The first solution to setting limits on allocating care to the elderly is a political one whose realization is hardly inconceivable. The astonishing growth in the number of elderly persons may be sufficient for them to summon the requisite degree of political will discussed earlier to secure government monies for rehabilitation and chronic care services for all elderly persons. This solution would entail that no one would go without needed services and would assert a generous comprehension of what needed would include. To the extent, however, that this solution would represent the will of the people as expressed through their state and federal legislatures, one would obviously anticipate numerous worries about the degree to which such an allocation of resources might deprive or diminish other social services from special interest groups and the extent to which conflicts between generations might ensue. Nevertheless, one out of every four persons in our society will be 65 years of age or over by the year 2040 (7); their political presence and power will be as formidable as their social agenda will be apparent.

A second solution is a scientific-technologic one. While superior health habits emphasizing diet, exercise, and wellness may result in longer life in the future, scientific breakthroughs and the utilization of increasingly sophisticated technologies may extend those years even further. While the prospects of increasing the life span to perhaps 125 years or 150 years may seem appealing, one can confidently predict that such prospects will be accompanied by a host of unprecedented ethical dilemmas. One dilemma, of course, would be the health care costs associated with caring for a much larger population of older individuals. Persons over 65 years of age in 1984 consumed over three dollars in health care costs for every one dollar consumed by persons under 65 years of age (33). It seems fair to assume, therefore, that the economic prospects of reimbursing care for persons routinely living well over 100 years would be staggering. Such individuals could experience numerous and discrete rehabilitations in their lifetimes as might be connected with multiple joint replacements, cardiac disease, and recurring strokes. Another problem that might eventually arise would be a need to control the number of births. In a country like the United States, which touts reproductive freedom, it is impossible to consider how such problems would be managed without massive cultural upheaval.

In the absence of either a political or scientific solution for certain problems associated with the allocation of health care and rehabilitation services for the elderly, one might suggest a return to the ethical drawing board to contemplate a position that most satisfactorily addresses the values of our liberal society so as to best maintain the general welfare. Preserving the welfare of all concerned, not just the elderly's, is imperative in our society since the demands of justice, fairness, and equal access must govern the allocation of socially available goods to all potential consumers—not just to a discrete group of persons with specific needs. However, this imperative returns our analysis to the seemingly intractable need to examine our social policy and, if not carve out a public philosophy on the intrinsic worth of human life and the value of function relative to that life, at least locate a socially meaningful place for physical decline and disability in the life span.

The passage of the Americans with Disabilities Act in 1990 illustrates the extent to which our society continues to resist articulating anything beyond a series of sanctions and penalties for discriminating against disabled persons' access to employment, public accommodations, transportation, and communication. The thrust of this legislation is one of reminding social forces of their duties to take reasonable steps to eradicate attitudinal or physical barriers that frustrate a disabled person's mainstreaming into society. Consequently, this Act advocates the negative rights of disabled persons in the form of assuring their confidence about anticipating physical or attitudinal noninterference in exercising their rights of equal access and opportunity (34). The Act, however, does not token a social empathy for disabled persons nor does it address disability per se as an obstacle or handicap to a meaningful life. The Act exists for those disabled persons who have persevered through their handicaps and wish to engage in social and communal life despite their disabilities. The Act does not focus social resources on the causes and nature of disabilities themselves in order to prevent their occurrence or diminish their effect.

To find a meaningful place for disability and aging within the context of our culture, the following considerations are worth contemplating. First, the political commentator George Will (15) has written that "all of us are, potentially, in the antechamber of the disability community." His point is that a communal or social sensitivity towards the needs of disabled persons can be best achieved not through alleging common law or statutory rights, but rather by encouraging a realization that "no one of us, handicapped or not, is independent of the community on which we depend for our moral fulfillment" (15). Will is concerned that pleading the language of legal rights and constitutional entitlements to advance the causes connected with disability may very well result in antagonizing and polarizing the nondisabled community since such pleading predictably tends to be contentious and adversarial. On the other hand, fostering social attitudes that understand disability not as a devastating and irreversible loss, but rather as an unfortunate but familiar occurrence within the course of protracted longevity may more effectively diminish the awkwardness or reluctance among nondisabled persons in addressing the needs of the disabled. It is important for society to continue to remind itself of the humanity that is shared and continuous from that stage of being temporarily able bodied to becoming disabled. Sustained reflection on the meaningfulness of being temporarily able bodied may yield deep and moving insights that uncover the benevolence and what Will calls the moral fitness necessary for overcoming the socially alienating forces of disability (15).

Second, even if the disabled elderly do not achieve a compelling political activism or presence, they ought to consider developing a coherent and visible social activism. The elderly disabled must aspire to make a social difference that defines their membership within a moral community. If the disengagement theory of aging is a hopeless anachronism, then the elderly themselves must prove that case by evidencing their preferences, energies, and civic commitment. One would be justifiably suspicious of, and probably miserly toward, any group's pleas to the moral sympathies of a society without that group's demonstrating any energy or interest in a meaningful engagement with that society's interests and aspirations.

The pressures to constrain costs in medicine are not likely to disappear. With regard to rehabilitating elderly persons, a third moral imperative exists to utilize such resources with a clear view and understanding of the good they are to achieve. As such, rehabilitationists need to examine the impact of rehabilitation services from a variety of ethical parameters. Rehabilitation providers should conduct a sustained professional examination of the kind of benefit that is presumed to accrue from rehabilitation services because the restoration of function does not necessarily imply a significant or meaningful improvement in one's quality of life. If rehabilitation is a social resource, then its providers need to assess and determine those instances wherein benefits may be maximized, not only for the patient, but for the family, other health care providers, third party payors, and so forth. It will doubtlessly be seen that benefits yields a variety of meanings given the multiple contexts in which it is understood. On the other hand, many instances can reliably be identified wherein rehabilitation does not improve a person's quality of life even though financial resources may be present. If the rationing of health care, including rehabilitation services, ever becomes a reality in the United States, then these kinds of utilitarian calculations of benefits will become not only familiar, but also influential in allocating services justly and wisely.

Fourth, our society remains confused and often unrealistic about the extent to which health care can alleviate suffering and decline in life. A considerable locus of this confusion appears to reside within health care's resistance to acknowledging the inevitability of dying and death. Death continues to be perceived as an insult to the efforts of health providers, while its conquest continues to be the ultimate goal of health research. Longevity has long been pursued without due consideration to its quality. Rehabilitation should focus its attention on the importance of locating a meaningful place for death within its self-understanding. This has clearly not yet occurred, as evidenced by the paucity of rehabilitation literature focusing on that period between rehabilitation discharge and the experience of death. Understandably, rehabilitation must harbor and convey to its elderly consumers an optimism about the utility of functional restoration and the meaningfulness and attainability of independence. Reflecting upon death at admission to rehabilitation seems oxymoronic or, at least, counterproductive to the rehabilitation effort. Yet, the occurrence of death is obviously an absolute limiting point on whatever success may have occurred with the rehabilitation of an elderly person. The prospect of death must qualify the perception and worth of rehabilitation's utility to its elderly consumers, thus encouraging its study among rehabilitation providers. While it is preposterous to think that rehabilitation can mean all things to all persons, its availability for consumers with adequate reimbursement may occasionally result in its impulsive and unwise distribution. The degree to which rehabilitation makes a meaningful difference in the elderly disabled person's quality of life after discharge must be assessed. Rehabilitation providers must contribute to this dialogue or another group with a nonrehabilitation agenda may prevail.

SUMMARY

The rehabilitation of elderly persons constitutes a remarkable moral gesture and manifestation of our society's understanding of itself and the status of older citizens. The provision of rehabilitation signifies a social disposition toward respecting an elderly person's right to regain the enjoyment and utility of functional independence and, thus, the right to continue to enjoy access to social goods and benefits. In signifying that life does not end with disability, the opportunity of rehabilitation connotes not only society's refusal to capitulate to a pessimistic view of the elderly persons' prospects for meaningful life, but also society's expectations that rehabilitation consumers will avail themselves of the social and communal life that rehabilitation attempts to make possible for them.

The existence of rehabilitation stands as medicine's most remarkable affirmation of our country's libertarian ideals of freedom, self-determination, and personal choice. Consequently, to the extent that the life span continues to increase, the presumption of rehabilitation will be that citizens should continue to enjoy their independence for as long as possible. However, to the extent that greater accountability continues to be demanded in health care, rehabilitationists will be compelled to allocate their services more judiciously than ever before. Therefore, one can expect that the future of rehabilitation services for elderly persons will be marked by serious reflection on society's moral commitments to our basic human freedoms, especially as they are punctuated by a communal notion of dignity and self-respect. A dimension of that reflection will inevitably include resolving our national ambivalence as to whether health care efforts for the elderly ought to focus on simply adding years to life or life to years.

References

1. Relman AS. Is rationing inevitable? *N Engl J Med.* 322:1809–1810, 1990.
2. Callahan D. Rationing medical progress. *N Engl J Med.* 322:1810–1813, 1990.
3. Levinsky N. Age as a criterion for rationing health care. *N Engl J Med.* 322:1813–1816, 1990.
4. Radovskuy S. U.S. medical practice before Medicare and now—differences and consequences. *N Engl J Med.* 322:263–267, 1990.
5. Morreim EH. The MD and the DRG. *Hastings Center Rep.* 15:30–38, 1985.
6. McGinnis GE, Osberg JS, DeJong G, Seward ML, Branch LG. Predicting charges for inpatient medical rehabilitation using severity, DRG, age and function. *Am J Public Health.* 77:826–829, 1987.
7. Callahan D. *Setting Limits: Medical Goals in an Aging Society.* Simon and Schuster; New York, NY, 1987.
8. Outka G. Social justice and equal access to health care. In: Mappes TA, Zembaty JS, eds. *Biomedical Ethics.* 1st ed. New York, NY: McGraw-Hill; 1981:523–531.
9. Smith GP. Death be not proud; medical, ethical and legal dilemmas in resource allocation. *J Contemporary Health Law Policy.* 3:47–63, 1987.
10. MacIntyre A. *After Virtue.* Notre Dame, Ind: University of Notre Dame Press; 1981.
11. Sandel M. *Liberalism and the Limits of Justice.* Cambridge: Cambridge University Press; 1982.
12. Rorty R. The contingency of community. *London Rev Books.* 24 July 1986:10–14.
13. Rorty R. The priority of democracy to philosophy. In: Malachowski A. *Reading Rorty.* Cambridge, Mass: Basil Blackwell; 1990:279–302.
14. Hospers J. The libertarian manifesto. In: Klemke ED, Kline AD, Hollinger R, eds. *Philosophy—The Basic Issues.* 3rd ed. New York, NY: St. Martin's Press; 1990:528–535.
15. Will GF. For the handicapped, rights but no welcome. *Hastings Center Rep.* 16:5–8, 1986.
16. Pawlson LG. Financing long-term care. *J Am Geriatr Soc.* 37:631–638, 1989.
17. Beauchamp TL, Childress JF. *Principles of Biomedical Ethics.* 3rd ed. New York, NY: Oxford University Press; 1989:55–66.
18. Curran WJ. The constitutional right to health care. *N Engl J Med.* 320:788–789, 1989.
19. Rosoff AJ. *Informed Consent: A Guide for Health Care Providers.* Rockville, Md: Aspen Publications; 1981:233–245.
20. Roth LH, Meisel A, Lidz CW. Tests of competency to consent to treatment. *Am J Psychiatry.* 134:279–284, 1977.
21. Banja J. Proxy consent to medical treatment: implications for rehabilitation. *Arch Phys Med Rehabil.* 67:790–792, 1986.
22. *In the Matter of Claire C. Conroy,* 486 A2d 1209 (NJ1985).
23. Iris MA. Guardianship and the elderly: a multi-perspective view of the decisionmaking process. *Gerontologist.* 28(special suppl):39–45, 1988.
24. High DM. All in the family: extended autonomy and expectations in surrogate health care decision-making. *Gerontologist.* 28(special suppl):46–51, 1988.
25. Haug M. Doctor patient relationships and the older patient. *J Gerontol.* 34:852–860, 1979.
26. Stanley B, Stanley M, Guido J, Garvin L. The functional competency of elderly at risk. *Gerontologist.* 28(special suppl):54–58, 1988.
27. Tymchuk AJ, Ouslander JG, Rahbar B, Fitten J. Medical decision-making among elderly people in long term care. *Gerontologist.* 28(special suppl):59–63, 1988.
28. Collopy BJ. Autonomy in long term care: some crucial distinctions. *Gerontologist.* 28(special suppl):10–17, 1988.
29. Banja J. Independence and rehabilitation: a philosophic perspective. *Arch Phys Med Rehabil* 69:381–382, 1988.
30. Haas J. Admission to rehabilitation centers: selection of patients. *Arch Phys Med Rehabil.* 609:329–332, 1988.
31. Cumming E, Henry WC. *Growing Old: The Process of Disengagement.* New York, NY: Basic Books; 1961.
32. Riley MH, Riley JW. The lives of older people and changing social roles. *Ann AAPSS.* 503:14–28, 1989.
33. Somers AR. Insurance for long-term care. *N Engl J Med.* 317:23–29, 1987.
34. Verville RE. The Americans with Disabilities Act: an analysis. *Arch Phys Med Rehabil.* 71:1010–1013, 1990.

Index